ANNALS OF THE NEW YORK ACADEMY OF SCIENCES

Volume 465

The New York Academy of Sciences
2 East 63rd Street
New York, New York 10021

TENTH INTERNATIONAL CONFERENCE ON SARCOIDOSIS AND OTHER GRANULOMATOUS DISORDERS

ANNALS OF THE NEW YORK ACADEMY OF SCIENCES
Volume 465

TENTH INTERNATIONAL CONFERENCE ON SARCOIDOSIS AND OTHER GRANULOMATOUS DISORDERS

Edited by Carol Johnson Johns

The New York Academy of Sciences
New York, New York
1986

Library of Congress Cataloging-in-Publication Data

International Conference on Sarcoidosis and Other
Granulomatous Disorders (10th: 1984 Baltimore,
Md.)
Tenth International Conference on Sarcoidosis
and Other Granulomatous Disorders.

(Annals of the New York Academy of Sciences; v. 465)
Bibliography: p.
Includes index.
1. Sarcoidosis—Congresses. 2. Granuloma—Congresses.
3. Lungs—Diseases—Congresses. I. Johns, Carol
Johnson. II. New York Academy of Sciences. III. Title.
IV. Series.
Q11.N5 vol. 465 500 s 86-12483
[RC182.S14] [616]

PCP
Printed in the United States of America
ISBN 0-89766-325-X (cloth)
ISBN 0-89766-326-8 (paper)
ISSN 0077-8923

ANNALS OF THE NEW YORK ACADEMY OF SCIENCES

Volume 465
June 6, 1986

TENTH INTERNATIONAL CONFERENCE ON SARCOIDOSIS AND OTHER GRANULOMATOUS DISORDERS[a]

Editor
CAROL JOHNSON JOHNS

International Committee on Sarcoidosis
F. BASSET, A. BLASI, J. S. CHAPMAN, J. CHRÉTIEN, R. G. CRYSTAL, M. M. CUMMINGS, A. C. DOUGLAS, Å. HANNGREN, Y. HOSODA, T. H. HURLEY, H. L. ISRAEL, D. G. JAMES (*Executive Secretary*), C. J. JOHNS, W. JONES WILLIAMS, L. LEVINSKÝ, R. MIKAMI, O. B. SELROOS, A. S. TEIRSTEIN, AND J. TURIAF

Local Organizing Committee
N. F. ADKINSON, JR., W. C. BALL, JR., R. G. CRYSTAL (*Vice-President*), H. L. ISRAEL (*Vice-President*), C. J. JOHNS (*President*), V. A. MCKUSICK (*Honorary Chairman*), J. R. MICHAEL, C. A. NEWILL, S. PERMUTT, A. S. TEIRSTEIN (*Vice-President*), P. B. TERRY, AND W. F. WILLOUGHBY

CONTENTS

[a]This volume is the result of the Tenth International Conference on Sarcoidosis and Other Granulomatous Disorders held by the International Committee on Sarcoidosis on September 17-22, 1984 in Baltimore, Maryland.

Louis E. Siltzbach Memorial Lecture

Part II. Other Granulomatous Disorders

Sven Löfgren Memorial Lecture

Part III. Clinical Studies of Sarcoidosis

Financial assistance was received from:

- FOGARTY INTERNATIONAL CENTER
- HOSPITAL FOR THE CONSUMPTIVES OF MARYLAND (EUDOWOOD)
- MIDDENDORF FOUNDATION
- NATIONAL HEART, LUNG, AND BLOOD INSTITUTE (NIH)

Preface

The Tenth International Conference on Sarcoidosis and Other Granulomatous Disorders was held at the Johns Hopkins University School of Medicine on September 17-22, 1984. Ronald Crystal, Harold Israel, and Alvin Teirstein served as vice-presidents and were invaluable in shaping and planning the program. In addition, the Local Organizing Committee of Hopkins faculty members included N. F. Adkinson, Jr., W. C. Ball, Jr., J. R. Michael, C. A. Newill, S. Permutt, P. B. Terry, and W. F. Willoughby. We had the constant advice and encouragement of the International Committee and especially the Executive Secretary, D. Geraint James.

Since Dr. James organized the first international sarcoidosis conference in London in 1958, triennial meetings have become a tradition. Jacques Chrétien, who chaired the 1981 conference in Paris, brought the "Sarcoid Olympic Torch" to Baltimore for the 1984 meeting.

This conference was attended by 305 delegates from 29 countries. It included 92 presentations, most of which are published in this volume. One hundred seventy-two posters were displayed. In all, 718 authors were represented.

At this meeting, two late members of the International Committee on Sarcoidosis were honored with memorial lectures: Herbert Y. Reynolds, of Yale-New Haven Hospital, presented the Louis E. Siltzbach Lecture, "Concepts of Pathogenesis and Lung Reactivity in Hypersensitivity Pneumonitis." Margaret Turner-Warwick, of Brompton Hospital, London, presented the Sven Löfgren Lecture, "Do Measurements of Bronchoalveolar Lymphocytes and Neutrophils, Serum Angiotensin-converting Enzyme, and Gallium Uptake Help the Clinician to Treat Patients With Sarcoidosis?"

The collegiality and friendships enjoyed at the sarcoidosis conferences set the stage for good communication and mutual understanding, conditions that will help us improve our knowledge of the intriguing disorders of sarcoidosis. The theme of the 1984 conference would well be described as that of clinicians and basic scientists coming together. Rapid advances in techniques of modern biology provide opportunities for significant new understandings. Bronchoalveolar lavage studies have opened some windows on the disease processes and provide a peek into the cracks of the interstitial tissues. Studies of the cellular and immunologic mechanisms and mediators, however, must be coupled with astute clinical observations. Both clinicians and basic scientists have important roles to play in unraveling the puzzles of sarcoidosis.

We welcome our readers to this publication of the proceedings of the conference, made possible by the New York Academy of Sciences. We thank Kevin M. Mayer of the Academy's Editorial Department for his careful work in the production of this volume.

This conference was supported in part by Grant 1R13HL31975-01 from the Heart, Lung, and Blood Institute and the Fogarty International Center, as well as by grants from the Hospital for the Consumptives of Maryland (Eudowood) and the Middendorf Foundation.

CAROL JOHNSON JOHNS

Sarcoidosis

A Case Study in Nosology

VICTOR A. McKUSICK[a]

Johns Hopkins Hospital
Baltimore, Maryland 21205

In entitling these brief remarks as I did, I had nothing very profound in mind. The history of the nosology and nosography of sarcoidosis has been well reviewed in earlier sarcoidosis conferences[1,2] and has been nicely summarized by D. Geraint James.[3]

Both the substance of nosology[4] and nosology as a process[5] have interested me for some time. The nosology of genetic disorders, genetic nosology, has concerned me particularly. It may be of interest to contrast the nosology of a disorder such as sarcoidosis with the nosology of hereditary diseases. Kurt H. Farber, in a monograph published over fifty years ago,[6] attributed to Mendelism and to bacteriology leading roles in nosology—quite an improvement over the thinking of scarcely a century and a half ago, when dropsy, jaundice, and anemia were viewed as specific, distinct disease entities. In sarcoidosis, neither the Mendelian[7] nor the microbiological paradigm has been proved to be adequate, however, and other paradigms have had to be explored.

Nosologists tend to be either "lumpers" or "splitters,"[5] but sometimes the nosologist straddles the issue. In medical genetics splitting has been the order of the day for the last quarter-century. Repeatedly, phenotypes that had been considered to represent a single entity have ultimately been found to represent several distinct entities. This has happened, for example, in familial amyloid neuropathy, hereditary intestinal polyposis, retinitis pigmentosa, congenital deafness, the mucopolysaccharidoses, and the Ehlers-Danlos syndromes.

The nosology of sarcoidosis has involved more of a lumping process: this is most evident when the early stages of sarcoidosis are considered. Skin lesions, which were described in the previous century, and uveoparotid fever and visceral involvement, which were described in the first two decades this century, were lumped together in the 1930's; that is, they were considered different expressions of one disease with a presumably unique etiology, a disease, in the jargon of genetics, with variable expressivity. The nosology of sarcoidosis has been similar to that of systemic lupus erythematosus, another disease of unknown etiology, seemingly complicated pathogenesis, and variable expression. I would not exclude the possibility that in both sarcoidosis and systemic lupus erythematosus, as the full story of their etiology and pathogenesis unfolds, nosologic subsets, multiple partially distinct entities, may become evident.

I would like to call your attention to two Johns Hopkins connections with the nosography of sarcoidosis, in the persons of Jonathan Hutchinson and Warfield T.

[a]Honorary Chairman of the Local Organizing Committee.

Longcope, and give a Johns Hopkins-related footnote to the history of sarcoidosis, in the person of Robert H. Williams.

Hutchinson (1828-1913) has been credited with the earliest descriptions of sarcoid skin lesions, as well as many other phenomena of clinical medicine. He was, of course, a London surgeon, but his large clinical collection was acquired by the medical school of Johns Hopkins shortly after his death, through the agency of Sir William Osler and the financial generosity of W. A. Marburg of Baltimore.[8]

Longcope (1877-1953) was professor of medicine at Johns Hopkins from 1922 to 1946. He graduated from the medical school of Johns Hopkins in 1901, was a student of Osler, and was a profound student of disease in the Oslerian tradition.[9] His papers, which began to appear in 1936,[10–13] on Boeck's sarcoidosis did more than any other publication, in this country at least, to establish sarcoidosis, in all of its various manifestations, as a distinct entity.

As James pointed out in his chronologic table,[2] Williams and Nickerson in 1935 preceded Kveim in the use of ground-up sarcoid tissue for skin testing.[14] Williams (1909-1979) graduated from the medical school of Johns Hopkins in 1934, was a pathology intern in Boston when he did the work with Nickerson, and was later a resident under Longcope. Williams is best known as the author of a widely used textbook of endocrinology and as the distinguished founding professor of medicine at the University of Washington School of Medicine in Seattle.

REFERENCES

1. Levinský, L. & F. Macholda, Eds. 1971. Proceedings of the Fifth International Conference on Sarcoidosis. Universita Karlova Praha. Prague.
2. James, D. G. 1976. The centenary of sarcoidosis. Ann. N.Y. Acad. Sci. **278:** 736-741.
3. James. D. G. 1984. The sarcoidosis movement. Sarcoidosis **1:** 4-10.
4. McKusick, V. A. 1983. Mendelian Inheritance in Man: Catalogs of Autosomal Dominant, Autosomal Recessive and X-linked Phenotypes. 6th edit. Johns Hopkins University Press. Baltimore, MD.
5. McKusick, V. A. 1969. On lumpers and splitters, or the nosology of genetic disease. Perspect. Biol. Med. **12:** 298-318.
6. Farber, K. H. 1930. Nosography: The Evolution of Clinical Medicine in Modern Times. P. B. Hoeber. New York, NY.
7. Buck, A. A. & V. A. McKusick. 1961. Epidemiologic investigations of sarcoidosis. III. Serum proteins; syphilis; association with tuberculosis; familial aggregation. Am. J. Hyg. **74:** 152-173.
8. McKusick, V. A. 1952. The clinical observations of Jonathan Hutchinson. Am. J. Syph. **36:** 101-126.
9. Harvey, A. M. 1975. Classical descriptions of disease. Johns Hopkins Med. J. **136:** 254-267.
10. Longcope, W. T. 1936. The generalized form of Boeck's sarcoid. Trans. Assoc. Am. Physicians **51:** 94-102.
11. Longcope, W. T. & J. W. Pierson. 1937. Boeck's sarcoid (sarcoidosis). Bull. Johns Hopkins Hosp. **60:** 223-296.
12. Longcope, W. T. 1941. Sarcoidosis, or Besnier-Boeck-Schaumann disease. J. Am. Med. Assoc. **117:** 1321-1327.
13. Longcope, W. T. & D. G. Freiman. 1952. A study of sarcoidosis, based on a combined investigation of 160 cases including 30 autopsies from the Johns Hopkins Hospital and Massachusetts General Hospital. Medicine **31:** 1-132.
14. Williams, R. H. & D. A. Nickerson. 1935. Skin reactions in sarcoid. Proc. Soc. Exp. Biol. Med. **33:** 402-405.

Triennial Report of the International Committee on Sarcoidosis

D. GERAINT JAMES[a]

Royal Northern Hospital
London N7 6LD, England

The First International Conference on Sarcoidosis was held in 1958 at the Brompton Hospital in London. There can be no doubt that the sarcoidosis movement has flourished since then: an international conference has been held every three years thereafter.

The success of the international conferences has stimulated Europe to organize its own series of conferences. These conferences have been equally successful, particularly the most recent one, which was held in Naples in September 1983.

INTERNATIONAL COMMITTEE ON SARCOIDOSIS

The International Committee on Sarcoidosis comprises nineteen doctors representing eight countries: T. H. Hurley, Australia; L. Levinský, Czechoslovakia; F. Basset, J. Chrétien, and J. Turiaf, France; A. Blasi, Italy; Y. Hosoda and R. Mikami, Japan; Å. Hanngren and O. B. Selroos, Sweden; A. C. Douglas, D. G. James, and W. Jones Williams, the United Kingdom; and J. S. Chapman, R. G. Crystal, M. M. Cummings, H. L. Israel, C. J. Johns, and A. S. Teirstein, the United States. This list includes organizers of past conferences, veterans of the first conference, several participants who have attended most of the conferences, and two participants who have attended all of the conferences. We are continuing to add new sarcoidologists to this committee, particularly those who come forward and make themselves responsible for organizing international or European conferences.

There have been three deaths—all were of distinguished sarcoidologists who made seminal contributions to the study of sarcoidosis and who were particulary active in this committee.

Louis E. Siltzbach

Louis E. Siltzbach was my predecessor as Executive Secretary. He was a New Yorker with a combination of rare intellect, generosity of mind, and an unswerving

[a] Executive Secretary of the International Committee on Sarcoidosis.

devotion to the study of sarcoidosis. His writings influenced thought throughout the world on all aspects of sarcoidosis. His contributions culminated in his editorship of the authoratative 751-page monograph based on the seventh international conference. This monograph was published in 1976 as volume 278 of the *Annals of the New York Academy of Sciences.*

A festschrift in his honor was published in 1977 as volume 44 of his hospital's journal, the *Mount Sinai Journal of Medicine.* It appeared when he was still well and able to enjoy this salute to his international contributions to sarcoidosis.

Sven Löfgren

Sven Löfgren's lifework was at St. Goran's Hospital, Stockholm, where he was influenced by Westergren and Schaumann. His most important contributions, the classic studies on erythema nodosum and hilar adenopathy, are set securely alongside the milestones demarcating the history of sarcoidosis. Other contributions include his superb organization of the conference held in Stockholm, and his editing of the volume based on this conference.

Erwin Uehlinger

Erwin Uehlinger was a Zurich pathologist who was faithful to the sarcoidosis movement throughout the years. His long experience on the histology of sarcoid tissue illuminated every conference.

INTERNATIONAL REVIEW OF SARCOIDOSIS AND OTHER GRANULOMATOUS DISORDERS

The International Committee on Sarcoidosis has given unanimous support to this new Italian-inspired Journal, for we wish to extend information, knowledge, and interest in sarcoidosis and other granulomatous disorders to an ever-widening audience around the world.

The idea for this new venture is that of Gianfranco Rizzato, who had nourished the notion for some time before bringing it to fruition by obtaining the necessary sponsorship from Giovanni Tosi of Camillo Corvi. They are to be congratulated on their initiative.

This new journal will be another landmark in the history of sarcoidosis and other granulomatous disorders. It will be of interst to clinicians of every discipline and to radiologists, pathologists, immunologists, epidemiologists, and geneticists—all of whom are now endeavouring to unravel our beloved enigma. It will appear twice each year, in the autumn and in the spring, and will contain new articles, reviews, and case presentations.

FUTURE EVENTS

The Eleventh International Conference on Sarcoidosis will be held in September 1987 in Milan, Italy. The organizers, Antonio Blasi and Gianfranco Rizzato, are good friends of the sarcoidosis movement.

The next European conference on sarcoidosis will be held in the last week of August 1986 in Vienna, Austria. It will be organized by Heinrich Klech.

Functional Aspects of Mononuclear Phagocyte Involvement in Lung Inflammation[a]

DAVID W. H. RICHES AND PETER M. HENSON

Department of Pediatrics
National Jewish Hospital and Research Center
Denver, Colorado 80206

INTRODUCTION

Macrophages, which constitute part of the mononuclear phagocyte system, are found in varying numbers in almost all mammalian tissues and organs. Elements of the mononuclear phagocyte system include the fixed macrophages that line the vascular beds of such organs as the liver and spleen, and the mobile resident macrophages that reside on the serous membrane of the peritoneum and in the alveoli and airways of the lung. Another element of the mononuclear phagocyte system is the mobile, pluripotent, blood-borne monocyte which can leave the circulation either randomly, under steady state conditions to populate specific tissues such as the spleen, or selectively, under the influence of a chemotactic gradient to infiltrate an inflammatory site.[1] Once in the tissues, monocytes acquire the generic morphological and functional characteristics of mature macrophages yet adapt to the specific local environment of the tissue into which they have migrated.

In view of this potential ubiquity of macrophages, it is perhaps not too surprising to find that these cells have been implicated in a plethora of human diseases ranging from a nonimmunological involvement in atheroma[2] to a strong immunological involvement in rheumatoid arthritis.[3] The objective of this review is to illustrate the pluripotential nature of the macrophage's responses to its environment and to stimuli in these environments with which it is known to interact. Rather than embark on a lengthy description of the many diverse responses ascribed to macrophages (some of which are summarized in FIG. 1), however, we will limit our discussion to one aspect of mononuclear phagocyte function, namely its adaptability (that is, its responsiveness) to its environment, particularly in the lung. This adaptability, we believe, contributes importantly to the role the cell plays in the initiation, continuation, and resolution of inflammation.

[a]This work was supported by United States Public Health Service-National Institutes of Health Grants HL-21565 and GM-24834.

EMIGRATION, SUBPOPULATIONS, MATURATION, AND PROLIFERATION

Mononuclear phagocytes are continually being turned over in all tissues and organs in which they are found. In the lung, the majority of these cells is believed to exit the alveoli via the terminal airways and to be expelled via the mucociliary pathway.[4] Under steady state conditions the mononuclear phagocytes are replaced by cells resulting from the division of bone marrow-derived precursor cells; thus the net mononuclear phagocyte equilibrium in the lung is maintained. Several hypotheses have been presented to explain the origin of the pulmonary macrophage. In one hypothesis, it has been speculated that a bone marrow-derived precursor pool exists in the interstitium and that local division of this population could produce the pulmonary macrophages.[5] A second hypothesis proposes that monocytes or promonocytes undergo a final division cycle in the lung capillary bed before populating, and maturing in, the alveoli.[6] [^{3}H]Thymidine incorporation studies, however, conducted both *in vivo* and *in vitro,* have overwhelmingly failed to demonstrate an indiginous dividing population of mononuclear phagocytes under steady state conditions.

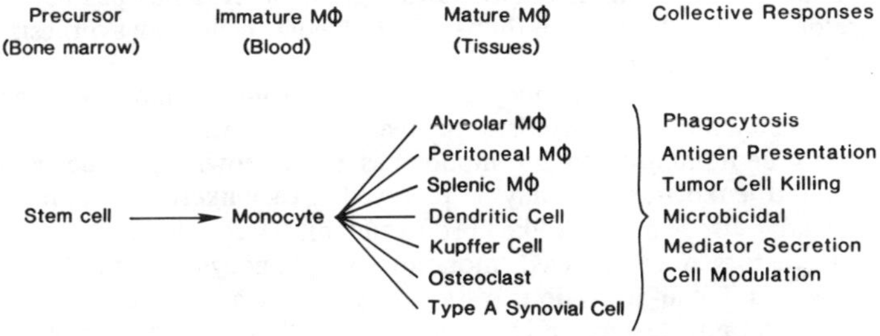

FIGURE 1. Origin, transport, maturation, and collective responses of the mononuclear phagocyte system.

Perhaps the most convincing and mechanistically simplistic view, however, has been put forward by van Furth and his colleagues, who propose that blood monocytes leave the circulation in a random fashion to populate extravascular sites in all tissues and organs. In the mouse, calculations based on the distribution of [^{3}H]thymidine-labeled monocytes indicate that after circulating in the blood with a mean half-time of 17.4 hours, 56% of the monocytes accumulate in the liver, while 15% accumulate in the lung.[7] It has been speculated that lung accumulation of monocytes may be related to the chemotactic properties of a pulmonary surfactant.[8] The implication of this hypothesis is that if cells are drawn from the circulating population into the lung in a random fashion by a chemotactic factor, the circulating blood monocyte population is likely to be relatively homogeneous in its functional properties, and that the differences seen in mature macrophages sampled from different organs, such as those between the alveolar macrophage and the Kupffer cell, must be due to conditioning of their functional properties after emigration from the blood, and not due to the infiltration of specific organs with specific subpopulations of preprogrammed stem cells or monocytes. A corollary to this conclusion is that contact of infiltrating monocytes either with specific chemoattractants or with specific tissue or organ components is sufficient to trigger the maturation of monocytes into the mature macrophages that characteristically inhabit a given tissue or organ. Although human peripheral blood monocyte subsets have been identified by both functional and structural criteria,[9–11] the hypothesis of a relatively homogeneous population of circulating cells is not at variance with these data because there is no evidence that these subsets are derived from separate stem cells. The differences observed may be explained simply by attributing them to differences in the maturation status between responsive cells freshly released from the bone marrow and unresponsive cells which are near the end of the circulating period.

During an inflammatory response in the lung, for example, mononuclear phagocyte numbers increase significantly both in the alveoli and in the interstitium. This response has been shown to be due in large part to an increased sequestration of monocytes from the blood.[12] A small, though significant, component of the increase under inflammatory conditions, however, appears to be due to local mitosis of mononuclear phagocytes. Whilst this phenomenon was originally thought to be due to proliferation of mature alveolar and interstitial macrophages, more recent data based on the disappearance of dividing cells following systemic hydrocortisone treatment (which produces a rapid and extensive monocytopenia) would suggest that the dividing population of mononuclear phagocytes is relatively immature.[12] The stimulus for increased mitosis under inflammatory conditions is unclear although some evidence has been obtained in our laboratory *in vitro* to indicate that type II alveolar cells may synthesize growth factors for mononuclear phagocytes.[13]

The stimulus for increased monocyte emigration from the blood into an inflammatory site is clearly not a characteristic of steady state conditions. The major chemotactic stimulus in inflammation for monocytes is unknown, but the complement fragment C5a and leukotriene B4 may be involved. Other likely factors include fragments of connective-tissue proteins like fibronectin[14] and T cell-derived lymphokines;[15] if indeed these factors were involved, mononuclear phagocyte accumulation at sites of tissue injury and T cell activation, respectively, could be explained. The problem of demonstrating monocyte-specific chemoattractants that are active *in vivo* is significant, and it requires further investigation. Again, the question arises as to the origin and phenotype of the infiltrating monocytes under inflammatory conditions. Bursuker[16] has speculated that during an inflammatory reaction a subpopulation of macrophage precursors, different from those of resident macrophages, is induced in the bone marrow and that these cells, which show normal monocyte kinetics, are the precursors of inflammatory tissue macrophages. The theme which we are developing in this discussion, however, is that the mononuclear phagocyte adapts to its environment, and we would thus suggest that C5a, a generic chemotactic factor that may attract neutrophils and monocytes to any site in the body where complement activation or C5 cleavage has occurred, merely enhances the sequestration of monocytes at an inflammatory site, and that the subsequent interaction of monocytes with material within the inflammatory site such as damaged connective-tissue components, lymphocyte-derived factors, bacterial/parasite products, etc., directs the monocyte to mature into a macrophage with a particular inflammatory phenotype.

MACROPHAGES AT INFLAMMATORY SITES

When considering the migration of the macrophages from the blood into an inflammatory site, the question arises as to what the macrophages does to influence the course of an inflammatory response. We wish to reemphasize our view that a phagocytotic interaction between the macrophage and material within the inflammatory site, or in the course of moving through the vessel wall itself, is instrumental in directing the monocyte to mature into an inflammatory macrophage. Whilst inflammatory macrophages have certain functional characteristics in common, however, such as enhanced superoxide anion production, neutral proteinase secretion, and C3b-receptor-mediated erythrophagocytosis, it is becoming clear that individual stimuli induce the expression of unique phenotypes indicating subtle changes in the induction and repression of certain gene products.

MACROPHAGE PROTEIN PHENOTYPIC CHANGES

An approach that we have taken to study the diversity of macrophage responses is to expose macrophages *in vitro* to stimuli for various periods of time and then to pulse the cells with [^{35}S]methionine to biosynthetically label cellular proteins. By employing a chase with unlabeled methionine, the secretion of labeled proteins to the cells' exteriors can also be measured. Supernatants and cell lysates are then subjected to sodium dodecylsulfate polyacrylamide gel electrophoresis (SDS-PAGE) and autoradiography to analyze the total protein biosynthetic profiles. FIGURE 2 illustrates the biosynthetic profiles of mouse macrophages exposed *in vitro* to either bacterial lipopolysaccharide or dextran sulfate, two stimuli which act similarly in many respects; for example, they both stimulate interferon synthesis by macrophages, and they both induce macrophages to become nonspecifically cytolytic towards tumor cells. The biosynthetic profiles, however, are markedly different from one another, and from unstimulated controls. Similarly, when the [^{35}S]methionine is "chased" with unlabeled methionine for 18 hr, marked differences are noted in the secreted-protein profiles (FIG. 3). More specifically, by examining the levels of individual labeled proteins by immunoprecipitation with specific antisera and by analyzing their abundance by SDS-PAGE, autoradiography, and scanning densitometry, we have found that LPS stimulates the synthesis of complement component C3 yet, at the same time, suppresses the synthesis of the lysosomal enzyme β-glucuronidase. Dextran sulfate, on the other hand, has the reverse effect in that it inhibits C3 biosynthesis by macrophages but stimulates β-glucuronidase synthesis. Although the identity of most of these products is unknown, functional assays of macrophage products indicate that they include factors that are involved in the degradation of the connective tissue matrix in preparation for tissue remodeling, and of growth factors which influence the division of cells (fibroblasts and type II alveolar cells) involved in deposition of a new connective tissue matrix.

DEGRADATION

The phagocytosis by mononuclear phagocytes of material within an inflammatory site—immune complexes in the rheumatoid synovium, bacteria in infectious foci, and tissue debris in other sites—induces the elaboration of many degradative enzymes as well as of factors which induce other cells such as fibroblasts to synthesize and secrete such proteins.

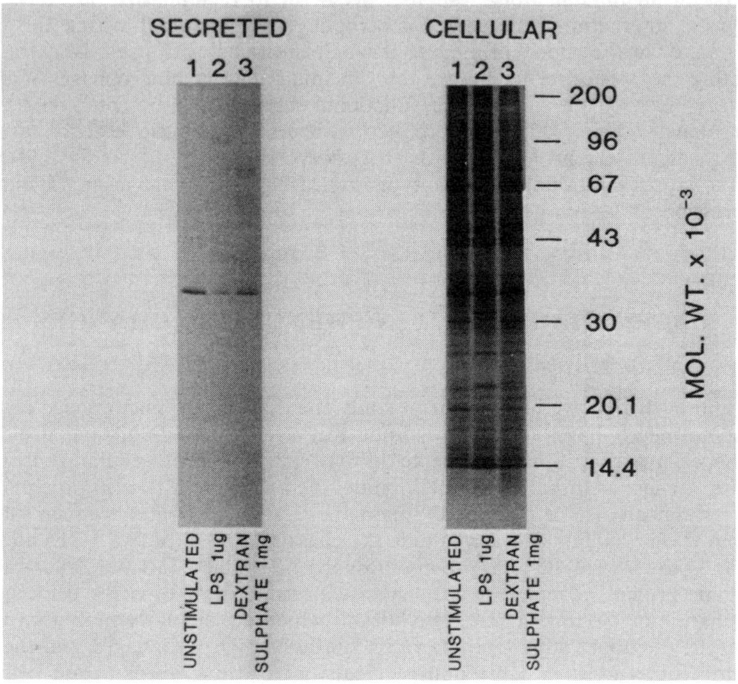

FIGURE 2. Protein biosynthetic profiles of resident mouse peritoneal macrophages after their exposure to bacterial lipopolysaccharide (0111:B4; 1 μg) and dextran sulfate (1 mg) for 24 hr. Cells were labeled with [^{35}S]methionine (200 μCi) for 1 hr and then lysed in a detergent/enzyme-inhibitor cocktail composed of Triton X-100 (0.5%), sodium deoxycholate (0.25%), EDTA (10 mM), and phenylmethane-sulfonyl fluoride (2 mM). Labeled proteins were separated by SDS-polyacrylamide gel electrophoresis through a 5-15% acrylamide gel under reducing conditions and then visualized by fluorography.

PROTEIN SYNTHESIS-INDEPENDENT SECRETION

Studies conducted a decade ago showed quite conclusively that macrophages that were engaged in the phagocytosis of inflammatory stimuli such as group A streptococcal cell walls[17] and zymosan particles[18] secreted a proportion of their intracellular lysosomal enzymes (hexosaminidase, β-glucuronidase, and acid phosphatase) to their exteriors by a process that was selective in that it did not result in cell death. Kinetic analyses revealed that the secretory process was, in most cases, complete within 12 hr of exposure to stimuli, and, since secretion occurred even in the presence of the protein synthesis inhibitor cycloheximide, the response is clearly a mobilization of preformed enzymes. The contribution of the response to an inflammatory episode, however, is not entirely clear since the enzymes are secreted over a relatively short time. Moreover, more recent studies have indicated that monocytes are also capable of this type of immediate secretory process.[19] Still, it is conceivable that the immediate secretory process, together with that of neutrophils, may provide an initially high local concentration of potentially degradative enzymes within the inflammatory site. The mechanism of secretion was originally thought to involve fusion of lysosomes with incompletely closed phagosomes. In view of the temporal displacement between phagocytosis and secretion,[19] however, the secretion is more likely to involve some form of microvesicular transport.

PROTEIN SYNTHESIS-DEPENDENT SECRETION

Following the short-term protein synthesis-independent secretion of lysosomal enzymes in response to the phagocytosis of inflammatory stimuli, mononuclear phagocytes start synthesizing a number of new lysosomal enzymes by a process that is clearly protein synthesis dependent.[20] A large proportion of these enzymes is secreted directly to the exterior of the cells. Soluble stimuli such as C5a also initiate the synthesis of lysosomal enzymes by macrophages. Here, the secretory process is entirely dependent on protein synthesis and lacks the short-term protein synthesis-independent

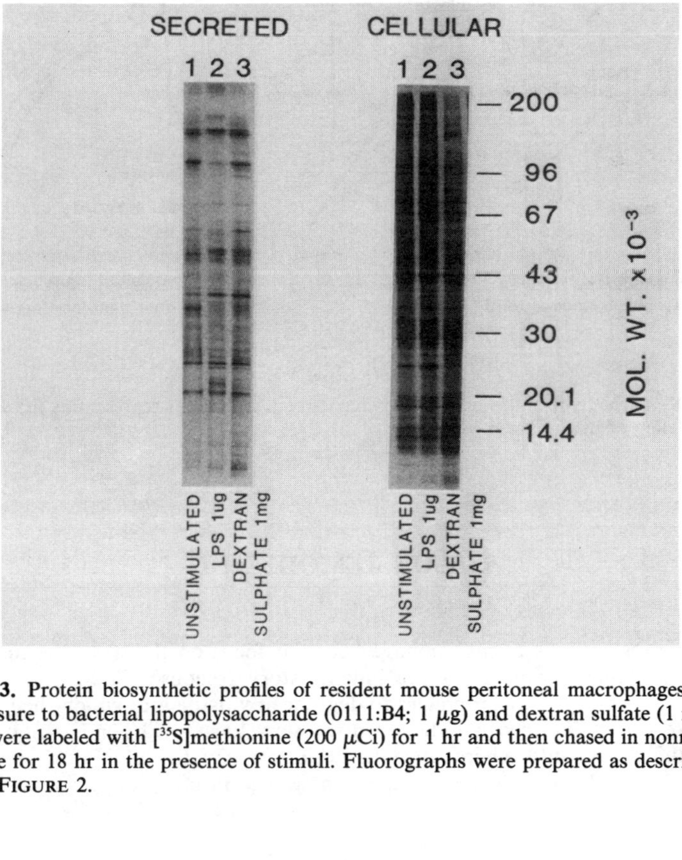

FIGURE 3. Protein biosynthetic profiles of resident mouse peritoneal macrophages following their exposure to bacterial lipopolysaccharide (0111:B4; 1 μg) and dextran sulfate (1 mg) for 24 hr. Cells were labeled with [^{35}S]methionine (200 μCi) for 1 hr and then chased in nonradioactive methionine for 18 hr in the presence of stimuli. Fluorographs were prepared as described in the legend to FIGURE 2.

component.[21] Not all macrophage stimuli, however, enhance the synthesis of lysosomal enzymes. Lipopolysaccharide, for example, a traditional macrophage stimulant, appears to inhibit the synthesis of lysosomal enzymes such as β-glucuronidase, although C3 and fibroblast growth factor[22] synthesis is markedly stimulated.

Many other degradative enzymes are also synthesized by macrophages in response to exposure to inflammatory stimuli. Most noticeable among these enzymes are a group of neutral proteinases characterized by plasminogen activator, elastase, and collagenase.[23-25] Unlike the lysosomal hydrolases, these enzymes are not stored within the cells and, furthermore, are only secreted in sizable quantities in response to specific types of macrophage-activating agents presented either *in vitro* or *in vivo.*

Mononuclear phagocytes also promote tissue degradation by influencing the functions of other cell types. It is known, for example, that macrophages and possibly osteoclasts (which are thought to be monocyte derived) secrete factor(s) which trigger fibroblasts and chondrocytes to synthesize and secrete collagenase and other neutral proteinases[26] which may be instrumental in initiating connective tissue breakdown. A schematic representation of the ways the macrophage participates in the degradation of the connective tissue matrix is illustrated in FIGURE 4.

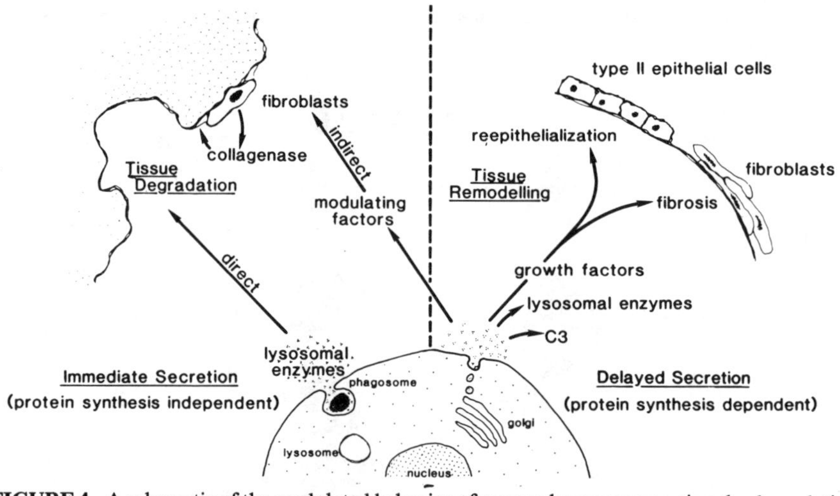

FIGURE 4. A schematic of the modulated behavior of macrophages representing the degradation and remodeling of the inflamed lung.

TISSUE REMODELING

Many investigations of macrophage behavior focus on the ways the macrophage can damage tissue during a chronic inflammatory response. These studies tend to emphasize the ability of macrophages to degrade any tissue into which they have been drawn. We would like to conclude this discussion, however, by indicating that macrophage infiltration into an inflamed tissue is essential to that tissue's remodeling. Monocytes not only degrade and remove damaged connective tissue components, they act as a source of growth factors that influence the restructuring of inflamed tissue and the healing of wounds.

Macrophages are known to produce protein factors that stimulate the growth of mesenchymal and parenchymal cells such as fibroblasts,[22] smooth muscle cells,[27] and endothelial cells.[28] In the lung, it is significant that the proliferation of rat type II alveolar cells (cells which serve to repopulate the denuded alveolar surface and from which pulmonary surfactant is derived) is also potentiated by medium conditioned by human monocyte-derived macrophages.[29] Thus, as graphically illustrated in FIGURE 4, the macrophage may greatly contribute to the remodeling of the lung after lung injury. It is not clear whether the growth factor for fibroblasts, which recent evidence suggests is interleukin-1,[30] is identical to that which stimulates type II alveolar cell proliferation. If indeed different factors are found to exist for each of these two types of cells, there are two possibilities which would have to be considered. Differential factor synthesis and secretion may establish a remodeling based mainly on fibroblast proliferation; this remodeling would ultimately lead to fibrosis of the lung. Alternatively, preferential type II alveolar cell proliferation may lead to reepithelialization of the lung. The latter possibility is, of course, the more desirable one.

SUMMARY

The theme we have presented herein is that of the adaptability of the mononuclear phagocyte. This has been illustrated by discussing the mechanisms underlying the emigration of blood monocytes into peripheral tissues and organs under steady state and inflammatory conditions. Our basic tenet is that monocytes represent a relatively homogenous cell population which migrates, either randomly or selectively, into a tissue and matures, following interaction with tissue components (be they normal or inflammatory), into macrophages characteristic of that tissue. Thus it is the interaction of a mononuclear phagocyte with an inflammatory stimulus that directs the phagocyte to mature into an inflammatory macrophage. Finally, we have also discussed how stimulus impingement on macrophages influences the products these cells secrete. We conclude that macrophages are essential to both the degradative and remodeling phases of an inflammatory response.

REFERENCES

1. VAN FURTH, R., F. DIESSELHOFF, M. M. C. DER DULK, J. A. RASBURN, T. L. VAN ZWET, R. DROFTON & A. BLUSSÉ VAN OUD ALBLAS. 1980. *In* Mononuclear Phagocytes: Functional Aspects. R. van Furth, Ed.: 279-295. Martinus Nijhoff. The Hague.
2. BROWN, M. S., S. K. BASU, J. R. FALCK, Y. K. YO & J. L. GOLDSTEIN. J. Supramol. Struct. **13:** 67-81.
3. ALLISON, A. C., C. CARDELLA & P. DAVIES. 1975. Rheumatology **6:** 251-266.
4. SPRITZER, A. A., J. A. WATSON, J. A. AULD & M. GUETHOFF. 1968. Arch. Environ. Health **17:** 726-730.
5. BOWDEN, D. & J. ADAMSON. 1972. Am. J. Pathol. **68:** 521-528.
6. MASSE, R., P. FRITSCH, D. NOLIBE, J. LAFUMA & J. CHRÉTIEN. 1977. ERDA Symp. Ser. **43:** 859.
7. BLUSSÉ VAN OUD ALBLAS, A. & R. VAN FURTH. 1979. J. Exp. Med. **149:** 1504-1518.

8. Blussé van Oud Alblas, A. 1980. *In* Heterogeneity of Mononuclear Phagocytes. O. Forster & M. Landy, Eds.: 21. Academic Press. London.
9. Shen, H. H., M. A. Talle, G. Goldstein & L. Chess. 1983. J. Immunol. **130:** 698-705.
10. Schreiber, A. D., M. Kelley, A. Dziarski & A. I. Levinson. 1983. Immunology 231-238.
11. McCarley, D. L., V. O. Shah & R. S. Weiner. 1983. J. Immunol. **131:** 1780-1783.
12. Blussé van Oud Alblas, A., B. van der Linden-Schrever & R. van Furth. 1981. J. Exp. Med. **154:** 235-252.
13. Leslie, C. C., R. J. Mason, D. R. Voelker, J. E. Henson & P. M. Henson. 1983. Am. Rev. Respir. Dis. **127:** 267A.
14. Norris, D. A., R. A. F. Clark, L. M. Swigert, C. Huff, W. L. Weston & S. E. Howell. 1982. J. Immunol. **129:** 1612-1618.
15. Harita, S., K. Sugimara & T. Watanabe. 1984. Eur. J. Immunol. **14:** 692-696.
16. Bursuker, I. 1980. *In* Heterogeneity of Mononuclear Phagocytes. O. Forster & M. Landy, Eds.: 25. Academic Press. London.
17. Davies, P., R. C. Page & A. C. Allison. 1974. J. Exp. Med. **139:** 1262-1282.
18. Schorlemmer, H. U., J. H. Edwards, P. Davies & A. C. Allison. 1977. Clin. Exp. Immunol. **27:** 198-207.
19. Henson, P. M. 1980. Am. J. Pathol. **101:** 494-511.
20. McCarthy, K., R. A. Musson & P. M. Henson. 1982. J. Reticuloendothel. Soc. **31:** 131-144.
21. McCarthy, K. & P. M. Henson. 1979. J. Immunol. **123:** 2511-2517.
22. Leslie, C. C., R. A. Musson & P. M. Henson. 1984. J. Leukocyte Biol. **36:** 143-160.
23. Unkeless, J., S. Gordon & E. Reich. 1974. J. Exp. Med. **139:** 834-850.
24. Werb, Z. & S. Gordon. 1975. J. Exp. Med. **142:** 346-360.
25. Werb, Z. & S. Gordon. 1975. J. Exp. Med. **142:** 361-377.
26. Krane, S. M., J. M. Dayer, S. R. Goldring & D. R. Robinson. 1981. *In* Research Monographs in Cell and Tissue Physiology. J. T. Dingle & J. L. Gordon, Eds.: 231-239.
27. Glenn, K. C. & R. Ross. 1981. Cell **25:** 603-615.
28. Martin, B. M., M. A. Gimbrone, E. R. Unanue & R. S. Cotran. 1981. J. Immunol. **126:** 1510-1515.
29. Leslie, C. C., P. C. Robinson, R. J. Mason, J. E. Henson & P. M. Henson. 1983. Am. Rev. Respir. Dis. **127:** 289A.
30. Schmidt, J. A., C. N. Oliver, J. L. Lepe-Zuniga, I. Green & I. Grey. 1984. J. Clin. Invest. **73:** 462-1472.

Genetic Control of Macrophage Responses[a]

R. VAN FURTH, W. SLUITER, AND J. T. VAN DISSEL

Department of Infectious Diseases
University Hospital
2333 AA Leiden, the Netherlands

INTRODUCTION

Sarcoidosis is a multisystem disease whose etiology is unknown. Histologically, the lesions are noncaseating granulomas in which the predominant cells are mononuclear phagocytes (macrophages, epithelioid cells, and multinucleated giant cells), but T lymphocytes also occur. Information about the origin, kinetics, and functions of macrophages has increased enormously in recent years. Although most of the research has been done in animals (the mouse, for example), the results provide some insight into the role of macrophages in chronic inflammatory diseases in man.

It may be assumed that some of the host factors that determine the degree of susceptibility to the development of sarcoidosis are genetically determined. To assess the contribution of these factors, information can be obtained from studies performed on genetically divergent strains of the same species of animal. For example, several inbred strains of mice differ in their relative susceptibility to infection with a number of intracellular pathogens including *Mycobacterium bovis* (bacillus Calmette Guérin), *Salmonella typhimurium, Listeria monocytogenes,* and *Leishmania donovani.*[1–4] These differences might be due to genetically determined differences in 1) the handling of microorganisms (phagocytosis, intracellular killing, and antigen presentation) by macrophages in the early phase of infection before the establishment of an immune response, that is, antibody formation and T lymphocyte-mediated macrophage activation; 2) the inflammatory response to the proliferation of certain microorganisms, characterized by an increase in the number of granulocytes and the exudation of macrophages at the site of infection; and 3) the development of humoral immunity and T lymphocyte-mediated immunity.

The preimmune phase of resistance to mycobacterial infection, defined as the inhibition of bacterial proliferation in the infected animal, is genetically controlled at the level of macrophage function. Macrophages from resistant mouse strains reduce the metabolic activity of intracellular bacilli more effectively than do macrophages from susceptible mouse strains.[5] With respect to the phase of cell-mediated immunity to mycobacterial infection, the potential of mice to develop granulomata has been

[a]This work was supported in part by the Netherlands Asthma Foundation and by the Foundation for Medical Research FUNGO, which is subsidized by the Netherlands Organization for the Advancement of Pure Research (ZWO).

shown to be under genetic control as well.[6] Low responsiveness is primarily due to impaired macrophage function, that is, to defective antigen presentation of T lymphocytes, rather than to impaired T lymphocyte function.[7] If the preimmune resistance of the host is adequate, the specific immune response involving macrophages activated by T lymphocyte products will play a relatively insignificant role as a host defense mechanism.

Since studies on genetic differences in the response to microorganisms or other agents are impossible or very difficult to perform in human subjects, information concerning the pathogenesis of certain human diseases must be obtained experimentally in animals. Research on the origin and kinetics of macrophages in mice led us to study the humoral regulation of monocyte production during inflammation, the monocyte being the precursor of the macrophage. Recently, we investigated the differences between two genetically divergent mouse strains with respect to the humoral regulation of monocytopoiesis and phagocytic functions.

ORIGIN AND KINETICS OF MONONUCLEAR PHAGOCYTES

Views on the origin of macrophages in the tissues and serous cavities under normal steady state conditions have differed, but at present it is generally agreed that during an inflammatory reaction, exudate macrophages arise from circulating monocytes. At one time, macrophages were thought to arise from fibroblasts or lymphocytes by transformation, but these concepts have been abandoned. Some authors, however, still adhere to the view that macrophages in normal tissues and body cavities are only renewed by local division,[8,9] despite the publication of evidence that under these conditions most of the macrophages originate from circulating monocytes.[10–13]

Our studies have shown that mononuclear phagocytes constitute a cell line that originates from a pluripotent stem cell in the bone marrow. The monoblast is the most immature cell of this cell line, and division of a monoblast gives rise to two promonocytes; the promonocyte too divides only once, giving rise to two monocytes (FIG. 1). Thus, from monoblast to monocyte there is a fourfold amplification. Monocytes do not divide again; they leave the bone marrow within 24 hr after they are formed and enter the circulattion, which they leave randomly within the next 24 hr to migrate to the tissues and serous cavities, where they differentiate into macrophages (FIG. 1).

Quantitative kinetic studies in normal mice have provided information about the percentage of monocytes that migrate from the circulation to various organs and serous cavities (TABLE 1).

In a new mathematical approach to the compartmental analysis of macrophage kinetics, the influx of monocytes, the local division of immature mononuclear phagocytes, and the efflux of macrophages from the tissues or serous cavities are taken into account.[14] The mononuclear phagocytes that divide locally have been shown to be cells that were labeled *in vitro* and had recently (less than 24-48 hr) entered the tissues.[15] These cells also originate in the bone marrow and thus in all probability divide only once within 24 hr after arriving in the tissues or serous cavities. Application of this approach to the data collected for Kupffer cells,[11] pulmonary macrophages,[12] spleen macrophages,[13] and peritoneal macrophages[10] showed that local division contributes appreciably to the size of the macrophage population of mice in the normal steady state (TABLE 1). According to this approach, the mean turnover time of macrophages, that is, the average time spent in a compartment, is rather short (TABLE 1), much shorter than the duration estimated in previous studies,[10–12] but we are of the opinion that the results obtained with the present mathematical approach are more accurate.[16]

Under normal steady state conditions, a constant influx of monocytes into the tissues where they become macrophages requires a constant efflux of macrophages from the tissue compartments and/or a constant cell death in the tissues. Little is known about this point. Various studies have shown that the afferent lymph of lymph nodes contains many macrophages whereas the efferent lymph has none. This means that macrophages migrate from the tissues to the local lymph nodes and suggests that they remain in the nodes and die there. Lung macrophages are exceptional in this respect because they can also leave the body via air spaces. If it occurs at all, recirculation of macrophages from tissues or serous cavities into the peripheral blood is probably minimal (FIG. 1).

TABLE 1. Data on the Kinetics of Monocytes and Macrophages in Different Tissues[a]

	Monocytes		Macrophages	
Tissue	Efflux from Circulation (%)	Influx into Tissue ($\times 10^3$/hr)	Local Production ($\times 10^3$/hr)	Mean Turnover Time (hr)
Liver[b]	71.8	93.3 (92%)	7.7 (8%)	3.8
Spleen	24.7	15.2 (55%)	12.2 (45%)	6.0
Lungs	14.7	9.1 (67%)	4.4 (33%)	6.0
Peritoneal cavity	6.7	4.1 (61%)	2.7 (39%)	14.9

[a] Adapted from R. van Furth.[16]
[b] Kupffer cells.

HUMORAL REGULATION OF MONOCYTE PRODUCTION

During an inflammatory reaction the number of macrophages increases at the site of inflammation, and this is accompanied by an increase in the number of monocytes[17–19] due to increased division of monoblasts and promonocytes in the bone marrow.[17] Recent investigations have shown that during the onset of an inflammatory reaction the circulating blood contains a factor that stimulates monocytopoiesis; this factor is called the factor increasing monocytopoiesis (FIM). The characteristics of FIM are summarized in TABLE 2.[20,21] Furthermore, it has been shown that FIM is not related to complement factors or clotting factors, has no chemotactic effect on macrophages, and has no colony-stimulating activity. These studies led to the following conclusion: FIM is synthesized and secreted by macrophages at the site of inflammation and is then transported via the circulation to the bone marrow where it exerts its stimulatory action (FIG. 2).

Although the available assay methods do not permit detection of FIM in the serum of mice under steady state conditions, it is conceivable that this factor regulates

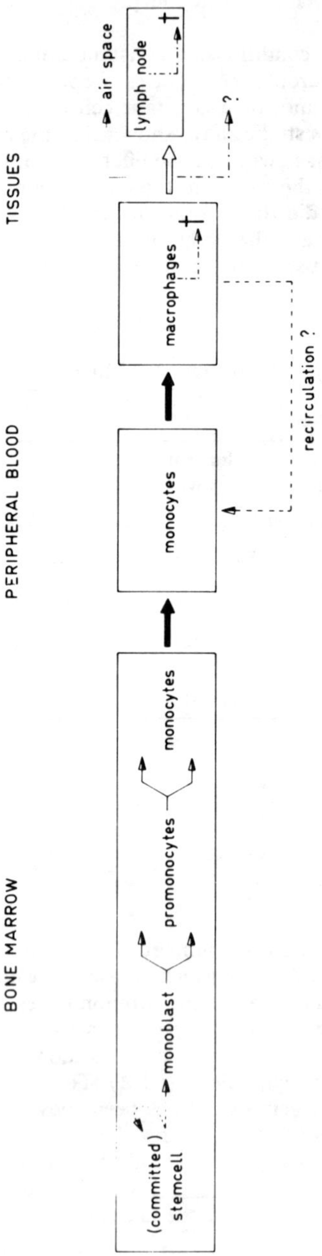

FIGURE 1. Schematic representation of the origin, kinetics, and fate of the mononuclear phagocytes.

TABLE 2. Characteristics of FIM in the Mouse and Rabbit

	Murine FIM[a]	Rabbit FIM[b]
Biological activity		
Monocyte production	Stimulation	Stimulation
Granulocyte production	No effect	No effect
Lymphocyte production	No effect	No effect
Origin	Macrophages	Macrophages
Species specificity	No	No
Concentration-effect relationship	Yes	Yes
Chemical nature	Protein	Protein
Molecular weight	18-24.5 kD	10-25 kD

[a] Adapted from van Waarde *et al.*[20]
[b] Adapted from Sluiter *et al.*[21]

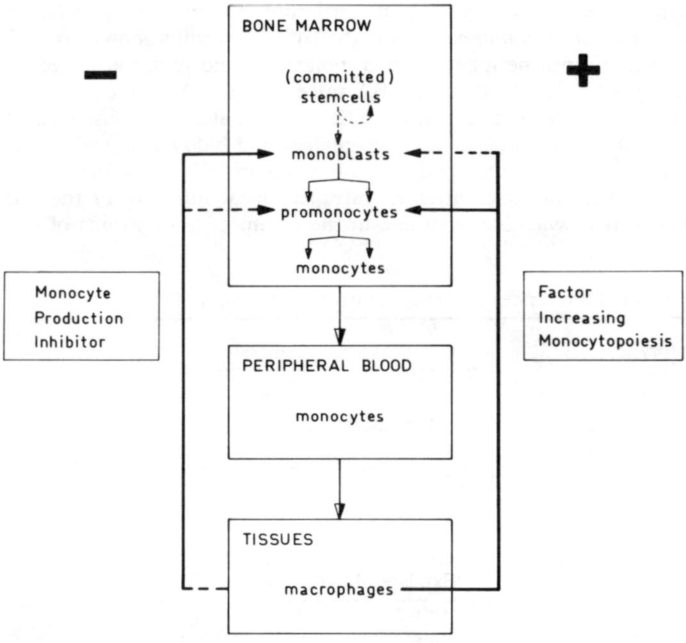

FIGURE 2. Schematic representation of the humoral control of monocytopoiesis. Macrophages at the site of inflammation synthesize and secrete FIM upon stimulation by an inflammatory agent. FIM is then transported via the circulation to the bone marrow, where it stimulates monocyte production at the level of the monoblasts and promonocytes. A second factor, MPI, inhibits monocyte production.

monocytopoiesis under these conditions as well. During a later phase of the inflammatory response the serum contains a factor that inhibits monocytopoiesis (FIG. 2). This factor, the monocyte-production inhibitor (MPI), has a molecular weight of 50 kD or more, but it has yet to be further characterized.[22]

GENETIC CONTROL OF MONOCYTE PRODUCTION

The increase in the number of macrophages in the inflammatory exudate in response to a variety of stimuli has been shown to be genetically controlled in mice.[23] Since monocyte production during an acute inflammation is stimulated by FIM, which in turn gives rise to increased numbers of macrophages in the inflammatory exudate, high- and low-responder mouse strains seemed likely to differ with respect to the production of FIM or the sensitivity of their monocyte precursor cells to this protein. This question was studied in specific pathogen-free, female low-responder CBA mice and high-responder C57BL/10 (B10) mice.

Studies on differences between these two strains showed that the number of blood monocytes was slightly higher in B10 mice (0.25×10^6 cells/ml) than in CBA mice (0.19×10^6 cells/ml) ($p < .0005$). The number of macrophages in the peritoneal cavity did not differ significantly between these two strains. For comparison of the magnitude of the cellular reaction in B10 and CBA mice, an inflammation was induced in the peritoneal cavity by injection of sterile polystyrene latex particles or a saline-soluble extract of *Listeria monocytogenes* (SEL).[24] The results showed that the increase in the numbers of both peripheral-blood monocytes and peritoneal macrophages was significantly greater in B10 than in CBA mice (TABLE 3).

To find out whether the difference in the inflammatory response of B10 and CBA mice, expressed in the numbers of macrophages and blood monocytes, was based on a difference in FIM production, the serum levels of FIM were determined in an *in vitro* assay[24] at various times after an intraperitoneal injection of the inflammatory agent. FIM activity was demonstrable in the serum of both strains of mice after an

TABLE 3. Strain Differences in Inflammatory Responses[a]

Inflammatory Stimulus	B10 Mice	CBA Mice	Difference
	Increase in the Number of Blood Monocytes ($\times 10^6$)		
Listeria extract[b]	2.0	-3.6	$p < .005$
Latex particles[c]	19.5	3.0	$p < .0005$
	Increase in the Number of Exudate Macrophages ($\times 10^5$)		
Listeria extract[b]	118.1	-5.6	$p < .0005$
Latex particles[c]	106.5	11.2	$p < .027$

[a] Adapted from Sluiter *et al.*[24] The increase in the number of cells is expressed as the area under the curve drawn for mice given intraperitoneal injections of inflammatory stimuli, minus the area under the curve drawn for control mice. Mice were observed for 72 hr after injection.

[b] A 0.1-ml saline-soluble extract (10 mg/ml) of *Listeria monocytogenes.*

[c] A 1-ml aliquot of a 1:40 dilution of polystyrene latex. The beads had diameters of 0.81 μm.

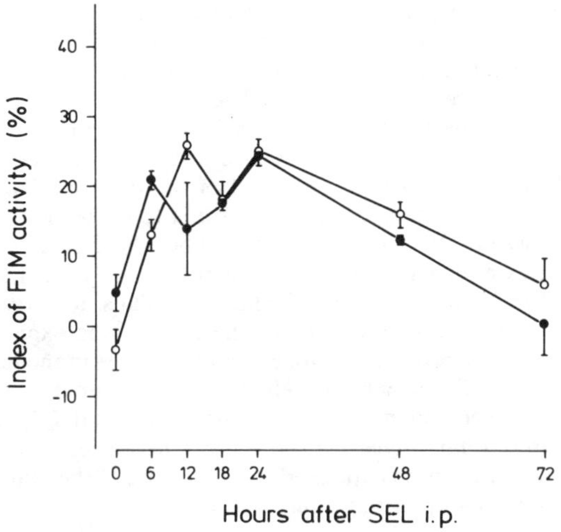

FIGURE 3. Course of the index of FIM activity in serum of B10 (●) and CBA mice (○) at various times after intraperitoneal injection of 0.1 ml of SEL, determined by an *in vitro* bioassay. The procedure used was the one described by Sluiter *et al.*[24]

intraperitoneal injection of latex (data not shown) or SEL (FIG. 3). The course of FIM activity and the maximum values were roughly the same in both mouse strains.

The finding that both low- and high-responder mice can produce FIM in similar amounts raised the question of whether the response to FIM might differ between these strains. To investigate this point, sera from B10 and CBA mice with maximal FIM activity were injected intravenously into normal B10 and CBA recipient mice in serial twofold dilutions in saline, and counts of circulating leukocytes were performed 24 hr later. In B10 recipient mice the number of blood monocytes increased with increasing doses of FIM-containing serum from high-responder (B10) and low-responder (CBA) mice; injection of these sera into CBA recipient mice did not induce monocytosis (FIG. 4). Apparently, CBA mice differ from B10 mice in the response of their monocytes to an injection of serum with FIM activity. The course of the numbers of granulocytes and lymphocytes in the two strains did not change significantly after injection of any of the sera under study.[24]

Thus, both mouse strains showed FIM in the peripheral blood during the initial phase of an inflammatory response, but low-responder CBA mice did not react by developing monocytosis after an intravenous injection of serum containing FIM, whereas in high-responder B10 mice FIM evoked monocytosis. The absence of a change in the numbers of granulocytes and lymphocytes after injection of serum containing FIM is consistent with the cell lineage-specific character of FIM.[19,21] Since the increase of the number of monocytes after the injection of FIM reflects the stimulation of monocyte production,[19,21] it may be concluded that only high-responder mice are able to respond to FIM by increased monocyte production.

GENETIC CONTROL OF PHAGOCYTOSIS AND INTRACELLULAR KILLING BY MACROPHAGES

To find out whether, in addition to the genetic differences in monocyte production, there are genetic differences in macrophage function in the preimmune phase of resistance between B10 and CBA mice, the phagocytosis and killing of *Listeria mono-*

cytogenes and *Salmonella typhimurium* by resident macrophages of these mouse strains have been studied. In these studies it must be kept in mind that B10 mice are susceptible to infection by *Salmonella typhimurium* but resistant to *Listeria monocytogenes* and that the reverse holds for CBA mice.[2,3]

The results show that resident macrophages of both B10 and CBA mice phagocytosed opsonized Salmonellae and Listeriae very effectively and to the same degree (data not shown). Assessment of the intracellular killing of *Salmonella typhimurium* by resident macrophages, according to three methods,[25] showed a consistent difference between CBA and B10 mice.[25] The initial rate of intracellular killing was about 1.7 times higher for the former than for the latter, but this difference was not found for *Listeria monocytogenes* (TABLE 4).[25] Thus, for *Salmonella typhimurium* the difference in the natural resistance of these mice was expressed in the efficacy of intracellular killing by resident peritoneal macrophages immediately upon ingestion of the bacteria. This finding might be relevant for the innate resistance of mice to Salmonellae, a resistance which does not require functional T lymphocytes.[26] This is not the case for *Listeria monocytogenes,* however, where other mechanisms (a difference in the inflammatory reaction expressed in an increase of the number of phagocytic cells, for instance) are probably of more importance.

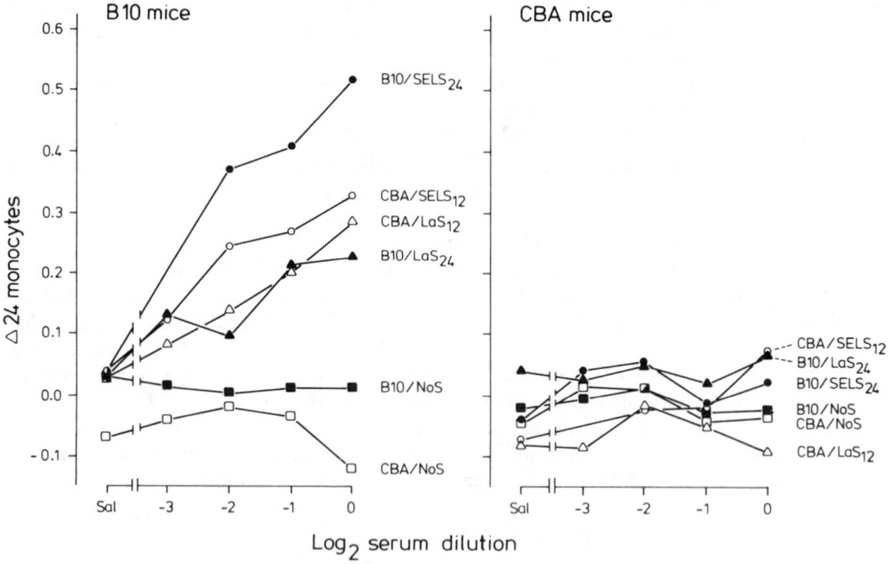

FIGURE 4. Monocyte response of B10 mice (left panel) and CBA mice (right panel) expressed as the difference between the number of blood monocytes at the time of and 24 hr after intravenous injection (Δ24) of normal serum (■—■), LaS_{24} (▲ — ▲), and $SELS_{24}$ (●—●) from B10 mice, and normal serum (□—□), LaS_{12} (△—△), and $SELS_{12}$ (○ — ○) from CBA mice. LaS_{12} and LaS_{24}: serum from mice 12 and 24 hr after an intraperitoneal injection of latex; $SELS_{12}$ and $SELS_{24}$: serum of mice 12 and 24 hr after an intraperitoneal injection of SEL.

TABLE 4. Rate Constants of the Intracellular Killing of Two Pathogens by Resident Peritoneal Macrophages[a]

	Rate Constant of Intracellular Killing	
Mouse Strain	*Salmonella typhimurium*	*Listeria monocytogenes*
B10	0.031 (± 0.013)	0.033 (± 0.009)
CBA	0.055 (± 0.017)	0.032 (± 0.011)

[a] The rate of intracellular killing was determined *in vitro* after phagocytosis of bacteria *in vivo*.[25] All data are mean values (± SD) of rates determined over a 60-min period. The significance level of the differences in rate constants of the two mouse strains is lower than 1%.

DISCUSSION

What is the relevance of our findings for the pathogenesis of sarcoidosis? Sarcoidosis is a granulomatous disease, the granulomas being composed of T lymphocytes and mononuclear phagocytes, that is, exudate macrophages, epithelioid cells, and multinucleated giant cells, all of which arise from circulating monocytes. It is conceivable that genetically controlled factors play a role in the genesis of a sarcoid lesion. The present results point to at least two mechanisms for the induction of a granulomatous response to an unknown agent which induces a sarcoid lesion and to which sarcoidosis patients may be high responders. These mechanisms involve 1) reactivity to the humoral regulator FIM, which stimulates the precursor cells in the bone marrow to form monocytes, and 2) the functional reactivity of the patient's macrophages. Sarcoidosis patients then dispose of an adequate supply of monocytes to maintain migration of these cells to the lesion and their transformation into macrophages, and macrophages of sarcoidosis patients may handle the antigen effectively and mount a cellular immune response by stimulating T lymphocytes. Other genetically controlled mechanisms unquestionably will play a role in the pathogenesis of sarcoidosis as well.

SUMMARY

A short review of current concepts concerning the origin and kinetics of monocytes and macrophages is given, and the humoral regulation of monocyte production by FIM, a factor synthesized and secreted by macrophages, is discussed. Genetic control of the responsiveness of monocyte precursors to FIM and that of the phagocytosis and intracellular killing of bacteria is dealt with.

REFERENCES

1. GROS, P., E. SKAMENE & A. FORGET. 1981. Genetic control of natural resistance to *Mycobacterium bovis* (BCG) in mice. J. Immunol. **127:** 2417-2421.

2. HORMEACHE, C. E. 1979. Natural resistance to *Salmonella typhimurium* in different inbred strains of mice. Immunology **37:** 311-318.
3. CHEERS, C. & I. F. C. MCKENZIE. 1978. Resistance and susceptibility of mice to bacterial infection: Genetics of listeriosis. Infect. Immun. **19:** 755-762.
4. BRADLEY, D. J. 1974. Genetic control of natural resistace to *Leishmania donovani.* Nature **250:** 353.
5. STACH, J. L., P. GROS, A. FORGET & E. SKAMENE. 1984. Phenotypic expression of genetically controlled natural resistance to *Mycobacterium bovis* (BCG). J. Immunol. **132:** 888-892.
6. YAMAMOTO, K. & K. KAKINUMA. 1978. Genetic control of granuloma response to oil-associated BCG cell wall vaccine in mice. Microbiol. Immunol. **22:** 335-348.
7. KAKINUMA, M., K. ONOÉ, R. YASUMIZU & K. YAMAMOTO. 1983. Strain differences in lung granuloma formation in response to a BCG cell wall vaccine in mice: Failure of antigen presentation by low-responder macrophages. Immunology **50:** 423-431.
8. VOLKMAN, A. 1976. Disparity in origin of mononuclear phagocyte populations. J. Reticuloendothel. Soc. **19:** 249-268.
9. DAEMS, W. T. 1980. Peritoneal macrophages. *In* The Reticuloendothelial System: A Comprehensive Treatise. I. Carr & W. T. Daems, Eds. Vol. **1:** 57-127. Plenum. New York, NY.
10. VAN FURTH, R. & Z. A. COHN. 1968. The origin and kinetics of mononuclear phagocytes. J. Exp. Med. **128:** 415-435.
11. CROFTON, R. W., M. M. C. DIESSELHOFF-DEN DULK & R. VAN FURTH. 1978. The origin, kinetics, and characteristics of the Kupffer cells in the normal steady state. J. Exp. Med. **148:** 1-17.
12. BLUSSÉ VAN OUD ALBLAS, A. & R. VAN FURTH. 1979. The origin, kinetics, and characteristics of pulmonary macrophages in the normal steady state. J. Exp. Med. **22:** 118-122.
13. VAN FURTH. R. & M. M. C. DIESSELHOFF-DEN DULK. 1984. Dual origin of mouse spleen macrophages. J. Exp. Med. **160:** 1274-1283.
14. BLUSSÉ VAN OUD ALBLAS, A., H. MATTIE & R. VAN FURTH. 1983. A quantitative evaluation of pulmonary macrophage kinetics. Cell Tissue Kinet. **16:** 211-219.
15. THOMPSON, J. & R. VAN FURTH. 1970. The effect of glucocorticosteroids on the kinetics of mononuclear phagocytes. J. Exp. Med. **131:** 429-442.
16. VAN FURTH, R. 1985. New perspectives on the kinetics of mononuclear phagocytes. *In* Mononuclear Phagocytes: Characteristics, Physiology and Function. R. van Furth, Ed. Martinus Nijhoff. Boston, MA.
17. VAN FURTH, R., M. M. C. DIESSELHOFF-DEN DULK & H. MATTIE. 1973. Quantitative study on the production and kinetics of mononuclear phagocytes during an acute inflammatory reaction. J. Exp. Med. **138:** 1314-1340.
18. VAN WAARDE, D., E. HULSING-HESSELINK & R. VAN FURTH. 1976. A serum factor inducing monocytopoiesis during an acute inflammatory reaction caused by newborn calf serum. Cell Tissue Kinet. **9:** 51-63.
19. VAN WAARDE, D., E. HULSING-HESSELINK & R. VAN FURTH. 1977. Humoral regulation of monocytopoiesis during the early phase of an inflammatory reaction caused by particulate substances. Blood **50:** 141-153.
20. VAN WAARDE, D., E. HULSING-HESSELINK & R. VAN FURTH. 1977. Properties of a factor increasing monocytopoiesis (FIM) occurring in the serum during the early phase of an inflammatory reaction. Blood **50:** 727-742.
21. SLUITER, W., I. ELZENGA-CLAASEN, E. HULSING-HESSELINK & R. VAN FURTH. 1983. Presence of the factor increasing monocytopoiesis (FIM) in rabbit peripheral blood during an acute inflammation. J. Reticuloendothel. Soc. **34:** 235-252.
22. VAN WAARDE, D., E. HULSING-HESSELINK & R. VAN FURTH. 1978. Humoral control of monocytopoiesis by an activator and an inhibitor. Agents Actions **8:** 432-437.
23. STEVENSON, M. M., P. A. L. KONGSHAVN & E. SKAMENE. 1981. Genetic linkage of resistance to *Listeria monocytogenes* with macrophage inflammatory responses. J. Immunol. **127:** 402-407.

24. SLUITER, W., I. ELZENGA-CLAASEN, A. VAN DER VOORT VAN DER KLEY-VAN ANDEL & R. VAN FURTH. 1984. Differences in the response of inbred mouse strains to the factor increasing monocytopoiesis. J. Exp. Med. **159:** 524-536.
25. VAN DISSEL, J. T., P. C. J. LEIJH & R. VAN FURTH. Differences in initial rate from various mouse strains. J. Immunol. **134:** 3404-3410.
26. O'BRIEN, A. D. & E. S. METCALF. 1982. Control of early *Salmonella typhimurium* growth in innately Salmonella-resistant mice does not require functional T lymphocytes. J. Immunol. **129:** 1349-1351.

Oxygen Radicals and Arachidonate Metabolites in Lung Injury[a]

PETER A. WARD, KENT J. JOHNSON,
AND GERD O. TILL

Department of Pathology
The University of Michigan Medical School
Ann Arbor, Michigan 48109

There is an increasing amount of evidence that oxygen radicals produced by activated phagocytic cells play an important role in the induction of acute lung injury, which in some cases leads to progressive lung injury. The bulk of work in the past several years deals with models of acute lung injury in experimental animals. The findings of many of these studies have recently been extrapolated to considerations of the adult respiratory distress syndome (ARDS) in humans.

Oxygen radical production by activated phagocytic cells is now a well-known fact,[1] and it is known that a variety of cells, such as neutrophils, eosinophils, monocytes, and macrophages, have the ability to produce oxygen radicals upon stimulation. There is more evidence that nonphagocytic cells may, under very special circumstances, also have the ability to produce oxygen radicals.[2] There is little evidence, however, that either platelets or basophils can, upon activation with a variety of stimuli, generate these oxygen products, even though secretion of granule products is known to occur.

Oxygen radical production by phagocytic cells is stimulated by a variety of agonists. These agonists include chemotactic peptides and lipids; complement activation products such as anaphylatoxins and C3b; phorbol myristate acetate; and phagocytic stimuli including immune complexes, zymosan particles, and other insoluble materials. Cell surface interaction with any of these agonists leads to a cascade of chemical reactions which appears to initially involve activation of a cell membrane associated NADPH oxidase. This results in the progressive reduction of molecular oxygen, by a sequential addition of electrons, to a series of products, as shown in the scheme below:

$$O_2 \xrightarrow{e^-} \cdot O_2^- \xrightarrow{e^-} H_2O_2 \xrightarrow[Fe^{2+}]{e^-} \cdot OH \xrightarrow{e^-} H_2O$$

The sequential addition of four electrons to molecular oxygen ultimately results in the production of water. It is important to note that the intermediate oxygen radicals from the series described above are always present. The most unstable one is the hydroxyl radical ($\cdot OH$), the superoxide anion ($\cdot O_2^-$) is moderately unstable, and hydrogen peroxide (H_2O_2) is very stable. It should be emphasized that the conversion of hydrogen peroxide to the hydroxyl radical is greatly facilitated by the presence of

[a] This work was supported in part by Grants GM18832, GM29507, HL28442, and HL31936 from the National Institutes of Health.

ionic iron. It has been known for some time that in lipid peroxidation reactions iron plays a key role.[3] Iron may be effective in these reactions because of its ability to facilitate the production of hydroxyl radical, although this is a controversial point at present. The recognition of a series of products appearing during the progressive reduction of molecular oxygen implies that in a given reaction at a given moment there will be a mixture of oxygen reduction products, which makes it difficult to implicate a single product in a reaction related to tissue injury. Evidence will be presented below that hydrogen peroxide and the hydroxyl radical may be the most important oxygen products that can be directly linked to tissue injury.

ARACHIDONATE PRODUCTS AND PHAGOCYTIC CELLS

Activation of phagocytic cells by chemotactic factors or phagocytic stimuli usually leads to a cascade of reactions ultimately resulting in the production of metabolic products from arachidonic acid (FIG. 1). Receptor-ligand interaction on the surface

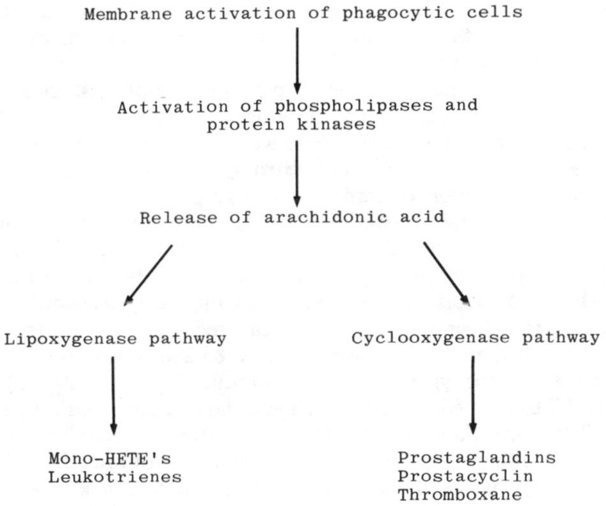

FIGURE 1. Arachidonate pathways in phagocytic cells.

of the phagocytic cell leads to activation of phospholipases, especially phospholipase A_2, which results in the cleavage of arachidonic acid from the second carbon position in the glycerol backbone of a phospholipid. There is some evidence that these reactions are also associated concomitantly with the activation of one or more protein kinases, which results in phosphorylation of lipomodulin, a naturally occurring inhibitor of phospholipases. The ultimate outcome of these reactions is the unrestrained activity of phospholipase A_2, which causes the appearance of free arachidonic acid within the cell. This fatty acid can then undergo metabolism by the cyclooxygenase and the lipoxygenase pathways. The former pathway results in the production of the classical prostaglandins and prostacyclin and thromboxane. The extent to which one or more classes of these cyclooxygenase products will be formed depends upon the cell type. In the neutrophil, for instance, large amounts of both classical prostaglandins (PGE_2 and $PGF_{2\alpha}$) and thromboxane (TxA_2) are formed, with little or no production of prostacyclin (PGI_2). In macrophages large amounts of prostaglandins are formed with little production of thromboxane. Metabolism of arachidonic acid via the lipoxygenase pathway results in the production of a series of mono-HETE compounds and often the simultaneous appearance of leukotrienes. Neutrophils tend to produce relatively large amounts of leukotriene B_4 (LTB_4) whereas macrophages tend to produce little in the way of LTB_4 and large amounts of the sulfidopeptide leukotrienes LTC_4, D_4, and E_4.[4,5]

The relationship between the appearance of these products of arachidonate metabolism and the functional response of the phagocytic cell is not very clear at present. Studies in different laboratories have produced conflicting results. The experimental approach has usually been either to measure the various arachidonate metabolites and correlate their presence with a functional response of the cell or to employ inhibitors, the specificity of which is often implied, in order to block either the lipoxygenase pathway or the cyclooxygenase pathway and to infer the role of products of each of these pathways in the functional response of the stimulated cell.

Our own studies on the production of arachidonate metabolites in stimulated rat neutrophils and the relationship of these products to the cell response are summarized in TABLE 1. Neutrophils were prelabeled with tritiated arachidonic acid which was fully incorporated into the phospholipid fraction. The cells were then stimulated with a variety of agonists: immune complexes, calcium ionophores, zymosan particles, chemotactic peptides, and phorbol myristate acetate. The cyclooxygenase inhibitors indomethacin, ibuprofen, and piroxicam, as well as the lipoxygenase inhibitors nordihydroguaiaretic acid (NDGA) and nafazatrom were employed. With reference to the specificity of these inhibitors (determined by high pressure liquid chromatography), it can be seen that the cyclooxygenase inhibitors reduced the generation of cyclooxygenase products between 40 and 50%. The effectiveness of the different lipoxygenase inhibitors varied; the production of cyclooxygenase products was reduced between 1.4 and 25.8%. When the effects of the same drugs on the generation of lipoxygenase products (chiefly 5-HETE and LTB_4) were measured, it was found that the cyclooxygenase inhibitors substantially increased (32.5 to 83.2%) the amount of leukotrienes produced, whereas the lipoxygenase inhibitors reduced (42.9 to 69.5%) the amounts of 5-HETE and LTB_4 formed. Based upon these data, it appears that cyclooxygenase products may "down-regulate" the lipoxygenase pathway; when the cyclooxygenase pathway is blocked, either through "substrate shunting" of arachidonic acid into the lipoxygenase pathway or via the loss of the negative feedback, there is a marked potentiation in the amount of lipoxygenase pathway products formed.

The effects of these inhibitors on the functional responses of rat neutrophils are summarized in TABLE 1. Oxygen radical production was reduced 15 to 43%, and, a consistent pattern was demonstrated in the enzyme release response: cyclooxygenase pathway inhibitors enhanced it 14 to 18% whereas the lipoxygenase pathway inhibitors reduced it 28 to 78%. These data can be interpreted to suggest that there is a linkage between lipoxygenase pathway product formation and enzyme secretion in activated rat neutrophils and that cyclooxygenase products tend to negatively affect this response. On the other hand, no such pattern has been noted with oxygen radical production. All inhibitors tend to have inhibitory effects, suggesting that there is a fundamental difference between the effects of arachidonate metabolites and their effects in the neutrophil responses of enzyme release and oxygen radical generation. These studies are described in detail in a recent report[4] and are summarized in TABLES 2 & 3.

TABLE 1. Relationship between Arachidonate Metabolite Production and Functional Responses in Stimulated Rat Neutrophils[a]

	Arachidonate Metabolites (Percent Reduction)		Functional Responses (Percent Reduction)	
Inhibitor Employed (5-10 μM)	Cyclooxygenase Products	Leukotrienes	$\cdot O_2^-$ Generation	Enzyme Release
Cyclooxygenase inhibitors				
Indomethacin	50.6	-83.2[b]	15	-14
Ibuprofen	40.5	-35.7	19	-15
Piroxicam	43.8	-32.5	17	-18
Lipoxygenase inhibitors				
Nordihydroguaiaretic acid	25.8	69.5		78
Nafazatrom	1.4	42.9	43	28

[a] Neutrophils were stimulated with immune complexes of BSA and of rabbit IgG to BSA; this stimulation elicited the functional responses and production of arachidonates.

[b] Negative numbers indicate enhancement of cell response.

Some interesting parallels have been noted when arachidonate metabolite production is studied in rat neutrophils undergoing stimulation by a variety of different agonists. For instance, stimulation of rat neutrophils by phorbol myristate acetate leads to maximal $\cdot O_2^-$ generation but with only trivial amounts of arachidonic products being formed, whereas stimulation of rat neutrophils by the chemotactic peptide *N*-formyl-methionyl-leucyl-phenylalanine (FMLP) results in substantial enzyme release coupled with substantial arachidonate product formation but with virtually no $\cdot O_2^-$ production. Again, these data suggest that there is a dissociation between $\cdot O_2^-$ generation and enzyme release and that if arachidonate metabolites are directly involved in the cell response, it is in the enzyme secretion reaction but not in the response of $\cdot O_2^-$ generation.

Although macrophages in general tend to produce prostaglandins as well as the leukotrienes C_4, D_4, and E_4, there is good evidence that a similar parallelism exists between cell activation and arachidonate product formation.[5] In studies in mice in

TABLE 2. Neutrophil Activation, Functional Responses, and Arachidonate Metabolism

	Functional Response		
Agonist	$\cdot O_2^-$ Generation	Enzyme Release	Arachidonate Metabolites
Phorbol myristate acetate	Yes	Little	Few, if any
Chemotactic peptide (FMLP)	No	Yes	TxB_2, 5-HETE, and LTB_4[a]
Calcium ionophores	Little	Yes	Similar to those elicited by FMLP
IgG-immune complexes	Yes	Yes	Similar to those elicited by FMLP

[a] ng quantities.

TABLE 3. Role of Arachidonate Metabolites in Functional Responses of Rat Neutrophils

	Functional Response	
	Enzyme Secretion	$\cdot O_2^-$ Generation
$\cdot O_2^-$	No correlation	—
Enzyme secretion	—	No correlation
Production of arachidonate metabolites[a]	Correlation	No correlation
Cyclooxygenase inhibitors	Enhancement	Inhibition
Lipoxygenase inhibitors	Inhibition	Inhibition

[a] PGE_2, TxB_2, 5-HETE, and LTB_4.

which T cell-dependent pulmonary granulomas have been investigated, it has been demonstrated that the *in vivo* application of lipoxygenase pathway inhibitors greatly diminishes granuloma formation whereas the treatment of animals with cyclooxygenase inhibitors of the type described above greatly increases the size of the granulomas. As might be expected, treatment of mice with prostaglandin E_2 markedly diminishes the size of the granulomas. Although these studies have been confined to the mouse, the interpretation of the role of arachidonate metabolites is similar to that in the study of the rat neutrophil (described above). That is to say, cyclooxygenase pathway products tend to be inhibitory whereas lipoxygenase pathway products enhance the ultimate biological response of the activated neutrophil or macrophage.

MODELS OF ACUTE LUNG INJURY DEPENDENT UPON OXYGEN RADICAL FORMATION

Mediator pathways in models of acute lung injury in which oxygen radical formation appears to be importantly involved in the ultimate expression of lung injury have been studied in a variety of experimental model systems: these are summarized in TABLE 4. Three general classifications of model systems can be made. The first involves reactions in which neutrophils and complement are both required for the ultimate outcome. The second involves reactions in which complement is but neutrophils are not required for the development of tissue damage. The third involves a reaction in which neither complement nor neutrophil participation is required for acute lung injury.

Acute lung injury mediated by complement and neutrophils has been well demonstrated in the case of immune complex deposition involving immunoglobulin G (IgG). Whether by the use of rabbit polyclonal antibody to bovine serum albumin (BSA) or mouse IgG monoclonal antibody to dinitrophenol (DNP), the resulting alveolar and vascular injury associated with deposition of immune complexes requires the availability of complement (presumably through its chemotactic factor C5a peptide and perhaps other neutrophil-activating products) and neutrophils[6] which, through the formation of oxygen radicals, bring about acute tissue injury.[7] Superoxide anion which can be intercepted by the presence of superoxide dismutase (SOD) results in an amplification of the early phases of the inflammatory response, causing the accumulation of increased numbers of neutrophils at the site of the immune complex deposition.[8] Additional studies have demonstrated that $\cdot O_2^-$ and H_2O_2 as well as iron participate in the outcome of immune complex-mediated tissue injury.[9] It is likely that iron is required because of its ability to facilitate conversion of H_2O_2 to $\cdot OH$. The basis for this conclusion is the recent demonstration that scavengers of hydroxyl radical as well as iron chelators will greatly attenuate the damage after IgG immune complex deposition in dermal vessels and lungs of rats.[9] Leukocytic myeloperoxidase may also contribute to the development of injury through the conversion of H_2O_2 to a halide-dependent product such as hypochlorous acid; however, this has not been directly demonstrated *in vivo.*

The second model of acute lung injury involving the role of neutrophils and complement is that of systemic complement activation: injection of the C3 activator isolated from cobra venom into rats produces a prompt and profound activation of the complement system, which results in the stimulation of neutrophils and in the aggregation and entrapment of neutrophils within the pulmonary interstitial capillary network. Neutrophil activation with oxygen radical production results in the injury of, and sometimes causes the necrosis of, pulmonary endothelial cells.[10] It has recently been demonstrated that the mechanism of injury is probably via hydroxyl radical formation; this seems likely because the endothelial cell damage can be greatly attenuated by the presence of catalase, hydroxyl radical scavengers (such as dimethyl sulfoxide), and iron chelators (apolactoferrin derived from human breast milk or deferoxamine).[11]

It has recently been demonstrated that another type of immune complex deposition leading to acute lung injury in rat follows a different immunopathogenic mechanism. The use of mouse monoclonal immunoglobulin A (IgA) antibody with reactivity to DNP has made it possible to demonstrate that immune complex deposition in rat lungs leads, in a manner in which neutrophils are not involved, to acute alveolar and vascular injury. The reaction, however, is clearly complement dependent.[6] Evidence that this is an oxygen radical-related form of injury is emerging even though the source of the oxygen radical production has not been determined (K. J. Johnson, B. Wilson, and P. A. Ward, unpublished observations). It could be that IgA immune complexes acting through some complement activation product are causing oxygen radical production from alveolar macrophages, interstitial macrophages, and, perhaps, recruited blood monocytes. This remains to be demonstrated.

The third model system of oxygen radical-dependent acute lung injury involves a system that is both complement and neutrophil independent. Phorbol myristate acetate

TABLE 4. Model Systems of Oxygen Radical-dependent Acute Lung Injury

Neutrophil- and Complement-dependent Lung Injury
Acute immune complex injury by deposition of rabbit polyclonal IgG antibody to BSA or mouse monoclonal IgG antibody to DNP
Systemic complement activation by injection of C3 activator from cobra venom
Neutrophil-dependent and Complement-independent Lung Injury
Acute immune complex injury by deposition of mouse monoclonal IgA antibody to DNP
Neutrophil- and Complement-independent Lung Injury
Acute and progressive lung injury by instillation of phorbol myristate acetate

instilled into the distal airways causes an intense and acute lung injury with the alveolar compartment being denuded of the epithelial lining cells. This results not only in acute injury with severe intraalveolar hemorrhage and edema but also in progressive pulmonary interstitial fibrosis.[12] It has been demonstrated that neither complement nor neutrophil depletion will alter either the acute or the chronic outcome of this reaction. On the other hand, the coinstillation of catalase with phorbol myristate acetate will prevent both the acute and the progressive damage found in this model system.

The various experimental models described above suggest that oxygen radical production from activated phagocytic cells plays an important role in lung injury. Interventions designed to intercept these radicals are markedly protective. What determines chronicity and irreversibility of the lung responses in these models of injury is not known, but the observations to date have important implications in a variety of lung inflammatory reactions in humans, perhaps the most obvious example being the adult respiratory distress syndrome. Extensive additional studies will have to be completed before these reactions are fully understood and effective clinical therapeutic interventions are developed.

REFERENCES

1. Fantone, J. C. & P. A. Ward. 1982. Review article: Role of oxygen-derived free radicals and metabolites in leukocyte-dependent inflammatory reactions. Am. J. Pathol. **107:** 395-418.
2. Freeman, B. A. & J. D. Crapo. 1982. Biology of disease: Free radicals and tissue injury. Lab. Invest. **47:** 412-426.
3. Aust, S. D. & B. A. Svingen. 1982. The role of iron in enzymatic lipid peroxidation. *In* Free Radicals in Biology. W. A. Pryor, Ed. Vol. **5:** 1-28. Academic Press. New York, NY.
4. Ward, P. A., M. C. Sulavik & K. J. Johnson. 1984. Role of lipoxygenase and cyclooxygenase products in neutrophil activation. Fed. Proc. **43:** 1803.
5. Kunkel, S. L., S. W. Chensue, C. Mouton & G. I. Higashi. 1984. Role of lipoxygenase products in murine pulmonary granuloma formation. J. Clin. Invest. **74:** 514-524.
6. Johnson, K. J., B. S. Wilson, G. O. Till & P. A. Ward. 1984. Acute lung injury in rat caused by immunoglobulin A immune complexes. J. Clin. Invest. **74:** 358-369.
7. Johnson, K. J. & P. A. Ward. 1981. Role of oxygen metabolites in immune complex injury of lung. J. Immunol. **126:** 2365-2369.
8. McCormick, J. R., M. M. Harkin, K. J. Johnson & P. A. Ward. 1981. Suppression by superoxide dismutase of immune complex-induced pulmonary alveolitis and dermal inflammation. Am. J. Pathol. **102:** 55-61.
9. Fligiel, S. E. G., P. A. Ward, K. J. Johnson & G. O. Till. 1984. Evidence for role of hydroxyl radical in immune complex-induced vasculitis. Am. J. Pathol. **115:** 375-382.
10. Till, G. O., K. J. Johnson, R. Kunkel & P. A. Ward. 1982. Intravascular activation of complement and acute lung injury: Dependency on neutrophilis and toxic oxygen metabolites. J. Clin. Invest. **69:** 1126-1135.
11. Ward, P. A., G. O. Till, R. Kunkel & C. Beauchamp. 1983. Evidence for role of hydroxyl radical in complement and neutrophil-dependent tissue injury. J. Clin. Invest. **72:** 789-801.
12. Johnson, K. J. & P. A. Ward. 1982. Acute and progressive lung injury after contact with phorbol myristate acetate. Am. J. Pathol. **107:** 29-35.

Assessment of Respiratory Epithelial Permeability by Bronchoalveolar Lavage and Aerosolized ^{99m}Tc-DTPA in Patients with Sarcoidosis[a]

DANIEL DUSSER, MADELEINE MORDELET-DAMBRINE, MARIE-ANNE COLLIGNON, GISÈLE STANISLAS-LEGUERN, JACQUES CHRÉTIEN, AND GÉRARD HUCHON[b]

Institut National de la Santé
et de la Recherche Médicale Unité 214
Hôpital Laennec
75340 Paris Cédex 07, France

INTRODUCTION

The increased permeability of the respiratory epithelium in many pulmonary diseases has already been described.[1-6] Endothelial permeability may be assessed by several different methods: by using indicator dilution curves and a range of tracer molecules in a single pass through the vascular bed,[7] by the measurement of the pulmonary transvascular flux of a radioactive protein using an external scintillation detector,[8] and by the study of transendothelial transport material after osmotic bolus.[9] These methods have limited application to studies in man, and they measure only the pulmonary endothelial permeability. Other techniques have recently been developed for measuring pulmonary endothelial and epithelial permeability that may be applicable to studies in patients: the determination of albumin flux by the measurement of albumin concentration in alveolar fluid obtained by a bronchoalveolar lavage (BAL),[10-12] and the determination of the flux of a radioactive solute introduced into respiratory spaces as an aerosol. The transfer of the radioactive solute from alveolar spaces to pulmonary blood circulation may be assessed by taking repeated venous blood samples[13] or using an external scintillation detector which counts the decay of radioactivity in the lung fields.[1,5] The purpose of this study was to compare two methods for assessing the

[a]This work was supported by NATO Research Grant 12482 and by a grant from René Descartes University.

[b]Address for correspondence and reprint requests: Hôpital Laennec, 42 rue de Sévres, 75340 Paris Cédex 07, France.

respiratory epithelial permeability in pulmonary sarcoidosis: the measurement of albumin flux through the alveolocapillary membrane using the ratio of the albumin concentration found in a BAL to that found in the serum (S) and the determination of clearance of an aerosolized radioactive solute.

MATERIALS AND METHODS

Subjects

We studied 59 healthy, nonsmoking subjects and 20 nonsmoking patients with sarcoidosis.

Control Subjects

The control subjects, healthy nonsmokers, were volunteers free of any symptom of pulmonary disease and who had normal results from pulmonary function tests. These subjects were divided into two groups: group C1 and group C2. A BAL was performed on each of the 21 subjects in group C1; respiratory epithelial permeability was assessed by the clearance of aerosolized ^{99m}Tc-labeled diethylenetriamine-pentaacetic acid (^{99m}Tc-DTPA) in each of the 38 subjects in group C2.

Patient Population

The patient group, group S, was comprised of 20 nonsmokers with pulmonary sarcoidosis. The diagnosis of sarcoidosis was established by demonstrating the presence of noncaseating epithelioid granulomas on bronchial biopsies or by a positive Kveim test using the Swiss antigen of Favez.[14] Five of these patients (group S1) had isolated bilateral hilar adenopathy, and the 15 others (group S2) had parenchymal abnormalities on their lung roentgenograms. Pulmonary function tests were performed in all patients and are shown in TABLE 1.

Both methods for assessing the respiratory epithelial permeability (the determination of the clearance of aerosolized ^{99m}Tc-DTPA and determination of the BAL/S albumin ratio) were successively performed in each of the patients. The aerosol was applied an average of 11 days before the BAL was performed.

Methods

Determination of BAL/S Albumin Ratio

The concentration of albumin was measured in the fluid of a BAL obtained during a bronchial fibroscopy by a technique previously described.[15] The fibroscope was introduced by the nasal or oral route in patients sitting upright who had received a premedication of 1 mg of atropine sulfate and who had undergone locoregional anesthesia with 2% xylocaine. After examination of the tracheobronchial tree and bronchial biopsies in the left lung, BAL was performed in a subsegmental bronchus of the middle lobe. The lavage was performed by instillation of 300 ml of sterile saline solution (0.15 M NaCl) at 37° C. The liquid was introduced in 100-ml fractions. Each fraction was recovered after instillation by simple siphoning initiated by the application of a pressure depression of 5 to 10 cm of water. The liquid was recovered in a sterile siliconized glass flask in order to reduce the adherence of cells to the walls of the flask.

The volume of fluid recovered was measured, then the liquid was filtered over sterile gauze to remove the mucus. After homogenizing, a small volume was removed for cell enumeration and differential cell counts. The remaining volume of BAL fluid was centrifuged in plastic conical centrifuge tubes at 500 g for 10 min. The albumin assay was performed on the supernatant fluid. The BAL fluid was stored at −20° C when the assays were not performed immediately after the lavage. Storage at −20° C does not alter the concentration of albumin.

A venous blood sample was taken at the same time, and the concentration of albumin in the serum in nonconcentrated BAL fluid was determined with a laser

TABLE 1. Results of Pulmonary Function Tests in Patients with Sarcoidosis[a]

Test	Percentage of Predicted Value
Total lung capacity	87 ± 14
Forced vital capacity	87 ± 17
Forced expiratory volume	80 ± 17
Carbon monoxide diffusing capacity (DL_{CO})	89 ± 14

[a] Each value is a mean ± SD.

nephelometer (Hoechst-Behring, Paris). This assay measures the turbidity induced by the formation of immune complexes in the presence of antihuman albumin antiserum (Hoechst-Behring).[16] A reference curve was constructed using the following serial dilutions of a standard albumin solution: 1:400, 1:800, 1:1600, 1:3200, 1:6400. The results are expressed as mg/100 ml, and the BAL/S albumin ratio was calculated and expressed in mg/g.

Determination of the Clearance of ^{99m}Tc-DTPA

Respiratory epithelial permeability was assessed in each patient by the determination of the clearance of aerosolized ^{99m}Tc-DTPA (the details concerning this technique have been described before[1,5]): a 50-mCi sample of sodium pertechnetate ($^{99m}TcO_4^-$) was introduced into a vial containing 3.3 mg of DTPA to produce ^{99m}Tc-DTPA (molecular weight: 492 daltons); aerosol was generated with a nebulizer by compressed air at flow rate of 9 l/min and stored in a 30-l balloon before inhalation to settle the largest particles; particles inhaled were measured with a cascade impactor.[17] The mass median diameter was 1 μm with a geometric standard deviation of 2.4.

This size of particle allows deposition in small airways and alveoli. The subjects inhaled the aerosol at their normal tidal volume through a non-rebreathing T valve for 3 minutes.

A gamma scintillation camera (Nuclear Chicago) was placed behind the thorax. Lung field radioactivity was framed at 30-second intervals for 20 minutes after inhalation. Six regions of equal size were selected over the peripheral portions of upper, middle, and lower fields. The counts obtained were corrected for the radionuclide decay, and the data were plotted on a logarithmic scale against time. The regression lines of the logarithm of the counts were calculated in the summed regions and in the region where the BAL was performed separately. The clearance values were the negative slopes of these lines expressed in percent per minute (%/min).

Statistical Analysis

The data are listed in TABLE 1 as means ± SD's. Mean values were compared using Student's t test. Fourfold tables were analyzed by the chi-square test with Yates' correction, if necessary, or by Fisher's exact probability test. Correlation coefficients were calculated by the least-squares method.[18]

RESULTS

In group C1 the BAL/S albumin ratio was 0.67 ± 0.31 mg/g, and the upper limit of the 95% confidence interval of normal subjects was 1.33 mg/g; in group C2 the mean value of the ^{99m}Tc-DTPA clearance was 1.16 ± 0.40 %/min, and the upper limit of normal value was 1.96 %/min.

The BAL/S albumin ratio and the clearance of ^{99m}Tc-DTPA in groups C1 and C2, respectively, were significantly lower than they were in group S: in group S the ratio was 3.4 ± 2.6 mg/g ($p < .001$) and the clearance was 2.00 ± 1.4%/min ($p < .001$). As shown in FIGURE 1, no correlation was observed between the values obtained for the BAL/S albumin ratio and those obtained for the ^{99m}Tc-DTPA clearance in any patient ($r = .14$; df = 18; NS), even when the clearance was determined in the region where the BAL was performed ($r = .38$; df = 18; NS). The BAL/S albumin ratio exceeded the normal value in 16 of the 20 patients (80%) with the same percentage for both group S1 (4/5 = 80%) and group S2 (12/15 = 80%). ^{99m}Tc-DTPA clearance, however, exceeded the normal value in 9 of the 20 group S patients (45%); all of these 9 patients were in group S2.

DISCUSSION

Patients with pulmonary sarcoidosis may have an increased respiratory epithelial permeability that is detectable by either method used in this study. No correlation was observed between the results obtained with these two methods. An increase in respiratory permeability was demonstrated more often by assessing BAL/S albumin ratios than by assessing ^{99m}Tc-DTPA clearance: increases were shown in 80% and 45% of patients by these two techniques, respectively. These results were surprising because the molecular weight of albumin (69 000 daltons) is much greater than that of ^{99m}Tc-DTPA (492 daltons). There may be several reasons for these results (one possibility that has been excluded was that of a change in the state of permeability between the two investigations; the mean delay was 11 days, and the ^{99m}Tc-DTPA clearance was performed prior to BAL so that no epithelial injury due to the lavage itself could have modified the result obtained with the ^{99m}Tc-DTPA clearance). Problems related to the techniques themselves are certainly important to consider.

BAL

In the lung, albumin is neither secreted nor metabolized, and its clearance via the lymphatic system is negligible.[19–22] Thus albumin concentration in alveolar fluid may

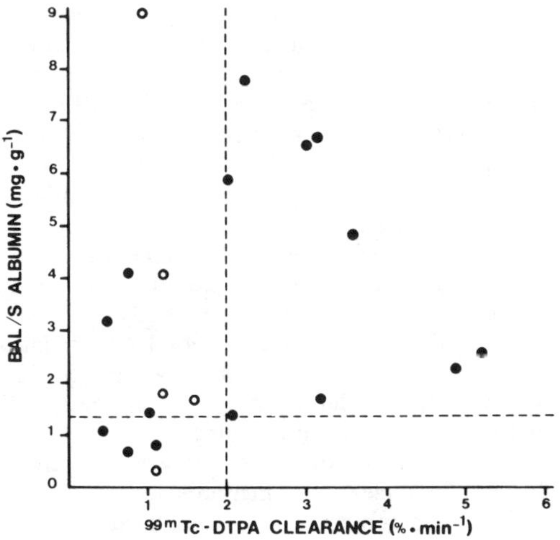

FIGURE 1. Individual values of ^{99m}Tc-DTPA clearance and BAL/S albumin ratios in patients with pulmonary sarcoidosis. Interrupted lines indicate the upper limit of the normal values. ○ = sarcoidosis without radiographic parenchymal abnormality; ● = sarcoidosis with radiographic parenchymal abnormalities.

be assumed to be proportional to the respiratory membrane permeability and to albumin concentration in the serum. Previous studies, however, have demonstrated that albumin concentration used in BAL is dependent on the volume of the lavage solution introduced:[23] that is, the more the alveolar surface is washed, the greater the amount of albumin that may be collected in the fluid; albumin concentrations decrease progressively in successive aliquots of instilled fluid.[24] In our study all BAL were performed with the same technique, and we assume that results between subjects are comparable.

On the other hand, it has been demonstrated that in diffuse sarcoidosis segmental lavage of the lung gives differences in results which prove that lung involvement is not homogeneous.[25,26] Still, the coefficient of correlation between the two methods we used was not improved when the BAL/S albumin ratio and the ^{99m}Tc-DTPA clearance were determined at the same site. This can be attributed to the preferential sampling of airway rather than alveolar fluid in the first aspirated aliquots of recovered BAL, as suggested by the presence of the free secretory component in the lavage.[12,27,28] Therefore, BAL/S albumin ratios also depend on the bronchial permeability which may be increased in pulmonary sarcoidosis.

^{99m}Tc-DTPA Clearance

The method using the clearance of aerosolized ^{99m}Tc-DTPA is based on animal studies which demonstrated an increased clearance of various small molecular weight solutes when the respiratory permeability was increased by different experimental injuries of the alveolocapillary membrane.[13] The most critical point of this technique is the site of deposition of the aerosolized particles. In normal subjects, extensive studies show that aerosolized particles with aerodynamic diameters of less than 2 μm are deposited almost exclusively in the alveolar region of the lung.[29,30] In this study, there are reasons for believing that the deposition of particles was not appreciably modified by ventilation disorders in patients: no deposition was seen in large airways on the chest scintigrams. As shown in TABLE 1, pulmonary function was not greatly impaired in these patients; moreover, recent work has demonstrated that airflow limitation does not increase the ^{99m}Tc-DTPA clearance.[31] Because smoking increases the respiratory epithelial permeability assessed by the ^{99m}Tc-DTPA clearance,[32–34] we excluded all smokers from this study.

Finally, respiratory epithelial permeability is not only related to the state of the alveolocapillary membrane, but it is also dependent on the substances used to determine it.[35,36] Differences in the mechanisms of transfer across the alveolocapillary membrane probably exist between albumin and ^{99m}Tc-DTPA which may also explain the lack of correlation between the two methods.

Recently, Jacobs *et al.*[37] found a correlation between albumin concentration in BAL fluid and ^{99m}Tc-DTPA clearance in 23 subjects. Nine of these 23 subjects, however, did not have pulmonary sarcoidosis (3 were normal control subjects, and 6 had nonspecified localized lung disease).

In conclusion, our objective was to compare the BAL/S albumin ratio and the ^{99m}Tc-DTPA clearance methods for assessing respiratory epithelial permeability in pulmonary sarcoidosis. We demonstrated that this permeability is increased in patients with pulmonary sarcoidosis compared to control subjects irrespective of which method is used. An increase in the respiratory epithelial permeability was demonstrated more often by assessing BAL/S albumin ratios than by assessing ^{99m}Tc-DTPA clearance. No correlation was observed between the results obtained with these two methods.

We believe that the ^{99m}Tc-DTPA clearance method is a better way to assess the permeability of the respiratory epithelium than the BAL/S albumin ratio method because BAL/S albumin ratios only reflect permeability in region of the lavage and because they also reflect the permeability of the bronchial epithelium. The permeability observed with each method in groups S1 and S2 suggests that ^{99m}Tc-DTPA clearance was affected by the severity of parenchymal involvement of sarcoidosis but BAL/S albumin ratios were not. Moreover, aerosolized ^{99m}Tc-DTPA is a noninvasive, easily repeated technique, and may assess permeability in whole lung fields, as well as in parts of them.

ACKNOWLEDGMENT

We are indebted to O. Peronne for the technical assistance he provided.

REFERENCES

1. CHOPRA, S. K., G. V. TAPLIN, D. P. TASHKIN & D. ELAM. 1979. Lung clearance of soluble radioaerosols of different molecular weights in systemic sclerosis. Thorax **34:** 63-67.
2. FEIN, A., R. F. GROSSMAN, J. G. JONES, E. OVERLAND, L. PITTS, J. F. MURRAY & N. C. STAUB. 1979. The value of edema fluid protein measurement in patients with pulmonary edema. Am. J. Med. **67:** 32-38.
3. HUCHON, G. J., L. G. BARRITAULT & J. CHRÉTIEN. 1983. Increased alveolar-capillary membrane permeability in patients with pulmonary sarcoidosis. Am. Rev. Respir. Dis. **127:**(Suppl.): 75.
4. HUNNINGHAKE, G. W., J. E. GADEK, O. KAWANAMI, J. FERRANS & R. G. CRYSTAL. 1979. Inflammatory and immune processes in the human lung in health and disease: Evaluation by bronchoalveolar lavage. Am. J. Pathol. **97:** 149-198.
5. RINDERKNECHT, J., L. SHAPIRO, M. KRAUTHAMMER, G. TAPLIN, K. WASSERMAN, J. M. USZLER & R. M. EFFROS. 1980. Accelerated clearance of small solutes from the lungs in interstitial lung disease. Am. Rev. Respir. Dis. **121:** 105-117.
6. STAUB, N.C. 1978. Pulmonary edema due to increased microvascular permeability to fluid and protein. Circ. Res. **43:** 134-151.
7. BRIGHAM, K. L., J. D. SNELL, JR., T. R. HARRIS, S. MARSHALL, J. HAYNES, R. E. BOWERS & J. PERRY. 1979. Indicator dilution lung water and vascular permeability in humans: Effects of pulmonary vasculature pressure. Circ. Res. **44:** 523-530.
8. GORIN, A. B., W. J. WEIDNER, R. H. DEMLING & N. C. STAUB. 1978. Noninvasive measurement of pulmonary transvascular protein flux in sheep. J. Appl. Physiol. **45:** 225-233.
9. QUEMADA, D., A. SYROIA & D. THEVEN. 1979. Méthode de transition osmotique rapide pour l'étude des échanges transcapillaires pulmonaires: Modèle théorique. C. R. Acad. Sci. Ser. D (Paris) **288:** 113-116.
10. LOW, R. B., G. S. DAVIS & M. S. GIANCOLA. 1978. Biochemical analyses of bronchoalveolar lavage fluid of healthy human volunteer smokers and nonsmokers. Am. Rev. Respir. Dis. **118:** 863-875.
11. MORDELET-DAMBRINE, M. S., G. M. STANISLAS-LEGUERN, G. J. HUCHON, F. C. BAUMANN, J. H. MARSAC & J. CHRÉTIEN. 1982. Elevation of the bronchoalveolar concentration of angiotensin I-converting enzyme in sarcoidosis. Am. Rev. Respir. Dis. **126:** 472-475.
12. REYNOLDS, H. Y., J. D. FULMER, J. A. KAZMIEROWSKI, W. C. ROBERTS, M. M. FRANK & R. G. CRYSTAL. 1977. Analysis of cellular and protein content of bronchoalveolar lavage fluid from patients with idiopathic pulmonary fibrosis and chronic hypersensitivity pneumonitis. J. Clin. Invest. **59:** 165-175.
13. HUCHON, G. J., J. W. LITTLE & J. F. MURRAY. 1981. Assessment of alveolar-capillary membrane permeability of dogs by aerosolization. J. Appl. Physiol. **51:** 955-962.
14. SILZBACH, L. E. 1980. Current world supply of Kveim test suspension. *In* Eighth International Conference on Sarcoidosis and Other Granulomatous Diseases. W. Jones Williams & B. H. Davies, Eds.: 679-681. Alpha Omega. Cardiff.
15. ROTH, C., A. ARNOUX, G. HUCHON, J. LACRONIQUE, J. MARSAC & J. CHRÉTIEN. 1981. Effet du tabagisme sur les cellules bronchoalvéolaires chez l'homme. Bull. Eur. Physiopathol. Respir. **17:** 767-773.

16. SCHLIER, G. & K. FELGENHAUER. 1978. Rapid determination of proteins in serum and cerebrospinal fluid by laser nephelometry. J. Clin. Chem. Clin. Biochem. **16:** 631-635.
17. MERCER, T. T., M. I. TILLERY & G. J. NEWTON. 1970. A multistage low flow rate cascade impactor. Aerosol Sci. **1:** 9-15.
18. ZAR, J. M. 1974. Biostatistical Analysis. Prentice-Hall. Englewood Cliffs, NJ.
19. GORIN, A. B. & P. A. STEWART. 1979. Differential permeability of endothelial and epithelial barriers to albumin flux. J. Appl. Physiol. **47:** 1315-1324.
20. MATTHAY, M. A., C. C. LANDOLT & N. C. STAUB. 1982. Differential liquid and protein clearance from the alveoli of anesthetized sheep. J. Appl. Physiol. **53:** 96-104.
21. MEYER, E. C., R. OTTAVIANO & J. J. HIGGINS. 1977. Albumin clearance from alveoli: Tissue permeation vs. airway displacement. J. Appl. Physiol. **43:** 487-497.
22. SCHNEEBERGER-KEELEY, E. E. & M. J. KARNOVSKY. 1971. The influence of intravascular fluid volume on the permeability of newborn and adult mouse lungs to ultrastructural protein tracers. J. Cell Biol. **49:** 319-334.
23. ATASSI, K., O. WASSEF, G. DE L'HOMME, P. GESLIN, R. SOLLE, C. HOLLER, M. PAHLAVAN & J. BIGNON. 1979. Influence de la technique du lavage bronchoalvéolaire sur les constituants cellulaires et protéiques recueillis. *In* Les Colloques de l'INSERM. Le Lavage Bronchoalvéolaire Chez l'Homme. G. Biserte, J. Chrétien & C. Voisin, Eds. Vol. **84:** 263-270. INSERM. Paris.
24. MERRILL, E., E. O'HEARN, J. RANKIN, G. NAEGEL, R. A. MATTHAY & H. Y. REYNOLDS. 1982. Kinetic analysis of respiratory tract proteins recovered during a sequential lavage protocol. Am. Rev. Respir. Dis. **126:** 617-620.
25. CANTIN, A., R. BEGIN, M. ROLA-PLESZCZYNSKI & R. BOILEAU. 1983. Heterogeneity of bronchoalveolar lavage cellularity in stage III pulmonary sarcoidosis. Chest **3:** 485-486.
26. TONNEL, A. B., C. VOISIN, J. J. LAFITTE, P. RAMON & C. AERTS. 1979. Variations des populations cellulaires recueillies par lavage bronchoalvéolaire en fonction de la topographie des lésions et de l'étage exploré. *In* Les Colloques de l'INSERM. Le Lavage Bronchoalvéolaire Chez l'Homme. G. Biserte, J. Chrétien & C. Voisin, Eds. Vol. **84:** 271-280. INSERM. Paris.
27. BIOT, N., A. REVOL, R. HARF, B. MONTAGNON, Y. PACHECO & M. PERRIN-FAYOLLE. 1980. Les immunoglobulines du liquide de lavage bronchoalvéolaire chez le sujet normal et en pathologie respiratoire. Poumon Coeur. **36:** 263-269.
28. MERRILL, W. W., D. GOODENBERGER, W. STROBER, R. A. MATTHAY, G. P. NAEGEL & H. Y. REYNOLDS. 1980. Free secretory component and other proteins in human lung lavage. Am. Rev. Respir. Dis. **122:** 156-161.
29. BATES, D. V., B. R. FISH, T. F. HATCH, T. T. MERCER & P. E. MORROW. 1966. Deposition and retention models for internal dosimetry of the human respiratory tract: Task group of lung dynamics. Health Phys. **12:** 173-207.
30. GERRITY, T. R., P. S. LEE, F. J. HASS, A. MARINELLI, P. WERNER & R. V. LOURENCO. 1979. Calculated deposition of inhaled particles in the airway generations of normal subjects. J. Appl. Physiol. **47:** 867-873.
31. HUCHON, G. J., J. A. RUSSELL, L. G. BARRITAULT, A. LIPAVSKY & J. F. MURRAY. 1984. Chronic airflow limitation does not increase respiratory epithelial permeability assessed by aerosolized solute, but smoking does. Am. Rev. Respir. Dis. **130:** 457-460.
32. JONES, J. G., B. D. MINTY, P. LAWLER, G. HULANDS, J. C. W. CRAWLEY & N. VEALL. 1980. Increased alveolar epithelial permeability in cigarette smokers. Lancet **i:** 66-68.
33. MASON, G. P., J. M. USZLER, R. M. EFFROS & E. REID. 1983. Rapidly reversible alterations of pulmonary epithelial permeability induced by smoking. Chest **83:** 6-11.
34. MINTY, B. D., C. JORDAN & J. G. JONES. 1981. Rapid improvement in abnormal pulmonary epithelial permeability after stopping cigarettes. Br. Med. J. **282:** 1183-1186.
35. TAYLOR, A. E., A. C. GUYTON & V. S. BISHOP. 1965. Permeability of the alveolar membrane to solutes. Circ. Res. **16:** 353-362.
36. WANGENSTEEN, D. & R. YANKOVICH. 1979. Alveolar epithelium transport of albumin and sucrose: Concentration difference effect. J. Appl. Physiol. **47:** 846-850.
37. JACOBS, M. L., R. P. BAUGHMAN, J. HUGHES & M. FERNANDEZ-ULLOA. 1985. Radioaerosol lung clearance in patients with active pulmonary sarcoidosis. Am. Rev. Respir. Dis. **131:** 687-689.

Prostaglandins in the Bronchoalveolar Lavage Fluid

Possible Block of Immunoregulation in Sarcoidosis[a]

ROBERT P. BAUGHMAN, LOIS S. GALLON, AND UNO BARCELLI

Department of Internal Medicine
University of Cincinnati Medical Center
Cincinnati, Ohio 45267

Prostaglandins are naturally occurring substances that act as local, potent hormones.[1] The lung is one of the major sites for prostaglandin synthesis and degradation. Various stimuli cause the release of prostaglandins from the lung, but the role of these released substances is only beginning to unfold.

Prostaglandins are involved in many physiological events. Traditionally, prostaglandins have been characterized as a major cause of the initiation and perpetuation of inflammatory responses. Recently, some classes of prostaglandins have been shown to have anti-inflammatory properties. This is particularly true for prostaglandin of the E class (PGE). PGE has been shown to be immunoregulatory, acting as a feedback inhibitor of T cell aggregation and an inhibitor of macrophage cytotoxicity.[2] For example, increased activity of PGE-producing cells in the peripheral blood has been shown to be a contributing cause of anergy in some patients with sarcoidosis.[3]

The role of PGE in granuloma formation is beginning to be understood. PGE is decreased in concentration in granulomas.[4] The exogenous administration of PGE inhibits the induction and elicitation phase of the cell-mediated response of *Schistosoma mansoni* egg-induced pulmonary granulomas.[5]

Bronchoalveolar lavage (BAL) is a widely used technique for sampling lung fluid in the distal airways. Recently, we described a technique that allowed us to quantitate the volume of lung fluid retrieved and to thus report lavage results per ml of lung fluid.[6] We measured the amounts of PGE in normal volunteers and patients with active pulmonary sarcoidosis.

[a]This research was supported in part by Grant R00068-21 from the National Institutes of Health General Clinical Research Center at the University of Cincinnati, by Grant NIH-AN 17196 from the National Institutes of Health, and by the Dialysis Clinic, Inc., Cincinnati, Ohio.

METHODS

We studied patients undergoing fiberoptic bronchoscopy for evaluation of pulmonary sarcoidosis at the University of Cincinnati Medical Center. No patient was on steroid therapy at the time of the study. The control group consisted of normal, healthy, nonsmoking volunteers. All patients signed an informed consent form approved by the Human Research Review Committee of the University of Cincinnati, after having had the purposes, methods, and risks of the study explained. None of the subjects had received a nonsteroidal anti-inflammatory agent in the two weeks prior to bronchoscopy.

Bronchoscopy and BAL were performed in the manner previously described.[6] Briefly, the patients were premedicated, and lidocaine was used for topical anesthesia. The bronchoscope was advanced to the wedge position in either the lingula or the right middle lobe. Then 60 ml of normal saline solution with a known concentration of methylene blue was introduced. Gentle suction was applied with a hand-held syringe and the aspirated fluid collected. Another 60 to 180 ml of fluid, in 60-ml aliquots, was added and aspirated, and then the total aspirated fluid was pooled. Methylene blue concentrations were calculated by measuring the absorbance at 660 nm of the introduced and aspirated fluid samples. Total and differential cell counts were performed on a sample of unspun fluid. The remaining fluid was centrifuged at 500 rpm for 5 min and the supernatant stored at −20° C for subsequent tests. Albumin was measured in the supernatant using the rate nephelometry technique (Auto ICS, Beckman, Fullerton, CA).[6]

Prostaglandins

The supernatants of all samples were assayed for PGE. The supernatant was thawed and centrifuged at 1000 rpm for 5 min. Then 10 ml of each sample were acidified to pH 3.1 using 5% formic acid. The sample was applied to an octadecylsilyl silica cartridge (SEP-PAK C-18, Waters Associates, Milford, MA) which had been primed with 20 ml of ethanol and 20 ml of water. The sample was then washed with 20 ml of water, 20 ml of 10% ethanol, and 20 ml of petroleum ether. The PGE was then eluted with 20 ml of an ethyl acetate-methanol mixture (9:1; v:v). This sample was dried under negative pressure, redissolved in acetonitrile, and added to a silica column (Bond Elut, Analytichem International, Harbor City, CA) which had been prepared with 6 ml of benzene. The sample was washed with 10 ml of benzene, and the PGE was eluted with 20 ml of an acetonitrile-methanol mixture (10:1; v:v) and evaporated with a rotary evaporator (Rotavapor R-110, Brinkman Instruments, Westbury, NY). The volume of the final extract was increased to 1.0 ml with phosphate buffer (pH 7.3), and 0.1-ml aliquots were assayed. PGE was measured with a competitive antibody technique using precipitation.[7] Known quantities of radiolabeled PGE were added to each sample to permit the quantitation of the amount of extracted lipids; all results were corrected for percent recovery.

Pulmonary function tests, including lung volume tests, were performed using a 7-L water seal spirometer (W.E. Collins, Braintree, MA). These tests were repeated on those patients treated with 40 mg of prednisone/day two months after said treatment began.

Statistics

Linear correlations were performed using the least-squares technique. Most of the data from the sarcoid group were not normally distributed, so comparisons were made using nonparametric tests including the Mann-Whitney *U* test and the Wilcoxon rank-sum test as appropriate.[8] A p value of less than .05 was considered an indication of significance.

RESULTS

We studied 11 patients with pulmonary sarcoidosis (which was diagnosed if a given patient had the appropriate clinical history and chest roentgenogram and a lung biopsy showing noncaseating granulomas with cultures negative for fungus and mycobacteria).[8,9] The patients' mean age was 35.8 with a range of 27 to 55. Eight of the patients were female; eight were black; and four were cigarette smokers.

TABLE 1. Results of Bronchoalveolar Lavage[a]

	Control Patients (N = 7)	Sarcoidosis Patients (N = 11)
PGE		
pg/ml lung fluid	2112.2 (1037.9-3626.7)	2019.2 (723.3-4909.0
pg/macrophage	4.85 (2.812-10.930)	1.549[b] (.393-5.1)
Lymphocytes in BAL (%)	6.4 (2-12)	30.8[c] (9-72)

[a] The table entries are means; the range for each mean is indicated in parentheses.
[b] $p < .05$ compared to control.
[c] $p < .002$ compared to control.

The control group consisted of seven nonsmoking male volunteers who had normal pulmonary function tests. Their mean age was 32.4 with a range of 27 to 53.

In the control group, we retrieved 554 cells/ml lung fluid (range: 267-1167 cells/ml) of which 93.6% (range: 88-98%) were macrophages. The sarcoid patients had a marked increase in the number of cells: a mean of 2316 cells/ml (range: 1424-8811 cells/ml; $p < .02$) was retrieved. Although the percentage of macrophages in the sarcoid group was decreased to 65.0% (range: 22-89%), there was a significant increase in the number of macrophages: a mean of 1827 macrophages/ml (range: 168-5483 macrophages/ml; $p < .02$) was retrieved. The major new cell in the lavage fluid was the lymphocyte: a mean of 30.8% (range: 9-72%; $p < .002$) of the cells retrieved by lavage were lymphocytes.

The results of the PGE measurements in all patients are shown in TABLE 1. We did not find a significant increase in the amount of PGE in the sarcoid group when expressed per ml of lung fluid. The amount of PGE/macrophage (1.55 pg) was significantly lower than that (4.85 pg; $p < .05$) in the control group.

We measured the amount of albumin/ml of lung fluid. There was a significant positive correlation between the amount of albumin in the lavage fluid and the amount of PGE found ($r = .64$; $p < .01$).

There was a significant correlation between the amount of PGE in the lavage fluid and the number of lymphocytes in the BAL of the sarcoid patients ($r = .71$; $p < .01$). There was no significant correlation between the amount of PGE and the number of lymphocytes in the control patients. There was also no significant correlation between the amount of PGE and the number of macrophages in either the control group or the sarcoid group.

We compared the pulmonary test results and the amounts of PGE present before and after the two-month prednisone treatment. There was a significant correlation between the improvement in vital capacity and the amount of PGE/ml of lung fluid ($r = .81$; $p < .01$).

DISCUSSION

The production site of the PGE found in the lavage fluid is unknown. The lung is a major site of production, synthesis, and degradation of prostaglandins within the body.[10] There may be secretion of PGE from endothelial cells in the lung into the fluid lining the alveolus and bronchus. Cells in the lavage fluid may also secrete PGE, however. Monocytes and macrophages have also been shown to secrete PGE.[11] Monocytes isolated from the peripheral blood secrete PGE.[12] In sarcoidosis, lymphocytes in the peripheral blood cause an increased secretion of PGE, thus blocking normal cellular response. Treatment with indomethacin, a prostaglandin inhibitor, will restore delayed immune response in the anergic sarcoid patients.[3]

In our study it appeared that the sarcoid group as a whole had a decreased amount of PGE/cell and that there was no relationship between the number of macrophages in the BAL and the amount of PGE measured. In patients with sarcoidosis, the greater the number of lymphocytes in the BAL fluid, the larger the amount of PGE. As in the peripheral blood, the lymphocyte may be enhancing release of PGE from macrophages.

PGE has been shown by several investigators to have immunosuppressive effects, which include decreased granuloma formation.[2,3] The mechanism of action appears to be feedback inhibition of macrophage cytotoxicity and T helper cells.

In patients with early pulmonary sarcoidosis, a bimodal pattern has been described.[13] The percentage of lymphocytes in the BAL fluid increases in the first 8 weeks of disease and thereafter levels off or begins decreasing. A rise in serum angiotensin-converting enzyme (ACE), however, is not seen until after 6-8 weeks of disease. ACE is associated with the granulomas of sarcoidosis, especially those seen in the lung. The early influx of lymphocytes into the alveolar fluid may diminish the initial granuloma formation. Eventual granuloma formation may be due to other, undetermined factors.

Steroids are potent drugs with many effects, which include blocking the release of PGE from cells.[2,14] Although their long-term effectiveness in sarcoidosis is contested, steroids clearly improve pulmonary function in some patients.[15] A correlation was found between steroid response and PGE levels in the BAL. This would suggest that

PGE or some other arachidonate metabolite, a lipoxygenase product, for example, has some unexplained effect.[16] Another possibility is a paraphenomenon: steroids may act on sarcoidosis independently of the effect of steroids on prostaglandin synthesis. A rigorous trial of more specific prostaglandin inhibitors in sarcoidosis may be useful in distinguishing between these two possibilities.

In conclusion, we found measurable levels of PGE in the bronchoalveolar lavage fluid of healthy volunteers and patients with pulmonary sarcoidosis. We found little difference between the absolute amount of PGE/ml of lung fluid in sarcoid and control patients; however, we found less PGE/macrophage in the lung fluid of sarcoid patients.

REFERENCES

1. HIGGINS, C. B. & E. BRAUNWALD. 1972. The prostaglandins: Biochemical, physiologic, and clinical considerations. Am. J. Med. **53:** 92-109.
2. GOODWIN, J. S. & J. CEUPPENS. 1983. Regulation of the immune response by prostaglandins. J. Clin. Immunol. **3:** 295-314.
3. GOODWIN, J. S., R. DEHORATIUS, L. H. ISRAE, G. T. PEAKE & R. P. MESSNER. 1979. Suppressor cell function in sarcoidosis. Ann. Intern. Med. **90:** 169-173.
4. OHUCHI, K., A. SATO & S. TSURUFUJI. 1976. The content of prostaglandin $F_{2\alpha}$ in the exudate of carrageenin granuloma of rats. Biochim. Biophys. Acta **424:** 239-248.
5. CHENSUE, S. W., S. L. KUNKEL, P. A. WARD & G. I. HIGASHI. 1983. Exogenously administered prostaglandins modulate pulmonary granulomas induced by *Schistosoma mansoni* eggs. Am. J. Pathol. **111:** 78-87.
6. BAUGHMAN, R. P., C. H. BOSKEN, R. G. LOUDON, P. HURTUBISE & T. WESSELER. 1983. Quantitation of bronchoalveolar lavage with methylene blue. Am. Rev. Respir. Dis. **128:** 266-270.
7. GRANSSTROM, E. & H. KINDAHL. 1978. Radioimmunoassay of prostaglandins and thromboxanes. Adv. Prost. Thrombox. Res. **5:** 119-125.
8. BRUNING, J. L. & B. L. KINTZ. 1977. Computational Handbook of Statistics. Scott Foresman and Company, Glenview, IL.
9. MITCHELL, D. N. & J. G. SCADDING. 1974. Sarcoidosis. Am. Rev. Respir. Dis. **110:** 774-802.
10. MATHE, A. A., P. HEDQVIST, G. K. STRANDBER & C. A. LESLIE. 1977. Aspects of prostaglandin function in the lung. N. Engl. J. Med. **296:** 850-855.
11. ROUZER, C. A., W. A. SCOTT, A. L. HAMILL & Z. A. COHN. 1982. Synthesis of leukotriene C and other arachidonic acid metabolites by mouse pulmonary macrophages. J. Exp. Med. **155:** 720-733.
12. FISCHER, A., A. DURANDY & GRISCELLIC. 1981. Role of prostaglandin E_2 in the induction of nonspecific T lymphocyte suppressor activity. J. Immunol. **126:** 1452-1455.
13. VALEYRE, D., G. SAUMON, R. GEORGES, J. L. KEMENY, D. BLADIER, J. AMOUROUX, J. PRE & J. P. BATTESTI. 1984. The relationship between disease duration and noninvasive pulmonary explorations in sarcoidosis with erythema nodosum. Am. Rev. Respir. Dis. **129:** 938-943.
14. FAUCI, A. S., D. C. DALE & J. E. BALOW. 1977. Glucocorticosteroid therapy: Mechanisms of action and clinical considerations. Ann. Intern. Med. **84:** 304-315.
15. DEREMEE, R. A. 1977. The present status of treatment of pulmonary sarcoidosis: A house divided. Chest **71:** 388-392.
16. KUNKEL, S. L., S. W. CHENSUE, C. MOUTON & G I. HIGASHI. 1984. Role of lipoxygenase products in murine pulmonary granuloma formation. J. Clin. Invest. **74:** 514-524.

The Stimulation of Angiotensin-converting Enzyme Induction in Cultured Monocytes by T4$^+$ and T8$^+$ Lymphocytes[a]

BRADLEY LAUDERDALE AND
MICHAEL S. ROHRBACH[b]

Thoracic Diseases Research Unit
Mayo Clinic and Foundation
Rochester, Minnesota 55905

INTRODUCTION

The sarcoid granuloma is composed of an organized collection of macrophages, epithelioid cells, multinucleated giant cells, thymus-derived (T) lymphocytes, and other cells.[1] Maintenance of the granuloma is believed to require constant recruitment of circulating blood monocytes, which differentiate into macrophages, epithelioid cells, and multinucleated giant cells. Recent evidence suggests a critical role for T lymphocytes in monocyte recruitment.[2] A better understanding of the sarcoid granuloma requires investigation into features specific to this disease. Increased concentrations of circulating angiotensin-converting enzyme (ACE) is one feature which commonly distinguishes sarcoidosis from several morphologically similar granulomatous diseases.[3] ACE has been demonstrated to be present on granuloma cells of monocytic origin in sarcoidosis but not in those of other granulomatous diseases.[4] Circulating monocytes from sarcoidosis patients, however, contain very little ACE (unpublished observation). This suggests that induction of ACE synthesis must take place during or after the transformation of monocytes to granuloma epithelioid cells.

Although the mechanism of this *in vivo* induction is unknown, an *in vitro* induction by normal T lymphocytes of ACE in normal blood monocytes in monocyte-T lymphocyte co-cultures has been found.[5,6] This event is the basis of an *in vitro* model of the *in vivo* induction of ACE in the monocyte-derived epithelioid cells of the sarcoid granuloma. Investigations by others into the T lymphocyte composition of bronchoalveolar lavage fluid have revealed an increase in the T4:T8 ratio in sarcoidosis[7] and a decrease in this T4:T8 ratio in chronic hypersensitivity pneumonitis,[8] a granulomatous disease not associated with elevated serum ACE.[9] The present study was designed to

[a] This work was supported in part by Grant HL-28482 from the National Institutes of Health and by funds from the Mayo Foundation.

[b] To whom correspondence should be addressed.

determine if an identifiable T lymphocyte subpopulation is responsible for ACE induction in monocytes *in vitro*.

MATERIALS

Ficoll-Paque and Percoll were obtained from Pharmacia, Piscataway, NJ and from Uppsala, Sweden. Essentially fat-free bovine and human serum albumins were obtained from Sigma, St. Louis, MO. RPMI 1640 and Earle's media 199 were obtained from KC Biological, Lenexa, KA. OKT4 and OKT8 monoclonal antibodies and fluorescein isothiocyanate conjugate goat antimouse immunoglobulin G (IgG) were obtained from Ortho, Raritan, NJ. Anti-Leu 7 was obtained from Becton-Dickinson, Mountain View, CA. Affinity-purified goat antimouse IgG was obtained from Cappel, Malvern, PA. Forty-eight well culture-plates were obtained from Costar, Cambridge, MA. Falcon 3003 tissue culture dishes, which were used in depletion experiments, were obtained from Falcon, Cockeysville, MD. All other reagents and chemicals were of analytical grade.

METHODS

Monocyte and T Lymphocyte Preparation

For each experiment monocytes and T lymphocytes were isolated from the buffy coat of one 500-ml unit of blood from a normal human donor as previously described.[10] Briefly, mononuclear cells were separated from granulocytes and erythrocytes using a modification of the Ficoll-Paque gradient centrifugation technique described by Boyum.[11] Platelets were removed by centrifugation of mononuclear cells through 5% bovine serum albumin (BSA) in Hanks' balanced salt solution (HBSS).

T lymphocytes were bound to sheep red blood cells (SRBC); the resulting rosettes were separated by Ficoll-Paque gradient centrifugation, using a modification of the technique described by Gmelig-Meyling and Ballieux.[12] SRBC were lysed with ammonium chloride. Cells from the interface layer, mostly monocytes and bone marrow-derived (B) lymphocytes, were separated by centrifugation on a continuous Percoll gradient using a modification of the technique described by Gmelig-Meyling and Waldmann.[13] Monocytes were collected from this gradient and washed before use. The techniques mentioned above were used to determine the purity of the T lymphocyte preparation (97 ± 1%) and of the monocyte preparation (94 ± 2%); Wright-Giemsa and myeloperoxidase stains were used, respectively.

Monocyte and T Lymphocyte Culture

Cells were cultured, in triplicate, in 11.3-mm flat-bottomed wells, in 0.5 ml of a 1:1 mixture of RPMI 1640 and Earle's media 199 supplemented with glutamine, penicillin, and streptomycin. The final monocyte and T lymphocyte concentrations were 6 × 10^5 cells/ml and 0-4 × 10^6 cells/ml, respectively. Cells were cultured for 6 days at 37° C in a 5% CO_2, 95% air atmosphere. The wells were then centrifuged for 10 minutes at 1000 g. The media were aspirated and, in some experiments, filter sterilized, frozen at −20° C, and saved for later use as conditioned media. Then, 75 μl 2% Triton X-100 in water was added to lyse the cells and solubilize the ACE. This was frozen at −20° C for later assay.

Assay of ACE

ACE was quantitated by examining the cleavage of the substrate [1-^{14}C]-glycylhippurylhistidylleucine in a radiochemical assay.[14] Duplicate samples were taken from each culture well. Results were expressed as milli-Units enzyme/1 × 10^6 monocytes originally cultured.

Irradiation of T Lymphocytes

T lymphocytes at a concentration of 20 × 10^6 cells/ml in media were irradiated with 2000 rad in a Mark 1-Model 25 ^{137}Ce Irradiator (J.L. Shepherd & Associates, Glendale, CA). The cells were washed once, resuspended in media at 20 × 10^6 cells/ml, and cultured with monocytes as described above for unirradiated T lymphocytes. Irradiation had no effect on viability as determined by trypan blue exclusion.

Separation of T Lymphocyte Subsets with Monoclonal Antibodies

Negative selection of T lymphocyte subsets was accomplished by selective antibody-mediated adherence to plastic dishes, using a modification of the methods described by Reinherz *et al.*[15] and Payne *et al.*[16] OKT4, OKT8, and anti-Leu 7 monoclonal antibodies were used.

Isolated T lymphocytes in HBSS + 0.25% human serum albumin (HSA) at 25 × 10^6 cells/ml were incubated for 30 min with monoclonal antibodies (1 μl/1 × 10^6 cells). After two washes the cells were resuspended in streptomycin + 0.25% HSA + 25 mM HEPES at 8-18 × 10^6 cells/ml. Then, 5-ml aliquots were layered onto freshly rinsed tissue culture dishes which had been incubated for 24-48 hr with 5 ml of affinity-purified goat antimouse IgG (50 μg/ml). After 60 min nonadherent cells were aspirated, combined with two 5-ml washes of the culture dish, and washed twice before use. The incubations and intervening washes were performed at 4° C.

Flow Cytometry

After incubation with monoclonal antibodies, duplicate samples, of 0.5-1.0 × 10^6 cells, were taken before and after the monoclonal antibody-binding cells were removed. These cells were stained with fluorescein isothiocyanate conjugate goat antimouse IgG, treated for several minutes with 0.5% formalin in 0.01 M phosphate-buffered saline, and analyzed within 3 days. This analysis was performed with a FACS IV flow cytometer (Becton-Dickinson, Mountain View, CA); 2500-5000 cells were counted. Positive cells were counted as a percentage of total cells with lymphocytic light-scattering properties. Negative controls using cells without monoclonal antibodies were less than 1% positive. Reincubating depleted cell populations with monoclonal antibodies did not change the results.

Statistical Analysis

Comparisons were made using paired *t* tests with significance accepted at $p \leq .05$.

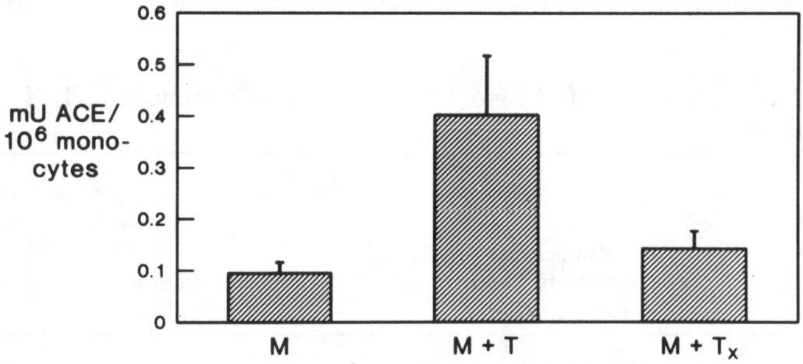

FIGURE 1. The effect of T lymphocyte irradiation on the induction of monocyte ACE. The amount of ACE induced (mU/1 $\times$ 10^6 monocytes) is shown for 6-day cultures of monocytes alone (M), monocytes with control T lymphocytes (M + T), and monocytes with irradiated T lymphocytes ($M+T_x$). The means of five experiments ± SEM are shown. The final concentrations of monocytes and T lymphocytes were 6 $\times$ 10^5 cells/ml and 4 $\times$ 10^6 cells/ml, respectively.

RESULTS

Effect of T Lymphocyte Irradiation on Monocyte ACE Induction

It was necessary to co-culture autologous monocytes and purified T lymphocytes irradiated with 2000 rad in order to examine the radiosensitivity of the T lymphocyte population. Unirradiated T lymphocytes cultured with monocytes and monocytes cultured alone served as controls. The mean results from five experiments are shown in FIGURE 1. Clearly, the induction of monocyte ACE was greater with the unirradiated T lymphocytes than it was with the irradiated T lymphocytes that were irradiated before culturing ($p < .05$). This loss of ACE-inducing activity upon irradiation was not due to the complete loss of T lymphocyte function because T lymphocytes irradiated under the same conditions retained their ability to enhance the induction of a second monocyte enzyme, leucine aminopeptidase (data not shown).

ACE-inducing Activity of T4$^+$ Cell- and T8$^+$ Cell-enriched Populations

Results of the depletion process are shown in TABLE 1. The average T4:T8 ratio before subset separation was 1.64. Among individuals, who were screened only by standard blood bank methods for blood donations, the ratio varied considerably, from 0.85 to 3.31. Because OKT4 and OKT8 are used to identify mutually exclusive subsets which together include most T cells,[17] T8$^+$ cell-depleted T cell populations are T4$^+$ cell enriched, and T4$^+$ cell-depleted T cell populations are T8$^+$ cell enriched. The percentages of contaminating monoclonal antibody-binding cells in each depleted population are shown in TABLE 1. These averaged 2.8% and 9.5% in the T4$^+$ cell- and T8$^+$ cell-enriched populations, respectively. In addition, an average of 7.0 ±2.2% of the T cells bound neither OKT4 nor OKT8; these cells would be expected to remain in both of the depleted nonadherent populations, but were not directly measured.

For each experiment T4$^+$ cell- and T8$^+$ cell-enriched populations were prepared simultaneously from a single donor's T cells. The results of one such experiment are illustrated in FIGURE 2. T4$^+$ cells had more ACE-inducing activity than did T8$^+$ cells at each of the three concentrations of lymphocytes used. Mean results are expressed as a stimulation index (SI):

TABLE 1. Characteristics of Monoclonal Antibody-fractionated T Lymphocyte Subpopulations

Final Cell Population	Monoclonal Antibody Used for Depletion	*N*	Percentage of Monoclonal Antibody-positive Cells[a]: Before Depletion	After Depletion
T4$^+$ enriched	OKT8	7	35.2 ± 4.1	2.8 ± 1.5
T8$^+$ enriched	OKT4	7	57.8 ± 2.9	9.5 ± 3.5
Leu 7$^+$ depleted	Anti-Leu 7	3	13.2 ± 4.2	6.0 ± 2.8

[a] The results are expressed as means ± SEM.

$$SI = \frac{mU_{m\,+\,Test} - mU_M}{mU_{M\,+\,Control} - mU_M}$$

The subscripts indicate the conditions under which a given amount of ACE, in milliUnits (mU), was induced. M + Test, monocytes and a T cell subset were used; M + Control, monocytes and control T cells; M, monocytes alone. Thus, the SI represents the ratio of ACE induced by a T cell subset to ACE induced by untreated, control T cells. Isolated, but unfractionated T cells from the same blood donation were used as a control population. Mean results for seven experiments are shown in FIGURE 3. On average, both T4$^+$ cell- and T8$^+$ cell-enriched populations had ACE-inducing activity comparable to that seen with control T cells. A trend is noted toward greater ACE-inducing activity with the T4$^+$ cell-enriched populations, but the difference is not statistically significant.

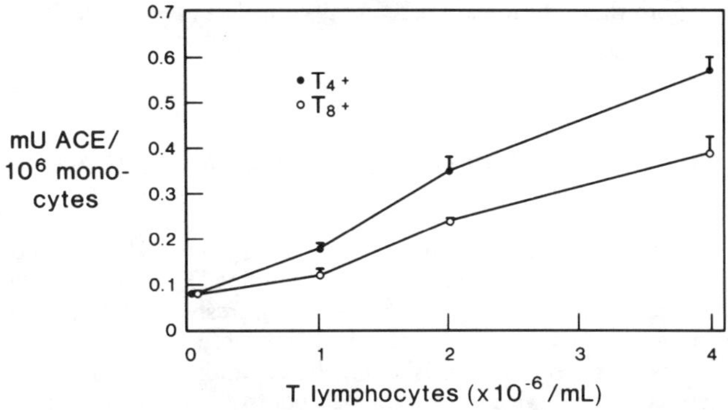

FIGURE 2. The induction of ACE in monocytes by $T4^+$ and $T8^+$ lymphocytes. Closed circles represent the amount of ACE induced by a co-culture of monocytes and $T4^+$ lymphocytes; open circles represent the amount of ACE induced by a co-culture of monocytes and $T8^+$ lymphocytes. The monocyte concentration was 6×10^5 cells/ml; the T lymphocyte concentration varied as shown. Results of one experiment are shown as means of triplicate culture with ± SEM.

ACE-inducing Activity of Conditioned Media

Conditioned media from a monocyte-T lymphocyte co-culture have been shown to contain a cellular, soluble factor which enhances the induction of ACE in fresh cultured monocytes.[18] We examined the relative activities of conditioned media from monocyte-T lymphocyte co-cultures containing $T4^+$ cell- and $T8^+$ cell-enriched populations. Means of three experiments, expressed as stimulation indices, are shown in FIGURE 4. Conditioned media from a culture of monocytes and cells from a $T4^+$ cell-enriched population show a more obvious trend toward greater ACE-inducing activity than conditioned media from a culture of monocytes and cells from a $T8^+$ cell-

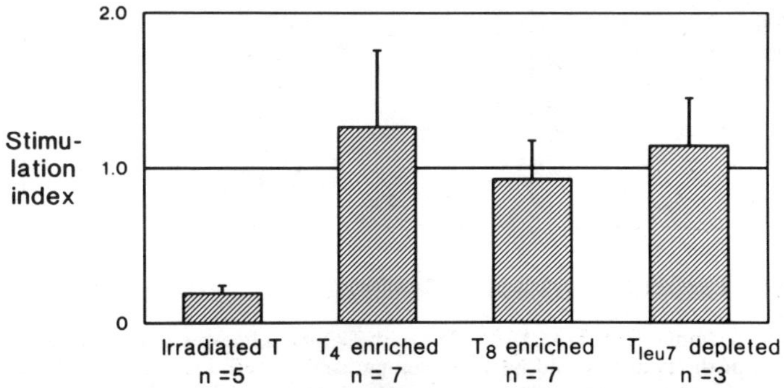

FIGURE 3. A comparison of the stimulation indices for ACE induction by T lymphocyte subsets. The ACE-inducing activity of each treated T lymphocyte population is compared to that of the corresponding control T lymphocytes by means of a stimulation index. See FIGURE 1 for the final cell concentrations. The results are shown as means ± SEM.

enriched population; these results are consistent with those seen with the original cell cultures.

ACE-inducing Activity of Leu 7⁺ Cell-depleted Populations

Anti-Leu 7 is used to identify some of the cells in the $T4^+$ cell- and $T8^+$ cell-depleted populations.[19] The effect of anti-Leu 7-binding T (Leu 7^+) cells on ACE induction in monocytes was investigated by depleting fresh T cell populations of Leu 7^+ cells by using anti-Leu 7. Results of the depletion process are shown in TABLE 1. Depletion was less complete with this monoclonal antibody. Leu 7^+ cell-depleted populations were compared with unfractionated control T cells from the same blood donation. The results of one experiment are shown in FIGURE 5. Populations depleted of Leu 7^+ cells did not exhibit reduced ACE-inducing activity. The mean results of three experiments, expressed in stimulation indexes, are shown in FIGURE 3. The Leu 7^+ cell-depleted populations show a statistically insignificant increase in activity.

DISCUSSION

The increased quantity of serum ACE which is found in many patients with sarcoidosis is believed to originate in monocyte-derived cells in granulomas.[4] Since most other morphologically similar granulomatous diseases are not associated with increased ACE,[9] the generation of this enzyme may serve as a marker of cellular interactions specific to sarcoidosis. *In vitro* studies of cells isolated from normal

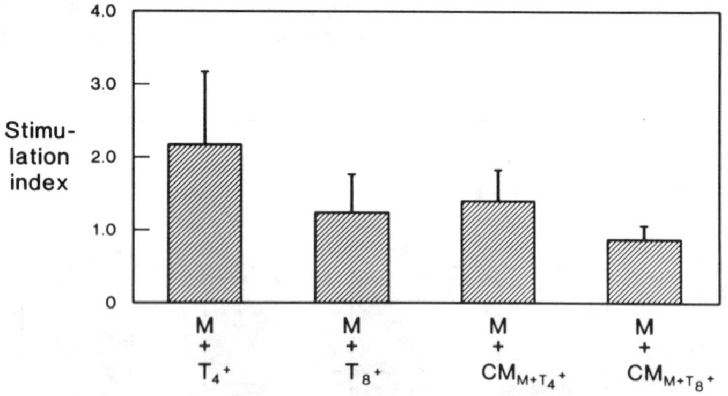

FIGURE 4. The induction of ACE by $T4^+$ and $T8^+$ lymphocytes and derived conditioned media. Shown in the two left-hand bars is a comparison of ACE induction, expressed as stimulation indices, for cultures of monocytes and $T4^+$ lymphocytes ($M + T4^+$) and of monocytes and $T8^+$ lymphocytes ($M + T8^+$). The induction of ACE in monocytes by the conditioned media (CM) derived from these cultures ($M + CM_{M+T4}{}^+$ and $M + CM_{M+T8}{}^+$) is illustrated in the two right-hand bars. See FIGURE 1 for the final cell concentrations. The means of three experiments ± SEM are shown.

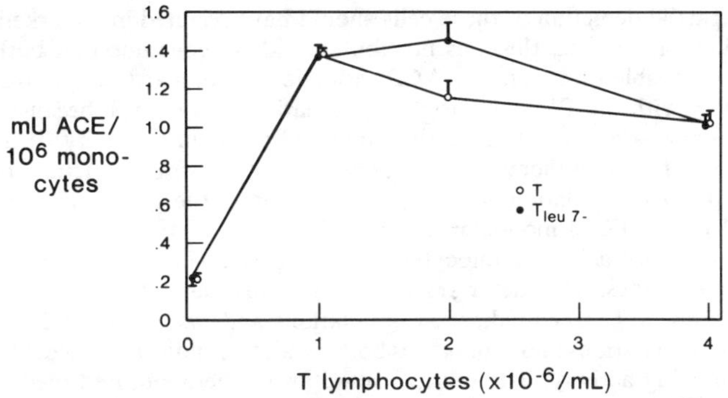

FIGURE 5. The induction of ACE in monocytes by a Leu 7$^+$ cell-depleted population of T lymphocytes. Closed circles represent ACE induced by a co-culture of monocytes and a Leu 7$^+$ cell-depleted T lymphocyte population; open circles represent ACE induced by a co-culture of monocytes and control T lymphocytes. See FIGURE 2 for more details.

peripheral blood have shown that T lymphocytes enhance the induction of ACE in monocytes.[5,6] This finding is of particular interest because T lymphocyte-monocyte interactions have been proposed by Hunninghake and others as key events in the development of sarcoid granulomas.[2] Bronchoalveolar lavage (BAL) has been used to study the alveolitis of sarcoidosis, which is believed to precede granuloma formation.[20] A marked increase in T lymphocytes is found in this BAL fluid, and these cells have been shown to release substances chemotactic for monocytes.[7] Other granulomatous diseases are associated with a T lymphocyte-predominant alveolitis,[8] but not with elevated ACE activity.[9] This suggests that only certain T lymphocytes, which are present in increased numbers in sarcoidosis, are capable of inducing ACE in monocyte-derived cells. Several studies of BAL fluid indirectly support this hypothesis; that is, they suggest that certain types of T lymphocytes are increased in the sarcoid alveolitis. These studies have demonstrated an increase in the T4:T8 ratio,[7] and cloning experiments suggest that lymphokine production is restricted to subpopulations of T lymphocytes.[21] If an ACE-inducing subpopulation of T lymphocytes could be identified *in vitro,* attention could be directed toward this potentially biologically significant subpopulation in *in vivo* studies.

The results of our T cell-irradiation experiments indicate that T cell-mediated induction of ACE in monocytes is a radiosensitive event, requiring more than simply the physical presence of T cells. The dose used, 2000 rad, has been shown to have selective inhibitory effects in other studies.[22] The lack of an irradiation effect on leucine aminopeptidase induction is additional evidence that this is a specific effect in our *in vitro* system. Because of uncertainty over which cells or functions are radiosensitive,[23,24] we sought to isolate T cell subpopulations and measure their ACE-inducing activity individually.

We prepared T cell subpopulations by depletion, using monoclonal antibodies directed toward the unwanted cells. This method provided the large number (1×10^7) of sterile cells needed for each experiment. The depletion was incomplete in that some monoclonal antibody-labeled cells were still present. The degree of contamination was considered acceptable because the function we were studying, enhancement of ACE induction, was strongly dependent on the concentration of T cells present. If only one subpopulation of T cells were able to enhance ACE induction in monocytes, then even a partial depletion of those cells should have resulted in a marked reduction in ACE induction. In fact, this was not found, and we conclude that both T4$^+$ and T8$^+$ cells are capable of enhancing ACE induction in monocytes. The trend toward greater activity with the T4$^+$ cell-enriched population is of interest because it suggests that T lymphocytes do not all have the same ACE-inducing activity. If a particular subpopulation of T lymphocytes is responsible for *in vitro* induction of ACE in monocytes, that subpopulation would appear to overlap the subpopulations identified by the OKT4 and OKT8 monoclonal antibodies.

Conditioned media from monocyte-T lymphocyte co-cultures enhance induction of ACE in monocytes. The factor responsible for this has not yet been well characterized. Cultures of T4$^+$ cell-enhanced populations and monocytes and those of T8$^+$ cell-enhanced populations and monocytes both result in conditioned media that contain this ACE-inducing activity. The relative activities of these cultured media appear to reflect the trend toward greater activity with the T4$^+$ subpopulation. Although we have not demonstrated that the two cultured media contain the same factor, results do suggest that T4$^+$ and T8$^+$ lymphocytes enhance the induction of ACE in monocytes through similar mechanisms.

The effect of the depletion of populations of Leu 7$^+$ cells was examined for several reasons. We assumed that T4$^-$T8$^-$ cells were left in both the T4$^+$ cell- and T8$^+$ cell-enriched populations. If these T cells were important in inducing ACE, they could have accounted for the activity seen with both enriched populations. Anti-Leu 7 is used to identify some of these T4$^-$T8$^-$ cells.[19] Leu 7$^+$ cells have also been reported in increasing numbers in blood and BAL fluid in patients with sarcoidosis.[25] Depletion of Leu 7$^+$ cells did not affect ACE-inducing activity, and we conclude that the ability to enhance induction of ACE in monocytes is not restricted to the Leu 7$^+$ cells. The design of the experiments did not allow us to determine if Leu 7$^+$ cells have any ACE-inducing activity.

A subpopulation of T cells uniquely capable of enhancing ACE induction in monocytes was not identified in these *in vitro* studies. The irradiation effect, and the trend toward a difference between T4$^+$ and T8$^+$ cells, suggest that such a subpopulation may exist. These results also suggest that the proportions of T cell subtypes present in the alveolitis and granulomas of sarcoidosis patients may be abnormal in more ways than in just the T4:T8 ratio.

REFERENCES

1. JAMES, D. G. & W. JONES WILLIAMS. 1983. Aetiology of sarcoidosis. *In* Fourth European Conference on Sarcoidosis and Other Granulomatous Disorders. A. Blasi, D. Olivieri & A. Pezza, Eds.: 79-85.
2. HUNNINGHAKE, G. W., J. E. GADEK, R. C. YOUNG, O. KAWANAMI, V. J. FERRANS & R. G. CRYSTAL. 1980. Maintenance of granuloma formation in pulmonary sarcoidosis by T lymphocytes within the lung. N. Engl. J. Med. **302:** 594-598.
3. ROHRBACH, M. S. & R. A. DEREMEE. 1982. Pulmonary sarcoidosis and serum angiotensin-converting enzyme. Mayo Clin. Proc. **57:** 64-66.
4. SILVERSTEIN, E., L. P. PERTSCHUK & J. FRIEDLAND. 1979. Immunofluorescent localization of angiotensin-converting enzyme in epithelioid and giant cells of sarcoidosis granulomas. Proc. Natl. Acad. Sci. USA **76:** 6646-6648.
5. SILVERSTEIN, E., J. FRIEDLAND & L. P. PERTSCHUK. 1980. Mechanism of angiotensin-converting enzyme elevation: Epithelioid cell localisation and induction in macrophages and monocytes in culture. *In* Eighth International Conference on Sarcoidosis and Other

Granulomatous Diseases. W. Jones Williams & B. H. Davies, Eds.: 246-258. Alpha Omega. Cardiff.

6. ROHRBACH, M. S. & R. A. ROLSTAD. 1983. Comparison of the induction of angiotensin-converting enzyme and leucine aminopeptidase in cultured human monocytes. Fed. Proc. **42:** 2130.
7. HUNNINGHAKE, G. W. & R. G. CRYSTAL. 1981. Pulmonary sarcoidosis: A disorder mediated by excess helper T lymphocyte activity at sites of disease activity. N. Engl. J. Med. **305:** 429-434.
8. LEATHERMAN, J. W., A. F. MICHAEL, B. A. SCHWARTZ & J. R. HOIDAL. 1984. Lung T cells in hypersensitivity pneumonitis. Ann. Intern. Med. **100:** 390-392.
9. LEIBERMAN, J., A. NOSAL, L. A. SCHLESSNER & A. SASTRE-FOKEN. 1979. Serum angiotensin-converting enzyme for diagnosis and therapeutic evaluation of sarcoidosis. Am. Rev. Respir. Dis. **120:** 329-335.
10. TRACY, P. B., M. S. ROHRBACH & K. G. MANN. 1983. Functional prothrombinase complex assembly on isolated monocytes and lymphocytes. J. Biol. Chem. **258:** 7264-7267.
11. BOYUM, A. 1968. Isolation of mononuclear cells and granulocytes from human blood. Scand. J. Clin. Lab. Invest. Suppl. **97:** 77-89.
12. GMELIG-MEYLING, F. & R. E. BALLIEUX. 1977. Simplified procedure for the separation of human T and non-T cells. Vox Sang. **33:** 5-8.
13. GMELIG-MEYLING, F. & T. A. WALDMANN. 1980. Separation of human blood monocytes and lymphocytes on a continuous Percoll gradient. J. Immunol. Methods **33:** 1-9.
14. ROHRBACH, M. S. 1978. [Glycine-1-^{14}C]hippuryl-L-histidyl-L-leucine: A substrate for the radiochemical assay of angiotensin-converting enzyme. Anal. Biochem. **84:** 272-276.
15. REINHERZ, E. L., A. C. PENTA, R. E. HUSSER & S. F. SCHLOSSMAN. 1981. A rapid method for separating functionally intact human T lymphocytes with monoclonal antibodies. Clin. Immunol. Immunopathol. **21:** 257-266.
16. PAYNE, S. M., S. O. SHARROW, G. M. SHEARER & W. E. BIDDISON. 1981. Preparative separation of human T cells reactive with the OKT4 monoclonal antibody. Int. J. Immunopharmacol. **3:** 227-232.
17. REINHERZ, E. L. & S. F. SCHLOSSMAN. 1980. Regulation of the immune response inducer and suppressor T lymphocyte subsets in human beings. N. Engl. J. Med. **303:** 370-373.
18. CONRAD, A. K. & M. S. ROHRBACH. 1983. Detection of a factor in conditioned media which enhances ACE induction in cultured human monocytes. Clin. Res. **31:** 744A.
19. LANIER, L. I., E. G. ENGLEMAN, P. GATENBY, G. F. BABCOCK, N. L. WARNER & L. A. HERZENBERG. 1983. Correlation of functional properties of human lymphoid cell subsets and surface marker phenotypes using multiparameter analysis and flow cytometry. Immunol. Rev. **74:** 143-160.
20. CRYSTAL, R. G., W. C. ROBERTS, G. W. HUNNINGHAKE, J. E. GADEK, J. D. FULMER & B. R. LINE. 1981. Pulmonary sarcoidosis: A disease characterized and perpetuated by activated lung T lymphocytes. Ann. Intern. Med. **94:** 73-94.
21. GLAZIER, A. J., M. SUNDELL & G. W. HUNNINGHAKE. 1984. Production of human-human lung T cell hybridomas from patients with interstitial lung disease. Clin. Res. **32:** 429A.
22. SIEGAL, F. P. & M. SIEGAL. 1977. Enhancement by irradiated T cells of human plasma cell production: Dissection of helper and suppressor functions *in vitro*. J. Immunol. **118:** 642-647.
23. AGAROSSI, G., C. MANCINI & G. DORIA. 1981. Synergism between two helper cell subpopulations characterized by different radiosensitivity and nylon adherence. J. Immunol. **126:** 955-960.
24. GUALDE, N. & J. S. GOODWIN. 1984. Effect of irradiation on human T cell proliferation: Low dose irradiation stimulates mitogen-induced proliferation and function of the suppressor/cytotoxic T cell subset. Cell. Immunol. **84:** 439-445.
25. SEMENZATO, G., C. AGOSTINI, A. PEZZUTTO, G. GASPAROTTO, A. CIPRIANI, M. CHILOSI, & G. PIZZOLO. 1984. Distribution of natural killer cells in sarcoidosis. J. Clin. Lab. Immunol. **13:** 25-28.

Activated T Cells with Immunoregulatory Functions at Different Sites of Involvement in Sarcoidosis

Phenotypic and Functional Evaluations

G. SEMENZATO,[a,b] C. AGOSTINI,[b] R. ZAMBELLO,[b] L. TRENTIN,[b] M. CHILOSI,[c] M. R. ANGI,[b] E. OSSI,[b] A. CIPRIANI,[b] AND G. PIZZOLO[c]

[b]*University of Padua School of Medicine Padua, Italy*

[c]*University of Verona School of Medicine Verona, Italy*

INTRODUCTION

The development of hybridoma technology and the consequent introduction of monoclonal antibodies (MoAb's) in clinical research has recently provided new possibilities in immunological studies of sarcoidosis. Findings based on studies of peripheral blood could merely reflect epiphenomena of events occurring in involved tissues, but the use of MoAb's allows the evaluation of cellular phenotypes at different sites of disease activity. Thus, in the last few years several labs have demonstrated an increased number of thymus-derived (T) cells with the "helper" phenotype (that is, T cells identified by the T4 MoAb) both in bronchoalveolar lavage (BAL) fluid[1-3] and at different sites of involvement[4-6] in patients with sarcoidosis; furthermore, several authors are trying to develop a clinical application of this knowledge, to relate prognoses, or predictions of the responsiveness to treatment, to the $T4^+$ cell levels in BAL fluid.[7-9]

The aim of the present study, however, does not address the issue of clinical applications but deals with the more basic problem of the nature and significance of $T4^+$ cells in sarcoidosis. To this end, in addition to the OKT4 MoAb, we used other, more specific reagents, and we often used a double-staining technique to better define

[a]Address for correspondence: Instituto di Medicina Clinica, via Giustiniani 2, 35128 Padua, Italy.

the precise phenotype and the possible heterogeneity of the $T4^+$ cell population. In fact, we now know that the cells which actually display helper functions in a control group are restricted to a minor subset within the whole $T4^+$ cell population. Cells of this subset account for approximately 20% of peripheral blood $T4^+$ cells and can be identified with the following MoAb's: Leu 8, OKT17, and 5/9.[10–12] In order to provide a direct demonstration of the function of these cells, we correlated the cellular phenotype with functional *in vitro* activity by evaluating the ability of cells under study to regulate a pokeweed mitogen (PWM)-driven differentiation assay of bone marrow-derived (B) cells. In addition, the ability of $T4^+$ cells to produce interleukin-2 (IL-2) and to respond in an autologous mixed lymphocyte reaction (AMLR) have been evaluated. Finally, taking advantage of immunohistological techniques we studied the precise topographic distribution of $T4^+$ cells, with particular regard to their relationship to antigen-presenting cells. In fact, $T4^+$ and $T8^+$ lymphocyte subsets have been found to be associated with the cell's capacity to recognize particular products of the major histocompatibility complex (MHC). While $T8^+$ cells can differentiate into cytotoxic cells with specificity for Class I (HLA-A and -B) molecules, $T4^+$ cells are capable of proliferating in response to MHC Class II (HLA-DR) alloantigens and soluble antigens presented in association with Class II determinants.

MATERIALS AND METHODS

Patients

Twenty-two patients with active sarcoidosis (14 women and 8 men; mean age: 33 ± 6 years) were studied. In every case, provided there was no evidence of inorganic material known to cause granulomatous diseases, the diagnosis depended on whether a biopsy (obtained from the lungs, lymph nodes, or liver) showed noncaseating epithelioid granulomas. The stage of each patient's disease was determined according to the radiological pulmonary changes that were observed. Twelve patients had stage I, eight patients had stage II, and two patients had stage III sarcoidosis. Disease activity was evaluated according to 1) the clinical features and laboratory findings, including the percentage of T cells in BAL fluid; 2) the positivity of the gallium-67 scan; and 3) the level of serum angiotensin-converting enzyme (SACE) activity. All patients were studied at the time of diagnosis and before any treatment was given.

Ten normal nonsmoking volunteers (six women and four men; mean age: 32 ± 5 years) were used as controls in studies of BAL specimens. For ethical reasons, biopsies (of lung, lymph node, conjunctiva, liver, and skin tissue) were only taken from volunteers suspected of having some disorder other than sarcoidosis, but who were ultimately found to be normal, or from volunteers with no clinical signs of sarcoidosis, during cardiac surgery.

Healthy patients could not be used as controls in studies of IL-2 production or in AMLR tests because an adequate number of T cells could not be obtained by BAL. Instead, 10 patients with inactive sarcoidosis (6 women and 4 men; mean age: 38 ± 4 years) were used. These patients were diagnosed as having inactive sarcoidosis according to the criteria mentioned above and were studied at the time of diagnosis and before any treatment was given.

Evaluation with MoAb's

Mononuclear cells obtained from BAL (performed with a total of 100 to 150 ml of sterile saline solution) were washed three times with phosphate-buffered saline solution (PBS) and resuspended in RPMI 1640 (Grand Island Biological, Grand Island, NY). Adherent cells were removed by incubating them at 37° C for 45 min in plastic petri dishes. T cells were identified either by their ability to spontaneously form rosettes with sheep erythrocytes, as previously described,[13] or by their reactivity with MoAb's such as OKT3 (Ortho Pharmaceutical, Raritan, NJ) or UCHT-1 (provided by Dr. P. Beverley, London),[14,15] using an indirect immunofluorescence technique.[6] T cell subpopulations were further characterized by different groups of MoAb's, most of them belonging to the OKT (Ortho Pharmaceutical) or the Leu (Becton Dickinson, Sunnyvale, CA) series.

Markers of Helper Cells and Suppressor Cells

The OKT4 and Leu 3 MoAb's have been used to define helper/inducer cells, and the OKT8 and Leu 2 MoAb's have reportedly been used to roughly define supressor/cytotoxic cells.[15,16] For convenience, these kinds of cells will be referred to as being $T4^+$ and $T8^+$, respectively.

Markers of Subsets of T4⁺ Cells Which Display in Vitro *Functions*

Some reagents mark cells of different $T4^+$ subsets and, it has been claimed, cells which actually display *in vitro* functions. These reagents are the OKT17, Leu 8, and 5/9 MoAb's.[10–12]

The OKT17 MoAb (Ortho Pharmaceutical) reacts with most resting T cells; however, $T4^+$ cells lose their reactivity with OKT17 after being cultured for 7 days at 37° C with PWM (Grand Island Biological) supplemented with 10% heat-inactivated fetal calf serum (FCS) (Microbiological Associates, Bethesda, MD).[10] This loss of reactivity reflects the OKT17 MoAb's most interesting aspect: the $T4^+$ $T17^+$ subset contains helper cells but is devoid of suppressor cells, which are confined to the $T4^+$ $T17^-$ subset.

The Leu 8 MoAb reacts with about 80% of all T cells, and these T cells may be either $T4^+$ or $T8^+$. Using a fluoresceine-conjugated Leu 8 MoAb and a phycoerythrin-conjugated Leu 3 MoAb, simultaneous analyses of the same cell can be done. It has been found that the Leu 3^+ Leu 8^- phenotype provides maximum helper *in vitro* activity.[11]

The subset reactive with the 5/9 MoAb (Technogenetic, Turin) appears to be associated with the helper activity of PWM-driven cell differentiation.[12]

Markers of IL-2 and Transferrin Receptors on Cell Membranes

The anti-Tac MoAb (provided by Dr. T. Uchiyama, Kyoto), originally described as a marker of activation,[17] has been found to recognize the membrane receptor for

IL-2 on activated T[18] and B[19] cells. Robb and Greene[20] have recently identified the IL-2-binding protein and described the recognition of this protein by the anti-Tac antigen. Bettens *et al.*[21] demonstrated that two IL-2 receptor types exist, and that anti-Tac recognizes one of them. One receptor type is for exogenous IL-2, and is recognized by anti-Tac, and the other receptor type is for endogenous IL-2. The latter type is not recognized by anti-Tac and perhaps never appears on the outer surface of the lymphocyte membrane.

The OKT9 MoAb (Ortho Parmaceutical), originally described as a marker of immature thymic lymphocytes and their corresponding leukemias,[22] has been found to be directed against the transferrin receptors.[23,24] These receptors seem to mediate, at least in part, the IL-2-dependent T cell proliferation.[25]

Markers of Natural Killer Cells

MoAb's that may be directed against natural killer (NK) cells have been associated with cells having the appearance of large granular lymphocytes (LGL's).[26] HNK-1 (Leu 7, Becton Dickinson) reacts with almost all LGL's.[27] NKP-15 (Leu 11, Becton Dickinson); VEP.13 (provided by Dr. H. Rumpold, Vienna); B73.1 (provided by Dr. B. Perussia, Philadelphia, PA); and Ab8.28 (provided by Dr. F. Malavasi, Turin) might react with the Fc receptor for immunoglobulin G or with some related structure of LGL's and seems to be better associated than the HNK-1 MoAb with killer and NK activity.[28–31]

Markers of B Cells

OKB2/OKB7 (Ortho Pharmaceutical) and Leu 12 (Becton Dickinson) were directed against mature B cells,[32,33] and BA-1 (Hybritech, La Jolla, CA) was directed against both immature and mature B cells.[34]

Functional in Vitro *Activities*

Analysis of Helper and Suppressor Activity of Cell Subsets in PWM-stimulated Cultures

The effect of total T or $T4^+$ cell-enriched populations on *in vitro* PWM-driven B cell differentiation was evaluated in a mixture of T cells depleted of cells bearing Fc receptors for immunoglobulin G (T_G) and normal B cell populations (5×10^4 and 10×10^5 cells/well, respectively). The basic procedure has already been described.[13] Cultures were performed in flat-bottomed microtiter plates (Falcon, Rockville, MD). Lymphocytes were cultured in 200 μl of RPMI 1640 supplemented with 20% autologous serum, 2 mM glutamine, and 50 μg/ml gentamycin. Control cultures were B cell fractions alone (10^5 cells/well) cultured in the presence of PWM. Total T cell populations were purified by the rosette-formation technique, as previously described.[13] T cell populations were enriched with $T4^+$ cells by using a negative selection technique in which the OKT8 MoAb was used. Briefly, 10×10^6 unfractioned T cells were resuspended in 1 ml of RPMI 1640 medium which contained 10% heat-inactivated FCS and 10 μg of the OKT8 MoAb and were incubated for 1 hr at 4° C. Fresh rabbit complement was added at a final dilution of 1:2, and the incubation was continued for 1 hr at 37° C. Analysis of the resulting population showed that fewer than 3% of the cells were $T8^+$. The various cell combinations were cultured at 37° C in a 5% CO_2 atmosphere for 7 days. The cells were then harvested and counted, and the cell suspensions were cytocentrifuged. The viability of the cells in these suspensions was assessed using the trypan blue exclusion test. The slides were fixed in methanol which contained 5% acetic acid, were rehydrated in PBS, and were stained at room temperature for 20 min with polyvalent or class-specific goat antihuman immunoglobulin antibodies (Meloy Laboratories, Springfield, IL). The percentage of cells with detectable amounts of cytoplasmatic immunoglobulins (that is, of cIg^+ cells) was determined, and the absolute number of plasma cells per well was determined as a function of the number of viable cells per well.

IL-2 Production Tests

Lymphocytes recovered by BAL at a concentration of 10^6 cells/ml were cultured with 1 μg/ml phytohemagglutinin (PHA) (Difco Laboratories, Detroit, MI) in RPMI supplemented with 1% heat-inactivated FCS, 4 mM glutamine, 50 U/ml penicillin, and 50 μg/ml streptomycin at 37° C in a humidified atmosphere of 5% CO_2 and 95% air. The supernatants were then collected by centrifugation and stored at −20° C until they were tested. Supernatants were assayed for IL-2 activity by their ability to induce the incorporation of [^{3}H]thymidine in IL-2-dependent cells.[35] To prepare this T cell growth assay, mononuclear cells from the blood of healthy volunteers were suspended in RPMI 1640 (1×10^6 cells/ml) and were stimulated for 48 hr in this suspension, which contained 1% heat-inactivated FCS and 1 μg/ml PHA. These cells were then recultured, for at least 15 days at 37° C in a 5% CO_2 atmosphere, in RPMI 1640 (0.5×10^6 cells/ml) which contained 20% heat-inactivated FCS, 30% of the IL-2-containing supernatants, and 4 mM glutamine. The culture medium was changed every 3 days, and the cell concentration was adjusted to 0.5×10^6 cells/ml. After 15 days 95% of the cultured cells formed E rosettes and reacted with monoclonal anti-T antisera. Then, 5×10^4 of these cultured cells were plated in microtiter wells (Limbro, Hamden, CT) with or without the addition of test supernatants (at different dilutions) for 72 hr in a 5% CO_2 atmosphere. The cells were pulsed for the final 6 hr with [^{3}H]thymidine (0.5 μCi; specific activity: 26 mCi/mM) (Cea Ire Sorin) and then harvested as previously described.[36] Each result is a mean of the values for the cases expressed in counts per minute (cpm). Each case was studied in triplicate.

IL-2-containing supernatants were received as gifts (from Dr. Gramatzki, Erlangen) and were generated as previously described.[37] Supernatants were obtained after 48 hr from a culture that contained a mixture of lymphocytes (1×10^6 cells/ml) and B lymphoblastoid cells (2×10^5 irradiated cells/ml)—the former were obtained by draining the thoracic ducts of patients that were about to have kidney transplants; the latter from the RM-1 B lymphoblastoid cell line—in RPMI 1640 medium supplemented with 2% heat-inactivated FCS and 0.5 μg/ml purified PHA (Wellcome, Research Triangle Park, NC).

AMLR Tests

AMLR tests were set up in round-bottomed microtiter plates (Griener, Nurtingen). Part of the test procedure has already been described.[38] T cell-enriched populations were obtained from BAL fluid as reported above. Some of these populations were co-cultured with autologous B cell-enriched populations obtained from peripheral blood; others were co-cultured with autologous alveolar macrophage suspensions (at different dilutions). The T cells were used as responders; the B cells and alveolar macrophages, after being treated with 50 μg of mitomycin C for 30 min at 37° C, were used as stimulators. DNA synthesis was quantified by determining the extent of [^{3}H]thymidine incorporation in cultured cells after 7 days, as described above.[36,38] Each result is expressed in cpm and is a mean ± SEM of the values for the cases. Each case was studied in triplicate.

Immunohistological Studies at Different Sites of Disease Activity

Biopsy specimens were obtained from the lung in 18 patients by transbronchial lung bronchoscopy, from the lymph nodes in 8 patients by mediastinoscopy, from the liver and the spleen in 1 patient, from the skin in 3 patients, and from the conjunctiva in 9 patients. After excision the specimen was divided: one half was fixed in 10% formalin and processed by paraffin embedding, and the other half was embedded in Ames OCT Compound (Miles Laboratories, Elkhart, IN) and snap frozen in liquid N_2 within 1 hr of excision. Five-micron sections were cut in a cryostat, transferred onto albuminized glass slides, air dried, and fixed in a 1:1 chloroform-acetone mixture for 5 min at 4° C before staining.

Immunohistological studies with the MoAb's described above were performed using immunoperoxidase procedures as previously described.[39,40] Briefly, sections were covered in a moist chamber with MoAb in 5-10 μl of fluid for 30 min, washed three times in PBS, and stained for 30 min with rabbit antimouse immunoglobulin coupled to peroxidase. The histochemical reaction for peroxidase was performed as previously described using H_2O_2 and 3,3′-diaminobenzidine.[39]

Due to technical reasons, we were unable to evaluate tissue specimens with the OKT17 and 5/9 MoAb's.

The possibility that cells under study bind MoAb's via Fc receptors was ruled out by evaluating suspensions and histological sections after incubation with γ-globulin Cohn fraction II and further washing.

Analysis of Data

All data were presented as means ± SEM's, and comparisons between values were made using the Cockran-Cox test.

RESULTS

As shown in FIGURE 1, most lymphocytes in BAL fluid recovered from patients with active sarcoidosis were T cells. Few lymphocytes expressed the T8 phenotype; indeed, most expressed the T4 phenotype. The resulting T4/T8 ratio (7.1 ± 1.5), with respect to that of controls (2.0 ± 0.4), was highly statistically significant ($p < .001$). The frequency of 5/9$^+$ cells (62 ± 5.8%), with respect to that of controls (32 ± 4.6%), was also significant ($p < .001$). Using a double-staining technique, we found that the majority of T4$^+$ cells are Leu 8$^-$ (92 ± 4.3%) and that T4$^+$ cells lose their T17 determinants after *in vivo* PWM culture. Even though we found a high frequency of T4$^+$ Leu 8$^-$ cells in controls (76 ± 4.0%), the frequency in sarcoidosis patients, in terms of absolute numbers, was markedly greater ($p < .001$) because of lymphocytosis. Unfortunately, we were unable to obtain enough BAL cells from healthy subjects to assess PWM cultures of T4$^+$ cells in order to evaluate the reactivity with the OKT17 MoAb.

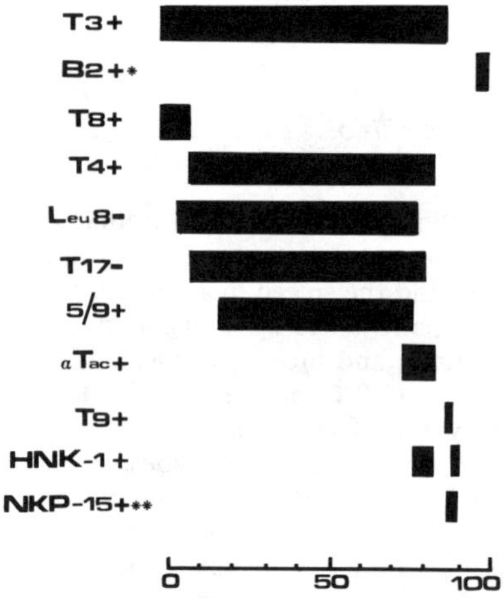

FIGURE 1. Surface phenotype of lymphocytes in BAL fluid recovered from patients with active sarcoidosis. * = Anti-B cell MoAb's (B7, BA1, and Leu 12) in addition to B2. ** = Anti-NK cell MoAb's (B73.1, VEP 13, and Ab8.28) in addition to NKP-15. The frequency of T17$^+$ cells was determined following a culture with PWM.

Anti-Tac$^+$ cells make up 11.1 ± 2.2% of the BAL cells in sarcoidosis patients but only 2.4 ± 2.0% of the BAL cells in controls ($p < .001$), and T9$^+$ cells make up less than 5% of the BAL cells in sarcoidosis patients and controls. On the other hand, 64 ± 5.4% of all macrophages express T9 determinants; that is, the transferrin receptors on some macrophages express T9 determinants.

HNK-1$^+$ cells make up 6.7 ± 1.2% of the BAL cells in sarcoidosis patients and 7.6 ± 1.1% of the BAL cells in controls (NS). Using double-staining techniques, we showed that most HNK-1$^+$ cells express T4 determinants. Thus these cells express the HNK-1$^+$ T4$^+$ T8$^-$ phenotype. The frequencies of NKP-15$^+$, B73.1$^+$, VEP13$^+$, and AB8.28$^+$ cells were always less than 5%.

Only a few lymphocytes with B cell characteristics have been found, using the B2, B7, Leu 12, and BA-1 MoAb's, among the BAL cells of our patients and controls.

Functional analyses of T cells from BAL fluid are shown in FIGURE 2 and TABLE 1. The ability of lung T cells from sarcoidosis patients to display helper activity has

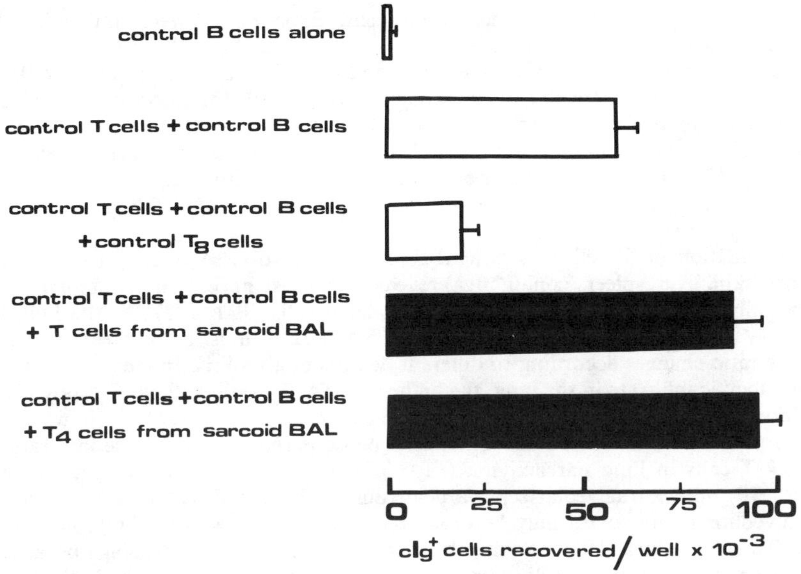

FIGURE 2. Helper *in vitro* activity on PWM-driven B cell differentiation by total and $T4^+$ cell-enriched T cell populations from BAL fluid recovered from patients with active sarcoidosis. Activities in cultures of mixed T_G-depleted (5×10^4 cells) and normal (10×10^5 cells) B cell populations were assessed with (open bars) and without (closed bars) the addition of total T or $T4^+$ cell-enriched T cell populations (5×10^{-4} cells) from sarcoidosis patients. Each result is the mean ± SEM of six experiments.

been assessed by *in vitro* PWM assay (FIG. 2). When either total or $T4^+$ cell-enriched T cell populations were added to a combination of T and B cells from normal volunteers (the basic combination in our tests, one which allows the optimal production of plasma cells), the number of plasma cells recovered per well increased; thus we have direct evidence that BAL $T4^+$ cells display helper activity in sarcoidosis.

As shown in TABLE 1, supernatants from cultures of lymphocytes from recovered BAL fluid were assayed to induce [^{3}H]thymidine incorporation in IL-2-dependent cells. Compared to the BAL supernatants from a group of patients with inactive sarcoidosis, those from patients with active sarcoidosis displayed, at several dilutions,

TABLE 1. Effect of IL-2-containing Supernatants from Cultures of Lung T Cells on T Cell Growth Assays

Source of Supernatants	*N*	[^{3}H]Thymidine Uptake at Different Supernatant Dilutions		
		1:2	1:4	1:8
Medium alone		472 ± 26	—	—
Sarcoidosis patients	3	8174 ± 794	5698 ± 597	4054 ± 492
Controls[a]	3	741 ± 138	604 ± 146	479 ± 107

[a]Three patients with inactive sarcoidosis were used as controls.

a better ability to grow IL-2-dependent cells. Experiments were limited to three patients.

Data obtained from AMLR's are reported in TABLE 2. The response of BAL T cells to mitomycin C-treated B lymphocytes from peripheral blood was significantly increased in patients with active sarcoidosis with respect to that in control patients ($p < .001$). [^{3}H]Thymidine uptake of BAL T lymphocytes from active sarcoidosis patients, when the lymphocytes were co-cultured with mitomycin C-treated alveolar macrophages, was higher than the [^{3}H]thymidine uptake of BAL T lymphocytes from control patients ($p < .001$).

Evaluation of T cell subsets at different sites of disease activity (lungs, lymph nodes, skin, liver, spleen, conjunctiva) revealed a consistent pattern in different organs, especially concerning infiltrates of helper-related cells (TABLE 3). At the lung level the T4/T8 ratio is 9, with a range between 5 and 22. It must be pointed out that the above ratio changes according to different degrees of alveolitis. In fact, the higher the lymphocytic infiltrate in the lung, the higher the T4/T8 ratio will be. FIGURE 3 shows different patterns of lymphocytic infiltration in sarcoid lung, that is, shows the life history of sarcoidosis alveolitis. The initial phase is represented by the infiltration of a few T cells in lung parenchyma (FIG. 3A). Progressively this infiltrate increases (FIG. 3B) until intraalveolar septa are surrounded by T cells (FIG. 3C). At the peak of alveolitis lymphocytes may be organized into aggregates (FIG. 3D). The highest T4/T8 ratio values (18 ± 4) have been found in the lung at this stage because the infiltrate is almost exclusively represented by $T4^+$ cells. Following the high-intensity alveolitis phase, the organization of follicles in the granulomas can be observed. At this time, however, the number of T cells begins to decrease (FIG. 3E), and T cells nearly disappear when fibrosis develops (FIG. 3F). It is interesting to note that in these patients $T4^+$ cells both surround and enter the granulomas (FIG. 3E).

$T4^+$ cells within granulomas are more evident in FIGURE 4, in a tissue section from a sarcoidosis lymph node. In addition to the great number of cells in the surrounding mantle, numerous $T4^+$ cells are evident in intimate contact with antigen-presenting cells in the central core of each granuloma. No $T8^+$ cells have been found

TABLE 2. AMLR's in Sarcoidosis

Culture Combination	Dilution	[^{3}H]Thymidine Uptake: Sarcoidosis Patients[a]	[^{3}H]Thymidine Uptake: Controls[b]	Significance
BAL T cells and mitomycin C-treated peripheral blood B cells	1:1	1109 ± 360	381 ± 77	$p < .001$
BAL T cells and mitomycin C-treated alveolar macrophages	1:1	911 ± 304	174 ± 45	$p < .005$
	1:0.5	795 ± 144	239 ± 34	$p < .005$
	1:0.2	759 ± 213	451 ± 67	NS
	1:0.1	820 ± 223	381 ± 146	NS

[a]Nine cases were studied with the one dilution of the first culture combination; seven cases were studied with each of the four dilutions of the second culture combination. Each individual case was studied in triplicate.

[b]Ten cases with inactive sarcoidosis were studied for each result below. Each individual case was studied in triplicate.

TABLE 3. T4/T8 Ratio at Different Sites of Involvement in Sarcoidosis[a]

Tissue	Number of Biopsies	T4/T8 Ratio[b]
Lungs[c]	18	9 (5-22)
Lymph nodes	8	24 (10-65)
Skin	3	20 (14-28)
Liver	1	18
Spleen	1	22
Conjunctiva	9	15 (7-34)

[a]In lymph nodes from controls the T4/T8 ratio was 5 (range: 2-7). The malpighian follicles of the spleen showed reactivity similar to that seen in the lymph nodes. In the lung and liver biopsies (both taken from the lobules and portal areas) from controls the ratios were similar to that found in the blood (2.1). In the skin and conjunctiva of controls lymphoid infiltrates were not detected.

[b]Results are expressed as means. Ranges are shown in parentheses.

[c]Tissue obtained by transbronchial lung biopsy.

in the middle of the follicle, and the mean T4/T8 ratio is 24 (TABLE 3). It must be pointed out that these $T4^+$ cells inside the granulomas are Leu 8^- (FIG. 5B), and thus bear the phenotype of cells from recovered BAL fluid.

A discrete number of Tac^+ cells have been observed in tissue sections from the lungs (FIG. 6A), lymph nodes (FIG. 6B), and conjunctiva.

DISCUSSION

The present study shows that lymphocytes in BAL fluid and among cells which infiltrate all the sites of disease activity in sarcoidosis are activated T cells with discrete immunoregulatory functions. This is evident because these lymphocytes express the $T4^+$ Leu 8^- $5/9^+$ $T17^-$ phenotype characteristic of cells with helper activity and the ability to spontaneously release IL-2 and because these lymphocytes react in AMLR's. The microanatomic location of activated T cells, as determined by immunohistological analysis, demonstrated that the state of activation of these T cells could be a consequence of intimate contact between $T4^+$ cells and macrophages and/or antigen-presenting cells within the sarcoidosis granuloma.

Because $T4^+$ lymphocytes are a heterogeneous population,[41,42] the definitive evidence we provide herein, with phenotypic and functional analyses, that cells at sites of ongoing inflammation belong to a discrete subset with helper properties, provides an important framework for understanding immunological phenomena in sarcoidosis. For one thing, the anergy of cell-mediated immunity observed in peripheral blood using different tests (including a test that showed a decrease in the frequency of helper cells[1-3] and a test that showed defective secretion of immunoglobulin in response to PWM[13,43]) can be interpreted as being a consequence of a compartmentalization of immunocompetent cells from the blood to different sites of involvement. In fact, we found that BAL T lymphocytes were committed to providing a helper function in a

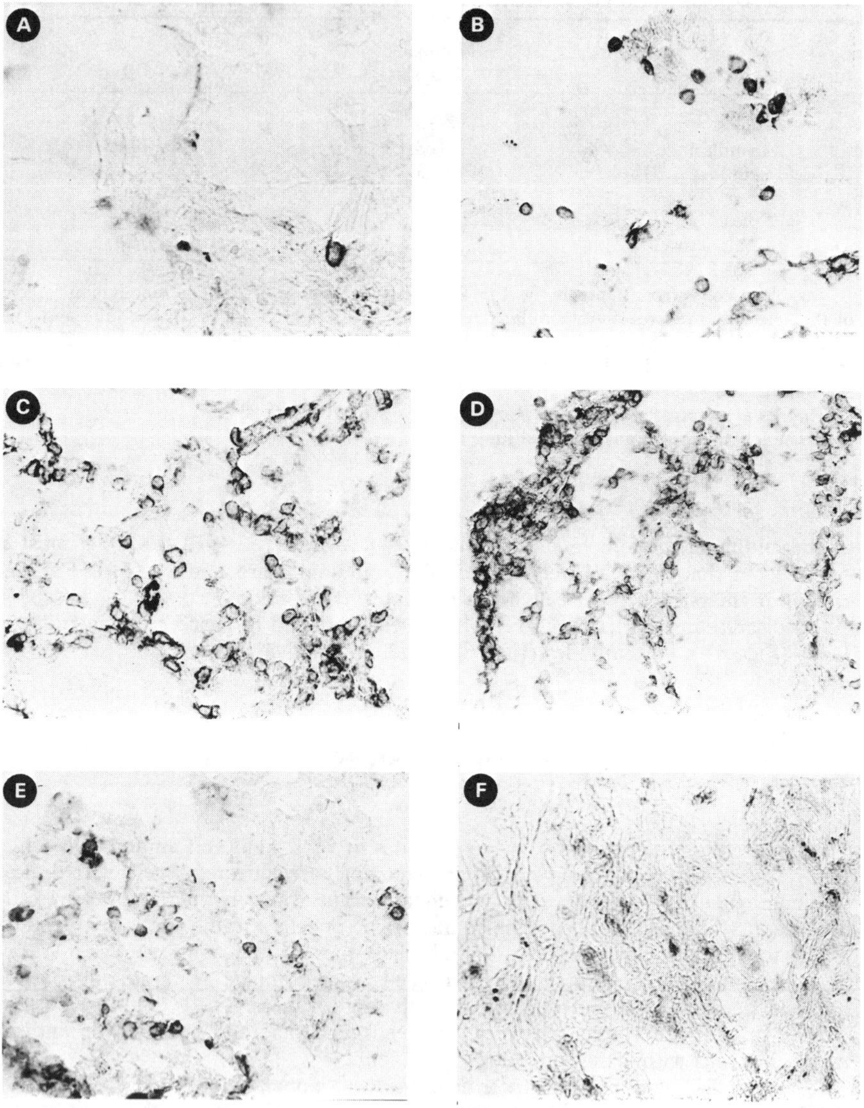

FIGURE 3. Cryostat sections, from the lung of patient with active sarcoidosis, stained using an immunoperoxidase method: the UCHT-1 MoAb was used, and there was no nuclear counter-staining. The sequence shows the different stages of alveolitis in sarcoidosis. **(A)** Only a few cells infiltrate lung parenchyma. Then, **(B)** the amount of infiltrate increases. Eventually, **(C)** alveolar septa are surrounded by T cells, and **(D)** lymphoid aggregates can be observed. **(E)** Sarcoid granulomas can be seen in the lung parenchyma, but the number of T cells begins to decrease until **(F)** T cells are virtually absent. Original magnification: ×400; reduced to 75% of original size.

PWM-driven B cell differentiation assay and, strikingly, that T4$^+$ cells were present at all sites of disease activity, that is, at the lungs, lymph nodes, conjunctiva, liver, spleen, and skin. It has been proposed[44] that lymphokines produced at sites of ongoing inflammation account for the migration of T4$^+$ cells from the blood to granulomatous lesions; however, the precise mechanism which controls these processes remains to be elucidated. All these findings taken together substantiate the concept already proposed[1,2,5,6,45,46] of a redistribution of helper cells in these patients and further stress the idea that sarcoidosis is a multisystem disease, thus emphasizing the necessity of evaluating different organs as possible sites of disease activity.

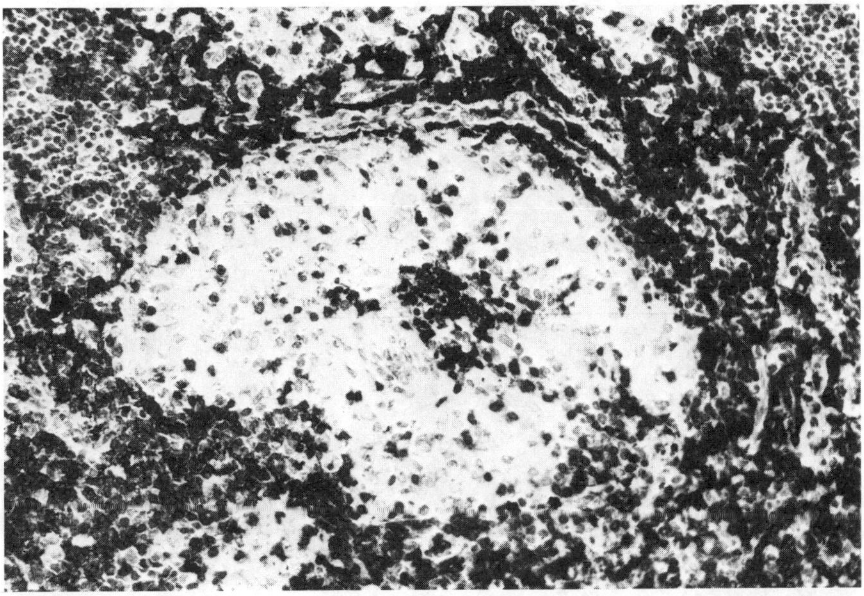

FIGURE 4. Cryostat section, from the lymph node of a patient with active sarcoidosis, stained using an immunoperoxidase method: the OKT4 MoAb and light hematoxylin staining were used. T4$^+$ cells surround the granuloma and are present in the middle of the follicle, in intimate contact with antigen-presenting cells. Original magnification: ×250; reduced to 95% of original size.

A redistribution of T cells, however, does not represent the only event accounting for the accumulation of inflammatory and immunocompetent cells at sites of involvement. In fact, the increased production of IL-2 by BAL T cells[47,48] (TABLE 1) associated with the presence of Tac$^+$ cells in different tissues[49] suggests that T cells are able to proliferate *in situ*. The major T cell subset responsible for the release of IL-2 seems to be the T4$^+$ Leu 8$^-$ subset (data not shown), and this finding is in line with the surface phenotype of activated T cells in sarcoidosis described above. IL-2 may act as a stimulating factor not only for T cells, but for B cells, via specific receptors.[19,50] In this connection, an infiltrate with helper activity may account for the presence of

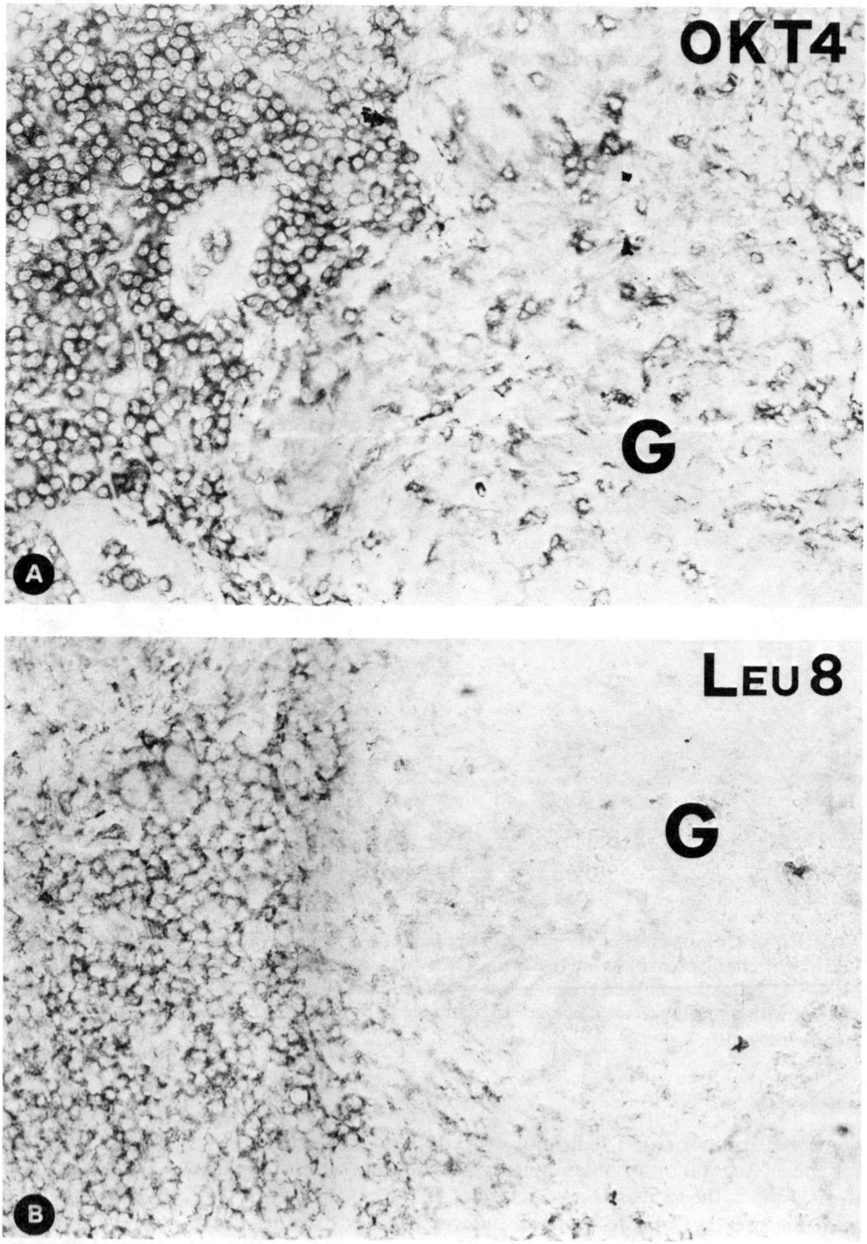

FIGURE 5. Cryostat sections, from the lymph node of a patient with active sarcoidosis, stained using an immunoperoxidase method: the (**A**) OKT4 and (**B**) Leu 8 MoAb's were used, and there was no nuclear counterstaining. In **A**, numerous T4$^+$ cells surround and are present inside the granuloma (G). In **B**, Leu 8$^+$ cells are present in the surrounding mantle of the granuloma but represent a mixed lymphocyte population (see Lanier *et al.*[77] for details). The crucial aspect, however, is that those cells which express the OKT4 MoAb do not express the Leu 8 MoAb.

plasma cells observed in the mantle surrounding sarcoidosis granulomas;[6] for the B cell hyperreactivity and the polyclonal hypergammaglobulinemia;[51] and, in particular, for the presence of immunoglobulin-releasing cells in the lungs of sarcoidosis patients.[52] In addition, peripheral blood studies in sarcoidosis which showed an impaired *in vitro* production of IL-2[47,53] and the lack of cells precommitted to respond to IL-2[49] are consistent with the concept of compartmentalization discussed above.

Thus, cellular redistribution and local proliferation lead to an accumulation of T cells in involved tissues. Different stages of this infiltration can only be monitored in the lung because of the possibility of performing serial transbronchial biopsies. Carrington *et al.*[54] and Rosen *et al.*[55] demonstrated that lymphocytic infiltration represents

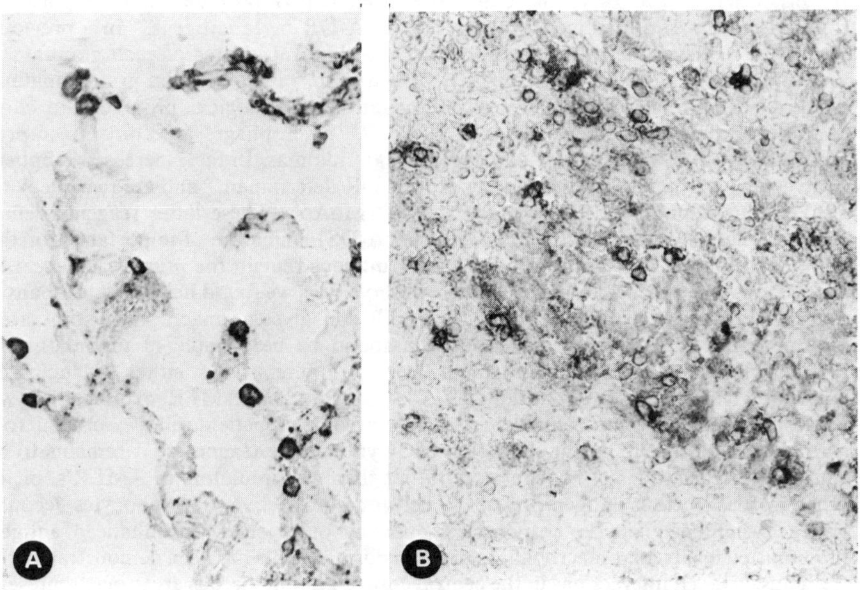

FIGURE 6. Cryostat sections, from the **(A)** lung and **(B)** lymph node of a patient with active sarcoidosis, stained using an immunoperoxidase method: the anti-Tac MoAb was used. Several Tac$^+$ cells can be seen in both the lung and lymph node sections. Original magnification for **A** was ×450 and that for **B** was ×300; both **A** and **B** were reduced to 87% of their original sizes.

the earliest lesion of the lung in sarcoidosis. In the sequence we presented in FIGURE 3, we extended the above observations[54,55] by providing immunohistological evidence of the life history of the sarcoidosis alveolitis, which is mediated by T cells of the helper type.

Because the alveolitis precedes the appearance of granulomas, the helper nature of the lymphocytic infiltration may be crucial, as well as in other granulomatous reactions,[56] in the regulation of the formation and maintenance of granulomas. Perhaps different components of the so-called lymphokine cascade, including IL-1, IL-2, and the interferons (the main substances involved in controlling these mechanisms), are released by different cellular subsets.[57,58] In this regard it is worth mentioning that the alveolitis of hypersensitivity pneumonitis, which is mediated by cells with the suppressor/cytotoxic phenotype,[59–61] develops in a different way than the alveolitis of sarcoidosis.[62] This emphasizes the importance of carefully characterizing the phenotype and functions of interstitial infiltrates not only in different disorders but at different stages of the disease. This can be done quite easily due to the availability of BAL techniques. Because, as we have demonstrated, the nature of the lymphocytic infiltrate is the same at different sites of involvement, we suggest that the evolution of granulomatous lesions is likely to be regulated at these sites in a similar way; one must, of course, keep in mind the different possibilities of cellular traffic in different organs. We have tried to evaluate this hypothesis in studies of the conjunctival follicles.[63] For ethical reasons, however, it is impossible to obtain tissue for complete serial demonstrations other than from the lung.

The major question now arises as to how $T4^+$ cells are triggered to initiate the mechanisms described above. In this regard, the focus must be placed on the role recently attributed to $T4^+$ cells. This subset is capable of proliferating in response to the MHC Class II alloantigens, that is, the HLA-DR or Ia antigens.[64] In a previous paper[4] we reported the presence of $T4^+$ cells in the central area of each granuloma, and this finding has been confirmed by Mishra *et al.*[65] in the Kveim granulomatous reaction. We provide in the present study immunohistological proof of the close relationship between helper cells and $HLA\text{-}DR^+$ macrophages and/or antigen-presenting cells in the central area of sarcoidosis granulomas. In fact, increased numbers of alveolar macrophages in sarcoidosis express DR determinant[66] and are reactive with Leu 10 (our unpublished data) and Mac-120[67] MoAb's. These latter reagents define the HLA antigens of the second D locus (HLA-DS) which are of importance for the antigen-presenting function.[68] The HLA-DR antigens remain the primary inducers of mitogenesis in AMLR's. In line with these observations we found heightened responses of BAL T cells in an AMLR, both in B cell- and alveolar macrophage-stimulated cultures. Alveolar macrophages have been found to be capable of modulating T lymphocyte responses to conventional antigens in different ways, either enhancing or inhibiting lymphocyte proliferation.[69,70] According to our AMLR experiments, we suggest that alveolar macrophages in active sarcoidosis patients play a crucial role acting as potent agents in the induction of T lymphocyte responses. It remains to be clarified whether they act as regulators rather than as stimulators in AMLR's, or, in other words, whether antigen-presenting cells or self-reactive T lymphocytes account for the heightened *in vitro* response. Supporting our results, an enhanced antigen presentation by alveolar macrophages in sarcoidosis patients has been demonstrated.[71,72]

Thus, cell-cell interactions in the central core of granulomatous areas may represent the essential event that initiates and maintains the state of inflammation via the production of different lymphokines. The relevance of these interactions is emphasized by the evidence of the presence of both $T4^+$ and Tac^+ cells within the granulomas.[4,49,65] Further studies, especially in the area of lymphokines, are needed in order to better define the precise steps by which the host-against-invader battle proceeds at the granuloma level. In this context, the findings of spontaneously released γ-interferon from the lung in active sarcoidosis patients[73] and of the presence in the sarcoidosis granulomas of cells reactive with an anti-γ-interferon MoAb (unpublished results) provide a basis for further investigation. In fact, other than representing a mechanism for amplifying the immune response as a part of the cascade of lymphokine-cell interactions, γ-interferon has been demonstrated to stimulate macrophages to synthesize and release IL-1,[74] to increase the HLA-DR expression, and, in turn, to increase their accessory Ia antigen-mediated function.[75] In addition, the presence of receptors for transferrin on alveolar macrophages represents another intriguing topic, considering that receptors for transferrin may act as a target structure for NK cells.[76] Definitive advances of our understanding of sarcoidosis will, perhaps, only be made after we identify the antigen(s) responsible for this disease.

SUMMARY

Cells from recovered BAL fluid and from infiltrates in different involved tissues (lungs, lymph nodes, conjunctiva, liver, spleen, and skin) were studied in 22 patients with active sarcoidosis in order to define the surface phenotype, functional *in vitro* properties, and topographic distribution of the cells in granulomatous lesions.

Our data demonstrated a compartmentalization of activated T cells with immunoregulatory functions from the blood to all sites of disease activity. In fact, these cells were found to express the $T4^+$ Leu 8^- $5/9^+$ $T17^-$ phenotype, which belongs to cells with helper activity, and that provide heightened responses in functional assays of helper activity, IL-2 release, and the ability to respond in AMLR's. Both a cellular redistribution and a local *in vitro* replication account for this tissue compartmentalization in sarcoidosis. The microanatomic location of activated T cells, as defined by immunohistological evaluation, showed that the state of activation in these T cells may be a consequence of an intimate contact between helper cells and macrophages within the sarcoidosis granulomas.

REFERENCES

1. HUNNINGHAKE, G. W. & R. G. CRYSTAL. 1981. N. Engl. J. Med. **305:** 429-439.
2. SEMENZATO, G. & A. PEZZUTTO. 1982. Immunol. Clin. Sper. **1:** 35-44.
3. GINNS, L. C., C. HURWITZ & H. KAZEMI. 1982. Clin. Immunol. Immunopathol. **25:** 11-20.
4. SEMENZATO, G., A. PEZZUTTO, M. CHILOSI & G. PIZZOLO. 1982. N. Engl. J. Med. **306:** 48-49.
5. MODLIN, R. L., F. M. HOFMAN, P. R. MEYER, O. P. SHARMA, C. R. TAYLOR & T. H. REA. 1983. Clin. Exp. Immunol. **51:** 430-438.
6. SEMENZATO, G., A. PEZZUTTO, G. PIZZOLO, M. CHILOSI, E. OSSI, M. R. ANGI & A. CIPRIANI. 1984. Clin. Immunol. Immunopathol. **30:** 29-40.
7. COSTABEL, U., K. J. BROSS & H. MATTHYS. 1983. Klin. Wochenschr. **61:** 349-356.
8. BAUGHMAN, R. P., M. FERNANDEZ, C. H. BOSKEN, J. MANTIL & P. HURTUBISE. 1984. Am. Rev. Respir. Dis. **129:** 676-681.
9. CEUPPENS, J. L., L. M. LACQUET, G. MARIEN, M. DEMEDTS, A. VAN DEN EECKHOUT & E. STEVENS. 1984. Am. Rev. Respir. Dis. **129:** 563-568.
10. THOMAS, J., L. ROGOZINSKI, O. H. IRIGOYEN, H. H. SHEN, M. A. TALLE, G. GOLDSTEIN & L. CHESS. 1982. J. Immunol. **128:** 1386-1390.
11. GATENBY, P. A., G. S. KANSAS, Y. C. XIAN, R. L. EVANS & E. G. ENGLEMAN. 1982. J. Immunol. **129:** 1997-2000.
12. CORTE, G., M. C. MINGARI, A. MORETTA, G. DAMIANI, L. MORETTA & A. BARGELLESI. 1982. J. Immunol. **128:** 16-19.
13. SEMENZATO, G., A. PEZZUTTO, C. AGOSTINI, G. GASPAROTTO & A. CIPRIANI. 1981. Clin. Immunol. Immunopathol. **19:** 416-427.
14. REINHERZ, E. L. & S. F. SCHLOSSMAN. 1980. N. Engl. J. Med. **303:** 370-373.
15. BEVERLEY, P. C. L. & R. E. CALLARD. 1981. Eur. J. Immunol. **11:** 329-334.
16. LEDBETTER, J. A., R. L. EVANS, M. LIPINSKI, C. CUNNINGHAM-RUNDLES, R. A. GOOD & L. A. HERZENBERG. 1981. J. Exp. Med. **153:** 310-323.
17. UCHIYAMA, T., S. BRODER & T. A. WALDMANN. 1981. J. Immunol. **126:** 1393-1397.
18. LEONARD, W. J., J. M. DEPPER, T. UCHIYAMA, K. A. SMITH, T. A. WALDMANN & W. C. GREENE. 1982. Nature **300:** 267-269.
19. TSUDO, M., T. UCHIYAMA & H. UCHINO. 1984. J. Exp. Med. **160:** 612-617.
20. ROBB, R. J. & W. C. GREENE. 1983. J. Exp. Med. **158:** 1332-1337.

21. Bettens, F., F. Kristensen, C. Walker, U. Schwulera, G. D. Bonnard & A. L. De Weck. 1984. J. Immunol. **132:** 261-265.
22. Reinherz, E. L., P. C. Kung, G. Goldstein, R. H. Levey & S. F. Schlossman. 1980. Proc. Natl. Acad. Sci. USA **77:** 1588-1592.
23. Sutherland, R., D. Delia, C. Schneider, R. Newman, J. Kemshead & M. Greaves. 1981. Proc. Natl. Acad. Sci. USA **78:** 4515-4519.
24. Goding, J. W. & G. F. Burns. 1981. J. Immunol. **127:** 1256-1258.
25. Neckers, L. M. & J. Cossman. 1983. Proc. Natl. Acad. Sci. USA **80:** 3494-3498.
26. Timonen, T., J. R. Ortaldo & R. B. Herberman. 1981. J. Exp. Med. **153:** 569-582.
27. Abo, T. & C. M. Balch. 1981. J. Immunol. **127:** 1024-1029.
28. Lanier, L. L., A. My Le, J. H. Phillips, N. L. Warner & G. F. Babcock. 1983. J. Immunol. **131:** 1789-1796.
29. Rumpold, H. D., D. Kraft, G. Obexer, G. Bock & W. Gebhart. 1982. J. Immunol. **129:** 1458-1463.
30. Perussia, B., S. Starr, S. Abraham, V. Fanning & G. Trinchieri. 1983. J. Immunol. **130:** 2133-2141.
31. Malavasi, F., G. Bellone, L. Matera, C. Milanese, E. Ferrero, A. Funaro, S. DeMaria, F. Caligaris-Cappio, G. Camussi & P. Dellabona. 1985. Hum. Immunol. **14:** 87-102.
32. Knowles II, D. M., L. D. Dodson, R. Raab, R. S. Mittler, M. A. Talle & G. Goldstein. 1983. Diagn. Immunol. **1:** 142-149.
33. Meeker, T. C., R. Miller, M. Link, J. Bindl, R. Warnke & R. Levy. 1984. Submitted for publication.
34. Abramson, C. S., J. H. Kersey & T. W. Le Bien. 1981. J. Immunol. **126:** 83-88.
35. Gillis, S., M. W. Ferm, W. Ou & K. A. Smith. 1978. J. Immunol. **120:** 2027-2032.
36. Semenzato, G., A. Cipriani, M. Colombatti, G. Amadori, G. Gasparotto & M. Serembe. 1980. *In* Sarcoidosis. W. Jones Williams & B. H. Davies, Eds.: 466-471. Alpha Omega. Cardiff.
37. Bonnard, G. D., K. Yasaka & R. D. Maca. 1980. Cell. Immunol. **51:** 390-401.
38. Semenzato, G., G. Amadori, I. Piazza, A. Pezzutto, M. Colombatti & G. Gasparotto. 1979. Transplant. Proc. **11:** 1373-1374.
39. Chilosi, M., F. Bonetti & A. Iannucci. 1981. Am. J. Clin. Pathol. **75:** 638.
40. Chilosi, M., G. Pizzolo, L. Fiore-Donati, M. Bofill & G. Janossy. 1983. Br. J. Cancer. **48:** 763-775.
41. Thomas, Y., L. Rogozinski, O. H. Irigoyen, S. M. Friedman, P. C. Kung, G. Goldstein & L. Chess. 1981. J. Exp. Med. **154:** 459-467.
42. Moretta, L., M. C. Mingari, P. R. Sekaly, A. Moretta, B. Chapuis & J. C. Cerottini. 1981. J. Exp. Med. **154:** 569-574.
43. Lawrence, E. C., B. J. Theodore, R. B. Teague & M. S. Gottlieb. 1982. Clin. Exp. Immunol. **49:** 96-104.
44. Glazier, A. J., M. Monick & G. W. Hunninghake. 1984. Clin. Res. **32:** 347A.
45. Semenzato, G., A. Pezzutto, A. Cipriani, C. Agostini, M. Colombatti, E. Mari, R. Raimondi & G. Gasparotto. 1983. *In* Sarcoidosis. J. Chrétien, J. Marsac & J. C. Saltiel, Eds.: 156-161. Pergamon Press. Paris.
46. Rossi, G. A., O. Sacco, E. Cosulich, G. Damiani, G. Corte, A. Bargellesi & C. Ravazzoni. 1984. Thorax **39:** 143-149.
47. Pinkston, P., P. B. Bitterman & R. G. Crystal. 1983. N. Engl. J. Med. **308:** 793-800.
48. Hunninghake, G. W., G. N. Bedell, D. C. Zavala, M. Monick & M. Brady. 1983. Am. Rev. Respir. Dis. **128:** 634-638.
49. Semenzato, G., C. Agostini, L. Trentin, R. Zambello, M. Chilosi, A. Cipriani, E. Ossi, M. R. Angi, L. Morittu & G. Pizzolo. 1984. Clin. Exp. Immunol. **57:** 331-337.
50. Parker, D. C. 1982. J. Immunol. **129:** 469-474.
51. James, D. G., E. Neville & A. Walker. 1975. Am. J. Med. **59:** 388-394.
52. Hunninghake, G. W. & R. G. Crystal. 1981. J. Clin. Invest. **67:** 86-92.
53. Agostini, C., G. Semenzato, R. Zambello, L. Trentin, A. Cipriani, A. Tommasini, M. Benetollo & G. Gasparotto. 1985. Boll. Ist. Sieroter. Milan **64:** 226-231.

54. CARRINGTON, C. B., E. A. GAENSLER, J. P. MIKUS, A. W. SCHACHTER, G. W. BURKE & A. M. GOFF. 1976. Ann. N. Y. Acad. Sci. **278:** 265-283.
55. ROSEN, Y., T. J. ATHANASSIADES, S. MOON & H. A. LYONS. 1978. Clin. Invest. **74:** 122-125.
56. CHENSUE, S. W., S. R. WELLHAUSEN & D. L. BOROS. 1981. J. Immunol. **127:** 363-367.
57. LAUGER, T. A., J. S. SMOLEN, T. M. CHUSED, A. D. STEINBERG & J. J. OPPENHEIM. 1982. J. Clin. Invest. **70:** 470-473.
58. KASAHARA, T., J. J. HOOKS, S. F. DOUGHERTY & J. J. OPPENHEIM. 1983. J. Immunol. **130:** 1784-1789.
59. LEATHERMAN, J. W., A. F. MICHAEL, B. A. SCHWARTZ & J. R. HOIDAL. 1984. Ann. Intern. Med. **100:** 390-392.
60. COSTABEL, U., K. J. BROSS, J. MARXEN & H. MATTHYS. 1984. Chest. **85:** 514-518.
61. AGOSTINI, C., L. TRENTIN, R. ZAMBELLO, G. MARCER, L. SIMIONI, A. CIPRIANI, A. TOMMASINI, E. OSSI, M. CHILOSI, G. PIZZOLO & G. SEMENZATO. 1984. Immunol. Clin. Sper. **3:** 283-293.
62. REYES, C. N., F. J. WENZEL, B. R. LAWTON & D. A. EMANUEL. 1982. Chest. **81:** 142-146.
63. ANGI, M. R., P. GERHARDINGER, P. CAPELLI & G. SEMENZATO. 1986. Submitted for publication.
64. MEUER, S. C., S. F. SCHLOSSMAN & E. L. REINHERZ. 1982. Proc. Natl. Acad. Sci. USA **79:** 4395-4399.
65. MISHRA, B. B., L. W. POULTER, G. JANOSSY & D. JAMES. 1983. Clin. Exp. Immunol. **54:** 705-715.
66. RAZMA, A. G., P. LYNCH III, B. S. WILSON, P. A. WARD & S. L. KUNKEL. 1984. Am. Rev. Respir. Dis. **129:** 419-424.
67. SEMENZATO, G., A. CIPRIANI, C. AGOSTINI, L. TRENTIN, R. ZAMBELLO, M. CHILOSI, G. PIZZOLO, E. OSSI & G. GASPAROTTO. 1984. International Conference on Bronchoalveolar Lavage. Columbia, MD.
68. GONWA, T. A., L. J. PICKER, H. V. RAFF, S. M. GOYERT, J. SILVER & J. D. STOBO. 1983. J. Immunol. **130:** 706-711.
69. LIU, M. C., D. PROUD, R. P. SCHLEIMER & M. PLAUT. 1984. J. Immunol. **132:** 2895-2903.
70. TOEWS, G. B., W. C. VIAL, M. M. DUNN, P. GUZETTA, G. NUNEZ, P. STASTNY & M. F. LIPSCOMB. 1984. J. Immunol. **132:** 181-186.
71. VENET, A. R., G. W. HUNNINGHAKE, J. CHRETIEN & R. G. CRYSTAL. 1981. Bull. Eur. Physiopathol. Respir. **17:** 32.
72. TOEWS, G. B., V. LEM, G. NUNEZ, T. BALL, P. STASTNY & M. F. LIPSCOMB. 1984. International Conference on Bronchoalveolar Lavage. Columbia, MD.
73. NUGENT, K., M. MONIK & G. W. HUNNINGHAKE. 1984. Clin. Res. **32:** 434A.
74. BORASCHI, D., S. CENSINI & A. TAGLIABUE. 1984. J. Immunol. **133:** 764-768.
75. BECKER, S. 1984. J. Immunol. **132:** 1249-1254.
76. VODINELICH, L., R. SUTHERLAND, C. SCHNEIDER, R. NEWMAN & M. GREAVES. 1983. Proc. Natl. Acad. Sci. USA **80:** 835-839.
77. LANIER, L. L., E. G. ENGLEMAN, P. GATENBY, G. F. BABCOCK, N. L. WARNER & L. A. HERZENBERG. 1983. Immunol. Rev. **74:** 143-160.

Antigen Presentation by Alveolar Macrophages in Patients with Sarcoidosis[a]

GALEN B. TOEWS,[b] VINCENT M. LEM,[b]
JONATHAN C. WEISSLER,[b] GABRIEL NUNEZ-OLLERO,[b]
EDWARD J. BALL,[b] PETER STASTNY,[b]
AND MARY F. LIPSCOMB[c]

[b]*Department of Internal Medicine*
and
[c]*Department of Pathology*
University of Texas Health Science Center at Dallas
Southwestern Medical School
Dallas, Texas 75235

INTRODUCTION

Pulmonary sarcoidosis is characterized by the presence of noncaseating granulomas in the pulmonary parenchyma and by the presence of increased numbers of alveolar macrophages (AM) and activated thymus-derived (T) lymphocytes.[1–8] Activated T lymphocytes are believed to be important in the formation of sarcoid granulomas. Bronchoalveolar lymphocytes obtained from sarcoid patients secrete the lymphokines interleukin-2,[9–11] monocyte chemotactic factor, and migration inhibition factor.[6] Interleukin-2 is probably involved in the previously observed spontaneous *in vitro* proliferation of isolated pulmonary T cells, and the latter two lymphokines may attract and immobilize peripheral blood monocytes (Mo) in the lung. It has been postulated that the recruited mononuclear phagocytes form granulomas[6] and stimulate fibroblast proliferation.[11,12]

The mechanisms of T cell recruitment and activation in sarcoidosis are unknown. Macrophages or other antigen-presenting cells are required to initiate lymphocyte responses to antigens.[13–16] AM might serve as antigen-presenting cells and initiate the alveolitis of sarcoidosis by presenting some as yet undefined antigen to local and recruited lymphocytes. It has been shown previously, however, that AM from normal individuals fail to function as antigen-presenting cells.[17–19] Thus, it was important to determine whether AM from patients with sarcoidosis could present antigen.

[a]This research was supported by Grants HL29543, 23870, and AI21278 from the National Institutes of Health. The facilities at the General Clinical Research Center were supported by Grant MO1RR00633 from the National Institutes of Health.

In these studies, the antigen-presenting capacity of bronchoalveolar cells (BAC) from sarcoid patients and normal volunteers were compared. Additionally, the requirement for histocompatibility between antigen-presenting cells and responding T cells was examined using T cell lines.

MATERIALS AND METHODS

Human Volunteers

Two groups of volunteers were studied. The first group consisted of three men and four women (age range: 27-53 years) with sarcoidosis whose conditions were being followed in the pulmonary clinics at Parkland Memorial Hospital and the Dallas Veterans Administration Medical Center. Each patient was required to fulfill the following criteria before being included in the study: 1) a lung or skin biopsy revealing noncaseating epithelioid granulomas; 2) the absence of mycobacterial, fungal, parasitic, or bacterial infection; 3) no known history of exposure to materials known to cause granulomatous disease; and 4) a chest roentgenogram demonstrating bilateral hilar enlargement and/or diffuse interstitial infiltrates.

The second group served as the control population. Seven young, healthy, nonsmoking normal individuals (age range: 20-35 years) were studied. The results of a chest roentgenogram, physical examination, and complete blood count were within normal limits in all normal volunteers. No normal volunteers had a history of viral illness in the preceding two weeks or a past history of lung disease.

Cell Preparation

Bronchoalveolar Cells

Bronchoalveolar lavage was performed utilizing a fiberoptic bronchoscope as previously described.[18] BAC were passed through gauze to remove particulate matter and excess mucus before being centrifuged. Cells were resuspended in complete medium, that is, RPMI 1640 with 25 mM HEPES, 2 mM glutamine, 100 U/ml penicillin, and 100 μg/ml streptomycin (Grand Island Biological, Grand Island, NY), with 20% heat-inactivated pooled human serum (PHS). The population of BAC from sarcoid patients consisted of 72% (range: 48-88%) AM and 26% (range: 12-52%) lymphocytes. The BAC population from normal volunteers consisted of 90% (range: 78-97%) AM and 8% (range: 3-22%) lymphocytes.

In some experiments, AM were purified from BAC by allowing BAC to adhere to plastic culture dishes and removing nonadherent cells by washing. Adherent cells were washed in cold phosphate-buffered saline (PBS), incubated for 30 min at 4° C, and removed from the dishes by gentle scraping with a rubber policeman. The procedure increased the numbers of cells morphologically compatible with AM to greater than 95%.

Peripheral Blood Cells

Autologous venous blood (120 ml) was obtained from sarcoid patients and normal volunteers. Peripheral blood mononuclear cells were separated on a Ficoll-Hypaque gradient[20] and washed. These cells were separated by adherence for 1 hr on plastic culture dishes into a nonadherent population of peripheral blood lymphocytes and an adherent monocyte population. Peripheral blood lymphocytes were collected by washing the plastic culture dishes. Purified T lymphocytes were obtained by binding the peripheral blood lymphocytes to 2-aminoethylisothiouronium bromide-treated sheep red blood cells[21] at 4° C; the resulting rosettes underwent sedimentation through a Ficoll-Hypaque gradient. The sheep red blood cells were lysed with 0.15 M NH_4Cl, and the lymphocytes were passed through a nylon-wool column to remove residual bone marrow-derived (B) cells and monocytes. The purified T cells were resuspended in complete medium with 20% PHS.

HLA-DR Typing

HLA-DR typing was performed with B lymphocytes obtained from peripheral blood by adherence to nylon wool. The cells were typed for all the HLA nomenclature committee-designated HLA-DR specificities including DRw52 and DRw53; the HLA-DQw1-3 antigens were typed using the NIH microcytotoxicity method with prolonged incubation.[22]

T Cell Proliferation Assays

Autologous T Cells

Cultures were performed in triplicate in flat-bottomed microtiter plates in 200 μl of complete media and 20% PHS. Purified T cells (10^5) were cultured alone and with various numbers of Mo and BAC, both with and without soluble antigen. Soluble antigen was added to separate cultures of T cells alone to assure the completeness of accessory cell depletion. Purified diphtheria toxoid or tetanus toxoid (Biologic Laboratories, Beverly, MA) diluted 1:10 in RPMI 1640 were added to cultures in 10-μl volumes. Cultures were incubated for six days at 37° C in 5% CO_2. Then, 18 hr before termination of cultures, 0.5 μCi of [^{3}H]thymidine ([^{3}H]TdR) was added to the cultures. Cultures were collected with an automated cell harvester and placed in a scintillation counter where [^{3}H]TdR was counted. Data were expressed as the difference in counts per minute (Δcpm) between experimental and control samples.

T Cell Lines

T cell lines that proliferate in response to specific antigen in conjunction with appropriate HLA-DR-matched antigen-presenting cells were prepared as previously described.[23] BAC and Mo from sarcoid patients and normal volunteers were cultured with HLA-DR-matched and -mismatched T cell lines (2×10^4). Culture conditions were exactly as described above except that cultures were incubated for 72 hr at 37° C in 5% CO_2.

RESULTS

Bronchoalveolar Cells from Sarcoid Patients as Accessory Cells in Antigen-induced T Cell Proliferation

BAC from normal volunteers are poor accessory cells for the induction of antigen-dependent T cell proliferation.[18] It was important to determine if, in contrast, BAC

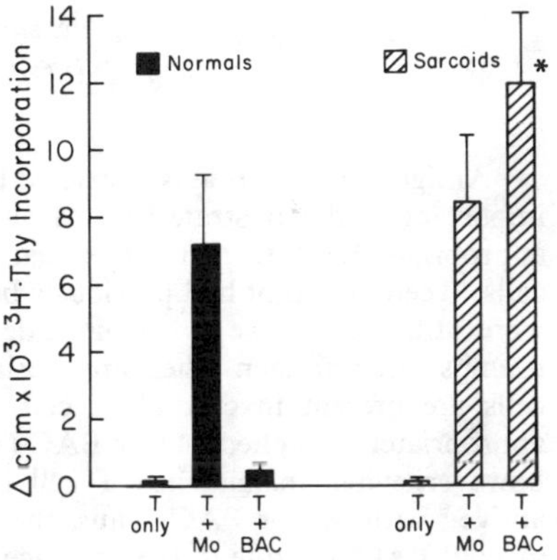

FIGURE 1. The effect of Mo and BAC from normal volunteers and sarcoid patients on antigen-induced proliferation of autologous T cells. Either no accessory cells or 2.5×10^4 irradiated Mo or BAC were added to 1×10^5 T cells per well, both with and without diphtheria toxoid. [^{3}H]TdR incorporation was assayed after six days, and Δcpm was calculated. The results are shown as means ± SEM. Values for [^{3}H]TdR incorporation in cultures without antigen utilizing accessory cells from normal volunteers were 98 ± 15 for T cells alone, 142 ± 20 for T cells and monocytes, and 172 ± 14 for T cells and BAC. [^{3}H]TdR incorporation in cultures without antigen utilizing accessory cells from sarcoid patients were 102 ± 15 for T cells only, 132 for T cells and monocytes, and 189 ± 30 for T cells and BAC. Seven normal volunteers and seven sarcoid patients were studied. *$p < .05$ compared to normal T cells + BAC.

from sarcoid patients could serve as accessory cells in facilitating antigen stimulation of T cells. As is shown in FIGURE 1, T cells depleted of Mo fail to respond to specific antigen. In normal volunteers, Mo were effective in reconstituting a proliferative response, but BAC were not. In contrast, T cell proliferation could be reconstituted with both Mo and BAC from sarcoid patients. Thus, sarcoid BAC, unlike normal BAC, are effective accessory cells for antigen-induced T cell proliferation. The data shown were obtained with diphtheria toxoid as the antigen. Comparable data were obtained using tetanus toxoid (data not shown).

In order to determine which cell population in the sarcoid BAC was responsible for the observed accessory cell function, AM were separated from BAC by adhesion on plastic dishes, and the effects of BAC and AM on antigen-induced T cell proliferation were compared (FIG. 2). T cell proliferation with AM was not statistically different from that obtained with BAC. Thus, the accessory cell function of sarcoid BAC was at least partially due to an adherent cell population, most likely one of AM.

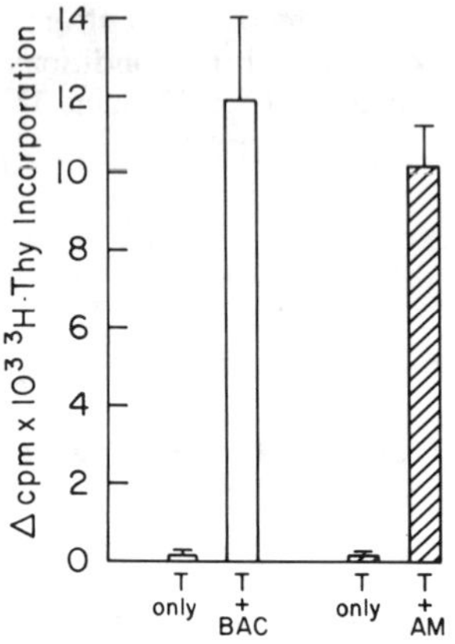

FIGURE 2. A comparison of BAC with AM on antigen-induced T cell proliferation in sarcoid patients. In each experiment, either no accessory cells or 2.5×10^4 irradiated BAC or AM purified by adherence on plastic were added to 1×10^5 T cells per well, both with and without diphtheria toxoid. [^{3}H]TdR incorporation was assayed after six days, and Δcpm was calculated. The results are shown as means ± SEM. Values for [^{3}H]TdR incorporation in cultures without antigen were 101 ± 12 for T cells alone, 153 ± 30 for T cells and BAC, and 139 ± 16 for T cells and AM. BAC and AM from seven sarcoid patients were studied. There was no significant difference in the reconstitution of T cell responses by AM and BAC.

Dependency of Antigen-dependent Proliferation on Histocompatibility between BAC and T Cells

Antigen presentation is restricted by HLA-D region determinants.[24,25] Thus, it was important to demonstrate that Mo and BAC from sarcoid patients could stimulate appropriate HLA-D region-matched T cells but not HLA-D region-mismatched T cells. T cell lines that had previously been shown to lack responsiveness to alloantigens were utilized.[23] These T cell lines demonstrate significant proliferative responses to mumps virus antigen when appropriate HLA-D region-matched antigen-presenting cells are present in culture. T cell lines responded to antigen in the presence of appropriately matched Mo or BAC (TABLE 1). No proliferative response was noted, however, when mismatched T cell lines were cultured in the presence of mumps antigen with Mo or BAC. Thus, the T cell response to antigen in the cultures with sarcoid BAC was due to the presence of histocompatible antigen-presenting cells and not due to the release by BAC of nonspecific enhancing factors.

TABLE 1. Effect of Histocompatibility on Antigen-induced T Cell Line Proliferation in Sarcoid Patients

T Cell Lines	*N*	[^{3}H]TdR Incorporation[a] (Δcpm ± SEM) Mo	AM
HLA-D region matched	2	6807 ± 332	4899 ± 156
HLA-D region mismatched	2	89 ± 6	33 ± 10

[a][^{3}H]TdR incorporation after 72 hr.

DISCUSSION

The major finding to emerge from the current studies is that BAC from sarcoid patients are more efficient than BAC from normal volunteers in acting as antigen-presenting cells for T cell proliferative responses. Suggestions that AM might play a role in the pathogenesis of sarcoidosis have been made in the past. AM bear HLA-D region antigens[18,26] which are required for antigen-presenting cells and T cells to interact.[24,25] Recent studies have reported an increase in the number of these antigens on AM obtained from patients with sarcoidosis.[27] Furthermore, in addition to displaying exogenous antigen in combination with HLA-D region antigens, antigen-presenting cells must deliver a second proliferative signal, that is, interleukin-1.[24,28–33] AM from patients with sarcoidosis have recently been reported to secrete interleukin-1.[34]

Our results clearly demonstrate that sarcoid BAC are true antigen-presenting cells rather than nonspecific accessory cells. Sarcoid BAC reconstituted antigen-induced proliferation of T cell lines, cells that are essentially free of monocytes. More importantly, HLA-D region compatibility was required between BAC and T cells for this reconstitution to occur. The enhanced ability of sarcoid BAC to induce a cell-mediated response could have important implications. Our studies suggest that AM may be important in initiating and/or perpetuating the disease process by processing and presenting an exogenous antigen to T lymphocytes within the parenchyma of the lung.

The mechanism for enhanced antigen presentation by BAC in pulmonary sarcoidosis is unknown. Normal AM have been shown to suppress T cell proliferative responses *in vitro.*[17–19,35,36] The observed enhancement may reflect an absence of suppression in patients with sarcoidosis. Alternately, it may reflect an alteration in the differentiation of AM. Finally, the enhancement might be the result of an increase in the number of newly recruited monocytes which have retained their antigen-presenting ability.

Although the etiology of sarcoidosis remains unknown, it is thought that the enhanced antigen presentation by AM may play an important role in the development of the characteristic pulmonary lesions. Antigen-presenting sarcoid alveolar macrophages might mediate the selective accumulation of circulating specific T lymphocytes, trigger secondary lymphoproliferation, and/or induce local production of lymphokines leading to a mononuclear alveolitis and granuloma formation. It is likely that the maintenance of normal lung homeostasis is dependent upon the balance of enhancement and suppressor functions of AM. A dominance of enhancement may result in local cell-mediated injury. The identification of a functionally active antigen-presenting cell within alveolar spaces provides additional evidence that sarcoidosis is an immune-mediated disease.

ACKNOWLEDGMENTS

The authors are indebted to Nadja Hauff and Lezlie Miller for their expert technical assistance and to Janet Maclin for her excellent secretarial help.

REFERENCES

1. SPENCER, H. 1977. Pulmonary diseases of uncertain aetiology. *In* Pathology of the Lung. H. Spencer, Ed.: 761-768. Pergamon Press. New York, NY.
2. MAYOCK, R. L., P. BERTRAND, C. E. MORRISON & J. H. SCOTT. 1963. Manifestations of sarcoidosis: Analysis of 145 patients with a review of 9 series selected from the literature. Am. J. Med. **35:** 67-89.
3. HUNNINGHAKE, G. W. & R. G. CRYSTAL. 1981. Pulmonary sarcoidosis: A disorder mediated by excessive helper T-lymphocyte activity at sites of disease activity. N. Engl. J. Med. **35:** 429-434.
4. HUNNINGHAKE, G. W., J. D. FULMER, R. C. YOUNG, JR., J. E. GADEK & R. G. CRYSTAL. 1979. Localization of the immune response in sarcoidosis. Am. Rev. Respir. Dis. **120:** 49-57.
5. HUNNINGHAKE, G. W. & R. G. CRYSTAL. 1981. Mechanisms of hypergammaglobulinemia in pulmonary sarcoidosis: Site of increased antibody production and the role of T-lymphocytes. J. Clin. Invest. **67:** 86-92.
6. HUNNINGHAKE, G. W., J. E. GADEK, R. E. YOUNG, O. KAWANAMI, V. J. FERRANS & R. G. CRYSTAL. 1980. Maintenance of granuloma formation in pulmonary sarcoidosis by T-lymphocytes within the lung. N. Engl. J. Med. **302:** 594-598.
7. CARRINGTON, C. B., E. A. GAENSLER, J. P. MIKUS, A. W. SCHACHTER, G. W. BURKE & A. M. GOFF. 1976. Structure and function in sarcoidosis. Ann. N.Y. Acad. Sci. **278:** 265-282.
8. SOLER, P. & F. BASSET. 1976. Morphology and distribution of the cells of a sarcoid granuloma: Ultrastructural study of serial sections. Ann. N.Y. Acad. Sci. **278:** 147-160.
9. PINKSTON, P., P. B. BITTERMAN & R. G. CRYSTAL. 1983. Spontaneous release of interleukin-2 by lung T-lymphocytes in active pulmonary sarcoidosis. N. Engl. J. Med. **308:** 793-800.
10. HUNNINGHAKE, G. W., G. W. BEDELL, D. C. ZAVALA, N. MONICH & M. BRADY. 1983. Role of interleukin-2 release by lung T-cells in active pulmonary sarcoidosis. Am. Rev. Respir. Dis. **128:** 634-638.
11. BITTERMAN, P. B., S. I. RENNARD, G. W. HUNNINGHAKE & R. G. CRYSTAL. 1982. Human alveolar macrophage growth factor for fibroblasts: Regulation and partial characterization. J. Clin. Invest. **70:** 806-822.
12. BITTERMAN, P. B., S. ADELBERG & R. G. CRYSTAL. 1983. Mechanisms of pulmonary fibrosis: Spontaneous release of the alveolar macrophage-derived growth factor in the interstitial lung disorders. J. Clin. Invest. **72:** 1801-1813.
13. OPPENHEIM, J. J., B. G. LEVENTHAL & E. M. HERSH. 1968. The transformation of column-purified lymphocytes with nonspecific and specific antigen stimuli. J. Immunol. **101**(2): 262-270.
14. SHORTMAN, K. & J. PALMER. 1971. The requirement for macrophages in the *in vitro* immune response. Cell. Immunol. **2:** 399-410.
15. UNANUE, E. R. 1981. The regulatory role of macrophages in antigenic stimulation. II. Symbiotic relationship between lymphocytes and macrophages. Adv. Immunol. **31:** 1-137.
16. SEEGER, R. C. & J. J. OPPENHEIM. 1970. Synergistic interaction of macrophages and lymphocytes in antigen-induced transformation of lymphocytes. J. Exp. Med. **132:** 44-65.
17. ETTENSOHN, D. B. & N. J. ROBERTS, JR. 1981. Human alveolar macrophage's support of lymphocyte responses to mitogen and antigen. Am. Rev. Respir. Dis. **128:** 516-522.
18. TOEWS, G. B., W. C. VIAL, M. M. DUNN, P. GUZETTA, G. NUNEZ, P. STASTNY & M. F. LIPSCOMB. 1984. The accessory cell function of human alveolar macrophages in specific T-cell proliferation. J. Immunol. **132:** 181-186.
19. YEAGER, H., JR., J. A. SWEENEY, H. B. HERSCOWITZ, I. S. BARSOUM & E. KAGAN. 1982. Modulation of mitogen-induced proliferation of autologous peripheral blood lymphocytes by human alveolar macrophages. Infect. Immun. **38**(1): 260-266.
20. BOYUM, A. 1968. Isolation of mononuclear cells and granulocytes from human blood. Scand. J. Clin. Lab. Invest. Suppl. **21:** 77-89.
21. KAPLAN, M. E. & C. CLARK. 1974. An improved rosetting assay for detection of human T lymphocytes. J. Immunol. Methods **5:** 131-135.

22. DANILOVS, J., G. AYOUB & P. TERASKI. 1980. B lymphocyte isolation by thrombin-nylon wool. *In* Histocompatibility Testing. P. Teraski, Ed.: 287-288. UCLA Tissue Typing Laboratory. Los Angeles, CA.
23. BALL, E. J. & P. STASTNY. 1984. Antigen-specific HLA-restricted human T-cell lines. Immunogenetics **19:** 13-26.
24. HANSEN, G., B. RUBIN, S. SORENSEN & A. SVEJGAARD. 1978. Importance of HLA-D antigens for the cooperation between human monocytes and T lymphocytes. Eur. J. Immunol. **8:** 520-525.
25. BERGHOLTZ, B. & E. THORSBY. 1977. Macrophage-dependent response of immune human T lymphocytes to PPD *in vitro*: Influence of HLA-D histocompatibility. Scand. J. Immunol. **6:** 779-786.
26. MASON, R., J. AUSTYN, F. BRODSKY & S. GORDON. 1982. Monoclonal anti-macrophage antibodies: Human pulmonary macrophages express HLA-DR (Ia-like) antigens in culture. Am. Rev. Respir. Dis. **125:** 586-593.
27. RAZMA, A. G., J. P. LYNCH, B. S. WILSON, P. A. WARD & S. L. KUNKEL. 1984. Expression of Ia-like (DR) antigen on human alveolar macrophages isolated by bronchoalveolar lavage. Am. Rev. Respir. Des. **129**(3): 419-424.
28. GEHA, R. S., M. E. JONSEN, B. H. AULT, E. YUNIS & M. D. BROFF. 1981. Macrophage T cell interaction in man: Binding of antigen-specific human proliferating and helper T cells to antigen-pulsed macrophages. J. Immunol. **126:** 781-786.
29. GERMAIN, R. 1981. Accessory cell stimulation of T cell proliferation requires active antigen processing: Ia-restricted antigen presentation, and a separate nonspecific second signal. J. Immunol. **127:** 1964-1966.
30. MAIZEL, A. L., S. R. MEHTA, R. J. FORD & L. B. LACHMAN. 1981. Effect of interleukin 1 on human thymocytes and purified human T cells. J. Exp. Med. **153:** 470-475.
31. TOGAWA, A., J. J. OPPENHEIM & S. B. MIZEL. 1979. Characterization of lymphocyte-activating factor (LAF) produced by human mononuclear cells: Biochemical relationship of high and low molecular weight forms of LAF. J. Immunol. **122:** 2112-2118.
32. ROSENWASSER, L. J. & A. S. ROSENTHAL. 1978. Adherent cell function in murine T lymphocyte antigen recognition. II. Definition of genetically restricted and nonrestricted macrophage functions in T cell proliferation. J. Immunol. **121:** 2497-2501.
33. CALDERON, J., J. M. KIELY, J. L. LEFKO & E. R. UNANUE. 1975. The modulation of lymphocyte functions by macrophages. I. Description and partial biochemical analysis. J. Exp. Med. **142:** 151-164.
34. HUNNINGHAKE, G. W. 1984. Release of interleukin-1 by alveolar macrophages of patients with active pulmonary sarcoidosis. Am. Rev. Respir. Dis. **129:** 569-572.
35. MCCOMBS, C. C., J. P. MICHALSKI, B. T. WESTERFIELD & R. W. LIGHT. 1982. Human alveolar macrophages suppress the proliferative response of peripheral blood lymphocytes. Chest **82:** 266-271.
36. DE SHAZO, R. D., D. E. BANKS, J. E. DIEM, J. A. NORDBERG, Y. BASER, D. BEVIER & J. E. SALVAGGIO. 1983. Bronchoalveolar lavage cell-lymphocyte interactions in normal non-smokers and smokers. Am. Rev. Respir. Dis. **127:** 545-548.

Role of Alveolar Macrophage- and Lung T Cell-derived Mediators in Pulmonary Sarcoidosis

GARY W. HUNNINGHAKE[a]

Pulmonary Disease Division
Department of Medicine
Veterans Administration Hospital
and
University of Iowa College of Medicine
Iowa City, Iowa 52242

INTRODUCTION

Pulmonary sarcoidosis is a disorder of unknown etiology characterized by the presence of granulomata in the lung.[1–9] Although granulomata are the hallmark of this disease, recent studies have demonstrated that the initial lesion which occurs in the lung is an inflammatory process.[1,10–14] When this inflammatory process occurs in the alveolar structures, it is termed an "alveolitis." This inflammatory process appears to set the stage for granuloma formation; that is, the cells which compose the alveolitis are utilized to form granulomata. The most prominent cells which constitute the alveolitis of pulmonary sarcoidosis are macrophages and thymus-derived (T) lymphocytes. This is not surprising because granulomata are composed, primarily, of macrophages, epithelioid cells, and multinucleated giant cells. Each of these cells is ultimately derived from monocytes/macrophages. In patients with active sarcoidosis, the granulomata are also surrounded by a rim of T lymphocytes. These observations suggest that pulmonary sarcoidosis is mediated by an intense interaction between macrophages and T lymphocytes. We will focus on the role of alveolar macrophage- and lung T cell-derived mediators which modulate the granulomatous process in the lung (TABLES 1 & 2).

INTERLEUKIN-1

Interleukin-1 (IL-1) is a monocyte/macrophage-derived mediator with an approximate molecular mass of 15 000 daltons.[15–17] The factor demonstrates a change heterogeneity with several pI values in the range of 4.5-5.5 and 6.8-7.4. Normal human alveolar macrophages do not spontaneously release this mediator, but they

[a] Address for correspondence: Room E 325-1, GH, University of Iowa Hospitals and Clinics, Iowa City, Iowa 52242.

TABLE 1. Macrophage-derived Mediators

Mediator	Function
Interleukin-1	Initiate lymphocyte activation and/or cell division ↑Fever ↑Prostaglandin synthesis ↑Collagenase (fibroblasts) ↑Synthesis of acute-phase reactants ↑Catabolic rate Growth factor for fibroblasts Chemotactic factor for T cells
Immune interferons	Augment or inhibit lymphocyte activation and/or cell division ↑Fever ↑Prostaglandin synthesis ↑Collagenase (fibroblasts) Induction of antiviral state Macrophage activation Growth factor for fibroblasts

can be stimulated to do so by a variety of agents.[18] Alveolar macrophages isolated from some patients with pulmonary sarcoidosis, however, spontaneously release this mediator *in vitro* without stimulation, presumably because they have been stimulated *in vivo* as a result of the underlying disease process.[18] This release of IL-1 appears to be associated with active disease because alveolar macrophages from patients with active disease spontaneously release large amounts of this mediator; those with relatively inactive disease release only small amounts of IL-1.

IL-1 can have a variety of effects on different organ systems. Fever is frequently present in patients with acute (early) sarcoidosis. Recent studies have shown that IL-1 is identical to leukocyte pyrogen, a factor which is thought to cause fever in immune-mediated disorders.[19,20] IL-1 appears to cause fever by interacting with the hypothalamic thermoregulatory center to increase the thermostatic point by increasing

TABLE 2. T Cell-derived Mediators

Mediator	Function
Monocyte chemotactic factor	Chemotactic activity for and activation of monocytes
Immune interferons	Augment or inhibit lymphocyte activation and/or cell division ↑Fever ↑Prostaglandin synthesis ↑Collagenase (fibroblasts) Induction of antiviral state Macrophage activation Growth factor for fibroblasts
Interleukin-2	Proliferation of activated T cells Chemotactic factor for T cells
B cell-growth factor	Proliferation of B cells
B cell-differentiation factor	Differentiation of B cells

the levels of prostaglandins, especially prostaglandin E_2 (PGE_2).[21,22] This observation is consistent with the clinical observation that antipyretics, which inhibit the production of prostaglandins, reduce fever.

Patients with active sarcoidosis also have increased serum levels of acute-phase reactant proteins such as fibrinogen, haptoglobin, ceruloplasmin, and C-reactive protein. IL-1 appears to be an important regulator of the synthesis of these proteins.[23–26]

An additional characteristic of patients with active sarcoidosis may be muscle weakness and weight loss. IL-1 may mediate these effects via its effects on protein degradation in muscle cells.[27–34] This effect of IL-1 on muscle cells also appears to be mediated by an increased production of prostaglandins, including PGE_2. Both IL-1-induced muscle proteolysis and PGE_2 production by muscle cells are prevented by indomethacin *in vitro*.

Pulmonary sarcoidosis is characterized by heightened cellular immune processes at sites of the disease as well as by a polyclonal hypergammaglobulinemia.[1–4] IL-1 is also associated with a number of important effects on the immune system. One of the predominant immune effects of IL-1 is its effect on T cells.[35–42] IL-1 itself does not function as a growth factor for T cells, but it increases the numbers of IL-2 receptors on T cells and also stimulates T cells to release IL-2. IL-2 subsequently induces a proliferation and a differentiation of these T lymphocytes. This capacity of IL-1 to act as a first signal for T lymphocyte proliferation and activation is a key process in most cellular immune responses.

Although the above observations suggest that IL-1 increases the numbers of T lymphocytes at sites of disease in the lung via its effect on the proliferation of these cells, recent studies have also shown that IL-1 is a potent chemotactic factor for blood T cells.[43] These observations suggest that IL-1 may also increase the number of lung T cells in patients with sarcoidosis by attracting T cells from blood into the lung.

IL-1 also appears to play an important role in immunoglobulin synthesis.[44–49] The proliferation and differentiation of bone marrow-derived (B) lymphocytes appears to be controlled, primarily, by B cell-specific factors.[50–53] IL-1 may be required for the synthesis of these factors by T cells. IL-1 also appears to have a direct effect on B cells to increase antibody production when the concentrations of antigens or mitogens are suboptimal.[48,49]

Patients with sarcoidosis also are characterized by fibrotic response in the lung, especially at sites of granuloma formation. Recent studies by Schmidt *et al.* have demonstrated that IL-1 is a potent growth factor for fibroblasts (cells which produce collagen).[54,55] In addition, other studies have demonstrated that IL-1 can stimulate synovial cells to increase their production of PGE_2 and collagenase.[56–58] These studies suggest that IL-1 may exert significant effects on fibroblasts which are relevant to the fibrotic process in the lung.

IMMUNE INTERFERONS

Immune interferons comprise a family of molecules which exerts nonspecific, antiviral activity in various types of cells.[59] While this antiviral effect was the biological activity originally identified with interferon, it is now known that these molecules also have potent additional effects on various types of cells, including macrophages and T and B lymphocytes.[60–66] Immune interferon can be produced by both lung T lymphocytes and alveolar macrophages following exposure to a variety of stimuli.[67] In marked contrast, alveolar macrophages and lung T cells from patients with active sarcoidosis spontaneously release this mediator *in vitro.*[67]

Alveolar macrophages from patients with sarcoidosis appear to be activated compared to macrophages from normal individuals. One of the most important effects of immune interferon is the activation of macrophages.[60–66] In this regard, macrophages that have been exposed to immune interferon exhibit an increased phagocytic capacity, an increased number of receptors for the crystallizable fragment (Fc) of immunoglobulin G (IgG), and an enhancement of antibody-dependent cellular cytotoxicity. Macrophages that have been exposed to interferon also have an increased tumoricidal capacity. Alveolar macrophages from patients with sarcoidosis resemble macrophages that have been exposed to interferon.

Interferon also has a potent effect on the antigen-presenting capacity of alveolar macrophages.[68–84] For most cellular immune responses in man, monocytes/macrophages and T lymphocytes must physically interact to initiate the immune response. The monocyte/macrophage which interacts with these T cells displays I-associated (Ia) antigens on its cell surface, which is thus Ia^+, and releases IL-1. In man, monocytes/macrophages may express two types of Ia antigens: HLA-DR and HLA-DS. Almost all monocytes/macrophages express HLA-DR antigens, but only a portion of these cells express the HLA-DS cell-surface antigen.[79,80] This is an important observation because only $HLA\text{-}DS^+$ monocytes/macrophages appear to be able to interact with specific T cells to initiate an immune response.[80]

A number of lines of evidence suggest that monocytes/macrophages play a similar role in initiating the immune response in sarcoidosis. In humans, it has been demonstrated that almost all alveolar macrophages, including those from patients with sarcoidosis, are $HLA\text{-}DR^+$ and $HLA\text{-}DS^+$.[81,82] In addition, as was noted above, alveolar macrophages from patients with active pulmonary sarcoidosis spontaneously release IL-1, the other macrophage product essential for the initiation of T lymphocyte activation.[18] Thus, in patients with active sarcoidosis, the macrophages are particularly primed to interact with T cells in order to initiate and maintain the cellular immune response and, thus, granuloma formation. Interferon appears to increase the expression of HLA-DR and HLA-DS antigens on macrophages as well as to enhance their ability to release IL-1.[68–84]

Interferon is also capable of both activating and suppressing B and T cell responses.[85] The activation or suppression of these responses depends upon the dose, timing, and administration of the mediator. These observations demonstrate that interferon may have potent immunoregulatory effects on both humoral and cellular immune processes.

Recent studies by Dinarello *et al.* have also shown that interferon is a pyrogen and can produce fever.[86] In this respect, the molecule appears to mimic the effects of IL-1. Thus, immune interferon may augment the effects of IL-1 to produce fever in patients with sarcoidosis.

Interferon also appears to be a very potent growth factor for human lung fibroblasts.[87,88] It has been shown that growth factors for fibroblasts can be divided into two categories: competence factors and progression factors. Competence factors act early in the G_1 phase of the cell cycle and prime the fibroblast to undergo cell division. Progression factors, on the other hand, act later in the cell cycle and stimulate cells which have already been exposed to a competence factor to undergo cell division. Interferon appears to act as a progression growth factor for human lung fibroblasts. These observations suggest that interferon may also interact with IL-1 to augment the fibrotic process at sites of granuloma formation in the lungs of patients with sarcoidosis.

INTERLEUKIN-2

Several reports have shown that the release of IL-2 by lung T cells is associated with active disease in pulmonary sarcoidosis.[89,90] Although normal lung T cells do not spontaneously release IL-2, various stimuli can induce the release of IL-2 from these cells. The mediator has a molecular mass of approximately 15 000 daltons and appears to function as a direct mitogenic factor for T cell proliferation.[91–96] The capacity of T cells to respond to IL-2 appears to correspond to their acquisition of receptors for this molecule. In addition to T lymphocytes, large granular lymphocytes also may express IL-2 receptors and will proliferate in response to IL-2. Purified IL-2 appears to have little direct effect on antibody production by B cells.

IL-2 also appears to have effects other than those on T cell proliferation.[90–96] In this regard, recent studies have suggested that IL-2 can stimulate subsets of T cells to release immune interferons and can also enhance cytotoxic responses of T cells. This observation suggests that IL-2 not only enhances the proliferation of T cells but also stimulates an activation of various types of T cells.

IL-2 is also a chemotactic factor for blood T cells.[97] This latter observation suggests that IL-1 and IL-2 may act in a synergistic manner to increase the migration of T cells from blood into the lung. Consistent with this hypothesis is the observation that supernatants of unstimulated bronchoalveolar cells from patients with active pulmonary sarcoidosis contain IL-1, IL-2, and substance(s) with chemotactic activity for blood T cells.[98] The IL-1 is released by sarcoid alveolar macrophages, and IL-2 is released by the sarcoid alveolar T cells. The chemotactic activity is due to the presence of IL-1 and IL-2 in the supernatants. Thus, the numbers of T lymphocytes at sites of disease in patients with pulmonary sarcoidosis may be increased by both attracting T cells from the circulation and by stimulating these cells to divide. These observations not only explain the presence of increased numbers of T cells at sites of granuloma formation but may also explain one additional feature of patients with sarcoidosis, that is, the decreased proportion of T cells in peripheral blood. This T cell lymphopenia may result simply from the migration of T cells out of the blood and into the lung.

B CELL FACTORS

Hypergammaglobulinemia is frequently found in patients with sarcoidosis. These immunoglobulins are polyclonal and are directed at multiple antigens. Lung T cells from patients with active sarcoidosis also release various factors which stimulate normal B cells to differentiate into immunoglobulin-secreting cells.[90,99–101] Although the identity of these factors is unknown, it is likely that two of these factors are B cell-growth factor (BCGF) and B cell-differentiation factor (BCDF).[50–53] BCGF functions to mediate B cell proliferation. The cellular source of BCGF has not been definitely proven; however, several lines of evidence suggest that the source of this factor is human T cells. BCGF has a number of biochemical properties that are similar to IL-2, and both factors migrate on gels with a molecular mass of 15 000-20 000 daltons. BCDF functions to stimulate the terminal differentiation of proliferating B cells into immunoglobulin-secreting cells. The cellular source of BCDF, like that of BCGF, is thought to be mature T cells. The molecular mass of this factor also appears to be in the range of 15 000-20 000 daltons.

These observations suggest that immunoglobulin production in pulmonary sarcoidosis may be, in part, a by-product of granuloma formation; that is, lung T cells activated as a result of the process of granuloma formation are releasing mediators, such as BCGF and BCDF, which nonspecifically stimulate the production of immunoglobulin by lung B cells in the vicinity of the developing granuloma. This hypothesis is supported by the following observations in patients with active sarcoidosis: 1) the number of plasma cells is increased at sites of granuloma formation in the lung; 2) immunoglobulin production appears to occur primarily at sites of active disease; 3) purified lung T lymphocytes, but not blood T lymphocytes, from patients with active disease can spontaneously (that is, without added antigens or mitogens) activate normal B cells to differentiate into immunoglobulin-secreting cells; and 4) there is a direct correlation between the numbers of activated T lymphocytes and the numbers of immunoglobulin-secreting cells that are present at sites of disease (that is, in bronchoalveolar lavage fluid).[101]

MONOCYTE CHEMOTACTIC FACTOR

An additional lymphokine which is associated with active disease in pulmonary sarcoidosis is monocyte chemotactic factor.[102,103] Monocyte chemotactic factor is produced by activated T cells and may function to attract monocytes to the lung in sarcoidosis. This is a crucial feature of granuloma formation since granulomata are comprised, primarily, of macrophages, epithelioid cells, and multinucleated giant cells: cells ultimately derived from blood monocytes. In patients with active sarcoidosis, it has been demonstrated that lung T cells release approximately 25 times more monocyte chemotactic factor, on a per cell basis, than do blood T cells from these same patients. This observation, together with the findings that there are increased numbers of T cells in the lung and decreased numbers of T cells in the peripheral blood, suggests that there exists a gradient of monocyte chemotactic factor between lung and blood which attracts monocytes into the lung.

Another potential mechanism to increase the numbers of macrophages in the lung is by the process of *in situ* cell division.[104–110] Although it is possible that lung macrophages are increased somewhat by this method, it is generally felt that the majority of cells which are present in lung granulomata are derived from blood monocytes.

The lung T lymphocyte also releases other lymphokines, such as macrophage migration-inhibitory factor (MIF) and various macrophage-activating factors, which interact with monocytes/macrophages to assist in the formation of the structure we recognize as a granuloma.[4,5]

SUMMARY

The process of granuloma formation in the lung is mediated by an intimate interaction between macrophages and T cells, and this interaction provides the appropriate environment for granuloma formation and the development of fibrosis. Much of this process of granuloma formation and fibrosis appears to be triggered by the release of immune mediators by alveolar macrophages and lung T cells.

REFERENCES

1. Hunninghake, G. W., K. C. Garrett, H. B. Richerson, J. C. Fantone, P. A. Ward, S. I. Rennard, P. B. Bitterman & R. G. Crystal. 1984. Am. Rev. Respir. Dis. 476-496.
2. Hunninghake, G. W., J. E. Gadek, O. Kawanami, V. J. Ferrans & R. G. Crystal. 1979. Am. J. Pathol. **97:** 149-206.
3. Hunninghake, G. W. & J. E. Gadek. Am. J. Pathol. **97:** 149-206.
4. Hunninghake, G. W. & P. L. Moseley. *In* Immunology of Lung Diseases. J. Bienenstock, Ed. In press. McGraw Hill. New York, NY.
5. Hunninghake, G. W., B. A. Keogh, B. R. Line, J. E. Gadek, O. Kawanami, V. J. Ferrans & R. G. Crystal. 1980. *In* Basic and Clinical Aspects of Granulomatous Diseases. D. L. Boros & T. Yoshida, Eds.: 275-290. Elsevier/North-Holland. New York, NY.
6. Crystal, R. G., G. W. Hunninghake, J. E. Gadek, B. A. Keogh, S. I. Rennard & P. B. Bitterman. 1981. *In* Sarcoidosis and Other Granulomatous Disorders. J. Chrétien, J. Marsac & J. C. Saltiel, Eds.: 13-35. Pergamon Press. Paris.
7. Mitchell, D. N. & J. G. Scadding. 1974. Am. Rev. Respir. Dis. **110:** 774-802.
8. Boros, D. L. 1978. Prog. Allergy **24:** 183-267.
9. Carrington, C. B., E. A. Gaensler & J. P. Mikus. 1976. Ann. N.Y. Acad. Sci. **278:** 265-282.
10. Rosen, Y., T. J. Athanassiades, S. Moon & H. A. Lyons. 1978. Chest **74:** 122-125.
11. Teilum, G. 1964. Acta Med. Scand. Suppl. **425:** 14-18.
12. Takahashi, M. 1970. Acta Pathol. **20:** 171-182.
13. Bernaudin, J. F., J. Lacronique, P. Soler, F. Lange, O. Kawanami & F. Basset. 1981. Bull. Eur. Physiopathol. Respir. **17:** 27P.
14. Lacronique, J., J. F. Bernaudin, P. Soler, F. Lange, O. Kawanami, G. Saumon, R. Georges & F. Basset. 1981. *In* Sarcoidosis and Other Granulomatous Disorders. J. Chrétien, J. Marsac & J. C. Saltiel, Eds.: 36-42. Pergamon Press. Paris.
15. Lachman, L. B., S. O. Page & R. S. Metzgar. 1980. Prep. Biochem. **10:** 387-403.
16. Lachman, L. B., S. O. Page & R. S. Metzgar. 1980. J. Supramol. Struct. **13:** 457-466.
17. Oppenheim, J. J., B. M. Stadler & B. Mathieson. 1982. Fed. Proc. **4:** 257-262.
18. Hunninghake, G. W. 1984. Am. Rev. Respir. Dis. **129:** 569-572.
19. Bernheim, H. A., L. H. Block & E. Atkins. 1979. Ann. Intern. Med. **91:** 261-270.
20. Dinarello, C. A. & S. M. Wolff. 1982. Am. J. Med. **72:** 799-819.
21. Bernheim, H. A., T. M. Gilbert & J. T. Stitt. 1980. J. Physiol. **301:** 69-78.
22. Coceani, F., I. Bishai, C. A. Dinarello & F. A. Fitzpatrick. 1983. Am. J. Physiol. **244:** R785-R793.
23. Merriman, C. R., L. A. Pulliam & R. F. Kampschmidt. 1975. Proc. Soc. Exp. Biol. Med. **149:** 782-784.
24. McAdam, K. P. W. J., J. Li, N. T. Foss, C. A. Dinarello, L. J. Rosenwasser, M. J. Selinger, M. M. Kaplan, R. Goodman, P. N. Herbert, L. L. Bausserman & L. M. Nadler. 1982. Ann. N.Y. Acad. Sci. **389:** 126-136.
25. McAdam, K. P. W. J. & C. A. Dinarello. 1980. *In* Bacterial Endotoxins and Host Response. M. D. Agawal, Ed.: 167-178. Elsevier/North-Holland. Amsterdam.
26. Sztein, M. B., S. N. Vogel, J. D. Sipe, P. A. Murphy, S. B. Mizel, J. J. Oppenheim & D. L. Rosenstreich. 1981. Cell. Immunol. **63:** 164-176.
27. Yang, R. D., L. L. Moldawer, A. Sakamoto, R. A. Keenan, D. E. Matthews, V. R. Young, R. W. Wannemacher, Jr., G. L. Blackburn & B. R. Bistrian. 1983. Metabolism **32:** 654-660.
28. Wannemacher, R. W., Jr., R. S. Pekarek, W. L. Thompson, R. T. Curnow, F. A. Beall, T. V. Zenser, F. R. Derubertis & W. R. Beisel. 1975. Endocrinology **96:** 651-661.
29. Powanda, M.C. 1977. Am. J. Clin. Nutr. **30:** 1254-1268.
30. Sobrado, J., L. L. Moldawer, C. A. Dinarello, G. L. Blackburn & B. R. Bistrian. 1983. Fed. Proc. **42:** 669.

31. Goldberg, A. L., V. Baracos, P. Rodemann, L. Waxman & C. A. Dinarello. 1984. Fed. Proc. In press.
32. Rodemann, H. P., L. Waxman & A. L. Goldberg. 1982. J. Biol. Chem. **257:** 8716-8723.
33. Rodemann, H. P. & A. L. Goldberg. 1982. J. Biol. Chem. **257:** 1632-1638.
34. Baracos, V., H. P. Rodemann, C. A. Dinarello & A. L. Goldberg. 1983. N. Engl. J. Med. **308:** 553-558.
35. Mizel, S. B. 1982. Immunol. Rev. **63:** 51-72.
36. Rao, A., S. B. Mizel & H. Cantor. 1983. J. Immunol. **130:** 1743-1748.
37. Irle, C., P. F. Piguet & P. Vassali. 1978. J. Exp. Med. **148:** 32-45.
38. Wagner, H., C. Hardt, R. Bartlett, M. Rollinghoff & K. Pfienmaier. 1980. J. Immunol. **125:** 2532-2538.
39. Kelso, A. & H. R. MacDonald. 1982. J. Exp. Med. **156:** 1366-1379.
40. Farrar, W. L., S. B. Mizel & J. J. Farrar. 1980. J. Immunol. **124:** 1371-1377.
41. Mizel, S. B. & A. Ben-Zvi. 1980. Cell. Immunol. **54:** 382-389.
42. Puri, J., M. Shinitzky & P. Lonai. 1980. J. Immunol. **124:** 1937-1942.
43. Hunninghake, G. W., C. Dinarello & M. Monick. Submitted for publication.
44. Wood, D. D., P. M. Cameron, M. T. Poe & C. A. Morris. 1976. Cell. Immunol. **21:** 88-96.
45. Wood, D. D. & P. M. Cameron. 1976. Cell. Immunol. **21:** 133-145.
46. Wood, D. D. 1979. J. Immunol. **123:** 2395-2399.
47. Wood, D. D. 1979. J. Immunol. **123:** 2400-2407.
48. Falkoff, R. J. M., A. Muraguchi, J-X. Hong, J. L. Butler, C. A. Dinarello & A. S. Fauci. 1983. J. Immunol. **131:** 801-805.
49. Lipsky, P. E., P. A. Thompson, L. J. Rosenwasser & C. A. Dinarello. 1983. J. Immunol. **130:** 2708-2714.
50. Howard, M., J. Farrar, M. Hilfiker, B. Johnson, K. Takatsu, T. Hamaoka & W. E. Paul. 1982. J. Exp. Med. **155:** 914-923.
51. Muraguchi, A., T. Kasahara, J. J. Oppenheim & A. S. Fauci. 1982. J. Immunol. **129:** 2486-2489.
52. Muraguchi, A. & A. S. Fauci. 1982. J. Immunol. **129:** 1104-1108.
53. Okada, M., N. Sakaguchi, N. Yoshimura, H. Hara, K. Shimizu, N. Yoshida, K. Yoshizaki, S. Kishimoto, Y. Yamamura & T. Kishimoto. 1983. J. Exp. Med. **157:** 583-590.
54. Schmidt, J. A., S. B. Mizel, D. Cohen & I. Green. 1982. J. Immunol. **128:** 2177-2182.
55. Schmidt, J. A., C. N. Oliver, J. L. Lepe-Zuninga, I. Green & I. Gery. J. Clin. Invest. **73:** 1462.
56. Krane, S. M., S. R. Goldring & J-M. Dayer. 1982. *In* Lymphokines: A Forum for Immunoregulatory Cell Products. E. Pick & M. Landy, Eds. Vol. **7:** 75-136. Academic Press. New York, NY.
57. Dayer, J-M., S. M. Krane, R. G. G. Russell & D. R. Robinson. 1976. Proc. Natl. Acad. Sci. USA **73:** 945-949.
58. Sauder, D. N., C. S. Carter, S. I. Katz & J. J. Oppenheim. 1982. J. Invest. Dermatol. **79:** 34-39.
59. Isaacs, A. & J. Lindenmann. 1957. Proc. R. Soc. London, Ser. B **147:** 258-267.
60. Huang, K-Y., R. M. Donahoe, F. B. Gordon & H. R. Dressler. 1971. Infect. Immun. **4:** 581-588.
61. Schultz, R. M., J. D. Papamatheakis & M. A. Chirigos. 1977. Science **197:** 674-676.
62. Oehler, J. R., L. R. Lindsay, M. E. Nunn, H. T. Holden & R. B. Herberman. 1978. Int. J. Cancer **21:** 210-220.
63. Schultz, W. W., K-Y. Huang & F. B. Gordon. 1968. Nature (London) **220:** 709-710.
64. Kazar, J., P. A. Krautwurst & F. B. Gordon. 1971. Infect. Immun. **3:** 819-824.
65. Kazar, J., J. D. Gillmore & F. B. Gordon. 1971. Infect. Immun. **3:** 825-832.
66. Gober, L. L., A. E. Friedman-Kien, E. A. Kavell & J. Vilcek, 1972. Infect. Immun. **5:** 370-376.
67. Nugent, K., M. Monick & G. W. Hunninghake. 1984. Clin. Res. **32:** 434A.
68. Steeg, P. S., R. N. Moore, H. M. Johnson & J. J. Oppenheim. 1982. J. Exp. Med. **156:** 1780-1793.

69. Basham, T. Y. & T. C. Merigan. 1983. J. Immunol. **130:** 1492-1494.
70. King, D. P. & P. P. Jones. 1983. J. Immunol. **131:** 315-318.
71. Vogel, S. N., L. L. Weedon, R. N. Moore & D. L. Rosenstreich. 1982. J. Immunol. **128:** 380-387.
72. Vogel, S. N., D. S. Finbloom, K. E. English, D. L. Rosenstreich & S. G. Langreth. 1983. J. Immunol. **130:** 1210-1214.
73. Schultz, R. M., J. D. Papamatheakis & M. A. Chirigos. 1977. Science **197:** 674-676.
74. Bordignon, C., R. Avallone, G. Peri, N. Polentarutti, C. Mangioni & A. Mantovani. 1980. Clin. Exp. Immunol. **41:** 336-342.
75. Shevach, E. M. & A. S. Rosenthal. 1973. J. Exp. Med. **138:** 1213-1229.
76. Unanue, E. R. 1980. N. Engl. J. Med. **303:** 977-985.
77. Rosenthal, A. S. 1980. N. Engl. J. Med. **303:** 1153-1156.
78. Unanue, E. R. 1981. Adv. Exp. Med. Biol. **155:** 49-63.
79. Goyert, S. M., J. E. Shively & J. Silver. 1982. J. Exp. Med. **156:** 550-566.
80. Gonwa, T. A., L. J. Picker, H. V. Raff, S. M. Goyert, J. Silver & J. D. Stobo. 1983. J. Immunol. **130:** 706-711.
81. Mason, R., J. Austyn, F. Brodsky & S. Gordon. 1982. Am. Rev. Respir. Dis. **125:** 586-593.
82. Glazier, A. J., Jr., M. Monick & G. W. Hunninghake. Submitted for publication.
83. Venet, A. R., G. W. Hunninghake & R. G. Crystal. 1982. Am. Rev. Respir. Dis. **125:** 178A.
84. Stadecker, M. J., D. J. Wyler & J. A. Wright. 1982. J. Immunol. **128:** 2739-2744.
85. Sonnenfeld, G. 1980. *In* Lymphokine Reports. E. Pick, Ed. Vol. **1.** Academic Press. New York, NY.
86. Dinarello, C. A., H. A. Bernheim, G. W. Duff, H. V. Le, T. L. Nagabhushan, N. C. Hamilton & F. Coceani. 1984. J. Clin. Invest. **74:** 906-913.
87. Hunninghake, G. W., C. Hemken, M. Brady & M. Monick. Submitted for publication.
88. Hunninghake, G. W., C. Hemken, M. Brady & M. Monick. 1984. Trans. Assoc. Am. Physicians. In press.
89. Pinkston, P., P. B. Bitterman & R. G. Crystal. 1983. N. Engl. J. Med. **308:** 793-800.
90. Hunninghake, G. W., G. H. Bedell, D. C. Zavala, M. Monick & M. Brady. 1983. Am. Rev. Respir. Dis. **128:** 634-638.
91. Gillis, S. & J. Watson. 1980. J. Exp. Med. **152:** 1709-1719.
92. Mier, J. W. & R. C. Gallo. 1980. Proc. Natl. Acad. Sci. USA **77:** 6134-6138.
93. Mier, J. W. & R. C. Gallo. 1982. J. Immunol. **128:** 1122-1127.
94. Smith, K. A. 1980. Immunol. Rev. **51:** 337-357.
95. Farrar, J. J., S. B. Mizel, J. Fuller-Farrar, W. L. Farrar & M. L. Hilfiker. 1980. J. Immunol. **125:** 793-798.
96. Ruscetti, F. W. & R. C. Gallo. 1981. Blood **57:** 379-394.
97. Hunninghake, G. W. & M. Monick. Submitted for publication.
98. Hunninghake, G. W. & M. Monick. 1983. Clin. Res. **31:** 512A.
99. Hunninghake, G. W. & R. G. Crystal. 1981. N. Engl. J. Med. **305:** 429-434.
100. Hunninghake, G. W. & G. N. Bedell. 1984. Semin. Respir. Med. **6:** 31-39.
101. Hunninghake, G. W. & R. G. Crystal. 1981. J. Clin. Invest. **67:** 86-92.
102. Hunninghake, G. W., J. E. Gadek, R. C. Young, O. Kawanami, V. J. Ferrans & R. G. Crystal. 1980. N. Engl. J. Med. **302:** 594-598.
103. Altman, L. C., R. Snyderman, J. J. Oppenheim & S. E. Mergenhagen. 1973. J. Immunol. **110:** 801-810.
104. Volkman, A. & J. L. Gowans. 1965. Br. J. Exp. Pathol. **46:** 62-70.
105. van Furth, R. 1970. Semin. Hematol. **7:** 125-141.
106. Mariano, M. & W. G. Spector. 1974. J. Pathol. **113:** 1-19.
107. Spector, W. G. 1976. Ann. N.Y. Acad. Sci. **278:** 3-6.
108. Turk, J. L. & R. B. Narayanan. 1982. Immunobiology **161:** 274-282.
109. Hadden, J. W., J. R. Sadlik & E. M. Hadden. 1975. Nature (London) **257:** 483-485.
110. Hadden, J. W., J. R. Sadlik & E. M. Hadden. 1978. J. Immunol. **121:** 231-238.

Interleukin-1 Production by Blood Monocytes and Bronchoalveolar Cells in Sarcoidosis

MARY ELLEN KLEINHENZ,[a] HIROSHI FUJIWARA,[b] AND ELIZABETH A. RICH[c]

Department of Medicine
Case Western Reserve University
Cleveland, Ohio 44106

INTRODUCTION

Hypersensitivity to antigen is a cell-mediated immune response that is readily assessed *in vivo* by skin testing and *in vitro* by observing lymphocyte blastogenesis. In sarcoidosis depressed antigen reactivity is frequently observed both in *in vivo*[1] and *in vitro*[2] studies and contrasts with local activation of cellular immune responses in the lung, skin, and other organs as evidenced by lymphocytic infiltration and granuloma formation.[3] The immune mechanisms underlying systemic anergy in sarcoidosis are poorly understood. Immunosuppressive serum factors have been demonstrated in some sarcoidosis patients,[4] and excessive production of immunosuppressive cyclooxygenase products of arachidonic acid by blood monocytes has been reported.[5] Although these observations suggest that anergy in sarcoidosis is caused by suppressor factors, alterations in antigen-responding thymus-derived (T) cells or mononuclear phagocyte immune accessory function may have contributory effects. A deficiency of circulating T lymphocytes has been reported by some investigators,[6] and recent studies demonstrating a reciprocal distribution of the T helper-inducer subpopulation in the lung and peripheral blood suggests that T helper-inducer cells may be selectively recruited from the circulation.[7] Mononuclear phagocytes have a pivotal role in the induction of the immune response to antigen, and production of the growth factor interleukin-1 (IL-1) is critical to the ability of monocytes/macrophages to function as immune accessory cells.[8] The objective of this study of sarcoidosis was to examine IL-1 production by blood monocytes and alveolar macrophages in order to determine if a deficiency in the production of this growth factor could contribute to the depression of antigen responses.

[a] A recipient of Clinical Investigator Award HL00907 from the National Heart, Lung, and Blood Institute.

[b] A Rockefeller Foundation Fellow.

[c] A recipient of a training fellowship from the American Lung Association.

MATERIALS AND METHODS

Study Population

Samples of venous blood and bronchoalveolar fluid were obtained from nine patients with histologically proven sarcoidosis; there were three males and six females. Each patient was untreated at the time of study. The mean age (± SD) of the patients was 38 ± 11 years. The mean duration (± SD) of symptoms prior to the study was 5 ± 3 months. Five patients had radiographic stage II sarcoidosis; the remaining patients had radiographic stage III sarcoidosis. Studies of blood monocytes were performed on samples from nine age- and sex-matched healthy volunteers and on bronchoalveolar lavage from three healthy subjects. Informed consent was obtained from each subject prior to his/her participation in this study.

Bronchoalveolar Lavage

Bronchoalveolar lavage was accomplished through a fiberoptic bronchoscope wedged in a segmental or subsegmental bronchus of the right middle lobe or lingula. Sterile 0.9% saline solution was instilled in 20-ml aliquots and recovered by gentle aspiration. A total of 150 ml of saline solution was instilled in each lavage, and only specimens having a return exceeding 50% were analyzed. Specimens of bronchoalveolar lavage fluid were filtered through sterile gauze to remove respiratory mucus prior to *in vitro* analysis.

Preparation of Mononuclear Cell Populations

The peripheral blood mononuclear cell (PBMC) fraction was separated from whole blood by Ficoll-Hypaque sedimentation.[9] Peripheral blood monocytes were recovered as a monolayer of cells that adhered to plastic petri dishes after a 60-min incubation at 37° C; these monocytes were removed by gentle scraping.[10] More than 90% of these plastic-adherent cells were identifiable as monocytes by peroxidase cytochemistry.[11] Bronchoalveolar mononuclear cells (BAMC) were recovered from the bronchoalveolar lavage fluid by centrifugation. The fractions of mononuclear cells and granulocytes were estimated from Wright-Giemsa-stained cytocentrifuge preparations. T cells among the BAMC were identified by their ability to form E-rosettes, and a procedure that involved the staining of cytocentrifuge preparations with nonspecific esterase[12] was used to identify alveolar macrophages. Only 44 ± 11% of the BAMC obtained from the sarcoid patients were E-rosette-forming T cells; 50 ± 16% were esterase-staining alveolar macrophages; and 8 ± 4% were granulocytes. In some experiments BAMC were depleted of T cells by preparative E-rosette formation. The resultant, T cell-depleted fractions were analyzed by esterase criteria and tested for more rosette-forming T cells; 91 ± 4% and 4 ± 3% of these cells were found to be alveolar macrophages and rosette-forming T cells, respectively.

Generation of IL-1 Supernatants

Monocytes or BAMC were suspended at 0.5-1.0 × 10^6 cells/ml in RPMI-1640 tissue culture medium (Bioproducts, Walkersville, MD) fortified with pooled human serum (2%, v:v) and antibiotics. Then, 1-ml aliquots were distributed in 16-mm Linbro plate wells (Falcon, Oxnard, CA). Cells were cultured alone or with *Escherichia coli* lipopolysaccharide (LPS) (Difco, Detroit, MI) at 10 μg/ml. Supernatants of cell cultures were collected after a 24-hr incubation at 37° C in 5% CO_2; filtered through 0.22-micron millipore membranes; and stored at −20° C until assayed for IL-1 activity.

IL-1 Assay

The IL-1 activity of culture supernatants was determined in a direct mitogenic assay.[13] Thymocytes were prepared from 8-10-week-old female C3H/HeJ mice (Jackson Labs, Bar Harbor, ME) and cultured at 7.5 × 10^6 cells/ml. An IL-1 standard and the experimental IL-1 supernatants were diluted serially in RPMI supplemented with antibiotics, glutamine, 5 × 10^{-5} M mercaptoethanol, and fetal calf serum. Aliquots of supernatants were added to thymocytes with triplicate wells set for each variable. The thymocytes were cultured at 37° C in 5% CO_2 for 3 days with 1.0 μCi of [^{3}H]methylthymidine (Amersham, Arlington Heights, IL) added 6 hr prior to termination of cell culture. The cultures were harvested onto filter-paper discs and the ^{3}H assayed by liquid scintillation spectrophotometry. The IL-1 activity was calculated by modified probit analysis and expressed in units/ml.[14]

Statistical Analysis

The significance of the results was determined by Student's *t* test.

RESULTS

Supernatants of blood monocytes or BAMC cultured alone or with LPS 10 μg/ml were collected after 24 hr and assayed for IL-1 activity in a direct mitogenesis assay. In our laboratory this direct assay of IL-1-induced mitogenesis is as sensitive to low concentrations of IL-1 as the comitogenic assay (TABLE 1) and is highly reproducible.

The IL-1 activities present in supernatants of monocyte cultures and BAMC cultures from control subjects are compared to those from sarcoid patients in TABLE 2. No significant IL-1 activity was detected in the supernatants of cultures of unstimulated monocytes or BAMC from either study population. The addition of 10 μg of LPS to cell cultures stimulated significant IL-1 production by blood monocytes ($p <$ .01) and BAMC ($p < .05$) from the control subjects. LPS induced significant IL-1

TABLE 1. Comparison of IL-1 Activity in Direct and Comitogenic Assays

Source of IL-1 Supernatant	Assay of IL-1 (units/ml) Direct	Comitogenic
Monocytes	< 1.6	2.0
Monocytes + LPS	61.2	60.1

production by blood monocytes from sarcoid patients ($p < .01$); however, BAMC (obtained from only three of nine sarcoid patients) produced significant IL-1 activity (12-28 units/ml) when stimulated by LPS. The mean IL-1 activity detected in supernatants of LPS-stimulated BAMC from the patients was not different from the IL-1 activity present in supernatants of unstimulated BAMC and was consistently and significantly less than the IL-1 activity produced by LPS-stimulated blood monocytes from the same patients ($p < .05$).

To understand this unanticipated finding, additional experiments were performed. First, IL-1 production by E-rosette-depleted BAMC was examined to assess whether the increased numbers of T cells present in the BAMC of sarcoid patients influenced IL-1 production. IL-1 production by unseparated and E-rosette-depleted BAMC from four patients is compared in TABLE 3. In these experiments, IL-1 activity detected in supernatants of unstimulated or LPS-stimulated E-rosette-depleted BAMC was not different from that present in supernatants of unseparated BAMC.

To examine the possibility that an inhibitor of IL-1 might be present in the supernatants of the BAMC from sarcoid patients, the effect of these supernatants on mouse thymocyte response to a standard preparation of IL-1 was assayed. In these experiments mouse thymocytes were incubated with the BAMC supernatants in the presence of tissue culture medium (control) or a 1:16 dilution of IL-1 standard. The results of these experiments, determinations of the extent of [^{3}H]thymidine ([^{3}H]TdR) incorporation, are expressed in counts per minute (CPM). Supernatants from seven sarcoid patients were assayed at a 1:2 dilution to determine the extent of the inhibition of the IL-1 responses (TABLE 4). [^{3}H]TdR incorporation by thymocytes cultured with supernatants of unstimulated BAMC was not different from that seen with controls; in a co-culture, however, the supernatants of unstimulated BAMC reduced the response to IL-1 standard from 30 864 ± 2403 to 17 370 ± 4009 CPM. A culture with the supernatants of LPS-stimulated BAMC increased the [^{3}H]TdR incorporation of thymocytes to a mean of 9040 ± 3375 CPM; this level of [^{3}H]TdR incorporation reflects

TABLE 2. IL-1 Activity of Monocytes and BAMC from Control Subjects and Sarcoid Patients

Study Population	Stimulus to IL-1 Production	IL-1 Activity (mean units/ml ± SD) Monocytes	BAMC
Control	None	0.8 ± 0.2	0.2 ± 0.1
	LPS	48.2 ± 13.0	54.6 ± 23.0
Sarcoid	None	2.4 ± 0.7	0.6 ± 0.2
	LPS	60.4 ± 16	10.8 ± 4.9

TABLE 3. IL-1 Production by E-Rosette-depleted BAMC

Conditions of Supernatant Generation	IL-1 Activity of BAMC (units/ml ± SD) Without E-Rosette Depletion	With E-Rosette Depletion
Culture medium	0.6 ± 0.3	1.1 ± 0.3
Culture medium + LPS	2.0 ± 1.4	5.2 ± 2.8

the low concentrations of IL-1 present in some supernatants. The mean response observed when thymocytes were cultured with IL-1 standard and the supernatants of LPS-stimulated BAMC was 25 276 ± 5388 CPM. The response, that is, the extent of [^{3}H]TdR incorporation, to these two stimuli is not significantly different from the one to the stimulus of the IL-1 standard alone; however, it is less than the one that would be predicted if the effects of these stimuli were assumed to be additive.

Consistent suppression of IL-1 responses by supernatants of BAMC was not observed when the dilution of supernatant in co-culture was less than 1:8. No IL-1 activity was present in diluted supernatants from unstimulated or LPS-stimulated BAMC of sarcoidosis patients.

DISCUSSION

These studies demonstrate the efficient production of the mononuclear phagocyte-derived growth factor IL-1 by blood monocytes and alveolar macrophages from healthy subjects. In sarcoidosis the vigorous production of IL-1 by blood monocytes contrasts with the low levels of IL-1 activity detected in supernatants of cultures of BAMC taken from the same patients. The depressed IL-1 activity of BAMC culture supernatants cannot be attributed to the dilution of IL-1-producing alveolar macrophages by T cells because supernatants of cultures that were enriched with alveolar macrophages did not produce amounts of IL-1 comparable to those generated by BAMC from controls. IL-1 production was not augmented by removing the E-rosette-forming T cell population; this indicates that *in vitro* IL-1 production was not modulated by T cells present among the BAMC. Rather, it appears that these culture supernatants contain a soluble factor produced by BAMC which suppresses *in vitro* responses to

TABLE 4. Effect of BAMC Supernatants on the Response of Mouse Thymocytes to IL-1

	[^{3}H]TdR Incorporated (CPM ± SD) No Supernatant Added	BAMC Supernatant Added	BAMC and LPS Supernatants Added
Control	707 ± 377	818 ± 170	9040 ± 3375
IL-1 standard	30 864 ± 2403	17 370 ± 4009	25 276 ± 5338

IL-1. Although this inhibitory activity of BAMC culture supernatants may be construed to mask IL-1 activity in the supernatants, dilutions of supernatant (1:8) which no longer suppressed IL-1 responses did not induce significant or consistent [^{3}H]TdR incorporation in mouse thymocytes.

The findings of the current study contrast with published reports of spontaneous IL-1 production by alveolar macrophages from sarcoid patients with high-intensity alveolitis.[15] While heterogeneity of disease activity in populations of patients with sarcoidosis is well recognized, patients in the current study all had untreated, biopsy-proven sarcoidosis of brief duration. In addition, the cellular analysis of bronchoalveolar lavage from our patients is consistent with high-intensity alveolitis,[3] and at least 28% of the BAMC were lymphocytes in all but one of the subjects. Several methodologic differences, then, may contribute to the apparent discrepancy in results. In an earlier study alveolar macrophages were selected from the BAMC according to their ability to adhere to plastic dishes; this adherence is known to induce IL-1 production by mononuclear phagocytes.[16] In the current study plastic adherence did not induce spontaneous IL-1 production by blood monocytes because alveolar macrophages were isolated by negative selection using E-rosette depletion. In addition, supernatants assayed for IL-1 content were harvested after different intervals of cell culture. The 24-hr interval used in the current study was selected as the optimal duration for IL-1 production from time-course studies of blood monocyte and alveolar macrophages taken from controls (M. E. Kleinhenz, unpublished observation). It is notable that, in each study of sarcoidosis, supernatants of BAMC cultures collected after 24 hr inhibited thymocyte response to IL-1.

The regulation of IL-1 production by mononuclear phagocytes is incompletely understood. Although IL-1 is not present in cell lysates of freshly isolated human mononuclear phagocytes, IL-1 can be detected in these cells after they undergo brief adherence to plastic and short intervals of *in vitro* culture.[16] Furthermore, the stimuli which influence IL-1 production *in vitro* may in fact have independent effects on synthesis and release of this polypeptide growth factor.[16] The experimental evidence available at present indicates that the immunosuppressive cyclooxygenase products of mononuclear phagocytes such as E-series prostaglandins may limit *in vitro* production of IL-1[17] and directly inhibit IL-1-induced thymocyte blastogenesis.[18] These inhibitory effects of prostaglandins are not specific for IL-1. Supernatants of human monocyte-derived tumor cell U937 cultures also inhibit mouse thymocyte response to IL-1; further analysis, however, indicates that the U937 suppressor factor inhibits IL-1-induced [^{3}H]TdR incorporation by blocking thymocyte production of IL-2.[19] In contrast, an inhibitor of IL-1 recovered from the urine of febrile patients[20] is specific for IL-1 and does not act through effects on IL-2. The cellular source of the 20-40 kD molecule suppressor has not been established. The nature and the cellular source of the IL-1 inhibitor produced by BAMC in sarcoidosis is currently under investigation. The *in vitro* production of such an inhibitor contrasts with the lymphocytic alveolitis and granulomatous inflammation documented in these patients. The suppressor activity may be a by-product of intense cell-mediated immune reactions resulting in an accumulation of cytostatic or cytotoxic molecules such as E-series prostaglandins. Alternatively, production of a specific inhibitor of IL-1 may reflect local regulatory mechanisms to limit the immune response.

The current study suggests that the immune accessory function of circulating mononuclear phagocytes is preserved in sarcoidosis. Thus, deficient production of IL-1 by blood monocytes cannot be implicated as a cause of anergy. The possibility exists, however, that the inhibitor of IL-1 produced by bronchoalveolar immune effector cells may leak into the peripheral circulation and thereby depress systemic immune reactivity.

REFERENCES

1. Friou, C. J. 1952. Yale J. Biol. Med. **24:** 533-539.
2. Tannenbaum, H., R. E. Rocklin, P. N. Schur & A. L. Sheffer. 1976. Clin. Exp. Immunol. **26:** 511-519.
3. Crystal, R. G., W. C. Roberts, G. W. Hunninghake, J. E. Gadek, J. D. Fulmer & B. R. Line. 1981. Ann. Intern. Med. **94:** 73-94.
4. Spagnuolo, P. J., J. J. Ellner, R. Bouknight, J. W. Tomford, M. E. Kleinhenz & K. L. Edmonds. 1980. J. Immunol. **125:** 1071-1077.
5. Goodwin, J. S., R. Dehoratius, H. Israel, G. T. Peak & R. P. Messner. 1979. Ann. Intern. Med. **90:** 169-173.
6. Daniele, R. P. & D. T. Rowlands. 1976. Ann. Intern. Med. **85:** 593-600.
7. Ceuppens, J. L., L. M. Lacquet, G. Mariën, M. Demedts, A. van den Eeckhout & E. Stevens. 1984. Am. Rev. Respir. Dis. **129:** 563-568.
8. Mizel, S. B. 1982. Immunol. Rev. **63:** 51-73.
9. Böyum, A. 1968. Scand. J. Clin. Lab. Invest. **21**(Suppl. 97): 77-89.
10. Kleinhenz, M. E., J. J. Ellner, P. J. Spagnuolo & T. M. Daniel. 1981. J. Clin. Invest. **68:** 153-162.
11. Kaplow, L. S. 1965. Blood **26:** 215-219.
12. Li, C. Y., K. W. Lam & L. T. Yaw. 1973. J. Histochem. Cytochem. **21:** 1-12.
13. Meltzer, M. A. & J. J. Oppenheim. 1977. J. Immunol. **118:** 77-82.
14. Stadler, B. M., S. F. Dougherty, J. J. Farrar & J. J. Oppenheim. 1981. J. Immunol. **127:** 1936-1940.
15. Hunninghake, G. W. 1984. Am. Rev. Respir. Dis. **129:** 569-572.
16. Lepe-Zuniga, J. L. & I. Gery. 1984. Clin. Immunol. Immunopathol. **31:** 222-230.
17. Farrar, W. L., S. B. Mizel, J. J. Farrar. 1980. J. Immunol. **124:** 1371-1377.
18. Dinarello, C. A., S. O. Marnoy & L. J. Rosenwaser. 1983. J. Immunol. **130:** 890-895.
19. Fujiwara, H., Z. Toossi & J. J. Ellner. 1984. Clin. Res. **32:** 346A.
20. Liao, Z., R. S. Grimshaw & R. L. Rosentreich. 1984. J. Exp. Med. **159:** 126-136.

A Proposed Model for the Accumulation of Helper/Inducer Lymphocytes in Sarcoidosis

The Role of Lymphocyte Subset-specific Chemoattractant Lymphokines

JEFFREY S. BERMAN, DENNIS J. BEER,
JOHN BERNARDO, HARDY KORNFELD, AND
DAVID M. CENTER[a]

Pulmonary Center
Boston University School of Medicine
Boston, Massachusetts 02118

INTRODUCTION

The secretory products of lymphocytes, monocytes/macrophages, and fibroblasts are all instrumental in the pathogenesis of pulmonary sarcoidosis. In sarcoidosis, as in granulomatous leprosy,[1] there appears to be a redistribution of a subset of thymus-derived (T) lymphocytes, more specifically, a subset identified by the OKT4 (helper/inducer) phenotype, from the blood to the target organ.[2] Once there, these lymphocytes elaborate several important regulatory proteins (lymphokines) including interleukin-2 (IL-2),[3,4] which promotes expansion of the lymphocyte pool; a monocyte chemoattractant factor[5] which promotes granuloma formation; and a fibroblast-activating factor[6] which promotes collagen synthesis. The mechanisms by which these circulating helper/inducer lymphocytes are recruited to inflammatory sites in lung parenchyma are unknown. Over the past several years, our laboratory has been investigating lymphocyte-derived factors which influence T cell motility.[7-10] This monograph describes two lymphocyte subset-specific chemoattractant lymphokines and provides a model for helper/inducer lymphocyte accumulation in the lung.

[a] Address for correspondence: Pulmonary Center, K-600, Boston University School of Medicine, 80 East Concord Street, Boston, Massachusetts 02118.

MATERIALS AND METHODS

Isolation of Mononuclear Cells

Human peripheral blood mononuclear cells (PBMC) were isolated from heparinized venous blood of healthy adult volunteers by density centrifugation on a Ficoll-Paque gradient.[11] Cells were recovered from the interface and washed three times in medium 199 supplemented with 25 mM HEPES buffer, 100 U/ml penicillin, and 100 μg/ml of streptomycin (M199-HPS).

For some experiments, nylon wool-nonadherent (NWNA) human T cell-enriched populations were prepared by a modification of the method of Julius *et al.*;[12] 95% of the cells obtained by this method were T lymphocytes, as assessed by immunofluorescent staining with OKT3 monoclonal antibody. Human T lymphocytes were further separated into helper/inducer ($OKT4^+$) or cytotoxic/suppressor ($OKT8^+$) subset-enriched populations by negative selection utilizing monoclonal antibody directed against cell membrane glycoproteins and complement. More than 95% of the cells in depleted cell populations were viable, as assessed by their ability to exclude trypan blue dye. More than 90% of the cells remaining after monoclonal antibody and complement treatment stained with the appropriate FITC-conjugated monoclonal antibody identifying the desired cell population. These subset-enriched T lymphocyte populations were then used to generate lymphokines or employed as target cells in the chemotaxis assay.

Generation of Supernatants

Normal human PBMC or NWNA T lymphocytes were employed as the source of lymphocyte chemoattractant lymphokines. Mononuclear cell populations were suspended at a concentration of 2×10^6 cells/ml of M199-HPS in the absence or presence of histamine dihydrochloride (1×10^{-4} M) or in the absence or presence of concanavalin A (con A) (10 μg/ml). Histamine-stimulated and con A-stimulated lymphocytes were incubated for 24 hr and 48 hr, respectively, at 37° C in a humidified 5% CO_2 atmosphere. The cell-free supernatants were harvested. Crude supernatants were dialyzed at 4° C against phosphate-buffered saline (PBS) at pH 7.4. In certain experiments, dialyzed culture supernatants were then concentrated to 1/15 to 1/30 of their original volumes by lyophilization. The functional and physicochemical properties of the chemoattractant lymphokines, whether derived from histamine- or con A-activated lymphocytes, were identical.

Cell Migration

Lymphocyte migration was assessed, employing a modification[7,13] of a Boyden chamber technique,[14] by utilizing a population of human blood or rat splenic T lymphocytes as the responding cell pool. To determine the effect on lymphocyte migration of an experimental sample, 50-μl aliquots of a lymphocyte suspension containing 10×10^6 cells/ml of M199-HPS enriched with 0.4% bovine serum albumin (BSA) were placed in the upper compartments of 48-well microchemotaxis chambers; these compartments were separated by 8-μm nitrocellulose micropore filters from the 25-μl control (M199-HPS alone) or experimental samples in the lower compartments. Lymphocyte migration experiments were carried out for 3 hr at 37° C in a moist 5% CO_2 atmosphere. The filters were fixed, stained, dehydrated, and quantitated by counting the total number of cells migrating beyond a fixed distance, with 10-μm increments used, in five high power fields (hpf) in duplicate micropore filters using an Optimax automated image analyzer. Counting depth was adjusted to give control numbers of 5 to 25 cells. Results were calculated as mean cells/hpf ± SD. Data from similar experiments underwent analyses of variance to determine their statistical significance; a p value of less then .05 was considered significant. In every figure each result is expressed as a mean percentage of migration under control conditions ± SD. It was convenient to use rat splenic lymphocytes as target cells in most of the experiments described in this paper because large quantities of these cells can be easily obtained. No qualitative differences were noted between the migratory responses of human T and rat splenic lymphocytes.

Characterization of Lymphokines

Concentrated supernatants of stimulated PBMC were dialyzed against PBS and applied to a Sephadex G-100 column. Chromatography was performed at 4° C in a 1.5 cm × 90 cm column eluted with PBS at 15 ml/hr; 2-ml fractions were collected in plastic tubes, and 30 μl of every other fraction were placed in the lower chambers only of microchemotaxis chambers and assessed for chemoattractant activity against human NWNA T cells or rat splenic lymphocytes. Fractions with chemoattractant activity were pooled and dialyzed against 0.01 M phosphate buffer at pH 7.8. This pooled material was then applied to a 10-ml Sephadex QAE anion exchange column and eluted with a linear 200-ml salt gradient to 1 M NaCl at 4° C. Conductance was measured at 4° C. Fractions were dialyzed against PBS and tested for chemoattractant activity.

Fractions with chemoattractant activity were pooled, dialyzed against distilled water, concentrated 10-fold by lyophilization, and then subjected to isoelectric focusing in sucrose. A Buchler gradient apparatus and a constant flow pump containing ampholytes in either the 3-10 or the 7-10 pH range were used to generate 10-40%, 3-ml sucrose gradients. Electrophoresis was carried out at a constant voltage until the current equilibrated, and then at a constant current for 120 min. Fractions containing 0.6 ml were eluted with a peristaltic pump, assessed for pH, and dialyzed against PBS for 48 hr to remove ampholytes and sucrose; 25-μl samples were assessed for lymphocyte chemoattractant activity in microchemotaxis chambers as described above.

RESULTS

The migratory responses of human blood and rat splenic T lymphocytes to con A- and histamine-stimulated human lymphocyte culture supernatants are shown in TABLE 1. Unfractionated supernatants (25 μl) derived from cells incubated with either

TABLE 1. Migratory Responses of Human Blood and Rat Splenic T Lymphocytes to Concanavalin A- or Histamine-stimulated Human Blood Mononuclear Cell Culture Supernatants

	Chemoattractant Activity[a]					
	Experiment 1		Experiment 2		Experiment 3	
Stimulant	Rat	Human	Rat	Human	Rat	Human
Buffer alone	9.2 ± 0.8	7.0 ± 0.9	7.8 ± 1.0	8.2 ± 1.4	10.5 ± 0.7	6.2 ± 0.5
Buffer + con A (10 μg/ml)	8.9 ± 1.0	7.5 ± 1.0	8.0 ± 0.8	9.0 ± 1.0	11.0 ± 0.6	7.1 ± 0.5
Buffer + histamine (10^{-4} M)	9.1 ± 1.2	8.0 ± 1.0	8.0 ± 1.2	7.6 ± 0.8	9.4 ± 1.0	7.6 ± 0.8
Cells[b]	10.3 ± 0.9	8.9 ± 1.2	10.2 ± 1.0	10.0 ± 1.1	12.0 ± 1.6	8.2 ± 0.6
Cells + con A (10 μg/ml)	19.3 ± 1.3[c]	24.1 ± 0.9	31.2 ± 2.0	24.6 ± 1.9	25.4 ± 2.1	14.8 ± 1.1
Cells + histamine (10^{-4} M)	23.9 ± 1.9	16.8 ± 2.0	17.8 ± 1.5	25.6 ± 3.1	22.7 ± 1.3	20.2 ± 3.0

[a]Mean cells/hpf ± SD.
[b]The unconcentrated culture supernatants were placed, in 25-μl aliquots, only in the lower compartments of the microchemotactic chambers.
[c]Significantly different from control groups ($p < .01$).

ligand enhanced the migration of rat cells from 2.10 to 4.0 times control migration and human T cells from 2.4 to 3.44 times control migration.

Although low doses of concentrated crude lymphocyte supernatants enhanced lymphocyte migration, higher doses inhibited lymphocyte migration (TABLE 2). In addition, a checkerboard analysis was performed employing partially purified lymphocyte chemoattractant factor (LCF) obtained after sequential molecular sieve and anion exchange chromatography (see below). The concentrations of the partially purified lymphokine placed on both sides of the micropore filters was varied from filter to filter. Thus it was possible to initiate a gradient across a filter, to eliminate any gradient, or to create a gradient away from a filter. The degree of enhancement of lymphocyte migration was found to be independent of the placement of partially purified lymphokine, whether it was above or below or on both sides of the filter. This activity was thus identified as a predominantly chemokinetic factor (data not shown).

The nature of the lymphocyte migratory responses to increasing concentrations of crude supernatant is reflected by the findings of Sephadex G-100 molecular sieve chromatography of concentrated mononuclear cell supernatants. These findings reveal

TABLE 2. Lymphocyte Migratory Responses to Increasing Concentrations of Crude Supernatant

	Crude Supernatant Dilutions[a]					
	0[b]	1:10	1:3	1:1	3:2	Neat[c]
Chemoattractant activity[d]	100 ± 10	118 ± 18	235 ± 28[e]	252 ± 12[e]	102 ± 12	72 ± 6[e]

[a]Ratios of concentrated (15-fold) crude histamine-induced lymphocyte supernatants to buffer.
[b]Migration under control conditions.
[c]Undiluted material (25 μl).
[d]Mean cells/hpf ± SEM; N = 3-6. The control was 14.8 ± 1.6 cells.
[e]Significantly different from the control ($p < .01$).

three regions of interest (FIG. 1). A region of human blood and rat splenic T lymphocyte migration enhancement (an activity corresponding to a molecular mass of 56 000 daltons) flanked by two areas of T lymphocyte migration inhibition. These activities were found in the supernatants of activated cells but not in column fractions from control supernatants, whether assayed with human T cells (FIG. 1A) or rat splenic lymphocytes (FIG. 1B). One region of migration-inhibitory activity eluted just prior to bovine serum albumin and corresponded to a molecular mass of 70-80 000 daltons ($LyMIF_{75K}$). The second region of migration-inhibitory activity eluted just after ovalbumin and corresponded to a molecular mass of 30-40 000 daltons ($LyMIF_{35K}$). More than 95% of the lymphocytes incubated for 3 hr in $LyMIF_{75K}$ or $LyMIF_{35K}$ were viable, as assessed by exclusion of trypan blue dye. There were no differences noted between the migratory responses of human blood T lymphocytes or rat splenic lymphocytes.

To further characterize LCF and $LyMIF_{35K}$, pooled material from molecular sieve chromatography was applied to a QAE anion exchange column. LCF eluted early in the salt gradient, corresponding to an ionicity of 5 to 7 mS. $LyMIF_{35K}$ eluted very early in the gradient, corresponding to an ionicity of 1 to 4 mS (data not shown). Pooled activity from each QAE column was subjected to isoelectric focusing in sucrose

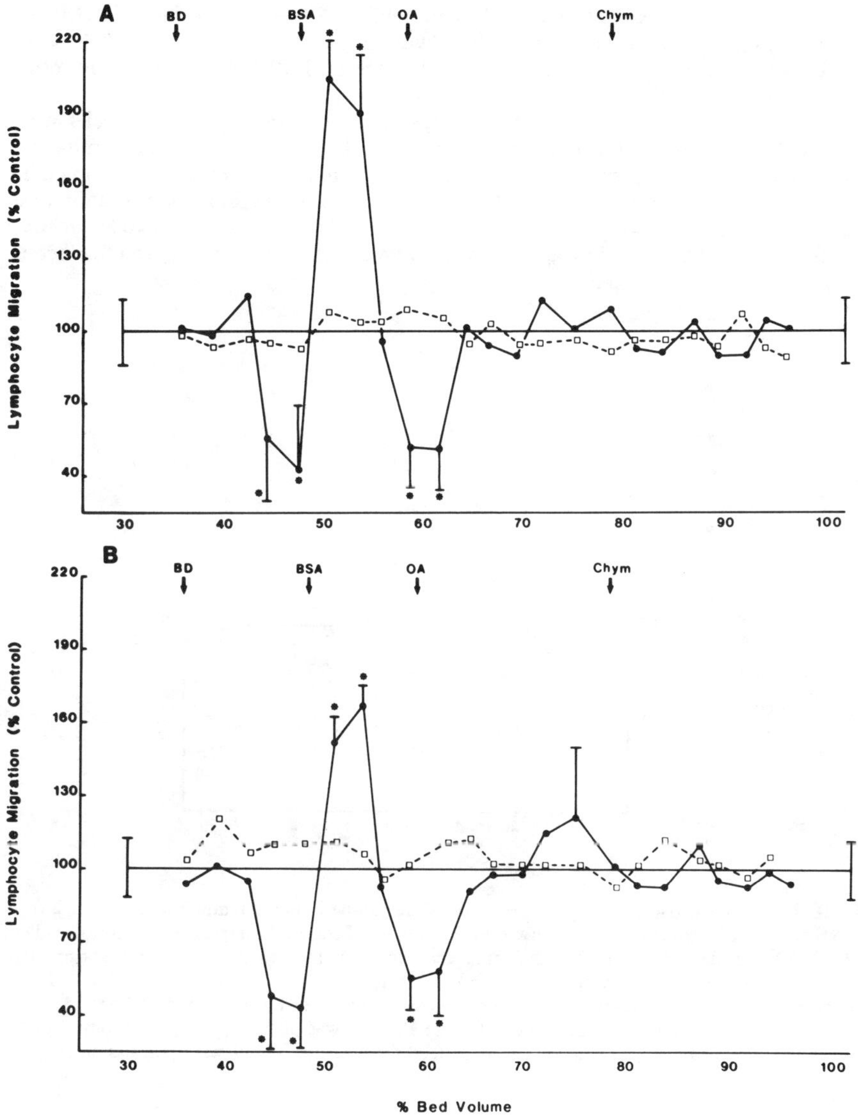

FIGURE 1. Representative Sephadex G-100 chromatograms (from three experiments) of histamine (10^{-4} M)-stimulated (●——●) mononuclear cell supernatants, or of supernatants of mononuclear cells incubated for 24 hr in medium alone (□- -□). Four molecular mass markers are indicated: blue dextran (BD), 2×10^6 daltons; bovine serum albumin (BSA), 68 000 daltons; ovalbumin (OA), 43 000 daltons; and chymotrypsin A (Chym), 25 000 daltons. Individual column fractions were assayed for their ability to alter the random migration of human blood NWNA T lymphocytes (**A**) or rat splenic lymphocytes (**B**). Results are expressed on the ordinate as percentage buffer control migration, where controls were 15.2 ± 2.2 cells (human NWNA T lymphocytes) and 18.6 ± 1.9 cells (rat splenic lymphocytes) (mean ± SEM). * = a migration that was different from that of the control ($p < .01$). (Reproduced from Berman *et al.*[10] with permission.)

(FIGS. 2 & 3). LCF had a single isoelectric point of 9.0-9.4. Focusing of $LyMIF_{35K}$ revealed a single area of inhibitory activity with an isoelectric point of 8.5-8.8. Wide-range focusing using ampholytes with a pH range of 3-10 did not reveal any other species possessing LCF or $LyMIF_{35K}$ activity.

In addition, separately pooled Sephadex G-100 LCF and $LyMIF_{35K}$ species were subjected to enzymatic degradation with trypsin (10^{-7} or 10^{-5} M) or neuraminidase (10^{-5} M) and to heat treatment (56° C) for 30 min. The results are shown in TABLE 3. The biological activity of LCF was sensitive to trypsin and neuraminidase but was resistant to heating. Trypsin digestion of $LyMIF_{35K}$ resulted in two fragments. The first was a 24 000-dalton fragment which retains biological activity, and the second

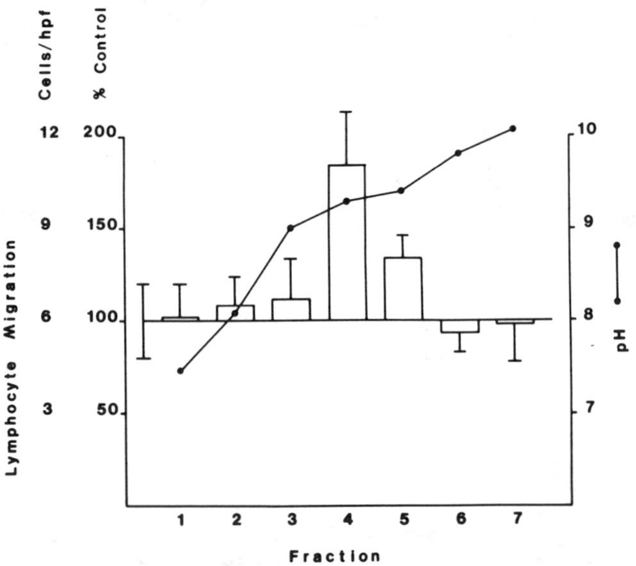

FIGURE 2. Isoelectric focusing of the peak of histamine-induced lymphotactic activity from QAE anion exchange chromatography of LCF. The pH of each 0.3-ml fraction of a 3-ml gradient (●——●) was determined before dialyzing each fraction to PBS, pH 7.4, for assessment of lymphocyte chemoattractant activity (LCA). LCA is expressed as cells/hpf ± SD and as a percentage of control migration in buffer (100% is indicated by a horizontal line). A 25-μl aliquot of each fraction was taken; each of these aliquots was placed in the lower compartment of a duplicate chemotactic chamber. (Reproduced from Center *et al.*[9] with permission.)

was a 10 000-dalton inactive fragment. $LyMIF_{35K}$ activity was resistant to neuraminidase treatment but was sensitive to heat.

To determine the cells of origin of LCF and $LyMIF_{35K}$, enriched mononuclear cell populations were incubated with either con A or histamine in the absence or the presence of specific histamine-type 1 (H_1) (diphenhydramine) or histamine-type 2 (H_2) (cimetidine) receptor antagonists. The supernatants were subjected to molecular sieve chromatography, and the column fractions were assayed for T cell chemoattractant activity. The results are presented in TABLE 4. Con A or histamine stimulation of unseparated T lymphocytes, but not of B lymphocytes or monocytes, resulted in the

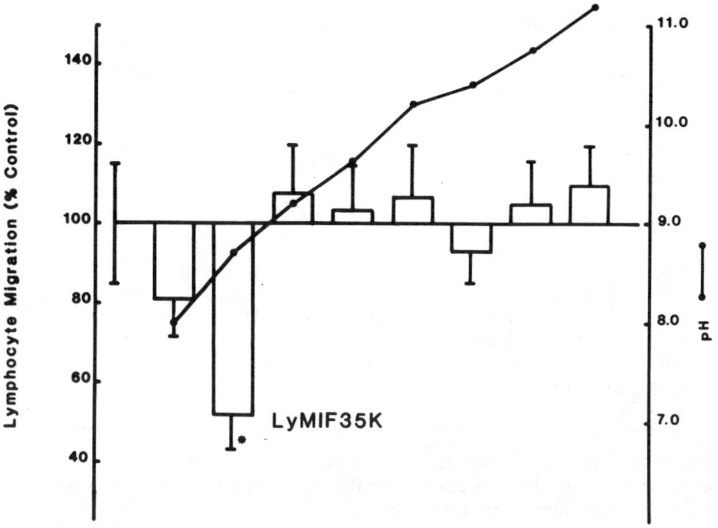

FIGURE 3. Isoelectric focusing of pooled active fractions from QAE anion exchange chromatography of $LyMIF_{35K}$. Ampholytes pH 7-10 were used. Rat splenic lymphocyte migratory responses are expressed on the ordinate as a percentage of migration in buffer control alone, where controls were 17.9 ± 2.5 cells. Expressed on the opposite ordinate is the pH measurement of the individual fractions (●——●). * = a migration that was different from that of the control ($p < .01$). (Reproduced from Berman *et al.*[10] with permission.)

production of both LCF and $LyMIF_{35K}$. Incubation of T cells with histamine plus diphenhydramine resulted in selective production of LCF; no $LyMIF_{35K}$ was produced. In contrast, supernatants generated by T cells incubated with histamine and cimetidine resulted in selective production of $LyMIF_{35K}$; no LCF was produced. The ability of con A to induce production of LCF and $LyMIF_{35K}$ was not affected by the addition of diphenhydramine and cimetidine. Finally, T lymphocyte subset-enriched populations were incubated with histamine and the supernatants fractionated on a Sephadex G-100 molecular sieve column. $OKT8^+$ cells produced only LCF and no $LyMIF_{35K}$ whereas $OKT4^+$ cells produced $LyMIF_{35K}$ and no LCF.

To determine the target cell specificity of these chemoattractant factors, enriched T lymphocyte subsets were employed as target cells for each of the lymphokines. As

TABLE 3. Physicochemical Characteristics of LCF and $LyMIF_{35K}$

	Molecular Mass (daltons)	pI	Trypsin	Neuraminidase	Heat
LCF	56 000[a]	9.0-9.4	Sensitive	Sensitive	Stable
$LyMIF_{35K}$	30-40 000	8.5-8.8	Stable	Sensitive	Sensitive

[a]Upon boiling with sodium dodecyl sulfate (SDS), LCF dissociates irreversibly into four biologically active subunits, each with a molecular mass of 14 000 daltons.

TABLE 4. Cell of Origin of LCF and $LyMIF_{35K}$[a]

Cell Population and Ligand	LCF	$LyMIF_{35K}$
PBMC + buffer	−	−
PBMC + con A (10 μg/ml)	+	+
PBMC + histamine (10^{-4} M)	+	+
Monocytes[b] + con A	−	−
Monocytes + histamine	−	−
B cells[c] + con A	−	−
NWNA T cells[d] + con A	+	+
NWNA T cells + histamine	+	+
NWNA T cells + histamine + diphenhydramine (10^{-5} M)	+	−
NWNA T cells + histamine + cimetidine (10^{-5} M)	−	+
NWNA T cells + con A + diphenhydramine + cimetidine	+	+
$OKT4^+$ cells + histamine	−	+
$OKT8^+$ cells + histamine	+	−

[a]Lymphokine activity is indicated as being either present (+) or absent (−).

[b]Monocytes were obtained by selecting those PBMC adherent to glass petri dishes. More than 95% of the monocytes were esterase positive.

[c]B cells were obtained by depleting PBMC of monocytes (glass adherence) and T cells (OKT3 monoclonal antibody and complement).

[d]More than 95% of these cells were OKT3 positive.

shown in FIGURE 4, LCF enhanced the motility of unseparated T lymphocytes and of $OKT4^+$ lymphocytes but had no effect on $OKT8^+$ lymphocytes. Likewise, $LyMIF_{35K}$ had a selective effect on $OKT4^+$ lymphocytes (FIG. 5). In separate experiments (data not shown), LCF and $LyMIF_{35K}$ had no effects on the motility of B cells or monocytes.

DISCUSSION

Our studies describe two lymphocyte chemoattractant lymphokines which are specific for the $OKT4^+$ (helper/inducer) subset. Lymphocyte chemoattractant factor (LCF), produced by H_2 receptor-bearing $OKT8^+$ lymphocytes, has been extensively characterized. It is a cationic (pI 9.0) sialoprotein with a molecular mass of 56 000 daltons.[7–9] It is selectively chemokinetic for the $OKT4^+$ lymphocyte subset. In contrast, a lymphocyte migration-inhibitory factor ($LyMIF_{35K}$) is produced by H_1 receptor-bearing $OKT4^+$ lymphocytes. $LyMIF_{35K}$ is a noncytotoxic cationic sialoprotein (pI 8.5-8.8) with a molecular mass of 30-40 000 daltons.[10] $LyMIF_{35K}$ selectively inhibits the random migration of $OKT4^+$ lymphocytes.

The observation that lymphocyte migration inhibition occurred with high concentrations of crude supernatants but not with partially purified LCF initially suggests that a lymphocyte-migration inhibitor is present in unseparated supernatants. A substance is said to be chemotactic if it enhances migration of the target cell along a concentration gradient. Chemotactic factors inhibit migration at high concentrations (high-dose inhibition). A chemokinetic factor enhances random cell migration and does not exhibit high-dose inhibition.[15] Therefore, chemokinetic substances cannot by themselves account for recruitment and immobilization of target cells at sites of inflammation because as the cells approach the source of the chemokinetic factor (high concentration) the motility of the cells increases. Immobilization in the presence of a chemokinetic factor requires the presence of a migration-inhibitory substance. Since $LyMIF_{35K}$ may reversibly inhibit or reverse LCF-induced chemokinesis, this lymphokine has the potential to interact with lymphocyte chemoattractants in a manner analogous to previously described migration-inhibitory factors for neutrophils and monocytes.[16] We postulate that activation of resident or infiltrating $OKT8^+$ and $OKT4^+$ lymphocytes to produce LCF and $LyMIF_{35K}$ by antigen, or by histamine released from tissue mast cells or basophils, may be one mechanism by which $OKT4^+$ (helper/inducer) cells are recruited to and immobilized at sites of granuloma formation.

The majority of lymphocytes recruited to sites of delayed hypersensitivity responses are not sensitized to the offending antigen.[17] Previously described chemoattractants for lymphocytes, most notably activated serum and casein,[18] act only on activated lymphocytes (lymphoblasts). LCF is a chemoattractant for unsensitized, unactivated T cells; target-cell activation is also unnecessary for the biological activity of $LyMIF_{35K}$. Thus, these lymphokines may be a means for the recruitment of nonsensitized, nonactivated T cells to sites of lymphocyte-mediated inflammatory responses.

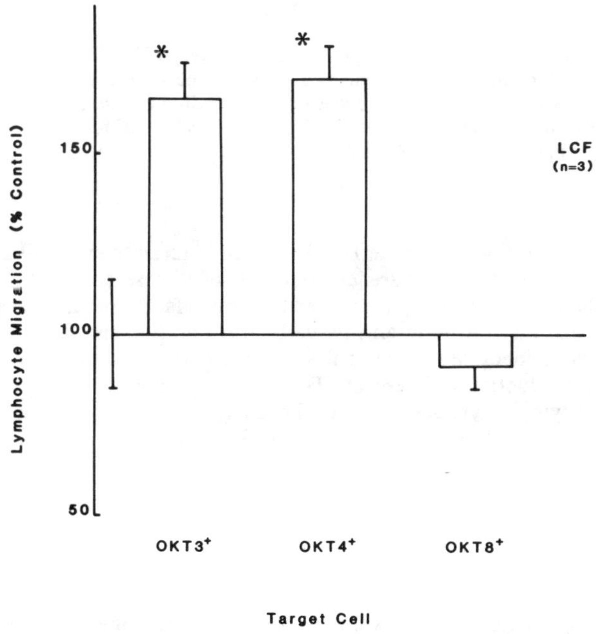

FIGURE 4. Migratory responses to partially purified LCF of nylon wool-purified human T lymphocytes (95% $OKT3^+$) or T cell subsets ($OKT4^+$ or $OKT8^+$) prepared from $T3^+$ cells were measured in a modified Boyden chamber assay. Lymphocyte migration is expressed on the ordinate as a percentage of migration under control conditions where control migration was 22.6 ± 3.6 cells/hpf for $OKT3^+$ ($N = 3$), 15.6 ± 2.7 cells/hpf for $OKT4^+$ ($N = 3$), and 17.6 ± 2.4 cells/hpf for $OKT8^+$ ($N = 3$). * = a significant difference from the control ($p < .05$).

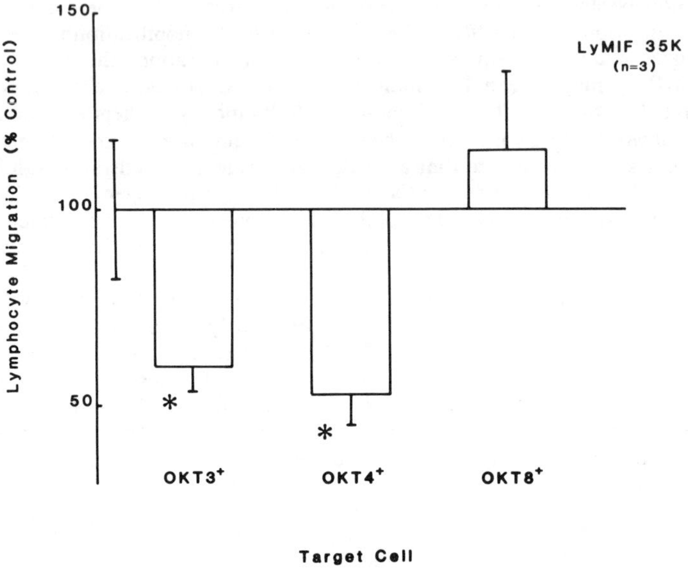

FIGURE 5. Lymphocyte migratory responses to partially purified $LyMIF_{35K}$ of nylon wool-purified human T lymphocytes or T cell subsets. Lymphocyte migration is expressed on the ordinate as a percentage of migration under control conditions where control migration was 22.6 ± 3.6 cells/hpf for $OKT3^+$ (N = 3), 15.6 ± 2.7 cells/hpf for $OKT4^+$ (N = 3), and 17.6 ± 2.4 cells/hpf for $OKT8^+$ (N = 3). * = a significant difference from the control (p < .05).

Sarcoidosis is a disease characterized by selective recruitment of $OKT4^+$ (helper/inducer) lymphocytes to lung parenchymal sites of disease activity.[2] Excess activity of helper/inducer cells is thought to mediate many facets of the disease, including granuloma formation[5] and lung and tissue injury[5] and fibrosis.[6] LCF and $LyMIF_{35K}$ have not yet been identified in clinical sarcoidosis. It is tempting, however, to hypothesize that production of these $OKT4^+$ subset-specific chemoattractant lymphokines at sites of lymphocyte activation in the early stages of sarcoidosis could account for the accumulation of resting, nonactivated T helper/inducer lymphocytes which participate in the pathogenesis of sarcoidosis.

REFERENCES

1. Van Voorhis, W. C., G. Kaplan, E. N. Savno, M. A. Horwitz, R. M. Steinman & W. R. Levis. 1982. The cutaneous infiltrates of leprosy: Cellular characteristics and predominant T-cell phenotypes. N. Engl. J. Med. **307:** 1593-1597.
2. Hunninghake, G. W. & R. G. Crystal. 1981. Pulmonary sarcoidosis: A disorder mediated by excess helper T-lymphocyte activity at sites of disease activity. N. Engl. J. Med. **305:** 429-433.
3. Pinkston, P., P. B. Bitterman & R. G. Crystal. 1983. Spontaneous release of interleukin-2 by lung T lymphocytes in active pulmonary sarcoidosis. N. Engl. J. Med. **308:** 793-800.

4. HUNNINGHAKE, G. W., G. H. BEDELL, D. C. ZAVALA, M. MONICK & M. BRADY. 1983. Role of interleukin-2 release by lung T-cells in active pulmonary sarcoidosis. Am. Rev. Respir. Dis. **128:** 634-639.
5. HUNNINGHAKE, G. W., J. E. GADEK, R. C. YOUNG, O. KAWANAMI, V. J. FERRANS & R. G. CRYSTAL. 1980. Maintenance of granuloma formation in pulmonary sarcoidosis by T lymphocytes within the lung. N. Engl. J. Med. **302:** 594-598.
6. WAHL, S. M., L. M. WAHL & J. S. MCCARTHY. 1978. Lymphocyte-mediated activation of fibroblast proliferation and collagen production. J. Immunol. **121:** 942-946.
7. CENTER, D. M. & W. W. CRUIKSHANK, 1982. Modulation of lymphocyte migration by human lymphokines. I. Identification and characterization of chemoattractant activity for lymphocytes from mitogen-stimulated mononuclear cells. J. Immunol. **128:** 2563-2568.
8. CRUIKSHANK, W. W. & D. M. CENTER. 1982. Modulation of lymphocyte migration by human lymphokines. II. Purification of a lymphotactic factor (LCF). J. Immunol. **128:** 2569-2573.
9. CENTER, D. M., W. W. CRUIKSHANK, J. S. BERMAN & D. J. BEER. 1983. Functional characteristics of histamine receptor-bearing human mononuclear cells. I. Selective production of lymphocyte chemoattractant lymphokines utilizing histamine as a ligand. J. Immunol. **131:** 1854-1859.
10. BERMAN, J. S., R. G. MCFADDEN, W. W. CRUIKSHANK, D. M. CENTER & D. J. BEER. 1984. Functional characteristics of histamine receptor-bearing human mononuclear cells. II. Identification and characterization of two histamine-induced human lymphokines that inhibit lymphocyte migration. J. Immunol. **133:** 1495-1504.
11. BOYUM, A. 1968. Separation of leukocytes from blood and bone marrow. Scand. J. Clin. Lab. Invest. **21**(Suppl. 97): 77-89.
12. JULIUS, M. H., E. SIMPSON & L. A. HERZENBERG. 1973. A rapid method for the isolation of functional thymus-derived murine lymphocytes. Eur. J. Immunol. **3:** 645-649.
13. CENTER, D. M., S. I. WASSERMAN & K. F. AUSTEN. 1978. Alteration of rat splenic lymphocyte migration *in vitro* by the state of microtubule integrity. Cell. Immunol. **39:** 325-335.
14. BOYDEN, S. 1962. The chemotactic effect of mixtures of antibody and antigen on polymorphonuclear leukocytes. J. Exp. Med. **115:** 453-464.
15. WILKINSON, P. C. 1982. Chemotaxis and Inflammation. Churchill Livingstone. New York, NY.
16. ALTMAN, L. C. 1978. Chemotactic lymphokines: A review. *In* Leukocyte Chemotaxis: Methods, Physiology and Implications. J. I. Gallin & P. G. Quie, Eds.: 267-287. Raven Press. New York, NY.
17. COHEN, S., R. T. MCCLUSKEY & B. BENACERRAF. 1967. Studies on the specificity of the cellular infiltrate of delayed hypersensitivity reactions. J. Immunol. **98:** 269-273.
18. RUSSELL, R. J., P. C. WILKINSON, F. SLESS & D. M. V. PARROTT. 1975. Chemotaxis of lymphoblasts. Nature **256:** 646-648.

Alveolar Macrophage Phagocytosis in Sarcoidosis

The Role of Activated Lymphocytes

FRANÇOIS CLAVEL,[a] ANNE-MARIE LAVAL, ALAIN VENET, ELISE CAYROL, AND JACQUES CHRÉTIEN

Institut National de la Santé
et de la Recherche Médicale Unité 214
Hôpital Laennec
75007 Paris, France

INTRODUCTION

Pulmonary sarcoidosis is characterized by the presence of noncaseating granulomas within the lung structures. Analyses of cells recovered by bronchoalveolar lavage (BAL) in this disorder, however, suggest there is a mixed alveolitis, one comprised of activated lymphocytes[1] and alveolar macrophages. Many experimental arguments uphold the hypothesis that these macrophages are activated,[2–10] but phagocytosis, which is a major function of these cells, has not been extensively studied in sarcoidosis. We therefore investigated phagocytosis and microbicidal activity of alveolar macrophages in pulmonary sarcoidosis. Furthermore, since activated lymphocytes are known to modulate some important macrophage functions, we also evaluated the modulation of alveolar macrophage phagocytosis by lymphocyte supernatants, either from mitogen-stimulated blood lymphocytes, or from unstimulated alveolar lymphocytes from sarcoid patients, making the hypothesis of a spontaneous modulation of macrophage functions by these cells.

METHODS

Patient Populations

In the first part of the study, we compared phagocytosis by alveolar macrophages (AM) from eight sarcoid patients and seven controls. The patient population, which

[a] Address for correspondence and reprint requests: INSERM U214, Hôpital Laennec, 42 rue de Sèvres, 75007 Paris, France.

comprised four males and four females, had a mean age of 36 ± 10 years. One patient was a smoker; seven were nonsmokers. They all had biopsy-proven sarcoidosis with thoracic involvement. Analysis of BAL cellular data from these patients yielded a total cell count of 58 ± 40 × 10^6 cells. AM accounted for 60 ± 13% and lymphocytes for 38 ± 14% of these cells.

In the second part, we studied the production of a factor modulating AM phagocytosis by alveolar lymphocytes from 12 patients with sarcoidosis. This second patient population was comprised of seven males and five females and had a mean age of 35 ± 7 years. Four patients were smokers; eight were nonsmokers. They all, except one patient with a typical Löfgren syndrome, had biopsy-proven sarcoidosis. Analysis of their BAL cellular data yielded a total cell count of 63 ± 35 × 10^6 cells. AM accounted for 50 ± 11% and lymphocytes for 48 ± 11% of these cells.

The control populations of the first and second parts comprised 17 healthy volunteers, 10 males and 7 females, who had a mean age of 32 ± 9 years. Six of the controls were smokers; 11 were nonsmokers. Analysis of BAL cellular data from these controls yielded a total cell count of 77 ± 31 × 10^6 cells for smokers and 36 ± 25 × 10^6 for nonsmokers. The mean percentage of lymphocytes was 7.6 ± 6.4%, and that of AM was 88.6 ± 7.9%.

Bronchoalveolar Lavage Procedure

BAL was carried out with a fiberoptic bronchoscope wedged into the subsegmental bronchus. A total of 300 ml of warm, sterile saline solution was delivered in three 100-ml aliquots to the same site, as previously described.[11]

Processing of Bronchoalveolar Lavage Fluid

After filtration on sterile gauze for removal of mucus, native BAL fluid was centrifuged (500 × g for 10 min). The cells were washed sequentially in Hanks' balanced salt solution (HBSS) (Eurobio, Paris, France) and then resuspended in RPMI 1640 (Gibco, Paisley, England). Total cell counts were determined on native BAL fluid with a hemocytometer. Differential cell counts were determined by examining May-Grünwald-Giemsa-stained, cytocentrifuged smears.

Cell Cultures

Alveolar Macrophages

AM were suspended at a concentration of 5 × 10^5 cells/ml in "complete medium": RPMI 1640 supplemented with 10% heat-inactivated fetal calf serum (Flobio, Courbevoie, France), 4 mM glutamine, 100 U/ml penicillin, and 100 μg/ml streptomycin. The cells were plated in 16-mm-wide wells of 24-well tissue culture dishes (Costar,

Cambridge, MA). There were 2.5×10^5 AM suspended in complete medium per well at 37° C in a humidified 5% CO_2 atmosphere.

Lymphocyte-enriched Blood Mononuclear Cell Culture Supernatants

Mononuclear blood cells were isolated from blood by Ficoll-Hypaque centrifugation and were washed and resuspended in complete medium at 10^6 cells/ml. The cells were incubated overnight in 25-cm^2 tissue culture flasks (Corning, NY) to allow monocytes to adhere. Nonadherent cells were then recovered and cultured at 10^6 cells/ml in complete medium for 48 hr. These cells are referred to as "blood lymphocytes." When indicated, phytohemagglutinin (PHA) (Difco) was added at 1 μg/ml final dilution in the culture medium. After centrifugation, the supernatants were recovered, filtered on 0.22-μ millipore filters, and stored at −30° C until use.

Lymphocyte-enriched Bronchoalveolar Cell Culture Supernatants

BAL cells (10^6 cells/ml in complete medium) were cultured overnight to allow the adherence of AM. Nonadherent cells were then recovered, centrifuged, washed in HBSS, resuspended at 10^6 cells/ml in complete medium, and cultured for an additional 48 hr. These nonadherent cells are referred to as "alveolar lymphocytes." After centrifugation the supernatants were recovered, filtered on 0.22-μ millipore filters, and stored at −30° C until use.

Yeast Cells

Dessicated, viable *Saccharomyces cerevisiae* were suspended just before use in HBSS at 37° C. The suspension was vigorously shaken, and the yeast cells were then counted on a hemocytometer. Concentrations were adjusted at 5×10^7 cells/ml. The organisms were then opsonized for 1 hr at 37° C in 10% pooled normal human serum.

Alveolar Macrophage Phagocytosis and Microbicidal Assay

After a 2-hr adherence period and the subsequent removal of nonadherent cells, AM (2.5×10^5 cells/well) in complete medium were challenged with 100 μl of yeast suspension (yeast cell/AM ratio = 20:1) and incubated for 1 hr at 37° C in a 5% CO_2 atmosphere. The AM well was then washed thoroughly with HBSS. After a 1-hr incubation in fresh medium to allow yeast killing by AM, supernatants were removed; the plates were dried, methanol fixed, and stained with Giemsa. Optical counting of intracellular yeast cells was performed at × 500 with oil immersion after the removal of the bottom of the well with an appropriate dentate punch.

A total of 100 AM was examined, and the number of intracellular viable (blue stained) or killed (unstained)[12] yeast cells was counted for each AM examined. We defined the total phagocytic index (TPI) as the mean number of engulfed yeast cells/AM and the killing index (KI) as the percentage of killed intracellular yeast cells. We also determined whether the number of ingested yeast cells/AM was homogeneously distributed inside each AM population. We therefore divided each AM population into six subclasses according to the number of phagocytized yeast cells/AM: 0, 1-5, 6-10, 11-15, 16-20, and >20. The number of AM in each subclass was calculated as a percentage of the total AM count.

Modulation of Alveolar Macrophage Phagocytosis by Activated Lymphocyte Culture Supernatants

AM from normal controls (2.5×10^5 cells/well), after a 2-hr adherence period, a washing, and their separation from nonadherent cells, were incubated in culture supernatants of blood or lung lymphocytes for 24 hr, then washed and assayed for phagocytosis in fresh medium. The supernatants tested were 1) supernatants from blood lymphocytes cultured with or without PHA, 2) serial twofold dilutions of PHA-stimulated blood lymphocyte supernatants, or 3) unstimulated alveolar lymphocyte supernatants from sarcoid patients. Controls of these experiments were made by incubating AM with RPMI and with nonstimulated normal blood lymphocyte supernatants, with or without reconstitution with PHA just before incubation of AM in the supernatants.

Each result is expressed as a percentage, of cells which were nonphagocytic (out of a total of 200 cells), or as an inhibition index: the percentage of nonphagocytic cells after incubation in tested supernatant minus the percentage of nonphagocytic cells after incubation in RPMI.

Statistical Analysis

Each result is presented as a mean ± SD. All statistical comparisons were made using the Mann-Whitney *U* test.

RESULTS

Yeast Phagocytosis and Killing by Alveolar Macrophages in Sarcoidosis

Data from assays that determined the extent of yeast phagocytosis and killing by sarcoid and normal AM (that is, by AM of every subset) are shown in TABLE 1. The mean number of phagocytized yeast cells/AM was slightly but not significantly lower in sarcoidosis ($p > .05$). Similarly, there was no difference in the proportion of killed yeast cells between the two study groups ($p > .05$).

TABLE 1. Phagocytosis and Killing of Yeast Cells by AM

	Sarcoidosis ($N=8$)	Controls ($N=7$)	U test[a]
Total phagocytotic index[b]	7.8 ± 1.6	9.9 ± 0.8	$p > .05$
Killing index[c]	9.1 ± 1.1	9.2 ± 2.6	$p > .05$

NOTE: AM from sarcoidosis and control patients were challenged with viable *Saccharomyces cerevisia* (yeast cell/AM ratio = 20:1) for 1 hr of phagocytosis and for 1 hr of killing.
[a]No statistically significant differences were found.
[b]Mean number of phagocytosed yeast cells/AM ± SD.
[c]Percentage of killed intracellular yeast cells ± SD.

When the population of AM in both groups was divided in six subclasses according to the number of ingested yeast cells/AM, an important discrepancy between sarcoid patients and controls became apparent (FIG. 1): the proportion of AM in the first subclass (AM which had not phagocytized any yeast cells) was significantly higher in sarcoid AM (17.5 ± 1.4%) than in control AM (3.6 ± 1.4) ($p < .01$). On optical analysis, those nonphagocytic sarcoid AM appeared normal, viable, and evenly distributed over the preparation.

There were no significant differences between the two study groups in the proportions of AM in each of the other phagocytic subclasses. The distribution of the number of killed yeast cells/AM was not significantly different between sarcoid patients and controls (data not shown).

Modulation of Alveolar Macrophage Phagocytosis by Activated Lymphocytes

When AM from normal controls were incubated for 24 hr with culture supernatants from PHA-stimulated blood lymphocytes, the number of nonphagocytic AM was markedly increased. In some instances, incubation of AM in RPMI for 24 hr led to the appearance of a higher proportion of nonphagocytic cells than when the same AM were challenged with yeast cells immediately after the initial 2-hr adherence period. In these cases, incubation of AM in "activated" supernatants always induced a proportion of nonphagocytic cells that was higher than that induced in the same AM by incubation in RPMI: this difference was then accurately expressed as the inhibition index. Thus, in all these experiments, the inhibition index was significantly higher when AM were incubated in stimulated lymphocyte supernatants than when AM from the same controls were incubated in unstimulated normal blood lymphocyte supernatants ($p < .01$) (FIG. 2). Furthermore, not only was the number of nonphagocytic AM increased, the whole AM population phagocytized fewer yeast cells. Nevertheless, in these experiments the number of nonphagocytic AM and the inhibition index appeared as reliable and easily appreciable parameters.

Optical examination of stained preparations or of fresh cells after incubation and phagocytosis under an inverted microscope revealed some typical cell-disposition patterns. AM incubated for 24 hr in RPMI or unstimulated blood lymphocyte supernatants always showed a regular and even distribution over the preparation. AM incubated in "stimulated" supernatants, however, exhibited three typical disposition

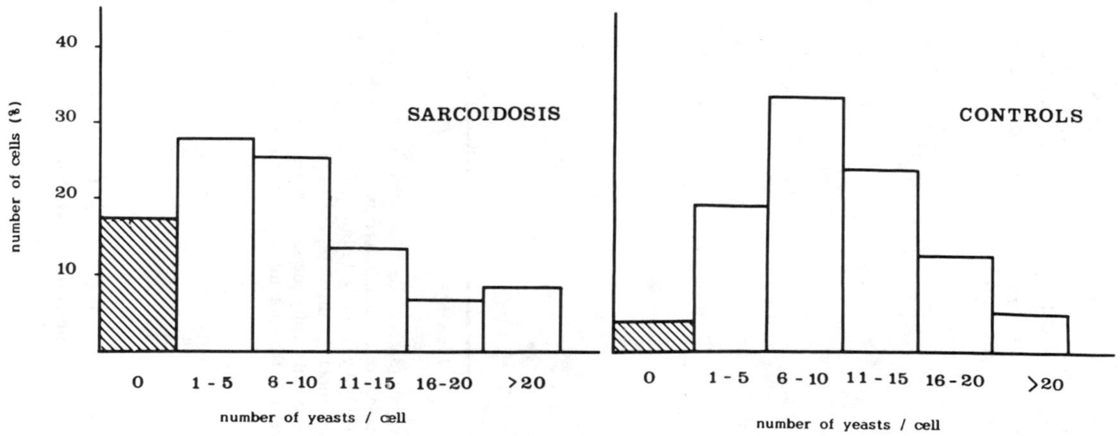

FIGURE 1. Distribution of the number of phagocytized yeast cells/AM in sarcoid and normal AM. AM from patients with sarcoidosis ($N=8$) and controls ($N=7$) were challenged with *Saccharomyces cerevisiae*. The AM population from each group was divided in six subclasses according to the number of ingested yeast cells/AM.

patterns: 1) clusters of mononucleated, and mainly phagocytic AM; 2) long, fusiform, fibroblast-like, and almost always phagocytic AM; 3) an even distribution of small, round, dense, refringent (hairy surrounding expansions and excentric nuclei), and mostly nonphagocytic AM.

When normal AM were incubated with serial twofold dilutions of five different "activated" supernatants, phagocytosis inhibition decreased strikingly with increasing dilutions. Thus the dose dependence of this phenomenon was demonstrated (FIG. 3).

The reconstitution of the control incubation media (RPMI or "unstimulated" supernatants) with PHA during the 24-hr incubation of AM did not significantly modify the number of nonphagocytic AM (data not shown).

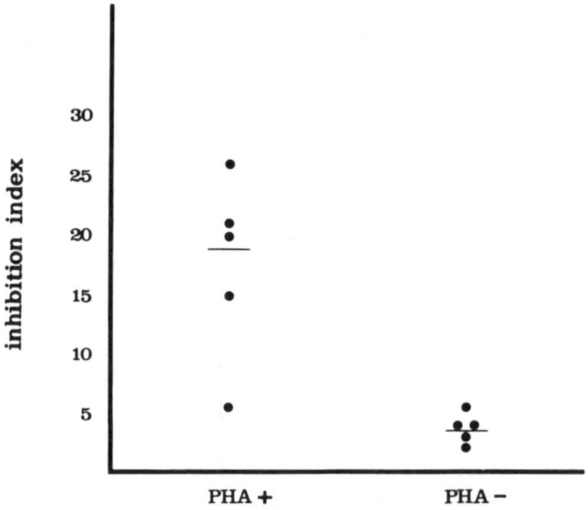

FIGURE 2. Modulation of alveolar macrophage phagocytosis by activated lymphocytes. Lymphocyte-enriched blood mononuclear cell populations from normal controls ($N=5$) were cultured for 48 hr with (+) or without (−) phytohemagglutinin (PHA). AM from normal controls were incubated for 24 hr in these supernatants, then allowed to phagocytize yeast cells. Each dot is the mean of three separate experiments using the same supernatant. The inhibition index is the percentage of nonphagocytic cells in supernatant minus the percentage of nonphagocytic cells in RPMI.

Ability of Alveolar Lymphocytes from Sarcoid Patients to Spontaneously Inhibit Phagocytosis by Normal Alveolar Macrophages

When AM from normal controls were incubated for 24 hr with culture supernatants of unstimulated alveolar lymphocytes from patients with pulmonary sarcoidosis, the number of nonphagocytic AM and the inhibition index were significantly higher than when normal AM were incubated in supernatants from unstimulated normal blood lymphocytes (FIG. 4). The mean inhibition index of phagocytosis by AM incubated

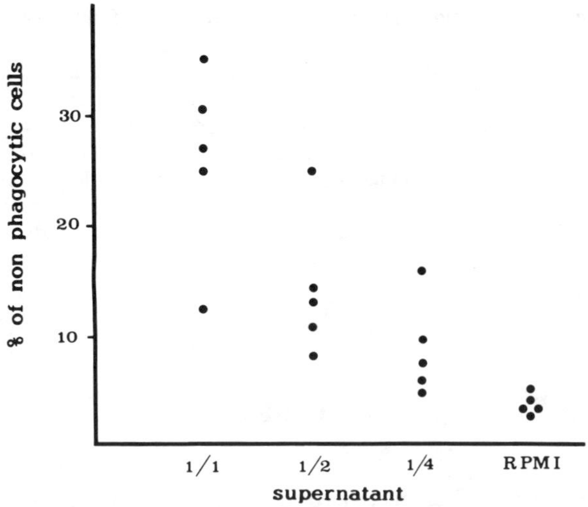

FIGURE 3. Dose dependence of the decrease of alveolar macrophage phagocytosis by activated lymphocyte supernatants. AM from one normal control were incubated with serial twofold dilutions of five different supernatants from PHA-activated normal blood lymphocytes. Results indicate the percentage of cells that were nonphagocytic.

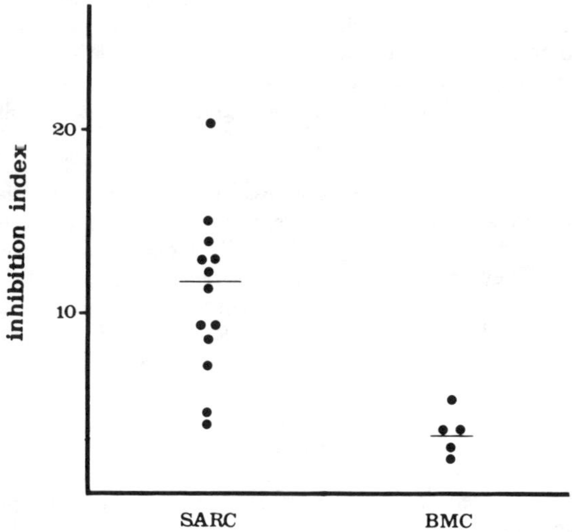

FIGURE 4. Ability of sarcoid alveolar lymphocytes to spontaneously decrease phagocytosis by alveolar macrophages. AM from normal controls were incubated with supernatants of alveolar lymphocytes from sarcoid patients (SARC) or of normal unstimulated blood mononuclear cells (BMS). Each result is expressed as an inhibition index, the percentage of AM in tested supernatant that were nonphagocytic minus the percentage of AM in RPMI that were nonphagocytic. Each dot is the mean of the values from two to four experiments using the same supernatant.

in sarcoidosis lung lymphocyte supernatants was 10.2 ± 5.6 whereas it was 3.7 ± 1.6 with unstimulated normal blood lymphocyte supernatants ($p < .01$). Nevertheless, supernatants from PHA-stimulated blood lymphocytes induced a significantly higher inhibition index (18.1 ± 7.4) than did supernatants from unstimulated sarcoid lung lymphocytes. We could find, however, a wide range of the inhibition index values, from 4.5 to 21%, from sarcoid lung lymphocyte supernatants. To further evaluate if these different inhibition index values were related to different degrees in the activity of the alveolitis, we tried to correlate these values to the lymphocyte percentages observed in the BAL. No statistical correlation could be found between these two parameters.

DISCUSSION

Pulmonary sarcoidosis is characterized by the presence within the lung structures of noncaseating granulomas, and by the existence of a mixed and mostly lymphocytic alveolitis. Mononuclear phagocytes are the precursors of epithelioid[13] and of multinucleated giant cells.[14] These cells are the main components of the granuloma and take an important part in the constitution of the alveolitis. In this study we demonstrated that when AM are challenged with opsonized yeast cells in sarcoidosis, the AM exhibit a qualitative phagocytic alteration; that is, the proportion of nonphagocytic AM increases. We also demonstrated that the same alteration can be reproduced *in vitro* among normal AM after incubation with supernatants from mitogen-activated blood lymphocytes, but not after incubation with supernatants from unstimulated lymphocytes. Furthermore, we have shown that AM from patients with pulmonary sarcoidosis spontaneously reduce phagocytosis by normal AM, suggesting that these sarcoid lung lymphocytes release a factor that gives rise to a nonphagocytic AM subset.

Several studies have argued that AM are activated in sarcoidosis. The absolute number of AM in BAL is increased in sarcoidosis.[2] Ultrastructural studies have shown that AM become larger.[3] AM seem to have a persistent high mitotic activity, as shown by flow cytometry[4] and by autoradiography.[5] They exhibit an increased antigen-presenting capacity.[6] They spontaneously release interleukin-1,[7] AM-derived growth factor for fibroblasts,[8] neutrophil chemotactic factor,[9] and increased amounts of fibronectin.[10] Few studies, however, concern phagocytosis, which is a major function of these lung effector cells.[5,15] Phagocytosis by sarcoid AM of nonopsonized zymosan has recently been shown to be lower than that by normal AM.[5] AM are also known to display, on their membranes, receptor sites for C3b and for the Fc fragment of immunoglobulin G (IgG):[16] molecules that mediate the phagocytosis of opsonized microorganisms. AM from sarcoid patients have been demonstrated to have a decreased number of C3b receptors,[17] which could lead to a decreased phagocytosis of C3b-opsonized organisms.

The contention that activated macrophages would have a decreased phagocytic activity has been emphasized by several studies. Macrophages from animals immunized with *Candida albicans* phagocytize fewer of these organisms.[18,19] Peritoneal macrophages from BCG-treated mice exhibit a reduced phagocytosis.[20] Activated lymphocytes decrease phagocytosis by normal human monocyte-macrophages.[21] Thioglycolate-activated mouse peritoneal macrophages phagocytize fewer cryptococci.[22]

Some other studies have described an increased phagocytosis by activated macrophages;[23–25] however, in these cases phagocytosis appears to be mediated by IgG, and the number of IgG Fc fragment receptors is known to be increased on activated macrophages.[25,26] Since normal human serum may contain only a very small amount of immune-specific antiyeast IgG, in our study, the uptake of yeast cells is likely to be mediated mostly by C3b receptors, or by mannose receptors. Mannose is an important constitutive hexose of the yeast cell wall, and some lectins from the membrane of phagocytic cells exhibit a specific affinity for this sugar and are thus able to mediate phagocytosis in the absence of any opsonin.[27] Activated macrophages display a lower number of such receptors.[28] Sarcoid AM, which are known to be activated, and which display a decreased number of C3b receptors, may also have a decreased number of mannose receptors. Thus, these mechanisms may be responsible for the phagocytic alteration of sarcoid AM and of lymphocyte-activated normal AM.

Decreased phagocytic activity parallels the increased microbicidal capacity of activated macrophages and monocytes[18,29] and may participate in the limitation by these activated cells of the spread of infections due to intracellular parasites.

Macrophage activation has been demonstrated to be mediated by a soluble factor. This factor was called the macrophage-activating factor (MAF), but it is now recognized as immune interferon (IFN-γ). IFN-γ is produced by activated T lymphocytes[30,31] and has been shown to activate oxidative metabolism and bactericidal activity of human macrophages,[32] as well as antiviral activity. Moreover, IFN-γ has also been shown to decrease the phagocytosis of opsonized zymosan by human monocyte-macrophages, as does IFN-α.[33] Since IFN-γ is produced by activated T lymphocytes and has been recently shown to be spontaneously produced by alveolar lymphocytes in sarcoidosis,[34] it is likely that IFN-γ is responsible for the phagocytic alteration shown in our study. We still do not know, however, whether IFN-γ-induced phagocytic alteration is mediated by a decrease in C3b or mannose receptors, or whether a decrease in both receptors is involved.

Activated lymphocytes, the main constitutive cells of the alveolitis in pulmonary sarcoidosis, are known to modulate granuloma formation.[35,36] Since they also induce a decrease in phagocytosis by AM, we raised the hypothesis that nonphagocytic AM may be involved in the constitution of the granuloma. The hypothesis of a relationship between activated nonphagocytic AM and epithelioid cells is supported by many arguments. Epithelioid cells have been shown to be weakly phagocytic, and to have a decreased number of C3b receptors and a normal number of Fc receptors on their membranes.[37] *In vitro,* we found these activated nonphagocytic AM to be dense, refringent, and to have hairy surrounding expansions. Ultrastructural examination of normal AM incubated in mitogen-activated lymphocyte culture supernatants reveals a larger rough endoplasmic reticulum, numerous vesicles, and interdigitating expansions:[36] morphologic attributes typical of epithelioid cells. More functional and ultrastructural studies are needed, however, to confirm the hypothesis that the increased proportion of nonphagocytic AM in sarcoidosis, which is likely to be the consequence of the release of IFN-γ by T lymphocytes, might be a step in the transformation of macrophages into epithelioid cells.

ACKNOWLEDGMENTS

We thank particularly G. Zarrindjam for the processing of the BAL, O. Peronne for the photographic work, and D. Guillemot for the secretarial assistance.

REFERENCES

1. Crystal, R. G., W. C. Roberts, G. W. Hunninghake, J. E. Gadek, J. D. Fulmer & B. R. Line. 1981. Pulmonary sarcoidosis: A disease characterized and perpetuated by T lymphocytes. Ann. Intern. Med. **94:** 73-94.
2. Crystal, R. G. 1981. State of the art: The pathogenesis of sarcoidosis. *In* Sarcoidosis and Other Granulomatous Disorders. J. Chrétien, J. Marsac & J. C. Saltiel. Eds.: 13-42. Pergamon Press. Paris.
3. Danel, C., A. Dewar, B. Corrin, M. Turner-Warwick & J. Chrétien. 1981. Ultrastructural findings in pulmonary sarcoidosis with particular reference to bronchoalveolar lavage cells. *In* Sarcoidosis and Other Granulomatous Disorders. J. Chrétien, J. Marsac & J. C. Saltiel, Eds.: 43-49. Pergamon Press. Paris.
4. Arnoux, A., R. Masse & J. Chrétien. 1981. Evidence for an increased persistant mitotic activity in cells recovered by BAL in sarcoidosis. *In* Sarcoidosis and Other Granulomatous Disorders. J. Chrétien, J. Marsac & J. C. Saltiel, Eds.: 50-54. Pergamon Press. Paris.
5. Bitterman, P. B., L. E. Saltzman, S. Adelberg, V. J. Ferrans & R. G. Crystal. 1984. One mechanism for the expansion of the mononuclear phagocyte population in the chronically inflamed lung. J. Clin. Invest. **74:** 460-469.
6. Venet, A., M. Wewers & R. Crystal. Enhanced antigen presentation by alveolar macrophages of patients with sarcoidosis. Clin. Res. **30:** 360A.
7. Hunninghake, G. W. 1984. Release of interleukin-1 by alveolar macrophages of patients with active pulmonary sarcoidosis. Am. Rev. Respir. Dis. **129:** 569-572.
8. Bitterman, P. B. & R. G. Crystal. 1984. Alveolar macrophages in idiopathic pulmonary fibrosis and sarcoidosis are spontaneously secreting a growth factor causing human lung fibroblasts to replicate. Clin. Res. **49:** 443A.
9. Roth-Fouret, C., H. Y. Reynolds, A. M. Laval, D. Sandron, G. Huchon & J. Chrétien. 1983. Facteur chemotactique pour les polynucléaires dans les macrophages alvéolaires et le fluide bronchoalvéolaire de patients atteints de sarcoïdose pulmonaire. Rev. Fr. Mal. Respir. **11:** 347.
10. Rennard, S. I., G. W. Hunninghake, P. B. Bitterman & R. G. Crystal. 1981. Production of fibronectin by the human alveolar macrophage: A mechanism for the recruitment of fibroblasts to sites of tissue injury in the interstitial lung diseases. Proc. Natl. Acad. Sci. USA **78:** 7147-7151.
11. Arnoux, A., J. Marsac, G. Stanislas-Leguern, G. Huchon & J. Chrétien. 1982. Bronchoalveolar lavage in sarcoidosis: Correlation between alveolar lymphocytosis and clinical data. Path. Respir. Pract. **175:** 62.
12. Zeligs, B. J. 1981. Bactericidal and fungicidal assay. *In* Manual of Macrophage Methodology. Immunology Series. H. B. Herscowite, H. T. Holden, J. A. Bellanti & A. Ghaffar, Eds. Vol. **13:** 271-287. Marcel Dekker. New York, NY.
13. Bernaudin, J. F., P. Soler & F. Basset. 1975. La cellule épithelioïde: Données ultrastructurales au cours des diverses entités pathologiques humaines. Pathol. Biol. **23:** 494-498.
14. Postlethwaite, A. E., B. K. Jackson, E. H. Beachey & A. H. Kang. 1982. Formation of multinucleated giant cells from human monocyte precursors. J. Exp. Med. **155:** 168-178.
15. Gee, J. B. L., P. T. Bodel, S. K. Zorn, L. M. Hinman, C. A. Stevens & R. A. Matthay. 1978. Sarcoidosis and mononuclear phagocytes. Lung **155:** 243-253.
16. Reynolds, H. Y., J. P. Atkinson, H. H. Newball & M. M. Franck. Receptors for immunoglobulin and complement on human alveolar macrophages. J. Immunol. **114:** 1813-1819.
17. du Bois, R. M. & M. Turner-Warwick. 1981. Bronchoalveolar macrophages in sarcoidosis. *In* Sarcoidosis and Other Granulomatous Disorders. J. Chrétien, J. Marsac & J. C. Saltiel, Eds.: 55-62. Pergamon Press. Paris.
18. Salvin, S. B. & S. L. Cheng. 1971. Lymphoid cells in delayed hypersensitivity. II. *In vitro* phagocytosis and cellular immunity. Infect. Immun. **3:** 548-552.
19. Neta, R. & S. B. Salvin. 1971. Cellular immunity *in vitro:* Migration inhibition and phagocytosis. Infect. Immun. **4:** 697-702.

20. NATHAN, C. F. & W. D. TERRY. 1977. Decreased phagocytosis by peritoneal macrophages from BCG-treated mice. Cell. Immunol. **29:** 295-311.
21. AL-IBRAHIM, M. S., F. T. VALENTINE & H. S. LAWRENCE. 1978. Activated lymphocytes depress phagocytosis of latex particles by human monocyte-macrophages. Cell. Immunol. **41:** 217-230.
22. SWENSON, F. J. & R. T. KOZEL. 1978. Phagocytosis of *Cryptococcus neoformans* by normal and thioglycolate-activated macrophages. Infect. Immun. **21:** 714-720.
23. NATHAN, C. F., M. L. KARNOWSKY & J. R. DAVID. 1971. Alterations of macrophage functions by mediators from lymphocytes. J. Exp. Med. **133:** 1356-1376.
24. MACKANESS, G. B. The mechanisms of macrophage activation. *In* Infectious Agents and Host Reactions. Mudd, Ed.: 62-67. W. B. Saunders. Philadelphia, PA.
25. SCHYLER, M. R. & D. STEINBERG. 1982. Activated alveolar macrophages: IgG and complement receptors. J. Lab. Clin. Med. **100:** 932-942.
26. GUYRE, P. M., P. M. MORGANELLI & R. MILLER. 1983. Recombinant immune interferon increases immunoglobulin G Fc receptors on cultured human mononuclear phagocytes. J. Clin. Invest. **72:** 393-397.
27. SUNG, S. S. J., R. S. NELSON & S. C. SILVERSTEIN. 1983. Yeast mannans inhibit binding and phagocytosis of zymosan by mouse peritoneal macrophage. J. Cell Biol. **96:** 160-166.
28. EZEKOWITZ, R. A. B., J. AUSTYN, P. D. STAHL & S. GORDON. 1981. Surface properties of BCG-activated mouse macrophages: Reduced expression of mannose-specific endocytosis, Fc receptors, and antigen F4/80 accompanies induction of Ia. J. Exp. Med. **154:** 60-76.
29. HORWITZ, M. A. & S. C. SILVERSTEIN. 1981. Activated human monocytes inhibit the intracellular multiplication of Legionnaires' disease bacteria. J. Exp. Med. **154:** 1618-1635.
30. WHEELOCK, E. F. 1985. Interferon-like virus inhibitor induced in human leukocytes by phytohemagglutinin. Science **149:** 310.
31. O'MALLEY, J. A., A. NOSSBAUM-BLUMENSON, D. SNEEDY, B. J. GROSSMAYER & H. OZER. 1982. Identification of the T cell subset that produces human gamma interferon. J. Immunol. **128:** 2522-2526.
32. NATHAN, C. F., H. W. MURRAY, M. E. WIEBE & B. Y. RUBIN. 1983. Identification of interferon gamma as the lymphokine that activates human macrophage oxidative metabolism and antimicrobial activity. J. Exp. Med. **158:** 670-689.
33. BECKER, S. 1984. Interferon as modulator of human monocyte-macrophage differentiation. I. Interferon gamma increases HLA-DR expression and inhibits phagocytosis of zymosan. J. Immunol. **132:** 1249-1254.
34. ROBINSON, B. W. F. & R. G. CRYSTAL. Gamma interferon is spontaneously released by alveolar macrophages and lung T lymphocytes in patients with pulmonary sarcoidosis. Submitted for publication.
35. HUNNINGHAKE, G. W., J. E. GADEK, R. C. YOUNG, O KAWANAMI, J. FERRANS & R. G. CRYSTAL. 1980. Maintenance of granuloma formation in pulmonary sarcoidosis by T lymphocytes within the lung. N. Engl. J. Med. **13:** 594-598.
36. VENET, A., E. CAYROL, A. M. LAVAL, F. CLAVEL & J. CHRÉTIEN. Activated lymphocytes modulate granuloma formation. First International Conference on Bronchoalveolar Lavage. May 1984. Columbia, MD.
37. WILLIAM, G. T. 1981. Functional studies and surface receptor characteristics of isolated epithelioid cells from experimental granulomas. *In* Sarcoidosis and Other Granulomatous Disorders. J. Chrétien, J. Marsac & J. C. Saltiel, Eds.: 76-83. Pergamon Press. Paris.

Immunoglobulin G Subclasses in Sarcoidosis

JOHN A. RANKIN,[a,b,c] JEANETTE OLCHOWSKI,[c]
GARY P. NAEGEL,[d] WILLIAM W. MERRILL,[c,e]
AND HERBERT Y. REYNOLDS[d,f]

[c]*Department of Pulmonary Medicine*
West Haven Veterans Administration Medical Center
West Haven, Connecticut

[d]*Department of Internal Medicine*
Pulmonary Section
Yale University School of Medicine
New Haven, Connecticut

INTRODUCTION

Human immunoglobulin G (IgG) is comprised of four different heavy-chain subtypes, IgG1-4. Currently, our knowledge about the respective roles of these subclasses in both health and disease states is incomplete. IgG1-4 differ considerably in many respects. For example, some data suggest that IgG1, IgG2, and IgG4 have half-lives of about 21 days whereas IgG3 has a half-life of approximately 7 days.[1-3] Biologic functions of IgG1-4 may differ also. Antipolysaccharide antibodies are preferentially of the IgG2 subclass,[1,4] and deficiencies of the subclasses, particularly IgG2 and IgG4, are associated with recurrent sinopulmonary infections.[5] IgG1 and IgG3 fix complement best, but IgG2 does so less well and IgG4 not at all.[6,7] Recently, our laboratory has demonstrated that alveolar macrophages from normal humans form rosettes with IgG1- and IgG3-coated red blood cells to a greater extent than with red cells coated with IgG2 and IgG4,[8] suggesting that receptors for IgG1 and IgG3 are the most abundant of IgG receptors on these cells. In addition, IgG1 and IgG3 interact with receptors on blood monocytes.[9] It is likely that IgG1 and IgG3 are particularly able to confer opsonic antibody activity.

IgG4 is particularly interesting. This subclass appears to have both a pathogenic role and a protective role,[10,11] depending on the disease and as yet undescribed genetic factors of the subject. Recently, Aalberse and co-workers showed that after an initial

[a] Address for correspondence: Yale University School of Medicine, Pulmonary Section, LCI 105, P.O. Box 3333, 333 Cedar Street, New Haven, Connecticut 06510.

[b] Fellow of the Puritan Bennett Foundation, and supported by the American Lung Association of Connecticut and by a Research Associate Career Development Award from the Veterans Administration.

[e] Supported by the Research Service of the Veterans Administration.

[f] Supported by Grant HL-22302 from the National Institutes of Health.

exposure to an antigen, bee venom, asymptomatic beekeepers developed an IgG1-dominated response.[12] In contrast, chronic exposure elicited an IgG4-dominated response. This change was reflected by a shift in the IgG4:IgG1 ratio. In addition, Iskander and co-workers reported that the relative contributions of IgG4 antibodies to the total IgG response to schistosomal antigens was considerably greater in patients chronically infected than in those recently infected with schistosomiasis.[13] One conclusion from these data is that this switch from an IgG1 to an IgG4 response may be one index of a normal immunoregulatory response.

Sarcoidosis is a chronic systemic disease of unknown etiology. Elevations in bronchoalveolar lavage (BAL) IgG levels and serum IgG levels occur frequently.[14–16] Evidence to date suggests that these elevated levels are due to increased IgG production at sites of disease activity, such as the lung.[16–18] This present work assesses the profile of IgG1-4 in the BAL fluid and serum of a group of patients with sarcoidosis and compares these values to those of a group of normal controls.

METHODS

Normal Controls

Nine normal subjects served as controls. All were nonsmokers. None had experienced an acute illness in the 4 weeks prior to study. Chest roentgenograms and pulmonary function tests were normal in all subjects on the day of testing.

Sarcoidosis Patients

This group included 39 individuals with sarcoidosis. All were nonsmokers. All but one patient had a tissue biopsy specimen which revealed noncaseating granulomata. The one remaining patient had a consistent clinical history but only giant cells evident in biopsy tissue. None had a significant occupational exposure to materials known to produce granulomatous lung disease, and infectious etiologies as a cause of disease were ruled out in all patients. Only two patients were on low-dose corticosteroid therapy at the time of study. Eight patients had not received corticosteroid therapy for at least 6 months prior to study; two patients had not for 6 weeks prior to study.

Bronchoalveolar Lavage and Processing of Lavage Fluid

Bronchoalveolar lavage was carried out in all patients using a standard technique described previously by us.[16] Approximately one-half of the lavage and serum samples from patients were obtained at neighboring hospitals and transported to our laboratory within 1 hr after being obtained. Processing a lavage fluid and the performance of differential cell counts were performed as reported.[16] Briefly, after filtering the fluid through a single layer of gauze, the fluid was centrifuged to separate cellular and sol phases. The cells were washed twice in Hanks' balanced salt solution, without Ca^{2+} and Mg^{2+} (Grand Island Biological, Grand Island, NY), and counted on a hemocytometer. Cell viability was assessed by trypan blue exclusion. Differential cell counts were performed on Wrights' stained cytocentrifuged preparations. The sol phase was concentrated by positive-pressure ultrafiltration through a UMO5 membrane (Amicon, Lexington, MA) to a 5-10-ml volume and stored at −70° C until assayed.

Immunochemical Analyses

On both concentrated BAL specimens and serum the total protein was determined by the method of Lowry and co-workers.[19] Albumin levels were determined using an enzyme-linked immunoassay or by radial immunodiffusion (Calbiochem Behring, La Jolla, CA).[16] IgG subclass determinations were performed using enzyme-linked immunoassays developed by us.[20]

Briefly, two methods were employed which depended on the source of the primary antibody. For quantitation of IgG1 and IgG4 (antibodies raised in primates), affinity-purified antibodies were coated on microelisa plates in alkaline buffer (pH 9.4). Standards of known concentration (purified IgG myeloma proteins) or samples of unknown concentration were diluted in phosphate-buffered saline with 0.5% Tween 20 (PBS-T) and mixed with IgG1 and IgG4 myeloma proteins which had been coupled covalently to horseradish peroxidase (HRP). The plates were incubated for 1 hr at 37° C and washed with PBS-T. Subsequently, substrate was added and the optical density read in an automated reader (Dynatech MR600). The concentrations of the samples were estimated by comparing the inhibition of color formation caused by the samples with that caused by the standards.

Purified monoclonal antibodies (the kind gift of Dr. Charles Rimers, CDC Atlanta, GA) were employed for analyses of IgG2 and IgG3. Unknown or known amounts of purified myeloma proteins were mixed with monoclonal antibodies (final dilution: 1:50 000) and incubated overnight at 4° C in PBS with 0.1% horse serum. The contents of the tubes were subsequently distributed to triplicate wells of microtiter plates previously coated with purified IgG2 or IgG3 myeloma proteins. Plates were incubated for 1 hr at 37° C and washed. Then biotinylated horse-antimouse antibody was added. After 1 hr the plates were again washed, and then Aviden-HRP was added. After 20 min the plates were washed; substrate was added; and the optical density was determined after a 30-min incubation. The concentrations of the samples were estimated by comparing the inhibition of color formation caused by the samples with that caused by purified subclass myeloma proteins of known concentrations.

Statistical Analyses

All data are presented as the means ± SD's. All statistical analyses were performed using the NIH-sponsored CLINFO project. Data were analyzed using the Wilcoxon two-group, ranked-sums test and the Wilcoxon signed-rank test for paired data (two tailed); p values less than or equal to .05 were considered significant.

RESULTS

All individuals tolerated the lavage procedure without major complications. Patients with sarcoidosis were significantly older than controls; their ages were 39.3 ± 12.1 years and 26.9 ± 5.1 years, respectively ($p = .002$). The volume of saline used for BAL in patients, 270 ± 59 ml, was less than that used in controls, 308 ± 10.5 ml ($p < .02$). The percent return in patients, 51.8 ± 19.5%, was similar to that in controls, 61.9 ± 9.4%. Despite this, the total number of cells retrieved from the patients, $36.8 \pm 27.3 \times 10^6$, was significantly greater than that retrieved from controls, $16.7 \pm 12.6 \times 10^6$ ($p < .03$). The percentage of BAL cells that were lymphocytes in sarcoidosis patients, 38.2 ± 16%, was significantly greater than that in controls, 9.5 ± 8.6% ($p < .001$)—results consistent with those published previously by others.[14] The percentages of polymorphonuclear cells in sarcoidosis and control patients, 1.5 ± 3.8% and 0.4 ± 0.2%, respectively, were similar ($p > .3$).

TABLE 1 shows the quantities of all four IgG subclasses, expressed as percentages of the quantity of albumin, in the lavage fluids of patients with sarcoidosis and of

TABLE 1. BAL IgG Subclass Levels

	Subclass Level[a]			
	IgG1	IgG2	IgG3	IgG4
Sarcoidosis patients ($N = 39$)	28.3 ± 23.1[b]	7.9 ± 6.3	1.9 ± 1.9[c]	0.17 ± 0.23[d]
Normal patients ($N = 9$)	7.1 ± 3.7	4.6 ± 3.6	0.1 ± 0.1	0.27 ± 0.24

[a] All subclass levels are expressed as IgG/albumin × 100.
[b] $p < .004$.
[c] $p < .001$.
[d] $p < .04$.

normal controls. IgG1 was the most abundant IgG subclass found in the lavage of patients with sarcoidosis; furthermore, its percentage in sarcoidosis patients, 28.3 ± 23.1%, was significantly greater than its percentage in normal controls, 7.1 ± 3.7% ($p < .004$). Levels of IgG2, the next most abundant IgG subclass, were similar in sarcoidosis patients (7.9 ± 6.3%) and normal controls (4.6 ± 3.6%). In addition to IgG1, IgG3 levels also were significantly greater in patients (1.9 ± 1.9%) than in normal controls (0.1 ± 0.1%) ($p < .001$). In contrast, BAL IgG4 levels were significantly lower for sarcoidosis patients, 0.17 ± 0.23%, than they were for controls, 0.27 ± 0.24% ($p = .04$). Representation of BAL IgG subclasses as a percentage of the total amount of protein yielded similar results.

TABLE 2 presents the IgG subclass quantities determined in the serum of patients and controls. IgG1, as in BAL, was the most abundant IgG subclass found in the patients with sarcoidosis. The mean serum value of IgG1 for sarcoidosis patients, 6.1 ± 3.8 mg/ml, was greater than that for controls, 3.6 ± 1.9 mg/ml, but this difference was not quite significant statistically ($p = .08$). Serum IgG2 levels in patients, 2.4 ±

1.7 mg/ml, were similar to those in controls, 2.4 ± 1.4 mg/ml. Serum IgG3 levels in patients, 0.41 ± 0.34 mg/ml, were higher to a significant degree compared to those in controls, 0.03 ± 0.01 mg/ml (p = .003); serum IgG4 levels in patients, 0.02 ± 0.02 mg/ml, were significantly lower than control values, 0.07 ± 0.06 mg/ml (p = .005).

Previous work by others[17,18] and ourselves[16] has demonstrated that the numbers of IgG-releasing cells in BAL of patients with sarcoidosis exceeds the numbers of those in their blood, suggesting that some IgG production occurs locally in the lung-lining fluid of these patients. As an indirect assessment of whether or not local production of all IgG subclasses occurs in lung-lining fluid of patients with sarcoidosis, we compared IgG subclass:albumin ratios in BAL with blood ratios. As shown in TABLE 3, IgG subclass:albumin ratios for all four subclasses in BAL of patients exceeded their respective serum ratios to a significant degree. BAL IgG1/Alb% of patients, 28.3 ± 23.1%, exceeded the serum value, 15.7 ± 9.9% ($p \leq .001$); BAL IgG2/Alb% of patients, 7.9 ± 6.3%, exceeded the serum value, 6.1 ± 4.3% ($p \leq .005$); BAL IgG3/Alb% of patients, 1.9 ± 1.9%, exceeded the serum value, 1.0 ± 0.8% ($p \leq .002$); and BAL IgG4/Alb% of patients, 0.17 ± 0.13%, exceeded the serum value, 0.06 ± 0.06% ($p \leq .001$).

DISCUSSION

These studies reveal that IgG1 and IgG3 levels are elevated to a significant degree in a large group of patients with sarcoidosis who have elevated levels of total IgG in lung lavage fluid and serum. BAL and serum IgG2 levels were similar in patients and normals. In contrast, IgG4 levels were significantly lower in BAL and serum of patients. The precise significance of these findings is unclear. Several points, however, are worthy of discussion.

Sarcoidosis is a disease associated with heightened bone marrow-derived (B) cell activity.[21] The single most frequently reported indicator of this fact is the presence of polyclonal hypergammaglobulinemia in many patients with this disease.[14,16,21] Immunoglobulin levels—most commonly those of IgG—also are elevated in the BAL of patients with sarcoidosis.[14–16] Coupled with the finding of hypergammaglobulinemia

TABLE 2. Serum IgG Subclass Levels

	Subclass Level[a]			
	IgG1	IgG2	IgG3	IgG4
Sarcoidosis patients (N = 39)	6.1 ± 3.8	2.4 ± 1.7	0.41 ± 0.34[b]	0.02 ± 0.02[c]
Normal patients (N = 9)	3.6 ± 1.9	2.4 ± 1.4	0.03 ± 0.01	0.07 ± 0.06

[a]All subclass levels are expressed in mg/ml.
[b]p = .003.
[c]p = .005.

TABLE 3. BAL and Serum IgG Subclass Levels in Sarcoidosis

	Subclass Level[a]			
	IgG1	IgG2	IgG3	IgG4
BAL	28.3 ± 23.1[b]	7.9 ± 6.3[c]	1.9 ± 1.9[d]	0.17 ± 0.13[e]
Serum	15.7 ± 9.9	6.1 ± 4.3	1.0 ± 0.8	0.06 ± 0.06

[a]All subclass levels expressed as IgG/albumin × 100.
[b]$p \leq .001$.
[c]$p \leq .005$.
[d]$p \leq .002$.
[e]$p \leq .001$.

is the observation that high titers of serum antibody to several antigens are observed frequently.[21] More recent studies have shown that increased numbers of IgG-releasing cells (presumably plasma cells) are present in both the blood and the lung-lining fluid of patients with sarcoidosis.[16–18] Indeed, it appears that increases in the number of IgG-releasing cells at sites of disease activity, such as the lung, are responsible for the elevations of IgG in BAL and serum.[16–18]

The data presented in this study suggest, but do not prove, that IgG1 and IgG3 production is elevated in patients with sarcoidosis and hypergammaglobulinemia, and that it is the elevations in these two subclasses which account for the overall increase in IgG levels. At least two additional factors must be examined before a more definitive statement can be made. First, binding studies of specific IgG subclasses to cells and/or tissue should be performed. Since pure preparations of IgG subclasses have become available only in the past several years, studies of subclass binding to receptors on cells such as alveolar macrophages have just begun to appear.[8] Naegel and co-workers examined alveolar macrophages from normal individuals and demonstrated that IgG1 and IgG3 became attached to a greater number of these cells than did the other two subclasses.[8] Similar studies using alveolar macrophages from patients with sarcoidosis are currently in progress.

Secondly, an additional component that will require investigation is the rate(s) of metabolism of the various IgG subclasses. Some evidence suggests that the serum half-lives of the IgG subclasses differ markedly. IgG1, IgG2, and IgG4 appear to have half-lives of about 21 days whereas the half-life of IgG3 is much shorter, approximately 7 days.[1–3] To what degree these half-lives differ, if at all, in patients with sarcoidosis is yet to be studied. But, it is conceivable that prolongations in selective subclass degradation could elevate IgG1 and IgG3 levels, and accelerated metabolism could explain the decrease in levels of IgG4. This possibility appears unlikely, however, because assays have detected an increased number of cells releasing IgG in the BAL and blood of patients with sarcoidosis.[16–18]

The presence of immune complexes in the serum of many patients with sarcoidosis[21] is another indicator of heightened B cell activity. In this regard our observation of elevations in the IgG1 and IgG3 levels in BAL and serum is of interest. These two IgG subclasses fix complement to a greater extent than IgG2, and IgG4 does not fix complement at all.[6,7] It appears likely that the immune complexes detected by the Raji cell assay (which detects immune complexes that fix complement) in sarcoidosis patients[22] are composed of IgG1 or IgG3 subclass immunoglobulin. The role of immune complexes in sarcoidosis is unknown. Current evidence suggests that the alveolar macrophage and lung thymus-derived (T) lymphocyte are the cells primarily responsible for the alveolitis seen in this disease.[23] If alveolar macrophages from patients with sarcoidosis possess receptors for IgG1 and IgG3, immune complexes containing these subclasses could bind to and assist in perpetuating this cell's activated state. One consequence of uncovering this sequence of events would be that a new therapeutic point of attack would become available.

The decreased levels of IgG4 in the BAL and serum of our patients is also of interest. Several pieces of evidence suggest that a normal immunologic response to chronic antigen stimulation is characterized by an elevation in serum IgG4 levels. Aalberse and co-workers have studied this response by performing longitudinal studies on beekeepers.[12] After a few initial stings in the novice beekeeper, the serum IgG antibody response to bee venom is located primarily within the IgG1 subclass. In contrast, after several years with repeated bee stings, there is a shift from an IgG1- to an IgG4-dominated response.[12] In another study Iskander and co-workers assessed IgG subclass levels in patients with recently contracted and chronic schistosomiasis. Patients with the chronic form of disease had significantly greater serum IgG4 levels than individuals who had recently contracted the disease.[13] Clearly, sarcoidosis is a chronic disorder. If this disease is due to continuous exposure to an as yet unidentified agent(s), then the depressed levels of IgG4 found in serum and BAL might indicate this disease is characterized by a disordered immune response. Merrill and co-workers recently presented data showing that patients with chronic hypersensitivity pneumonitis also have elevated IgG1 levels and decreased IgG4 levels in BAL and serum.[24] Of interest was their observation that four individuals treated with corticosteroids demonstrated increases in IgG4 levels to normal range. Longitudinal studies on both treated and untreated sarcoidosis patients are in progress.

In summary, the profile of IgG subclasses found in BAL and serum of a large group of patients with sarcoidosis consists of elevated levels of IgG1 and IgG3 and decreased levels of IgG4. It is likely that increases in the production of IgG1 and IgG3 by a hyperactive B cell system are responsible, at least in part, for the elevations in these two subclasses. The reason(s) for the depressed levels of IgG4 are not known. Future studies of IgG subclasses should provide important insights into the immunopathogenesis of sarcoidosis.

REFERENCES

1. YOUNT, W. J., M. M. DORNER, H. G. KUNKEL & E. A. KABAT. 1968. Studies on human antibodies. IV. Selective variations in subgroup composition and genetic marker. J. Exp. Med. **127:** 633-646.
2. SPIEGELBERG, H. L. & W. O. WEIGLE. 1965. The catabolism of homologous and heterologous 7S gammaglobulin fragments. J. Exp. Med. **121:** 323-338.
3. MORELL, A., W. D. TERRY & T. A. WALDMANN. 1970. Metabolic properties of IgG subclasses in man. J. Clin. Invest. **49:** 673-680.
4. RIESEN, W. F., F. SKVARIL & D. B. BROWN. 1976. Natural infection of man with group A streptococci: Levels; restriction in class, subclass, and type; and clonal appearance of polysaccharide-group-specific antibodies. Scand. J. Immunol. **5:** 383-390.
5. BECK, C. S. & D. C. HEINER. 1981. Selective immunoglobulin G4 deficiency and recurrent infections of the respiratory tract. Am. Rev. Respir. Dis. **124:** 94-96.
6. KURLANDER, R. J., W. F. ROSSE & G. L. LOGUE. 1977. Qualitative influence of antibody and complement coating of red cells on monocyte-mediated cell lysis. J. Clin. Invest. **61:** 1309-1319.

7. ABRAMSON, N., E. W. GELFAND, J. H. JANDI & F. S. ROSEN. 1970. The interaction between human monocytes and red cells. Specificity for IgG subclasses and IgG fragments. J. Exp. Med. **132:** 1207-1215.
8. NAEGEL, G. P., K. R. YOUNG, JR. & H. Y. REYNOLDS. 1984. Receptors for human IgG subclass on human alveolar macrophages. Am. Rev. Respir. Dis. **129:** 413-418.
9. HUBER, H., S. D. DOUGLAS, J. NUSBACHER, S. KOCKWA & R. E. ROSENFIELD. 1971. IgG subclass specificity of human monocyte receptor sites. Nature **229:** 419-420.
10. HEINER, D. C. 1984. Significance of immunoglobulin G subclasses. Am. J. Med. **76:** 1-6.
11. PERLMUTTER, L. 1984. IgG4: Non-IgE-mediated atopic disease. Ann. Allergy **52:** 64-69.
12. AALBERSE, R. C., R. VAN DERGOOG & J. VAN LEEWEN. 1983. Serologic aspects of IgG4 antibodies. I. Prolonged immunization results in a IgG4-restricted response. J. Immunol. **130:** 722-726.
13. ISKANDER, R., P. K. DAS & R. C. AALBERSE. 1981. IgG4 antibodies in Egyptian patients with schistosomiasis. Int. Arch. Allergy Appl. Immunol. **66:** 200-207.
14. HUNNINGHAKE, G. W., J. E. GADEK, O. KAWANAMI, J. FERRANS & R. G. CRYSTAL. 1979. Inflammatory and immune processes in the human lung in health and disease: Evaluation by bronchoalveolar lavage. Am. J. Pathol. **97:** 149-206.
15. VALEYRE, D., G. SAUMAN, D. BLADIER, J. AMOUROUX, J. PRE, J.-P. BATTESTI & R. GEORGES. 1982. The relationship between noninvasive explorations in pulmonary sarcoidosis of recent origin, as shown in bronchoalveolar lavage, serum and pulmonary function tests. Am. Rev. Respir. Dis. **126:** 41-45.
16. RANKIN, J. A., G. P. NAEGEL, C. E. SCHRADER, R. A. MATTHAY & H. Y. REYNOLDS. 1983. Airspace immunoglobulin production and levels in bronchoalveolar lavage fluid (BAL) of normals and patients with sarcoidosis. Am. Rev. Respir. Dis. **127:** 442-448.
17. LAWRENCE, E. C., R. R. MARTIN, R. M. BLAESE, R. B. TEAGUE, R. J. AWE, R. K. WILSON, W. J. DEATON, K. BLOOM, S. D. GREENBURG & P. M. STEVENS. 1980. Increased bronchoalveolar IgG-secreting cells in interstitial lung diseases. N. Engl. J. Med. **302:** 1186-1188.
18. HUNNINGHAKE, G. W. & R. G. CRYSTAL. 1981. Mechanisms of hypergammaglobulinemia in pulmonary sarcoidosis. J. Clin. Invest. **67:** 86-92.
19. LOWRY, O. H., N. J. ROSENBROUGH, A. L. FARR & R. J. RANDALL. 1951. Protein measurement with the Folin phenol reagent. J. Biol. Chem. **193:** 265-275.
20. MERRILL, W. W., G. P. NAEGEL, J. OLCHOWSKI & H. Y. REYNOLDS. 1985. Immunoglobulin G subclass proteins in serum and lavage fluid of normal subjects: Quantitation and comparison to immunoglobulins A and E. Am. Rev. Respir. Dis. **131:** 584-587.
21. DANIELE, R. P., J. H. DAUBER & M. D. ROSSMAN. 1980. Immunologic abnormalities in sarcoidosis. Ann. Intern. Med. **92:** 406-416.
22. DANIELE, R. P., P. M. HENSON, J. C. FANTONE III, P. A. WARD & R. B. DREISIN. 1981. Immune complex injury of the lung. Am. Rev. Respir. Dis. **124:** 738-755.
23. CRYSTAL, R. G., P. B. BITTERMAN, S. I. RENNARD, A. J. HANCE & B. A. KEOGH. 1984. Interstitial lung diseases of unknown cause. N. Engl. J. Med. **310:** 154-166, 235-244.
24. MERRILL, W. W., G. P. NAEGEL, J. OLCHOWSKI & H. Y. REYNOLDS. 1984. Immunoglobulin G subclasses in blood and lavage fluid of patients with hypersensitivity pneumonitis. Clin. Res. **32:** 427A.

Different Expansions of T Lymphocyte Subpopulations in the Lung and Corticosteroid-induced Changes in Patients with Active Pulmonary Sarcoidosis[a]

GIOVANNI A. ROSSI,[b,c] OLIVIERO SACCO,[d]
ELISABETTA COSULICH,[d] BRUNO BALBI,[c]
ANGELA RISSO,[d] AND CESARE RAVAZZONI[c]

[c]*First Division of Pneumology*
San Martino Hospital
Genoa, Italy

[d]*University Institute of Biochemistry*
Genoa, Italy

INTRODUCTION

Pulmonary sarcoidosis is a chronic disorder characterized by a mononuclear cell inflammation ("alveolitis"); interstitial noncaseating granulomata; changes in alveolar epithelial, endothelial, and mesenchymal cells; and interstitial fibrosis.[1–3] Although the granulomata have been considered to be central to the pathogenesis of pulmonary sarcoidosis, it is now recognized that the alveolitis is the first manifestation of the disease and causes the disarrangement of the alveolar structures.[4–5] The alveolitis in active untreated sarcoidosis is characterized by a marked increase in the number of thymus-derived (T) lymphocytes and, to a lesser degree, of alveolar macrophages.[5–7] Current concepts of the pathogenesis of this disease suggest that the T lymphocytes play an important role in 1) modulating the formation of granulomata,[8] 2) inducing the expansion of responsive T cells,[9,10] 3) providing nonspecific "help" for immunoglobulin production by bone marrow-derived (B) cells,[11] and 4) activating alveolar macrophages through the release of gamma interferon.[12]

The increased numbers of T lymphocytes in the alveolar structures and the enhanced immune effector functions of these cells are associated to marked changes in the proportions of subpopulations of T cells present. Patients with active, untreated sarcoidosis have increased percentages of lung helper T cells recognized by the OKT4 monoclonal antibody and have decreased percentages of the lung suppressor T cells

[a]Supported by Grants 83.00469.04 and 83.028404.56 from the Consiglio Nazionale delle Ricerche, Rome, Italy.

[b]Address for correspondence and reprint requests: First Division of Pneumology, San Martino Hospital, Viale Benedetto XV, 10, 16132 Genoa, Italy.

recognized by the OKT8 monoclonal antibody; thus the T helper to T suppressor cell ratio is markedly increased at sites of disease activity in this disorder.[13] Using monoclonal antibodies specific for helper T cell subpopulations with different functions, it is possible to analyze the different expansions of helper T cell subtypes and to speculate on the roles of the different subpopulations in the pathogenesis of pulmonary sarcoidosis. Recently, a monoclonal antibody named 5/9 has been used to identify a small T cell subpopulation with helper functions.[14] The surface antigen recognized by the 5/9 monoclonal antibody is present on about the 30% of the OKT4$^+$ cells and reacts with only 15-20% of peripheral T cells from normal subjects. The 5/9$^+$ lymphocytes are responsible for many T cell activities, such as T cell proliferation in response to allogenic cells or to soluble antigens and T cell helper function for the pokeweed mitogen-driven bone marrow-derived (B) cells.[14,15] In addition, the presence of the 5/9$^+$ T cells is necessary to induce the 5/9$^-$ cells to develop cytolytic activity.[15]

The purpose of the present study is to describe the expansion and the functional characteristics of the 5/9$^+$ T lymphocytes in pulmonary sarcoidosis and to evaluate the sensitivity to corticosteroid treatment of this T cell subset in patients with active lung disease.

MATERIALS AND METHODS

Study Population

Patients with biopsy-proven pulmonary sarcoidosis that had not been treated in the 12 months prior to this study were divided into two groups according to the activity of the lung disease assessed from the percentages of T lymphocytes in bronchoalveolar lavage fluid and from gallium-67 (^{67}Ga) lung scans. Patients were considered to have high-intensity alveolitis if they had 28% or more T lymphocytes in bronchoalveolar lavage fluid and a positive ^{67}Ga lung scan, and to have low-intensity alveolitis if they had less than 28% T lymphocytes in the lavage fluid and a negative ^{67}Ga lung scan.[16] The above criteria were used to characterize the activity of the lung disease because most untreated patients with high-intensity alveolitis have functional deteriorations within 6 months whereas most patients with low-intensity alveolitis remain in stable condition.[17,18]

Normal Controls

Normal nonsmokers were used as controls. The results of pulmonary function tests and chest radiographs were within normal limits in all normal subjects.

Preparation of Inflammatory and Immune Effector Cells

Cells were obtained from the lower respiratory tract by bronchoalveolar lavage, as previously described,[19] by infusing 100 ml of sterile saline solution in five 20-ml aliquots into segments of the lingula or of the middle lobe. In each subject one or two segments were lavaged. Heparinized venous blood was obtained immediately before the lavage procedure. Differential cell counts were carried out on cytocentrifuge preparations.[20,21] Mononuclear cells were isolated by Hypaque-Ficoll centrifugation.[22]

Purification of Lung and Blood T Lymphocytes

T lymphocytes were identified by their ability to form rosettes with neuraminidase-treated sheep red blood cells (N-SRBC's) at 4° C.[23] Purified T lymphocytes were obtained after rosette formation: mononuclear cell suspensions from blood and lavage were supplemented with N-SRBC's twice at 4° C and subsequently subjected to Hypaque-Ficoll centrifugation.[20]

Identification of T Lymphocyte Subpopulations

T lymphocyte suspensions from lung and blood were tested with the murine monoclonal antibodies OKT4 (Ortho Diagnostic Systems, Milan) and 5/9, as previously described.[13,19] Briefly, the monoclonal antibodies OKT4 or 5/9 were added to the T cell suspensions at 4° C for 30 min; the cells were then washed, and a fluorescein-conjugated $F(ab')_2$ goat antimouse immunoglobulin reagent was added to the T cell suspensions at 4° C for an additional 30 min. The cells were then washed three times and examined by fluorescence microscopy.

Isolation of the 5/9⁺ T Cell Subset

The $5/9^+$ T cell subset was isolated from lung T cell suspensions by the chromium chloride rosette-formation method.[24] Briefly, ox red blood cells (ORBE's) coated with the 5/9 monoclonal antibody were added to the T cell suspensions and the rosette-forming T cells separated by Hypaque-Ficoll centrifugation, as previously described.[25]

Spontaneous Secretion of Monocyte Chemotactic Factor

Supernatants of unseparated $5/9^+$ and $5/9^-$ lung T cells, from patients with pulmonary sarcoidosis and high-intensity alveolitis, were obtained by culturing the unstimulated cells in sterile microtiter plates, as previously described.[8,25] The cells were cultured for 48 hr, and then the supernatants were harvested and filtered. Assays to determine the amount of monocyte chemotactic factor in the supernatants were performed using a Blindwell micropore filter chamber technique with normal blood mononuclear cells. Chemotactic activity was expressed as cells per high-power field reaching the lower surface of the filter in the presence of supernatants, minus the cells per high-power field reaching the lower surface of the filter in presence of RPMI-1640 alone.

Polyclonal Activation of B Lymphocytes

Unseparated $5/9^+$ and $5/9^-$ lung T cell populations from patients with active pulmonary sarcoidosis were co-cultured with autologous peripheral blood non-T cells in the presence of pokeweed mitogen, as previously described.[25] After 7 days the supernatants were harvested, and the amounts of the immunoglobulins present were determined by solid-phase immunoassay, using ^{125}I-labeled goat antihuman immunoglobulins and measuring the amount of radioactivity present with an autogamma scintillation spectrometer.

Spontaneous Release of Interleukin-2

Unseparated $5/9^+$ and $5/9^-$ lung T cells from patients with active pulmonary sarcoidosis were cultured for 48 hr in RPMI-1640 with 1% fetal calf serum.[9,10,26] The supernatants were then assayed for interleukin-2 activity by their ability to stimulate the incorporation of [^{3}H]thymidine in the CTL-L T cells, a murine interleukin-2-dependent cell line (kindly provided by L. Moretta), as previously described.[26]

Treatment Protocol

After proven diagnosis of active pulmonary sarcoidosis, patients received oral prednisone at the dose of 0.75 mg/kg daily for 6 weeks. The prednisone dose was then lowered by 0.25 mg/kg each week until a maintenance dose of 0.25 mg/kg daily was reached.[27]

Bronchoalveolar lavage was repeated after 3 and 6 months of therapy.

RESULTS

Bronchoalveolar lavage was performed without difficulty or complications in normal controls and in patients with sarcoidosis. The total amounts of fluid recovered were similar in the three groups of subjects, although the total numbers of bronchoalveolar cells were, compared to normals, about twofold higher in patients with sarcoidosis and low-intensity alveolitis and fourfold higher in patients with sarcoidosis and high-intensity alveolitis (TABLE 1).[19] The proportions of cells from lavage fluid that were T lymphocytes were significantly higher in patients with high-intensity alveolitis than in patients with low-intensity alveolitis or in control subjects ($p < .05$

TABLE 1. Total Numbers and Proportions of Cells Present in Bronchoalveolar Lavage[a]

Patient Groups	Total Number of Cells[b] (× 10^6)	Lymphocytes (% of Lavage Cells)	T Lymphocytes (% of Lymphocytes)	T Lymphocyte Subpopulations (% of T Lymphocytes) OKT4$^+$	5/9$^+$
Normal controls	9±2	7±2	72±4	48±3	13±2
Sarcoidosis					
High-intensity alveolitis	36±5	55±9	93±2	85±5	85±6
Low-intensity alveolitis	22±4	16±4	85±3	55±4	38±4

[a]All results are means ± SEM's.
[b]Number of cells recovered from 100 ml of lavage fluid.

for each comparison). In addition patients with high-intensity alveolitis had significantly higher proportions of OKT4$^+$ and 5/9$^+$ T cells in bronchoalveolar lavage fluid than patients with low-intensity alveolitis or normal controls ($p < .05$ for each comparison). Interestingly, patients with low-intensity alveolitis had, compared to normal controls, similar proportions of OKT4$^+$ T cells ($p > .2$) but increased percentages of 5/9$^+$ T cells ($p < .05$). In addition, compared to normal controls, patients with high-intensity alveolitis had an approximately twofold increase in the percentages of lung OKT4$^+$ T cells, but a fivefold increase in the percentages of 5/9$^+$ T cells; these data suggest a preferential expansion of the 5/9$^+$ T cell subpopulation at sites of disease activity in pulmonary sarcoidosis.[19]

Functional Evaluation of the 5/9$^+$ Lung T Cells in Patients with High-intensity Alveolitis

Unfractionated T cells, the 5/9$^+$ T cell fractions, and the 5/9$^-$ T cell fractions recovered by bronchoalveolar lavage from patients with pulmonary sarcoidosis and high-intensity alveolitis have been evaluated for secretion of mediators relevant to the pathogenesis of the disease.[25,26]

The supernatants of unfractionated lung T cells cultured for 48 hr contained large amounts of chemotactic factor for blood mononuclear cells, and this activity appeared to be related to the 5/9$^+$ T cell fraction because the supernatants from the purified 5/9$^+$ T cells showed similar levels of chemotactic activity whereas the supernatants from the 5/9$^-$ T cells did not have significant levels of monocyte chemotactic factor (TABLE 2).[25]

Similarly unfractionated lung T lymphocytes and the 5/9$^+$ lung T cell fractions from patients with pulmonary sarcoidosis and high-intensity alveolitis were able to induce autologous peripheral blood B cell differentiation and immunoglobulin production with pokeweed mitogen stimulation (TABLE 2). In contrast, no immunoglobulin production was detected when autologous B cells were co-cultured with the 5/9$^-$ lung T cell fractions.[25] When the supernatants from unfractionated lung T cells, the 5/9$^+$ and the 5/9$^-$ lung T cell fractions, were tested for the spontaneous release of interleukin-2 (TABLE 2), the unfractionated T cells and the $5/9^+$ T cell fractions from patients with sarcoidosis and high-intensity alveolitis were found to release interleukin-2 whereas no or very little interleukin-2 activity was found in the supernatants of the $5/9^-$ T cell fractions.[26]

Corticosteroid-induced Effects on the T Cell Alveolitis

All patients tolerated the corticosteroid therapy well, and in no case were major side effects noted. Bronchoalveolar lavage analyses showed improvement of the lymphocytic alveolitis in all patients after the 3 months of prednisone therapy. Interestingly, although there was only a slight decrease in the percentage of lung T lymphocytes present (52 ± 5% of the bronchoalveolar cells before treatment, 43 ± 3% after treatment; $p < .05$) (FIG. 1A), corticosteroid treatment caused a marked reduction in the percentage of the helper T cell subset recognized by the 5/9 monoclonal antibody (40 ± 4% of the bronchoalveolar cells before treatment, 17 ± 2% after treatment; $p < .01$) (FIG. 1B). After 6 months of therapy both the proportions of lymphocytes and of $5/9^+$ T cells were decreased in a similar fashion compared to the pretreatment values ($p < .001$ for each comparison).

DISCUSSION

Pulmonary sarcoidosis is a disease characterized by a heightened cellular immune response within the lung involving T lymphocytes and alveolar macrophages.[1–7] This macrophage-lymphocyte alveolitis is associated with increased numbers of T lymphocytes in the alveolar structure that result in an imbalance of T cell subpopulations that are recognized by different monoclonal antibodies: the proportion of the $OKT8^+$ suppressor/inducer lung T cells is markedly decreased whereas the percentage of the $OKT4^+$ helper/suppressor lung T cells is increased.[13] Within the helper T cell subtypes, however, the subpopulation recognized by the 5/9 monoclonal antibody appears to be preferentially expanded in the lungs of patients with active disease.[19] Moreover, in normal subjects the 5/9 monoclonal antibody reacts with only 30% of the $OKT4^+$ T cells and 20% of the total T cells[14] whereas in pulmonary sarcoidosis most of the

TABLE 2. Functions of Unfractionated T Cells and of T Cell Subpopulations[a]

Secretion of Mediators	Total T Cells	$5/9^+$ T Cells	$5/9^-$ T Cells
Monocyte chemotactic factor	Yes	Yes	No
Help for immunoglobulin production	Yes	Yes	No
Interleukin-2	Yes	Yes	No

[a]The T cells were recovered by bronchoalveolar lavage from patients with pulmonary sarcoidosis and high-intensity alveolitis. See Rossi *et al.*[25,26] for details.

lung T cells express both the OKT4 and the 5/9 surface antigens.[19] Although caution must be used in evaluating T lymphocyte subsets only by surface antigens, the proliferation of the T lymphocytes within the alveolar structures in this disorder seems to preferentially involve the OKT4$^+$ 5/9$^+$ T cell subset. This hypothesis is supported by the functional studies on the 5/9$^+$ lung T cells isolated from bronchoalveolar lavage in patients with sarcoidosis and high-intensity alveolitis.[25,26] These studies have demonstrated that the T cell subset recognized by the 5/9 monoclonal antibody is responsible in pulmonary sarcoidosis for attracting blood monocytes into the alveolar structures, for immunoglobulin production by B lymphocytes, and for the secretion of interleukin-2, the mediator which stimulates the proliferation of responsive T lymphocytes.[25,26]

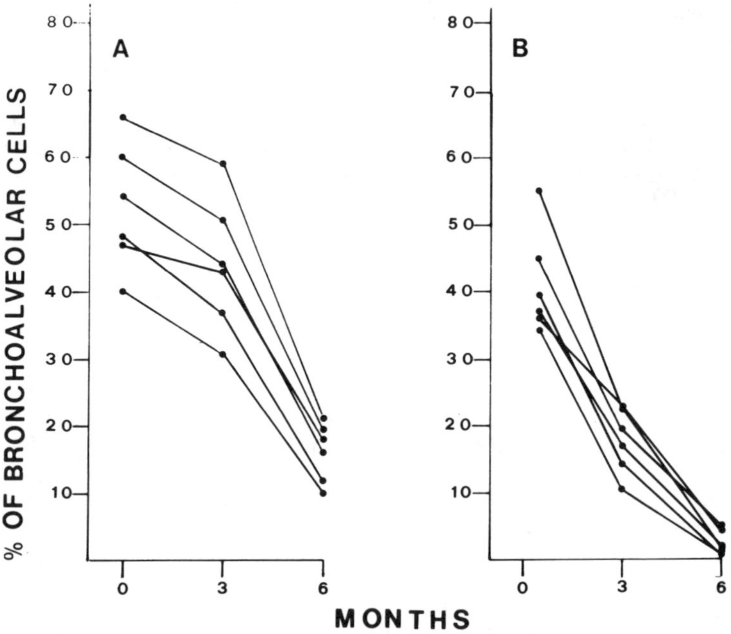

FIGURE 1. Sequential evaluation of patients with active pulmonary sarcoidosis by bronchoalveolar lavage. (**A**) Percentages of T lymphocytes recovered. (**B**) Percentages of 5/9$^+$ T lymphocytes recovered. The data represent the results obtained in six patients.

Although the mechanisms responsible for T lymphocyte activation and for the proliferation and/or attraction to the lung of T lymphocytes have not been entirely clarified, the available evidence suggests that the evaluation of the T cell proportions in bronchoalveolar lavage, together with the ^{67}Ga uptake, accurately reflects the alveolitis of pulmonary sarcoidosis, predicts the functional outcome of the patients, and accurately evaluates the response to treatment.[17,18,27]

Analysis of T cell subpopulations after 3 and 6 months of oral prednisone therapy suggests that the suppression of the T cell alveolitis is modulated, at an earlier stage, by the marked decrease in the percentages of the 5/9$^+$ T lymphocytes when the numbers of T cells present in the alveolar structures are still elevated. This finding is consistent with a recent report by Pinkston and Crystal[28] that shows a suppression of interleukin-2 release by oral prednisone therapy prior to the decrease of the percentages of lung T cells.

These data show that the studies of the T cell subpopulations, their state of activation, and their functions may not only be a more sensitive monitor of disease activity but also a useful tool to evaluate the early response to therapy and to find the minimal dose of corticosteroids necessary to suppress the exaggerated inflammatory and immune processes that characterize this disorder.

In this context the 5/9 monoclonal antibody seems to be a reliable marker of activity in pulmonary sarcoidosis.

SUMMARY

Pulmonary sarcoidosis is a disease characterized by increased numbers of T lymphocytes within the alveolar structures and the consequent spontaneous release of a variety of mediators relevant to the pathogenesis of this disorder. This phenomenon is associated with a different expansion of the T cell subpopulations present in the lung. Using monoclonal antibodies specific for T cell subsets with helper functions, we have evaluated the different T lymphocyte subpopulations present in patients with active and inactive pulmonary sarcoidosis. The small fraction of helper T cells recognized by the 5/9 monoclonal antibody appear to be preferentially expanded in the lung of patients with active disease. The functions of the $5/9^+$ lung T cells in pulmonary sarcoidosis were evaluated by considering the spontaneous release of monocyte chemotactic factor, the help in immunoglobulin production, and the spontaneous production of interleukin-2 by the $5/9^+$ lung T cells from patients with active disease. These T cell functions appeared to be restricted to the $5/9^+$ T cell subset.

The sensitivity of the $5/9^+$ lung T cells to corticosteroid treatment in pulmonary sarcoidosis was studied by performing bronchoalveolar lavage in patients with active disease before and after oral prednisone therapy. Evaluation of lymphocyte subsets after 3 months of therapy showed a marked reduction of $5/9^+$ T cell percentages even though the overall proportion of lavage cells that were T lymphocytes was still elevated.

Thus the 5/9 monoclonal antibody may be considered a good marker in gauging the activity of the alveolitis in pulmonary sarcoidosis because it recognizes the T cell subsets responsible for many activities relevant to the pathogenesis of this disorder.

In addition, analysis of the proportions of $5/9^+$ lung T cells may result in a useful means to evaluate the early response to therapy.

REFERENCES

1. Scadding, J. G. 1967. Sarcoidosis. Eyre and Spottiswoode. London.
2. Mitchell, D. N. & J. G. Scadding. 1974. Sarcoidosis. Am. Rev. Respir. Dis. **110:** 774-802.
3. Carrington, C. B., E. A. Gaensler, J. P. Mikus, A. W. Schacter, G. W. Burke & A. M. Goff. 1976. Structure and function in sarcoidosis. Ann. N.Y. Acad. Sci. **278:** 265-278.

4. Rosen, Y., T. J. Athanassiades, S. Moon & H. A. Lyons. 1978. Nongranulomatous interstitial pneumonitis in sarcoidosis: Relationship to development of epithelioid granulomas. Chest **74:** 122-125.
5. Crystal, R. G., W. C. Roberts, G. W. Hunninghake, J. E. Gadek, J. D. Fulmer & B. R. Line. 1981. Pulmonary sarcoidosis: A disease characterized and perpetuated by activated lung T lymphocytes. Ann. Intern. Med. **94:** 73-94.
6. Hunninghake, G. W., B. A. Keogh, B. R. Line, J. E. Gadek, O. Kawanami, V. J. Ferrans & R. G. Crystal. 1981. Pulmonary sarcoidosis: Pathogenesis and therapy. *In* Basic and Clinical Aspects of Granulomatous Disease. D. Boros & T. Yoshida, Eds.: 275-290. Elsevier/North-Holland, New York, NY.
7. Crystal, R. G., G. W. Hunninghake, J. E. Gadek, B. A. Keogh, S. I. Rennard & P. B. Bitterman. 1983. State of the art: The pathogenesis of sarcoidosis. *In* Sarcoidosis and Other Granulomatous Disorders. J. Chrétien, J. Marsac & J. C. Saltiel, Eds.: 13-35. Pergamon Press. Paris.
8. Hunninghake, G. W., J. E. Gadek, R. C. Young, Jr., O. Kawanami, V. J. Ferrans & R. G. Crystal. 1980. Maintenance of granuloma formation in pulmonary sarcoidosis by T lymphocytes within the lung. N. Engl. J. Med. **302:** 594-598.
9. Pinkston, P., P. B. Bitterman & R. G. Crystal. 1983. Spontaneous release of interleukin-2 by lung T lymphocytes in active pulmonary sarcoidosis. N. Engl. J. Med. **308:** 793-800.
10. Hunninghake, G. W., G. N. Bedell, D. C. Zavala, M. Monick & M. Brady. 1983. Role of interleukin-2 release by lung T cells in active pulmonary sarcoidosis. Am. Rev. Respir. Dis. **128:** 634-638.
11. Hunninghake, G. W. & R. G. Crystal. 1981. Mechanisms of hypergammaglobulinemia in pulmonary sarcoidosis: Site of increased antibody production and role of T lymphocytes. J. Clin. Invest. **67:** 86-92.
12. Robinson, B. W. & R. G. Crystal. 1985. Gamma interferon is spontaneously released by alveolar macrophages and lung T lymphocytes in patients with pulmonary sarcoidosis. J. Clin. Invest. **75:** 1488-1495.
13. Hunninghake, G. W. & R. G. Crystal. 1981. Pulmonary sarcoidosis: A disorder mediated by excess helper T lymphocyte at sites of disease activity. N. Engl. J. Med. **305:** 429-434.
14. Corte, G., M. C. Mingari, A. Moretta, G. Damiani, L. Moretta & A. Bargellesi. 1982. Human T cell subpopulations defined by a monoclonal antibody. I. A small subset is responsible for proliferation to allogenic cells or to soluble antigens and for helper activity for B cell differentiation. J. Immunol. **128:** 16-19.
15. Moretta, A., G. Corte, M. C. Mingari & L. Moretta. 1982. Human T cell subpopulations defined by a monoclonal antibody. II. Evidence for cell cooperation in response to alloantigens and generation of cytolitic cells. J. Immunol. **128:** 20-24.
16. Line, B. R., G. W. Hunninghake, B. A. Keogh, A. E. Jones, G. S. Johnston & R. G. Crystal. 1981. Gallium-67 scanning to stage the alveolitis in sarcoidosis: Correlation with clinical studies, pulmonary function studies and bronchoalveolar lavage. Am. Rev. Respir. Dis. **123:** 440-446.
17. B. A. Keogh, G. W. Hunninghake, B. R. Line, D. Price, R. Young & R. G. Crystal. 1980. Therapy decisions in sarcoidosis: Prospective use of bronchoalveolar lavage and gallium-67 scanning. Am. Rev. Respir. Dis. **121:** 155.
18. Keogh, B. A., G. W. Hunninghake, B. R. Line & R. G. Crystal. 1983. The alveolitis of pulmonary sarcoidosis: Evaluation of natural history and alveolitis-dependent changes in lung functions. Am. Rev. Respir. Dis. **128:** 256-265.
19. Rossi, G. A., O. Sacco, E. Cosulich, G. Damini, G. Corte, A. Bargellesi & C. Ravazzoni. 1984. Pulmonary sarcoidosis: Excess of helper T lymphocytes and T cell subset imbalance at sites of disease activity. Thorax **39:** 143-149.
20. Hunninghake, G. W., J. E. Gadek, O. Kawanami, V. J. Ferrans, R. G. Crystal. 1979. Inflammatory and immune processes in the human lung in health and in disease: Evaluation by bronchoalveolar lavage. Am. J. Pathol. **97:** 149-206.
21. Rossi, G. A., G. W. Hunninghake & R. G. Crystal. 1981. Evaluation of inflammatory and immune processes in the interstitial lung disorders: Use of bronchoalveolar lavage.

In Cellular Biology of the Lung. G. Cumming & G. Bonsignore, Eds.: 107-126. Plenum. New York, NY.

22. Böyum, A. 1968. Isolation of mononuclear cells and granulocytes from human blood. Scand. J. Clin. Inv. **21**(Suppl 97): 77-89.
23. Weiner, M. S., C. Bianco & V. Nussenweig. 1976. Enhanced binding erythrocytes of neuroaminidase-treated sheep to human T lymphocytes. Blood **42:** 939-946.
24. Linz, M. R., S. Bishop & R. Jefferis. 1977. Use of antibody-coated red blood cells for the sensitive detection of antigens and in rosette tests for cells bearing surface immunoglobulins. J. Immunol. Methods **15:** 279-281.
25. Rossi, G. A., E. Cosulich, O. Sacco, A. Risso, B. Balbi, G. Damiani, A. Bargellesi & C. Ravazzoni. 1983. Pulmonary sarcoidosis: A T cell subpopulation is responsible for blood monocyte attraction and increased antibody production. *In* Proceedings of the Fourth European Conference on Sarcoidosis and Other Granulomatous Disorders. A. Blasi, D. Olivieri & A. Pezza, Eds.: 57-67. Naples.
26. Rossi, G. A., O. Sacco, E. Cosulich, A. Risso, B. Balbi & C. Ravazzoni. 1985. Helper T lymphocytes in pulmonary sarcoidosis: Functional analysis of a lung T cell subpopulation in patients with active disease. In press.
27. Rossi, G. A., G. Bernabo Di' Negro, E. Balzano, E. Cerri, O. Sacco, B. Balbi, A. Venturini, R. Ramoino & C. Ravazzoni. 1985. Suppression of the alveolitis in pulmonary sarcoidosis by oral corticosteroids. Lung **163:** 83-93.
28. Pinkston, P. & R. G. Crystal. Corticosteroid suppression of interleukin-2 release from sarcoid lung T cells. First International Conference on Bronchoalveolar Lavage. May 1984. Columbia, MD.

Alveolar Lymphocyte Activation during Sarcoidosis[a]

G. CORDIER,[b,c] J. BRUNE,[c,d] AND J. P. REVILLARD[c]

[c] *Centre de Cytofluorométrie*
Unité d'Enseignement et de Recherche de Biologie Humaine
Institut National de la Santé et de la Recherche Médicale Unité 80
and
Equipe de Recherche Associée 782
du Centre National de la Recherche Scientifique
Hôpital E. Herriot
Lyons, France

[d] *Service de Pneumologie*
Hôpital L. Pradel
Lyons, France

INTRODUCTION

Pulmonary sarcoidosis is a chronic interstitial lung disease characterized by the presence of noncaseating granulomas within alveolar structures.[1] The first manifestation of sarcoidosis is an alveolitis[2–4] which comprises an increase in the density of alveolar macrophages and lymphocytes. These cells, when activated, modulate the granuloma formation, maintain the alveolitis process, and disorganize the normal architecture of the lung parenchyma; these activities lead to fibrosis.[2–4]

Thymus-derived (T) lymphocytes play a key role in sarcoidosis alveolitis. Alveolar T lymphocytes from sarcoidosis patients have been shown to release a leukocyte inhibitory factor[5] and a monocyte chemotactic factor which attracts and activates blood monocytes.[6] Lung T cells were also shown to release interleukin-2 and to thus control local T cell proliferation.[7] In addition, T cells are likely to induce and to control local polyclonal bone marrow-derived (B) cell activation.[8] It has recently been demonstrated that an evaluation of the parameters of the intensity of the alveolitis (that is, alveolar T cell numbers and macrophage activation) can give an accurate assessment of pulmonary sarcoidosis.[9] Since activated T lymphocytes play a major role in this disease, the direct measurement of the number of activated alveolar T cells should be a useful parameter in determining the intensity of the alveolitis. The activation of alveolar T cells in sarcoidosis is associated with their local proliferation, and this proliferation can be evaluated by flow cytometric analysis of the cell cycle.[10] Although several studies have focused on the imbalance of the alveolar T cell sub-

[a] The work was supported by Contrat de Recherche Libre INSERM 82.5.033.

[b] Address for correspondence: INSERM U80, Hôpital E. Herriot, Pavillon P, 69374 Lyon Cédex 08, France.

sets,[11,12] the expression of new antigenic membrane markers by T cells upon activation has not been yet analyzed.

In this study we have used flow cytometry analysis of T lymphocytes to evaluate membrane-marker expression and to determine the distribution of lymphocytes within the phases of the cell cycle. For the former, the immunofluorescence of the antigens was considered; for the latter, the DNA and RNA contained in the cells.

PATIENTS AND METHODS

Patients

Thirty patients (18 men and 12 women), each with a diagnosis of pulmonary sarcoidosis, were investigated. Twenty-two of the diagnoses depended on organ biopsies that demonstrated noncaseating epithelioid cell granulomas and other features of sarcoidosis.[13] The other eight were based on 2-year histories: each history showed an asymptomatic course through stage I and stage II radiologic patterns.

Mycobacterial, fungal, and parasitic infections were ruled out by history, pathology, and culture. The possibility of exposure to organic or inorganic material associated with granulomatous disease was excluded by clinical history. As a group, these patients had no functional abnormalities. Forced vital capacity, single-breath diffusing capacity, and resting and exercise arterial O_2 pressures were within normal limits.

Bronchoalveolar Lavage Cells

A flexible fiberoptic bronchoscope (Olympus BF2T or BFB2) was passed transnasally and wedged into the middle bronchus lobe while the patient was under local anesthesia. Bronchoalveolar lavage began with the infusion of 0.9% sterile saline solution; after discarding the first 20 ml, 50–120 ml were recovered from each patient. The cell suspensions were filtered through sterile gauze and placed in a hemocytometer in which the cells were counted. A differential count was performed on cytocentrifuge smears. The cells were washed twice in phosphate-buffered saline that was Ca^{2+} and Mg^{2+} free. No further separation was performed.

Peripheral Blood

Blood leukocytes were obtained from heparinized blood after lysis of red blood cells.[14] Peripheral blood leukocytes from 34 healthy controls were used for immunofluorescence studies, and those from 15 of these healthy controls were used for lymphocyte cell cycle analysis.

Membrane Marker Expression

Membrane markers were identified by their immunofluorescence using flow cytometry analysis of cells labeled with monoclonal antibodies. Staining and flow cytometry analysis have been detailed elsewhere.[15] Briefly, cell suspensions from blood and BAL were analyzed in a Cytofluorograf 50H (Ortho Instruments, Westwood, MA). Lymphocytes were gated according to their light-scattering properties. As a control more than 90% of the cells within the gated region were shown to be stained by BL16 (raised by J. Brochier), which recognizes all lymphocytes but does not recognize monocytes. Conversely, less than 5% of the cells were labeled with Mo2 (Coultronics, France), which specifically recognizes monocytes.[16] Fluorescence profiles were determinated for each monoclonal antibody within the gated area for lymphocytes. Ten thousand cells were analyzed for each sample.

T lymphocytes and their subsets were identified with OKT3, OKT4, and OKT8 antibodies (Ortho Diagnostic Systems, France) and with Leu 2a and Leu 3a antibodies (Becton Dickinson, France).[17–19] Several monoclonal antibodies directed against HLA-DR I-associated (Ia)-like antigens were used: OKIal (Ortho Diagnostic Systems, France),[20] BL2 (raised by J. Brochier),[21] and I_2 (Coultronics, France).[22] Membrane markers of lymphocyte activation were detected using MLR1, MLR2, and MLR3 (kindly provided by G. Corte and L. Moretta).[23,24] Dual-staining experiments were performed using phycoerythrin-conjugated Leu2a or Leu3a, and BL2 was revealed by a fluoresceinated goat IgG antimouse IgG and IgM.

Cell Cycle Analysis

Simultaneous measurement of the amounts of DNA and RNA contained in the cells was done after acridine orange staining as previously described.[10,15] The distribution of lymphocytes within the phases of the cell cycle was determined. For each sample 10 000 cells were analyzed.

Statistical Analysis

Data were analyzed using either the two-tailed *t* test or the Wilcoxon *t* test. Significance was determined at the $p < .05$ level.

RESULTS

Blood and Lung T Lymphocyte Subsets

Blood lymphocytes from sarcoidosis patients showed no major imbalance between the T cell subsets; the OKT4:OKT8 ratio, for example, was within the normal range. The percentage of $OKT3^+$ cells and especially that of $OKT4^+$ cells, however, were markedly decreased in blood as compared to normal controls (TABLE 1). In contrast, lymphocytes from the bronchoalveolar lavage of sarcoidosis patients had a high proportion of T lymphocytes, and these T lymphocytes had a low percentage of $OKT8^+$ lymphocytes ($p < .05$ when compared to normal blood) and a high OKT4:OKT8 ratio (TABLE 1).

Expression of Activation Markers by Alveolar Lymphocytes

The percentage of $HLA\text{-}DR^+$ lymphocytes was much higher in the bronchoalveolar lavage (26.8 ± 3.8) than in the blood samples of the patients (18.3 ± 2.0). In 6 out of 14 bronchoalveolar lavage samples the sum of the percentages of $OKT3^+$ and DR^+ cells exceeded 100%, indicating the presence of cells expressing both antigens. Since

TABLE 1. Distribution of Peripheral T Cell Subsets according to Their Clusters of Differentiation (CD).[a]

	Percentage of T Cells[b]			
	CD3	CD4	CD8	CD4/CD8
Normal blood	73 (34)	55 (34)	31 (34)	1.9 ± 0.7 (34)
Patient blood	63 ± 3.9 (18)	38.5 ± 2.8* (18)	27 ± 2.3 (19)	1.89 ± 0.36 (18)
Bronchoalveolar lavage	74 ± 4.1 (23)	57 ± 4.8 (20)	22 ± 2.7* (21)	4.50 ± 0.83* (20)

[a] CD3 was recognized by OKT3 antibody; CD4, by OKT4 and/or Leu 3a; and CD8, by OKT8 and/or Leu 2a.

[b] Values are expressed as means ± SEM. The number of patients is indicated in parentheses. Asterisks indicate $p < .05$.

percentages of DR^+ $OKT3^+$ cells are liable to be underestimated by this method of calculation, we performed double-staining experiments in three patients in order to quantify more accurately the percentage of DR^+ $OTK3^+$ cells and to identify the subset of T cells involved. In these patients 20-30% of the alveolar T lymphocytes express DR, and most of these DR^+ cells are part of the Leu $3a^+$ subset (FIG. 1).

A marked increased of lymphocytes expressing MLR1, MLR2, and MLR3 was found in the bronchoalveolar lavages of five out of seven patients (FIG. 2). In addition, MLR^+ lymphocytes were found in increased numbers in the blood of these patients (data not shown).

Cell Cycle Analysis

The DNA content of blood lymphocytes was elevated in only three patients, and the overall percentage of lymphocytes in the S + (G2 + M) phases of the cell cycle

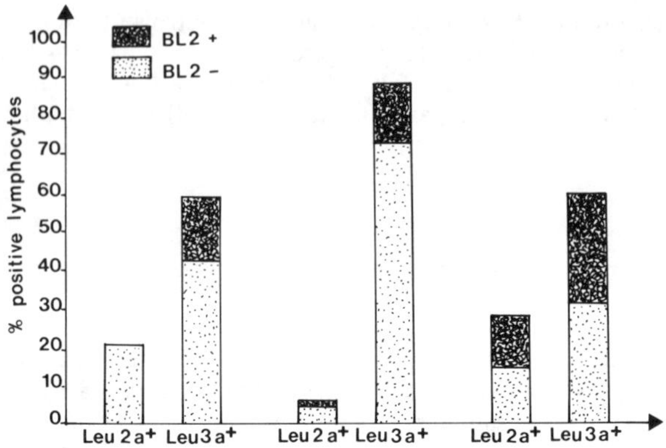

FIGURE 1. Dual staining of lymphocytes from bronchoalveolar lavage of three sarcoidosis patients. Percentages of cells expressing HLA-DR ($BL2^+$) are shown by heavily shaded bars.

was not significantly different from that observed in normal controls (FIG. 3). In contrast, the percentage of lymphocytes in the S + (G2 + M) phases was higher in bronchoalveolar lavage samples than it was in the blood samples (FIG. 3).

DISCUSSION

In the present study lung lymphocyte activation was assessed in sarcoidosis by flow cytometry analysis of membrane markers and of the cell cycle. Flow cytometry, unlike estimation of mediator release, provides a direct quantification of the number of activated T cells. As shown by *in vitro* models using mitogens, allogeneic cells, or specific antigens for stimulation, T cell activation can be regarded as a multistep phenomenon controlled by sequential signals.[25] Upon a first signal the resting G0 cells may enter the G1 phase, release mediators, and express new surface antigens.[26–28] A second signal provided by interleukin-2 is required for the cell to proceed in the mitotic cycle.[29,30] A variety of surface structures on T cells may be detected by identifying

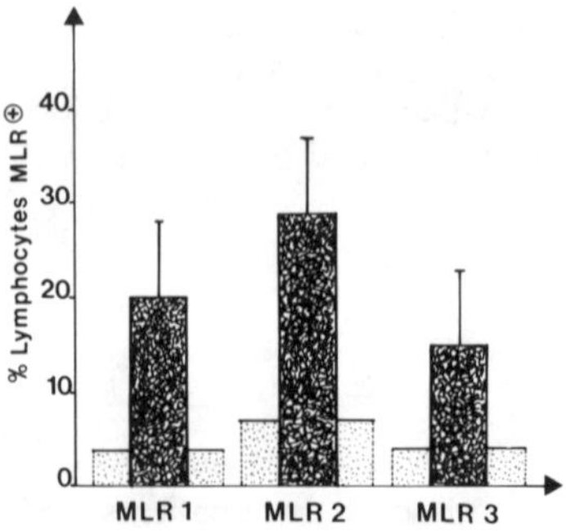

FIGURE 2. Percentages of cells expressing MLR1, MLR2, or MLR3 antigens among alveolar lymphocytes in sarcoidosis patients.

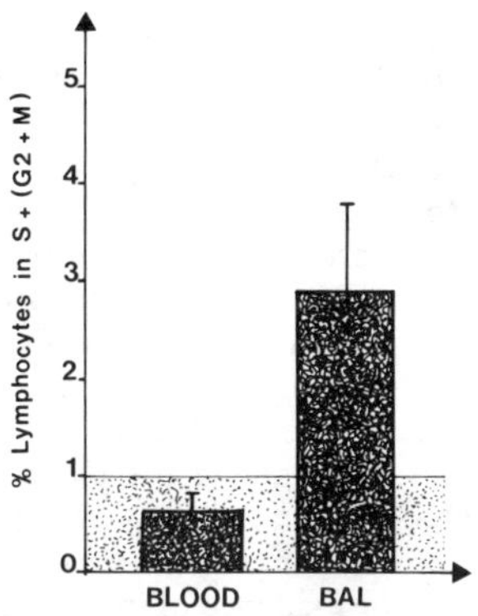

FIGURE 3. Percentages of lymphocytes in the S + (G2 + M) phases of the cell cycle among alveolar lymphocytes in sarcoidosis patients.

which monoclonal antibodies the T cells bind. Some of these structures are only detectable once the T cells have been activated. Some antigens, such as interleukin-2 receptors, are expressed before the cell enters the S phase; others, DR (Ia-like) antigens, for example, are expressed after the cells have completed one cycle. The exact time course of membrane marker expression during the activation phase of the cell cycle is known only for a few antigens (FIG. 4).[28,29,31–40] We studied two groups of markers that were expressed late in the cell cycle: HLA-DR and MLR antigens. Histocompatibility class II antigens are expressed by T cells only after *in vitro* or *in vivo* activation. Bronchoalveolar lavage T lymphocytes from at least half of the patients expressed HLA-DR. Furthermore, the number of DR^+ cells could be quantified among the different T cell subsets. Preliminary observations showed that there were more T cells that expressed DR within the "helper-inducer" subset than within the "suppressor-cytotoxic" subset. Such a result is consistent with the current concepts of the pathogenesis of sarcoidosis.[2–4,7,12] Indeed, it is assumed that $OKT4^+$ cells are involved in the production of the lymphokines (including the macrophage activating factor) responsible for the delayed hypersensitivity reaction.

Antigens recognized by monoclonal antibodies MLR1 and MLR2 are detectable on T cells following *in vitro* activation but not on resting T cells nor on any other

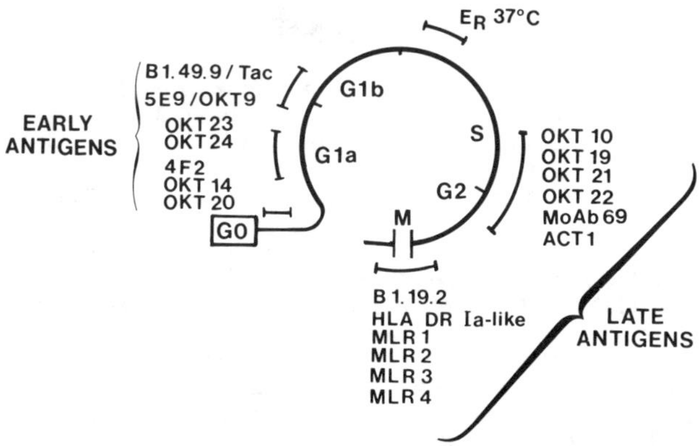

FIGURE 4. Membrane antigen expression during T lymphocyte activation.

cell types.[23] Those two markers of activated T cells were present in the blood and the bronchoalveolar lavage of most of the patients in whom they have been investigated. Enumeration of $MLR1^+$ and $MLR2^+$ cells is a direct and easy way of quantifying activated T lymphocytes in the bronchoalveolar lavage of sarcoidosis patients. On the other hand, the MLR3 antigen is expressed by B or T cells upon activation.[23,24] Therefore its expression by some blood and alveolar lymphocytes might reflect B as well as T lymphocyte activation. The presence of $MLR1^+$ and $MLR2^+$ cells in patients' blood would suggest that T cell activation is not restricted to the alveolar inflammatory reaction but may also occur in other sites such as lymph nodes. It has not yet been studied whether $MLR1^+$ or $MLR2^+$ cells were also HLA-DR^+. The mere comparison of percentages in the blood would suggest the presence of MLR^+ HLA-DR^- cells. The discrepancy may reflect a difference in sensitivity between the two assays or a more prolonged expression of MLR than that of HLA-DR after T cell activation.

The evidence of increased numbers of lavage and, to a much lesser extent, of blood cells in the S + (G2 + M) phases of the cell cycle is consistent with the presence of cells expressing "late antigens" specific for activated lymphocytes. In addition, it extends the demonstration of the presence of a pool of actively replicating lymphocytes within the alveolar space.[2,7,10] Cell cycle analysis after acridine orange staining allows a quantification of these replicating cells.

In conclusion, the enumeration of activated T cells in the bronchoalveolar lavage of sarcoidosis patients gives a direct measure of cells playing a key role in the disease. Association of cell cycle analysis and detection of membrane markers specific for activated T cells is useful in assessing the degree of activation of lung lymphocytes. Therefore these assays can be used as a part of the staging of the alveolitis in sarcoidosis.[3,9,41]

ACKNOWLEDGMENTS

J. F. Mornex initiated this study and contributed to the first part of this study until July 1983. We wish to thank C. Molina for the antibody precipitation determinations; J. Brochier, G. Corte, and L. Moretta for the monoclonal antibodies; B. Lahnèche for the gallium-67 scans; and S. Alfano for the secretarial assistance.

REFERENCES

1. Mitchell, D. N. & J. G. Scadding. 1974. Am. Rev. Respir. Dis. **110:** 774-802.
2. Crystal, R. G., W. C. Roberts, G. W. Hunninghake, J. E. Gadek, J. D. Fulmer & B. R. Line. 1981. Ann. Intern. Med. **94:** 73-94.
3. Keogh, B. A. & R. G. Crystal. 1982. Thorax **37:** 1-10.
4. Crystal, R. G. 1983. *In* Sarcoidosis and Other Granulomatous Disorders. J. Chrétien, J. Marsac & J. C. Saltiel, Eds.: 13-35. Pergamon Press. Paris.
5. Hunninghake, G. W., J. D. Fulmer, R. C. Young, J. E. Gadek & R. G. Crystal. 1979. Am. Rev. Respir. Dis. **129:** 49-57.
6. Hunninghake, G. W., J. F. Gadek, R. C. Young, O. Kawanami, V. J. Ferrans & R. G. Crystal. 1980. N. Engl. J. Med. **302:** 594-598.
7. Pinkston, P., P. B. Bitterman & R. G. Crystal. 1983. N. Engl. J. Med. **308:** 793-800.
8. Hunninghake, G. W. & R. G. Crystal. 1981. J. Clin. Invest. **67:** 86-92.
9. Keogh, B. A., G. W. Hunninghake, B. R. Line & R. G. Crystal. 1983. Am. Rev. Respir. Dis. **128:** 256-265.
10. Pacheco, Y., G. Cordier, M. Perrin-Fayolle & J. P. Revillard. 1982. Am. J. Med. **73:** 82-88.

11. Ginns, L. C., P. D. Goldenheim, R. C. Burton, R. D. Colvin, L. G. Miller, G. Goldstein, C. Hurwitz & H. Kazerni. 1982. Clin. Immunol. Immunopathol. **25:** 11-20.
12. Hunninghake, G. W. & R. G. Crystal. 1981. N. Engl. J. Med. **305:** 429-434.
13. Mitchell, D. N., J. G. Scadding, B. E. Heard & K. F. W. Hinson. 1977. J. Clin. Pathol. **30:** 395-408.
14. Hoffman, R. A., P. C. Kung, W. P. Hansen & G. Goldstein. 1980. Proc. Natl. Acad. Sci. USA **77:** 4914-4917.
15. Mornex, J. F., G. Cordier, J. Pages, R. Lefebvre, J. P. Revillard, J. M. Vergnon, M. Vincent, J. F. Cordier & J. Brune. 1985. J. Lab. Clin. Med. **105:** 70-76.
16. Todd, R. F., L. M. Nadler & S. F. Schlossman. 1981. J. Immunol. **126:** 1435-1442.
17. Kung, P. C., F. Goldstein, E. L. Reinherz & S. F. Schlossman. 1979. Science **206:** 347-349.
18. Reinherz, E. L. & S. F. Schlossmann. 1980. N. Engl. J. Med. **303:** 307-373.
19. Ledbetter, J. A., A. E. Frankel & L. A. Herzenberg. 1981. *In* Monoclonal Antibodies and T Cell Hybridomas: Perspectives and Technical Notes. G. Hammerling, Ü. Hammerling & J. Kernery, Eds. Elsevier/North-Holland. New York, NY.
20. Reinherz, E. L., P. C. Kung, J. M. Pesando, J. Ritz, F. Goldstein & S. F. Schlossman. 1982. J. Exp. Med. **150:** 1472-1482.
21. Yonish-Rouach, E., G. Cordier, J. Cohen, C. Vincent & J. Brochier. 1983. *In* Protides of the Biological Fluids. H. Peeters, Ed. Vol. **30:** 487-490. Pergamon Press. Oxford.
22. Pesando, J. M., L. M. Nadler, H. Lazarus, K. J. Tomaselli, P. Stashenko, J. Ritz, E. J. Lev Yunis & S. F. Schlossman. 1981. Hum. Immunol. **3:** 67-69.
23. Corte, G., L. Moretta, F. Damiani, M. C. Mingari & A. Bargellesi. 1981. Eur. J. Immunol. **11:** 162-164.
24. Canonica, G. W., M. Bagnasco, C. Corte, S. Ferrini, O. Ferrini & G. Giordano. 1982. Clin. Immunol. Immunopathol. **23:** 616-625.
25. Mornex, J. F., G. Cordier & J. P. Revillard. 1983. Rev. Fr. Mal. Respir. **11:** 787-812.
26. Bettens, F., F. Kristensen, C. Walker & A. L. de Weck. 1982. Eur. J. Immunol. **12:** 948-952.
27. Kristensen, F., C. Walker, F. Bettens, F. Joncourt & A. L. de Weck. 1982. Cell. Immunol. **74:** 140-149.
28. Cotner, T., J. M. Williams, L. Christenson, H. M. Shapiro, T. B. Strom & J. L. Strominger. 1983. J. Exp. Med. **157:** 461-472.
29. Sekaly, R. P., H. R. MacDonald, P. Zaecii & M. Nabholz. 1982. J. Immunol. **129:** 1407-1415.
30. Brown, R. L., R. L. Griffith, R. H. Neubauer & H. Rabin. 1982. J. Immunol. **129:** 1849-1852.
31. Burns, G. F. B., F. L. Battye & G. Goldstein. 1982. Cell. Immunol. **71:** 12-26.
32. Charron, D. J. 1981. Immunol. Commun. **10:** 293-311.
33. Hercend, T., J. Ritz, S. F. Schlossman & E. L. Reinherz. 1981. Hum. Immunol. **3:** 247-259.
34. Haynes, B. F., M. Hemler, T. Cotner, D. L. Mann, G. S. Eisenbarth, J. L. Strominger & A. S. Fauci. 1981. J. Immunol. **127:** 342-351.
35. Sutherland, R., D. Delia, C. Schneider, R. Newman, J. Kemsluad & M. Greaves. 1981. Proc. Natl. Acad. Sci. USA. **78:** 4515-4519.
36. Lazarovits, A., R. Moscicki, J. Kurnick & R. B. Colvin. 1984. J. Allerg. Clin. Immunol. **73**(1, part 2): 187.
37. Talle, M. A., N. Allegar, M. Makowski & G. Goldstein. 1984. Cell. Immunol. **84:** 285-298.
38. Williams, J. M., R. Loertscher, T. Cotner, M. Reddish, H. M. Shapiro, C. B. Carpenter, J. L. Strominger & T. B. Strom. 1984. J. Immunol. **132:** 2330-2337.
39. Hemler, M. E., M. B. Brenner, J. M. McLean & J. L. Strominger. 1984. Proc. Natl. Acad. Sci. USA **81:** 2172-2175.
40. Galili, U. & M. Schlesinger. 1976. J. Immunol. **117:** 730-735.
41. Mornex, J. F., G. Cordier, J. Pages & J. P. Revillard. 1983. Monogr. Allergy **18:** 178-180.

Lymphocyte Phenotypes in Bronchoalveolar Lavage and Lung Tissue in Sarcoidosis

IRVIN L. PARADIS,[a,b] ROBERT M. ROGERS,[b]
BRUCE S. RABIN,[c] AND JAMES H. DAUBER[b]

[b]*Department of Medicine*
and
[c]*Department of Pathology*
University of Pittsburgh
Pittsburgh, Pennsylvania 15261
and
Oakland Veterans Administration Medical Center
Pittsburgh, Pennsylvania 15240

INTRODUCTION

Pulmonary sarcoidosis is characterized by an accumulation of immune effector cells and by alterations in parenchymal cells within the lung (the alveolitis) that often result in the derangement of structure and function of alveolar-capillary units. The standard approach in the evaluation of this disorder is to perform biopsies of the lung parenchyma and qualitatively describe the cellular infiltrate by standard histologic methods.[1,2] Understanding the pathogenesis of this disorder, however, requires knowledge of the type and function of the cells constituting the alveolitis: information that is not available from the routine histologic evaluation.

Immune effector cells that line the epithelial surface of the lung can be obtained by bronchoalveolar lavage (BAL).[3] Analysis of the type and function of these cells has provided insight into the pathogenesis of this disorder, but information from these studies would be more reassuring if it could be demonstrated that the types and functions of the cells recovered by BAL are representative of the types and functions of the cells within the pulmonary interstitium. A previous study demonstrated a relationship between the percentages of the cell types recovered by BAL and those extracted from open lung biopsy specimens in six patients with sarcoidosis.[4]

A drawback to this approach is that extraction of cells from tissue may damage them and fail to recover all cells.[5,6] To avoid the problems associated with extraction, we used monoclonal antibodies and a sensitive avidin-biotin immunoperoxidase method to identify and enumerate T cell phenotypes *in situ* and in lavage fluid.[7,8] We found that there was excellent agreement between the numbers of immunostained cells within each T cell subset recovered by lavage and those present in biopsy specimens. These

[a]Address for correspondence: Oakland Veterans Administration Medical Center, University Drive C, Pittsburgh, Pennsylvania 15240.

results support the concept that the cells recovered by lavage reflect the types of cells present in the lung interstitium in pulmonary sarcoidosis.

MATERIALS AND METHODS

Population

The study population consisted of six patients with newly diagnosed, untreated sarcoidosis (five of the patients had acute sarcoidosis; one had chronic sarcoidosis). The diagnosis of sarcoidosis was established by 1) a lung biopsy (two biopsies were open; four were transbronchial) demonstrating noncaseating epithelioid granulomas; 2) a compatible clinical picture without evidence of mycobacterial or fungal infection; and 3) a history indicating the patient had no exposure to inorganic or organic material known to cause granulomatous lung disease. Informed consent for BAL was obtained from all patients according to a protocol approved by the institutional review board for biomedical research of the University of Pittsburgh.

Bronchoalveolar Lavage

Patients were premedicated intramuscularly with atropine (0.8 mg) and sometimes intravenously with Valium (5-10 mg). After topical xylocaine anesthesia, a flexible fiberoptic bronchoscope was introduced into the lungs via the nares and wedged in a subsegment of the right middle lobe. A sterile saline solution lavage of 200 ml was performed by the sequential instillation of 50-ml aliquots of saline solution which were subsequently removed by aspiration with a negative pressure of 100 cm H_2O. The lavage fluid was filtered through two layers of surgical gauze, and the volume was measured. The cells were separated from the lavage fluid by centrifugation (500 g for 10 min), washed twice, and resuspended in Hanks' balanced salt solution (HBSS) without Ca^{2+} or Mg^{2+}. The cells were evaluated for total number with an automated particle counter (Coulter Electronics, Hialeah, FL), for viability by trypan blue dye exclusion, and for cell types by a differential cell count of a cytocentrifuge preparation (Cytospin II, Shandon Instruments, Sewickley, PA) stained with Wright-Giemsa. Macrophages were distinguished from lymphocytes by nonspecific esterase stains. Additional cytocentrifuge smears for lymphocyte immunostaining were prepared by spinning 5×10^4 cells at 1000 rpm for 5 min. Smears were fixed in acetone for 10 min at room temperature immediately after preparation and stored at 4° C for up to 2 weeks before being immunostained.

Lung Tissue

Two transbronchial biopsies from each of the four patients and a portion of an open lung biopsy from the two remaining patients were embedded in O.C.T. Compound

(Miles, Naperville, OH) and frozen at −40° C. Sections 4-μ thick were cut on a cryostat microtome, fixed in acetone for 10 min at −20° C, and stored at −20° C for up to 1 week before being immunostained.

Lymphocyte Immunostaining

Cytocentrifuge smears of BAL and tissue sections were warmed to room temperature in sealed containers. The specimens were rehydrated in modified phosphate-buffered saline (PBS) and then incubated with monoclonal antibody diluted in PBS. The monoclonal antibodies employed were Leu 4 for total T cells at a 1:200 dilution, Leu 3a for T helper cells at a 1:150 dilution, and Leu 2a for T suppressor/cytotoxic cells at a 1:100 dilution (Becton Dickinson, Sunnyvale, CA). The specimens were rinsed in PBS and incubated for 15 min with a biotinylated horse antimouse antibody solution (Vector Labs, Burlingame, CA) at a 1:80 dilution in PBS. The specimens were rinsed in PBS and incubated for 15 min with an avidin-biotinylated horseradish peroxidase solution (ABC) (Vector Labs, Burlingame, CA) at a 1:80 dilution for the avidin and at a 1:80 dilution for the biotinylated horseradish peroxidase. The specimens were rinsed in PBS, and the color reaction product was developed with the chromogen 3-amino-9-ethylcarbazole (AEC) (Sigma, St. Louis, MO) as follows. A 0.001 M AEC solution in *N, N*-dimethylformamide (Sigma, St. Louis, MO) was added to a 0.01% H_2O_2 solution in 0.02 M sodium acetate buffer, pH 5.2. The specimens were incubated in this peroxidase substrate solution for 10 min, counterstained with Mayer's hematoxylin (Sigma, St. Louis, MO) for 10 min, and washed under tap water for 10 min. Coverslips were then placed over the specimens with Aquamount (Lerner Labs, New Haven, CT).

Specificity of immunostaining was determined by omitting the primary monoclonal antibody step from one section of each tissue specimen. Sensitivity of immunostaining was monitored by staining tonsil tissue with each monoclonal antibody along with the tissue sections. Tonsil staining patterns were compared with known patterns of lymphocyte staining in this tissue.[9] From previous reagent titration experiments, the antibody and ABC dilutions chosen were those that demonstrated optimum immunostaining.

Lymphocyte Enumeration

For each lymphocyte phenotype in lavage fluid, 400 immunostained and unstained lymphocytes were counted at a magnification of × 1000 on the cytocentrifuge preparations, and the percentage of immunostained cells was determined. The total number of immunostained cells and the number of immunostained cells/ml recovered lavage fluid for each phenotype were calculated. For lymphocyte phenotypes in tissue, immunostained cells were enumerated over a representative 2-8-mm^2 area of tissue. This area chosen for enumeration included granulomata and adjacent lung tissue where there was no evidence of distortion from the sectioning procedure. Immunostained cells were enumerated by using a 7 × 7-mm^2 counting grid in the ocular of a light microscope at a magnification of × 400, and the number of immunostained cells/mm^2 of tissue was calculated. Different lymphocyte phenotypes were enumerated on serial sections from the same area of each specimen. For BAL and tissue specimens, the total number of immunostained cells for a particular phenotype divided by the total number of immunostained cells from another phenotype defined the Leu 3/Leu 4, Leu 2/Leu 4, and Leu 3/Leu 2 ratios.

Statistics

Immunostained cell populations in lavage fluid and tissue were compared by the Spearman rank-correlation test, Wilcoxon signed-rank test, and Mann-Whitney rank-sum test. A p value of less than or equal to .05 was regarded as significant.

RESULTS

Pattern of Immunostaining

Immunostained cells in lavage fluid (FIG. 1A) and tissue (FIG. 1B) developed a reddish-brown reaction product which was confined to the cell surface. There was no staining of the cytoplasm of any of the lymphocyte phenotypes. The Leu 4 and Leu 2 monoclonal antibodies stained only cells which resembled lymphocytes by morphologic criteria. Some cells having the morphologic features of macrophages stained with the Leu 3 monoclonal antibody, but the staining pattern differed from that of lymphocytes in that the reaction product was confined to the cytoplasm and was irregularly distributed. Thus Leu 3-immunostained lymphocytes in BAL were distinguished from nonspecifically stained macrophages by morphologic criteria and by the pattern of immunostaining (intense reddish-brown rim vs. light stipled red color). In tissue, lymphocytes bearing the Leu 3 marker could be identified because of their rim pattern of immunostaining.

Comparison of Lymphocyte Phenotypes in Tissue and Bronchoalveolar Lavage

The total number and the number of immunostained cells/ml of recovered lavage fluid were compared to the number of immunostained cells in tissue by the Spearman rank-correlation test. There was a statistically significant correlation between the total number of Leu 4^+, Leu 3^+, and Leu 2^+ cells in lavage fluid and the corresponding number of cells/mm^2 of tissue, that is, between columns A and C, D and F, and G and I, respectively (TABLE 1). When cell recovery was expressed as cells/ml of recovered lavage fluid, significant correlations were found between lavage and tissue for Leu 4 and Leu 3 phenotypes (between columns B and C and columns E and F, respectively) but not for Leu 2 (between columns H and I). The ratios of Leu 3^+ to Leu 4^+ cells and Leu 2^+ to Leu 4^+ cells were nearly identical in lavage fluid and

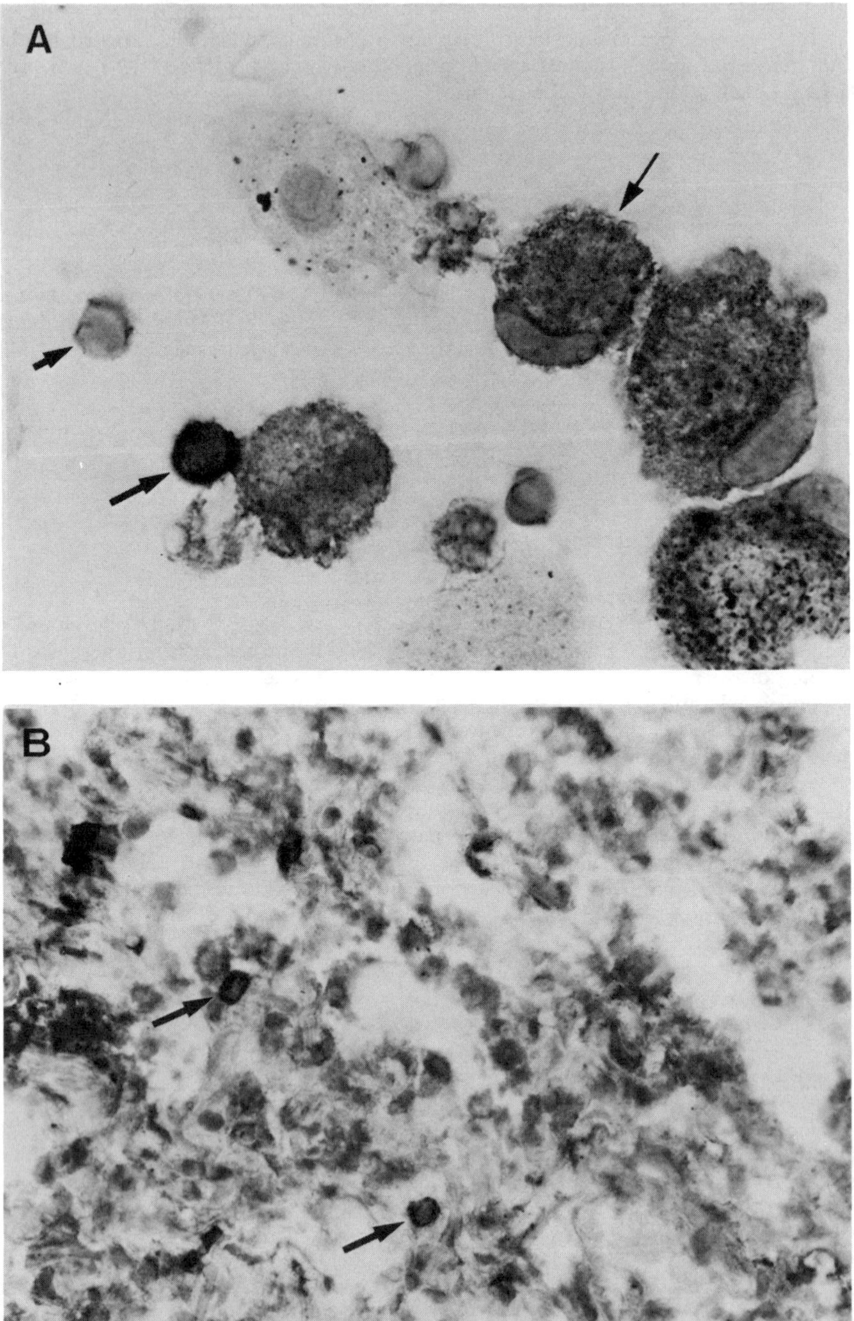
A
B

tissue (TABLE 2). Although the ratio of Leu 3^+ to Leu 2^+ cells in lavage fluid was greater than that for cells in tissue, the difference was not significant ($p > .05$, the Mann-Whitney rank-sum test). The sums of the total numbers of cells of the Leu 3 and Leu 2 phenotypes (TABLE 1) for BAL total cells (columns D and G), for BAL cells/ml of recovered fluid (columns E and H), and for cells in tissue (columns F and I) were greater than the corresponding values for the Leu 4 phenotype (columns A, B, and C), but the differences were not statistically significant for any of the comparisons ($p > .06$, the Wilcoxon signed-rank test).

DISCUSSION

In this comparison of lymphocyte phenotypes in lung tissue and in lavage fluid from six patients with sarcoidosis, we found that the number of immunostained lymphocytes in tissue was positively correlated to the absolute number of immunostained lymphocytes and the number of immunostained lymphocytes/ml of recovered lavage fluid (TABLE 1). The greater the number of cells of a given lymphocyte phenotype in lavage fluid, the greater the number of cells of the corresponding phenotype in tissue. In addition, the proportions or ratios of these lymphocyte phenotypes in BAL and tissue were also similar (TABLE 2). These findings support the notion that for the lymphocyte phenotypes studied, the cells recovered by lavage are representative of interstitial cells in pulmonary sarcoidosis.

The results for patient 2, the only patient with chronic disease (dyspnea and the presence of pulmonary infiltrates for more than 2 years), seemed to be different from those for the patients with acute disease. The lung tissue obtained by open biopsy had a mild increase in interstitial cellularity but only a few granulomas. No granulomas had been found on previous transbronchial lung biopsies. Results for cell phenotypes in tissue reported in TABLES 1 & 2 were derived from counting cells in areas which included these rare granulomas adjacent to which there was mild diffuse interstitial inflammation. The open biopsy specimen, however, also contained a few large coalesced granulomas which were very fibrotic. The number of immunostained cells at the border of these granulomas was much greater than that in adjacent areas of the lung (Leu 4: 274 vs. 62 cells/mm^2; Leu 3: 162 vs. 50 cells/mm^2; Leu 2: 75 vs. 19 cells/mm^2) because the entire enumerated area consisted of granuloma tissue. Despite this, the proportions of the different phenotypes in these two areas of the biopsy specimen were similar (Leu 3/Leu 4: 81 vs. 59; Leu 2/Leu 4: 31 vs. 27; Leu 3/Leu 2: 2.6 vs. 2.2). We enumerated cells in the area containing the rare granulomas because this area was more representative of the entire biopsy specimen and was probably more

FIGURE 1. **(A)** A BAL smear stained by the ABC method and the Leu 3 monoclonal antibody. Immunostained lymphocytes (arrow) are distinguished from unstained lymphocytes (short arrow) by morphologic criteria and by an intense reddish-brown rim of color on the cell surface. With the Leu 3 monoclonal antibody, but not the Leu 4 or Leu 2 monoclonal antibodies, some cells having the morphologic features of alveolar macrophages (thin arrow) were stained with irregular deposits of light pink color confined to the cell cytoplasm. Original magnification: $\times$ 1000; reduced to 98% of original size. **(B)** Lung tissue stained by the ABC method and the Leu 3 monoclonal antibody. This lung tissue is from a representative area of lung parenchyma chosen for cell enumeration. Immunostained cells (arrows) are identified by the specific pattern of rim staining. Original magnification: $\times$ 400; reduced to 98% of original size.

TABLE 1. Lymphocyte Phenotypes in Bronchoalveolar Lavage and Lung Tissue

	Leu 4			Leu 3			Leu 2		
	Lavage		Tissue	Lavage		Tissue	Lavage		Tissue
Patient	(A) Total Cells ($\times 10^6$)	(B) Cells/ml ($\times 10^3$)	(C) Cells/mm^2	(D) Total Cells ($\times 10^6$)	(E) Cells/ml ($\times 10^3$)	(F) Cells/mm^2	(G) Total Cells ($\times 10^6$)	(H) Cells/ml ($\times 10^3$)	(I) Cells/mm^2
1	18.1*	125*	69	17.1*	118*	64	1.8*	12	11
2	4.4	33	62	2.2	16	50	2.6	19	19
3	12.6	84	159	10.2	68	116	2.6	17	43
4	2.7	10	61	2.3	9	53	0.6	2	16
5	1.3	8	44	0.4	6	38	0.3	2	11
6	31.7	159	229	28.4	142	181	3.7	18	35
Mean ± SD	11.8 ± 11.7	70 ± 63	104 ± 74	10.1 ± 10.9	60 ± 60	84 ± 55	1.9 ± 1.3	12 ± 8	23 ± 13

NOTE: Asterisks indicate BAL results that are significantly related ($p < .05$) to tissue results for each lymphocyte phenotype by the Spearman rank correlation coefficient.

similar to the area of the lung sampled by lavage. The percentage of Leu 3^+ cells in the lavage fluid from patient 2 was low compared to that of the other patients whereas the fraction of Leu 2^+ cells seemed high. This resulted in a relatively low Leu 3/Leu 2 ratio in lavage fluid compared to the patients with more acute disease (TABLE 2). It may be that lavage does not accurately reflect the lymphocyte phenotypes in tissue in chronic disease. More patients with chronic disease need to be studied if this possibility is to be confirmed or refuted.

The sum of the numbers of Leu 2^+ and Leu 3^+ cells was always higher than the number of Leu 4^+ cells in BAL and tissue (TABLE 1). This has also been observed by other investigators and may be due to inaccuracies in enumeration methods or to the presence of cells with markers for both the Leu 3 and Leu 2 phenotypes.[10] The explanation for why there was a statistically significant correlation for the number of Leu 2^+ cells in tissue and the total number of cells in lavage fluid but not for the number of Leu 2^+ cells/ml of lavage fluid recovered is unclear. One possibility is that the recovery of cells of the Leu 3 and Leu 2 phenotypes by lavage differs, but further studies are required to clarify this point.

TABLE 2. Ratios of Lymphocyte Phenotypes in Bronchoalveolar Lavage and Lung Tissue

	Leu 3/Leu 4		Leu 2/Leu 4		Leu 3/Leu 2	
Patients	Lavage	Tissue	Lavage	Tissue	Lavage	Tissue
1	94*	93	10*	16	9.7*	5.8
2	50	81	59	31	0.9	2.6
3	81	73	21	27	3.9	2.7
4	85	87	22	26	3.8	3.3
5	77	86	25	25	3.1	3.5
6	89	79	12	15	7.7	5.2
Mean ± SD	79±16	83±7	25±18	23±6	4.9±3.2	3.9±1.3

NOTE: Asterisks indicate BAL results that are not significantly different from tissue results for each ratio by the Mann-Whitney rank-sum test.

We have observed that in pulmonary sarcoidosis, the distribution among the different phenotypes of lymphocytes from BAL fluid is similar to that of lymphocytes seen in tissue by *in situ* analysis; that is, a given phenotype may be shown to be composed of a similar number of lymphocytes and to constitute a similar proportion of the entire lymphocyte population by both BAL and tissue analysis. Thus, previous observations which utilized extraction of cells from tissue[4] have been extended, and the concept that BAL is a useful technique to characterize the alveolitis of sarcoidosis has been further supported. Since the phenotypes of lymphocytes recovered by lavage are similar to those present in the pulmonary interstitium, it is possible that the function of lavaged lymphocytes reflects the function of their phenotypic counterparts *in situ,* but this possibility must be confirmed by appropriate studies.

REFERENCES

1. MITCHELL, D. N. & J. G. SCADDING. 1974. Sarcoidosis. Am. Rev. Respir. Dis. **110:** 774-802.

2. Crystal, R. G., W. C. Roberts, G. W. Hunninghake, J. E. Gadek, J. D. Fulmer & B. R. Line. 1981. Pulmonary sarcoidosis: A disease characterized and perpetuated by activated T-lymphocytes. Ann. Intern. Med. **94:** 73-94.
3. Hunninghake, G. W., J. E. Gadek, O. Kawanami, V. J. Ferrans & R. G. Crystal. 1979. Inflammatory and immune processes in the human lung in health and disease: Evaluation by bronchoalveolar lavage. Am. J. Pathol. **97:** 149-206.
4. Hunninghake, G. W., O. Kawanami, V. J. Ferrans, R. C. Young, W. C. Roberts & R. G. Crystal. 1981. Characterization of the inflammatory and immune effector cells in the lung parenchyma of patients with interstitial lung disease. Am. Rev. Respir. Dis. **123:** 407-412.
5. Tilney, N. L., M. R. Garovoy, G. J. Busch, T. B. Strom, M. J. Graves & C. B. Carpenter. 1979. Rejected human renal allografts: Recovery and characteristics of infiltrating cells and antibody. Transplantation **128:** 421-426.
6. Haslam, P. L., C. W. G. Turton, P. Heard, A. Lukoszek, J. V. Collins, A. J. Salsbury & M. Turner-Warwick. 1980. Bronchoalveolar lavage in pulmonary fibrosis: Comparison of cells obtained with lung biopsy and clinical features. Thorax **35:** 9-18.
7. Warnke, R. & R. Levy. 1980. Detection of T and B cell antigens with hybridoma monoclonal antibodies: A biotin-avidin-horseradish peroxidase method. J. Histochem. Cytochem. **28:** 771-776.
8. Hsu, S., L. Raine & H. Fanger. 1981. A comparative study of the peroxidase-antiperoxidase method and an avidin-biotin complex method for studying polypeptide hormones with radioimmunoassay antibodies. Am. J. Clin. Pathol. **75:** 734-738.
9. Si, L., G. Roscoe & T. L. Whiteside. 1983. Distribution and quantitation of T lymphocyte subsets in human tonsils as defined by monoclonal antibodies. Arch. Pathol. Lab. Med. **107:** 228-231.
10. Bach, M. & J. F. Bach. 1981. The use of monoclonal anti-T cell antibodies to study T cell imbalances in human disease. Clin. Exp. Immunol. **45:** 449-456.

Spontaneous Production of Interleukin-2 in the Supernatants of Cultured Cutaneous Sarcoidal Granulomas

Y. P. KATARIA,[a,b] R. C. PADGETT,[c] AND
L. S. ENGLISH[d]

[b]*Pulmonary Diseases Section*
Department of Medicine
East Carolina University School of Medicine
Greenville, North Carolina

[c]*University of North Carolina School of Medicine*
Chapel Hill, North Carolina

[d]*Department of Microbiology*
East Carolina University School of Medicine
Greenville, North Carolina

INTRODUCTION

Sarcoidosis is a multisystemic disease of unknown etiology. It is accompanied by disparate immunologic alterations suggestive of both depressed and hyperactive cell-mediated immunity. The evidence on the whole, however, points towards a hyper-reactive immune system that is both cellular and humoral.[1] The hallmark of this disease is granuloma formation, the pathogenesis of which remains undetermined. Recent evidence from the analysis of bronchoalveolar lavage has demonstrated the presence of increased numbers of lymphocytes, the majority of which are thymus-derived (T) lymphocytes with an increased proportion of activated T cells.[2] These lymphocytes have been shown to produce lymphokines such as chemotactic factor.[3]

Although the morphology and function of the mononuclear cells present in the bronchoalveolar spaces or lavage in patients with pulmonary sarcoidosis point towards an active process of cellular immunity, these observations may not reflect what might be going on at the actual site of granulomatous inflammation. We cannot be certain if the cells present in the bronchoalveolar lavage have actually been eluted from the sarcoidal granulomas present in the alveolar septa or have immigrated from the peripheral blood into the bronchoalveolar spaces. If the latter is the case, these cells would show quantitative and qualitative changes in response to soluble factors secreted by adjacent sarcoidal granulomas. Thus, it becomes imperative to examine the granulomas *per se* in order to determine the nature of immunologic processes which might contribute to their formation and evolution. We have recently demonstrated the

[a]To whom correspondence and reprint requests should be addressed.

spontaneous production of monocytic chemotactic factor in the supernatants of cultured cutaneous sarcoidal granulomas.[4] In response to chemotactic factor, the monocytes are attracted toward the site of its production and, in the presence of other lymphokines, may lead to induction of granulomatous inflammation. The accumulation of these cells, however, does not occur all at once because in sarcoidosis there are continuously inflammatory processes that require an uninterrupted supply of mononuclear cells. There has to be a constant stimulus to the proliferation of activated T lymphocytes which would produce lymphokines continuously at the site of the granulomatous inflammation. Interleukin-2 (IL-2) appears to serve that function.[5–7] The purpose of this study was to examine the cutaneous sarcoidal granulomas in culture for the spontaneous production of IL-2.

MATERIALS AND METHODS

Cutaneous Biopsy Cultures

Four-millimeter biopsies of sarcoidal skin lesions obtained from patients under local anesthetic and sterile conditions were cultured in RPMI 1640 medium supplemented with 1% heat-inactivated fetal calf serum (FCS) and antibiotics at 37° C in a humidified atmosphere of 5% CO_2 in air. The cell-free supernatants were harvested after 24 hr of culturing by centrifugation and stored at −70° C until assayed. Control supernatants were prepared in a similar manner, and these consisted of biopsies of normal-looking skin either from patients with sarcoidosis (normal sarcoid skin) or from surgical patients free of sarcoidosis (normal nonsarcoid skin) and culture medium alone incubated concurrently with biopsy cultures.

Cultured T Lymphocytes

Ficoll-Hypaque-separated human peripheral blood lymphocytes (PBL) were resuspended at 10^6 cells/ml in RPMI 1640-10% FCS containing 2 μg/ml purified phytohemagglutinin (PHA-P) (Wellcome Reagents, Bechenham, England) and cultured for 3 days at 37° C in a humidified atmosphere of 5% CO_2 in air.[8–10] After this culture period the viable cells were counted and resuspended in fresh media at 10^5 cells/ml in the presence of 10% commercial human IL-2 (Cellular Products, Buffalo, NY). To maintain long-term growth of these cultures, the cells were harvested every 4 days and were resuspended at 10^5 cells/ml in fresh media supplemented with the commercial IL-2. These cells were routinely used to assay the test samples for IL-2.[11,12]

Interleukin-2 Assay

Cultured T cells (CTC) were harvested from the long-term growth medium, washed, and resuspended at 5×10^5 cells/ml in medium-10% FCS containing various concentrations of the test samples. Triplicate 0.2-ml samples of suspension were dispensed into wells of microtiter plates, and the plates were incubated for 72 hr at 37° C in a humidified atmosphere of 5% CO_2 in air. The cells were pulsed 4 hr before harvest with 1 μCi [^{3}H]thymidine (New England Nuclear, Boston, MA) in 25 μl of medium. At the end of the culture period the cells were harvested onto glass-fiber filters using a semiautomated cell harvester.[11,12] The oven-dried filters were placed in 5 ml Scintilene scintillation fluid (Fisher Scientific, Pittsburgh, PA), and the cells on the filters were counted in a Packard Tricarb 4530 counter. The counts were expressed as the mean counts per minute (cpm) of the triplicate cultures, the standard error being less than 15% of the mean in all reported results.

In a long-term growth assay[13] the test samples were assessed for their ability to support the growth of activated T cells (cells that had been cultured with PHA-P for 3 days) over a period of 12 days. In this assay duplicate samples, of 10^5 cells each, were resuspended in 1 ml of medium containing either media or sarcoid supernatant, or nonsarcoid supernatant, of the commercial human IL-2 and dispensed into replicate wells of a four-well plate (Nunclon, Intermed, Denmark). Increases in cell numbers were assessed every 2 days over the 12-day period, and the cells were resuspended at 10^5 cells/ml in fresh media supplemented with the test samples when the cell concentration reached 4-5 $\times$ 10^5 cells/ml.

Exclusion Chromatography of Sarcoidal Supernatants

Concentrated samples of crude sarcoidal supernatants were applied to a 1.5 $\times$ 100-cm Biogel P-60 column (Pharmacia Fine Chemicals, Piscataway, NJ) that had been previously calibrated with blue dextran (2 $\times$ 10^6 daltons), ovalbumin (44 000 daltons), chymotrypsinogen (24 400 daltons), and ribonuclease-A (13 700 daltons). The fractionations were performed at 4° C, and the eluting buffer was 0.04 M sodium phosphate, pH 7.0. Two-milliliter fractions were collected, lyophilized, and reconstituted in 0.5 ml of medium prior to assay for IL-2. Both the applied sample and the eluting buffer contained 0.1 mg/ml of polyethylene glycol 6000 to improve the recovery of the IL-2.

RESULTS

Supernatants derived from cultures of sarcoidal skin biopsies were examined for release of IL-2-like activity during the 24-hr culture period. In three separate experiments low levels of IL-2-like activity were detected in these supernatants, the [^{3}H]thymidine uptake by 10^5 CTC averaging about 3500 cpm compared with 100 000 cpm by cells cultured in the presence of commercial human IL-2 (TABLE 1). Supernatants derived from normal nonsarcoid and normal sarcoid skin biopsies did not contain any detectable IL-2-like activity based on this assay.

In a further assay for the presence of IL-2 in sarcoidal supernatants the test samples were examined for their ability to support the continued growth of stimulated PBL (these cells had been cultured with PHA-P for 3 days) over a 12-day period. FIGURE 1 shows the results of one of three experiments indicating growth of lymphocytes when cultured in the presence of undiluted sarcoidal supernatant. A

TABLE 1. IL-2-like Activity in the Supernatants of Cutaneous Sarcoidal Granulomata[a]

Experiment Number	Test Sample	[³H]Thymidine Uptake (cpm) Undiluted	1:1	1:2	1:4
1	Sarcoid supernatant	4223	3230	2643	430
	Culture medium	1793	146	16	0
2	Sarcoid supernatant	3973	3510	3020	3193
	Culture medium	1398	573	10	26
3	Sarcoid supernatant	4951	3681	1400	0
	Culture medium	1363	1100	0	0
4	Normal nonsarcoid skin supernatant	1286	450	96	26
	Culture medium	883	348	0	0
5	Normal sarcoid skin supernatant	26	23	16	24
	Culture medium	30	16	9	16
	Partially purified IL-2	94 217	102 070	39 584	22 367

[a]The activities are expressed as net counts per minute (cpm) by [³H]thymidine uptake of cultured T cells.

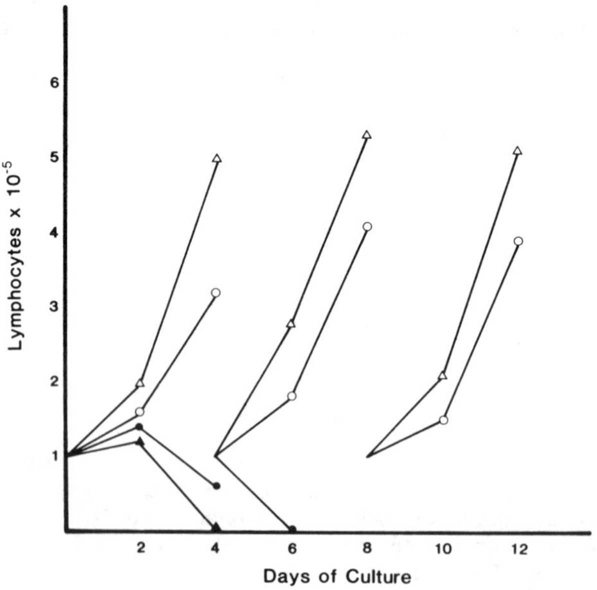

FIGURE 1. IL-2-dependent growth of cultured T cells. The peripheral blood mononuclear cells were stimulated with PHA-P for 72 hr, washed, and placed in cultures with partially purified IL-2 (△), cutaneous sarcoidal supernatant (○), nonsarcoidal skin supernatant (●), and culture medium (▲). Cultures containing cutaneous sarcoidal supernatant and IL-2 show continued proliferation of T cells.

300-400% increase in cell numbers was routinely observed over three consecutive 4-day periods in these experiments. Cultures exposed to 10% commercial human IL-2 regularly exhibited cells that were increased in number, from 1×10^5 to 5×10^5 cells/ml culture medium, whereas cells grown in medium alone were not increased in number.

When fourfold-concentrated sarcoidal supernatant was subjected to gel exclusion chromatography, the TCGF activity was found to be restricted to a narrow peak corresponding to an apparent molecular mass of about 14 900 daltons (FIG. 2).

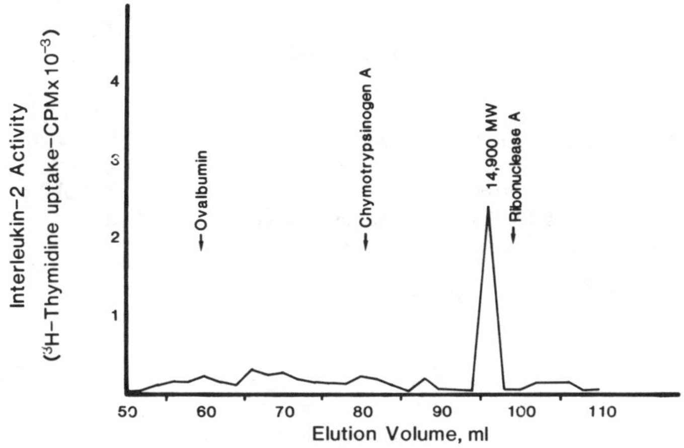

FIGURE 2. P-60 Bio-gel column chromatography of cutaneous sarcoidal supernatant showing a fraction with IL-2-like activity with an apparent molecular mass of 14 900 daltons.

DISCUSSION

The data presented clearly demonstrate the production of small amounts of IL-2-like activity by cells contained within biopsies of cutaneous sarcoidal granulomata when cultured *in vitro*. This is evidenced by continued support of growth of CTC by these supernatants and the molecular mass of the active component (approximately 14 900 daltons), which corresponds to the reported molecular mass of IL-2 produced conventionally *in vitro*.[14]

It is recognized that the antigenic stimulation of immune T lymphocytes induces differentiation of these cells into a variety of subsets.[15,16] These include a subset of cells bearing receptors for IL-2 and cells responding to IL-2. The latter group includes a variety of clones suited for different functions: cytotoxic and suppressive functions and lymphokine production. It has been demonstrated that activated T lymphocytes present in the bronchoalveolar lavage of patients with active pulmonary sarcoidosis spontaneously produce IL-2.[17] Although the nature of antigen in sarcoidosis remains unknown, T cell differentiation does seem to occur. It is supported by the spontaneous production of lymphokines by T cells from the peripheral blood, bronchoalveolar lavage, and sarcoidal granulomata.[1,4,17] Further, it has been shown that clones produced by human-human lung T cell hybridomas in sarcoidosis produce either IL-2 or monocytic chemotactic factor, suggesting that monocytic chemotactic factor and IL-2 are distinct factors and are produced by distinct subsets of lung T cells.[18] As the granulomas of sarcoidosis in any part of the body have similar morphologic characteristics, the presence of predominant helper cells in these granulomas may play a key role in regulating the granulomatous inflammation in sarcoidosis. IL-2 produced at the site of granulomatous inflammation will lead to continuous proliferation of clones of activated T lymphocytes responsible for the production of a variety of lymphokines. This could explain the induction and perpetual formation of granulomas in sarcoidosis.

SUMMARY

Biopsies of cutaneous sarcoidal lesions were cultured for 24 hr *in vitro,* and the cell-free supernatants were examined for the presence of T cell growth factor (IL-2). Low levels of IL-2 were detected in these supernatants based on their ability to support the growth of cultured T cells. The apparent molecular mass of the active component in these supernatants, as assessed by exclusion chromatography, was 14 900 daltons. These findings suggest that IL-2 production within these sarcoidal lesions may be partly responsible for their evolution and maintenance.

REFERENCES

1. KATARIA, Y. P., R. A. SHAW & P. B. CAMPBELL. 1982. Sarcoidosis: An overview II. Clin. Notes Respir. Dis. **20:** 3-16.
2. DOMBY, W. R., Y. P. KATARIA, M. MCSHANE & M. E. WHITCOMB. 1980. Immunological and diagnostic characteristics of bronchoalveolar cells in pulmonary sarcoidosis. *In* Eighth International Conference on Sarcoidosis and Other Granulomatous Diseases. W. Jones Williams & B. H. Davies, Eds.: 436-441. Alpha Omega. Cardiff.
3. HUNNINGHAKE, G. W., J. E. GADEK, R. C. YOUNG, JR., O. KAWANAMI, V. J. FERRANS & R. G. CRYSTAL. 1980. Mechanisms of granuloma formation in pulmonary sarcoidosis by T-lymphocytes within the lung. N. Engl. J. Med. **302:** 594-598.
4. KATARIA, Y. P., P. B. CAMPBELL, H. K. PARK & K. C. KALMUS. 1983. *In vitro* observations on intact granulomas of sarcoidosis. *In* Sarcoidosis and Other Granulomatous Disorders. J. Chrétien, J. Marsac & J. C. Saltiel, Eds.: 126-131. Pergamon Press. Paris.
5. SMITH, K. A., S. GILLIS, P. E. BAKER, D. MCKENZIE & F. W. RUSCETTI. 1979. T-cell growth factor-mediated T-cell proliferation. Ann. N.Y. Acad. Sci. **332:** 423-432.
6. CHEEVER, M. A., P. D. GREENBERG, C. IRLE, J. A. THOMPSON, D. L. URDAL, D. Y. MOCHIZUKI, C. S. HENNEY & S. GILLIS. 1984. Interleukin-2 administered *in vivo* induces the growth of cultured T-cells *in vivo.* J. Immunol. **132:** 2259-2265.
7. KELSO, A., H. R. MACDONALD, K. A. SMITH, J. A. CEROTTINI & K. T. BRUNNER. 1984. Interleukin-2 enhancement of lymphokine secretion by T-lymphocytes: Analysis of established clones and primary limiting dilution microcultures. J. Immunol. **132:** 2932-2938.
8. PERPER, R. J., T. W. ZEE & M. M. MICKELSON. 1968. Purification of lymphocytes and platelets by centrifugation J. Lab. Clin. Med. **72:** 842-848.
9. NOBLE, P. B., J. H. CUTTS & K. K. CARROLL. 1968. Ficoll flotation for the separation of blood leukocyte types. Blood **31:** 66-73.

10. KATARIA, Y. P. & K. R. GLAUS. 1978. Sarcoidosis: Phytohemagglutinin response of lymphocyte fractions isolated by velocity sedimentation and enhanced helper cell activity. Am. Rev. Respir. Dis. **117:** 519-526.
11. GILLIS, S., M. E. FERM, W. OUJ & K. A. SMITH. 1978. T-cell growth factor: Parameters of production and a quantitive microassay for activity. J. Immunol. **120:** 2027-2032.
12. GULLBERG, M., F. IVARS, A. COUTINITO & E. LARSSON. 1981. Regulation of T-cell growth production: Arrest of TCGF production after 18 hours in normal lectin-stimulated mouse spleen cell cultures. J. Immunol. **127:** 407-411.
13. GRIMM, E. A. & S. A. ROSENBURG. 1982. Production and properties of human IL-2. *In* Isolation, Characterization, and Utilization of T-Lymphocyte Clones. G. Fathman & F. Fitch, Eds.: 57-82. Academic Press. New York, NY.
14. GILLIS, S., K. A. SMITH & J. WATSON. 1980. Biochemical characterization of lymphocyte regulation molecules. II. Purification of a class of rat and human lymphokines. J. Immunol. **124:** 1954-1962.
15. LARRSON, E. 1981. Mechanism of T-cell activation. II. Antigen- and lectin-dependent acquisition of responsiveness to TCGF is a nonmitogenic, active response of resting T-cells. J. Immunol. **126:** 1323-1326.
16. MANNEL, D. N., W. FALK & W. DROGE. 1983. Induction of cytotoxic T-cell function requires sequential action of three different lymphokines. J. Immunol. **130:** 2508-2510.
17. HUNNINGHAKE, G. W., G. N. BEDELL, D. C. ZAVALA, M. MONICK & M. BRADY. 1983. Role of interleukin-2 release by lung T-cells in active pulmonary sarcoidosis. Am. Rev. Respir. Dis. **128:** 634-638.
18. GLAZIER, A. J., M. SUNDELL & G. W. HUNNINGHAKE. 1984. Production of human-human lung T-cell hybridomas from patients with interstitial lung disease. Clin. Res. **32:** 429A.

The Kveim–Siltzbach Granuloma

A Model for Sarcoid Granuloma Formation[a]

B. B. MISHRA,[b] L. W. POULTER, G. JANOSSY, S. SHERLOCK, AND D. G. JAMES

The Royal Northern and Royal Free Hospitals
London, England

INTRODUCTION

The intradermal injection of a heat-treated suspension of sarcoid tissue homogenate produces microscopic epithelioid cell granulomas at the injection site in patients with active sarcoidosis.[1] This constitutes the positive Kveim test, and it can be elicited in about 75% of sarcoid patients with active disease.[2] Only 2% of nonsarcoid subjects develop positive Kveim reactions,[3] so it is a specific diagnostic test for active sarcoidosis.[3–5] Furthermore, it is the only currently known model of sarcoid granuloma formation. No other granuloma, produced in man, can appear specifically and synchronously during periods of disease activity as well as disappear during periods of inactivity.[5] Sarcoid granuloma formation may involve at least two basic processes: first, a systemic process that is responsible for the simultaneous production of granulomas at multiple sites, and second, a local process that allows the systemic process to act at discrete locations to produce granulomas.[6] The systemic pathogenic process that causes sarcoid granulomas to develop and grow in a patient with active sarcoidosis probably provides the background for the injection site granulomas. The Kveim reagent should be regarded as that required to produce the local granuloma when the systemic process is active.

The cellular composition of the Kveim and sarcoid granulomas are likely to be similar if the two are produced by the same process; the first aim of this study was to compare the cellular composition of these two kinds of granulomas, to examine this possibility. To this end, monoclonal antibodies specific for cell membrane antigens of particular lymphoid or nonlymphoid cells were used to identify various mononuclear cells by their phenotype in frozen sections of tissue biopsies.[7]

Two newly developed monoclonal reagents, RFD 1 and RFD 2, were used to label, respectively, dendritic interdigitating cells and macrophages. Indirect immunofluorescence was combined with histochemistry to provide a more detailed analysis

[a] This work was made possible by generous financial support from the Roger Gibbs Research Foundation; the E.B. Hutchinson Trust; and the Department of Neurology, Temple University School of Medicine.

[b] Present address: Department of Neurology, Temple University Hospital, 3401 North Broad Street, Philadelphia, Pennsylvania 19140.

of these macrophage cell types.[7,8] The early events in the evolution of the sarcoid tissue granuloma have been difficult to analyze because there is no reliable method of distinguishing between an early and late sarcoid granuloma. The evolution of the Kveim granuloma begins when the Kveim reagent is injected into the skin, and hence the early stages of the Kveim granuloma formation can be studied by examining the Kveim infiltrates sequentially. The second aim was to use this method of phenotypic analysis to compare the cellular phenotypes seen during the evolution of the Kveim granuloma with those seen in spontaneous sarcoid tissue granulomas, in an attempt to see if the variations seen in the sarcoid granuloma were analogous to well-defined stages in the evolution of the Kveim granuloma.

MATERIALS AND METHODS

Portions of skin biopsies were obtained from five patients; liver biopsies from six; a lymph node biopsy from one; a bronchial nodule from one; and a laryngeal nodule from one. Each of these 14 sarcoid patients had only one biopsy. All the skin biopsies were performed on patients with chronic skin lesions whereas the other biopsies were performed in the course of evaluating acute symptoms. Nine other sarcoid patients with proven positive Kveim reactions had biopsies of the Kveim reaction sites either 2 weeks or 4 weeks after a Kveim test. In two of these patients the Kveim reaction sites were subjected to biopsy both at the 2-week stage and at the 4-week stage. Two others had a biopsy of the Kveim reaction site only at the 2-week stage and five others had biopsies at the 4-week stage (TABLE 1). The biopsies were covered with Optimal Cutting Temperature (OCT) compound and snap-frozen in isopentane precooled in liquid nitrogen. Sections 6 μm-thick were cut using a cryostat at $-25°$ C, air-dried overnight at room temperature, and fixed for 7 min in a 1:1 mixture of chloroform-acetone fixative. Some sections from each specimen were stained with hematoxylin and eosin (H&E) to demonstrate and confirm pathology. Immunofluorescent, immunoperoxidase, and histochemical methods used are described elsewhere.[9] The antibody reagents used to study the nonlymphoid cell phenotypes were RFD 1, which labels mostly lymph node interdigitating cell phenotype, and RFD 2, which labels monocyte-macrophage cell phenotypes.[8,9] The helper-cytotoxic and the suppressor-cytotoxic lymphocyte phenotypes were identified by their reactivity with the monoclonal reagents similar to OKT4 and OKT8, respectively. Thymus-derived (T) lymphocytes were identified by the antibody label UCH T1 that labels most peripheral T cells.[9] The monoclonal reagent TO 15 was used to label bone marrow-derived (B) cells in the sections.[9]

Acid-phosphatase enzyme activity was demonstrated histochemically.[7] Immunofluorescent labeling and histochemistry were performed in combination on at least three sections of each biopsy specimen as previously described.[7] This demonstrated essentially two subtypes of the cells labeled by RFD 2 monoclonal antibody (RFD 2^+ cells). Some RFD 2^+ cell types demonstrated strong acid-phosphatase enzyme activity (RFD 2^+, ACP^+ cell types) while other RFD 2^+ cell types demonstrated weak acid-phosphatase activity under the conditions of the experiments (RFD 2^+, $ACP^{-/+}$ cell types).

Two kinds of counts were performed to quantify the differences in the predominant macrophage phenotype in the granulomas. At least three double-labeled sections of each biopsy specimen were examined, and the total number of cells in the granulomas

TABLE 1. Biopsies from Sarcoid Patients

Biopsy Material	Number of Patients
Liver	6
Skin	5
Lymph node	1
Bronchial nodule	1
Laryngeal nodule	1
Kveim-reaction granulomas	
4 weeks old	7
2 weeks old	4
Total number of patients studied	23

was counted. The number of RFD 2^+ cells that had strong acid-phosphatase enzyme activity (RFD 2^+, ACP^+ cell types) was counted and expressed as a percentage of the total number of all cells counted. The second kind of count was made by counting the number of granulomas in at least three sections from each biopsy specimen. If in more than half the granulomas a majority (greater than 66%) of the macrophage cell types (RFD 2^+ cell type) had strong acid-phosphatase enzyme activity, the biopsy specimen was classified as a predominantly RFD 2^+, ACP^+ type. The other variety of biopsy specimen was therefore the RFD 2^+, $ACP^{-/+}$ type wherein more than half the granulomas had a majority (greater than 66%) of RFD 2^+ cells with weak acid-phosphatase activity.

RESULTS

Two-week-old Kveim Granulomas

Histology

Kveim-positive biopsy specimens showed collections of epithelioid cells, giant cells, and lymphocytes (FIG. 1) similar to the sarcoid granuloma described below. In addition, three out of four biopsies had amorphous, eosinophilic particles of Kveim material of varying size bordered by large and small mononuclear cells, many epithelioid cells, and a few giant cells. The smaller mononuclear cells with the morphology of lymphocytes appeared mostly in the periphery of the collection of cells bordering the Kveim particle whereas the larger mononuclear cells, epithelioid cells, and giant cells were found adjacent to the Kveim particle. A few collections of mononuclear cells containing all the morphological cellular varieties described above were found unassociated with Kveim particles.

Lymphoid Cells

About 30% of the cells were lymphocytes and were labeled by the T lymphocyte marker, UCH T1. The B lymphocyte marker, TO 15, did not label any of the cells in the mononuclear cell infiltrate. About half the T cells were labeled by the helper-cytotoxic T cell label, OKT4, and hence were the $T4^+$ phenotype. Most of the $T4^+$ cells were amongst the collections not associated with the Kveim particle, although a few $T4^+$ subtypes did lie in the periphery of the collections around the Kveim particle (FIG. 2A). The suppressor-cytotoxic T cell label, RFT8, labeled approximately the other half of the T cells in the areas described above. In the collections not associated with the Kveim particle, these $T8^+$ cell types showed a tendency to be distributed in the periphery of the granuloma (FIG. 2B), a feature more characteristically seen in the sarcoid granulomas described below.

Nonlymphoid Cells

Except for the few cells labeled by UCH T1, the cells bordering the Kveim particle were all labeled by either RFD 1 or RFD 2, showing them all to be nonlymphoid cells. The cells with the morphological appearance of epithelioid cells and giant cells were also labeled by RFD 2 monoclonal reagent (FIG. 3A) and showed strong acid-phosphatase activity, confirming previous studies on sarcoid granulomas.[9] The Kveim

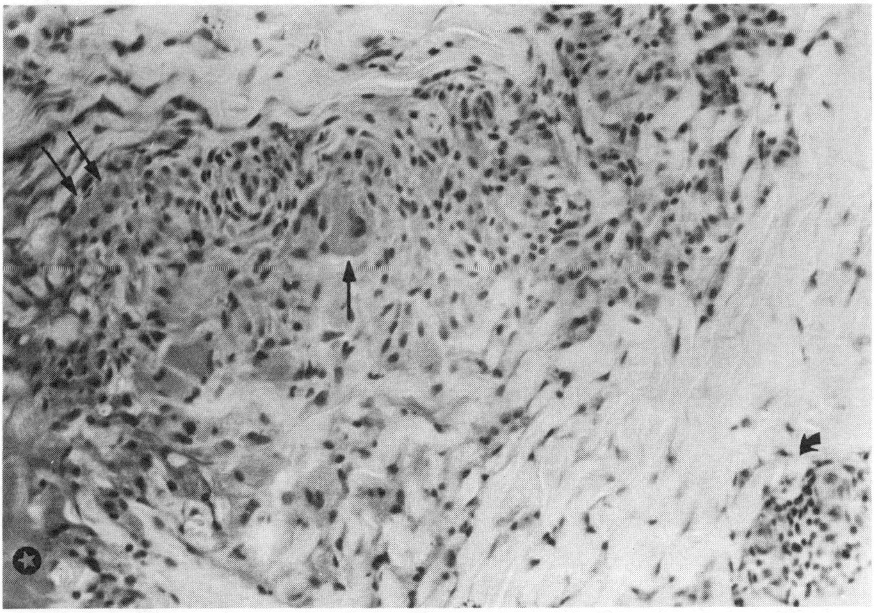

FIGURE 1. A 2-week-old, Kveim reagent-induced infiltrate in a biopsy of the 2-week-old intradermal Kveim injection site in a patient with active sarcoidosis and a histologically proven positive Kveim test. The infiltrate was stained with hematoxylin and eosin. The particulate Kveim material is seen (star) as homogenous eosinophilic material with a border made up of a mononuclear cell infiltrate. Large, nonlymphoid cells and epithelioid cells (thin arrows) are predominant; there are very few small, lymphoid-like cells. A second collection of large, morphologically nonlymphoid cells, along with a large proportion of small lymphoid cells, is seen some distance from the larger infiltrate (thick arrow).

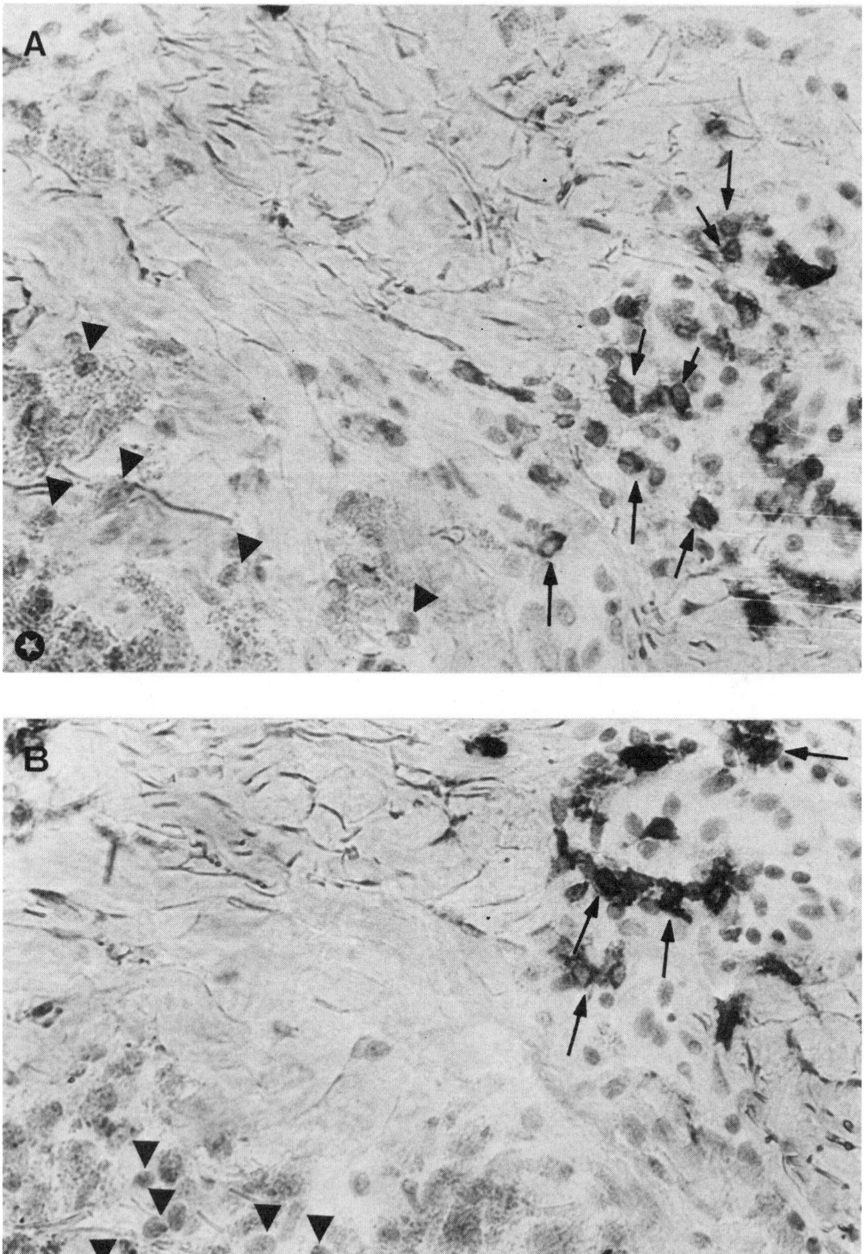
A
B

reagent particle itself produced a nonspecific fluorescence when illuminated with UV light and turned light brown during histochemical reactions used to demonstrate acid-phosphatase enzyme activity (FIG. 3B). The homogenous appearance of the nonspecific fluorescence easily distinguished it from the membrane fluorescence of the surrounding cells: the latter was broken up with dark spots of unstained nuclei surrounded by immunofluorescent membrane labels on UV microscopy. Counts revealed that 70% of the granulomas had a majority of the RFD 2^+, ACP^+ phenotype (TABLE 2). This was similar to the counts on sections of liver, lymph node, bronchial nodule, and laryngeal nodule biopsy specimens, and was clearly different from the sarcoid skin biopsy specimens.

Four-week-old Kveim Granulomas

Histology

Kveim reaction sites that were subjected to biopsy 4 weeks after the Kveim test injection showed noncaseating epithelioid cell granulomas. The particles of Kveim material that were observed in the 2-week-old Kveim reaction site biopsy specimens were not seen in the 4-week-old biopsies. Also, the collections of mostly nonlymphoid cells surrounding the Kveim particles were not seen in any of the biopsy specimens, including the ones performed sequentially 2 weeks after the first biopsy.

Lymphoid Cells

In the 4-week-old Kveim granulomas T lymphocytes labeled by UCH T1 (UCH $T1^+$ cells) were the only lymphoid cells seen. The B lymphocyte monoclonal antibody did not label any cells in the sections studied. There were slightly more T lymphocytes at the 4-week stage than there were at either the 2-week stage or the sarcoid granulomas. Approximately half the total number of cells counted were UCH $T1^+$ cells. The pattern of distribution of $T4^+$ cells and $T8^+$ cells approached the pattern seen in all sarcoid granulomas, with the $T4^+$ cells being distributed throughout the granulomas whereas the $T8^+$ cells showed a tendency to be restricted to the periphery.

FIGURE 2. (A) Analysis of the $T4^+$ cell (helper phenotype) in a consecutive section of the same 2-week-old Kveim test biopsy shown in FIGURE 1. The $T4^+$ cells are easily recognized because of the dark stains on their cell membranes (arrows), and are diffusely distributed in the collection of cells some distance from the Kveim particle (star). None of the cells bordering the Kveim particle (arrowheads) are labeled by the OKT4 monoclonal reagent. The latter cells are macrophages labeled by the RFD 2 monoclonal reagent as shown in FIGURE 3A. **(B)** Analysis of the $T8^+$ cells (suppressor-cytotoxic phenotype) in a consecutive section of the same biopsy shown in FIGURE 3A. The $T8^+$ cells may be recognized because of the black stains on their membranes (arrows), and are seen in the granuloma some distance from the Kveim particle (star). The $T8^+$ cells are restricted to the periphery of the granuloma. Again, there are no $T8^+$ cells bordering the Kveim particle (arrowheads).

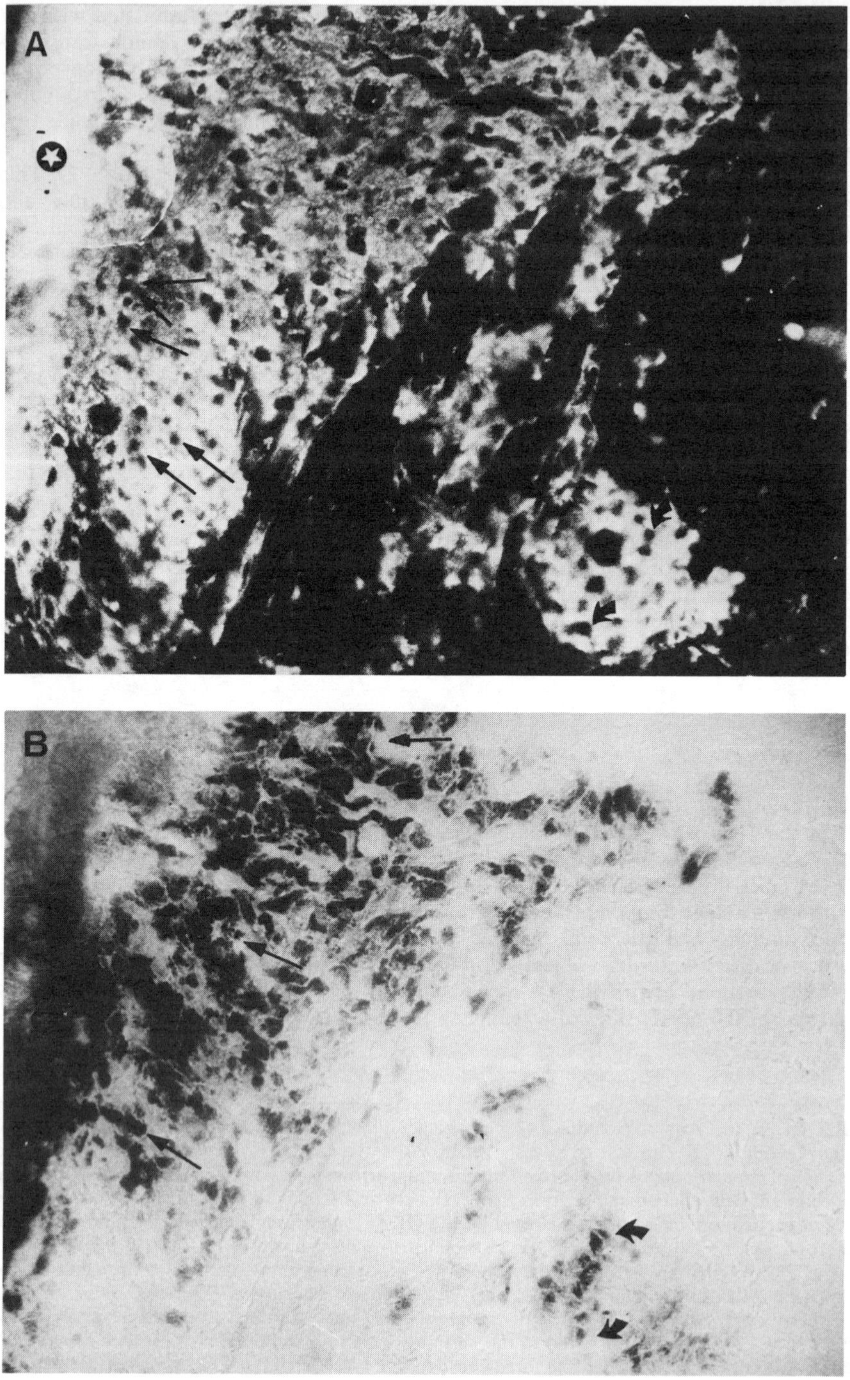
A
B

Nonlymphoid Cells

The various phenotypes of nonlymphoid cells that were seen in the 2-week-old Kveim granulomas and in the sarcoid granulomas were also seen in the 4-week-old Kveim granulomas. RFD 1 labeled about 60% of the nonlymphoid cells scattered throughout the small granulomas. Although the RFD 2 antibody labeled about 50% of the cells in the granulomas, only a minority of these cells (30% of the RFD 2^+ cells) showed strong acid-phosphatase enzyme activity. Only 15% of all cells in the sections examined were macrophage phenotypes with strong acid-phosphatase enzyme activity (RFD 2^+, ACP^+ cell type). Therefore the predominant phenotype in most of the granulomas was the RFD 2^+, $ACP^{-/+}$ phenotype. Only 5 to 10% of the granulomas had a majority of the RFD 2^+, ACP^+ phenotype.

In all these respects the 4-week-old Kveim granulomas were similar to the sarcoid skin granulomas but differed from the other sarcoid granulomas examined, which, as described below, demonstrated strong acid-phosphatase enzyme activity in most of the macrophage cell types (TABLE 2).

Sarcoid Tissue Biopsies

Histology

Characteristic noncaseating epithelioid cell granulomas were seen in the sarcoid tissue biopsies.

Lymphoid Cells

Most of the lymphocytes were labeled by UCH T1 and hence were T lymphocyte phenotypes (UCH $T1^+$). They constituted approximately a third of the total population of cells in the granuloma. Less than 1% of the cells were B cell phenotypes as detected by the B cell-specific monoclonal antibody, TO 15. Labeling with OKT4 monoclonal reagent demonstrated the characteristically diffused, scattered distribution of $T4^+$

FIGURE 3. (A) A section from the same 2-week-old Kveim reaction biopsy shown in FIGURE 1. Immunofluorescence outlines cells labeled by the macrophage-specific marker, RFD 2 (thin arrows). The Kveim particle shows a homogenous, nonspecific fluorescence (star). In the zone bordering the Kveim material, mostly RFD 2^+ cells are seen. The second collection of cells also demonstrates RFD 2^+ phenotype macrophages (thick arrows). The cell margins of the RFD 2^+ cells are blurred because of the interdigitations between processes of neighboring epithelioid cells and macrophages.[10] Individual cells may be identified because of their dark, unlabeled nuclei (thin arrows). **(B)** The same section shown in FIGURE 3A, showing histochemistry for acid-phosphatase. Almost all RFD 2^+ cells bordering the Kveim particle (star) show strong acid-phosphatase reactivity (thin arrows). The RFD 2^+ cells in the second collection also show strong acid-phosphatase reactivity (thick arrows).

TABLE 2. Distribution of Nonlymphoid Subsets

	Granulomas			
	Kveim (4 weeks old)	Sarcoid Skin	Kveim (2 weeks old)	Sarcoid Liver
Number of patients	6	5	4	6
Number of sections counted	18	15	12	18
Predominant phenotype in most granulomas[a]	RFD 2^+, $ACP^{+/-}$	RFD 2^+, $ACP^{+/-}$	RFD 2^+, ACP^+	RFD 2^+, ACP^+
Percentage of RFD 2^+, ACP^+ cells in the granulomas	15	30	66	66

[a] RFD 2^+ cells: cells labeled by the monocyte-macrophage-specific monoclonal RFD 2; $ACP^{+/-}$ cells: cells with weak acid-phosphatase enzyme activity; ACP^+ cells: cells with strong acid-phosphatase enzyme activity.

helper-cytotoxic T cell subtypes in the sarcoid granuloma. In contrast, the $T8^+$ suppressor-cytotoxic subtype labeled by OKT8 monoclonal reagent was restricted only to the periphery of the granulomas. This distribution of T cell subsets is characteristic of sarcoid tissue granulomas.[9]

Nonlymphoid Cells

About 66% of all cells in the sarcoid tissue granulomas were nonlymphoid cells, and were labeled either by RFD 2 or by RFD 1 monoclonal reagents. Analysis of nonlymphoid cells in sarcoid granulomas showed that a majority (66%) of the granuloma was made up of these cells. In the sarcoid granulomas, too, the cells labeled by RFD 2 monoclonal reagents were either strongly acid-phosphatase positive or weakly acid-phosphatase positive. The latter (RFD 2^+, $ACP^{-/+}$) predominated in the sarcoid skin biopsies whereas the former (RFD 2^+, ACP^+) predominated in the liver, bronchial nodule, and laryngeal nodule biopsy specimens. Counts revealed that more than 50% of the granulomas in sarcoid liver biopsy specimens had a majority (greater than 66%) of the RFD 2^+, ACP^+ cell type. The bronchial nodule and laryngeal nodule biopsy specimens were similar to the liver biopsy specimen in this regard. In contrast, only 10 to 20% of the sarcoid skin granulomas had a majority of the RFD 2^+, ACP^+ phenotype. The sarcoid skin biopsy was similar to the 4-week-old Kveim granuloma with regard to the predominant nonlymphoid cell phenotype. Other sarcoid granulomas in this study resembled the 2-week-old Kveim granulomas (TABLE 2).

The remaining phenotype of nonlymphoid cells were those labeled by RFD 1, which also labels the interdigitating cells of the lymph node interfollicular areas. These cells were seen either scattered in the periphery of some granulomas, as described before,[9] or were found scattered throughout the granuloma. They constituted about half of the nonlymphoid cells in most sarcoid granulomas.

DISCUSSION

The present study demonstrates that the phenotypes of lymphoid and nonlymphoid cells in 2-week-old Kveim granulomas and acute or active sarcoid granulomas are similar. The 2-week-old Kveim reaction sites demonstrate epithelioid cell granulomas in addition to collections of nonlymphoid cells around Kveim particles. In the later, 4-week-old Kveim reaction sites, however, the collections of nonlymphoid cells appear to have resolved leaving behind only the epithelioid cell granulomas that are made up of lymphoid and nonlymphoid cells just as in the sarcoid granulomas.

The predominance of the nonlymphoid cell type in all granulomas is striking and consistent with earlier observations of Kveim sarcoid granulomas.[9] Most of the nonlymphoid cells retain reactivity with the macrophage-specific monoclonal reagent, RFD 2. In this study the RFD 2^+ macrophage-type cells are divided into two subsets depending upon the acid-phosphatase enzyme activity demonstrated on combined immunofluorescence and histochemistry. Although all macrophage cell types possess acid-phosphatase enzyme activity,[8] some demonstrate strong reactivity (RFD 2^+,

ACP^+), and others demonstrate a weak reactivity (RFD 2^+, $ACP^{+/-}$). Both varieties are found in sarcoid granulomas as well as in early and late Kveim granulomas. It is significant that a predominance of RFD 2^+, ACP^+ phenotype was seen in the granulomas of sarcoid liver, lymph node, laryngeal nodule, and bronchial nodule biopsy specimens which were obtained in the course of evaluating acute symptoms. Strong acid-phosphatase enzyme activity may be a feature of RFD 2^+ cells in recently formed granulomas. This is definitely observed in the 2-week-old Kveim granulomas. The sarcoid skin granulomas are, however, more like the 4-week-old Kveim granulomas in that the RFD 2^+, $ACP^{+/-}$ phenotype predominates in the granulomas. It is significant that skin granulomas are chronic lesions whereas liver granulomas, which are phenotypically similar to young, 2-week-old Kveim granulomas, are more often associated with features of active sarcoidosis.[11]

The 2-week-old Kveim granulomas demonstrate some restriction of $T8^+$ cells to the periphery of the granulomas. This is seen in all sarcoid granulomas, which again suggests that the 2-week-old Kveim granuloma reflects early changes in the sarcoid granuloma. The distribution of $T4^+$ cells and $T8^+$ cells in the 4-week-old Kveim granulomas, which shows an even more striking resemblance to the sarcoid granuloma distribution, is consistent with the concept that the development of the Kveim granuloma reflects the development of the sarcoid granuloma.

Using the 2-week-old Kveim infiltrate as a model of the early stages of granuloma formation, it appears that the Kveim granuloma begins as collections of large nonlymphoid cells around particulate Kveim material. Experimental granulomas produced by injections of inert particulate matter into animals are characterized by collections of nonlymphoid cells.[12] These have been described as foreign body granulomas to distinguish them from larger hypersensitivity granulomas which are made up with lymphoid cells in addition to nonlymphoid cells and are produced by injections of particulate antigenic material into sensitized animals.

The later 4-week-old Kveim granulomas and sarcoid granulomas resemble the hypersensitivity granulomas. Unlike the spontaneous evolution of the Kveim granuloma from the 2-week stage to the 4-week stage, however, the experimental foreign body granulomas do not evolve spontaneously into hypersensitivity granulomas, although this development can be induced. This has been done by the intravenous injection of an allergen against which the animal with a foreign body granuloma can mount a hypersensitivity reaction. The antigenemia with a sensitizing antigen represents the "systemic process" that converts the foreign body granulomas in the early Kveim injection sites and in other tissues (the "local process") into a hypersensitivity-type sarcoid granuloma.[6]

ACKNOWLEDGMENTS

We are grateful to the Friends of the Royal Northern Hospital for their help and to Dr. J. I. Greenstein for his help in preparing this manuscript.

REFERENCES

1. KVEIM, A. 1941. En ny og spesifikk kutan reaksjon ved Boeck's sarcoid. Nord. Med. **9:** 169.

2. JAMES, D. G., A. D. THOMSON & A. WILLCOX. 1956. Erythema nodosum as a manifestation of sarcoidosis. Lancet **ii:** 218.
3. SILTZBACH, L. E. 1961. The Kveim test in sarcoidosis. J. Am. Med. Assoc. **178:** 476-482.
4. DOUGLAS, A. C., A. WALLACE, J. CLARK, J. H. STEPHEN, I. E. SMITH & N. C. ALLAN. 1976. The Edinburgh spleen: Source of a validated Kveim-Siltzbach material. Ann. N.Y. Acad. Sci. **278:** 670.
5. ANDERSON, R., D. G. JAMES, P. M. PETERS & A. D. THOMSON. 1963. The Kveim test in sarcoidosis. Lancet **i:** 650-653.
6. MISHRA, B. B., J. I. GREENSTEIN & L. W. POULTER. 1984. Sarcoidosis: A disorder due to allergic granulomatous transformation. In preparation.
7. POULTER, L. W., M. CHILOSI, G. J. SEYMOUR, S. HOBBS & G. JANOSSY. 1983. Immunofluorescence membrane staining and cytochemistry applied in combination for analysing cell interactions *in situ. In* Immunochemistry: Practical Applications in Pathology and Biology. J. Polak & S. van Noorden, Eds.: 233-248. Wright. London.
8. POULTER, L. W. 1983. Antigen-presenting cells *in situ:* Their identification and involvement in immunopathology. Clin Exp. Immunol. **53:** 513.
9. MISHRA, B. B., L. W. POULTER, G. JANOSSY & D. G. JAMES. 1983. The distribution of lymphoid- and macrophage-like cell subsets of sarcoid and Kveim granulomata: Possible mechanism of negative PPD reaction in sarcoidosis. Clin. Exp. Immunol. **54:** 705-715.
10. PAPADIMITROU, J. M., J. M. FINLAY-JONES & M. N. WALTERS. 1973. Surface characteristics of macrophages and epithelioid and giant cells using scanning electron microscopy. Exp. Cell. Res. **76:** 353.
11. SCADDING, J. G. 1967. Sarcoidosis of the skin. *In* Sarcoidosis: 174-194. Eyre & Spottiswoode. London.
12. BOROS, D. L. & K. S. WARREN. 1973. The bentonite granuloma: Characterisation of a model system for infectious and foreign body granulomatous inflammation using soluble mycobacterial, histoplasma, and schistoma antigens. Immunology **24:** 511.

Enhanced Inflammatory Response with Histiocytes and Epithelioid Cells in Rabbits to the Intradermal Injection of Supernatants of Cultured Cutaneous Sarcoidal Granulomas

Y. P. KATARIA,[a,b] H. K. PARK,[c] AND L. D. MOUNTAIN[d]

[b] *Pulmonary Diseases Section*
Department of Medicine
[c] *Department of Clinical Pathology and Diagnostic Medicine*
and
[d] *Department of Medicine*
East Carolina University School of Medicine
Greenville, North Carolina 27834

INTRODUCTION

Sarcoidosis is a multisystemic granulomatous disease of unknown etiology. Its hallmark is the formation of noncaseating granulomas. Recent immunohistochemical studies on biopsy specimens obtained from a variety of organs from patients with sarcoidosis suggest that sarcoidosis has an immunologic origin.[1–3] These studies have shown the presence of large numbers of thymus-derived (T) cells: helper-inducer T lymphocytes predominate; there are only a few bone marrow-derived (B) cells and suppressor-cytotoxic cells; and, in the center of granulomas, a large number of epithelioid cells and a few multinucleated giant cells may be seen. The concept of an immunologic origin for sarcoidosis has been further supported by evidence of lymphokine production by the cultured cutaneous sarcoidal granulomas.[4] It is recognized that foreign body granulomas do not, and that granulomas of immunologic origin do, produce lymphokines.[5] More recently, production of interleukin-2 (IL-2) has been demonstrated in the cultures of cutaneous sarcoidal granulomas.[6] The chemotactic factor appears to attract the monocytes at the site of antigen deposition, possibly initiating the granulomatous inflammation. IL-2 has a continuous proliferative action on a variety of T lymphocyte clones which in turn produce lymphokines,[7,8] and this may explain the perpetual formation of granulomas in sarcoidosis. The purpose of

[a] To whom correspondence and reprint requests should be addressed.

this study was to examine the inflammatory response to intradermal injection of lymphokine-containing supernatants of cultured cutaneous sarcoidal granulomas in an experimental animal.

MATERIALS AND METHODS

Cutaneous Biopsies of Sarcoidal Skin Lesions and Cultures

Punch biopsies (4 mm) taken from patients with sarcoidosis were performed with local anesthetic under sterile conditions and were then cultured in RPMI 1640 with L-glutamine (Gibco) containing 100 units of penicillin and 100 μg of streptomycin per ml and 10% heat-inactivated donor calf serum. Tissue cultures were incubated at 37° C in a humidified atmosphere of 5% CO_2 and air. Cell-free supernatants were harvested every 72 hr by centrifugation at 400 g for 10 min and stored at −70° C. There were three controls: two were supernatants of normal-looking skin biopsy specimens, obtained from patients with sarcoidosis and from surgical patients free of sarcoidosis, and one was merely incubated media.

Selection of Experimental Animals

A comparative study of chemotactic response of monocytes obtained from rabbits, guinea pigs, rats, monkeys, and humans was carried out utilizing sarcoidal granuloma supernatants. Peripheral venous blood from these animals was fractionated on a Ficoll-Hypaque gradient to obtain mononuclear cells. The monocytes were used in the leukotactic assay as previously described.[4] Rabbit monocytes were found to be most responsive to the sarcoidal granuloma supernatants as shown in TABLE 1.

Selection of the Vehicle for Injection of Supernatants

Because of the lack of inflammatory response at the injection site with supernatants alone, some type of matrix was needed as a carrier for lymphokine-containing supernatant. The vehicle used as a matrix for the inoculation of test samples was chosen after pretesting a variety of inert sterile materials, such as teflon, and a variety of sponges implanted into the skin of the rabbit. Other materials tested consisted of inert gels (Sephadex and Sepharose), 0.81-μ bacto-latex beads (BLB), and Kveim-Siltzbach (K-S) antigen inactivated by boiling for 2 hr. Implants were not satisfactory because of the high incidence of infection, even with the administration of antibiotics. The BLB and inactivated K-S antigen produced the least inflammatory response and were therefore selected to be used in the experiments.

Preparation of Supernatants for Injection

Cell-free supernatants were tested for leukotactic activity as previously described to determine the presence of monocytic chemotactic factor.[4] Supernatants were dialyzed for 24 hr against distilled water at 4° C under sterile conditions. Test samples were lyophilized (Virtis) and reconstituted in sterile normal saline to 1/10 the original volume. Test samples were prepared by mixing 0.1 ml of reconstituted supernatant with an equal volume of 0.81-μ BLB (Difco) or inactivated K-S antigen.

Injection of Supernatants into the Rabbit's Skin

The rabbit was anesthetized with ketamine hydrochloride (25 mg/kg body weight), and the skin on its back was shaved and prepared with absolute alcohol before injection. Injections were made in duplicate on both sides of midline, approximately equidistant from the dorsal line and the injection site; 0.2 ml of test samples were injected intracutaneously. Antibiotics were administered every 48 hr until the animal was biopsied. After 3-5 days the injection sites were checked for reactivity, and a punch biopsy (6 mm) was performed from each injection site and put in 10% buffered formalin for histopathological examination. These specimens were processed in a routine fashion to prepare multiple serial sections and stained with hematoxylin and eosin.

TABLE 1. Chemotactic Response of Peripheral Blood Monocytes to Supernatants of Cultured Cutaneous Granulomas

Source of Monocytes	Number of Animals	Chemotactic Response[a] (%)	Significance[b]
Rabbit	4	241 ± 97	$p < .01$
Guinea pig	3	70 ± 5	NS
Rat	3	0	NS
Monkey	3	122 ± 42	$p < .05$
Human	10	66 ± 18	

[a] The chemotactic responses are expressed as percentages of the zymosan-activated human serum response. Each value is a mean ± SD. Results compared with human response.

[b] The levels of significance were calculated with Student's *t* test.

RESULTS

Monocytic Chemotactic Activity of Cutaneous Sarcoidal Supernatants

The monocytic chemotactic response of sarcoidal supernatants ranged from 39% to 210% of that produced in the zymosan-activated human serum; four supernatants had less than 60% and eight more than 60% of the monocytic chemotactic response.

Histiopathologic Examination of Biopsy Specimens From the Injection Sites

Injection of supernatants alone, control media, or normal saline solution produced no significant inflammatory reaction at the injection site.

Biopsy specimens obtained from the site injected with sarcoidal supernatants mixed with heat-inactivated K-S antigen revealed an increased histiocytic reaction in 9 out of 11 experiments, compared with control media containing K-S antigen. Well-formed granulomas were seen in six experiments with sarcoidal supernatants mixed with K-S antigen and in three with control media plus K-S antigen. The extent of cellular infiltration was much greater with sarcoidal supernatants (FIG. 1).

Similarly, sarcoidal supernatants mixed with BLB showed an enhanced histiocytic reaction at the injection site in 8 out of 10 experiments, compared with control media containing BLB. The histiocytes were foamy looking with little tendency toward epithelioid or multinucleated giant cell reaction. It was rather unique to observe a variable degree of necrosis in most experiments with sarcoidal supernatants or control media containing BLB. Lymphocytic response was also variable and did not appear to be significantly different with sarcoidal supernatant or control media (FIG. 2).

The supernatants from normal-looking skin specimens, sarcoidal or nonsarcoidal, showed a variable histiocytic response with or without K-S antigen or BLB, but their responses were not significantly different from those of their own controls. In these experiments there was no evidence of epithelioid or multinucleated giant cell response.

DISCUSSION

The data from these experiments demonstrate that the supernatants of cultured cutaneous sarcoidal granulomas mixed with K-S antigen and BLB caused a significant increase in infiltration with histiocytic epithelioid cells at the injection sites. The supernatants alone produced no response. This was probably due to the rapid absorption of injected material which was nonparticulate in nature. The supernatants of normal-looking skin specimens from sarcoid patients or patients free of sarcoidosis showed no significant differences in the amount of cellular infiltrates when compared with their own controls.

We have demonstrated spontaneous production of lymphokines in the supernatants of cultured cutaneous sarcoidal granulomas.[4,6] These lymphokines include monocytic chemotactic factor and IL-2. In a few experiments evidence for the production of macrophage aggregating factor and migration inhibition factor was also found (unpublished observations). It is well recognized that the granulomas of immune origin produce lymphokines whereas those of foreign body origin do not.[5] Thus it can be accepted that sarcoidal granulomas are of immune origin. This is further supported by the morphologic structure of these granulomas in terms of cell type.[1–3] It has been shown that lymphocyte populations seen in sarcoidal granulomas overwhelmingly consist of T cells, most of which are T helper cells; only a few suppressor T cells and B cells may be seen. The remaining series of cells are of the epithelioid type; there are few monocytes, histiocytes, and multinucleated giant cells. In the artificially induced foreign body granulomas the histiocytic type predominates.[5] This study demonstrates the role of lymphokine-containing sarcoidal supernatants in inducing the monocytic histiocytic reaction at the injection site. The inflammatory response is most likely maintained by continuous secretion of lymphokines. In the present study, an

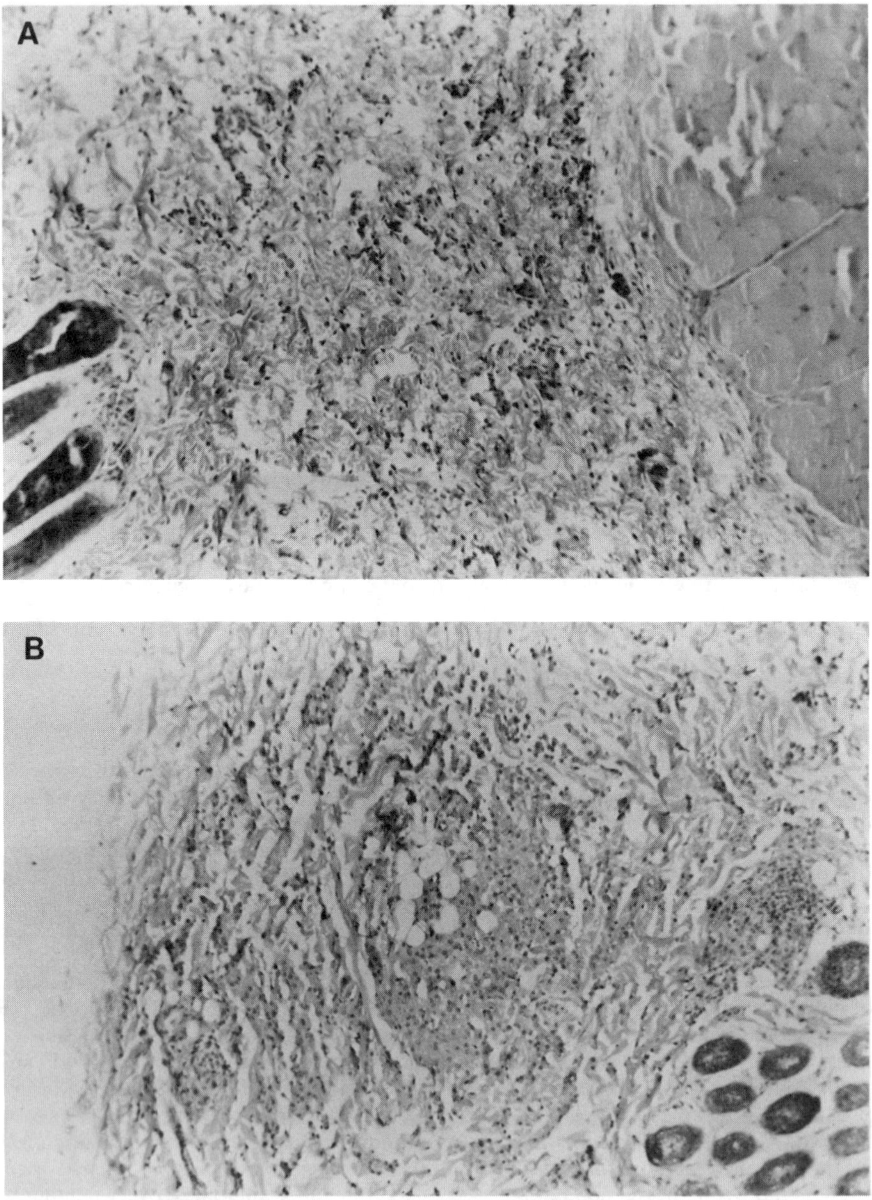

FIGURE 1. The cellular infiltrate in **A** exhibits scattered histiocytes and a few lymphocytes and eosinophils in response to control media plus heat-inactivated K-S antigen. A markedly increased histiocytic infiltration, in response to sarcoidal supernatant plus heat-inactivated K-S antigen at the injection site in the rabbit skin, is evident in **B**. The specimens shown in **A** and **B** were stained with hematoxylin and eosin. Original magnification: $\times$ 100; reduced to 68.8% of original size.

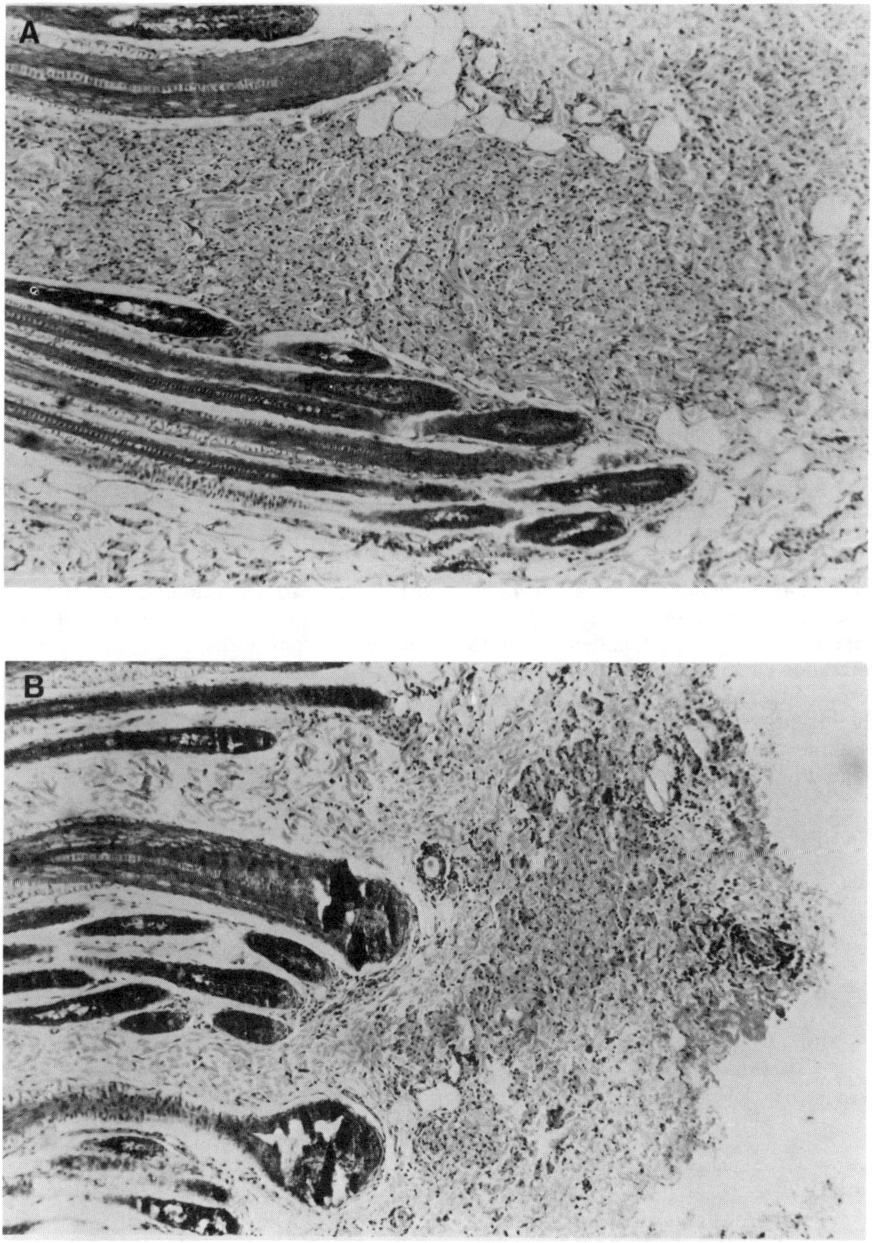

FIGURE 2. The histiocytic infiltration at the injection site in rabbit skin evident in **A,** in response to control media plus BLB, is not as great as that evident in **B,** in response to sarcoidal supernatant plus BLB. The specimens shown in **A** and **B** were stained with hematoxylin and eosin. Original magnification: × 100; reduced to 68.8% of original size.

enhanced inflammatory reaction was seen only when sarcoidal supernatants were mixed with K-S antigen or BLB, mixtures which probably lead to the slow release of lymphokines from the bound matrix. In sarcoidosis, the process of an inflammatory reaction is an immunogenic response, and it appears to be amplified and maintained by IL-2.

It may be concluded that the continuous secretion of lymphokines are probably responsible for the induction and maintenance of sarcoidal granulomas.

SUMMARY

This study was designed to examine the inflammatory response in rabbits to intradermal injections of lymphokine-containing supernatants from cultured cutaneous sarcoidal granulomas (sarcoidal supernatant). Cell-free sarcoidal supernatants and concurrently incubated culture medium controls, alone or mixed with heat-inactivated K-S antigen or BLB, were injected intradermally into rabbits. These were, compared to control results, increased inflammatory reactions with histiocytes and epithelioid cells at the injection sites in 9 out of 11 experiments using sarcoidal supernatants mixed with K-S antigen and in 8 out of 10 experiments with these supernatants mixed with BLB. Sarcoidal supernatant alone, control medium, or normal saline solution produced no inflammatory response. Supernatants from cultured normal skin tissues obtained from sarcoid patients and those obtained from surgical patients free of sarcoidosis, when mixed with K-S antigen or BLB, showed variable inflammatory responses similar to the response seen with sarcoidal supernatants, but these were not significantly different from those of their own controls. It was concluded that lymphokines released locally may initiate and maintain the formation of sarcoidal granulomata.

REFERENCES

1. SEMENZATO, G., A. PEZZUTTO, G. PIZZOLO, M. CHILOSI, E. OSSI, M. R. ANGI & A. CIPRIANI. 1984. Immunohistological study in sarcoidosis: Evaluation at different sites of disease activity. Clin. Immunol. Immunopathol. **30:** 29-40.
2. BUECHNER, S. A., R. K. WINKELMANN & P. M. BANKS. 1983. T-cell subsets in cutaneous sarcoidosis. Arch. Dermatol. **119:** 728-732.
3. BJERKE, J. R., R. MATRE & R. NILSEN. 1983. Characterization of mononuclear cells in sarcoid skin lesions using monoclonal antibodies. Acta Pathol. Microbiol. Scand. Sect. B **91:** 233-236.
4. KATARIA, Y. P., P. B. CAMPBELL, H. K. PARK & K. C. KALMUS. 1983. *In vitro* observations on intact granulomas of sarcoidosis. *In* Sarcoidosis and Other Granulomatous Disorders. J. Chrétien, J. Marsac & J. C. Saltiel, Eds.: 126-131. Pergamon Press. Paris.
5. CARRICK, L., JR. & D. L. BOROS. 1980. The artificial granuloma. I. *In vitro* lymphokine production by pulmonary artificial hypersensitivity granulomas. Clin. Immunol. Immunopathol. **17:** 415-426.
6. KATARIA, Y. P., R. C. PADGETT & L. S. ENGLISH. Ann. N.Y. Acad. Sci. This volume.
7. SMITH, K. A., S. GILLIS, P. E. BAKER, D. MCKENZIE & F. W. RUSCETTI. 1979. T-cell growth factor-mediated T-cell proliferation. Ann. N.Y. Acad. Sci. **332:** 423-432.
8. KELSO, A., H. R. MACDONALD, K. A. SMITH, J. C. CEROTTINI & K. T. BRUNNER. 1984. Interleukin-2 enhancement of lymphokine secretion by T-lymphocytes: Analysis of established clones and primary limiting dilution microcultures. J. Immunol. **132:** 2932-2938.

In Vitro Granuloma-like Formations in Bronchoalveolar Cell Cultures from Patients with Sarcoidosis

ANNIE G. ARNOUX, FRANÇIS JAUBERT,
GISÈLE STANISLAS-LEGUERN,
CLAIRE DANEL, AND JACQUES CHRÉTIEN

Institut National de la Santé
et de la Recherche Médicale Unité 214
Hôpital Laennec
75007 Paris, France

INTRODUCTION

We have previously demonstrated that bronchoalveolar cells (BAC's) recovered from patients with sarcoidosis exhibit mitotic activity consistent with morphologic and autoradiographic criteria,[1] and this fact has recently been confirmed.[2]

In the present work, the behavior of BAC's in long-term cell cultures (8 to 10 weeks) was investigated in order to compare the BAC cultures from sarcoidosis patients to those from control subjects.

METHODS

Study Population

Patients with Sarcoidosis

The diagnosis of sarcoidosis was established in patients according to the classical clinical criteria and was always associated with the presence of noncaseating epithelioid cell granulomas in biopsy material from at least one involved organ.

None of the sarcoid patients ($N = 30$) included in this study had ever been treated. Their mean age, ± SD, was 33 ± 9 years. Twenty-one of the patients were male; nine were female. Eight patients were smokers.

Control Group

Eight subjects served as controls. All had normal chest radiographs. Their mean age, ± SD, was 41 ± 15 years. Seven of the patients were male. Five patients were smokers.

Bronchoalveolar Lavage

All of the subjects underwent bronchoalveolar lavage (BAL) during fiberoptic bronchoscopy, as previously described.[3] BAL was performed by the instillation and the immediate recovery, using gravity flow of three 100-ml boluses, of a sterile 0.15 M NaCl solution. The BAL was usually performed in a subsegmental bronchus of the right middle lobe in both sarcoid patients and controls. The fluid was strained through loose gauze to remove mucus immediately after the BAL procedure.

After the recovery of the lavage fluid, a cell count, a viability test, and a differential cell count (on 1000 cells) on May-Grünwald-Giemsa-stained cytocentrifuged preparations were routinely performed.

Bronchoalveolar Cell Culture

After recovery, the lavage fluid was centrifuged (500 g) for 10 min at 4° C. The cell pellets were pooled and washed three times with Hanks' balanced saline solution without Ca^{2+} and Mg^{2+}; the resulting fluid was centrifuged (400 g) for 10 min at 4° C. RPMI 1640 supplemented with 10% heat-inactivated fetal calf serum, 2 mM glutamine, and antibiotics was used as the standard tissue culture medium. Alveolar cells were resuspended in tissue culture medium and counted. Alveolar macrophages (5×10^6 cells) were dispensed into plastic tissue culture flasks (25 cm^2) irrespective of the lymphocyte differential. Cultures were incubated at 37° C in a humidified atmosphere of 5% CO_2 and air. After 18 hr, the nonadherent cells were removed. Fresh culture medium (10 ml) was added to the adherent cells, and afterwards the medium was changed at least weekly. The BAC cultures were maintained as long as possible (8 to 10 weeks).

Differentiation of Fibroblasts from Alveolar Macrophages

Several methods were used to differentiate fibroblasts from alveolar macrophages (AM's): 1) Inverted-stage light and phase-contrast microscopy; 2) Autoradiographic analysis after [^{3}H]thymidine incorporation in cells, for 3 hr, as previously described;[1] 3) Nonspecific esterase staining;[4] 4) Enzymatic dissociation by trypsin (0.25%) to permit the removal of fibroblast cells from the original lavage culture and the subsequent transfer of the fibroblasts to a new flask; 5) Establishment of a fibroblast line by trypsinization, and subcultures, after at least five passages; and 6) Transmission electron microscopy: Fibroblast cells were fixed either in suspensions, after recovery by trypsinization, or directly in culture flasks. The different steps currently used in electron microscopy for processing samples were then performed.[1,5]

RESULTS

Evidence for the Presence of Fibroblasts in Bronchoalveolar Cell Cultures

Inverted-Stage Light and Phase-Contrast Microscopy

Clones of proliferating fibroblasts appeared between 2 and 4 weeks of culture within the AM monolayer. The AM's were more refractive than the fibroblasts, which appeared more finely pointed and less granular (FIG. 1).

Autoradiographic Analysis after [^{3}H]Thymidine Incorporation in Cell Nuclei

Fibroblasts exhibit a high labeling index in nuclei. Many fibroblasts, close together, replicated at the same time in BAC cultures. No evidence of the label, however, was seen in the nuclei of AM's.

Nonspecific Esterase Staining on Bronchoalveolar Cell Cultures

AM's appeared strongly positive (red-brown) compared to fibroblasts, which were only pink colored.

Transmission Electron Microscopy

Bronchoalveolar macrophages recovered by lavage exhibited some differences from lavage fibroblasts. The fibroblast shown in FIGURE 2A was obtained by trypsinization from a fibroblast line monolayer. Each fibroblast had an abundant and distended endoplasmic reticulum; furthermore, the fibroblasts had no phagolysosomes but were replete with intracytoplasmic fibrils. The AM's (FIG. 2B), however, did exhibit phagolysosomes, and microvilli were present on the AM cell surface, particularly in sarcoid patients, as previously reported.[1,5]

In addition, it is important to note that lavage fibroblasts exhibit characteristics similar to those of a human fetal lung fibroblast line (MRC 5). These characteristics are evident by both phase-contrast and electron microscopies.

In Vitro Follow-up of the Bronchoalveolar Cell Cultures

At day 30, fibroblasts were observed in only one culture among the BAC cultures of the control subjects. Fibroblasts appeared in 27 cultures of sarcoidosis patients by day 30, or even earlier. A fibroblast line could be established in 19 out of 27 cultures in which the development of fibroblasts was first observed. Moreover, we have observed formations that mimicked jellyfish (on the bottoms of the flasks) in half the cultures of the sarcoid patients by inverted-stage light and phase-contrast microscopy (FIG. 3). The ultrastructures of these formations resembled granulomas.

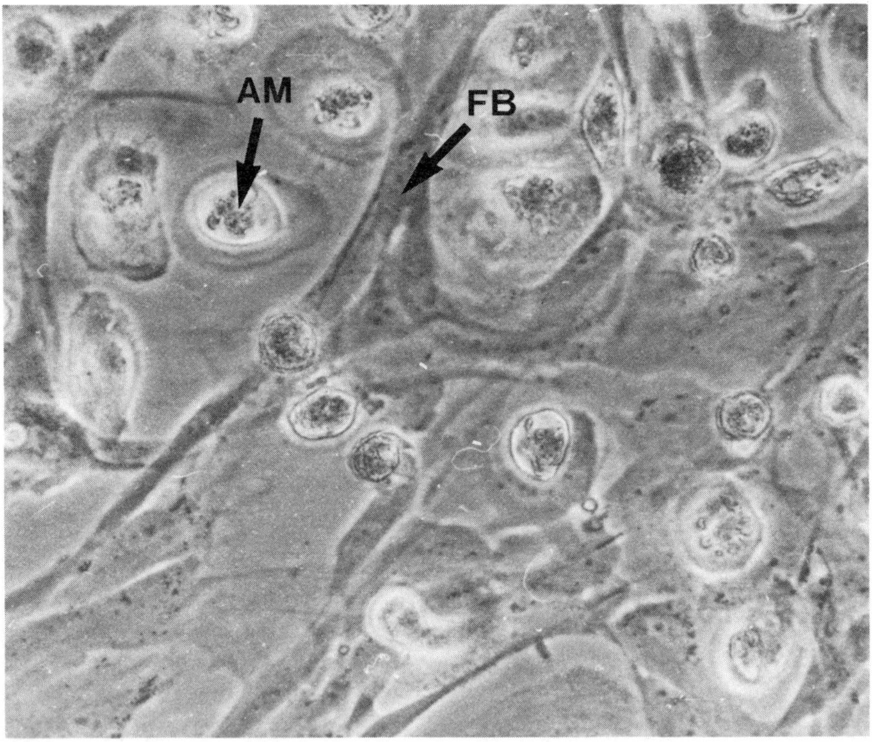

FIGURE 1. Inverted-stage light and phase-contrast micrograph of BAC's in culture. Alveolar macrophages (AM) appear more refractive than fibroblasts (FB), which are finely pointed and less granular. Original magnification: $\times$ 200; reduced to 88.5% of original size.

Correlation between Lavage Data and Culture Results

A trend becomes apparent when lavage specimens which allowed the establishment of fibroblast lines are compared to those which did not: the former had a significantly higher percentage of lymphocytes (40.8 $\pm$ 12.1%, mean $\pm$ SD) than did the latter

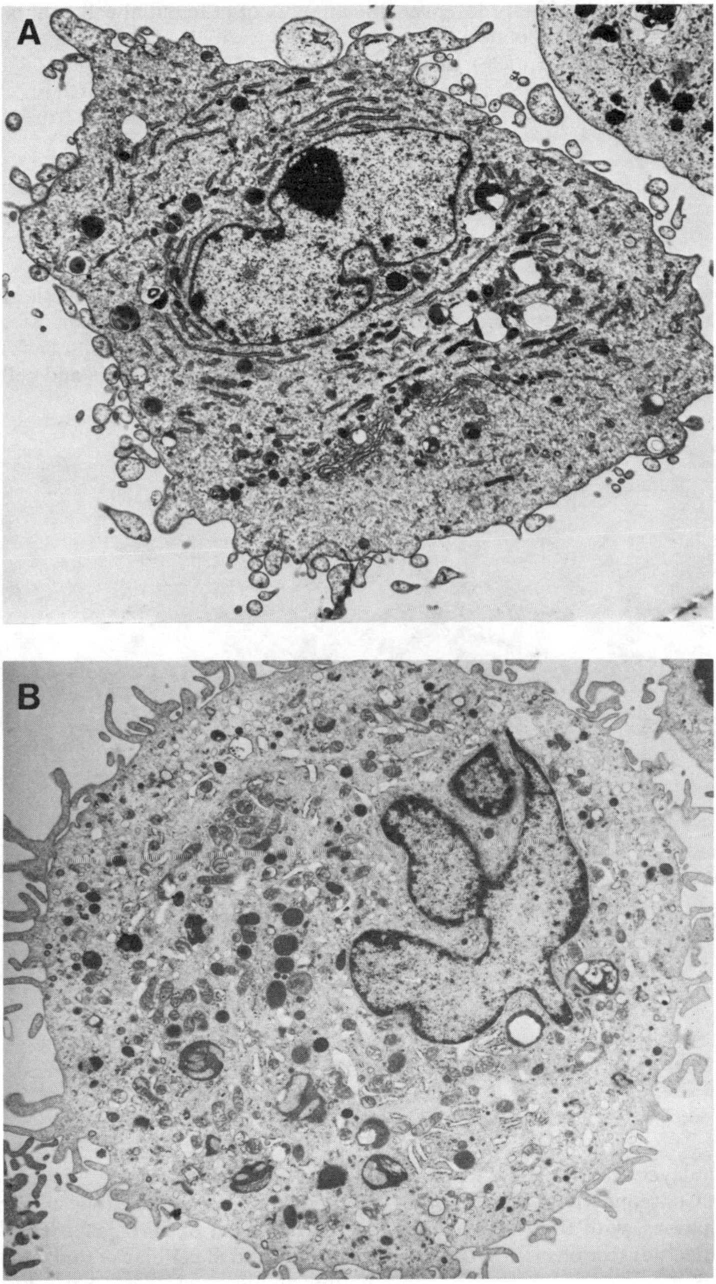

FIGURE 2. Ultrastructural features of a fibroblast in cell suspension **(A)** and of an AM **(B)** obtained from the BAL of sarcoid patients. Original magnification: × 7000; reduced to 77.5% of original size.

(20.9 ± 11.5%) ($p < .001$). Moreover, the analysis of differential cell counts showed a higher percentage of polymorphonuclear leucocytes in BAL which gave rise to a fibroblast line (2.65 ± 1.85%) than that in BAL which did not (1.25 ± 0.78%) ($p < .05$). No correlation was observed with the number of macrophages.

Electron Microscopy of Granuloma-like Formations

The examination of a vertical 1-μm section of one typical formation shows AM's and fibroblasts stacked together (FIG. 4A). By studying serial sections of different formations, it appears that fibroblasts will usually cover the bottom of a flask and not the cells of the AM monolayer, at least at first. Eventually fibroblasts and cells of the

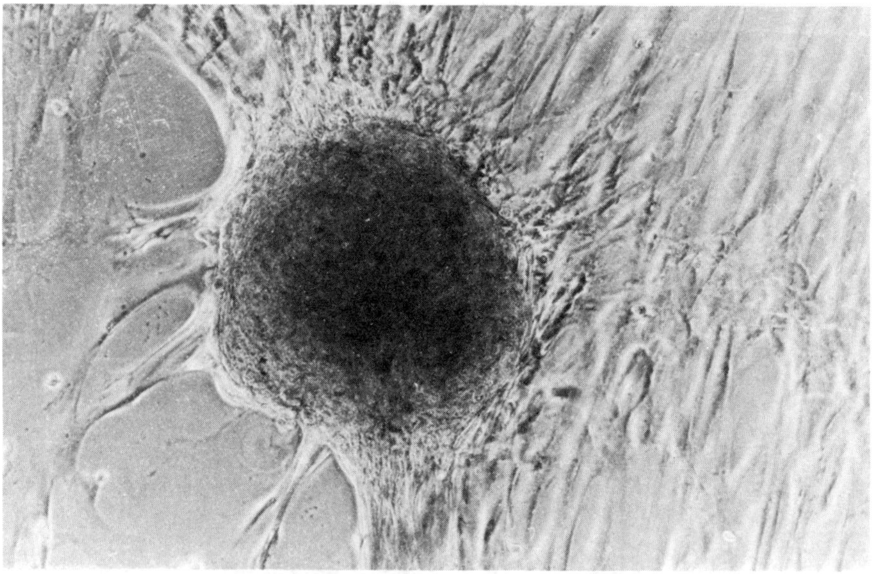

FIGURE 3. Inverted-stage light and phase-contrast micrograph of a jellyfish-like formation observed in BAC cultures of sarcoid patients. Original magnification: × 100; reduced to 84.5% of original size.

AM monolayer intermingle, with fibroblasts and AM rolling up the sides of the flask together. Consequently, AM and fibroblasts appear on the 1-μm sections in granuloma-like formations, with the AM's always covered by a coat of fibroblasts. The study of serial horizontal sections (FIG. 4B) shows the same kind of cellular organization. Some fibroblasts are intermingled with AM's in the middle, and these AM's are always encircled by a ring of fibroblasts. Between the different cells in the middle of the formation the presence of a matrix can be observed. Fibroblasts often exhibit a big nucleolus in their nuclei.

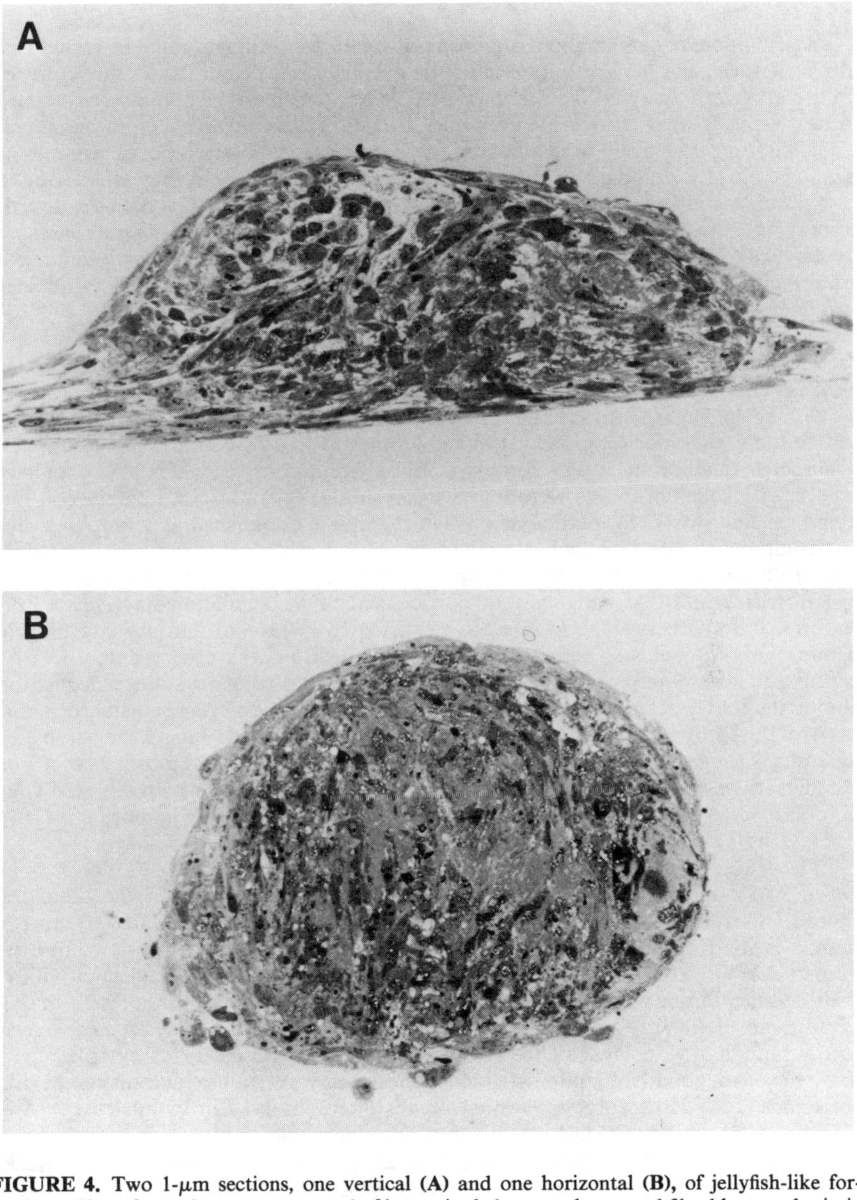

FIGURE 4. Two 1-μm sections, one vertical **(A)** and one horizontal **(B)**, of jellyfish-like formations. These formations are composed of intermingled macrophages and fibroblasts and mimic a granuloma in its recovery phase. Original magnification: $\times$ 200; reduced to 85% of original size.

DISCUSSION

Based upon a combination of morphological, autoradiographic, histochemical, ultrastructural, and *in vitro* culture data, the present study demonstrates that cultured, proliferating cells derived from human BAC's are fibroblasts. These findings appear to be related to the chronic inflammatory process which involved the lungs in sarcoidosis, and particularly with an acute lymphocyte alveolitis. Moreover, granuloma-like formations were observed in some sarcoid BAC cultures, and they arose after the first fibroblast layers. These results confirm a previous study that documented the recovery of lavage fibroblasts from patients with diffuse interstitial lung disease.[6]

Lavage fibroblasts were easily recognized within the AM monolayer when proliferating clones had been grown in BAC cultures. These enlarging groups of adjacent and finely pointed cells were assumed to be clones representing the progeny of single lavage cells. The small number of clones obtained per flask (generally less than five) explains why fibroblasts were not identified in the BAL cell population by light and electron microscopies.

Since AM's are the most important cells recovered by bronchoalveolar lavage, and can be maintained for long periods in cell culture (8 to 10 weeks), it was essential to distinguish them from lavage fibroblasts by differential criteria. The morphological aspects of lavage fibroblasts were found to be similar to those of a human fetal lung fibroblast line (MRC 5), particularly when they were established as a fibroblast line.

Compared to AM's which remained viable but were not observed to multiply, fibroblasts proliferated rapidly and showed many cells replicating at the same time by autoradiography. Although a small portion of the AM population may show mitotic features and synthetize DNA *in vitro,* particularly in sarcoid and chronic lung inflammation,[1,2] no cluster formation by AM replication was observed in the BAC cultures. It would be practically impossible, however, to recognize cluster formations among the BAC cultures because the culture conditions for observing cluster formation by AM's used by Bitterman *et al.*[2] in the chronically inflamed lung were completely different. Lavage fibroblasts appeared negative when tested for the presence of non-specific acid esterase with the appropriate stain. The difference between AM's and fibroblasts was easy to see because AM's were rapidly colored in intense red-brown whereas fibroblasts were pink colored and kept their finely pointed shape.

The study by transmission electron microscopy demonstrated the differences between AM's and lavage fibroblasts. These fibroblasts had characteristics similar to those of fibroblasts from a human fetal lung fibroblast line. The ultrastructure of human AM's from normal and sarcoid patients has been studied before.[1,5,7] In brief, human AM's recovered by lavage were round and had well-developed microvilli on their cell membranes. Numerous lysosomes and phagolysosomes were present in their cytoplasms; fewer were present on their endoplasmic reticulums (FIG. 2A). In contrast to the human AM, a lavage fibroblast has no phagolysosomes in its cytoplasm, but does have an abundant and distended endoplasmic reticulum and many fibrillar secretions (FIG. 2B). Moreover, a nucleolus is often observed in its nucleus.

Lavage fibroblasts could be trypsinized from a surface monolayer, transferred to a new flask, and then maintained in a proliferative state over a period of many weeks. All this is essential to differentiate fibroblasts from AM's, which are not sensitive to trypsin dissociation.

The *in vitro* follow-up of the BAC cultures has shown that lavage fibroblasts were recovered from 90% of the lavage specimens from sarcoid patients but from only one of the eight controls. The high incidence of isolation of fibroblasts from patients with sarcoidosis compared to that from controls suggests that recovery of these cells may in some way be associated with the chronically inflamed state of this disease. This fact is strongly supported by the significant correlation found between the alveolar lymphocytosis in lavage specimens and the establishment of a fibroblast line in 70% of the patients with sarcoidosis (the 27 patients that exhibited some fibroblast clones at day 30). The same correlation exists with the percentage of polymorphonuclear leukocytes in BAL specimens.

From these results, it appears that the initial BAC cultures, particularly those from sarcoid patients, were composed not only of macrophages, lymphocytes, and polymorphonuclear leukocytes, but also of some fibroblasts. The cell culture conditions used represented a complex co-cultivation system involving these different types of cells, and consequently the different types of mediators that each cell was able to release in culture. Thus it remains possible that fibroblasts were present in all or most lavages, even in controls, and that the other cells present in sarcoid BAL specimens enhance fibroblast growth by releasing some mediators. AM's, although not correlated with the establishment of fibroblast lines, are always present, and are known for their ability to release factors which enhance fibroblast growth, such as the AM-derived growth factor,[8] interleukin-1,[9] and fibronectin,[10] but their state of activation is not determined. Lymphocytes and polymorphonuclear leukocytes, which are correlated with the establishment of fibroblast lines, may also release mediators; for example, lymphocytes may release gamma interferon.

We observed jellyfish-like formations on fibroblast layers in 15 BAC cultures from sarcoid patients by inverted-stage light and phase-contrast microscopy. These formations always appeared in BAC cultures which gave clones of fibroblasts but are not specifically related to the establishment of a fibroblast line. The ultrastructural analysis of these jellyfish-like formations showed a cellular organization that resembled that of a granuloma in a recovery phase. Epithelioid cells, however, were not found, and it was only the organization of the cells, macrophages, and fibroblasts that brought the granuloma analogy to mind. The absence of epithelioid cells may be due to the elimination of the nonadherent cells (mostly lymphocytes) from BAC cultures on day 1. Thus, the lymphocytes may play an important role in the immune mechanisms which lead to the granulomatous reaction *in vivo*.[11] Usually, lymphocytes are present in the sarcoid granuloma, the central area of which mainly consists of transformed cells of the mononuclear phagocytic system (epithelioid and multinucleated giant cells). This central area is surrounded mainly by thymus-derived (T) helper lymphocytes and plasma cells; T suppressor lymphocytes are less numerous and are confined to the border of granulomas.[12] These histologic features involving lymphocytes might explain why epithelioid cells are not observed in the granuloma-like formations.

The recovery of lavage fibroblasts from patients with sarcoidosis confirmed the previous study of patients with diffuse interstitial lung disease.[6] Thus the ability to obtain fibroblasts from human lung by lavage offers a new opportunity to examine the function of pulmonary cells involved in a granulomatous reaction. The *in vitro* observation of granuloma-like formations in BAC cultures might be a first step towards the study of epithelioid cells *in vitro,* if immune lymphocytes are kept in the complex co-cultivation system.

ACKNOWLEDGMENTS

The authors wish to thank L. Rousseau-Vaillant, D. Pechaud, and N. Colombet for their excellent technical assistance and D. Guillemot for her secretarial help. They also wish to thank R. Dufat and C. Roth-Fouret for performing the bronchoscopic examinations.

REFERENCES

1. ARNOUX, A., R. MASSE & J. CHRÉTIEN. 1983. Evidence of an increased persistent mitotic activity in cells recovered by bronchoalveolar lavage in sarcoidosis. *In* Sarcoidosis and Other Granulomatous Disorders. J. Chrétien, J. Marsac & J. C. Saltiel, Eds.: 50-54. Pergamon Press. Paris.
2. BITTERMAN, P. B., L. E. SALTZMAN, S. ADELBERG, V. J. FERRANS & R. G. CRYSTAL. 1984. Alveolar macrophage replication: One mechanism for the expansion of the mononuclear phagocyte population in the chronically inflamed lung. J. Clin. Invest. **74:** 460-469.
3. ARNOUX, A., J. MARSAC, G. STANISLAS-LEGUERN, C. HUCHON & J. CHRÉTIEN. 1982. Bronchoalveolar lavage in sarcoidosis: Correlation between alveolar lymphocytosis and clinical data. Pathol. Res. Pract. **175:** 62-79.
4. ELIAS, J. & F. MILLER. 1982. Factors affecting acid α-naphtyl acetate esterase activity in peripheral blood lymphocytes. Am. J. Clin. Pathol. **77:** 611-614.
5. DANEL, C., A. DEWAR, B. CORRIN, M. TURNER-WARWICK & J. CHRÉTIEN. 1983. Ultrastructural changes in bronchoalveolar lavage cells in sarcoidosis and comparison with the tissue granuloma. Am. J. Pathol. **112:** 7-17.
6. DAVIS, G. S., J. M. MOEHRING, P. M. ABSCHER, A. R. BRODY, J. KELLEY, R. B. LOW & G. M. GREEN. 1979. Isolation and characterization of fibroblasts obtained by pulmonary lavage of human subjects. In Vitro. **15:** 612-623.
7. HAWLEY, R. J., B. L. BEAMAN, M. C. WILLIAMS & H. YEAGER. 1979. The ultrastructure of bronchial macrophages and lymphocytes in sarcoidosis. Hum. Pathol. **10:** 155-163.
8. BITTERMAN, P. B., S. I. RENNARD, G. W. HUNNINGHAKE & R. G. CRYSTAL. 1982. Human alveolar growth factor for fibroblasts: Regulation and partial characterization. J. Clin. Invest. **70:** 806-822.
9. SCHMIDT, J. A., S. B. MIZEL, D. COHEN & I. GREEN. 1982. Interleukin-1: A potential regulator of fibroblast proliferation. J. Immunol. **128:** 2177-2182.
10. RENNARD, S. I., G. W. HUNNINGHAKE, P. B. BITTERMAN & R. G. CRYSTAL. 1981. Production of fibronectin by the human alveolar macrophage: Mechanism for the recruitment of fibroblasts to sites of tissue injury in interstitial lung diseases. Proc. Natl. Acad. Sci. USA **78:** 7147-7151.
11. SEMENZATO, G., A. PEZZUTO, M. CHILOSI & G. PIZZOLO. 1982. T lymphocyte redistribution in the lymph nodes of sarcoidosis patients. N. Engl. J. Med. **306:** 48.
12. MISHRA, B. B., L. W. POULTER, G. JANOSSY & D. G. JAMES. 1983. The distribution of lymphoid- and macrophage-like cell subsets of sarcoid and Kveim granulomata: Possible mechanism of negative PPD reaction in sarcoidosis. Clin. Exp. Immunol. **54:** 705-715.

Release of Superoxide Anion by Alveolar Macrophages in Pulmonary Sarcoidosis

C. AERTS, B. WALLAERT, J. M. GROSBOIS, AND C. VOISIN[a]

Département de Pneumologie
Hôpital A. Calmette et Institut Pasteur
Lille, France

INTRODUCTION

Although lung lymphocytes have been extensively evaluated in pulmonary sarcoidosis, it is likely that alveolar macrophages (AM's) also play a crucial role in the pathophysiology of this disease. AM's constitute an important component of the alveolitis in sarcoidosis and are precursors of the cells that constitute granulomas. AM's in sarcoidosis are in the activated state as judged by demonstration of *in vitro* gallium uptake and increased antigen presentation.[1,2]

It is known that activated AM's are capable of releasing several reactive oxidant species, including hydroxyl radical and superoxide anion.[3-5] The aim of this study was to determine if AM's from sarcoidosis patients release potentially toxic forms of O_2. Lucigenin-dependent chemiluminescence is a reliable method of measuring superoxide anion production.[6] We have investigated the chemiluminescence of alveolar cells obtained by bronchoalveolar lavage (BAL) in 50 patients with pulmonary sarcoidosis at various stages of the disease. An attempt is made herein to correlate our findings with radiological types and the activity of the disease as assessed by serum angiotensin-converting enzyme (SACE) levels,[7] gallium scanning,[8] and lymphocyte percentages in BAL.[9]

PATIENTS AND METHODS

Patients

Fifty patients with proved sarcoidosis were included in the study. There were 31 females and 19 males, their ages ranging from 20 to 61 years (mean: 43 ± 11.9 years). Five patients were cigarette smokers. Twenty-nine patients had active and recent

[a] Address for correspondence and reprint requests: Départment de Pneumologie, Hôpital A. Calmette, Boulevard J. Leclerq, 59037 Lille Cédex, France.

disease (< 2 years): type 0 in seven cases (normal chest roentgenogram); type 1 in eight cases (hilar adenopathy without pulmonary changes); type 2 in six cases (hilar adenopathy with pulmonary changes); and type 3 in eight cases (pulmonary changes only, without evidence of pulmonary fibrosis). Ten patients had received corticosteroid therapy at various doses (from 5 to 25 mg/day). The last 11 patients demonstrated spontaneous resolutive disease as judged by normalization of the clinical, radiological, and biological abnormalities, and they were considered cured.

Control Subjects

The control group (18 subjects) included hospital staff and healthy volunteers, their ages ranging from 19 to 46 years. Nine subjects were cigarette smokers. All were free of clinical pulmonary symptoms and had normal chest roentgenograms.

Bronchoalveolar Lavage

Informed consent was obtained from all subjects. BAL was performed after premedication with atropine under local anesthesia with lignocaine. A wedged fiberoptic bronchoscope (Olympus model BF-B_3, Olympus Corps of America, New Hyde Park, NY) was used, and 250 ml of sterile saline solution was applied in five 50-ml aliquots with immediate gentle vacuum aspiration after each aliquot. The aspirated fluid was collected into sterile siliconized jugs and immediately transported on ice to the laboratory. The first recovered sample was not considered because it was thought to reflect the bronchial level.[10] BAL fluid was filtered through several layers of sterile surgical gauze, and the cells were separated from the fluid by centrifugation at 800 g (10 min). After three washings, the cells were resuspended in 10 ml of Hanks' balanced salt solution (HBSS) and evaluated for their total number and for a differential cell count. Cellular viability of AM's was assessed by trypan blue exclusion.

Chemiluminescence of Alveolar Macrophages

The chemiluminescence of AM's was investigated using a lucigenin-dependent chemiluminescence method adapted from Williams and Cole.[6,11] Lucigenin (10^{-4} M) (Sigma) was dissolved in HBSS buffered with 18 mM HEPES (*N*-2-hydroxyethylpiperazine-*N*-2-ethanesulfonic acid). Phorbol myristate acetate (PMA) (Sigma) was dissolved in dimethylsulfoxide at a concentration of 0.5 mg/ml. PMA (10 μl) was dissolved just before use in 5 ml of HBSS-HEPES. Superoxide dismutase (SOD) (Sigma) was dissolved in HBSS-HEPES (120 μg/ml). Alveolar cells were washed with HBSS, centrifuged at 400 g (10 min, 4° C), and resuspended in HBSS-HEPES to a concentration of 1×10^6 viable AM's/ml. The suspension was kept on ice in a siliconized glass container until use.

Chemiluminescence was measured at 37° C using a nucleotimeter 107. AM suspension aliquots (500 μl) were added to vials containing lucigenin aliquots (900 μl) with or without PMA (100 μl) and/or SOD (100 μl). The total volume in each vial was brought to 1.650 ml by adding a 50-μl aliquot from a 3% gelatin solution and the appropriate amount of HBSS-HEPES. Intensity of luminescence was integrated for 60 sec after a 12-min incubation at 37° C. The results are expressed in relative luminescent units (RLU).

Blood Test

The assay for SACE activity was performed according to the method of Lieberman.[7] Activity was expressed in units (U)/ml. The normal value for healthy controls determined in our laboratory was 25.2 ± 4.7 U/ml.

Gallium Scanning

A gallium scan was carried out in each subject before the BAL procedure. Each patient received 35 μCi/kg of ^{67}Ga citrate IV 72 hr before scanning. Anterior and posterior scans were recorded using a whole-body imager. Accumulation of ^{67}Ga in the lungs, mediastinum, spleen, eyes, salivary glands, and superficial adenopathy was compared with the uptake of ^{67}Ga found in the liver and the soft tissue of the shoulders using a subjective score.[8]

RESULTS

The total cell count for sarcoidosis patients was higher than the one for controls. Differential counting of BAL cells showed an increased percentage of alveolar lymphocytes (36 ± 14.6%). The percentage of neutrophils and eosinophils did not differ between control and sarcoidosis patients. The cellular viability of AM's was 84 ± 5.4% in patients and 87 ± 5.1% in controls.

The chemiluminescence (CL) determinations for bronchoalveolar cells from controls and patients are shown in TABLE 1. Spontaneous and PMA-induced CL's of BAL cells were slightly higher in smoker controls than in nonsmoker controls, a result previously reported by Hoidal *et al.*[5] CL of BAL cells was significantly higher in patients with radiological evidence of sarcoidosis ($p < .05$); there were no CL differences corresponding to different radiological types of the disease. Surprisingly, CL was increased in patients with extrathoracic sarcoidosis and normal chest roentgenograms (type 0). CL was slightly increased in treated patients. The CL of BAL cells from cured patients, however, did not differ from that of healthy controls. It could be assumed that superoxide anion is involved in CL production because SOD inhibits 60 to 75% of spontaneous CL and 91 to 93% of PMA-induced CL.

Neither spontaneous CL nor PMA-induced CL could be correlated with SACE levels (FIG. 1) or gallium scores (FIG. 2). On the other hand, CL was significantly higher in patients with increased alveolar lymphocytosis (≥ 18%) than in patients with normal BAL ($p < .05$) (FIGS. 3 & 4).

TABLE 1. Spontaneous and PMA-induced Chemiluminescence of Bronchoalveolar Cells[a]

		Chemiluminescence of Alveolar Macrophages			
Patients	*N*	Spontaneous Chemiluminescence (RLU)	Inhibition by SOD (%)	PMA-induced Chemiluminescence (RLU)	Inhibition by SOD (%)
Healthy controls					
Nonsmokers	9	668 ± 246	64	13 280 ± 4123	92
Smokers	9	1095 ± 387	75	15 043 ± 5204	91
Untreated sarcoidosis patients					
Type 0	7	2672 ± 1839	60	20 560 ± 5557	93
Type 1	8	3826 ± 3209	64	34 872 ± 10 844	92
Type 2	6	4510 ± 3460	72	24 347 ± 7678	92
Type 3	8	2628 ± 1620	62	33 609 ± 7992	92
Treated sarcoidosis patients	10	2295 ± 1144	73	27 474 ± 10 480	93
Spontaneously cured patients	11	1129 ± 773	65	16 450 ± 6550	93

[a] The bronchoalveolar cells were obtained from 18 healthy controls and 50 sarcoidosis patients. CL is expressed in RLU/0.5 $\times$ 10^6 viable AM's. Inhibition of CL by SOD is expressed as the mean percentage of inhibition.

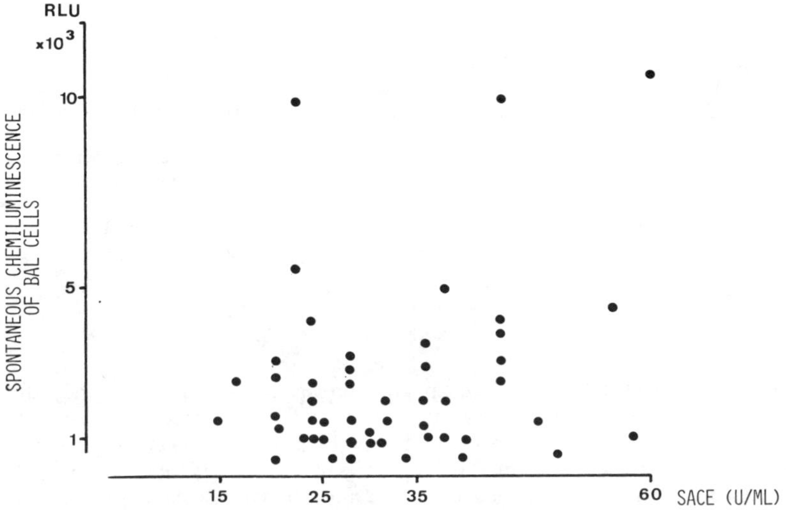

FIGURE 1. Correlation between SACE levels and spontaneous CL of BAL cells in 50 sarcoidosis patients.

DISCUSSION

Our study demonstrates that the CL of bronchoalveolar cells is greater in sarcoidosis patients than it is in controls. CL could not be correlated with clinical data, radiological type, SACE levels, or pulmonary gallium uptake. CL, however, was significantly greater in patients with increased alveolar lymphocytosis ($\geq$ 18%) than in patients with normal BAL.

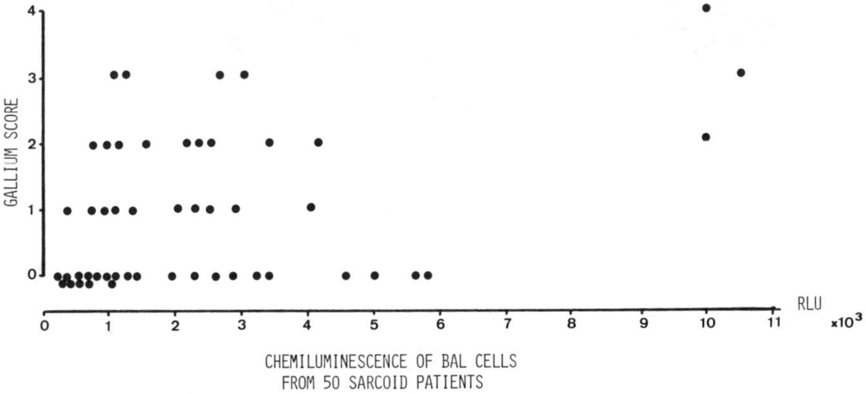

FIGURE 2. Correlation between ^{67}Ga scores and spontaneous CL of BAL cells in 50 sarcoidosis patients.

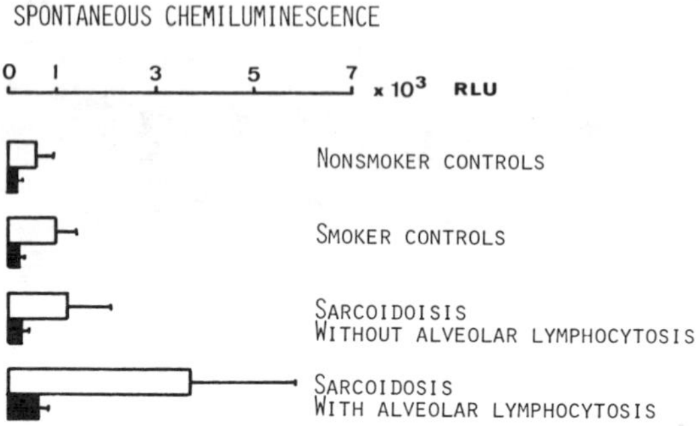

FIGURE 3. Spontaneous CL of BAL cells (□) and inhibition by SOD (■) in 18 healthy controls and 50 sarcoidosis patients according to alveolar lymphocytosis (≥ 18% or < 18%) in BAL. Results are expressed as RLU/0.5 × 10^6 viable AM's.

The CL of the total BAL cellular population was measured immediately after the cells were harvested from the respiratory tract; CL measurements obtained in this way were considered representative of the biological events occurring in the lung. Activated T lymphocytes from the lungs of sarcoidosis patients, however, do not produce any lucigenin-dependent CL (data not shown). Since there were neither polymorphonuclear neutrophils nor eosinophils in BAL from both patients and controls, it may be postulated that CL is produced by AM's. CL inhibition by SOD suggests that the superoxide anion ($\cdot O_2^-$) is involved in the production of CL. Moreover, lucigenin-dependent CL accurately reflects $\cdot O_2^-$ production as measured by ferrocytochrome *c* reduction.[6,11] Thus, we believe that the CL of BAL cells is related to superoxide anion generation by AM's.

The significance of our findings is unclear. It has been established that AM's from healthy smokers release more $\cdot O_2^-$ than AM's from nonsmokers.[5] It has been suggested, however, that this increase in $\cdot O_2^-$ is an adaptive and reversible response of AM's to toxic and stimulating substances of cigarettes.[12] In our studies increased $\cdot O_2^-$ production in sarcoidosis has been associated with persistent activity of the disease as assessed by alveolar lymphocytosis. On the other hand, in cured patients with normal BAL, $\cdot O_2^-$ generation did not differ from that in healthy controls.

Increased oxidant activity may reflect an activated state of AM's in sarcoidosis. Toxic forms of $\cdot O_2^-$, however, can induce cytotoxic reactions in lung parenchymal

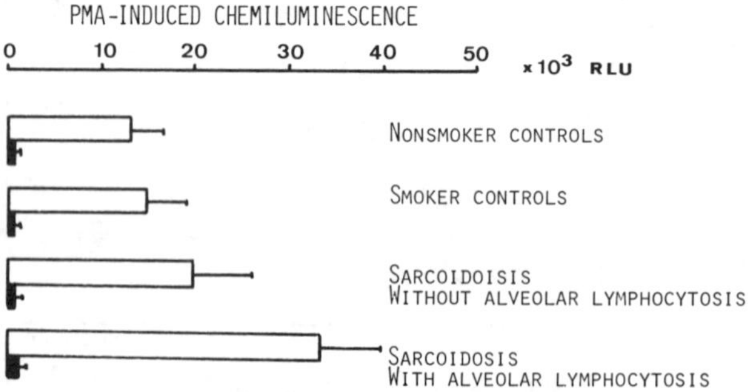

FIGURE 4. PMA-induced CL of BAL cells (□) and inhibition by SOD (■) in 18 healthy controls and 50 sarcoidosis patients according to alveolar lymphocytosis (≥ 18% or < 18%) in BAL. Results are expressed as RLU/0.5 × 10^6 viable AM's.

cells.[13–15] The release of both superoxide anion and related radicals may be of importance in the pathogenesis of pulmonary sarcoidosis.

SUMMARY

Biological mechanisms involving nonprotease factors mediate the alterations of the alveolar structures which lead to the interstitial fibrosis of pulmonary sarcoidosis. Thus, we have investigated the production of oxidant species by BAL cells from 50 sarcoidosis patients and 18 healthy controls using a lucigenin-dependent CL method. Spontaneous and PMA-induced CL's were significantly higher in untreated patients and treated patients than in spontaneously cured patients or healthy controls ($p < .05$). SOD inhibits 60 to 75% of spontaneous CL and 91 to 93% of PMA-induced CL. There was no apparent correlation between the CL of AM's and the radiological types, SACE levels, and gallium scans. In marked contrast, CL was significantly higher in patients with increased alveolar lymphocytosis ($\geq$ 18%) than in patients with normal BAL. Since there were neither neutrophils nor eosinophils in BAL and since lymphocytes do not produce lucigenin-dependent CL, we believe that CL is produced by AM's. CL inhibition by SOD suggests that superoxide anion is involved in the production of CL. The release of both superoxide anion and related radicals may be of importance in the pathogenesis of pulmonary sarcoidosis.

REFERENCES

1. Rossi, G. A., G. W. Hunninghake, B. R. Line, B. A. Keogh & R. G. Crystal. 1981. Mechanisms of gallium-67 uptake in the lung in pulmonary sarcoidosis. Bull. Eur. Physiopathol. Respir. **17:** 54.
2. Venet, A. R., G. W. Hunninghake & R. G. Crystal. 1982. Antigen presentation by human alveolar macrophages: Elevation in normals and interstitial lung disease. Am. Rev. Respir. Dis. **125:** 178A.
3. Hoidal, J. R., R. B. Fox & J. E. Repine. 1979. Defective oxidative metabolic responses *in vitro* of alveolar macrophages in chronic granulomatous disease. Am. Rev. Respir. Dis. **120:** 613-618.
4. Hoidal, J. R., G. D. Beall & J. E. Repine. 1979. Production of hydroxyl radical by human alveolar macrophages. Infect. Immun. **26:** 1088-1094.
5. Hoidal, J. R., R. B. Fox, P. A. Lemarbe, R. Perri & J. E. Repine. 1981. Altered oxidative metabolic responses *in vitro* of alveolar macrophages from asymptomatic cigarette smokers. Am. Rev. Respir. Dis. **123:** 85-89.
6. Williams, A. J. & P. J. Cole. 1981. Investigation of alveolar macrophage function using lucigenin-dependent chemiluminescence. Thorax **36:** 866-869.
7. Lieberman, J. 1975. Elevation of serum angiotensin-converting enzyme in sarcoidosis. Am. J. Med. **59:** 365-372.
8. Beaumont, D., S. Y. Herry, M. Sapene, P. Bourguet, J. S. Larzul & B. de Labarthe. 1982. Gallium-67 in the evaluation of sarcoidosis: Correlation with serum angiotensin-converting enzyme and bronchoalveolar lavage. Thorax **37:** 11-18.

9. Daniele, R. P. & D. T. Rowlands. 1976. Lymphocyte subpopulations in sarcoidosis: Correlation with disease activity and duration. Ann. Intern. Med. **85:** 593-600.
10. Voisin, C., B. Wallaert, E. Fournier, F. Steenhouwer, M. Guiselin & J. M. Grosbois. Cell population analysis of the first bronchoalveolar lavage sample in interstitial lung diseases. First International Conference on Bronchoalveolar Lavage. May 1984. Columbia, MD.
11. Williams, A. J. & P. J. Cole. 1981. *In vitro* stimulation of alveolar macrophage metabolic activity by polystyrene in the absence of phagocytosis. Br. J. Exp. Pathol. **62:** 1-7.
12. Hoidal, J. R. Reversible alterations in oxidant-antioxidant systems of alveolar machrophages from cigarette smokers. First International Conference on Bronchoalveolar Lavage. May 1984. Columbia, MD.
13. Fridovich, I. 1978. The biology of oxygen radicals. Science **201:** 875-880.
14. Nathan, C. F., L. H. Bruckner, S. C. Silverstein & Z. A. Cohn. 1979. Extracellular cytolysis by activated macrophages and granulocytes. II. Hydrogen peroxide as a mediator of cytotoxicity. J. Exp. Med. **149:** 100-113.
15. Sacks, T., F. Moldow, P. R. Craddock, T. K. Bowes & H. S. Jacob. 1978. Oxygen radicals mediate endothelial cell damage by complement-stimulated granulocytes: An *in vitro* model of immune vascular damage. J. Clin. Invest. **61:** 1161-1167.

Activated Alveolar Macrophage and Lymphocyte Alveolitis in Extrathoracic Sarcoidosis without Radiological Mediastinopulmonary Involvement

B. WALLAERT,[a,b] P. RAMON,[b] E. C. FOURNIER,[b]
L. PRIN,[c] A. B. TONNEL,[b] AND C. VOISIN[b]

[b] *Département de Pneumologie*
Hôpital A. Calmette et Institut Pasteur
Lille, France

[c] *Laboratoire d'Immunologie*
Faculté de Médecine
Lille, France

INTRODUCTION

Sarcoidosis is a chronic multisystem disorder characterized by an accumulation of inflammatory and immune effector cells, by noncaseating granulomas, and by fibrosis in affected organs. Although sarcoidosis is known as a granulomatous disorder, it is now evident that alveolitis precedes and is responsible for the formation of granulomas and for fibrosis.[1,2] Thus alveolitis plays a crucial role in the pathogenesis of the disease. Development of bronchoalveolar lavage (BAL) has increased our knowledge of alveolitis. The lymphocyte component of alveolitis is composed of activated thymus-derived (T) lymphocytes, and alveolitis formation involves a significant increase in the number of lung T helper cells: an increase reflected by a shift in the T helper:T suppressor ratio in the lung.[3] The alveolar macrophage (AM) component of alveolitis is composed of an activated AM population performing various functions (especially the release of interleukin-1, fibronectin, and fibroblast growth factor) that are critical to the pathogenesis of sarcoidosis.[4–6]

Lymphocyte alveolitis as assessed by BAL has been described in patients with extrathoracic sarcoidosis without clinical, functional, or radiological manifestations of mediastinopulmonary involvement.[7] We undertook this study to determine the characteristics of AM's and lymphocytes in BAL of patients with extrathoracic sarcoidosis. The state of activation of AM's was evaluated by spontaneous and by phorbol myristate acetate (PMA)-induced chemiluminescence, which reflects the oxidative

[a] Address for correspondence and reprint requests: Département de Pneumologie, Hôpital A. Calmette, Boulevard J. Leclercq, 59037 Lille Cédex, France.

metabolism and is related to the metabolic activity of AM's.[8] Lymphocyte-specific monoclonal antibodies, namely OKT3, OKT4, and OKT8, were used to determine the proportions of T cells, T helper cells, and T suppressor cells, respectively.[9,10] Three control groups were used: normal persons, patients with active pulmonary sarcoidosis, and patients with another extrathoracic granulomatous disease, that is, Crohn's disease.

PATIENTS AND METHODS

Patients

Eighteen patients with proved extrathoracic sarcoidosis were included in the study. There were 14 females and 4 males; their ages ranged from 14 to 69 years (mean: 45 ± 15.6 years). One patient was a cigarette smoker. Clinical characteristics of the patients are summarized in TABLE 1. Four patients (numbers 5 to 8) had undergone splenectomy for idiopathic thrombocytopenic purpura. The diagnosis of sarcoidosis was confirmed by the histologic study of the spleen. One patient (number 9) had

TABLE 1. Clinical Characteristics, Alveolar Lymphocytosis, and SACE Activity in Patients with Extrathoracic Sarcoidosis[a]

Patient Number	Age (years)	Sex	Clinical Manifestations	BAL Lymphocytes (%)	SACE Activity (U/ml)
1	48	M	skin sarcoidosis	36	25
2[b]	46	M	uveitis	12	32
3	55	F	uveitis	21	19
4	60	F	cervical adenopathy	19	26
5	19	F	purpura, splenomegaly	19	27[c]
6	34	F	purpura, splenomegaly	3	29[c]
7	46	F	purpura, splenomegaly	35	48[c]
8	35	F	purpura, splenomegaly	19	27[c]
9	45	F	hypercalcemia, nephritis, adenopathy, iridocyclitis	45	15
10	34	F	ulcer of stomach	87	37[d]
11	24	M	meningitis, adenopathy	25	28
12	57	F	parotitis	19	30
13	50	F	skin sarcoidosis involving the phalanges	57	26
14	14	F	uveitis	22	66
15	69	M	nasal mucosal sarcoidosis	58	27
16	52	F	parotitis	20	29
17	67	F	parotitis	49	34
18	62	F	cervical adenopathy	5	19

[a] All of the patients were free of clinical pulmonary symptoms and had normal chest roentgenograms.
[b] The only patient that was a smoker.
[c] The SACE activity was determined after a splenectomy.
[d] The SACE activity was determined after ulcer excision.

interstitial nephritis, hypercalcemia (125 mg/1), cervical adenopathy, and ocular changes (iritis). The diagnosis of sarcoidosis was established by minor salivary gland and cervical adenopathy biopsy examination. One patient (number 10) presented an ulcer of the stomach; the ulcer was excised after a 6-month trial of cimetidine therapy proved to be ineffective. This patient's diagnosis was based on pathological examination of the ulcer and adenopathy and on a positive Kveim test. One patient (number 11) had presented spontaneously resolving lymphocytic basal meningitis. A biopsy of a cervical adenopathy that appeared 4 months later confirmed the diagnosis. Three patients (numbers 2, 3, and 14) had a clinical history and ocular changes compatible with sarcoidosis. No known etiology was found. A Kveim test was positive in one of these patients (number 2); a Kveim test was not done in the two others. Eight patients had extrathoracic lesions easily accessible for biopsy: superficial adenopathy (numbers 4 and 18), skin sarcoidosis (numbers 1 and 13), chronic parotitis (numbers 12, 16, and 17), and nose (number 15) lesions.

Normal Controls

Eight normal nonsmokers (four men and four women) were used as controls. Their ages ranged from 19 to 52 years (mean: 34 ± 12.4 years). The results of pulmonary function tests and chest roentgenograms were within normal limits in all eight subjects.

Patients with Active Pulmonary Sarcoidosis

Pulmonary sarcoidosis was diagnosed in 10 untreated patients, all nonsmokers, according to established criteria such as whether a lung or bronchi biopsy could demonstrate noncaseating epithelioid cell granulomas. There were six women and four men. Their ages ranged from 18 to 57 years (mean: 41 ± 16 years). All these patients had acquired the disease recently, within the 2 years preceding the study, and it was evident, by increased alveolar lymphocytosis and abnormal pulmonary gallium uptake, that the disease was active.

Patients with Crohn's Disease

Eight patients, all nonsmokers, with proved Crohn's disease and with normal chest roentgenograms were used as controls with extrathoracic granulomatous disorder. There were five women and three men. Their ages ranged from 18 to 44 years (mean: 29 ± 8.4 years). Seven of the patients showed abnormal BAL with increased alveolar lymphocytosis, as previously described.[11]

Bronchoalveolar Lavage

Informed consent was obtained from all patients. BAL was performed after premedication with atropine under local anesthesia with lignocaine using a wedged fiberoptic bronchoscope (Olympus model BF-B_3, Olympus Corps of America, New Hyde Park, NY), and 250 ml of sterile saline solution was applied in five 50-ml aliquots with immediate gentle vacuum aspiration after each aliquot. The aspirated fluid was collected into sterile siliconized jugs and immediately transported on ice to the laboratory. The first recovered sample was not considered because it was thought to reflect the bronchial level. BAL fluid was filtered through several layers of sterile surgical gauze, and the cells were separated from the lavage fluid by centrifugation at 800 g (10 min). After three washings, the cells were resuspended in 5 ml of Hanks' balanced salt solution (HBSS) and evaluated for their total number and for a differential cell count. The cellular viability of AM's was assessed by trypan blue exclusion.

Identification of Lymphocyte Subsets

Lymphocytes were separated from AM's by centrifugation at 400 g (20 min, 4° C) on a continuous gradient of Percoll.[12] The resulting pellet was washed twice, and RPMI-SVF medium was added so that a lymphocyte-enriched suspension (5×10^6 cells/ml) could be obtained. Each of three 200-μl aliquots of the suspension was preincubated on ice for 30 min with a different murine monoclonal antibody, that is, with 5 μl of OKT3, OKT4, or OKT8 (Ortho Pharmaceutical, Raritan, NJ). Another aliquot was preincubated with 5 μl of medium alone.

Fluorescein-conjugated goat antimouse immunoglobulin reagent was added to each lymphocyte pellet, one that was washed twice with RPMI-SVF, and medium was added until the reagent was diluted 1:40 and the final volume of the suspension was 200 μl. The suspension was then preincubated on ice for 30 min. After two washings the cells were examined by epifluorescence microscopy; 200 lymphocytes were counted. Only 2% of the lymphocytes on the control slide (which was preincubated with medium alone) were fluorescent.

Chemiluminescence of Alveolar Macrophages

The chemiluminescence of AM's was investigated using a lucigenin-dependent chemiluminescence method adapted from Williams and Cole.[13] Lucigenin (10^{-4} M) (Sigma) was dissolved in HBSS buffered with 18 nM HEPES (*N*-2-hydroxyethylpiperazine-*N*-2-ethanesulfonic acid). PMA (Sigma) was dissolved in dimethylsulfoxide, and the resulting concentration was 0.5 mg/ml. Alveolar cells were washed with HBSS, centrifuged at 800 g (10 min, 4° C), and resuspended in HBSS-HEPES to a concentration of 1×10^6 viable AM's/ml. The suspension was kept on ice in a siliconized glass container until use.

Chemiluminescence was measured at 37° C using a nucleotimeter 107. A 500-μl aliquot of the AM suspension was added to each of four vials; each vial contained a 900-μl aliquot of the lucigenin solution. A 100-μl aliquot from a 1 μl/ml PMA solution was added to one of the vials; a 100-μl aliquot from a 120 μg/ml superoxide dismutase (SOD) solution was added to another; and one vial contained 100-μl aliquots of both PMA and SOD. The total volume in each vial was brought to 1.650 ml by adding a 50-μl aliquot from a 3% gelatin solution and the appropriate amount of HBSS-HEPES. All the vials were incubated in parallel. Intensity of luminescence was integrated for 60 sec after a 12-min incubation. The results are expressed in relative luminescent units (RLU).

Blood Tests

The assay for serum angiotensin-converting enzyme (SACE) was performed according to Lieberman's method.[14] Activity was expressed in units (U)/ml. The normal value for healthy controls determined in our laboratory was 25.2 ± 4.7 U/ml.

Gallium Scanning

A gallium scan was carried out in each subject before the BAL procedure. Each patient received 35 μCi/kg of ^{67}Ga citrate IV 72 hr before scanning. Anterior and posterior scans were recorded using a whole-body imager. Accumulation of ^{67}Ga in the lungs, mediastinum, spleen, eyes, salivary glands, and superficial adenopathy was compared with the uptake of ^{67}Ga in the liver and the soft tissue of the shoulders using a subjective score.[15]

RESULTS

All patients had normal chest roentgenograms: no mediastinal or pulmonary changes were apparent. Pulmonary function tests (TLC, FVC, DL_{CO}, and PO_2) were normal in the 18 patients. The total BAL cell count (10.8 ± 7 × 10^4 cells/ml) and cellular viability of the AM's (79.6 ± 8%) did not differ significantly between patients and controls. In 15 out 18 patients abnormal percentages of lymphocytes (from 18 to 87%) were noted (FIG. 1). No mediastinopulmonary gallium uptake was observed. The SACE levels were normal in 15 of the patients but were significantly increased (> 2 SD's) in the remaining three (37, 48, and 66 U/ml) (TABLE 1). Transbronchial biopsies were performed on five patients: lung parenchyma was normal in two of these patients but showed an accumulation of mononuclear cells within alveolar structures in the other three. Computed tomography of the thorax was performed in five patients: enlarged lymph nodes behind the vessels in the pretracheal region and under the carina were apparent in one patient.

The chemiluminescence of AM's was studied in seven patients. Five of these patients had greater spontaneous and PMA-induced chemiluminescence than did the controls (FIG. 2). The level of luminescence, however, was lower than that observed in patients with active pulmonary sarcoidosis or in patients with Crohn's disease. SOD inhibits both PMA-induced (−93%) and spontaneous (−60%) chemiluminescence of AM's. The proportions of lymphocyte subsets in the BAL of five patients with extrathoracic sarcoidosis were determined (TABLE 2). The percentage of $T3^+$ lymphocytes did not significantly differ from that of controls. The $T4^+$:$T8^+$ ratio was normal in four cases and slightly increased in one of the patients.

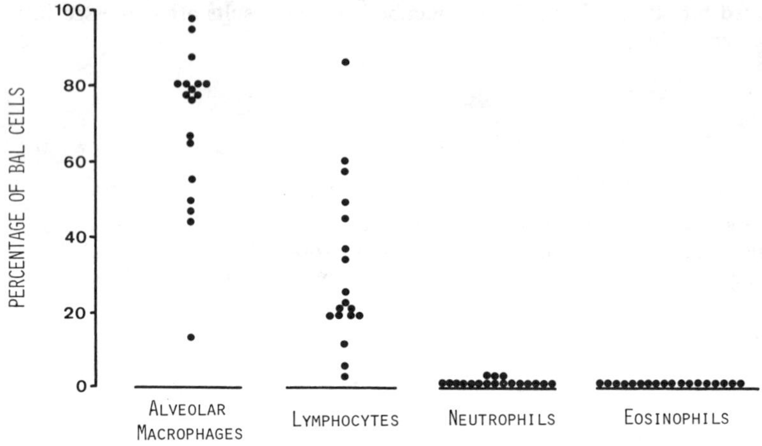

FIGURE 1. Cellular characteristics of BAL in 18 patients with extrathoracic sarcoidosis.

The evolution of clinical, functional, and BAL data was studied in 10 patients. The results of pulmonary function tests remained unchanged in all patients. In four untreated patients (numbers 5, 6, 7, and 11), the favorable course of the disease correlated with normal alveolar lymphocytosis. In patient 9, who received corticosteroid treatment, we noted a favorable course of the disease: regression of cervical

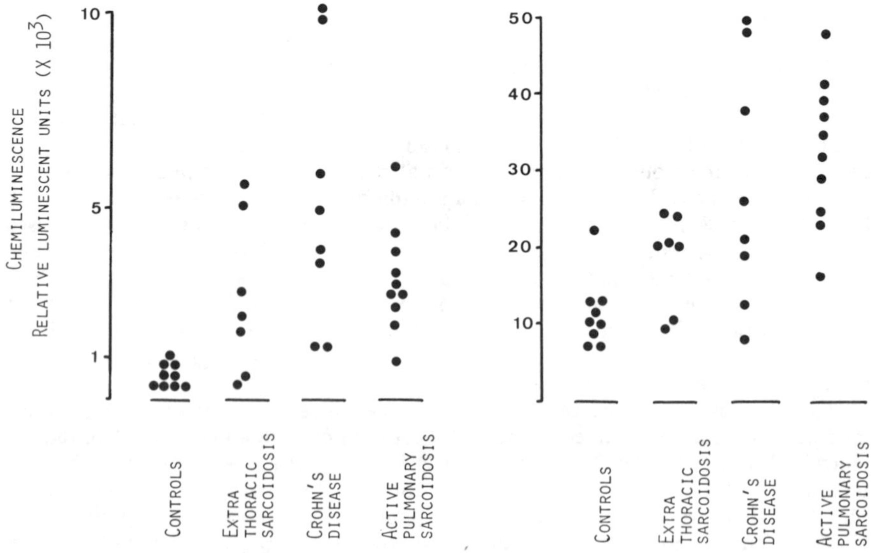

FIGURE 2. Spontaneous (left) and PMA-induced (right) chemiluminescence of bronchoalveolar cells of 9 nonsmoking, healthy controls; 7 nonsmoking patients with extrathoracic sarcoidosis; 8 nonsmoking patients with Crohn's disease; and 10 nonsmoking patients with pulmonary sarcoidosis.

TABLE 2. Characteristics of Bronchoalveolar Cells

Total Cell Count (10^{-4} cells/ml)	Lymphocytes (%)	Lymphocyte Subsets (% of lymphocytes) T3+	T4+	T8+	T4+:T8+
Control Subjects[a]					
9.6 ± 4.3	11.5 ± 6	64 ± 4.5	44 ± 2.7	30 ± 1.3	1.5 ± 0.15
Patients with Extrathoracic Sarcoidosis[b]					
13.1	52	61	48	30	1.6
1.5	66	68	53	25	2.1
5.0	35	65	57	36	1.6
6.5	19	59	42	27	1.55
6.5	3	62	45	27	1.66
Patients with Active Pulmonary Sarcoidosis[c]					
36.5 ± 16	44 ± 12.1	74 ± 2.5	47 ± 11.2	20.6 ± 5.7	2.7 ± 1.6
Patients with Crohn's Disease[d]					
19.4 ± 10.2	40.3 ± 21.7	68.6 ± 6.2	39.3 ± 15.6	29.3 ± 14	1.98 ± 1.14

[a] Mean ± SD for five nonsmoking subjects.
[b] Results for each patient shown individually.
[c] Mean ± SD for eight patients.
[d] Mean ± SD for six patients.

adenopathy and ocular changes and normalization of calcemia (101 mg/1). The clinical amelioration was associated with a decrease of the BAL lymphocytosis (from 45 to 9%). In patient 8, the lymphocyte increase was correlated with secondary bilateral hilar lymph node enlargement, mediastinal gallium uptake, and significantly increased SACE activity. In four untreated patients (numbers 4, 10, 12, and 13), unresolving extrathoracic manifestations were associated with a persistent or increased alveolar lymphocytosis (FIG. 3).

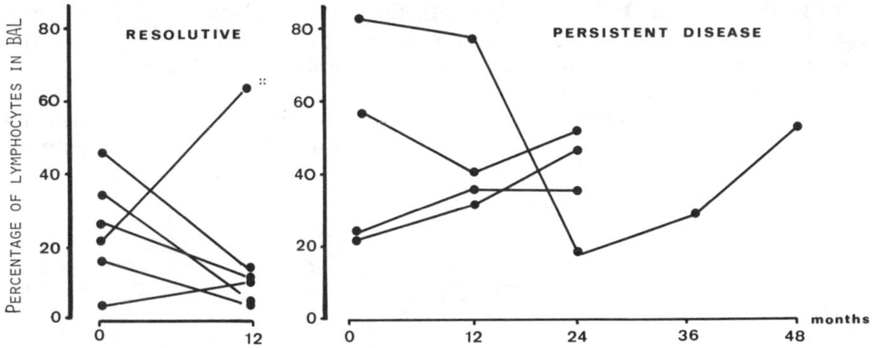

FIGURE 3. Bronchoalveolar lymphocytosis follow-up in six patients with resolutive extrathoracic sarcoidosis (left) and in four patients with persistent extrathoracic involvement (right). One patient (*) showed secondary hilar lymph node enlargement.

DISCUSSION

Our study determined two characteristics of bronchoalveolar cells in patients with extrathoracic sarcoidosis, no clinical pulmonary symptoms, and normal chest roentgenograms: 1) The lymphocyte component of alveolitis has neither an increased proportion of T lymphocytes nor an increased $T4^+:T8^+$ ratio; 2) AM's are activated, as indicated by the increased release of oxygen metabolites.

Increased alveolar lymphocytosis only reflects a shift in the relative proportion of effector cells in BAL. Previous studies, however, have demonstrated that the proportions of immune and inflammatory cells within the BAL accurately reflects those in the alveolar structures.[16] Moreover, three out of five transbronchial lung biopsies performed on patients with alveolar lymphocytosis showed an accumulation of mononuclear cells within the alveolar structures. So it is likely that alveolar lymphocytosis is associated with a lymphocyte alveolitis in our patients.

Bronchoalveolar cells are found to release increased quantities of oxygen metabolites. It is known that lymphocytes do not produce lucigenin-dependent chemiluminescence.[13] Moreover, there were neither polymorphonuclear neutrophils nor eosinophils in BAL of both our patients and controls. Thus it is likely that chemiluminescence is related to the metabolic activity of AM's, and, since SOD inhibits PMA-induced chemiluminescence (−93%) of AM's, it may be that PMA-induced chemiluminescence reflects increased production of superoxide anion by AM's. SOD, however, inhibits only 60% of spontaneous chemiluminescence, suggesting that other oxygen metabolites are produced and detected at rest by the lucigenin-dependent chemiluminescence method. The release of superoxide anion in sarcoidosis patients is slightly higher than that in healthy controls (FIG. 1) and may reflect an abnormal activation of AM's in extrathoracic sarcoidosis.

The clinical and radiological follow-up of patients with alveolar lymphocytosis is most striking. Although alveolar lymphocytosis persisted in 4 patients with persistent extrathoracic manifestation, only 1 out of 15 patients with initially abnormal BAL showed a secondary hilar lymph node enlargement. Moreover, lung biopsies performed in five patients never did show granulomas in the lung. Therefore, it was postulated that AM-lymphocyte alveolitis in patients with extrathoracic sarcoidosis could differ from that described in patients with active pulmonary sarcoidosis.[17] Our findings demonstrate that the percentages of $T3^+$, $T4^+$, and $T8^+$ cells in BAL did not differ significantly between patients and controls; in particular, there was no influx of helper ($T4^+$) lymphocytes in BAL of our patients. Since the development of granulomas depends on the secretion of lymphokines by lung helper T cells, it could be that the absence of lung granulomas in extrathoracic sarcoidosis is related to a normal proportion of effector lymphocytes in BAL.

The significance of our data remains unclear. Abnormalities of BAL cells in patients with extrathoracic sarcoidosis may be due to initial involvement of the respiratory tract in extrathoracic sarcoidosis or to the diffusion from an extrathoracic site into the lung of activated macrophages and lymphocytes.

SUMMARY

Cellular characteristics of BAL were investigated in 18 patients with proved extrathoracic sarcoidosis (that is, sarcoidosis that affected the skin, eyes, parotid glands, stomach, nose, kidneys, or meninges) without clinical or radiological mediastinopulmonary involvement. Computed tomography of the thorax was performed on five patients: four patients were normal, and one had enlarged lymph nodes (these enlargements were not detectable on the patient's chest roentgenogram). The results of pulmonary function tests were normal in all patients. The total BAL cell count did not differ significantly between controls and patients. Abnormal percentages of alveolar lymphocytes (from 18 to 87%) were noted in 15 out of 18 patients. SACE levels were normal in 15 patients. No pulmonary gallium uptake was detected. The chemiluminescence of AM's, whether spontaneous or PMA induced, was increased in five out of seven patients. The percentages of $T3^+$ lymphocytes in sarcoidosis patients did not significantly differ from those in controls. The $T4^+$:$T8^+$ ratio was normal in four patients and slightly increased in one. Follow-up of patients showed that alveolar lymphocytosis is as lasting as extrathoracic involvement. Our data demonstrate increased percentages of lymphocytes and activated AM's in the BAL of patients with extrathoracic sarcoidosis. This may be due to the initial involvement of the respiratory tract in extrathoracic sarcoidosis or to the diffusion of activated macrophages and lymphocytes from an extrathoracic site into the lung.

ACKNOWLEDGMENTS

We wish to thank E. Leleux and N. Duhautois for the technical assistance, E. Sarkis for the review of the manuscript, and C. Zeiske for the secretarial assistance.

REFERENCES

1. JUDD, P. A., P. FINNEGAN & R. C. CURREN. 1975. Pulmonary sarcoidosis: A clinicopathologic study. J. Pathol. **115:** 191-198.
2. ROSEN, Y., T. J. ATHANASSIADES, S. MOON & H. A. LYONS. 1978. Nongranulomatous interstitial pneumonitis in sarcoidosis: Relationship to the development of epithelioid granulomas. Chest **74:** 122-125.
3. HUNNINGHAKE, G. W. & R. G. CRYSTAL. 1981. Pulmonary sarcoidosis: A disorder mediated by excess helper T-lymphocyte activity at sites of disease activity. N. Engl. J. Med. **305:** 429-434.
4. HUNNINGHAKE, G. W. 1984. Release of interleukin-1 by alveolar macrophages of patients with active pulmonary sarcoidosis. Am. Rev. Respir. Dis. **129:** 569-572.
5. RENNARD, S. I., G. W. HUNNINGHAKE, P. B. BITTERMAN & R. G. CRYSTAL. 1981. Production of fibronectin by the human alveolar macrophage: A mechanism for the recruitment of fibroblasts to sites of tissue injury in the interstitial lung diseases. Proc. Natl. Acad. Sci. USA **78:** 7147-7151.
6. BITTERMAN, P. B., S. ADELBERG & R. G. CRYSTAL. 1983. Mechanism of pulmonary fibrosis: Spontaneous release of the alveolar macrophage-derived growth factor in the interstitial lung disorders. J. Clin. Invest. **72:** 1801-1813.
7. WALLAERT, B., P. RAMON, E. C. FOURNIER, A. B. TONNEL & C. VOISIN. 1982. Bronchoalveolar lavage, serum angiotensin-converting enzyme and gallium-67 in extrathoracic sarcoidosis. Chest **82:** 553-555.
8. JOHNSTON, R. B., C. A. GODZIK & Z. A. COHN. 1978. Increased superoxide anion production by immunologically activated and chemically elicited macrophages. J. Exp. Med. **148:** 115-127.

9. KUNG, P. C., G. GOLDSTEIN, E. L. REINHERZ & S. F. SCHOLSSMAN. 1979. Monoclonal antibodies defining distinctive human T-cell surface antigens. Science **206:** 347-349.

10. REINHERZ, E. L., P. C. KUNG, G. GOLDSTEIN & S. F. SCHOLSSMAN. 1979. Further characterization of the human inducer T-cell subset defined by a monoclonal antibody. J. Immunol. **123:** 2894-2896.

11. WALLAERT, B., J. F. COLOMBEL, A. B. TONNEL, P. BONNIERE, A. CORTOT, J. C. PARIS & C. VOISIN. 1985. Evidence of lymphocyte alveolitis in Crohn's disease. Chest **87:** 363-367.

12. DAUBER, J. H., A. HOLIAN, M. E. ROSEMILLER & R. P. DANIELE. 1983. Separation of bronchoalveolar cells from the guinea pig on continuous density gradient of Percoll: Morphology and cytochemical properties of fractionated lung macrophages. J. Reticuloendothel. Soc. **33:** 119-134.

13. WILLIAMS, A. J. & P. J. COLE. 1981. Investigation of alveolar macrophage function using lucigenin-dependent chemiluminescence. Thorax **36:** 866-869.

14. LIEBERMAN, J. 1975. Elevation of serum angiotensin-converting enzyme level in sarcoidosis. Am. J. Med. **59:** 365-372.

15. BEAUMONT, D., S. Y. HERRY, M. SAPENE, P. BOURGUET, J. S. LARZUL & B. DE LABARTHE. 1982. Gallium-67 in the evaluation of sarcoidosis: Correlation with serum angiotensin-converting enzyme and bronchoalveolar lavage. Thorax **37:** 11-18.

16. HUNNINGHAKE, G. W., O. KAWANAMI, V. J. FERRANS, R. C. YOUNG, JR., W. C. ROBERTS & R. G. CRYSTAL. 1981. Characterization of the inflammatory and immune effector cells in the lung parenchyma of patients with interstitial lung disease. Am. Rev. Respir. Dis. **123:** 407-412.

17. CRYSTAL, R. G., G. W. HUNNINGHAKE, J. E. GADEK, B. A. KEOGH, S. I. RENNARD & P. B. BITTERMAN. 1983. State of the art: The pathogenesis of sarcoidosis. *In* Sarcoidosis and Other Granulomatous Disorders. J. Chrétien, J. Marsac & J. C. Saltiel, Eds.: 13-35. Pergamon Press. Paris.

In Vitro Formation of Macrophage-Epithelioid Cells and Multinucleated Giant Cells by 1α,25-Dihydroxyvitamin D_3 from Human Circulating Monocytes[a]

MASATAKA OHTA, TETSURO OKABE, KEIYA OZAWA,
AKIO URABE, AND FUMIMARO TAKAKU

The Third Department of Internal Medicine
Faculty of Medicine
University of Tokyo
Tokyo 113, Japan

INTRODUCTION

Sarcoidosis is not infrequently associated with hypercalcemia.[1] Clinical observations suggest that hypercalcemia in sarcoidosis is caused by the elevated serum concentration of 1α,25-dihydroxyvitamin D_3 (calcitriol), a naturally occurring active form of vitamin D_3.[2-4] The abnormal elevation of the serum calcitriol concentration in sarcoidosis appears to be caused by its production by extrarenal tissues because an increased concentration of calcitriol has been observed in an anephric patient.[5] One paper reports that the sarcoid lymph node itself has *in vitro* potential to synthesize calcitriol from its precursor, 25-hydroxyvitamin D_3 (25(OH)D_3) whereas normal lymph nodes have failed to show such a capacity.[6] Moreover, it has been shown that alveolar macrophages from sarcoidosis patients have the ability to convert 25(OH)D_3 to an active metabolite indistinguishable from calcitriol, especially in cases with hypercalcemia and an elevated serum concentration of calcitriol.[7] These studies suggest that the abnormal production of calcitriol by the sarcoid lesion itself may be the cause of hypercalcemia in sarcoidosis patients.

Recent evidence shows that calcitriol induces human myeloid-malignant cell clones to become mature macrophages.[8-10] These studies suggest that this hormone is a promoter of differentiation in myelocyte-macrophage lineage. Furthermore, it has been shown that human circulating monocytes are endowed with calcitriol receptors.[11] Monocyte-macrophages are believed to be precursors of epithelioid cells, which are major constituents of the noncaseating granuloma of sarcoidosis.[12] These studies led us to infer an association between the biological effect of calcitriol on monocyte-

[a]This research was supported by grants-in-aid for cancer research from the Ministry of Education, Science, and Culture of Japan.

macrophage lineage and its role in the pathogenesis of the sarcoidosis granuloma. The role of calcitriol in the pathogenesis of sarcoidosis and the formation of sarcoidosis granulomas, however, has yet to be well investigated.

Our present study evaluates the biological effects of calcitriol on monocyte-macrophage lineage and the evidence that calcitriol plays a critical role in the formation of the sarcoid granuloma. Our results demonstrate that calcitriol is a potent stimulator of the mitotic activity of human circulating monocytes[13] and promotes the formation of macrophage-epithelioid cells and of multinucleated giant cells, a ubiquitous constituent of the noncaseating granuloma of sarcoidosis.

METHODS

Isolation of Monocytes

Monocytes were isolated and incubated as reported previously.[13] Mononuclear cells were isolated from heparinized whole blood of healthy young adult volunteers by Lymphoprep (Nyegaard), the density of which was 1.077. To obtain a purified fraction of monocytes, mononuclear cells were incubated overnight in 24-well tissue culture plates (Falcon), 2×10^6 cells per well, in RPMI 1640 medium containing 10% autologous serum. After the overnight incubation, which took place in a chamber that was continuously flushed with 5% CO_2-95% air at 37° C, the plates were rinsed with phosphate-buffered saline (PBS). Nonadherent cells were completely removed by trypsin treatment, that is, with 0.1% trypsin dissolved in Hanks' balanced salt solution (Gibco) at 37° C for 10 min, and washing. About 2-3% of the initially plated cells, or, $4\text{-}6 \times 10^4$ of the cells in each well, were harvested by these procedures. More than 97% of the adherent cells were shown to be monocytes by the positive α-naphtylbutyrate esterase reaction and the phagocytosis of latex particles; less than 0.5% of the adherent cells formed rosettes with neuraminidase-treated sheep red blood cells.

Incubation of Monocytes

The monocytes which adhered to the plates were incubated in RPMI 1640 medium supplemented with 10% autologous serum (0.5 ml medium/well) in the presence of various agents or vehicle (ethanol) alone for up to 12 days without changing medium. Calcitriol and other derivatives of vitamin D_3 were stored in ethanol at a concentration of 10^{-4} M until they were added to the cultures. The addition of vehicle alone to the culture (the final concentration of ethanol in the culture medium: 0.5%) had no significant effect on the DNA synthesis of monocytes.

Measurement of Mitotic Activity of Monocytes

The degree of DNA synthesis was reflected by the extent of [^{3}H]thymidine incorporation into the cultured monocytes. During the last 18 hr of incubation the cultured monocytes were pulse-labeled with 1.0 μCi/ml of [^{3}H]thymidine (specific activity: 6.7 Ci/mmole). At the end of the incubation the trichloroacetic acid (TCA)-insoluble fraction of the harvested cells was measured with a liquid scintillation counter as previously described.[13] The number of the nuclei of cultured monocytes was counted using the method of Nakagawara and Nathan.[14] After the medium was removed the culture wells were treated with 1% Cetavlon (Daiichi, Japan) in a 0.2 M citric acid solution for 20 min. After the vigorous pipetting the number of cell nuclei in the solution was counted with a hemocytometer under a phase-contrast microscope.

Measurement of Lysozyme Activity

Lysozyme activity of the culture medium was measured using the modified Litwack method described by Okabe *et al.* Lysozyme activity of the 0.5-ml samples, hen egg-white standard lysozyme preparation or culture medium, was assayed by measuring the initial rate of lysis of a suspension of *Micrococcus lysodietics.* The decrease in turbidity was measured at 540 nm and was correlated with lysozyme concentrations by means of a calibration curve.[15]

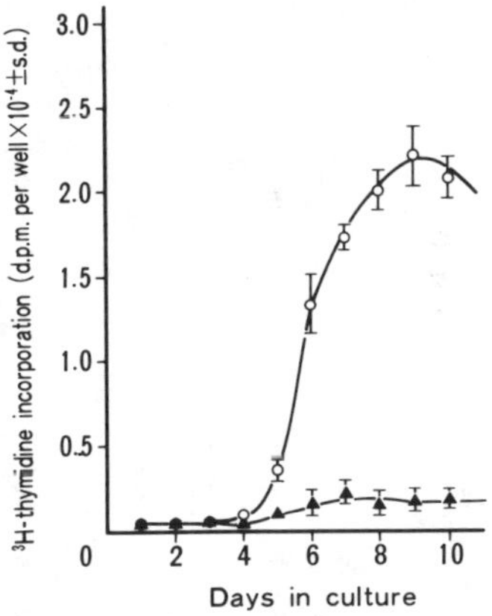

FIGURE 1. Time course of the [^{3}H]thymidine incorporation into the cultured monocytes. Monocytes were incubated in the presence of 10^{-8} M calcitriol (○) or 0.5% ethanol vehicle alone (△) in medium containing 10% autologous serum. [^{3}H]Thymidine incorporation into the monocytes was measured as described in the methods section. Each point represents a mean ± SD of three values from three identical cultures.

RESULTS

Calcitriol markedly stimulated the mitotic activity of monocytes. Monocytes incubated with 10^{-8} M calcitriol began to show marked [^{3}H]thymidine incorporation after day 5, and the DNA synthesis reached a plateau on day 9 (FIG. 1). The number of cell nuclei in the monocyte culture increased to about three times that in the control culture on day 11 (TABLE 1). More than 99.0% of these cultured cells were positive for α-naphthylbutyrate esterase (FIGS. 2A & 2B). Mitotic features of the large adherent cells were often observed during the second week of the culture with calcitriol (FIG. 2C). There was no significant increase in the number of cell nuclei in the control cultures; however, a small increase in [^{3}H]thymidine uptake was observed (FIG. 1).

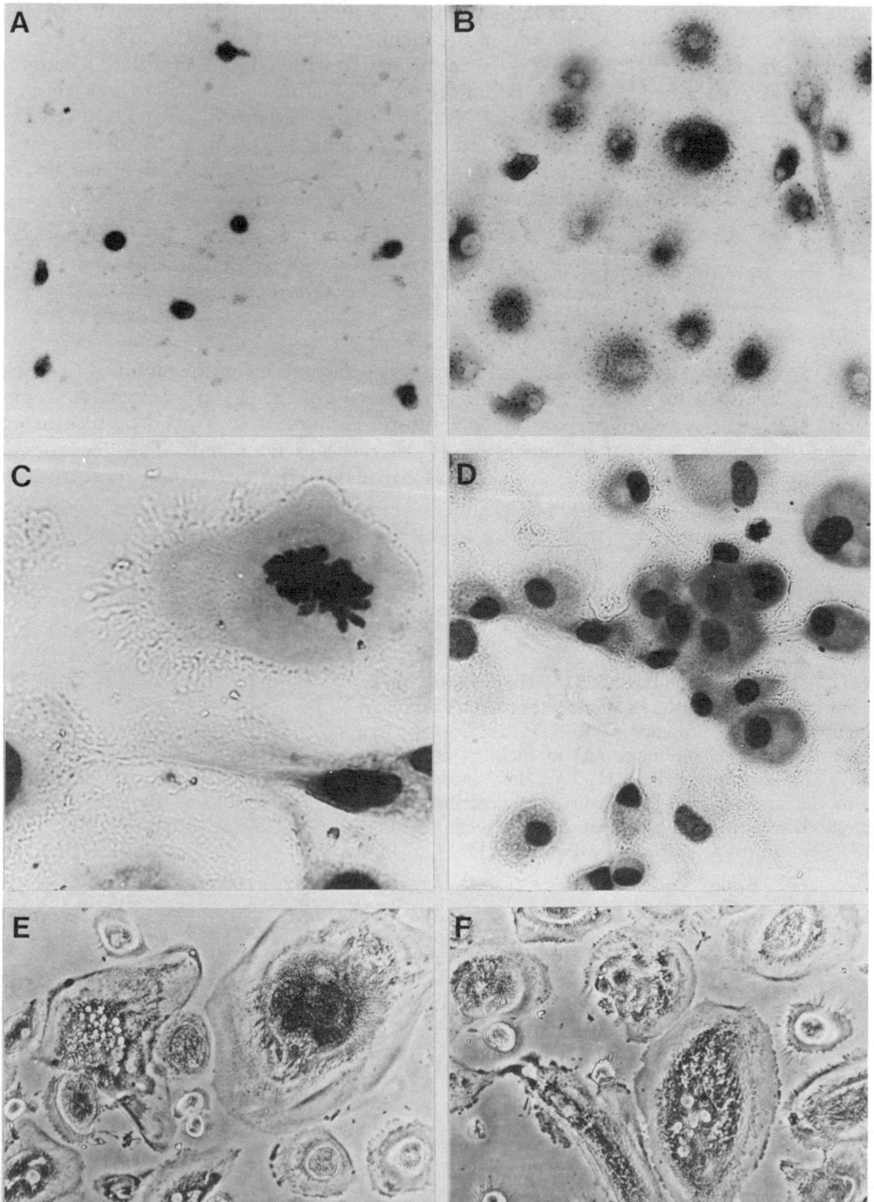
A
B
C
D
E
F

TABLE 1. Time Course of Changes in the Number of Cell Nuclei of Cultured Monocytes[a]

Days in Culture	Number of Nuclei[b]	
	Calcitriol (10^{-8} M)	Control
0	6.2 ± 0.4	6.0 ± 0.3
3	6.7 ± 0.6	4.7 ± 0.6
7	10.2 ± 1.5	4.6 ± 0.6
11	12.7 ± 1.4	4.7 ± 1.1

[a] Monocytes were incubated as described in the methods section. The number of cell nuclei was measured using the method described by Nakagawara and Nathan.[14]

[b] Entries indicate mean counts per well × 10^{-4} ± SD. Each entry is the mean of three values obtained from three identical cultures.

The cultured monocytes showed marked morphological changes. Monocytes incubated in the presence of 10^{-8} M calcitriol began to increase in size 3 or 4 days after the beginning of the incubation. The monocytes developed into large macrophages with ruffled borders, and large clumps of macrophages were often observed during the second week of incubation (FIG. 2D). These morphological changes were much less prominent in the control cultures, that is, in the cultures without calcitriol. The macrophages that had been grown in the medium with 10^{-8} M calcitriol, which was changed weekly, further developed into large epithelioid cells with cytoplasms that appeared dark under phase-contrast microscopy in 3 weeks (FIGS. 2E & 2F). Large epithelioid cells with many nuclei were frequently observed among these cells. These epithelioid cells could survive more than 3 months.

To evaluate whether calcitriol induces secretion of an enzyme specific for macrophages, the activity of lysozyme, one of the major lysosomal enzymes of macrophages, was measured. The enzyme activity released into the medium from the cells treated with 10^{-8} M calcitriol for 10 days was four to five times that from untreated monocytes (TABLE 2). This increase was greater than the increase in the number of cell nuclei described above. Furthermore, analysis of newly synthesized proteins by two-dimensional electrophoresis showed that the protein composition of the calcitriol-treated monocytes was somewhat different from that of untreated monocytes (data not shown).

FIGURE 2. Morphological changes of monocytes in culture. (**A**) Monocytes, before the incubation, that were stained with α-naphthylbutyrate esterase. (**B**) Monocytes that were incubated for 10 days in the presence of 10^{-8} M calcitriol and were then stained with α-naphthylbutyrate esterase. (**C**) A mitotic monocyte that was incubated in the presence of calcitriol and was then stained with Wright-Giemsa. (**D**) A clump of macrophages that were stained with Wright-Giemsa and were observed on day 9 of the incubation with calcitriol. (**E**) Large epithelioid cells, with phase-dense cytoplasms, that were observed on week 3 of the incubation. (**F**) A giant epithelioid cell, with seven nuclei, that was observed on week 3 of the incubation. The original magnification for **A, B,** and **C** was × 400; that for **C** was × 1000; and that for **E** and **F** (under phase-contrast microscopy) was × 280. Each part of this figure was reduced to 72% of its original size.

TABLE 2. Lysozyme Activity in Monocyte-conditioned Medium[a]

	Untreated Monocyte-conditioned Medium	Calcitriol-treated Monocyte-conditioned Medium
Lysozyme activity[b] (μg/ml)	1.4 ± 0.5	6.4 ± 0.6

[a] Monocytes were incubated for 10 days in RPMI 1640 medium supplemented with 10% autologous serum in the presence or absence of 10^{-8} M calcitriol. Lysozyme activity in each 0.5-ml sample of monocyte-conditioned medium was assayed using the modified Litwack method described by Okabe *et al.*[15]

[b] Entries indicate means ± SD. Each entry is the mean of three values.

Calcitriol stimulated the DNA synthesis of monocytes in a dose-related manner (FIG. 3). It stimulated the mitotic activity at concentrations as low as 1×10^{-11} M, at concentrations below the physiological concentration of serum calcitriol, and the maximal DNA synthesis was obtained at 1×10^{-8} M. Calcitriol is the most potent derivative of vitamin D_3 in its ability to promote the DNA synthesis of the cultured monocytes. Other steroid hormones, including testosterone or dexamethasone, failed to show a stimulatory effect on the proliferation of monocytes (data not shown).

DISCUSSION

Our results clearly show that calcitriol is a potent stimulator of the proliferation of circulating monocytes *in vitro* and induces the maturation of monocytes, as shown by the secretion of lysozyme activity and the marked morphological changes. The newly formed monocytes eventually developed into macrophage-epithelioid cells and multinucleated giant cells. Calcitriol stimulated the mitotic activity of monocytes in a dose-related manner, and the dose-response curve is most steep around the concentration of 10^{-10} M, the physiological concentration of calcitriol. This result raises the

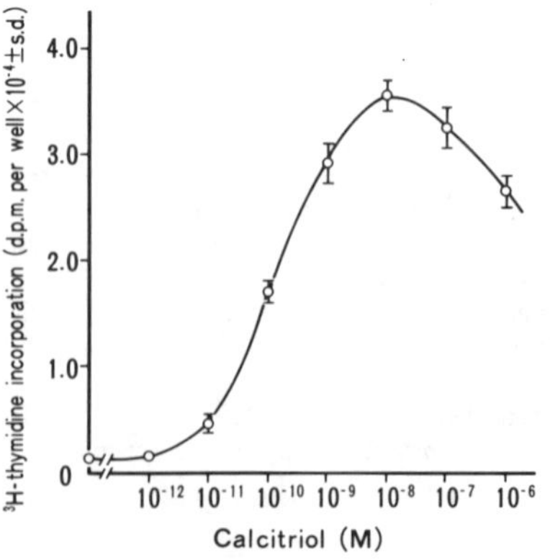

FIGURE 3. The effect of different calcitriol doses on [^{3}H]thymidine incorporation into cultured monocytes. Monocytes were incubated for 9 days in medium containing various concentrations of calcitriol or vehicle alone, and [^{3}H]thymidine incorporation into the cultures was measured as described in the methods section. Each point represents a mean ± SD of three values from three identical cultures.

possibility that the mitotic activity of monocytes may be regulated by the concentration of serum calcitriol. The stimulatory effect on the proliferation of monocytes was highly specific to the active form of vitamin D_3.

A much smaller increase in [^{3}H]thymidine incorporation into the monocytes was observed in the control culture, the culture that did not contain calcitriol. This may be due to the presence of calcitriol in the autologous serum because our results show that the mitotic activity of monocytes was induced by the addition of calcitriol at 10^{-11} M, a concentration well below the physiological concentration of serum calcitriol.

Sarcoidosis manifests itself in patients by the systemic formation of noncaseating granulomas. Macrophages are prominent in sarcoid lesion, and it is widely believed that the cellular origin of epithelioid cells or multinucleated giant cells which constitute the sarcoid granuloma is in monocyte-macrophage lineage.[12] The mechanism which leads monocytes or macrophages to form these granulomas has long been investigated. Some reports suggest that helper thymus-derived (T) cells, which exist in excess at the sarcoid lesion, activate the macrophages to clump into actively secreting epithelioid cells and multinucleated giant cells.[16] This accounts for the local formation of sarcoid lesions, where continuous antigen challenge stimulates T cell activity, but it does not explain why sarcoid lesions are distributed systemically. Sarcoidosis is frequently involved in the liver or spleen, and these organs do not seem to be in contact with antigen; furthermore, circulating T cell activity is decreased in sarcoidosis patients. Other reports suggest that prolonged antigenemia leads to the stimulation of macrophages, which in turn coalesce into epithelioid and multinucleated giant cells.[12] Although clinical findings show the nonspecific rise in immunoglobulins of all classes and immune complexes,[16–18] there are neither many demonstrations of any elevated antigen concentrations in circulating blood of sarcoidosis patients nor any direct demonstrations that the nonspecific elevation in circulating immune complexes or immunoglobulins promotes the formation of the epithelioid cells.

Recent studies suggest that abnormal production of calcitriol by sarcoid lymph nodes or sarcoid macrophages may cause elevated serum calcitriol concentrations.[6,7] It has been suggested that calcitriol plays a critical role in the differentiation of cells of myelocyte-monocyte lineage,[8–10] which are widely believed to be the ancestors of the macrophage-epithelioid cells of the sarcoid granuloma. Although these studies suggest that abnormal production of calcitriol by the sarcoid lesion is involved in the pathogenesis of the sarcoidosis granuloma, the demonstration of a possible role for calcitriol in the pathogenesis of sarcoidosis has not yet been well investigated. Our results provide evidence that calcitriol is a potent stimulator of the proliferation of human circulating monocytes and differentiates these monocytes into macrophage-epithelioid cells to form multinucleated giant cells, major cellular constituents of the sarcoidosis granuloma. The present study may be the first demonstration that calcitriol plays a critical role in the formation of the sarcoidosis granuloma.

Our results show that DNA synthesis by monocytes is promoted by calcitriol at its physiological concentration, but not by calcitriol at the physiological concentration of 25(OH)D_3. In view of studies that show that sarcoid macrophages convert 25(OH)D_3 to calcitriol,[6,7] our results support the idea that the active metabolite of vitamin D_3, which may be produced by macrophage-epithelioid cells, induces the proliferation and differentiation of circulating monocytes into macrophage-epithelioid cells, which in turn form sarcoidosis granulomas (FIG. 4). The autostimulation of macrophage growth, that is, the stimulation of macrophage growth mediated by the production of calcitriol by macrophages, may lead to the formation of the sarcoidosis granuloma.

Our hypothesis provides an explanation of some clinical observations; for example, if abnormally high calcitriol production does promote the formation of granulomas from monocytes, the systemic distribution of sarcoidosis granulomas, as exemplified by sarcoidosis of the liver or spleen (where antigen challenge is unlikely to occur but where cells of monocyte-macrophage lineage are abundant), could be explained. On the other hand, elevated serum calcitriol concentrations are not observed in all clinical cases. Still, clinical observations show that sarcoidosis patients almost invariably have an increased sensitivity to vitamin D_3 administration,[19] so there may yet be another factor that regulates sensitivity to calcitriol.

Another clinical finding is that of elevated serum concentrations of lysosomal enzymes in sarcoidosis.[20,21] Our result that calcitriol markedly induces the secretion of lysozyme, one of the major lysosomal enzymes of macrophage-epithelioid cells, provides a good explanation of these clinical observations.

Recently, Tsoukas *et al.* reported that calcitriol inhibited interleukin-2, the growth-promoting lymphokine which is produced by mitotically activated human T lymphocytes.[22] They also showed that the proliferation of mitogen-activated lymphocytes was inhibited by calcitriol. These results also give an explanation for the role of calcitriol in immunological alterations in sarcoidosis patients. The investigation of possible immunological abnormalities of sarcoidosis patients, such as anergy to tuberculin test, has revealed that the mitotic response of circulating T cells is diminished.[16] The decreased number of circulating helper T cells may be due, in part, to the continuous exposure of T cells to elevated serum concentrations of calcitriol.

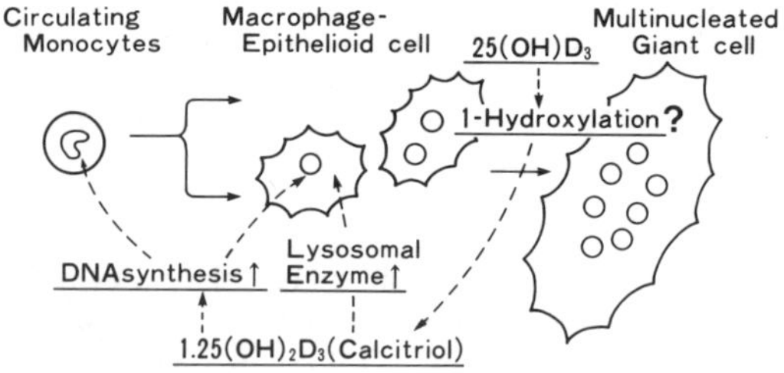

FIGURE 4. Schematic presentation of the possible role of calcitriol in the formation of the sarcoidosis granuloma.

We have presented evidence that calcitriol may play an important role in the pathogenesis of the sarcoid granuloma and in other clinical aspects of sarcoidosis. Abnormally high calcitriol production, however, does not explain the overall pathological processes. For example, our hypothesis of granuloma formation does not exclude the possibility that T cell activation is involved in the formation of sarcoid granulomas because our preliminary results show that the biological responses of monocytes to calcitriol described above are much enhanced in the presence of mitogen-induced human lymphokine.[23] Another outstanding abnormality of immunological systems of sarcoidosis patients is the overactivity of bone marrow-derived (B) cells, as exhibited by the nonspecific increases in the concentrations of serum immunoglobulins of all classes.[16] We are now in the process of elucidating the mechanism of B cell overactivity.

In addition to the results reported by Tsoukas *et al.*,[22] our results further strengthen the idea that calcitriol may be an immunoregulatory hormone in that calcitriol not only inhibits the mitotic activity of circulating T cells but also promotes both the mitotic activity and the differentiation of circulating monocytes.[13]

SUMMARY

1α,25-Dihydroxyvitamin D_3, the active form of vitamin D_3, induced maturation of circulating monocytes to form macrophage-epithelioid cells and multinucleated giant cells *in vitro*. Calcitriol not only promoted the differentiation of monocytes, as shown by the marked morphological changes and enhanced secretion of lysozyme, but also induced their prominent proliferation, as exhibited by enhanced DNA synthesis and the increased number of monocyte cell nuclei. The proliferation of monocytes was observed after the addition of physiological concentrations of calcitriol. Multinucleated giant cells were frequently observed among the monocytes. These marked morphological changes and the proliferation of monocytes were not observed in control cultures, which did not include calcitriol. These results indicate that calcitriol plays a critical role in the formation of the sarcoid granuloma and give an explanation of some of the clinical findings on sarcoidosis. In view of the evidence that sarcoid macrophages convert 25(OH)D_3 to calcitriol, our results raise the possibility that the active metabolite of vitamin D_3, which may be produced by macrophage-epithelioid cells, induces the differentiation and proliferation of circulating monocytes into macrophage-epithelioid cells, which in turn form sarcoidosis granulomas. This autostimulation mechanism of sarcoid granuloma formation may provide a model for future studies.

ACKNOWLEDGMENTS

We thank T. Suda of the Department of Biochemistry of Showa University and M. Kawakami of the Third Department of Internal Medicine of Tokyo University for their technical advice and Y. Nishii of Chugai Pharmaceutical for his gift of calcitriol and other vitamin D_3 derivatives.

REFERENCES

1. MAYOCK, R. L., P. BERTRAND, C. E. MORRISON & J. H. SCOTT. 1963. Manifestations of sarcoidosis: Analysis of 145 patients, with review of nine series selected from literature. Am. J. Med. **35:** 67-89.
2. PAPAPOULOS, S. E., T. L. CLEMENS, L. J. FRAHER, I. G. LEWIN, L. M. SANDLER & J. L. H. O'RIORDAN. 1979. 1,25-Dihydroxycholecalciferol in the pathogenesis of the hypercalcemia of sarcoidosis. Lancet **i:** 627-630.
3. BELL, N. H., P. H. STERN, E. PANTZER, T. K. SINHA & H. F. DELUCA. 1979. Evidence that increased circulating 1α,25-dihydroxyvitamin D is the probable cause for abnormal calcium metabolism in sarcoidosis. J. Clin. Invest. **64:** 218-225.
4. STERN, P. H., J. D. OLAZABAL & N. H. BELL. 1980. Evidence for abnormal regulation of circulating 1α,25-dihydroxyvitamin D in patients with sarcoidosis and normal calcium metabolism. J. Clin. Invest. **66:** 852-855.
5. BARBOUR, G. L., J. W. COBURN, E. SLATOPOLSKY, A. W. NORMAN & R. L. HORST. 1981. Hypercalcemia in an anephric patient with sarcoidosis: Evidence for extrarenal generation of 1,25-dihydroxyvitamin D. N. Engl. J. Med. **305:** 440-443.

6. MASON, R. S., T. FRANKEL, Y. L. CHAN, D. LISSNER & S. POSEN. 1984. Vitamin D conversion by sarcoid lymph node homogenate. Ann. Intern. Med. **100:** 59-61.
7. ADAMS, J. S., O. P. SHARMA, M. A. GACAD & F. R. SINGER. 1983. Metabolism of 25-hydroxyvitamin D_3 by cultured pulmonary alveolar macrophages in sarcoidosis. J. Clin. Invest. **72:** 1856-1860.
8. TANAKA, H., E. ABE, C. MIYAURA, Y. SHINA & T. SUDA. 1983. 1α,25-Dihydroxyvitamin D_3 induces differentiation of human promyelocytic leukemia cells (HL-60) into monocyte-macrophages, but not into granulocytes. Biochem. Biophys. Res. Commun. **117:** 86-92.
9. MCCARTHY, D. M., J. F. SAN MIGUEL, H. C. FREAKE, P. M. GREEN, H. ZOLA, D. CATOVSKY & J. M. GOLDMAN. 1983. 1,25-Dihydroxyvitamin D_3 inhibits proliferation of human promyelocytic leukemia (HL-60) cells and induces monocyte-macrophage differentiation in HL-60 and normal human bone marrow cells. Leukemia Res. **7**(1): 51-55.
10. BAR-SHAVIT, Z., S. L. TEITELBAUM, P. REITSMA, A. HALL, L. E. PEGG, J. TRIAL & A. J. KAHN. 1983. Induction of monocytic differentiation and bone resorption by 1,25-dihydroxyvitamin D_3. Proc. Natl. Acad. Sci. USA **80:** 5907-5911.
11. PROVVEDINI, D. M., C. D. TSOUKAS, L. J. DEFTOS & S. C. MANOLAGAS. 1983. 1,25-Dihydroxyvitamin D_3 receptors in human leukocytes. Science **221:** 1181-1183.
12. JAMES, D. G. 1982. Sarcoidosis. *In* Cecil Textbook of Medicine. 16th edit. J. B. Wyngaarden & L. H. Smith, Eds.: 1891-1898. Saunders. Philadelphia, PA.
13. OHTA, M., T. OKABE, K. OZAWA, A URABE & F. TAKAKU. 1985. 1α,25-Dihydroxyvitamin D_3 (calcitriol) stimulates proliferation of human circulating monocytes *in vitro*. FEBS Lett. **185**(1): 9-13.
14. NAKAGAWARA, A. & C. F. NATHAN. 1983. A simple method for counting adherent cells: Application to cultured human monocytes, macrophages and multinucleated giant cells. J. Immunol. Methods **56**(2): 261-268.
15. OKABE, T., A. SUZUKI, H. ISHIKAWA, H. YOTSUMOTO & N. OHSAWA. 1981. Cells originating from sarcoid granulomas *in vitro*. Am. Rev. Respir. Dis. **124**(5): 608-612.
16. JAMES, D. G. & W. JONES WILLIAMS. 1982. Immunology of sarcoidosis. Am. J. Med. **72:** 5-8.
17. JAMES, D. G., E. NEVILLE & A. N. WALKER. 1975. Immunology of sarcoidosis. Am. J. Med. **59:** 388-394.
18. GUPTA, R. C., F. KUEPPERS, R. A. DEREMEE, K. R. HUSTON & F. C. MCDUFFIE. 1977. Pulmonary and extrapulmonary sarcoidosis in relation to circulating immune complexes. Am. Rev. Respir. Dis. **116:** 261.
19. WINNACKER, J. L., K. L. BECKER & S. KATZ. 1968. Endocrine aspects of sarcoidosis. N. Engl. J. Med. **278:** 427-434.
20. PASCUAL, R. S., J. B. L. GEE & S. C. FRINCH. 1973. Usefulness of serum lysozyme measurement in diagnosis and evaluation of sarcoidosis. N. Engl. J. Med. **289:** 1074-1076.
21. SILVERSTEIN, E., J. FRIEDLAND & T. ACKERMAN. 1977. Elevation of granulomatous lymph node and serum lysozyme in sarcoidosis and correlation with angiotensin-converting enzyme. Am. J. Clin. Pathol. **68:** 219-224.
22. TSOUKAS, C. D., D. M. PROVVEDINI & S. C. MANOLAGAS. 1984. 1,25-Dihydroxyvitamin D_3: A novel immunoregulatory hormone. Science **224:** 1438-1439.
23. OHTA, M., K. OZAWA, T. OKABE, A. URABE & F. TAKAKU. 1985. Induction of proliferation of human circulating monocytes *in vitro* by lectin-induced factor(s) from lymphocytes. Biochem. Biophys. Res. Commun. **126**(2): 705-711.

Dynamics and Mechanism of the Sarcoidal Granuloma

Detecting T Cell Subsets, Non-T Cells, and Immunoglobulins in Biopsies at Varying Intervals of Kveim-Siltzbach Test Sites

YASH P. KATARIA[a,b] AND H. KIM PARK[c]

[b] *Pulmonary Diseases Section*
Department of Medicine
and
[c] *Department of Clinical Pathology and Diagnostic Medicine*
East Carolina University School of Medicine
Greenville, North Carolina 27834

INTRODUCTION

Sarcoidosis is a multisystemic disease of unknown etiology and is associated with disparate immunologic alterations.[1] Its hallmark is the presence of noncaseating granulomatous inflammation, the pathogenesis of which has not been clearly defined. Recent studies on lymphokine production by the cultured cutaneous sarcoidal granulomas point towards its immunologic origin.[2,3] This is further supported by immunohistochemical studies of sarcoidal lesions from a variety of organs in the body.[4-6] These studies demonstrate the presence of a large number of thymus-derived (T) cells in which T helper cells predominate and in which T suppressor cells and bone marrow-derived (B) cells are occasionally present. In the center of the granuloma varying numbers of macrophage-epithelioid cells and few giant cells are also found. No information is available, however, on the development of earlier phases of sarcoidal granulomas. The histologic examination of lung biopsy specimens from patients with sarcoidosis has suggested that the alveolitis with infiltration of mononuclear cells precedes the development of sarcoidal granulomas.[7,8] It is recognized that the granulomas induced in response to Kveim-Siltzbach (K-S) antigen and the naturally occurring sarcoidal granulomas found in a variety of organs in the body share similar histological, histochemical, immunofluorescent, and ultrastructural features.[9] Thus, it seemed appropriate to look upon K-S antigen-induced granulomas as an experimental model for the further study of sarcoidosis. This study examined the punch-biopsy specimens of K-S test sites in patients with sarcoidosis at varying intervals for the presence of T lymphocytes and their subsets, non-T cells, and immunoglobulins.

[a] To whom correspondence and reprint requests should be addressed.

MATERIALS AND METHODS

Kveim-Siltzbach Tests

K-S tests were performed in K-S-reactive patients with sarcoidosis using well-validated CR-1 antigen.[10] In each patient, two tests were performed on the lateral aspect of the left upper thigh, and full-thickness skin biopsies were taken under sterile conditions, from the site of injection, with a 4-mm punch-biopsy apparatus. Before the biopsy, the area around the injection site was infiltrated with 2% xylocaine. In each patient, a biopsy was taken of a K-S test site within 3 weeks. Each biopsy specimen was bisected: one portion was fixed in 10% formalin, and the other was snap-frozen in a cryobath and stored at −70° C until it was ready to be processed for further examination.

STUDIES ON TISSUE SECTIONS

Hematoxylin-Eosin Staining

Formalin-fixed biopsy specimens were imbedded in paraffin and processed in a routine fashion for hematoxylin-eosin (H-E) stains. The stained sections were examined under light microscopy in order to confirm the pathology and demonstrate the morphology.

Immunohistochemical Staining

Cryostat sections 5-6-μm thick were made from frozen specimens and were mounted on slides that had been precoated with a 0.2% gelatin solution. These slides were air dried for 10 min and then fixed in acetone for 10 min at room temperature. After this, the sections underwent two 5-min washings with phosphate-buffered saline (PBS) after being air dried.

The monoclonal antibody for indirect staining was Leu-1 for T lymphocytes, Leu-2a for suppressor-cytotoxic lymphocytes, Leu-3a for helper-inducer T lymphocytes, Leu-M3 for monocytes (Becton-Dickinson, Sunnyvale, CA), and BA-1 for B lymphocytes (Hybritech, San Diego, CA). Sections were incubated for 5 min in 5% normal horse serum diluted in 2% bovine serum albumin (BSA) to block the background staining with antibody. Excessive horse serum was drained from each section, and the area around each section was carefully wiped with a piece of gauze. Primary antibody diluted in 2% BSA to a predetermined dilution was placed on the sections and incubated for 12 min; afterwards, the slides were thoroughly rinsed by being flooded several times with PBS. The slides were drained again, and the area around each section was carefully wiped. Biotinylated secondary antibody diluted in PBS was then applied and incubated for 8 min, and the sections were well rinsed several times with PBS. Avidin-biotin complexes (ABC's) of avidin DH and biotinylated horseradish peroxidase H complex (Vector Lab, Burlingame, CA) were prepared by mixing equal amounts of these reagents diluted in PBS. The ABC's were mixed at least 30 min before they were to be applied to the slides for an 8-min incubation that was to be terminated by rinsing with PBS. The last incubation was in 3,3-diaminobenzidine hydrochloride (DAB) (Sigma Chemical Company, St. Louis, MO) that was prepared in tris buffer solution containing imidazole. Sections were incubated 1-2 min and were then washed for several minutes in running water. Counter staining was done with Mayer's hematoxylin for 3 min. The specimens were washed, dipped in ammonia water, washed again, dehydrated with alcohol, cleared in Amerclear, and mounted with the Krystalon resin-mounting media. The whole procedure was carried out on an Ortho Stainplate® (Ortho Diagnostic Systems, Raritan, NJ).

Some sections were stained with immunoglobulins (Ig's); the peroxidase-conjugated primary antibodies were diluted in PBS (goat antihuman IgG, IgM, IgA, and the kappa and lambda side chains were obtained from Tago, Burlingame, CA). The staining procedure was identical to the one outlined above, except that tris buffer without imidazole replaced normal horse serum, and DAB was used for direct staining.

RESULTS

Hematoxylin-Eosin Stain

FIGURE 1 shows biopsy specimens stained with H-E as they appear under light microscopy. A necrotic area of collagen with a few mononuclear cells at the injection site became apparent 6 hr after the K-S test. On day 1, necrotic collagen became more well defined, and, in addition to mononuclear cells, a few polymorphonuclear cells were present. On day 7, altered collagen was still seen, and an increased number of mononuclear cells and a rare eosinophil were present. From day 12 to day 21, altered collagen was beginning to become organized, and a dense infiltration of mononuclear cells and rare giant cells were present. On day 28, there was reduction in the amount of altered collagen, and the collagen was more organized; the mononuclear cell infiltration became denser, and there were well-formed granulomata. On day 34, apart from changes seen on day 28, altered collagen was seen being replaced by normal collagen.

Immunohistochemical Stain

Immunohistochemical stains of altered collagen were observed much the way H-E stains were observed (FIGS. 2-5). Several T lymphocytes (marked with Leu-1) were seen around the vessels and the necrotic collagen. A majority of these cells were helper T cells (Leu-3a), and a few were suppressor T cells (Leu-2a). Until day 7 there was a progressive increase in the number of T lymphocytes, a majority of which were helper cells. There were very few suppressor cells. Several Leu-M3-marked monocytes were also seen. These cells had shown a maximal increase in number in the day 2 biopsy specimen. Only a few B lymphocytes were seen. From day 12 to day 34, there

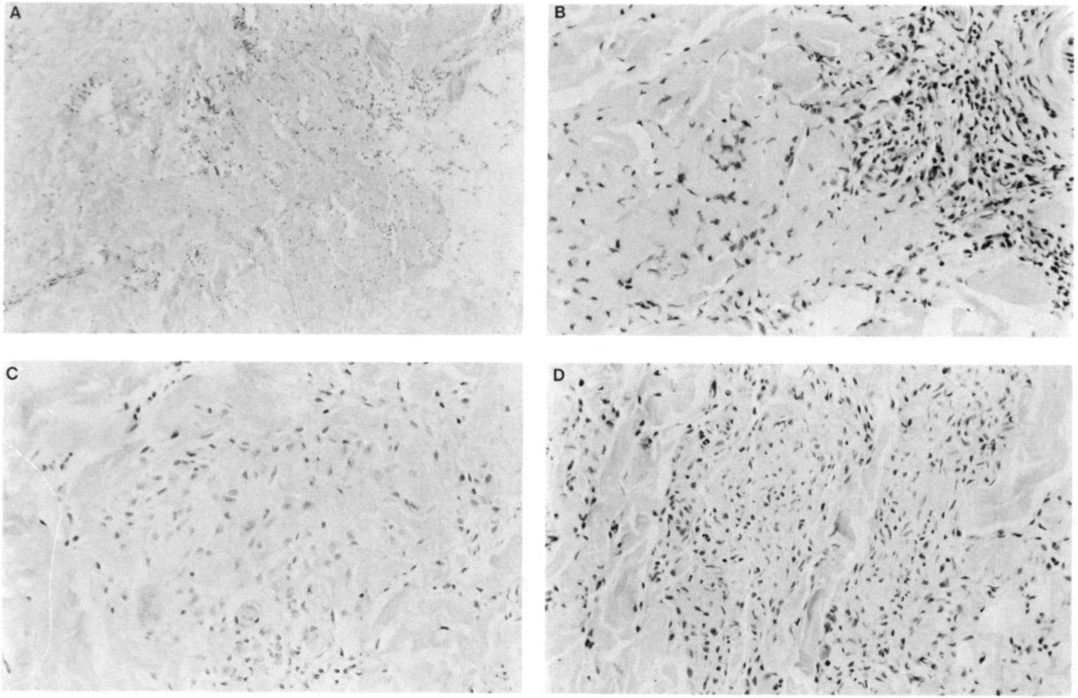

FIGURE 1. **(A)** A K-S test site specimen section at 6 hr showing a necrotic area of collagen at the injection site and a few mononuclear cells around the blood vessels and the necrotic collagen. **(B)** A K-S test site specimen section at 7 days showing an increased number of mononuclear cells, a few eosinophils, and altered collagen. **(C)** A K-S test site specimen section at 12 days showing organized collagen, mononuclear cells, epithelioid cells, and a few multinucleated giant cells. **(D)** A K-S test site specimen section at 34 days showing altered collagen being replaced by normal collagen, and multiple well-formed epithelioid cell granulomas. All stains were made with H-E. The original magnifications for **A** and for **B, C,** and **D** were ×100 and ×250, respectively; each part of the figure was reduced to 42% of its original size.

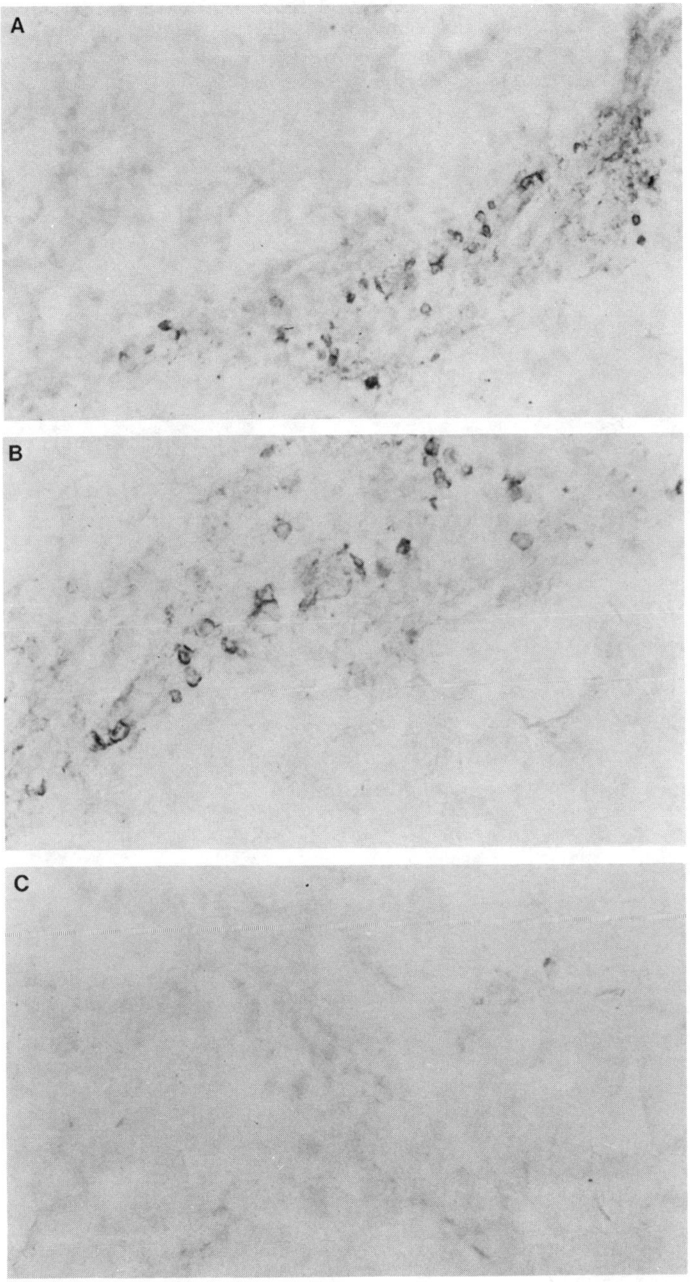

FIGURE 2. Frozen K-S test site specimen sections at 6 hr stained with monoclonal antibodies by the immunohistochemical technique. **(A)** Leu-1-stained T lymphocytes. **(B)** Many Leu-3a-stained helper T lymphocytes. **(C)** A few Leu-2a-stained suppressor T lymphocytes. The original magnifications for **A** and for **B** and **C** were ×250 and ×400, respectively; each part of the figure was reduced to 54% of its original size.

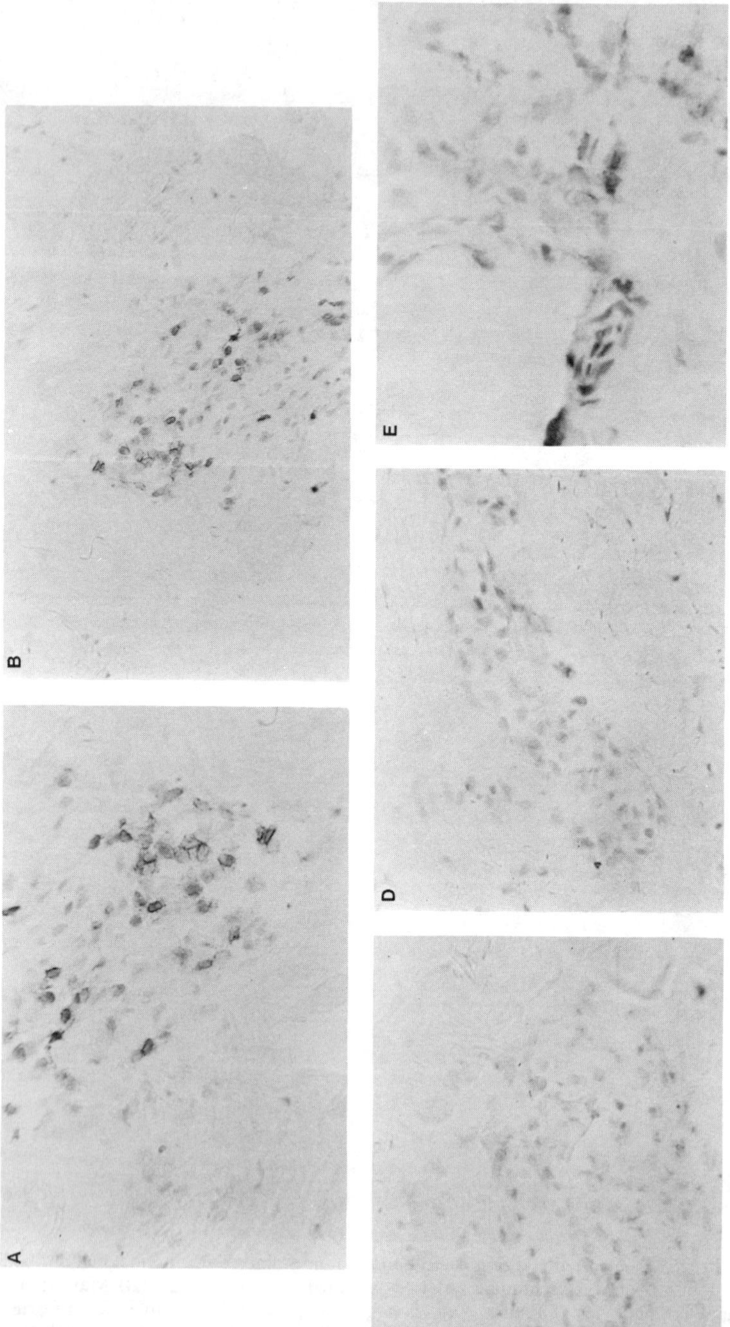

FIGURE 3. Frozen K–S test site specimen sections at 7 days stained with monoclonal antibodies by the immunohistochemical technique. **(A)** Leu-1-stained T lymphocytes. **(B)** Many Leu-3a-stained helper T lymphocytes. **(C)** A few Leu-2a-stained suppressor lymphocytes. **(D)** A few B-1-stained B lymphocytes. **(E)** A few Leu-M3-stained monocytes. The original magnifications for **B** and for **A, C,** and **D** were ×250 and ×400, respectively; each part of the figure was reduced to 46% of its original size.

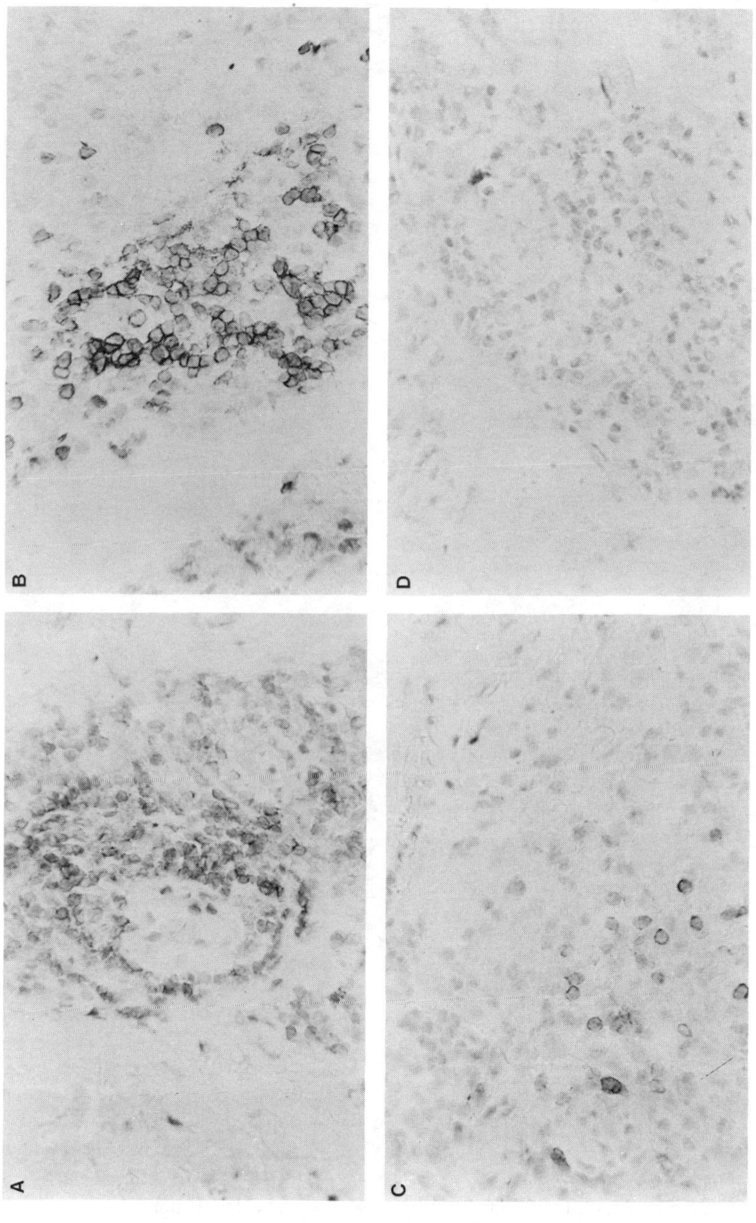

FIGURE 4. Frozen K-S test site specimen sections at 12 days stained with monoclonal antibodies by the immunohistochemical technique. **(A)** Leu-1-stained T lymphocytes. **(B)** Many Leu-3a-stained helper T lymphocytes. **(C)** A few Leu-2a-stained suppressor T lymphocytes. **(D)** A few Leu-M3-stained monocytes. Original magnification: ×400; reduced to 47% of original size.

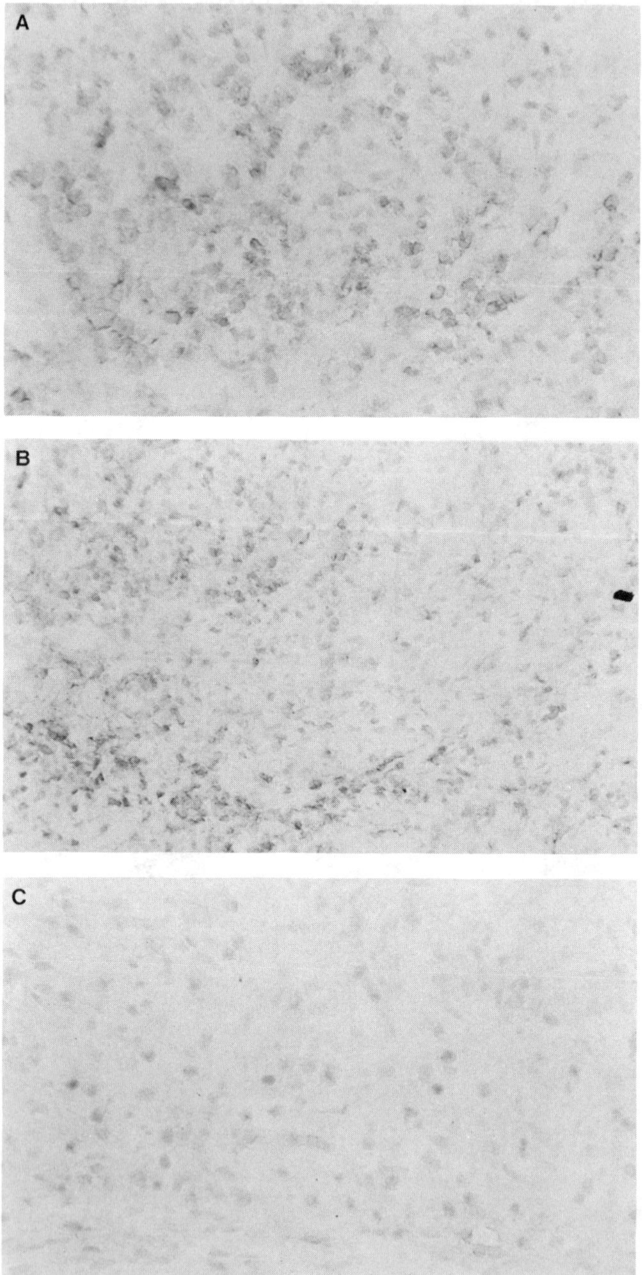

FIGURE 5. Frozen K-S test site specimen sections at 34 days stained with monoclonal antibodies by the immunohistochemical technique. **(A)** Leu-1-stained T lymphocytes. **(B)** Many Leu-3a-stained helper T lymphocytes. **(C)** A few T suppressor cells. Original magnification: ×400; reduced to 52% of original side.

was a progressive increase in the number of T lymphocytes, the majority of which were again helper cells; only a few were suppressor cells. On day 12, the first of several giant cells to appear was seen, but it did not stain with Leu-M3 antibody; only rarely was a monocyte or a B lymphocyte seen. Biopsy specimens taken on day 21, day 28, and day 34 showed the progressive changes of granulomas during their formation. Although epithelioid cells and multinucleated giant cells were easily identified, none were marked with the Leu-M3 antibody; hardly any B cells or monocytes were seen.

DISCUSSION

The etiology of sarcoidosis is unknown, and there is no experimental model for the study of the disease: the pathogenesis of granulomatous inflammation in sarcoidosis cannot be studied from its inception. Biopsy specimens of papules resulting from K-S tests demonstrate a similarity between the cellular elements of the granulomas of these papules and those of naturally occurring lesions of sarcoidosis in various parts of the body. Thus it seems worthwhile to examine the Kveim papule in order to study the pathogenesis and evolution of the sarcoidal granuloma. In the present study light microscopy revealed altered collagen at the injection site of K-S antigen. Initially, a necrotic area was seen which gradually became more organized, and, by day 34, the laying down of normal collagen was apparent. Altered collagen indicated the location of the injection site of K-S antigen and persisted until the development of a typical noncaseating granuloma. It is possible that the granuloma-inducing antigen present in the K-S suspension binds to collagen and is thus able to remain at the injection site for a prolonged period. Its nature, however, remains undetermined.

Regarding cellular infiltrates, a few lymphocytes were found around the blood vessels and altered collagen 6 hr after the injection of antigen. By day 2, there was an influx of monocytes as well. The mononuclear cell infiltrate became progressively denser by day 12, by which time granulomas began to form, as indicated by the appearance of a few multinucleated giant cells and some epithelioid cells. Subsequently the numbers of epithelioid cells increased; this increase indicated the granulomatous inflammation and reached its maximum by day 34. Thus, it became evident that in the initial phase of the development of the sarcoidal granuloma there is nonspecific inflammation with mononuclear cells, which is nondiagnostic for sarcoidosis and is equivalent to the alveolitis seen in lung biopsy specimens.[7]

The immunohistochemical staining method clearly demonstrated the early appearance of T lymphocytes. A majority of these lymphocytes were helper cells; a few were suppressor cells. From 6 hr to 34 days after injection of K-S antigen, there was a progressive increase in the total number of T lymphocytes, and of T lymphocyte subsets, but no alteration in their proportions was apparent. The influx of monocytes was recognized for the first time in the biopsy specimen taken on day 2. The influx continued until day 7. After that, few monocytes were seen, although the monoclonal antibody used remained the same. The antibody stained more than 95% of peripheral blood monocytes as well as monocytes from a patient with monocytic leukemia. In the granulomas, epithelioid cells and multinucleated giant cells were in abundance, but these cells were not stained with the Leu-M3 antibody. If these cells were considered to be transformed monocytes, these findings would suggest a change in their phenotype. Others using OKM1 monoclonal antibody have demonstrated staining of monocytes, epithelioid cells, and multinucleated giant cells.[11]

The presence of predominant helper-inducer cells is not unique to sarcoidosis. It has also been demonstrated in tissues of patients with rheumatoid arthritis.[12] In contrast, a number of diseases show a predominance of suppressor-cytotoxic cells in the afflicted tissues. These include viral diseases, toxoplasmosis, graft versus host disease, rejection of transplanted kidney, idiopathic pulmonary fibrosis, and pigeon breeder's disease.[4,13-17]

It is possible that both the nature of the antigen and host response would determine the type and course of the disease. This has been demonstrated in studies of leprosy patients.[18] In lepromatous leprosy the lymphocytic infiltrate almost exclusively consists of suppressor cells whereas in tuberculoid leprosy the predominant T cell is from the helper subset. The type of T lymphocyte which predominates seems to influence the course of the disease. Antigen-differentiated immune T lymphocytes are known to produce interleukin-2,[19] which in turn causes proliferation of clones of activated T lymphocytes, in the absence of any antigenic stimulation,[20] leading to the production of a variety of lymphokines.[20,21] These lymphokines appear to help in the induction of granulomatous inflammation. Interleukin-2 and other lymphokines have indeed been demonstrated in supernatants of cultured cutaneous sarcoidal granulomas.[2,3] The predominance of helper T lymphocytes and the lack of suppressor-cytotoxic lymphocytes could explain the perpetual formation of granulomas in sarcoidosis and the indolent nature of the disease.

The scarcity of B lymphocytes and lack of any immunoglobulin deposits in the biopsy specimens suggests that there is no role for humoral immunity in the development of sarcoidal granulomas. In the well-developed, naturally occurring sarcoidal lesions, some studies have reported the presence of plasma cells in the periphery of the granulomas,[4] suggesting that these cells arrive late at the site of granulomatous inflammation. It is possible that the activation of B lymphocytes is secondary to injury sustained by cell-mediated immunity and that the presence of dominant helper T lymphocytes would lead to the activation of B lymphocytes which cause hypergammaglobulinemia.

It is concluded that the development of sarcoidal granulomas in response to K-S antigen is a purely cell-mediated phenomenon, and the presence of predominant helper T lymphocytes leads to ineffective control and thus perpetual formation of granulomas in sarcoidosis.

SUMMARY

Punch biopsies of K-S test sites were studied by the use of monoclonal antibodies for the presence of T cells, T cell subsets, B cells, IgG, IgM, IgA, and kappa and lambda chains by an indirect and direct immunoperoxidase technique. A total of 10 biopsies were performed at intervals ranging from 6 hr to 34 days.

Results revealed that at 6 hr there was an influx of T cells, predominantly helper cells, at the injection site, followed by an infiltration of monocytes, an infiltration that was maximal at 48 hr. By day 7 there was a marked increase in the number of T lymphocytes, predominantly helper cells, and a few persistent monocytes were seen. By day 12 there was evidence of granuloma formation with the appearance of some epithelioid cells and a few giant cells. These cells, along with helper T cells, were seen to have progressively increased in number when the confluent granulomas on the day 34 biopsies were studied. Epithelioid cells, however, did not show any reactivity with

Leu-M3 monoclonal antibody, which stained the majority of peripheral blood monocytes. B cells were rarely present; immunoglobulins were absent in all biopsies.

It was concluded that the evolution of the sarcoidal granuloma in response to K-S antigen is a purely cell-mediated phenomenon. Helper-inducer T cells appear to play a dominant role in its evolution and maintenance. Lack of reactivity of epithelioid and giant cells with Leu-M3 monoclonal antibody indicates either a different lineage from monocytes or a change in their phenotype.

REFERENCES

1. KATARIA, Y. P., R. A. SHAW & P. B. CAMPBELL. 1982. Sarcoidosis: An overview. II. Clin. Notes Respir. Dis. **20:** 3-16.
2. KATARIA, Y. P., P. B. CAMPBELL, H. K. PARK & K. C. KALMUS. 1983. *In vitro* observations on intact granulomas of sarcoidosis. *In* Sarcoidosis and Other Granulomatous Disorders. J. Chrétien, J. Marsac & J. C. Saltiel, Eds.: 126-131. Pergamon Press. Paris.
3. KATARIA, Y. P., R. C. PADGETT & L. S. ENGLISH. Ann. N.Y. Acad. Sci. This volume.
4. SEMENZATO, G., A. PEZZUTTO, G. PIZZOLO, M. CHILOSI, E. OSSI, M. R. ANGI & A. CIPRIANI. 1984. Immunohistological study in sarcoidosis: Evaluation of different sites of disease activity. Clin. Immunol. Immunopathol. **30:** 29-40.
5. SEMENZATO, G., A. PEZZUTTO, M. CHILOSI & G. PIZZOLO. 1982. Redistribution of T lymphocytes in the lymph nodes of patients with sarcoidosis. N. Engl. J. Med. **306:** 48-49.
6. BUECHNER, S. A., R. K. WINKELMANN & P. M. BANKS. 1983. T-cell subsets in cutaneous sarcoidosis. Arch. Dermatol. **119:** 728-732.
7. ROSEN, Y., T. J. ATHANASSIADES, S. MOON & H. A. LYONS. 1978. Nongranulomatous interstitial pneumonitis in sarcoidosis. Chest **74**(2): 122-125.
8. CARRINGTON, C. B., E. A. GAENSLER, J. P. MIKUS, A. W. SCHACHTER, G. W. BURKE & A. M. GOFF. 1976. Structure and function in sarcoidosis. Ann. N.Y. Acad. Sci. **278:** 265-283.
9. SILTZBACH, L. E. 1967. Concepts of sarcoidosis in the light of the Kveim reaction. *In* Proceedings of the Fourth International Conference on Sarcoidosis. T. Turiaf & J. Chabot, Eds.: 129-140. Masson & Cie. Paris.
10. KATARIA, Y. P., O. P. SHARMA, L. ISRAEL & M. ROGERS. 1980. Kveim antigen CR-I: Its sensitivity and specificity in sarcoidosis. *In* Eighth International Conference on Sarcoidosis and Other Granulomatous Diseases. W. Jones Williams & B. H. Davies, Eds.: 660-667. Alpha Omega. Cardiff.
11. BJERKE, M. R., R. MATRE & R. NILSEN. 1983. Characterization of mononuclear cells in sarcoid skin lesions using monoclonal antibodies. Acta Pathol. Microbiol. Immunol. Scand. **91:** 233-236.
12. JANOSSY, G., O. DUKE, L. W. POULTER, G. PANAYI, M. BOFILL & G. GOLDSTEIN. 1981. Rheumatoid arthritis: A disease of T-lymphocyte/macrophage immunoregulation. Lancet **ii:** 839-842.
13. FENYK, J. R., P. I. WARKENTIN, R. Q. GOLTZ, M. E. NESBIT, P. F. COCCIA, C. M. SMITH, W. KRIVIT, J. E. NEELY, N. K. C. RAMSAY & J. H. KERSEY. 1978. Sclerodermatous graft-versus-host disease limited to an area of measles exanthema. Lancet **i:** 472-473.
14. CARNEY, W. P., P. H. RUBIN, R. A. HOFFMAN, W. P. HANSEN, K. HEALEY & M. S. HIRSCH. 1981. Analysis of T-lymphocyte subsets in cytomegalovirus mononucleosis. Immunology **126:** 2114-2116.
15. LAMPERT, I. A., A. J. SUITTERS, G. JANOSSY, J. A. THOMAS, S. PALMER & E. G. SMITH. 1981. Lymphoid infiltrates in skin in graft-versus-host disease. Lancet **ii:** 1352.
16. PLATT, J. L., T. W. LEBIEN & A. F. MICHAEL. 1982. Interstitial mononuclear cell populations in renal graft rejection. J. Exp. Med. **155:** 17-30.

17. MORITZ, E. D., J. M. SMIEJAN, B. A. KEOGH & R. G. CRYSTAL. 1982. Non-fibrotic pigeon breeder's syndrome: A disorder characterized by a chronic suppressor T-cell alveolitis. Clin. Res. **30**(2): 435A.
18. VAN VOORHIS, W. C., G. KAPLAN, E. N. SARNO, M. A. HORWITZ, R. M. STEINMAN, W. R. LEVIS, N. NOGUEIRA, L. S. HAIR, C. R. A. GATTASS, B. A. ARRICK & Z. A. COHN. 1982. The cutaneous infiltrates of leprosy: Cellular characteristics and the predominant T-cell phenotypes. N. Engl. J. Med. **307:** 1593-1642.
19. LARSSON, E. 1981. Mechanism of T cell activation. II. Antigen- and lectin-dependent acquisition of responsiveness to TCGF is a nonmitogenic, active response of resting T cells. J. Immunol. **126:** 1323-1326.
20. SMITH, K. A., S. GILLIS, P. E. BAKER, D. MCKENZIE & F. W. RUSCETTI. 1979. T-cell growth factor-mediated T-cell proliferation. Ann. N.Y. Acad. Sci. **332:** 423-432.
21. KELSO, A., H. R. MACDONALD, K. A. SMITH, J. C. CEROTTINI & K. T. BRUNNER. 1984. Interleukin-2 enhancement of lymphokine secretion by T lymphocytes: Analysis of established clones and primary limiting dilution microcultures. J. Immunol. **132:** 2932-2938.

Complement Activity in Pulmonary Fluid during Sarcoidosis

C. R. LAMBRÉ, S. LE MAHO, H. DE CRÉMOUX,
K. ATASSI, AND J. BIGNON

*Institut National de la Santé
et de la Recherche Médicale Unité 139
Centre Hospitalier Universitaire H. Mondor
94010 Créteil Cédex, France*

Complement is a complex system of proteins with numerous biological activities that can be either beneficial or baneful for the organism. Besides possessing a lytic activity that completes the antigen-antibody reaction, the complement system, in the course of its activation, releases numerous mediators that are involved in the clearance of pathogenic particles as well as in the appearance of an inflammatory reaction leading to tissue injury. The numerous possibilities for this system to be activated in the lung make complement an important factor to be considered in the normal physiology as well as in the pathology of the lung.

Mononuclear alveolitis with subsequent granulomatous formation appears to be the dynamic histopathological change characteristic of active pulmonary sarcoidosis.[1-4] In a small percentage of patients, this inflammatory process is perpetuated and leads to extensive alveolar derangement and deterioration of pulmonary functions. Pathogenic factors leading to such an unusual chronic course remain obscure. The current concept, however, is that alveolitis in active and chronic sarcoidosis is perpetuated by replicating thymus-derived (T) cells. Release of interleukin-2 (IL-2) by T lymphocytes has a key role in T cell proliferation.[3] Such a release has been demonstrated in active sarcoidosis.[5] Lasting antigenic activation and stimulation of resting T lymphocytes by macrophage interleukin-1 (IL-1) are the two factors that are necessary for IL-2 production, which in turn induces an increased antibody synthesis.[6] Other factors such as complement have not yet been extensively studied in sarcoidosis. It is conceivable that the complement system has a role in granuloma formation and maintenance because some of the numerous by-products released in the fluid phase during complement activation are potent modulators of the functions of macrophages, monocytes, and lymphocytes. For example, phagocytosis, lysosomal enzyme release, oxygen metabolite generation, and antibody synthesis are somehow under the control of cleavage fragments from C2, C3, C4, C5, and B appearing during complement activation.

MATERIALS AND METHODS

Subjects

This study included 46 subjects; each subject was either a volunteer or a hospitalized patient. The subjects were divided into two groups.

Pulmonary Sarcoidosis Group

The pulmonary sarcoidosis (S) group comprised 30 patients with biopsy-proved pulmonary sarcoidosis. Most of the patients had no extrathoracic sarcoidosis. The mean age was 31 years (range: 21 to 57 years); there were 16 men and 14 women.

Chest roentgenograms were classified as follows: Type 0, normal roentgenograms at the time of the bronchoalveolar lavage (BAL) in patients which had previously presented a typical feature of sarcoidosis or had returned to normal within the following 6 months (5 patients); Type 1, sarcoidosis with isolated bilateral hilar lymphadenopathy (8 patients); Type 2, parenchymal changes with bilateral hilar lymphadenopathy (10 patients, of which 4 were smokers); Type 3, diffuse parenchymal changes without hilar lymphadenopathy (7 patients, of which 4 were smokers).

Patients with a disease of more than a year's duration were classified as having chronic sarcoidosis; patients with a disease of less than a year's duration were classified as having recent sarcoidosis.

Control Groups

There were two control groups. The first comprised seven patients (six men and one woman), all of whom were smokers with idiopathic pulmonary fibrosis (IPF); the mean age of the patients in the IPF group was 54 years (range: 35 to 79 years). The second group comprised nine normal volunteers (eight men and one woman), five of whom were smokers; the mean age for the normal (N) group was 29 years (range: 20 to 43 years).

BAL

The BAL technique used in this study was a simple extension of a fiberoptic bronchoscopy technique used routinely in this institution. After local anesthesia was given to a patient, the fiberoptic bronchoscope was wedged into the patient's distal bronchus, usually in the lingula or the right middle lobe. Then, a total of 200 ml of 0.9% sterile saline solution was used applied in four successive 50-ml aliquots. Each aliquot of preheated saline solution was flushed through the bronchoscope and immediately aspirated using a conventional suction device. The BAL fluid was homogenized, and a small volume of it was removed for cell numeration and differential cell counts. Smears were stained with Wright-Giemsa; 200 cells were counted and the percentages of macrophages, lymphocytes, and polymorphonuclear leucocytes were determined. The remaining volume of BAL fluid was centrifuged at $300 \times g$ for 15 min at 20° C to separate the cellular and fluid phases. The supernatant underwent a 25-fold concentration, from 55 to 2.2 ml, on a Diaflo PM 10 membrane (Amicon, Paris) under 3.5 kg/cm^2 positive pressure at 4° C.

Serum

Samples of venous blood were allowed to clot at room temperature for 1 hr. The serum was then separated and used at once for complement titration, and aliquots were stored at −40° C for further analysis.

Protein Determination

The determination of the total protein concentration in the concentrated BAL fluid was performed by the method of Lowry *et al.*[7] and expressed in mg/ml.

Complement Activity

Total complement hemolytic activity (CH_{50}) was determined by functional hemolytic titration[8] by incubating 0.1 ml of a reagent containing 1.5×10^8 sensitized sheep red blood cells (EA)/ml in 0.1 ml of doubling dilutions of freshly concentrated BAL.

C2 hemolytic activity was measured in a simple one-step hemolytic assay in Veronal-buffered saline (VBS) containing Ca^{2+} and Mg^{2+} with a C2-deficient human serum as previously described.[9] Before the complement assay, BAL fluid was absorbed at 4° C for 30 min on unsensitized sheep red blood cells in order to remove heterophil antibodies.

VBS; VBS containing 0.15 mM Ca^{2+} and 0.5 mM Mg^{2+}; VBS containing 0.04 M ethylenediaminetetraacetic acid; VBS containing 0.1% gelatin; and VBS containing 0.1% gelatin, 2 mM magnesium, and 8 mM ethyleneglycoltetraacetic acid were prepared as previously described.[10,11]

Statistical Evaluations

The mean values were expressed ± SD. The differences between two groups were analyzed by the two-tailed *t* test.

RESULTS

Volume of Retrieved BAL Fluid

The mean retrieved volumes of BAL fluid were 115 ± 23 ml, 94 ± 36 ml, and 137 ± 16 ml in the S, IPF, and N groups, respectively. The volume of the retrieved fluid was not dependent on smoking habits.

Analysis of the Cellular Population of the BAL Fluid

Total cell counts in BAL fluid from the different groups revealed a significant ($p < .01$) increase of the total cell number in the S and IPF groups by comparison with the N group; furthermore, as is usually found, the mean percentage of lymphocytes in the S group and of polymorphonuclear neutrophils (PMN's) in the IPF group was markedly elevated (TABLE 1).

TABLE 1. Cell Populations in BAL Fluid

Population	Total Number of Cells ($\times$ 10^4/ml BAL fluid)	Macrophages (%)	Neutrophils (%)	Lymphocytes (%)
Normal volunteers	18 ± 10 (9-35)	89.5 ± 5	0.5 ± 0.2	9.8 ± 4
IPF patients	65 ± 30 (29-111)	78.2 ± 13	18.8 ± 10	3 ± 2
Sarcoidosis patients	45 ± 18 (16-97)	53.8 ± 13	1.2 ± 0.8	45 ± 12

NOTE: Each value is expressed as a mean ± SD. Ranges are expressed in parentheses.

Total Protein Determination in BAL Fluid

BAL fluid from the N group contained 1.65 ± 0.69 mg of protein/ml whereas BAL fluids from the IPF and S groups contained 2.05 ± 0.4 and 6.98 ± 3.93 mg/ml, respectively.

Modifications of the Complement Activity in Serum and in BAL Fluid

The serum complement hemolytic activity was not increased in IPF, but it was increased by 25% ($p < .01$) in sarcoidosis (FIG. 1).

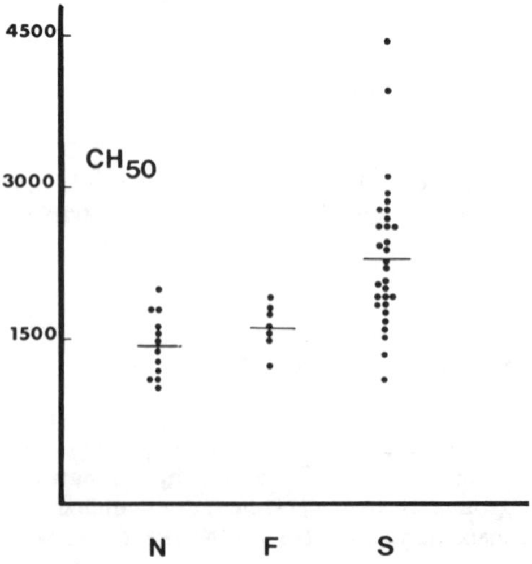

FIGURE 1. Complement hemolytic activities in serum samples from normal volunteers (N), patients with idiopathic pulmonary fibrosis (P), and patients with sarcoidosis (S).

In the N group, no complement activity was detected in BAL fluid from non-smokers, but two out of five smokers had a little activity. Only one patient with IPF had no complement activity whereas the six other IPF patients had a moderate complement activity. In all patients with sarcoidosis the complement activity was appreciable (FIG. 2); in some cases, activity was even detected in BAL fluid before the fluid was concentrated. The difference in the complement activity detected in BAL fluid from IPF and from S patients was significant ($p < .01$).

Upon examining the complement activity of the BAL fluid with respect to the onset of the disease (FIG. 2) it appeared, in the case of recent sarcoidosis where patients had Type 1 or Type 2 sarcoidosis, that there was a wide range of complement activity: CH_{50} values ranged from 20 to 554 units/ml BAL fluid. In the BAL fluid of patients

FIGURE 2. Complement hemolytic activities in BAL fluid samples from normal volunteers (N), patients with idiopathic pulmonary fibrosis (F), and patients with recent (○) or chronic (●) sarcoidosis (S).

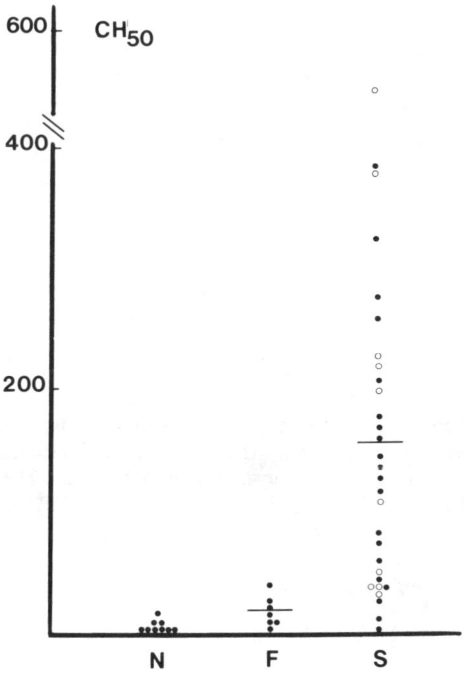

with Type 0 sarcoidosis; that is, with a resolutive or rapidly cured disease, the complement activity was very low. In cases where the disease lasted more than 1 year (chronic disease), there were high complement activities in BAL fluids. The difference between the results with chronic and resolutive sarcoidosis was highly significant. No correlation was found between the complement activity and the extent of alveolar lymphocytosis.

A marked decrease in CH_{50} activity in the BAL fluids from patients receiving corticotherapy (15 mg of cortisone every 2 days) was noted (FIG. 3).

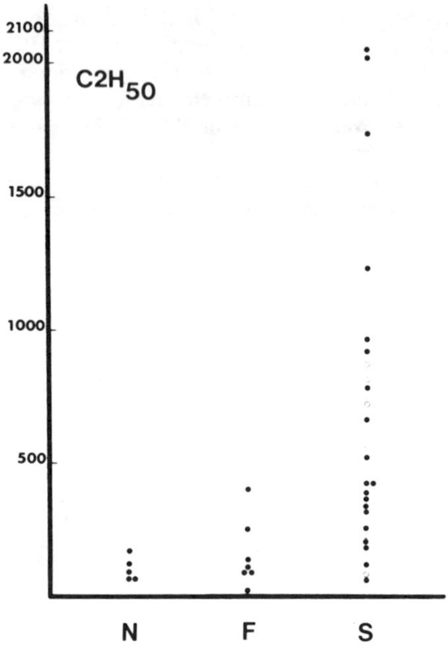

FIGURE 3. C2 hemolytic activity in BAL fluid samples from normal volunteers (N), patients with fibrosis (F), and patients with recent (○) or chronic (●) sarcoidosis (S).

C2 Activity in BAL

C2 hemolytic activity ($C2H_{50}$) was extremely high in sarcoidosis, except in the spontaneously resolutive individuals, when compared to other groups (FIG. 4). It is apparent, however, that a C2 hemolytic activity does exist in BAL from normal controls, even in those who do not smoke. Here again, we did not find any correlation between $C2H_{50}$ and the lymphocyte population in BAL.

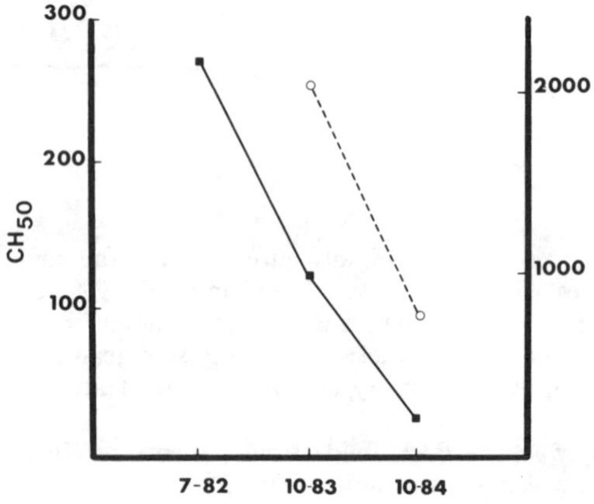

FIGURE 4. Changes in complement (■) and C2 (○) hemolytic activities in successive BAL fluid samples taken from a patient receiving corticotherapy. After 2 years CH_{50} was markedly reduced; $C2H_{50}$ remained elevated.

In patients with chronic sarcoidosis ($N = 14$), the $C2H_{50}/CH_{50}$ ratios were 1.41 ± 0.45 and 5.36 ± 1.7 in the serum and BAL, respectively. This difference demonstrates that the complement activity we detected in BAL does not simply reflect a passive transudation of serum proteins towards the pulmonary airways, that is, a transudation associated with a sarcoidal inflammatory process.

DISCUSSION

This study was undertaken in order to investigate the possible modification of the complement activity in serum and in BAL fluid and to evaluate the possible role of the complement system in the pathogenesis of sarcoidosis. We found that the serum complement activity was significantly increased ($p < .01$) in a group of sarcoidosis patients compared to that found in a group of IPF patients, as well as to that found in a group of normal volunteers. This slight increase (25%) of serum complement activity has already been described.[12] A specific increase in the production of complement components or a decrease in a function of the complement regulatory system could account for this enhanced activity.

We found very low complement activities in the BAL fluids of three out of five of the normal volunteers who smoked. This could reflect the increased permeability of the alveolar capillary membrane associated with smoking habits[13] or could correspond to an increased local synthesis, as has already been suggested.[14] In IPF the complement activity was slightly increased whereas in sarcoidosis it was strikingly elevated. Apparently complement activity is high in patients with recent active sarcoidosis whereas it is normal or rapidly returns to normal in diseases of short duration. In chronic diseases, the stable patients had a lower activity than those with progressive parenchymal derangements.

The origin of complement activity was not investigated in this study; however, two main mechanisms must be involved: 1) a transudation of serum proteins into the alveolar spaces, as indicated by the mean fourfold increase in the albumin concentration in BAL fluid from the sarcoidosis group; 2) a local increased synthesis and secretion rate of complement components by macrophages[15] or by other pulmonary cells.[16] The transudation of serum complement cannot be the only mechanism involved because there is no correlation between the albumin concentration and the complement activity in BAL fluid.

It is possible to speculate on the participation of the complement system in the pathogenesis of sarcoidosis because it is known that complement fragments released during complement activation are potent mediators of pulmonary injury[17–19] and have a strong leukoattractant activity (these fragments even bind to lymphocytes).[20] The response of lymphocytes to complement-derived chemotactic factors could account for the accumulation of lymphocytes within the alveolar spaces.

The possible causes of complement system activation in sarcoidosis are numerous, including secretory immunoglobulin A,[21] lysozomal enzymes,[22,23] and changes in the biochemical composition of the lung parenchyma; moreover, Type II collagen seems to be able to activate complement.[24] Circulating immune complexes and hypergammaglobulinemia,[12] which are often associated with sarcoidosis, could also be responsible for activation of the complement system; furthermore, we have demonstrated the presence of complement-activating autoantibodies with a membrane-antigen specificity in the serum of patients with active sarcoidosis.[25]

The activity of complement component C2 was also increased in BAL from sarcoidosis patients; however, the observation that C2 activity was detectable in BAL fluid from controls demonstrates that at least this component is locally synthesized. Alveolar macrophages are likely to be responsible for this local production.[15]

Based on the above and the observation of decreased BAL CH_{50} activity following corticotherapy, we suggest that the complement activity within the alveolar spaces could be a good marker of the activity of the disease. The answers to the questions concerning the origin of the complement activity, the significance of this activity, and the mechanisms able to activate this system would contribute much to the understanding of the pathogenesis of sarcoidosis.

REFERENCES

1. Katz, P., B. F. Haynes & A. S. Fauci. 1978. Alteration of T lymphocyte subpopulations in sarcoidosis. Clin. Immunol. Immunopathol. **10:** 350-354.
2. Crystal, R. G. 1981. Pulmonary sarcoidosis: A disease characterized and perpetuated by activated lung T lymphocytes. Ann. Intern. Med. **94:** 73-94.
3. Hunninghake, G. W. & R. G. Crystal. 1981. Pulmonary sarcoidosis: A disorder mediated by excess helper T lymphocyte activity at sites of disease activity. New Engl. J. Med. **305:** 429-434.
4. Keogh, B. A. & R. G. Crystal. 1982. Alveolitis: The key to the interstitial lung disorders. Thorax **37:** 1-10.
5. Pinkston, P., P. B. Bitterman & R. G. Crystal. 1983. Spontaneous release of interleukin-2 by lung T lymphocytes in active pulmonary sarcoidosis. New Engl. J. Med. **308:** 793-800.
6. Hunninghake, G. W. & R. G. Crystal. 1981. Mechanisms of hypergammaglobulinemia in pulmonary sarcoidosis. J. Clin. Invest. **67:** 86-92.
7. Lowry, O. H., N. J. Rosebrough, A. L. Farr & R. J. Randall. 1951. Protein measurement with the Folin phenol reagent. J. Biol. Chem. **193:** 265-275.
8. Mayer, M. M. 1971. Complement and complement fixation. *In* Experimental Immunochemistry. E. A. Kabat & M. M. Mayer, Eds. 2nd edit.: 133-240. Charles C. Thomas. Springfield, IL.
9. Ngan, B. Y., E. W. Gelfand & J. O. Minta. 1977. A simple one-step hemolytic assay for C2 with C2-deficient human serum. J. Immunol. **118:** 736-741.
10. Nelson, R. A., J. Jensen, I. Gigli & N. Tamura. 1966. Methods for the separation, purification and measurement of the nine components of hemolytic complement of guinea pig serum. Immunochemistry **3:** 111-135.
11. Nydegger, U. E., D. T. Fearon & K. F. Austen. 1978. The modulation of the alternative pathway of complement in C2-deficient human serum by changes in concentration of the component and control proteins. J. Immunol. **120:** 1404-1408.
12. Saint-Remy, J. M. R., D. N. Mitchell & P. J. Cole. 1983. Variation in immunoglobulin levels and circulating immune complexes in sarcoidosis. Am. Rev. Respir. Dis. **127:** 23-27.
13. Reynolds, H. Y. & H. H. Newball. 1974. Analysis of proteins and respiratory cells obtained from human lungs by bronchial lavage. J. Lab. Clin. Med. **84:** 559-573.
14. Bell, D. Y., J. A. Haseman, A. Spock, G. McLennan & G. E. R. Hook. 1981. Plasma protein of the bronchoalveolar surface of the lung of smokers and nonsmokers. Am. Rev. Respir. Dis. **124:** 72-79.
15. Cole, F. S., W. J. Matthews, T. H. Rossing, D. J. Gash, N. A. Lichtenberg & J. E. Pennington. 1983. Complement biosynthesis by human bronchoalveolar macrophages. Clin. Immunol. Immunopathol. **27:** 153-159.
16. Kreutzer, D. L., J. Varani, W. Douglas & D. E. Blazka. 1980. Elaboration of complement components by primary cultures and continuous lines of human type II pneumocytes. Am. Rev. Respir. Dis. **121:** 78.

17. DESAI, L., D. L. KREUTZER, H. SHOWELL, C. V. ARROYAVE & P. A. WARD. 1979. Acute inflammatory pulmonary reactions induced by chemotactic factors. Am. J. Pathol. **96:** 71-84.
18. STIMLER, N. P., T. E. HUGLI & C. M. BLOOR. 1980. Pulmonary injury induced by C3a and C5a anaphylatoxins. Am. J. Pathol. **100:** 327-348.
19. SHAW, J. O., J. HENSON & R. O. WEBSTER. 1980. Lung inflammation induced by complement-derived fragments in the alveolus. Lab. Invest. **42:** 545-558.
20. EL NAGGAR, A. R., D. E. VAN EPPS & R. C. WILLIAMS, JR. 1980. Human B and T lymphocyte locomotion in response to casein, C5a and F-Met-Leu-Phe. Cell. Immunol. **56:** 365-373.
21. ROBERTSON, J., J. R. CALDWELL, J. R. CASTLE & R. H. WALDMAN. 1976. Evidence for the presence of components of the alternative (properdin) pathway of complement activation in respiratory secretions. J. Immunol. **117:** 900-903.
22. JOHNSON, U., K. OHLSSON & I. OHLSSON. 1976. Effect of granulocyte neutral proteases on complement components. Scand. J. Immunol. **5:** 421-426.
23. TAYLOR, J. C., I. P. CRAWFORD & T. E. HUGLI. 1977. Limited degradation of the third component (C3) of human complement by human leukocyte elastase (HLE): Partial characterization of C3 fragments. Biochemistry **16:** 3390-3396.
24. PONTH, B. F., H. HANAUSKE-ABEL & H. U. SCHORLEMMER. 1979. Activation of the alternative pathway of the complement system by different collagen types. Immunobiology **156:** 239.
25. LAMBRÉ, C. R., S. LE MAHO, E. M. TISSERAND, G. DI BELLA, H. DE CRÉMOUX & J. BIGNON. 1984. Occurrence of complement-activating cytotoxic anti-T circulating antibodies in active sarcoidosis. Am. Rev. Respir. Dis. **129:** 21.

Angiotensin I-converting Enzyme

A Marker of Highly Differentiated Monocytic Cells

C. GRÖNHAGEN-RISKA,[a,b] F. FYHRQUIST,[b]
AND E. VON WILLEBRAND[c]

[b] *Minerva Foundation Institute for Medical Research*
Fourth Department of Medicine
and
[c] *Transplantation Laboratory*
University of Helsinki
Helsinki, Finland

INTRODUCTION

Angiotensin I-converting enzyme (ACE), or kininase II, is mainly located on the luminar surfaces of vascular endothelial cells,[1] which produce this enzyme and glycoprotein, but is also present in the circulation.[2] Its main site of action is the pulmonary vasculature, where it converts angiotensin I into angiotensin II. ACE can also inactivate bradykinin, a potent vasodilator and inflammation mediator. Serum ACE activity has been reported to be increased in some diseases associated with activation and/or proliferation of mature cells of the monocytic cell line, that is, macrophages, histiocytes, and epithelioid and giant cells. Such diseases include sarcoidosis,[3] Gaucher's disease,[4] leprosy,[5] silicosis, and asbestosis;[6] increased ACE activity has also been seen in histiocytic medullary reticulosis,[7] a disorder which is considered to involve a neoplasm of true histiocytes. Serum ACE activity was observed to reflect the dissemination of these cells.[7] On the other hand, normal serum ACE levels have been reported in monoblast leukemia.[7–9]

ACE has been histochemically indicated in macrophages and epithelioid cells of sarcoid granulomas,[10] and these cells are believed to produce this enzyme.

We suggest that ACE is produced by monocytic cells that have reached a mature stage. To test this hypothesis we studied two malignant human monocytic cell lines. U-937 cells are monocytoid cells frozen at a stage close to that of myelomonocytic stem cells[11] whereas RC-2A cells represent a more differentiated, macrophage-like cell line.[12] U-937 cells were also studied after induction with 12-*O*-tetradecanoylphorbol-13-acetate (TPA), which is known to induce both morphological and functional maturation of these cells.[13]

[a] Address for correspondence: Minerva Foundation Institute for Medical Research, P.O. Box 819, 00101 Helsinki 10, Finland.

METHODS

ACE was purified from human lung obtained at thoracotomy. Most of the purification procedure has been described before.[14] Briefly, after homogenization and ultracentrifugation for 90 min at 78 000 g, membrane proteins were solubilized with Triton X-100. After reultracentrifugation, ACE was in the supernatant, and further degrees of purification were obtained with DE-52 cellulose ion-exchange chromatography, Sepharose 4B gel filtration, and isoelectric focusing. After purification, the pooled samples were dialyzed under negative pressure against a neutral Cl^--containing potassium phosphate buffer, and then Sephadex G-75 gel filtration was performed to remove ampholyte impurities.

Sodium dodecylsulfate electrophoresis of the purified protein indicated there was one protein with a molecular mass of 165 000 daltons. The specific activity, as measured with the tripeptide hippuryl-histidyl-leucine as a substrate, was 18 500 U/mg protein.[3]

Antiserum against purified human lung ACE was raised in rabbit by repeated, multiple subcutaneous injections of pure ACE (100-400 μg) with complete Freund's adjuvant. The antiserum chosen precipitated ACE in countercurrent electrophoresis.

The U-937 and RC-2A cell lines were cultured, in a 5% CO_2 atmosphere, in RPMI medium supplemented with glutamine, antibiotics, and 10% fetal calf serum. TPA (PL Biochemicals) was used as an inducer at concentrations of 10^{-9}-10^{-7} M and was left with the cells for 1-3 days.

Viability tests and cell counts were carried out and compared with those of untreated controls. Cytocentrifuged cell smears were made of induced cells on days 0-3 and stained with May-Grünwald-Giemsa (MGG) to study cell maturation.

ACE expression on the cell surface was assessed by *Staphylococcus aureus* Cowan I rosette assay.[15] In short, the cells were treated first with anti-ACE antiserum that was diluted 1:20 (the most suitable dilution was found in tests with dilutions from 1:10 to 1:50). After a wash, another incubation was performed with staphylococci, and the number of rosette-forming cells was counted from MGG-stained cytocentrifuge cell smears. Results were expressed in two different ways, as the percentage of cells binding more than five staphylococci on their surface, or as the average number of staphylococci per positive rosette-forming cell. Normal rabbit serum, diluted 1:20, was used in the controls, that is, in the determinations of nonspecific membrane binding.

The density of receptors for crystallizable fragments (Fc) of immunoglobulin G (IgG) was assessed by IgG-coated human O red blood cell rosette assay.[16] After rosette formation, cytocentrifuge smears were made and stained with MGG. Cells which bound four or more erythrocytes were regarded as rosette-forming cells.

The chi-square test and Student's *t* test were used for statistical calculations.

RESULTS

The macrophage-like RC-2A cells expressed significantly more ACE than the monocyte-like U-937 cells (TABLE 1 & FIG. 1). ACE was bound to ACE-specific receptors on 1-8% of the uninduced U-937 cells: the U-937 cells that were in batches without TPA. The percentages shown in TABLES 1 & 2 were determined by making deductions that took nonspecific membrane binding into account; the percentage of

TABLE 1. Expression of ACE in Malignant Monocytic U-937 and RC-2A Cell Lines

Percentage of Staphylococcus Rosette-forming Cells[a]		
U-937	RC-2A	Significance
8	42	$p < .001$

[a] Values determined by subtracting the background, that is, the percentage of positive cells stained with control rabbit serum.

cells that expressed the control rabbit serum (via nonspecific receptors) was deducted from the percentage of cells that expressed ACE (via nonspecific and specific receptors).

U-937 cells changed appearance after they were activated by the addition of TPA to the culture medium, in which they were incubated for 1-3 days. They increased in size, their cytoplasms became more vacuolated, and their membranes became more villous. All the tested concentrations of TPA caused increased expression of ACE (TABLE 2 & FIG. 2), which varied somewhat depending on the original, uninduced expression of this glycoprotein; the TPA concentration used; and the length of induction.

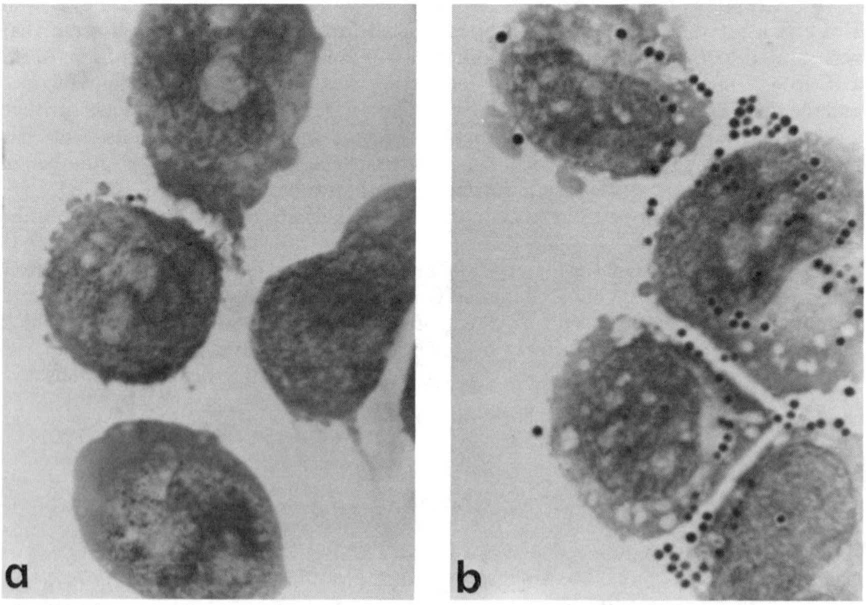

FIGURE 1. MGG-stained, cytocentrifuged smears showing staphylococci bound to (**a**) monocytic U-937 cells and (**b**) macrophage-like RC-2A cells that were treated with antihuman ACE antiserum.

TABLE 2. Expression of ACE in U-937 Cells before and after TPA Induction

TPA (M)	Percentage of Staphylococcus Rosette-forming Cells[a] Day 0	1	2	3
10^{-9}	8	—	—	40[b]
10^{-8}	1	18[b]	16[b]	10[c]
10^{-7}	8	0	44[b]	44[b]

[a] Values determined by subtracting the background, that is, the percentage of positive cells stained with control rabbit serum.

[b] $p < .001$.

[c] $p < .01$.

The mean number of staphylococci per rosette-forming cell for RC-2A cells was considerably greater than that for uninduced U-937 cells, but was not very different than that for TPA-induced U-937 cells (TABLE 3 & FIG. 3).

The induction also caused an increase in the number of Fc receptors, which increased from 50% to 68% in the 3 days following the addition of 10^{-8} M TPA ($p < .01$).

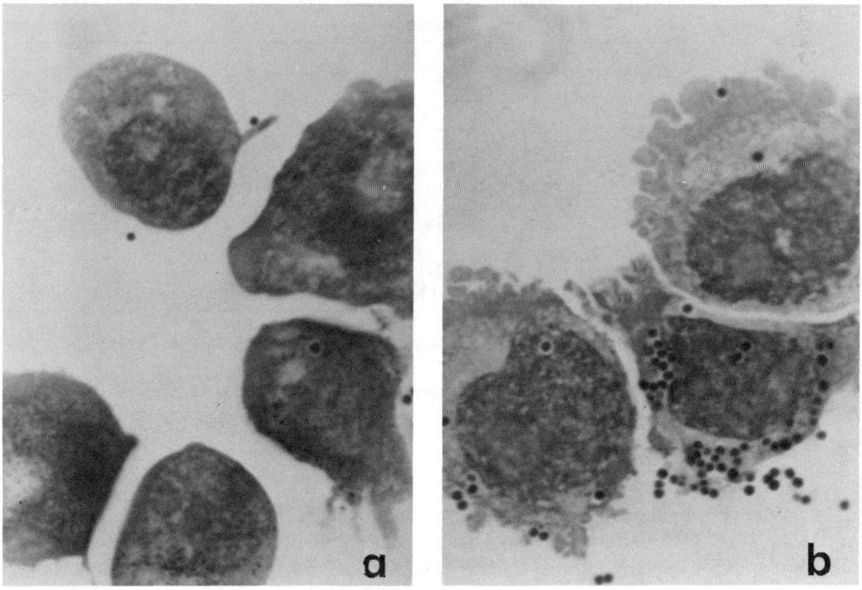

FIGURE 2. MGG-stained, cytocentrifuged smears showing staphylococci bound to (**a**) uninduced and (**b**) 10^{-7} M TPA-induced (day 3) U-937 cells that were treated with antihuman ACE antiserum.

DISCUSSION

Clinical observations that serum ACE levels are normal in monoblast leukemia[7-9] but are increased in histiocytic medullary reticulosis[7] suggest that ACE-producing cells of the monocytoid cell line must reach a certain degree of maturation before they express this glycoprotein. This assumption was, indeed, verified in this study. U-937 cells, which resemble the myelomonocytic stem cell,[11] did not express ACE whereas macrophage-like RC-2A cells[12] contained abundant amounts of this enzymatic glycoprotein.

Induction or activation of U-937 cells is achieved with the substance TPA,[13] with physiological substances present in supernatants of mixed lymphocyte cultures,[17] or with interferon.[18] In all cases the cells adapt characteristics of more differentiated monocytes or macrophages. In addition to morphological changes, indications of functional maturation, such as increased adhesiveness, phagocytic capacity, and potency as an effector cell in antibody-dependent cellular cytotoxicity tests *in vitro,* have been reported. Activated U-937 cells produce more lysozyme, and the number of Fc receptors and the amount of HLA-A, -B, -C and -DR and -B2 microglobulin are increased in 15-30% of these cells. Thus, it seems clear that a sizable fraction of U-937 cells undergoes the phenotypic changes expected for normal, maturing monocytic

TABLE 3. Number of Staphylococci per ACE-positive, Rosette-forming U-937 or RC-2A Cell

Type of Cell	Number of Staphylococci per Cell (mean ± SD)	Number
	Without TPA Induction	
U-937	9.5 ± 5.6	33
RC-2A	22.3 ± 11.0[a]	33
	With TPA Induction (Day 3)	
U-937		
10^{-9} M TPA	25.3 ± 20.6[a]	37
10^{-8} M TPA	15.1 ± 11.5[b]	21
10^{-7} M TPA	20.8 ± 15.8[a]	37

[a] $p < .001$, compared to the number of staphylococci per uninduced U-937 cell (9.5 ± 5.6, $N = 33$).

[b] $p < .001$, compared to the number of staphylococci per uninduced U-937 cell (5.5 ± 0.5, $N = 10$).

Against this background it was interesting to observe increased ACE expression in 15-36% of TPA-induced cells. This increase was mostly observed in cells that morphologically appeared more mature. An increase in the number of Fc receptors was also recorded as an objective sign of maturation.

Membrane-bound ACE is abundant, particularly in pulmonary vascular endothelial cells.[1] The origin of circulating ACE is unknown, but this ACE is believed to be the result of active or passive shedding from membranes. Increased concentration of ACE in granulomatous lymph nodes[20] and increased serum ACE activity in sarcoidosis[3] are probably due to the expression and shedding of ACE by granulomatous monocytoid cells, that is, by macrophages, epithelioid cells, and giant cells.

Upon induction U-937 cells change their surface glycoprotein (SGP) pattern.[21] This has been demonstrated by studies on the SGP composition using galactose oxidase-titrated NaB^3H_4 labeling.[22] Among the most prominent changes recorded was an increase in the amount of a 160 000-dalton SGP. ACE is about the size of this SGP, and the results of the present study suggest that ACE may be one of the SGP's whose amount is increased after induction. Experimental results suggest that the SGP changes are due to alterations in the carbohydrate portion of the molecule rather than to a *de novo* protein synthesis.[19] Functionally the surface modulations have been associated with several factors, including a decreased sensitivity to natural killer cells.[23] Monocytic cells change their SGP profile when activated. These surface antigens are recognized through receptor mechanisms by other inflammatory cells. Membrane-bound ACE may contribute to the interaction between these cell elements, and, on the other hand, free ACE may saturate hypothetical receptors. It is also possible, however, that circulating ACE differs from the membrane-bound molecule, especially with regard to the glycoprotein part of the molecule.[24]

In rabbit pulmonary ACE two glycoprotein (GP) fractions have been reported. GPII accounted for about one-quarter of the weight of the enzyme. The function of this oligosaccharide is unknown but is not expected to be associated with the catalytic function of ACE.[24]

Some experimental observations suggest there are undefined immunological functions of ACE. We have reported migration inhibition of leukocytes caused by purified human lung ACE.[25] This was a direct effect on neutrophils and not a lymphocyte-mediated phenomenon. Results did not change when the specific ACE inhibitors captopril or enalapril were added to the test. This suggests that the migration-inhibiting effect of ACE was not associated with the active center of the enzyme. Others have induced experimental granulomatous disorders in mice associated with ACE production by granulomatous cells.[26,27] Captopril in large doses seems to suppress or to reduce the induction of the granulomatous response.[27,28] Recently, salutatory effects of captopril treatment on rheumatoid arthritis were reported.[29] This was expected to be associated with molecular features of this drug, which resembles D-penicillamine. If this is so, other ACE inhibitors, which do not contain a thiol group, should not affect the course of rheumatoid arthritis.

Another explanation, however, should be considered for these observations. ACE inhibition causes an increase in the amounts of both membrane-bound and circulating ACE *in vivo* and in cultured endothelial and monocytic cells.[30–33] Thus, changes in the immunologic response associated with specific inhibition of the enzymatic activity of ACE, may, in fact, be due to an increase of this glycoprotein.

The immunological functions of ACE should be further elucidated. Malignant monocytic cell lines, which express this glycoprotein in variable amounts, depending upon degree of activation, can be used as easily manipulated tools for this research.

REFERENCES

1. RYAN, J. W., U. S. RYAN, D. R. SCHULTZ, C. WHITAKER & A. CHUNG. 1975. Subcellular localization of pulmonary angiotensin-converting enzyme (kininase II). Biochem. J. **146:** 497-499.

2. ONDETTI, M. A. & D. W. CUSHMAN. 1982. Enzymes of the renin-angiotensin system and their inhibitors. Annu. Rev. Biochem. **51:** 238-308.
3. LIEBERMAN, J. 1975. Elevation of serum angiotensin-converting enzyme (ACE) level in sarcoidosis. Am. J. Med. **59:** 365-372.
4. LIEBERMAN, J. & E. BEUTLER. 1976. Elevation of serum angiotensin-converting enzyme in Gaucher's disease. N. Engl. J. Med. **294:** 1442-1444.
5. LIEBERMAN, J. & T. H. REA. 1977. Serum angiotensin-converting enzyme in leprosy and coccidioidomycosis. Ann. Intern. Med. **87:** 422-425.
6. GRÖNHAGEN-RISKA, C., K. KURPPA, F. FYHRQUIST & O. SELROOS. 1978. Angiotensin-converting enzyme and lysozyme in silicosis and asbestosis. Scand. J. Respir. Dis. **59:** 228-231.
7. GRÖNHAGEN-RISKA, C., M. KLOCKARS & O. SELROOS. 1983. Elevated angiotensin I-converting enzyme in histiocytic medullary reticulosis. N. Engl. J. Med. **308:** 283-284.
8. LIEBERMAN, J., A. NOSAL, L. A. SCHLESSNER & A. SASTRE-FOKEN. 1979. Serum angiotensin-coverting enzyme for diagnosis and therapeutic evaluation of sarcoidosis. Am. Rev. Respir. Dis. **120:** 329-335.
9. SILVERSTEIN, E. & J. FRIEDLAND. 1979. Serum angiotensin-converting enzyme in sarcoidosis and other diseases. Lancet **i:** 382-383.
10. PERTSCHUK, L. P., E. SILVERSTEIN & J. FRIEDLAND. 1981. Immunohistologic diagnosis of sarcoidosis: Detection of angiotensin-converting enzyme in sarcoid granulomas. Am. J. Clin. Pathol. **75:** 350-354.
11. SUNDSTRÖM, C. & K. NILSSON. 1976. Establishment and characterization of a human histiocytic lymphoma cell line (U-937). Int. J. Cancer **17:** 565-577.
12. BRADLEY, T. R., G. PILKINGTON, M. GARSON, G. S. HODGSON & N. KRAFT. 1982. Cell lines derived from a human myelomonocytic leukemia. Br. J. Haematol. **51:** 595-604.
13. NILSSON, K., L. C. ANDERSSON, C. G. GAHMBERG & K. FORSBECK. 1980. Differentiation *in vitro* of human leukemia and lymphoma cell lines. *In* International Symposium on New Trends in Human Immunology and Cancer Immunotherapy. B. Serrou & C. Rosenfeld, Eds.: 271-282. Doin Éditeur. Paris.
14. GRÖNHAGEN-RISKA, C., F. FYHRQUIST, T. PETTERSSON, M. G. WELIN & T. H. WEBER. 1983. Leukocyte migration-inhibiting effect of purified human lung angiotensin I-converting enzyme. *In* Sarcoidosis and Other Granulomatous Disorders. J. Chrétien, J. Marsac & J. C. Saltiel, Eds.: 326-331. Pergamon Press. Paris.
15. GHETIE, V., K. NILSSON & J. SJÖQUIST. 1974. Identification of cell surface immunoglobulin markers by protein A-containing fluorescent staphylococci. Scand. J. Immunol. **3:** 397-403.
16. JONDAL, M., H. WIGZELL & F. AIUTI. 1973. Human lymphocyte subpopulations: Classification according to surface markers and/or functional characteristics. Transplant. Rev. **16:** 163-195.
17. KOREN, H. S., S. J. ANDERSON & J. W. LARRICK. 1979. *In vitro* activation of a human macrophage-like cell line. Nature **279:** 328-331.
18. HATTORI, T., M. PACK, P. BOUGNOUX, Z.-L. CHANG & T. HOFFMAN. 1983. Interferon-induced differentiation of U-937 cells. J. Clin. Invest. **72:** 237-244.
19. NILSSON, K. 1982. Phenotypic characterization and induced differentiation of established human non-Hodgkin lymphoma cell lines. *In* Malignant Lymphomas. S. A. Rosenberg & H. S. Kaplan, Eds.: 35-51. Academic Press. New York, NY.
20. SILVERSTEIN, E., J. FRIEDLAND, H. A. LYONS & A. GOURIN. 1976. Elevation of angiotensin-covering enzyme in granulomatous lymph nodes and serum in sarcoidosis: Clinical and possible pathogenic significance. Ann. N.Y. Acad. Sci. **278:** 498-513.
21. NILSSON, K., K. FORSBECK, M. GIDLUND, C. SUNDSTRÖM, T. TÖTTERMAN, J. SÄLLSTRÖM & P. VENGE. 1981. Surface characteristics of the U-937 human histiocytic lymphoma cell line: Specific changes during inducible morphologic and functional differentiation *in vitro*. *In* Modern Trends in Human Leukemia. R. Neth, R. C. Gallo, T. Graf, K. Mannweiler & K. Winkler, Eds. Vol. **4:** 215-221. Springer-Verlag. Berlin and Heidelberg.
22. GAHMBERG, C. G. & S. HAKOMORI. 1973. External labeling of cell surface galactose and galactosamine in glycolipid and glycoprotein of human erythrocytes. J. Biol. Chem. **248:** 4311-4317.

23. GIDLUND, M., A. ÖRN, P. K. PATTENGALE, M. JANSSON, H. WIGZELL & K. NILSSON. 1981. Natural killer cells kill tumour cells at a given stage of differentiation. Nature **292:** 848-850.
24. HARTLEY, J. L. & R. L. SOFFER. 1978. On the oligosaccharide moiety of angiotensin-converting enzyme. Biochem. Biophys. Res. Commun. **83:** 1545-1552.
25. GRÖNHAGEN-RISKA, C., F. FYHRQUIST, M.-G. WELIN & T. WEBER. 1982. Leukocyte migration inhibition effect of angiotensin I-converting enzyme. Immunobiology **163:** 282.
26. WEINSTOCK, J. V., D. L. BOROS & J. B. GEE. 1981. Enhanced granuloma angiotensin I-converting enzyme activity asssociated with modulation in murine schistosomiasis. Gastroenterology **81:** 48-53.
27. SCHRIER, D. J., L. M. RIPANI, A.-L. KATZENSTEIN & V. L. MOORE. 1982. Role of angiotensin-converting enzyme in bacille Calmette-Guérin-induced granulomatous inflammation. J. Clin. Invest. **69:** 651-657.
28. WEINSTOCK, J. V., N. M. EHRINPREIS, D. L. BOROS & J. B. GEE. 1981. Effect of SQ 14225, an inhibitor of angiotensin I-converting enzyme, on the granulomatous response to *Schistosoma mansoni* eggs in mice. J. Clin. Invest. **67:** 931-936.
29. MARTIN, M. F. R., F. MCKENNA, H. A. BIRD, K. E. SURRALL, J. S. DIXON & V. WRIGHT. 1984. Captopril: A new treatment for rheumatoid arthritis. Lancet **i:** 1325-1328.
30. FYHRQUIST, F., T. FORSLUND, I. TIKKANEN & C. GRÖNHAGEN-RISKA. 1980. Induction of angiotensin I-converting enzyme in rat lung with captopril (SQ 14225). Eur. J. Pharmacol. **67:** 473-475.
31. FORSLUND, T., F. FYHRQUIST, C. GRÖNHAGEN-RISKA & I. TIKKANEN. 1982. Induction of angiotensin-converting enzyme with the ACE-inhibitory compound MK-421 in rat lung. Eur. J. Pharmacol. **80:** 121-125.
32. FYHRQUIST, F., L. HORTLING & C. GRÖNHAGEN-RISKA. 1982. Induction of angiotensin I-coverting enzyme by captopril in cultured human endothelial cells. J. Clin. Endocrinol. Metab. **55:** 783-786.
33. FYHRQUIST, F., C. GRÖNHAGEN-RISKA, L. HORTLING, T. FORSLUND, I. TIKKANEN & M. KLOCKARS. 1983. The induction of angiotensin-converting enzyme by its inhibitors. Clin. Exp. Hyper. Theory Practice A **5:** 1319-1330.

Quantitation of Cutaneous Langerhans' Cells of Sarcoidosis Patients[a]

BRIAN BERMAN,[b,c] JOSHUA L. FOX,[d]
AND ALVIN S. TEIRSTEIN[e]

[c]*Department of Dermatology*
School of Medicine
University of California, Davis
Davis, California 95616
and
Veterans Administration Medical Center
Martinez, California 94553

[d]*Department of Dermatology*
New York University School of Medicine
New York, New York 10016

[e]*Department of Pulmonary Medicine*
Mount Sinai School of Medicine
New York, New York 10029

INTRODUCTION

Sarcoidosis is a systemic disease of unknown etiology in which cell-mediated immunity is often depressed.[1] Reduced delayed-type hypersensitivity to a wide variety of bacterial, fungal, and viral antigens is evident in sarcoidosis patients by hyporeactivity in skin tests.[2] Whereas 90-95% of healthy controls exhibit a positive intradermal skin test to *Candida albicans* extract, positive reactions occur in only 40-53% of sarcoidosis patients.[3,4] Further evidence of depressed cell-mediated immunity in sarcoidosis patients includes the reduced proliferative response of blood mononuclear cells to antigens and mitogens, and lower absolute numbers of peripheral blood thymus-derived (T) lymphocytes.[5-7] On the other hand, there is evidence that the depression in cell-mediated immunity is not absolute:[8] sarcoidal disease does not delay the rejection of skin homografts,[9] and increased numbers of "helper" T lymphocytes are localized within sarcoidal granulomas.[10]

Although the origin and function of Langerhans' cells have been matters for conjecture and theory ever since the discovery of these cells by Paul Langerhans,[11] similarities between Langerhans' cells and macrophages have recently been reported. Some of the similarities that have been found involve plasma membrane 5'-adenosine

[a]This work was supported in part by Grant OH 01955-02 from the National Institute for Occupational Safety and Health and by the Veterans Administration Medical Research Service.

[b]Address for correspondence: Veterans Administration Medical Center, 150 Muir Road, Martinez, California 94553.

triphosphatase (ATPase) activity,[12] the ability to migrate,[13] I-associated (Ia) histocompatibility antigens,[14,15] crystallizable fragment (Fc) receptors,[16] C3b receptors,[17] nonspecific esterase activity,[18] the ability *in vitro* to transfer antigen in lymphocyte stimulation,[19] and bone marrow derivation.[20] Langerhans' cells are immunocompetent cells that play a pivotal role in antigen-driven T lymphocyte proliferation, in allogeneic and syngeneic T lymphocyte proliferation, and in the generation of cytotoxic T lymphocytes: Langerhans' cells are also capable of synthesizing immunomodulatory products such as interleukin-1.[21]

Immunofluorescent detection of cells expressing HLA-DR and/or T6 antigenicity has been used to specifically enumerate Langerhans' cells within the normal epidermis.[22,23] We investigated 17 anergic patients with sarcoidosis to determine 1) whether the density of Langerhans' cells (as detected by DR and T6 antigenicity) within the epidermis, in noninvolved, sarcoidal, and Kveim-reactive skin, differs from that within the epidermis of healthy volunteers and 2) whether demographic and clinical features of sarcoidosis patients can be related to Langerhans' cell density.

PATIENTS

Seventeen of 18 patients who were consecutively admitted to the Sarcoidosis Clinic of the Mount Sinai Medical Center and considered for inclusion in this study qualified; the patient that did not qualify was pregnant. None of the 17 patients had received immunosuppressive medications other than glucocorticosteroids, which 6 of the patients had received, and none of the patients had applied topical steroids for at least 6 months. Each of the 17 patients had clinical features of sarcoidosis and histologic evidence of noncaseating epithelioid granulomas: 15 out of 16 patients had a positive Kveim test, and 9 out of 10 patients had tissue biopsies which showed granulomas with little or no necrosis. Other causes of noncaseating granuloma formation were excluded.

Demographic analysis of these patients revealed a population similar to that of a previous study conducted at this clinic (TABLE 1).[24] Ten healthy females who had an average age of 52.8 years (range: 36-65 years) served as control subjects. The Langerhans' cell densities in the skin of this control group (see Results) were similar to those of 10 other control subjects in another study in which no significant race, age, or sex differences in Langerhans' cell densities were detected.[25]

Six of the sarcoidosis patients (35%) were receiving oral prednisone; one of these six patients was receiving 60 mg/day, and the other five were receiving 7.5-10 mg/day. Four of these six patients were being treated with prednisone for more than 1 year. Five of the sarcoidosis patients (29%) had sarcoidal skin lesions. All of the sarcoidosis patients were found to be anergic to intracutaneously injected candidin extract.

MATERIALS AND METHODS

Skin Samples

Following receipt of written informed consent, skin biopsies 4 mm in diameter were performed on patients that were under 1% lidocaine local anesthesia. Twenty-four biopsies were obtained from the 17 patients and 10 from the control subjects. Biopsies were taken of "noninvolved skin" from the medial aspect of the right upper arm, that is, of skin that had not been exposed to the sun ($N = 14$); of "sarcoidal skin" from the extremities ($N = 5$); of clinically "Kveim-reactive skin" from the flexor of right forearm ($N = 5$); and of "control skin" from the arm ($N = 10$). Light microscopic examination of clinically noninvolved skin samples failed to reveal any granulomas.

Kveim Test

Kveim antigen was prepared, testing was carried out, and cutaneous reactions were histologically analyzed as previously described.[1,26]

TABLE 1. Demographics of and Disease Duration for Sarcoidosis Patients

Clinical Characteristics	Percent of Population[a]
Race	
Black	59
Caucasoid	25
Hispanic	16
Sex	
Female	71
Male	29
Age (years)	
22-49	71
50-76	29
Disease duration (years)	
≤ 2	53
> 2	47

[a]The population comprised 17 sarcoidosis patients who were anergic to candidin extract.

Immunofluorescent Detection of Epidermal Langerhans' Cells

The following antibodies were obtained commercially: monoclonal mouse antihuman T6 antigen IgG1 (50 mg/ml; Ortho Pharmaceuticals, Raritan, New Jersey), monoclonal mouse antihuman DR antigen IgG2b (1 mg/ml; New England Nuclear, Boston, Massachusetts), and goat antimouse IgG IgG-fluorescein isothiocyanate (FITC) (F/P = 4.7; Meloy Laboratories, Springfield, Virginia). Phosphate-buffered saline (PBS) was used for all dilutions and washings.

All samples were processed within 3 hr after biopsy. Separation of epidermis from dermis was carried out in 2 N NaBr at 37° C for 30 min. Epidermal blisters were removed intact with fine forceps and bisected. Half of each blister was bathed in 50 μl of either monoclonal mouse antihuman DR IgG2b (1:100 dilution) or antihuman

T6 IgG1 (1:100 dilution) at 37° C for 2 hr. After three 10-min washings at 20° C, the samples were incubated in 50 μl of rabbit antimouse IgG IgG-FITC (1:20 dilution) at 37° C for 1 hr and washed three times. The samples were then mounted between two glass coverslips with glycerol gelatin and examined with epifluorescence microscopy. The fluorescing dendritic cells were enumerated in at least 10 randomly chosen fields by an examiner who was unaware of the source of the specimen. The density of epidermal Langerhans' cells was expressed as the mean number (± SEM) of cells within a 0.05-mm^2 area.

Statistics

The mean number (± SEM) of Langerhans' cells within the epidermis of patient and control groups was determined. Comparisons of the mean epidermal Langerhans' cell densities of patient and control groups were performed using Student's t test, and p values of less than .05 were considered significant.

RESULTS

Comparison of the Langerhans' Cell Densities within Epidermis Overlying Noninvolved, Sarcoidal, Kveim-reactive, and Control Skin

The densities of DR-positive and T6-positive Langerhans' cells within the epidermis overlying the noninvolved skin of sarcoidosis patients (14.1 ± 1.8 and 31.5 ± 3.4 cells/0.05 mm^2, respectively) were significantly ($p < .05$) lower than those within the control epidermis (18.3 ± 1.1 and 39.5 ± 1.3 cells/0.05 mm^2, respectively); furthermore, as is shown in FIGURE 1, those within the epidermis overlying sarcoidal skin (6.7 ± 0.8 and 16.3 ± 3.7 cells/0.05 mm^2, respectively) were also significantly ($p < .025$) lower than those within the control epidermis. Similarly, epidermis overlying Kveim-reactive skin contained fewer DR-positive and T6-positive cells (7.4 ± 1.2 and 20.3 ± 9.0 cells/0.05 mm^2, respectively) than did the control epidermis ($p < .0005$ and $p < .005$, respectively), or, the epidermis overlying noninvolved skin ($p < .025$ and $p < .10$, respectively). In patients with sarcoidal skin, the epidermis overlying noninvolved skin contained only 83% (12.1 ± 1.1 cells/0.05 mm^2) of the number of DR-positive cells and 78% (29.0 ± 7.3 cells/0.05 mm^2) of the number of T6-positive cells that were present in the epidermis overlying the noninvolved skin of sarcoidosis patients without sarcoidal skin lesions; however, these differences were not significant.

Comparison of the Langerhans' Cell Densities within Epidermis of Steroid-treated and Untreated Sarcoidosis Patients

As is shown in TABLE 2, the epidermis overlying either noninvolved or sarcoidal skin for both steroid-treated and untreated patients contained significantly fewer Langerhans' cells than did the control epidermis. There are no significant differences, however, in the densities of epidermal Langerhans' cells of prednisone-treated and untreated patients. Furthermore, among untreated sarcoidosis patients, the epidermis overlying sarcoidal skin contained fewer DR and T6 antigen-bearing Langerhans' cells ($p < .05$ and $p < .0025$, respectively) than did the epidermis overlying noninvolved skin.

Comparison of Langerhans' Cell Densities within Epidermis Overlying Noninvolved and Sarcoidal Skin

Three patients underwent biopsies of both noninvolved and sarcoidal skin. As is shown in TABLE 3, the epidermis overlying their sarcoidal skin in each case contained fewer DR and T6 antigen-bearing Langerhans' cells than did the epidermis overlying their noninvolved skin.

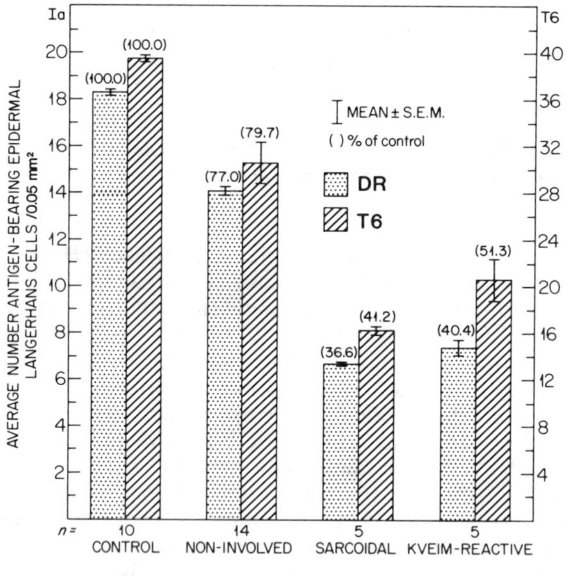

FIGURE 1. The density of DR and T6 antigen-bearing Langerhans' cells within noninvolved, sarcoidal, Kveim-reactive, and control skin.

Epidermal Langerhans' Cell Morphology

We did not detect any consistent differences in either the dendritic nature or fluorescent staining intensity of either DR or T6 antigen-bearing Langerhans' cells within epidermis overlying noninvolved, sarcoidal, Kveim-reactive, or control skin.

TABLE 2. Densities of Marked Epidermal Langerhans' Cells in Sarcoidosis Patients Compared to Those in Controls

Subjects/Source of Epidermis	Epidermal Langerhans' Cell Density[a] (cells/0.05 mm² ± SD) DR Positive: Untreated[b]	DR Positive: Sarcoid Treated[c]	T6 Positive: Untreated[b]	T6 Positive: Sarcoid Treated[c]
Sarcoid patients/Noninvolved skin	12.7 ± 1.8(8) $p < .01$	11.3 ± 1.4(6) $p < .0005$	29.5 ± 2.8(8) $p < .0025$	29.7 ± 3.9(6) $p < .01$
Sarcoid patients/Sarcoidal skin	5.6 ± 0.8(3) $p < .0005$	8.3 ± 0.4(2) $p < .0025$	10.8 ± 0.0(3) $p < .0005$	19.0 ± 9.1(2) $p < .0005$
Healthy controls/Normal skin	18.3 ± 1.1(10)		39.5 ± 1.3(10)	

NOTE: Skin biopsies 4 mm in diameter were obtained from 17 sarcoidosis patients and 10 controls. The number of biopsies taken for each subgroup is indicated in parentheses immediately following the corresponding cell density value. The *p* values refer to Student's *t* test comparisons of cell densities in healthy controls to those in sarcoidosis patient subgroups.

[a]Epidermal sheets that were separated from the dermis by 2 N NaBr were incubated in monoclonal mouse antihuman DR or T6 IgG followed by rabbit antimouse IgG IgG-FITC. DR and T6 antigen-bearing cells were enumerated under epifluorescence microscopy.

[b]Patients who had not received immunosuppressive therapy within 2 years.

[c]Patients who had been receiving oral prednisone (7.5-60 mg/day) for at least 3 months.

TABLE 3. Epidermal Langerhans' Cell Densities within Sarcoidal and Noninvolved Skin

Patient	Epidermal Langerhans' Cell Density[a] (cells/0.05 mm² ± SD) DR Positive: Noninvolved Skin	DR Positive: Sarcoidal Skin	T6 Positive: Noninvolved Skin	T6 Positive: Sarcoidal Skin
1	9.9 ± 0.9	4.6 ± 0.6	15.0 ± 1.5	10.7 ± 0.9
2	13.9 ± 1.4	8.8 ± 1.1	39.2 ± 2.0	28.1 ± 1.0
3	12.7 ± 0.5	7.9 ± 0.8	32.8 ± 0.5	9.9 ± 0.7

NOTE: Skin biopsies 4 mm in diameter of both noninvolved and sarcoidal skin were obtained from three sarcoidosis patients.

[a]Epidermal sheets that were separated from the dermis by 2 N NaBr were incubated in monoclonal mouse antihuman DR or T6 IgG followed by rabbit antimouse IgG IgG-FITC. DR and T6 antigen-bearing cells were enumerated under epifluorescence microscopy.

Correlation of Demographic and Clinical Characteristics with Epidermal Langerhans' Cell Densities in Sarcoidosis Patients

No significant differences in Langerhans' cell densities in noninvolved skin depended on any of the following clinical characteristics: whether a patient was < 50 or ≥ 50 years of age; was a male or a female; was a black, a Hispanic, or a Caucasian; was in or beyond stage I of the disease; had < 4800 or ≥ 4800 leukocyte counts/mm^3; had a lysozyme level > 13 or < 13 $\mu g/\mu l$; had an erythrocyte sedimentation rate > 20 or < 20 mm/hr; or had an angiotensin-converting enzyme level > 30 or ≤ 30 nmol/min. Patients in which the onset of sarcoidosis was recent (acute-subacute: ≤ 2 years), however, tended ($p < .15$) to have more DR-bearing Langerhans' cells in the epidermis of their noninvolved skin (17.9 ± 4.2 cells/0.05 mm^2) than did patients with chronic (> 2 years) disease (12.0 ± 2.0 cells/0.05 mm^2). Patients with biopsy-proven involvement, but an involvement not including the lymph nodes, of more than one organ system (that of the lung and some other system) had significantly ($p < .05$) fewer DR-bearing Langerhans' cells in the epidermis of their noninvolved skin (10.5 ± 1.4 cells/0.05 mm^2) than did patients who had only lung involvement (16.8 ± 2.6 cells/0.05 mm^2), whether or not the involvement included the lymph nodes.

DISCUSSION

The epidermis of patients with psoriasis,[27] hyperkeratotic verrucae,[28] and contact dermatitis[29,30] has been reported to contain fewer Langerhans' cells than are present in control skin. In this study, we have found the density of epidermal Langerhans' cells within the skin of sarcoidosis patients to be significantly lower than that within the skin of healthy volunteers. The reasons for the observed reductions are unclear. It is possible that the fewer numbers of Langerhans' cells in these anergic patients reflect a systemic reduction in cell-mediated immunity, a reduction which has been suggested to occur in these patients.[1,2,9,31] Langerhans' cells play a pivotal role in antigen presentation in contact sensitization, which has been reported to be reduced in patients with sarcoidosis.[32]

The lower densities of epidermal Langerhans' cells appear to parallel both the duration and extent of systemic sarcoidal involvement. Furthermore, the concept of systemic reductions in Langerhans' cells is consistent with the recent finding that Langerhans' cells were present within normal and fibrotic lungs but were not present within the alveolar epithelium of 41 sarcoidosis patients.[33] Local reductions in the number of epidermal Langerhans' cells have been reported in other diseases[27–30] and after exposure to certain agents.[34–36] This study demonstrated a general reduction in density of Langerhans' cells in sarcoidal skin as compared to control skin, and the finding of even lower densities of Langerhans' cells within the epidermis overlying sarcoidal and Kveim-reactive skin than that within the epidermis overlying noninvolved skin suggests there are localized reductions in areas of active disease. It is not known whether these changes are simply due to an obstruction of Langerhans' cell migration to the epidermis[37] or to the recruitment of Langerhans' cells within dermal infiltrates.[38]

Systemic or epicutaneous exposure to glucocorticosteroids has been reported to induce dose-dependent reductions in the density of epidermal Langerhans' cells.[39–43]

The densities of epidermal Langerhans' cells that were observed in steroid-treated and untreated sarcoidosis patients were both less than the density observed in controls; furthermore, parallel reductions were found in both the steroid-treated and untreated groups of patients, and no significant differences were noted between these two groups. These findings suggest that the lowered densities of Langerhans' cells in these patients were not secondary to a steroid effect. The most probable explanation for the lack of a more pronounced reduction of Langerhans' cells in the steroid-treated group is that five of the six patients in this group were receiving low systemic doses of prednisone (7.5-10 mg/day). Interestingly, the noninvolved skin of the patient that received 60 mg of prednisone daily had the lowest density of DR-bearing epidermal Langerhans' cells (4.2 cells/0.05 mm^2) of any skin type, from any patient, that was tested.

It has been our experience that the immunofluorescent assay for DR-positive Langerhans' cells using Ortho monoclonal antibodies detects 55-60% of the number of Langerhans' cells determined by immunofluorescent detection of human T6 antigen.[42,43] One could speculate that these antigens are present on two different subpopulations of Langerhans' cells: on indeterminate Langerhans' cells, which have been suggested to be an immature form, and on Birbeck granule cell-containing Langerhans' cells. T6 antigens are expressed by all Langerhans' cells,[23] and the possibility exists that the expression of DR antigens, Fc, and C3b receptors are restricted to differentiated Langerhans' cells. Differences in assay sensitivities as the basis for the differences in Langerhans' cell detection cannot be ruled out.

In conclusion, we have found the density of epidermal Langerhans' cells in sarcoidosis to be decreased; the degree to which this is seen appears to parallel the disease chronicity and multisystem involvement. Whether these abnormal numbers of Langerhans' cells are due to a local and/or a systemic effect of sarcoidosis or reflect the anergic state of these patients is unknown. Interestingly, not all patients with metastatic carcinomas who are anergic have reduced numbers of Langerhans' cells.[25,44] Although all patients included in that study were anergic, depletion of Langerhans' cells was observed only in patients with metastatic lung cancer and not in patients with metastatic breast carcinomas. Therefore we feel that the reduced number of Langerhans' cells in sarcoidosis patients may reflect the specific disease rather than the anergic state.

REFERENCES

1. SILTZBACH, L. E. 1971. Sarcoidosis. *In* Immunologic Diseases. M. Samter, Ed. Vol. **1:** 581-599. Little, Brown. Boston, MA.
2. SHARMA, O. P. 1975. The immunology of sarcoidosis. *In* Sarcoidosis: A Clinical Approach. O. P. Sharma, Ed.: 135-146. Charles C. Thomas. Springfield, IL.
3. FRIOU, G. J. 1952. A study of cutaneous reactions to oidiomycin trichophytin and mumps skin test antigens in patients with sarcoidosis. Yale J. Biol. Med. **24:** 533-539.
4. CITRON, K. M. 1957. Skin tests in sarcoidosis. Tubercle **38:** 33-41.
5. KATARIA, Y. P., A. L. SAGONE, A. F. LOBUGLIO & P. A. BOOMBERG. 1973. *In vitro* observations on sarcoid lymphocytes and their correlation with cutaneous anergy and clinical severity of disease. Am. Rev. Respir. Dis. **108:** 767-776.
6. ROSSMAN, M. D., J. N. DAUBER & R. P. DANIELE. 1978. Identification of activated T-cells in sarcoidosis. Am. Rev. Respir. Dis. **117:** 713-720.
7. TANNENBAUM, H., R. E. ROCKLIN, P. H. SCHUR & A. L. SHEFFER. 1976. Immunological identification of subpopulations of mononuclear cells in sarcoid granulomas. Ann. N.Y. Acad. Sci. **278:** 136-146.
8. SNYDER, G. B. 1964. The fate of skin homografts in patients with sarcoidosis. Bull. Johns Hopkins Hosp. **115:** 81-91.

9. CRYSTAL, R. G., W. C. ROBERTS, G. W. HUNNINGHAKE, J. E. GADEK, J. D. FULMER & B. R. LINE. 1981. Pulmonary sarcoidosis: A disease characterized and perpetuated by activated lung T-lymphocytes. Ann. Intern. Med. **94:** 73-94.
10. HUNNINGHAKE, G. W. & R. G. CRYSTAL. 1981. Pulmonary sarcoidosis: A disorder mediated by excess helper T-lymphocyte activity at sites of disease activity. N. Engl. J. Med. **305:** 429-434.
11. LANGERHANS, P. 1868. Uber die Nerven der menschlichen Haut. Virchows Arch. Pathol. Anat. Physiol. **44:** 325-327.
12. WOLFF, K. & R. K. WINKELMANN. 1967. Ultrastructural localization of nucleoside triphosphatase in Langerhans cells. J. Invest. Dermatol. **48:** 50-54.
13. SILBERBERG, I. 1973. Apposition of mononuclear cells to Langerhans cells in contact allergy. I. An ultrastructural study in actively induced contact dermatitis in guinea pigs. Acta. Derm. Venereol. (Stockholm) **53:** 1-12.
14. STINGL, G., S. I. KATZ, E. M. SHEVACH, E. WOLFF-SCHREINER & I. GREEN. 1978. Detection of Ia antigens of Langerhans cells in guinea pig skin. J. Immunol. **120:** 570-578.
15. ROWDEN, G., M. G. LEWIS & A. K. SULLIVAN. 1977. Ia antigen expression on human Langerhans cells. Nature **268:** 247-248.
16. STINGL, G., E. C. WOLFF-SCHREINER, W. J. PICHER, F. GSCHNAIT, W. KNAPP & K. WOLFF. 1977. Epidermal Langerhans cells bear Fc and C3b receptors. Nature **268:** 245-246.
17. BERMAN, B. & I. GIGLI. 1980. Complement receptors on guinea pig epidermal Langerhans cells. J. Immunol. **124:** 685-690.
18. BERMAN, B. & D. S. FRANCE. 1979. Histochemical analysis of Langerhans' cells. Am. J. Dermatopathol. **1:** 215-221.
19. STINGL, G., S. I. KATZ, L. CLEMENT, I. GREEN & E. M. SHEVACH. 1978. Immunological functions of Ia-bearing epidermal Langerhans cells. J. Immunol. **121:** 2005-2013.
20. KATZ, S. I., K. TAMAKI & D. H. SACHS. 1979. Epidermal Langerhans cells are derived from cells which originate in the bone marrow. Nature **282:** 324-326.
21. BERMAN, B. 1985. Langerhans cells. *In* Dermatologic Allergy and Immunology. J. Stone, Ed.: 217-236. C. V. Mosby. St. Louis, MO.
22. CHU, A., M. EISINGER, J. S. LEE, S. TAKEZAKI, P. KUNG & R. EDELSON. 1982. Immunoelectron microscopic identification of Langerhans cells using a new antigenic marker. J. Invest. Dermatol. **78:** 177-180.
23. BERMAN, B., V. L. CHEN, D. S. FRANCE, W. I. DOTZ & G. PETRONI. 1983. Anatomical mapping of epidermal Langerhans cell densities in adults. J. Invest. Dermatol. **80:** 472-475.
24. SILTZBACH, L. E., D. D. KRAKOFF & A. S. TEIRSTEIN. 1980. Elevated levels of serum angiotensin-converting enzyme (kininase IIJ) and lysozyme levels in sarcoidosis. Eighth International Conference on Sarcoidosis and Other Granulomatous Diseases. W. Jones Williams & B. H. Davies, Eds.: 298. Alpha Omega. Cardiff.
25. FOX, J. L., B. BERMAN & R. GOODMAN. 1985. Reduced epidermal Langerhans cell densities in patients with pulmonary malignancies does not correlate with anergy or nutritional status. J. Dermatol. Surg. Oncol. **11:** in press.
26. SILTZBACH, L. E. 1961. The Kveim test in sarcoidosis: A study of 750 patients. J. Am. Med. Assoc. **178:** 476-482.
27. MULLER, S. A., R. K. WINKELMANN & P. R. VANDERSTEIN. 1971. Langerhans cells and cutaneous nerves in psoriasis: A histochemical study. *In* Psoriasis. M. Farber & A. J. Cox, Eds.: 187-202. Stanford University Press. Stanford, CA.
28. FRITZ, P. & E. DIEM. 1972. Enzyme cytochemical studies on cell suspensions and primary cultures of guinea pig epidermis. Arch. Dermatol. Forsch. **243:** 364.
29. SILBERBERG, I., R. L. BAER & S. A. ROSENTHAL. 1974. The role of Langerhans cells in contact allergy. Acta Derm. Venereol. (Stockholm) **54:** 321-331.
30. SILBERBERG, I., R. L. BAER, S. A. ROSENTHAL, G. J. THORBECK & V. BEREZOWSKY. 1975. Langerhans cells at sites of passively induced allergic contact sensitivity. Cell. Immunol. **18:** 435-453.
31. SEMENZATO, G., A. PEZZUTTO, C. AGOSTINI, G. GASPAROTTO & A. CIPRIANI. 1981. Immunoregulation in sarcoidosis. Clin. Immunol. Immunopathol. **19:** 416-427.

32. COSEMANS, J. & A. C. LOUWAGIE. 1979. Tuberculin and DNCB skin tests and *in vitro* lymphocyte transformation in patients with sarcoidosis. Acta Clin. Belg. **34:** 353-359.
33. KAWANAMI, O., F. BASSET, V. J. FERRANS, P. SOLER & R. G. CRYSTAL. 1981. Pulmonary Langerhans cells in patients with fibrotic lung disorders. Lab. Invest. **44:** 227-233.
34. ABERER, W., G. SCHALER, G. STINGL, H. HONIGSMANN & K. WOLFF. 1981. Ultraviolet light depletes surface markers on Langerhans cells. J. Invest. Dermatol. **76:** 202-210.
35. STINGL, G., L. A. GAZZE-STINGL, W. ABERER & K. WOLFF. 1981. Antigen presentation by murine epidermal Langerhans cells and its alteration by ultraviolet B light. J. Immunol. **127:** 1707-1713.
36. WOLFF, K., R. J. LESSARD & R. K. WINKELMANN. 1971. Electron microscopic observations on Langerhans cells after epidermal trauma. Dermatol. Dig. **10:** 35.
37. MITCHELL, D. N., J. G. SCADDING & B. E. HEARD. 1977. Sarcoidosis: Histopathological definition and clinical diagnosis. J. Clin. Pathol. **30:** 395-408.
38. FOX, J. L., B. BERMAN & D. S. FRANCE. 1982. Abnormal numbers of Langerhans cells in sarcoidosis. J. Invest. Dermatol. **78:** 355.
39. NORDLUND, J. J., A. E. ACKLES & A. B. LERNER. 1981. The effects of ultraviolet light and certain drugs on Ia-bearing Langerhans cells in murine epidermis. Cell. Immunol. **60:** 50-63.
40. LYNCH, D. H., H. F. GURISH & R. A. DAYNES. 1981. Relationship between epidermal Langerhans cell density, ATPase activity and the induction of contact hypersensitivity. J. Immunol. **126:** 1892-1897.
41. BERMAN, B. & D. S. FRANCE. 1981. Modulation of epidermal Langerhans cell properties following *in vitro* and *in situ* exposure to glucocorticosteroids. J. Invest. Dermatol. **76:** 324-325.
42. BERMAN, B. & D. S. FRANCE. 1982. Effects of *in vitro* and *in situ* exposure to amcinonide on human Langerhans cells. Clin. Res. **30:** 154A.
43. BERMAN, B. & D. S. FRANCE. 1982. Effects of *in vitro* and *in situ* exposure to corticoids on human Langerhans cells. Clin. Res. **30:** 260A.
44. FOX, J. L., B. BERMAN, A. BATRA, R. GOODMAN & D. S. FRANCE. 1984. Epidermal Langerhans cell densities in patients with malignancies. Clin. Res. **32:** 17A.

Increased Monocyte Fc(IgG) Receptor Expression in Sarcoidosis[a]

MILTON D. ROSSMAN,[b] PAUL CHIEN,
ANGELICA CASSIZZI, JACK A. ELIAS, AND
ALAN D. SCHREIBER

Cardiovascular-Pulmonary Division
and
Hematology-Oncology Section
Department of Medicine
University of Pennsylvania School of Medicine
Philadelphia, Pennsylvania 19104

INTRODUCTION

Sarcoidosis is a systemic granulomatosis of unknown etiology. The hallmark of this disease, a noncaseating epithelioid granuloma, is believed to be a high-intensity granuloma,[1] that is, one into which monocytes from the blood are continually moving and in which these monocytes mature and/or differentiate into epithelioid cells. This theory suggests that there is an increased turnover of monocytes in sarcoidosis and that these monocytes might be in an activated state.

Early studies of monocyte/macrophage function are consistent with the possibility that circulating monocytes are activated in sarcoidosis. Monocytes from patients with sarcoidosis have been shown to bind increased numbers of immunoglobulin G (IgG)- and C3-coated red blood cells[2,3] and to migrate more effectively into skin windows.[4] Few studies, however, have compared the activity of sarcoid monocytes to that of tissue macrophages.

The human macrophage receptor for IgG, the Fc(IgG) receptor, has recently been shown to be modulated by inflammatory stimuli.[5] In this study the number and affinity of monocyte and alveolar macrophage IgG binding sites were measured in normal controls and in patients with active sarcoidosis; any differences that were found were examined for correlations with other markers of disease activity.

[a] This work was supported in part by Grants 5 R01-HL-31136 and 5 R01-HL-30715 (M.D.R.), 1 K08-HL-01064 (J.A.E.), and HL-27068, AI-22193, and HL-28207 (A.D.S.) from the National Institutes of Health; by a grant from the American Lung Association; and by the Edward Livingston Trudeau Scholar and Dalsemer Scholar Awards (J.A.E.).

[b] Address for correspondence: 811 East Gates Building, Box 678, Hospital of the University of Pennsylvania, 3400 Spruce Street, Philadelphia, Pennsylvania 19104.

METHODS

Preparation of Monocytes

Mononuclear cells were isolated from heparinized human blood by density centrifugation (LSM, Bionetics Laboratory Products, Kensington, Maryland). Between 40×10^6 and 60×10^6 cells were incubated for 1 hr at room temperature in tissue culture flasks that had been pretreated with heat-inactivated fetal calf serum (Gibco, Grand Island, New York). The nonadherent cells were washed from the flasks with RPMI-1640 (M.A. Bioproducts, Walkersville, Maryland) supplemented with 10% heat-inactivated fetal calf serum. The adherent cells were dislodged[6] by incubating the cells at 4° C for 15 min in Hanks' balanced salt solution, without calcium or magnesium (M.A. Bioproducts, Walkersville, Maryland), supplemented with 5% fetal calf serum, with or without 0.2% EDTA (Sigma, St. Louis, Missouri). The cells prepared in this manner, when stained with Diff-Quik (Dade Diagnostics, Aguada, Puerto Rico), had the appearance of monocytes, and more than 95% of the cells were shown to be esterase positive after nonspecific esterase staining.[7] More than 90% of the cells were able to phagocytose latex articles; more than 95% were viable as assessed by trypan blue exclusion.

Preparation of Alveolar Macrophages

Alveolar macrophages were obtained by a standard (300-500 ml) bronchopulmonary lavage.[8] Lavages were performed on five nonsmokers and four smokers (minimum of 3 pack years; range: 3-8 pack years). Cell yield from the nonsmokers averaged 171 000 ± 57 000 cells/ml of lavage fluid recovered. Cell yield from the smokers averaged 477 000 ± 196 000 cells/ml of lavage fluid recovered. In all cases, more than 90% of the recovered cells were alveolar macrophages as assessed by Diff-Quik and nonspecific esterase stains. The cells were filtered through gauze to remove mucus and washed three times in Hanks' balanced salt solution.

Clinical Specimens

Informed consent was obtained from all the patients listed in TABLE 1 before collecting blood and/or lavage specimens. All of the patients had biopsy-proven sarcoidosis. None of the patients had been treated with corticosteroids. Of the 11 patients studied, 8 were newly diagnosed cases of sarcoidosis. Of the three cases of chronic sarcoidosis, only one, GB, had clinically inactive disease. Only 2 of the 11 patients were smokers. Extrapulmonary disease was present in six patients. Angiotensin-converting enzyme levels were measured in 10 patients and were abnormal in 7 patients. Eight of the patients had stage II radiologic disease; two had stage I disease; and one had stage III disease. The vital capacity averaged 85.5 ± 4.4% of that predicted, and the diffusing capacity averaged 64.4 ± 5.2% of that predicted. Blood monocytes were obtained from 10 patients, and alveolar macrophages were obtained from 5 patients.

TABLE 1. Patient Profiles

Patient	Age	Sex	Radiographic Stage	Lavage (% lymphocytes)	ACE Level[a]	VC[b]	DL_{CO}[b]	Extrapulmonary Disease	Onset of Disease (years)
EB	27	M	II	10	160	93	72	No	< 1
GB	40	F	III	5	103	107	56	No	7
WL	26	F	II	ND	138	65	57	Cardiac	< 1
LW	26	F	II	ND	229	73	55	Uveitis	< 1
AB	36	F	II	7	23	74	62	No	< 1
SF	29	M	I	21	125	89	85	Arthralgia	< 1
PF	30	M	II	21	ND	103	90	Uveitis	< 1
SF	39	F	II	33	137	72	79	Uveitis (*E. nodosum*)	< 1
JJ	39	F	II	29	157	72	32	No	5
RB	28	M	I	18	87	99	76	No	< 1
SD	40	F	II	ND	223	94	48	Skin sarcoidosis	5
Mean ± SE	32.7 ± 1.8			18 ± 3.6	151 ± 16.2	85.5 ± 4.4	64.4 ± 5.2		

[a] Normal ACE level for any given patient (except AB): < 124 units; normal ACE level for AB (determined by Bio-Science): < 34 units.
[b] Values expressed as a percentage of the predicted value.

Preparation of IgG

Human IgG[9] was purified from fresh human serum by column-affinity chromatography with rabbit antihuman IgG (Miles-Yeda, Rehovat, Israel). IgG, in 0.2% Na_3N-supplemented phosphate-buffered saline (PBS) at pH 7.3, was stored at 4° C until it was used. IgG was labeled with ^{125}I (New England Nuclear, Boston, Massachusetts) by the chloramine-T method.[10] Just prior to each assay, the IgG was centrifuged in a Beckman airfuge at 100 000 × g to remove any potential aggregates. IgG fractionated as IgG monomer on Sephadex G-200 chromatography.

Binding Studies with Monomeric ^{125}I-IgG

All assays were performed in Delbecco's PBS (Gibco, Grand Island, New York) containing 0.1% gelatin, 10 mM EDTA, and 0.1% Na_3N-supplemented PBS. Before each binding assay, monocytes or alveolar macrophages were incubated for 30 min at 37° C in PBS to permit any cell-associated IgG to dissociate from the cell surface. The cells were centrifuged and resuspended at 2×10^6 cells/ml in PBS that contained varying amounts of radioiodinated monomeric IgG in the presence or absence of a 100-fold excess of unlabeled IgG. The amount of cell-associated ^{125}I-IgG was quantitated after rapidly centrifuging the cells through a layer of silicone oil in microfuge tubes using a Beckman B centrifuge. An aliquot of the supernatant was counted on a Beckman Bio-gamma counter to determine the "free" concentration of ^{125}I-IgG. After removing the supernatant, the microfuge tubes were cut through the oil layer, and the counts in the cell pellets (bound counts) were determined. Nonspecific binding was defined to be the total number of counts for cell-associated ^{125}I-IgG that occurred in the presence of a 100-fold excess of unlabeled IgG; nonspecific binding was usually less than 30% of the counts for cell-associated ^{125}I-IgG that occurred without an excess of unlabeled IgG (total bound counts). Specific binding was the total bound counts minus the nonspecifically bound counts.

Statistics

The best line describing the results of Scatchard plots of equilibrium binding data was derived from linear regression programs using a least-squares method. Student's *t* test was used to determine if the difference between two means was significant.

RESULTS

Characteristics of IgG Binding to Normal Blood Monocytes and Pulmonary Macrophages

Specific binding of IgG monomer was observed for both monocytes and alveolar macrophages at either 4° C or 37° C. Binding of ^{125}I-IgG equilibrated within 30 to 60 min for both cell types at 37° C. At 4° C, however, equilibrium binding was not observed until after 24 hr. At both temperatures maximum specific binding was similar. When an excess of cold IgG was added after equilibrium binding, more than 90% of the specifically bound IgG could be displaced from the cells. A similar degree of dissociation of specifically bound ^{125}I-IgG occurred when the cells were resuspended in IgG-free medium.

Specific binding at 37° C of monomeric IgG under equilibrium conditions was saturable. Scatchard plots[11] of the data were consistent with the possibility of a single class of receptors for monomeric IgG on both monocytes and alveolar macrophages at 37° C. Significantly more ($p < .001$) IgG binding sites were found, at 37° C, on alveolar macrophages than were found on blood monocytes (alveolar macrophages: 116 477 ± 29 236 binding sites/cell; monocytes: 24 968 ± 1361 binding sites/cell). For both cell types there was no significant difference between the number of binding sites for monomeric IgG that was measured at 4° C and that measured at 37° C. Monocytes and alveolar macrophages had similar affinities (K_d's) for monomeric IgG at 37° C ($p > .10$), as well as at 4° C.

IgG Binding Studies in Sarcoidosis

Significantly more ($p < .001$) IgG receptor sites/cell were observed on monocytes from sarcoidosis patients ($N = 10$) than were observed on monocytes from normal volunteers ($N = 23$); sarcoid monocytes and normal monocytes had 44 860 ± 6652 and 24 968 ± 1361 binding sites/cell, respectively (TABLE 2). Interestingly, only 2 of the 10 patients with sarcoidosis had a normal number of IgG binding sites/monocyte. One of these was the patient with chronic inactive sarcoidosis. No significant difference between the affinities determined for normal and sarcoid monocytes was observed.

We were also able to examine IgG binding to alveolar macrophages from patients with sarcoidosis ($N = 5$) and normal volunteers ($N = 9$). Although fewer binding sites were detected on sarcoid alveolar macrophages than on normal alveolar macrophages, this difference was not statistically significant ($p > .30$); sarcoid and normal alveolar macrophages had 61 800 ± 6694 and 88 653 ± 16 668 binding sites/cell, respectively (TABLE 3).

When the number of IgG binding sites/cell was measured simultaneously on blood monocytes and alveolar macrophages from the same individual, alveolar macrophages always had more IgG binding sites/cell than did the blood monocytes. In the individuals with sarcoidosis, whose blood monocytes had markedly elevated monocyte

TABLE 2. Monomeric IgG Binding to Monocytes[a]

Monocytes	Number of Patients	Number of Binding Sites/Cell	K_d (M/L × 10^{-9})
Normal	23	24 968 ± 1361	2.35 ± 0.155
Sarcoid	10	44 860 ± 6652[b]	2.21 ± 0.782

[a] The number of IgG binding sites and K_d's were calculated from Scatchard plots of data from equilibrium binding studies performed at 37° C.

[b] Significantly different from the result for normal monocytes.

TABLE 3. Monomeric IgG Binding to Human Alveolar Macrophages[a]

Alveolar Macrophages	Number of Patients	Number of Binding Sites/Cell	K_d (M/L × 10^{-9})
Normal	9	88 653 ± 16 668	5.0 ± 0.75
Sarcoid	5	61 800 ± 6694	7.6 ± 0.70

[a] The number of IgG binding sites and the K_d's were calculated from Scatchard plots of data from equilibrium binding studies performed at 4° C.

IgG binding, in all but one patient, EB, the alveolar macrophages had more binding sites for monomeric IgG than did the blood monocytes.

Monocyte IgG binding in sarcoidosis patients was evaluated in the presence or absence of extrapulmonary disease, in different radiologic stages, at various percentages of bronchoalveolar lymphocytosis, and at various angiotensin-converting enzyme levels; no correlations were observed ($r < .25$ for all comparisons).

DISCUSSION

We analyzed the expression of IgG binding sites on monocytes and alveolar macrophages from patients with sarcoidosis. Our data indicate that the number of binding sites for monomeric IgG is significantly greater on monocytes from patients with active sarcoidosis than on those from normal volunteers. The increase in the number of binding sites for monomeric IgG on monocytes that apparently occurs in sarcoidosis is consistent with other observations of the activation of blood monocytes in sarcoidosis.[2–4,12] Taken together, these data further support the notion of a high-intensity granuloma in sarcoidosis, that is, a granuloma with a constant influx of monocytes.[1]

The exact mechanism responsible for the increase in IgG receptor expression is not known. A role for the release of endogenous mediators, however, can be speculated upon. The inflammatory process in sarcoidosis causes the release of several mediators, some of which have the ability to influence macrophage function.[13–15] One such potent mediator known to be released in sarcoidosis is immune interferon.[13] Guyre *et al.* have previously demonstrated that recombinant immune interferon will increase the number of monocyte Fc receptors.[5] This increase in receptor number may facilitate the recognition and removal of immune complexes containing multivalent IgG ligands which appear during the course of sarcoidosis.[16,17]

No correlation was noted between the number of monocyte IgG binding sites and other measures of disease activity or extent in sarcoidosis. This may reflect the small number of patients in the study or a difference in activity between blood and tissues. Alternatively, the poor correlation may simply reflect differences in the rate of onset and resolution of the different parameters. It is known that angiotensin-converting enzyme and bronchoalveolar lymphocytosis levels may take weeks or even months to return to normal during spontaneous remission or steroid therapy. Abnormal monocyte Fc receptor activity levels may return to normal sooner.

In contrast to the greater than normal number of IgG binding sites noted on monocytes from patients with sarcoidosis, alveolar macrophages from these patients had a normal number of binding sites. There are several possible explanations for this unexpected observation. A population of alveolar macrophages which expresses an increase in receptor number may be present in the tissue but not in the air spaces because they are preferentially bound in the granuloma. Alternatively, such a population with an increased number of receptors may be unappreciated because of an influx of younger macrophages (monocyte-derived macrophages, for example) which express fewer IgG binding sites/cell. Finally, alveolar macrophages may be less responsive to stimulation from such inflammation-derived signals such as lymphokines, or perhaps the Fc(IgG) receptors on alveolar macrophages are down regulated because of the presence of immune complexes in the lung.

SUMMARY

Since the macrophage Fc(IgG) receptor appears to be modulated by inflammatory stimuli, we measured the binding of monomeric IgG to monocytes and alveolar macrophages from patients with pulmonary sarcoidosis. Equilibrium binding studies were performed, and the number and affinity of Fc(IgG) receptors were calculated from Scatchard plots of the data. Monocytes from patients with sarcoidosis had nearly twice the number of binding sites for monomeric IgG as did the monocytes from normals. In contrast to the findings with monocytes, alveolar macrophages from patients with sarcoidosis did not have a greater number of monomeric IgG binding sites than did normal alveolar macrophages. These findings are consistent with those on the activation of circulating monocytes in sarcoidosis. That the number of Fc(IgG) receptors on sarcoid alveolar macrophages was not greater than that on normal alveolar macrophages suggests that Fc(IgG) receptor activity on alveolar macrophages does not reflect the activated state of sarcoidosis.

REFERENCES

1. Warren, K. S. 1976. Functional classification of granulomatous inflammation. Ann. N. Y. Acad. Sci. **178:** 7-18.
2. Schmidt, M. E. & S. D. Douglas. 1977. Monocyte IgG receptor activity, dynamics and modulation: Normal individuals and patients with granulomatous diseases. J. Lab. Clin. Med. **89:** 332-340.
3. Douglas, S. D. 1976. Human monocyte spreading *in vitro:* Inducers and effects on Fc and C3 receptors. Cell. Immunol. **21:** 344-349.
4. Kohout, J. 1976. Macrophage reactivity in skin windows. Ann. N. Y. Acad. Sci. **278:** 201-203.
5. Guyre, P. M., P. M. Morganelli & R. Miller. 1983. Recombinant immune interferon increases immunoglobulin G Fc receptors on cultured human mononuclear phagocytes. J. Clin. Invest. **72:** 393-397.
6. Kumagai, K., K. Etoh, S. Hinuma & M. Tada. 1979. Pretreatment of plastic petri dishes with fetal calf serum: A simple method of macrophage isolation. J. Immunol. Methods **19:** 17-25.
7. Yam, L. T., C. Y. Li & W. H. Crosby. 1971. Cytochemical identification of monocytes and granulocytes. Am. J. Clin. Pathol. **55:** 283-287.
8. Dauber, J. H., M. D. Rossman & R. P. Daniele. 1979. Bronchoalveolar cell populations in acute sarcoidosis. J. Lab. Clin. Med. **94:** 862-871.

9. CUATRECASAS, P. & C. B. ANFINSEN. 1971. Affinity chromatography. *In* Methods in Enzymology. W. B. Jakobi, Ed. Vol. **22:** 345-378. Academic Press. New York, NY.
10. HUNTER, W. M. & F. C. GREENWOOD. 1962. Preparation of iodine-131-labeled human growth hormone of high specific activity. Nature **194:** 495-496.
11. SCATCHARD, G. 1949. The attraction of protein for small molecules and ions. Ann. N. Y. Acad. Sci. **51:** 660-663.
12. ELIAS, J. A., M. D. ROSSMAN & R. P. DANIELE. 1984. Blood and lung mononuclear cell inhibition of fibroblast growth in sarcoidosis. Am. Rev. Respir. Dis. **130:** 1050-1057.
13. NUGENT, K., M. MONICK & G. W. HUNNINGHAKE. 1984. Pulmonary macrophages from patients with active sarcoidosis spontaneously release immune interferon. Clin. Res. **32:** 434A.
14. HUNNINGHAKE, G. W. 1984. Release of interleukin-1 by alveolar macrophages of patients with active sarcoidosis. Am. Rev. Respir. Dis. **129:** 569-572.
15. HUNNINGHAKE, G. W., J. E. GADEK, R. C. YOUNG, JR., O. KAWANAMI, V. J. FERRANS & R. G. CRYSTAL. 1980. Maintenance of granuloma formation in pulmonary sarcoidosis by T lymphocytes within the lung. N. Eng. J. Med. **302:** 594-598.
16. DANIELE, R. P., L. J. MCMILLIAN, J. H. DAUBER & M. D. ROSSMAN. 1978. Immune complexes in sarcoidosis: A correlation with activity and duration of disease. Chest **74:** 261-264.
17. HEDFORS, E. & R. NORBERG. 1974. Evidence for circulating immune complexes in sarcoidosis. Clin. Exp. Immunol. **16:** 493-496.

Organization of the Connective Matrix of the Sarcoid Granuloma

Evolution and Cell-Matrix Interactions[a]

SIMONE PEYROL,[b] CHRISTINA TAKIYA,[c]
JEAN-FRANÇOIS CORDIER,[d]
AND JEAN-ALEXIS GRIMAUD[b]

[b]*Institut Pasteur*
Centre National de la Recherche Scientifique ERA 819
Lyons, France

[c]*Departamento de Patologia*
Universidade Federal do Rio de Janeiro
Rio de Janeiro, Brazil

[d]*Hôpital Louis Pradel*
Lyons, France

INTRODUCTION

Recovery from sarcoidosis can sometimes occur spontaneously. This may result from the involution of the sarcoid granuloma.[1]

The sarcoid granuloma is classically defined as a spherical, well-delimited epithelioid granuloma[2] modulated by immunocompetent cell populations which are present from the outset.[3] With time, a decrease of immunocompetent cells and a simultaneous expansion of the epithelioid cell population are associated with the development of a fine reticulin network within the granuloma. At the same time, the progressive concentric deposition of a connective matrix in the periphery results in an acellular fibrotic hyalin nodular lesion.[4]

Several recent studies investigated the mechanisms responsible for controlling the cellular secretion of connective matrix macromolecules.[5] In relation to the precise nature of hyalin fibrosis of sarcoid granuloma, few comprehensive studies have been performed. Despite the demonstration of its polymorphic character,[6,7] its ability to undergo histological regression, which clinical work suggests it has, remains an unexplained phenomenon. The aim of the present work was to study the changes in the connective tissue related to cell populations during the natural history of the sarcoid granuloma. Specific immunolabeling of connective components was done in order to identify cell-matrix interactions in the evolution of the sarcoid granuloma.

[a]This work was supported by a grant from the Comité National et Comités Départementaux contre les Maladies Respiratoire and a fellowship from the Société d'Hépatologie Expérimentale.

MATERIALS AND METHODS

Samples

Six patients with intrathoracic or abdominal sarcoidosis were selected. Two patients had only pulmonary lesions whereas the others presented both pulmonary and extrathoracic (splenic, cutaneous, ocular, and/or hepatic) lesions. Attention was focused on the granuloma reaction, that is, on the histological distribution of the granulomas. Organ-specific lesions were also noted. TABLE 1 summarizes clinical and histopathological findings.

Light Microscopy

Different connective tissue stains were performed in order to visualize the connective components of the sarcoid granuloma. Masson's trichrome staining, Gordon-Sweets' silver impregnation, and immunofluorescent labeling were performed on matrix proteins.

The preparation of immune reagents (specific antibodies against collagen types I, III, and IV; procollagen III; fibronectin; and laminin) and the histological immunofluorescent staining techniques have already been described.[9]

Electron Microscopy

After standard and immunoperoxidase processing for electron microscopy,[9] the examination of semithin sections allowed us to select granulomas of different aspects and of different hyalinized zones.

RESULTS

Histopathology

The light microscopic study of single granulomas concentrated not only on their cell populations but also on their relationship with the connective tissue content of the sarcoid granuloma during the different stages of the sarcoid granuloma's evolution. The connective tissue could be visualized as a Gordon-Sweet network or as a Masson trichrome-positive matrix (FIG. 1).

During the early stages, the sarcoid granuloma consisted of a focal accumulation of macrophages, monocytes, epithelioid cells, and lymphocytes (FIG. 1(1)). A fine condensation of reticulin fibers was seen around the granuloma (FIG. 1(2)). In mature

TABLE 1.

	Clinical Data						Histopathological Findings	
Patient	Sex	Age (years)	Duration of Disease (months)[a]	Intrathoracic Stage[b]	Extrathoracic Sarcoidosis	Site of Biopsy	Localization of Granulomas	Associated Findings
1	M	44	< 18	III	None	Lung	Interlobular septa, alveolar septa, bronchiole wall, vessel wall, and bronchovascular axis	Intraalveolar edema (focal), focal alveolitis, focal fibrotic thickening of alveolar wall, and focal and diffuse fibrosis of pleura
2	F	31	> 7, < 31	III	None	Lung	Pleura, intralobular septa, vascular axis, and alveolar septa	Intraalveolar edema (focal), focal alveolitis, fibrotic thickening of alveolar septa, and diffuse and focal fibrotic thickening of pleura
3	M	28	?	III	Spleen	Lung	Pleura, intralobular septa, vascular axis, and alveolar septa	Intraalveolar edema (focal), focal alveolitis, fibrotic thickening of alveolar septa, and diffuse and focal fibrotic thickening of pleura

4	F	24	?	I	Skin	Lymph node	Cortical and medullary sinus	Zones of diffuse lymphoreticular hisitocytosis and focal fibrotic thickening of the capsule
5	M	33	> 12	I	Eyes	Lymph node	Rare granulomas and isolated cells trapped within the hyalin matrix	Almost total substitution of tissue by a hyalin matrix
6	M	31	> 45	III	Spleen	Spleen	Splenic trabecular	
					Liver	Liver	Portal spaces and lobular localization	Fibrotic thickening of portal spaces

[a] The duration of disease until the time of biopsy.
[b] The intrathoracic staging of sarcoidosis was assessed according to roentgenographic findings: stage I, bilateral hilar lymphadenopathy; stage II, bilateral hilar lymphadenopathy and parenchymal infiltration; and stage III, parenchymal infiltration without bilateral hilar lymphadenopathy.[8]

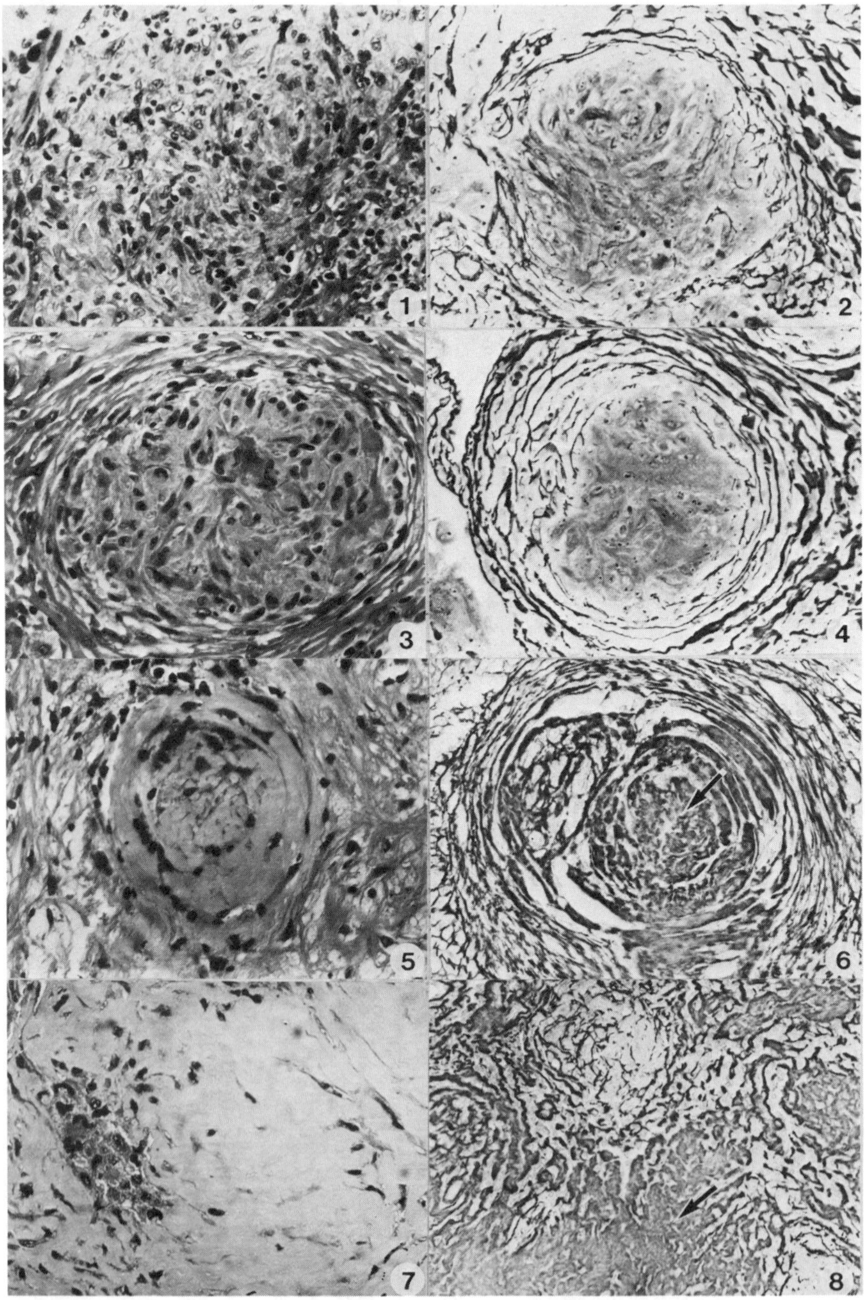
1
2
3
4
5
6
7
8

stages, all cell populations consisted mainly of epithelioid cells, but some giant cells and a few peripherally disposed lymphocytes and monocytes were present. The well-defined ring of connective tissue that had developed was composed of concentrically disposed reticulin fibers and a Masson trichrome-positive matrix (FIG. 1(3,4)). Fibroblasts were present within this capsule.

A progressive centripetal thickening of this peripheral fibrous ring associated with a decrease in the number of epithelioid cells was considered to represent the late-stage granuloma (FIG. 1(5,6)). The fibroblastic population increased at this stage.

The maximal extension of this Masson-positive, concentric matrix resulted in an acellular, amorphous hyalin formation (FIG. 1(7,8)).

Granulomas were generally confluent, mainly in the lung and in the spleen. In these cases they were connected by a dense, Masson-positive hyalin matrix.

In the case of pulmonary localization, focal alveolitis was always present, consisting of exogenous mononuclear cells in the alveolar septa. A fibrotic reaction of the alveolar septa was sometimes observed in the vicinity of granulomas (TABLE 1).

In lymph nodes, sarcoid granulomas did not exhibit a developed concentric capsule and thus were not well defined. It was interesting to note that young and mature granulomas coexisted in the same organ, even in confluent lesions.

Connective Matrix Components

Connective matrix components (CMC's) of the sarcoid granuloma included interstitial collagens (types I and III) and fibronectin, as shown by immunofluorescence labeling. All these components were present either around or within the granulomas; in the early stage, however, these components were only peripheral (FIG. 2(9-11)).

In the mature and late stages, these matrix proteins were detected both around and within the granulomas (FIG. 2(12-14)).

The immunolabeling of CMC's emphasizes the concentric pattern of the peripheral organization of the matrix and the irregular fibrillar pattern within the granuloma.

No basement membrane-associated proteins (collagen type IV or laminin) were detected.

In hyalin granulomas the clear-cut differences in CMC organization described above were not seen, but the same components were present as a diffuse framework (FIG. 2(15-17)). No particular localization was noted for any of the CMC's.

FIGURE 1. The connective matrix at different evolutionary stages of the sarcoid granuloma. The sections in the left-hand column underwent Masson's trichrome staining; those in the right-hand column underwent Gordon-Sweets' silver impregnation. All sections were studied under light microscopy. The original magnification for each section (unless otherwise indicated, in parentheses) was × 950; each part of the figure was reduced to 95% of its original size. Early stage granulomas: **(1)** a roughly delimited aggregation of inflammatory cells and **(2)** an almost absent reticulin network inside a granuloma. Mature granulomas: **(3)** a well-defined lesion surrounded by a concentric ring of connective tissue and **(4)** a concentric deposition of several layers of reticulin fibers. Late-stage granulomas: **(5)** concentric layers of connective tissue around a granuloma and **(6)** the substitution of almost an entire granuloma by a connective matrix negative for silver impregnation (see arrow). Hyalin matrix: **(7)** a hyalinized lymph node parenchyma (one that had contained a few isolated granulomas) composed of collagenous tissue and **(8)** its amorphous aspect (see arrow) (× 500).

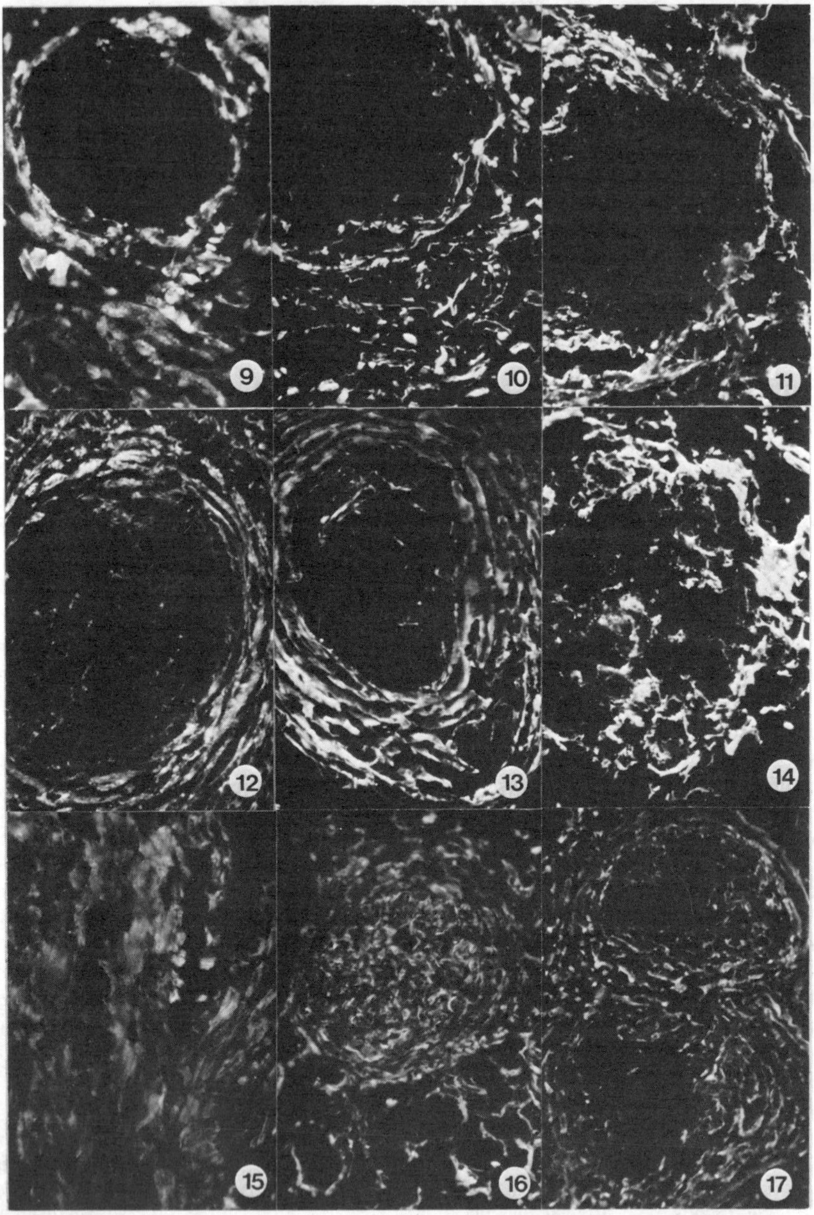

FIGURE 2. Immunofluorescence labeling of connective proteins. The original magnification for each section (unless otherwise indicated, in parentheses) was × 800; each part of the figure was reduced to 88% of its original size. The formation of fine networks around early-stage granulomas: **(9)** collagen type I, **(10)** collagen type III, and **(11)** fibronectin. The deposition of connective matrix proteins around mature granulomas: **(12)** collagen type I, **(13)** collagen type III, and **(14)** fibronectin. The focal or diffuse deposition of hyalin substance: **(15)** collagen type I in a diffuse deposition, **(16)** collagen type III in a hyalinized granuloma, and **(17)** fibronectin in a diffuse hyalin matrix around confluent granulomas (× 500).

In one of the cases, a diffuse hyalinization of the lymph node tissue was observed. No differences in CMC labeling were noted between this case and the one described before (FIG. 2(15)).

Ultrastructural Findings

A remodeling of the preexisting connective matrix of the alveolar septa seemed to be the initial change associated with migrating inflammatory cells. Regular, dense septal bundles of collagen fibers were disrupted by edema (FIGS. 3(18) & 4(20)), and there was a prominent local accumulation of fibronectin, one made evident by immunoperoxidase labeling (FIG. 3(19)). Fibronectin was found intermingled with collagen fibers and basement membranes (capillary and epithelial) facing the septal connective axis; it was also present inside some alveolar lumina.

The first stage of a sarcoid granuloma was identified as a collection of epithelioid cells and some macrophages. A few lymphocytes were found among the macrophages at the periphery. Epithelioid cells and macrophages exhibited long and numerous philopodial, interdigitating processes (FIG. 4(21)). Fibronectin was detected on limited areas of epithelioid cell membranes (FIG. 5(25)), as well as between philopodial processes of adjacent cells (FIG. 5(26)). The intercellular space appeared devoid of interstitial deposits. At the periphery, the granulomas were delimited by a preexisting connective matrix, composed of collagen bundles and fibronectin, that was made evident by immunoperoxidase labeling (FIG. 5(27)).

In mature granulomas, fibroblasts formed a concentric peripheral ring and increased in number from the periphery inwards (FIG. 4(22)). Interstitial matrix deposits associated with the fibroblasts were composed of an unusual compound that was both microfibrillar and fibrillar (FIG. 6(28)). Within the granuloma a similar matrix deposit was observed between epithelioid cells. Philopodial processes were less numerous. Differentiated junctions, however, were present between epithelioid cells (FIG. 6(29)).

Old granulomas were characterized by an extensive connective capsule composed of several concentric layers of fibroblasts associated with the matrix already described. This connective matrix extended throughout the whole granuloma and isolated the epithelioid cells. At this stage these cells had already become elongated (FIG. 6(30)).

Hyalinization was the result of a nearly complete substitution of the granuloma's cells by the connective matrix. The latter was a mixture of fibrous, fibrillar, and granular components associated in either loose or dense patterns (FIG. 7(31,32)).

Immunoperoxidase labeling of matrix proteins revealed that the disposition of each component (collagen types I and III and fibronectin) remained unchanged throughout all the maturative stages of the granuloma (FIG. 7(33-35)).

Labeling of collagen type I showed unusual deposits: fibrils and fibrillar components were disposed in a mixed pattern (FIG. 8(37)); labeling of collagen type III showed fibrils disposed between collagen type I deposits (FIG. 8(38)).

Fibronectin was always present, intermingled with deposits of collagen types I and III (FIG. 8(35,36)).

DISCUSSION

As in all granulomatous diseases, connective interstitial components in sarcoidosis might play an important mediative function between migrating cell populations and adjacent normal tissue during the course of the disease.

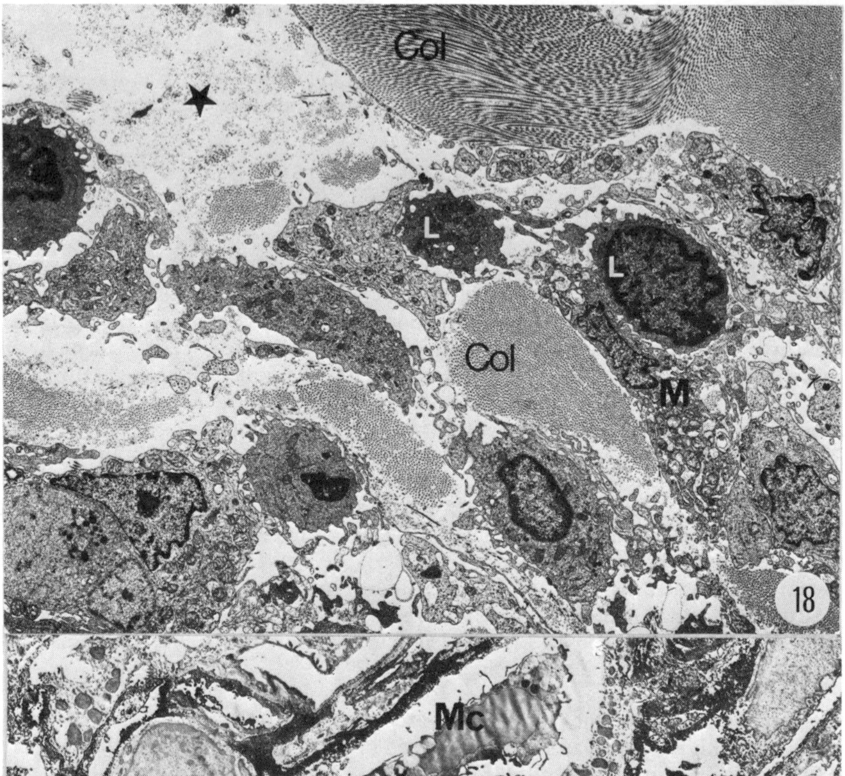

FIGURE 3. The connective matrix of the alveolar septa during alveolitis: (**18**) dense septal bundles of collagen fibers disrupted by edema (× 3500) and (**19**) a local accumulation of immunoperoxidase-labeled fibronectin (× 3000). The original magnifications are shown above in parentheses; each part of the figure was reduced to 92% of its original size. A = alveolus; BM = basement membrane; C = capillary; COL = bundles of collagen fibers; L = lymphocytes; M = macrophages; MC = mast cell; ★ = edema; + = peroxidase labeling linked to fibronectin.

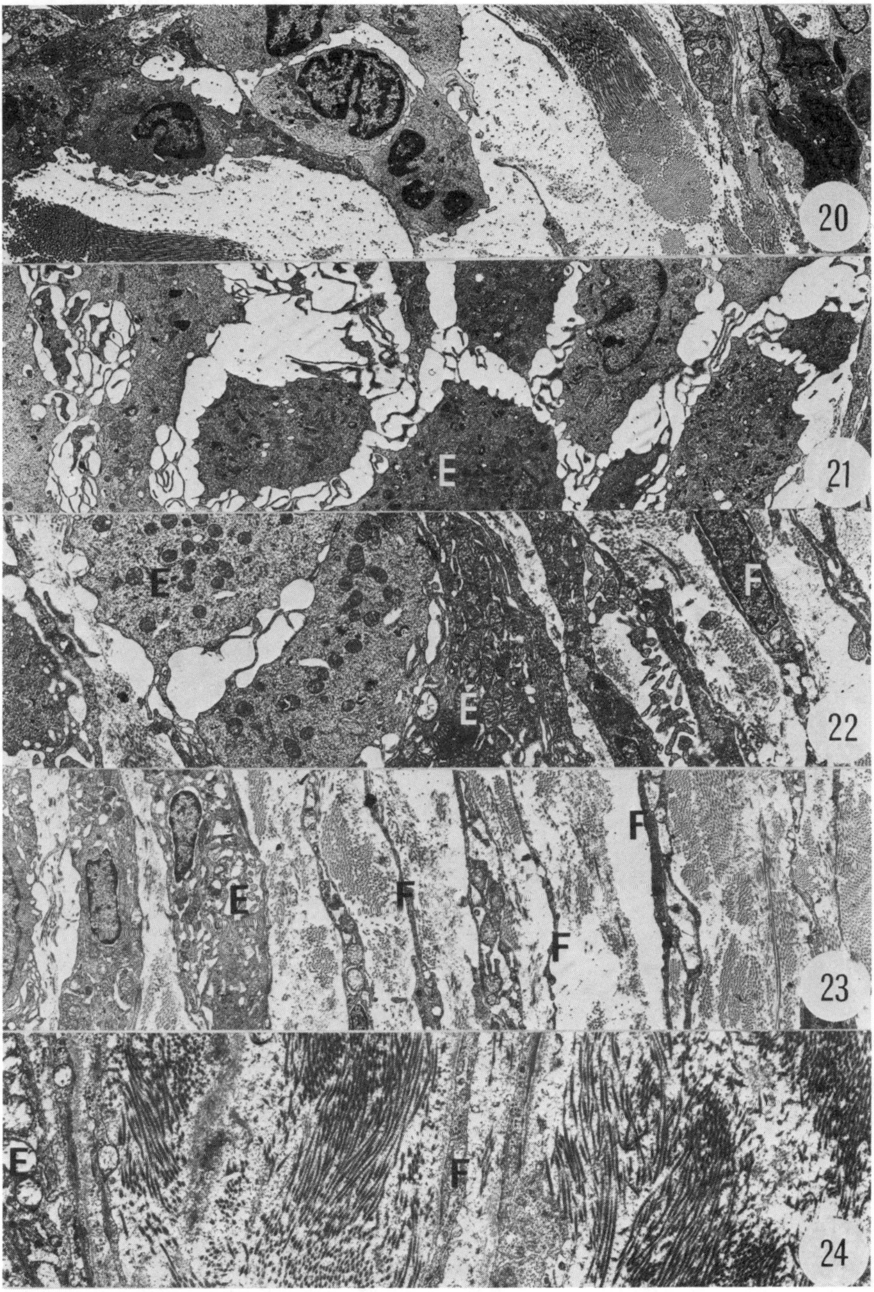

FIGURE 4. Changes in the connective matrix during maturation of the sarcoid granuloma: **(20)** during alveolitis (× 2000), **(21)** in the early-stage granuloma (× 3000), **(22)** in the mature granuloma (× 6000), **(23)** in the old granuloma (× 4000), and **(24)** in the hyalinized granuloma (× 8000). The original magnifications are shown above in parentheses; each part of the figure was reduced to 96.5% of its original size. E = epithelioid cell; F = fibroblast.

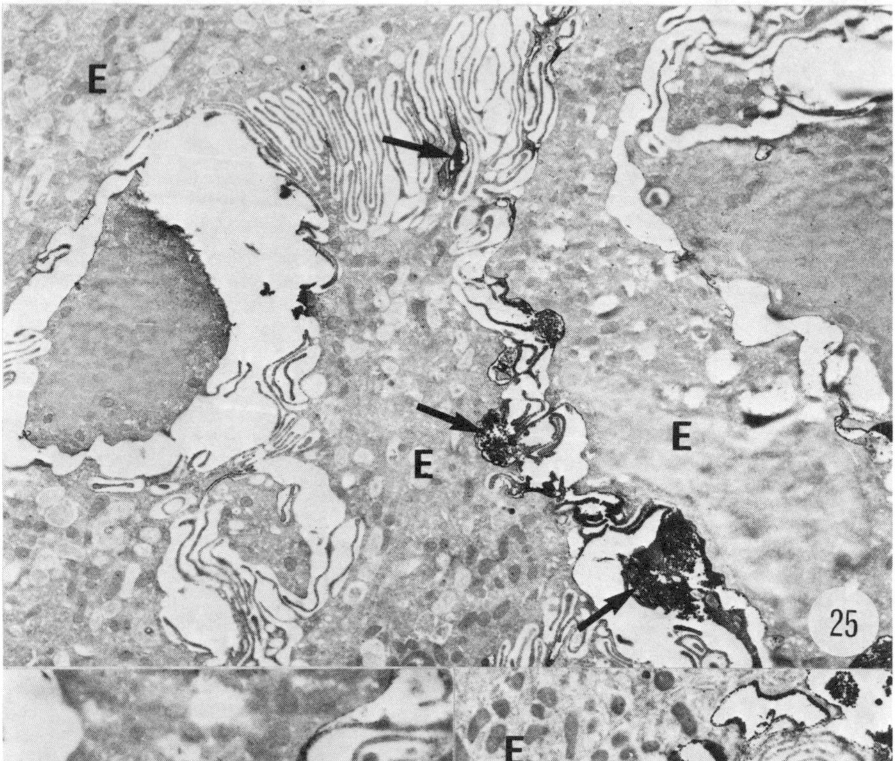
E
E
E
25
E
26
27

As already described in previous studies, a clear-cut difference exists in sarcoid granulomas between peripheral and central areas in cell composition and organization. Peripheral areas, which are composed of fibroblasts, form rings around granulomas; central zones consist of collections of epithelioid cells.[10]

Little attention has been given to interstitial connective tissue in these areas: light microscopic data have distinguished concentric layers of collagen in peripheral areas and a reticulin network in central areas.[4]

This structure disappears in older granulomas, in which the homogenization known as hyalinization is seen. Ultrastructural studies on hyalinized granulomas have demonstrated the distinct aspect of the matrix deposits when compared to classical reparative fibrosis.[6,7] In the former the close association between fibrillar-microfibrillar and granular components results in a polymorphic ground substance. It has been generally assumed that this appearance represents a modification of a previously deposited connective tissue by the addition of new proteins.[7,11–14] It has been claimed that this change is brought about by the binding of immunoglobulin to interstitial collagen fibers[15] because amyloid-like microfibrils have been recognized mixed with collagen components.[6,7] Such an interpretation supports the idea of a modification of a preexisting connective matrix by the addition of a new component. It has also been suggested that hyalin substance could be the result of a slow progressive transformation of the fibrotic matrix, a transformation that might be induced by local proteolytic activity.[16]

No precise and convincing morphological data have been offered, however, to illustrate these two concepts. In the present study, the reexamination by electron microscopy of the characteristic aspect of the sarcoid granuloma's connective matrix during the different evolutive stages leading to a so-called hyalin transformation provided new information. It seems clear that the typical aspect of the connective matrix from early fibrosis to the hyalin stage does not undergo any significant morphological changes. The polymorphic deposits of this matrix first appear around granulomas associated with fibroblasts. It seems significant that the same appearance is also seen in hyalinized ones.

Consequently, our results suggest that the hyalinization process is not a secondary phenomenon, induced either by addition of new substances or by transformation of the connective matrix, but results from a simple rearrangement and/or a more organized morphology, one unique to the sarcoid granuloma, of the different connective matrix components.

To our knowledge the precise site of connective macromolecules in the sarcoid granuloma has never been documented before the present study. Recent studies on these connective matrix macromolecules, however, have demonstrated the production of fibronectin by the human alveolar macrophage[17] and have suggested a mechanism for the recruitment of fibroblasts to sites of tissue injury in the interstitial lung diseases.[18]

In sarcoidosis a similar pathogenetic process may occur: elevations of fibronectin have been demonstrated,[19] and the macrophage appears to be one of the key cells in the progression of this disease.[3] Our results confirm the significant presence of fibronectin throughout the different stages of sarcoidosis. In this respect it was demonstrated

FIGURE 5. Localization of immunoperoxidase-labeled fibronectin in early-stage granulomas: **(25)** on epithelioid cell membranes (× 6000); **(26)** between adjacent epithelioid cells (× 15 000: a more magnified version of **25**); and **(27)** on the periphery of a granuloma, associated with the preexisting connective matrix (× 7800). Fibronectin deposits are indicated with arrows. The original magnifications are shown above in parentheses; each part of the figure was reduced to 96.5% of its original size. E = epithelioid cell.

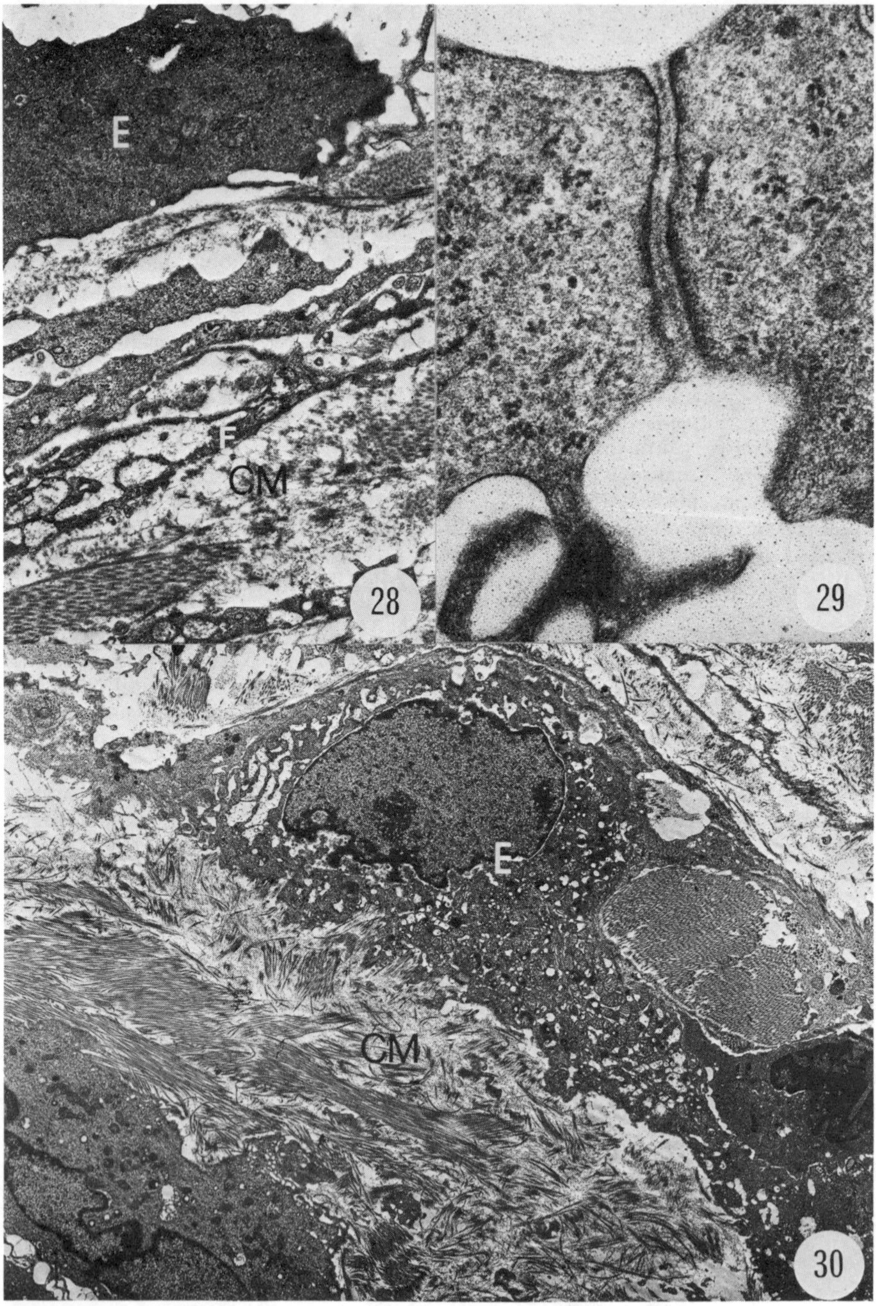

FIGURE 6. Mature and old granulomas: (**28**) matrix deposits on the periphery of a mature granuloma (× 10 000), (**29**) junction between epithelioid cells in mature granulomas (× 25 000), and (**30**) matrix deposits between elongated epithelioid cells in old granulomas (× 2100). The original magnifications are shown above in parentheses; each part of the figure was reduced to 96% of its original size. CM = connective matrix; E = epithelioid cell; F = fibroblastic cell process.

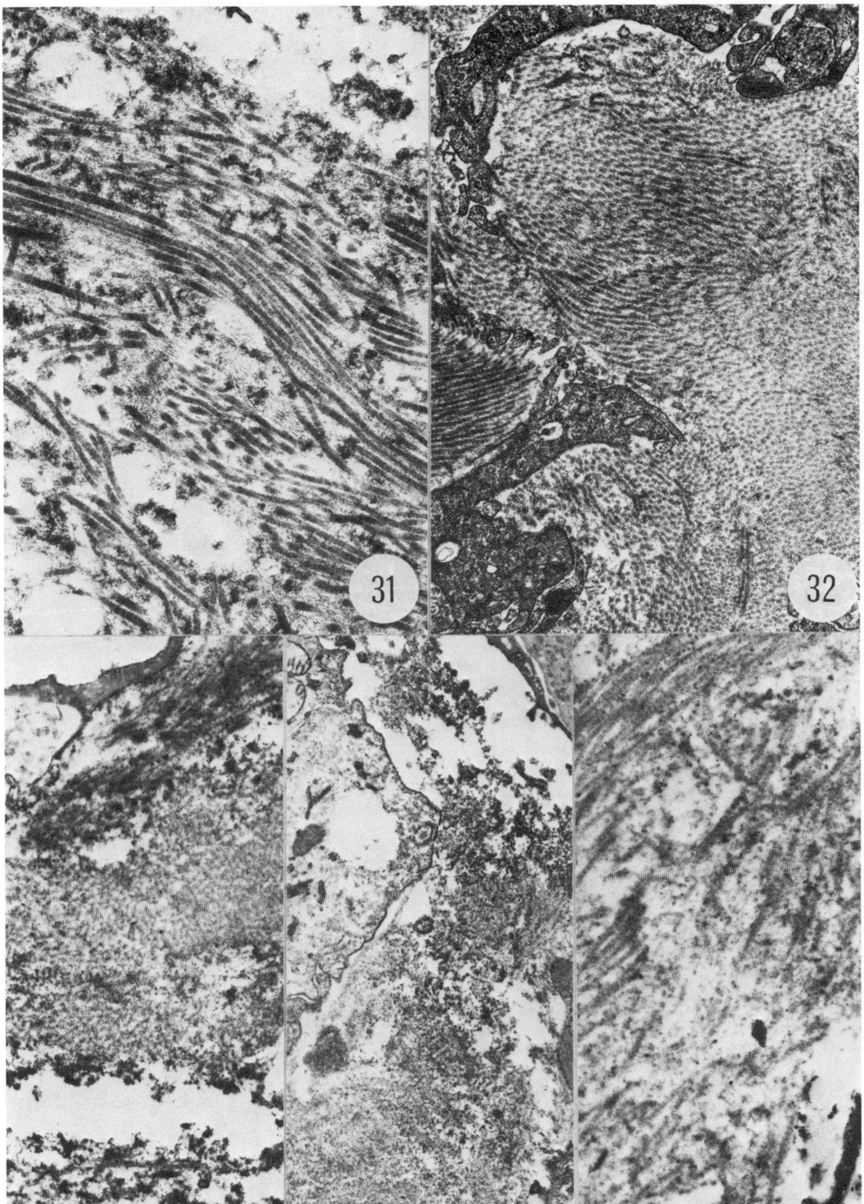

FIGURE 7. A hyalinized granuloma, both loose (**31**) and dense (**32**) aspects (× 25 000 and × 11 200, respectively). Immunoperoxidase-labeled matrix components: (**33**) collagen type I (× 7700), (**34**) collagen type III (× 6300), and (**35**) fibronectin (× 8200). The original magnifications are shown above in parentheses; each part of the figure was reduced to 95% of its original size.

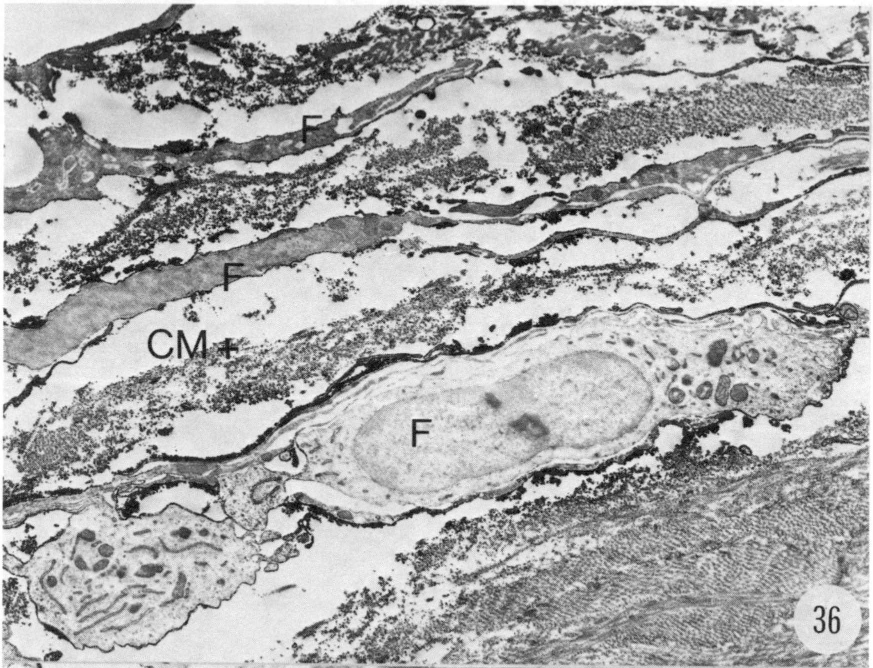
F
F
CM
F
36

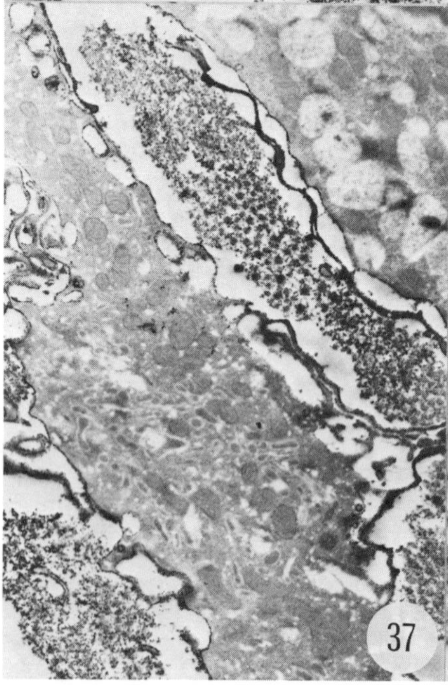
37

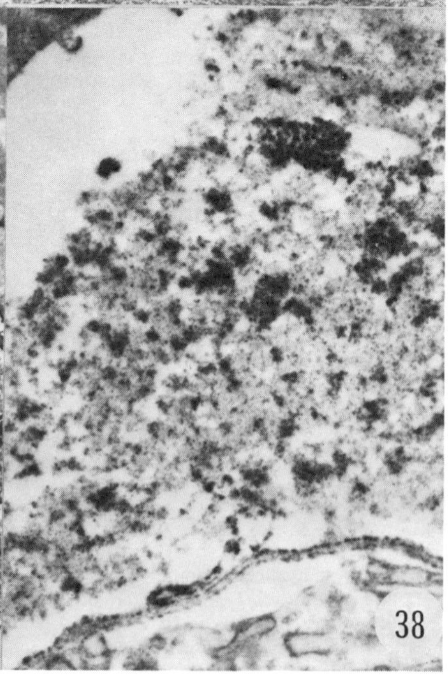
38

that in the early lesion (focal alveolitis) fibronectin was found in large amounts in the interstitium. It is difficult to assess the precise origin of fibronectin deposits at this stage. Two mechanisms seem to be involved simultaneously: following a loss of integrity of the alveolocapillary membrane, passive exudation of plasmatic fibronectin might occur, and local production might occur by inflammatory cells. Similar phenomena have already been documented in various pathological situations where the codistribution of plasmatic and cellular fibronectin appeared characteristic of the acute phase in local injury.[20–22]

Later on, when granulomas are constituted, less fibronectin is found between epithelioid cells. At this stage, numerous philopodial processes, a sign of a search for cell contact, are present on the surface of epithelioid cells. Immunoelectron labeling of fibronectin has shown irregular membranous and interphilopodial deposits. These results suggest a mediative role for fibronectin between different epithelioid cell populations at this stage and a probable local production by these cells. At the same time, it is interesting to note the absence of other matrix components, particularly the interstitial collagens. As the hyalinization of the fibrous deposit progresses, however, newly deposited collagen fibers, upon which fibronectin is bound, may be seen. It is difficult to identify the origin of fibronectin at this stage: recruited fibroblasts appear which probably actively participate in matrix expansion. Finally, fibronectin seems to be one of the basic components of the sarcoid hyalin matrix; our results indicate that the other basement membrane proteins (collagen type IV and laminin) are absent from this matrix. These facts reflect the distinct character of sarcoid hyalin compared to other fibrotic processes, including the hyalinized glomeruli.[23–25] In the latter all the components of the normal matrix are increased whereas in the former only some of them accumulate and form the interstitial excess.

In the sarcoid granuloma, hyalin deposits result from the association between certain connective matrix components. The precise interrelationship between these components remains unknown, but seems to result in an unstable framework. It should be interesting to study the inter- and intramolecular crosslinks. They may well be different from those in other fibrotic lesions.

The mechanism of cellular involvement in the connective matrix degradative process should also be investigated in the sarcoid granuloma: it represents an excellent model of a focal, immunologically dependent, and fully reversible lesion.

SUMMARY

The connective matrix of sarcoid granulomas is polymorphic. Immunolabeling techniques show that it is partly composed of fibronectin and collagen types I and III and is found at all stages of the granulomas' evolution. This suggests that the process known as hyalinization is not due to changes in the composition of the matrix but results from a gradual accumulation of connective tissue components. Fibronectin

FIGURE 8. Immunoperoxidase-labeled CMC's in mature granulomas: (**36**) fibronectin on the periphery of a granuloma (× 5000); (**37**) fibrous and fibrillar collagen type I inside a granuloma (× 12 000); and (**38**) fibrillar collagen type III inside a granuloma, between fibers of collagen type I (× 33 000). The original magnifications are shown above in parentheses; each part of the figure was reduced to 96% of its original size. CM+ = fibronectin associated with matrix deposits; F = fibroblast.

seems to play an essential role as mediator between different cell populations during the evolution of the granulomas.

REFERENCES

1. Jones Williams, W. 1983. State of the art: Granulomas to fibrosis. *In* Sarcoidosis and Other Granulomatous Disorders. J. Chrétien, J. Marsac & J. C. Saltiel, Eds.: 199-203. Pergamon Press. Paris.
2. Mitchell, D. N., J. G. Scadding, B. E. Heard & K. F. W. Hinson. 1977. Sarcoidosis: Histopathological definition and clinical diagnosis. J. Clin. Pathol. **30:** 395-408.
3. Crystal, R. G. 1981. Pulmonary sarcoidosis: A disease characterized and perpetuated by activated lung T lymphocytes. Ann. Intern. Med. **94:** 73-94.
4. Barrie, H. J. & A. Bogoch. 1953. The natural history of the sarcoid granuloma. Am. J. Pathol. **29:** 451-470.
5. Crystal, R. G. 1981. State of the art: The pathogenesis of sarcoidosis. *In* Sarcoidosis and Other Granulomatous Disorders. J. Chrétien, J. Marsac & J. C. Saltiel, Eds.: 13-55. Pergamon Press. Paris.
6. Gusek, W. 1968. Formale Pathogenese der hyalien Tranformation des Sarkoide-granulomas. Virchows Arch. A **345:** 264-275.
7. Kalifat, S. R., M. Bouteille & J. Delarue. 1969. Changes in connective tissue in sarcoid granuloma: Hyalin, paraamyloid and fibrinoid. Electron microscopic study of 11 cases. Virchows Arch. B **3:** 348-358.
8. DeRemee, R. A. The roentgenographic staging of sarcoidosis. Chest **83:** 128-133.
9. Takiya, C., S. Peyrol, J. F. Cordier & J. A. Grimaud. 1983. Connective matrix organization in human pulmonary fibrosis: Collagen polymorphism analysis in fibrotic deposits by immunohistological methods. Virchows Arch. B **44:** 223-240.
10. Soler, P., F. Basset, J. F. Bernaudin & J. Chrétien. 1976. Morphology and distribution of the cells of a sarcoid granuloma: Ultrastructural study of serial sections. Ann. N.Y. Acad. Sci. **278:** 147-160.
11. Teilum, G. 1948. Allergic hyperglobulinosis and hyalinosis (paramyloidosis) in the reticulo-endothelial system in Boeck's sarcoid and other conditions: A morphologic immunity reaction. Am. J. Pathol. **24:** 389-407.
12. Biava, C. G., I. Dyrda, J. Genest & S. A. Bencosme. 1964. Renal hyalin arteriosclerosis and electron microscope study. Am. J. Pathol. **44:** 349-368.
13. Wanstrup, J. & P. Elling. 1968. Immunochemistry of sarcoidosis. Acta Pathol. Microbiol. Scand. **73:** 37-48.
14. Ghose, T., P. Landrigan & A. Asif. 1974. Localization of immunoglobulin and complement in pulmonary sarcoid granulomas. Chest **66:** 264-268.
15. Schauenstein, E. & G. Rumpf. 1952. Physikochemische Befunde an Bindegenebigem hyalin. Z. Biol. **105:** 117-133.
16. Dubreuil, G. & M. Riviere, Eds. 1947. Morphologie et Histologie des Corps Progestatifs et Gestatifs (Corps Jaunes) de l'Ovaire Féminin: Modes de Dégénérescence et Reliquats. Vigot. Paris.
17. Villiger, B., D. G. Kelley, W. Engleman, C. Kuhn III & J. A. McDonald. 1981. Human alveolar macrophage fibronectin: Synthesis, secretion, and ultrastructural localization during gelatin-coated latex particle binding. J. Cell Biol. **90:** 711-720.
18. Rennard, S. I., G. W. Hunninghake, P. B. Bitterman & R. G. Crystal. 1981. Production of fibronectin by the human alveolar macrophage: Mechanism for the recruitment of fibroblasts to sites of tissue injury in interstitial lung diseases. Proc. Natl. Acad. Sci. USA **78:** 7147-7151.
19. Rennard, S. I. & R. G. Crystal. 1981. Fibronectin in human bronchopulmonary lavage fluid: Elevation in patients with interstitial lung disease. J. Clin. Invest. **69:** 113-122.
20. Grinnell, F., R. E. Billingham & L. Burgess. 1981. Distribution of fibronectin during wound healing *in vivo.* J. Invest. Dermatol. **76:** 181-189.

21. REESE, A. C., J. E. DORAN, B. D. CALLAWAY & A. R. MANSBERGER. 1982. Sequestration of fibronectin at the site of injury. Adv. Shock Res. **8:** 119-127.
22. REPESH, L. A., T. J. FITZGERALD & L. T. FURCHT. 1982. Fibronectin involvement in granulation tissue and wound healing in rabbits. J. Histochem. Cytochem. **30:** 351-358.
23. HAHN, E., G. WICK, D. PENCEV & R. TIMPL. 1980. Distribution of basement membrane proteins in normal and fibrotic human liver: Collagen type IV, laminin, and fibronectin. Gut **21:** 63-71.
24. MISRA, R. P. 1981. Recent studies on "hyalinized" glomeruli. Arch. Pathol. Lab. Med. **105:** 599-602.
25. FOIDART, J. M., D. NOCHY, B. NUSGENS, J. B. FOIDART, P. R. MAHIEU, C. M. LAPIERE, R. LAMBOTTE & J. BARIETY. 1983. Accumulation of several basement membrane proteins in glomeruli of patients with preeclampsia and other hypertensive syndromes of pregnancy: Possible role of renal prostaglandins and fibronectin. Lab. Invest. **49:** 250-259.

Introduction to the Louis E. Siltzbach Memorial Lecture

ALVIN S. TEIRSTEIN

Department of Medicine
Mount Sinai Medical Center
New York, New York 10029

It was my privilege and pleasure to introduce the first Louis E. Siltzbach Memorial Lecture, the first of two memorial lectures that were heard at the conference upon which this volume is based. I limited myself to only a few words about Dr. Siltzbach, which follow below, knowing that the excellence of the conference already stood as a fitting tribute to this man.

I first saw Dr. Siltzbach in 1953 when I arrived as an intern at the Mount Sinai Hospital. I found that every evening, someone would be sneaking around our floor with a peculiar, muddy looking material in a vial. He was always very careful not to touch the alcohol swab to the top of the vial, using, in those days, a glass syringe, which he washed with saline, and then performing what looked like a tuberculin skin test. Over the years, we have come to recognize, and revel in, Dr. Siltzbach's brilliance. But it is perhaps not so widely recognized that this brilliance was due in large measure to the diligence reflected by the care with which he handled that vial of antigen. His greatness was not only in his intellect, his scholarship, and his remarkable ability to inspire his students and colleagues, but in his meticulous and diligent attention to detail.

Concepts of Pathogenesis and Lung Reactivity in Hypersensitivity Pneumonitis[a]

HERBERT Y. REYNOLDS[b]

Pulmonary Section
Yale University School of Medicine
New Haven, Connecticut 06510

Among the forms of interstitial lung disease that affect alveolar walls and their supporting tissue, a prominent feature in some is the formation of granulomas, a host defense response that is considered to be part of a cell-mediated immune reaction and evidence of delayed hypersensitivity. Common diseases in this group of granulomatous diseases are sarcoidosis, eosinophilic granuloma, and lymphomatoid granulomatosis. Some diseases involve vascular (Wegener's) structures with necrotizing granulomas or exist as part of an asthmatic syndrome (such as the allergic granulomatous disease of Churg-Strauss). All are of unknown cause. Certain particles inhaled into the peripheral airways, such as those of beryllium or silica, can produce a granulomatous reaction, and a large variety of aerosolized organic dusts can do likewise. This latter group that can be associated with hypersensitivity pneumonitis will be my subject as we review pathologic and immunologic changes which contribute to the acute and chronic forms of alveolitis and interstitial inflammation that may cause respiratory symptoms.[1,2] Although the focus of this international conference is on sarcoidosis, the health impact of hypersensitivity pneumonitis may be even greater because of the occupational nature of many illnesses; the diversity of organic dusts that can sensitize the respiratory tract; the widespread, and even ubiquitous, exposure to antigen that is possible; and the chronicity of lung disease because the correct cause may not be recognized. Moreover, since specific antigens can be identified and used to immunize experimental animals, models of hypersensitivity disease can be created.

CLINICAL FEATURES

Repeated inhalation of a variety of organic dusts can cause hypersensitivity pneumonitis, that is, extrinsic allergic alveolitis. These dusts can be derived from animal dander; proteins from saprophytic fungi that contaminate vegetables, wood bark, or water reservoir vaporizers; and dairy and grain products. Colorful, descriptive names

[a] This work was supported by Grant NHLBI 22302 from the National Institutes of Health.

[b] Address for correspondence: Pulmonary Section, Yale University School of Medicine, P.O. Box 3333, 333 Cedar Street, New Haven, Connecticut 06510.

for the disease underscore the frequent occupational nature of exposure. Implied in the nosologic term is that the affected subject has acquired an abnormal sensitivity or heightened reactivity to the inciting agent and that the resulting host inflammatory response is located primarily in the alveolar air exchange portion of the lung and not in the larger conducting airways, which are usually involved in asthmatic diseases. The distinction is important, for certain asthma syndromes, notably extrinsic, immunoglobulin E (IgE)-mediated allergic asthma, are also forms of hypersensitivity lung disease and are often associated with airborne organic antigens.[3]

A fascinating thing about these hypersensitivity lung diseases is that many people can be exposed to common antigens and many can develop immune reactions to them, usually in the form of specific serum antibodies, yet relatively few people manifest overt respiratory disease. Obviously, a certain degree of unique host susceptibility, or resistance as the case may be, influences the individual response. This is especially true for younger subjects. Sensitization to an organic dust is usually insidious. In certain avocations such as bird handling, almost all people intimately involved in the care of birds develop serum-precipitating antibodies to some avial antigens, but this immune response is not associated with disease in most. Likewise, farm workers may have serum antibodies to certain thermophilic bacteria. The onset of respiratory symptoms may not occur at first but may appear only later, after an exposure pattern is well established.

Although the list of agents that cause hypersensitivity pneumonitis is lengthy, and new etiologies continue to appear, we will focus on two diseases: farmer's lung and bird fancier's or bird handler's lung. Large series of patients have been studied, and most of the recent immunologic research on lung secretions and tissue has been done on these patients.

Farmer's Lung

This was probably the first occupationally related form of hypersensitivity pneumonitis to be clearly described and is probably the most widely recognized form. In fact, it is often used as a synonym for the entire group of these diseases because rural dwellers and those with jobs in gardening or with animals constitute most of the patients. *Micropolyspora faeni* and *Thermoactinomyces vulgaris*, the most important antigens in farmer's lung, are found in moldy hay that has been improperly dried before storage. If the moisture content of the hay is about 40%, temperatures of 60° C or so can develop in the packed layers of vegetation, which is ideal for luxurious growth of thermophilic organisms. Based upon spore counts obtained after shaking moldy hay, theoretically a person working in an atmosphere of moldy hay could have as many as 750 000 spores (0.5×1.3 μm in size)/min deposited in the alveolar areas.[4]

In Campbell's description,[5] the workers had had noticeable shortness of breath for some weeks previously while conducting regular farm chores, including work with hay; such symptoms were accepted in the ordinary course of this farm work. Severe acute disease occurred only after an exceptional exposure, and extreme dyspnea developed within 36 hr. Clearly, antecedent exposure to the hay dust had occurred many times and was associated with tolerable respiratory symptoms. When Campbell actually examined the five reported cases some 3 weeks after the acute illness, dyspnea was still extreme and weight loss was noted in all the patients. Chest rales and sibilant rhonchi were audible over most of the lungs. Chest radiographs showed a generalized, very fine granular stippling and an increasing tendency to fibrosis. Thus, Campbell's cases emphasize the acute and episodic nature of the disease and also dramatize the chronic nature of the disease and its residual injury to the lung parenchyma. One of these farm workers had radiographic evidence of fibrosis and emphysema 18 years later, and another at autopsy had cystic disease of the lungs.[6,7]

Pigeon Breeder's Lung

This disease differs from farmer's lung in that it is caused by inhaled proteins rather than by inhaled microbial antigens and spores. Exposure to excreta and proteinaceous material from pigeons and other birds (geese, chickens, turkeys, and parakeets) provokes the disease. Symptoms follow inhalation of proteins found in bird excreta, which on drying can be easily dispersed as a fine dust.

The disease was described about 15 years ago by two groups of investigators[8,9] and has been extensively studied since. Hypersensitivity to avian proteins causes the two distinct syndromes characteristic of the farmer's lung group: 1) an acute reaction occurring 2-6 hr after heavy exposure and causing dyspnea, chills, fever, malaise, transient restrictive impairment of pulmonary function, and, in the absence of repeat exposure, spontaneous recovery, and, 2) with chronic exposure, persistent shortness of breath and progressive pneumonitis that leads to deteriorating, restrictive lung function. With time the chest radiograph will show a diffuse reticular pattern in the lung fields. The person's serum reveals precipitins against avian proteins found in serum and excreta or against feathers. Usually intimate contact with birds is apparent; this occurs from roosting them as part of a hobby or commercial venture, or through household exposure during caging. Although pigeon proteins (albumin) are the putative cause of sensitivity, excreta can contain various fungi, including *Histoplasma capsulatum* and *Cryptococcus neoformans*, and bacteria, so acute infection is a diagnostic possibility in some cases.

As is true for the other hypersensitivity diseases, persons with the same exposure history and titers of serum precipitins can be symptomatic or asymptomatic, and the individual host factors that determine this intrinsic resistance to overt disease remain unknown. This disease is especially important because it is the one most actively under study in terms of immunopathogenesis.

ACUTE OR EARLY STAGES OF DISEASE

Acute forms of the disease are not seen frequently nor diagnosed readily at this stage. A savvy person might make the connection between environmental exposure and subsequent respiratory symptoms, and voluntary avoidance may solve the problem. When the exposure is job related, this simple solution can be difficult, but the person may gradually develop more tolerable symptoms. Often the worker may not present with symptoms until a chronic stage, and initial inciting factors may then be difficult to identify. A considerable amount of medical detective work is usually required.

The diagnostic approach needed for these kinds of patients requires a thorough history and detailed probing of environmental factors. Finding serum precipitins to environmental antigens can provide a clue to the cause but does not make the diagnosis; a visit to the suspect area and cultures from contaminated appliances are usually needed. Although the patient may have radiographic lung changes and abnormal pulmonary function tests, an inhalational challenge with an appropriate antigen that reproduces the signs and symptoms is the most convincing proof. Skin test reactivity is not as reliable. For chronic forms of disease that may no longer cause acute symptoms, the challenge test is less useful. Open lung biopsy may ultimately be required for diagnosis, although lung lavage and transbronchial biopsy may be sufficient in some cases, as will be discussed. We found the diagnosis to be very difficult in a group of patients with chronic disease who basically had dyspnea and dry cough and on radiographic appearance and pulmonary function testing appeared to have idiopathic pulmonary fibrosis.[10]

Special note should be taken of the presence of precipitating serum antibodies, which have formed much of the epidemiologic basis for selecting potential cases of disease. These do not discriminate between those who are asymptomatic and may remain so (despite a comparable degree of exposure) and those destined to become ill.[11] Moreover, normal persons without ostensible exposure may have incidental precipitins. Such a distinction does not hold up as well in older workers exposed repeatedly for many years because few of these workers escape without some evidence of pulmonary involvement. This variation in the serum immune response following comparable exposure to *Micropolyspora faeni* antigens was studied by Solal-Céligny *et al.*[12] Some dairy farmers with precipitins had acute lung disease, others had positive serum precipitins but were free of respiratory symptoms, yet had evidence of alveolitis when lung lavage cellular and immunoglobulin components were analyzed (asymptomatic disease), and another group had negative serum antibodies and was asymptomatic (but two of the nine had alveolitis detected).

Few patients with acute forms of hypersensitivity pneumonitis have had systematic studies because these patients are rarely encountered; furthermore, once these patients leave the offending environment, and are no longer exposed to the antigen, their symptoms usually abate rapidly. Therefore, it is uncertain what immunologic changes are occurring in the airways during the interval in which the exposed subject is undergoing primary sensitization with an aerosol antigen. This may be a subclinical phase of illness or the subject reacts with acute symptoms of dyspnea, chills, and fever. Animal models can be utilized more precisely to monitor these induction phases of airway immunity: this will be discussed. For humans, before they have been investigated, there has been a considerable period of immunization, even though they may be classified as having "acute" disease. A systemic humoral response (specific serum-precipitating antibodies in the IgG class) is evident, and antibodies are usually present in alveolar secretions, as sampled by lung lavage. There have been few attempts in humans to document immediate changes that occur in the peripheral airways and alveoli of subjects challenged with organic dust antigens, and in those so studied it must be remembered that they are already sensitized and have existing humoral immunity.

Voisin and colleagues[13] compared the clinical and physiological responses in symptomatic patients having acute ($N = 6$) or chronic ($N = 3$) bird fancier's lung with asymptomatic patients (which had serum precipitins to pigeon antigens). For baseline immunologic values, analysis of bronchoalveolar lavage cells that were retrieved from the six patients in the acute category revealed that a high percentage of the cells were alveolar lymphocytes (mean: 72%; range: 56-90%); in concentrated lavage fluid, four out of five specimens that were tested had precipitating antibodies to pigeon serum and high values of immunoglobulins, including IgM, which was found in four out of four samples that were tested. In contrast, patients with chronic disease had a slightly lower percentage of lymphocytes in lavage (mean: 40%; range: 34-45%), less protein, and less immunoglobulin. Only one chronic disease specimen had antibody present; IgM was found in two out of three samples. In asymptomatic subjects (with serum precipitins against serum or pigeon dropping extracts), the lavage fluid cell counts indicated normal lymphocyte levels (range: 10-13%); lavage fluid precipitins were not assayed. These subjects were given an aerosol challenge with various dilutions of pigeon serum (total exposure was limited to 5 min) and observed for 30 hr. No symptoms or physiological changes occurred immediately, but some were noted within 5 hr after challenge. Clinical symptoms of malaise, dyspnea, and auscultation of lung crepitations were recorded in five out of six subjects in the acute group; in one out of three subjects in the chronic group; and in none of the subjects among the previously asymptomatic controls. Fever (> 38° C), leukocytosis, and changes in pulmonary function tests occurred in one-half to two-thirds of the patients in the acute group and in some of the chronic patients (pulmonary function decreased in all three), and no abnormalities were noted in the ostensibly asymptomatic controls.

As a follow-up to the previous challenge study, Fournier and colleagues[14] examined the actual lung cellular response by comparing bronchoalveolar lavage cells before aerosol antigen and after their exposure to aerosol antigens. They studied five acute-stage patients: two normal, previously exposed subjects (with serum antibodies) and one normal, unexposed person. All underwent lung lavage before and after (either at 24 hr or at 48 hr) bronchial provocation with pigeon serum. With antigen challenge, all five acute-stage subjects experienced fever, restrictive changes in lung function, and leukocytosis; these did not occur in the controls. Bronchoalveolar cellular analysis *before* challenge (bronchoscopy and lavage for baseline values had been done 2 weeks before subsequent challenge) for the "acute" subjects revealed an elevated cell recovery (mean: 40×10^6 cells), a high lymphocyte percentage (mean: 61%), and a low polymorphonuclear neutrophil leukocyte (PMN) percentage (about 4%). When four subjects were relavaged 24 hr after antigen challenge, however, the total cell recovery in lavage had increased appreciably (mean: 10×10^7 cells), and PMN's constituted a large percentage of the cells (mean: 44%; range: 18-71%). In two subjects lavaged at 48 hr, however, the respiratory cell count was back to baseline (mean: 44×10^6 cells), PMN's had disappeared (2.5% of the differential count), and lymphocytes were again predominant (71%). In the two normal but exposed subjects and the nonexposed control, lavage analysis after antigen challenge showed no changes from baseline values, that is, no increment in PMN's or total cells. No comments were given about how the "acute" subjects fared with having bronchoscopy and lavage after airway provocation that caused clinical and lung function changes, but presumably no adverse effects occurred with this investigative protocol.

These studies just reviewed represent clinical investigation that may be difficult to perform readily in larger groups of patient volunteers, so it is necessary to use these results as a precious and unique window to view the immunologic responsiveness of the alveolar milieu in immunized subjects, following a specific protein antigen stimulation. As these subjects already had precipitating antibodies in serum and lung secretions against pigeon serum, they probably manifested an Arthus reaction (type III hypersensitivity reaction) in their lungs. It would seem reasonable that antigen-antibody immune complexes were formed in the alveoli and that the subsequent stimulation of the PMN-inflammatory response was mediated by complement activation and/or cellular activation of resident alveolar macrophages whereby local chemotactic factors might attract inflammatory cells. These investigators[15] have indicated in preliminary work that a complement factor, probably C5, was involved in the acute PMN influx that occurred, but the origin of this phlogistic factor has not been determined.

Again, the troublesome question is raised about the asymptomatic person with evidence of alveolitis as reported by Solal-Céligny *et al.*[12] An immunologic response in lung tissue is present, yet clinical disease is suppressed, or, perhaps, is smoldering. Proper advice to give such a worker about job-related environmental exposure must await further longitudinal evaluation of such people. Chronic forms of disease can be quite severe and lung changes can progress to extensive fibrosis and restrictive lung function that characterize other interstitial diseases.

SUBCLINICAL DISEASE IN ASYMPTOMATIC SUBJECTS WITH PERSISTENT EXPOSURE

This situation must occur frequently, given the prevalence of serum precipitins (5-17%) against offending antigens associated with hypersensitivity lung diseases that occurs in apparently healthy farmers. The consequences of having serum precipitins to these antigens were studied by Solal-Céligny *et al.*[12] to see if asymptomatic subjects had any immune reactions in their lungs. Three groups of subjects were sampled by bronchoalveolar lavage, and alveolar secretions were analyzed for cells and immunoglobulins. Seven patients with acute farmer's lung were lavaged within 2 days after cessation of exposure; in the second group, 10 asymptomatic dairy farmers with serum precipitins to *Micropolyspora faeni* were sampled; and, as controls, 10 asymptomatic dairy farmers without serum precipitins were included. As expected, the symptomatic, recently exposed farmers had an increase in the number of cells recovered in lavage fluid, and most of these cells were lymphocytes (72%); furthermore, the levels of immunoglobulins A and G were elevated. In the group of asymptomatic but humorally immune farmers, however, the total yield of cells was somewhat increased (mean: 54×10^6 cells), but less of this total was attributable to lymphocytes (almost 40%). It is notable that the percentage of lymphocytes exceeded 30% in six out of the ten subjects (range: 30-85%). In two of the control farmers without humoral antibody, total cells and lymphocytes were increased in number in lavage. Thus, some asymptomatic farmers can have alveolitis. What to advise such a person in terms of disease progression, lung injury, and avoidance of continued exposure to putative antigens may present a difficult decision for the physician. Cormier *et al.*[16] have provided some long-term follow-up on the natural history of patients that had farmer's lung. Most of the subjects who remained on the farms had persisting alveolitis; 6 out of 15 subjects (about 40%) who left their farms for more than 1 year, and who thus ceased to have antigen contact, had persisting alveolitis, as sampled by bronchoalveolar lavage, but tended to have normal thymus-derived (T) cell helper/suppressor ratios.

CHRONIC DISEASE

If exposure is continuous and protracted, insidious symptoms may progress to a chronic form of disease that no longer features the acute exacerbations of respiratory symptoms, fever, etc. with antigen reexposure. Instead, patients may develop persistent breathlessness, dyspnea with exertion, and cough: symptoms which are indistinguishable from those noted in many other forms of interstitial pulmonary diseases. Fatigue, poor appetite, and loss of weight can be significant in this form of disease. Symptoms and evidence of constitutional effects of disease may be evident for months and occasionally for years before the patient presents them for evaluation. Unfortunately, many patients with hypersensitivity pneumonitis are not diagnosed until this more advanced stage of disease is present. Chest radiographs are abnormal and have telltale changes of interstitial markings and fibrosis. Pulmonary function is characterized by a restrictive ventilatory pattern and a deficit in diffusing capacity for carbon monoxide. Such patients with this chronic form of inhalational hypersensitivity disease can be difficult to separate clinically from other patients with unknown forms of interstitial lung diseases, unless the exposure history happens to be obvious. A serum screen for hypersensitivity antigen precipitins will not establish a diagnosis but, if positive, might orient the clinician toward a possible environmental exposure.

Most of the lung pathology and bronchoalveolar lavage analyses of cells and immunoglobulins have been obtained from patients with chronic disease. Even if the patients are labeled as being in an acute phase because of prominent respiratory symptoms, they in fact have well-established exposure and hallmarks of prior immunity. What is confusing in the sequence of disease is the comparably exposed but asymptomatic subject, perhaps with alveolitis and other airway changes that suggest a smoldering but subclinical stage. As addressed, individual host resistance and other compensating mechanisms must exist to subdue potential clinical manifestations of illness.

A review of lung pathology will be presented, before discussing some of the abnormalities in alveolar secretions, for two reasons: 1) Descriptions of lung biopsy pathology have preceded the more recent lavage fluid studies of cellular immunology. 2) Realization of what histologic changes exist in the interstitial and peribronchiolar areas of the lung will provide a comparison for the bronchoalveolar fluid results and focus the question of how faithful or representative they are of the parenchyma which is not sampled directly with lavage.

Histopathology of Lung Tissue

Although it was known for many years that people could develop chronic lung disease after prolonged exposure to moldy hay, grain, and silage, good descriptions of the pathology did not appear until about 25 years ago. Following the pathologic descriptions of Dickie and Rankin[17] and Totten and colleagues[18] which stressed the granulomatous response of farmer's lung, some other studies have added controversy because their emphasis on terminal airway involvement and on associated vasculitis have proved to be debatable or minor findings.

Seal and colleagues[6] described the pathology in five patients that had acute forms of farmer's lung and in six patients that had chronic disease determined at the time of autopsy. The acute cases usually had lung biopsies done at an average of 10 weeks (range: 3-28 weeks) after a severe attack that prompted evaluation and after about 3 weeks (range: 3-5 weeks) of corticosteroid therapy. These biopsies generally revealed interstitial pneumonia with mononuclear cell infiltration and featured lymphocytes and histiocytes (some with the appearance of foamy cytoplasm) and sarcoid-like granulomas. Bronchiolitis was described, and evidence of vascular thickening and infiltration suggested an element of vasculitis. Such biopsies might be considered representative of early lung changes in the course of the disease, but certainly not of "acute" pathologic changes, as was suggested in the paper, because of the interval before biopsies were obtained and because there were probably anti-inflammatory effects from the 3 weeks or so of corticosteroid therapy. In the chronic stages of disease the necropsy lung specimens showed interstitial pulmonary fibrosis, cystic changes, and residual lymphocytic infiltration of intraalveolar septa, but the noncaseating granuloma phase seemed to have resolved.

Human biopsy tissue is usually obtained from patients with established disease, hence at a time when chronic changes are present in lung tissue. In this context, the pathologic findings cited by Reyes *et al.*[19] should be recalled, which included 60 biopsies secured from patients with farmer's lung (caused by a variety of *Thermophilic actinomycetes*) and which perhaps gives the most careful analysis to date of the pathologic changes that occur. All biopsies contained interstitial pneumonitis described as a patchy infiltrate of the alveolar walls consisting primarily of lymphocytes along with plasma cells and occasionally other inflammatory cells. When the infiltrate was extensive, similar cells were seen within the alveolar spaces. The pathologic pattern was patchy, not uniform, and intervening pulmonary parenchyma did not appear to be involved. In 27 of the 60 biopsies, the degree of interstitial pneumonitis was graded extensive (3+), and all biopsies contained some evidence of it. Unresolved pneumonia, featuring a fibrinous exudate and PMN's, was observed in two-thirds of the specimens. Large histiocytes with foamy cytoplasm were observed in more than half the biopsies. Granulomas were usually present, but none were seen in 18 out of 60 biopsies. It may be difficult to distinguish between granulomas of sarcoidosis and those of hypersensitivity pneumonitis. Their histologies are similar. On the other hand, these granulomas do have different locations: sarcoid granulomas can be found in peribronchial and vascular structures, and hypersensitivity granulomas are usually found in intraalveolar walls and parenchyma. Other prominent findings in the specimens included interstitial fibrosis (65%); bronchiolitis obliterans (50%); foamy histiocytes (65%); granulomas that contained giant cells that in turn contained foreign body material, as determined by polarized light examination (70%); and pleural fibrosis (about 50%). Unfortunately, the biopsies were not separated on the basis of clinical stage of disease as to acute or early versus chronic. Biopsies from our patients showed similar histology: granuloma, interstitial infiltrate with lymphocytes, and foamy macrophages.[10]

Alveolar Milieu—As Sampled with Bronchoalveolar Lavage

As acute forms of these diseases rarely are investigated with bronchoscopy and lung lavage, little information exists about the initial phases of lung inflammation. As just reviewed, when organic antigens are inhaled and deposited in the airways of subjects who have already mounted a primary systemic antibody reponse to the inciting antigen(s), intraairway immune complexes may form to stimulate the cellular reaction, which consists of an immediate influx of PMN's. Several days after inhalational challenge, the lung response shifts to a lymphocytic one, which is characteristic of other granulomatous, delayed hypersensitivity lung diseases. Generally, most patients with a form of farmer's lung or pigeon breeder's disease (bird fancier's lung) have been investigated in subacute or chronic stages of disease. Principal changes in blood and lung secretions are given in TABLE 1.

Peripheral blood values are generally normal in contrast to cellular and protein changes in lung lavage fluid. This same dichotomy exists in sarcoidosis, emphasizing the fact that blood indices are not very accurate means of assessing airway-alveolar inflammatory changes. In bronchoalveolar lavage fluid recovered from patients with established hypersensitivity pneumonitis,[10] lymphocyte numbers are most impressive and account for about 50-60% of the recovered respiratory cells. Lymphocyte percentages are often higher in lung lavages from these patients than they are in those from patients with sarcoidosis, even in the most active phase of sarcoid alveolitis. The morphology of the stained lymphocytes is different. In sarcoidosis most lung lymphocytes are typically a small cell with scant cytoplasm and a large compact nucleus, but in hypersensitivity the lymphocytes are larger, have more voluminous cytoplasm, have a large irregular nucleus, and often resemble a blastic form of the cell.

We conducted an analysis of lung lavage cells and proteins from patients with chronic hypersensitivity pneumonitis.[10] The recovery of respiratory cells in bronchoalveolar lavage fluid (10 specimens) was considerably higher for these patients than it was for nonsmoking controls (1.8×10^7 cells and 6.3×10^6 cells, respectively,

TABLE 1. Immunologic Features of the Blood, Bronchoalveolar Lavage Fluid, and Lung Tissue in Hypersensitivity Pneumonitis

- Blood
  - Normal blood cell counts
  - Normal immunoglobulin levels
  - Positive serum precipitins
- Bronchoaleolar Lavage Fluid
  - Lung cell recovery increased
    - High lymphocyte percentages
      - T lymphocytes predominate
      - Possible to have an increased number of suppressor cells
    - Large and foamy macrophages, a minimal number of eosinophils, and an increased number (up to 1% of all lavage cells) of basophils
  - T cell division high (RNA)
  - Total protein increased
    - Elevated IgG and IgM levels
    - IgG and IgA antibodies present
    - Abnormal surfactant composition
- Lung Tissue
  - Alveolitis
    - Lymphocyte, plasma cells, granulomas, and foamy histiocytes
  - Bronchiolitis
  - Fibrosis

with comparable 100-ml lavages). Lymphocyte levels were quite high (mean: 60%; range: 50-75%); T lymphocytes predominated (80%), and there were few B lymphocytes (6%). The mean T cell/B cell ratio in lavage (14:1) was very different from the one in blood (3:1); the latter ratio is approximately the one found in normals. At the time (1977), T cell populations could not be divided into subpopulations, as can be done now with the currently available monoclonal antibodies. Flow cytometry analysis of lung lavage T cells, based on respective RNA and DNA content, showed that 10-15% of the T cells were in an actively dividing stage.[20] The number of cells in this subpopulation in chronic disease patients was somewhat higher than that noted in stage II sarcoidosis patients. T lymphocytes predominate and can respond to *in vitro* antigen challenges.[21]

In contrast to sarcoidosis, in which lung T helper cells may be increased, suppressor cells may be more numerous in hypersensitivity pneumonitis. Moritz and colleagues[22] studied three pigeon breeders who had been asymptomatic for at least 4 weeks before undergoing lung lavage. Lung function tests and gallium lung scans were normal. In the lavage fluid, all had a higher percentage of lymphocytes (mean: 50%) with an enhanced proportion of T cells (mean: 89%). Monoclonal antisera staining revealed that T helper cell levels were lower than in normals (means: 25 and 46%, respectively) and that T suppressor cell levels were higher (means: 68 and 25%, respectively). The resulting T_H/T_S ratio for these pigeon breeders was 0.4; the normal ratio is about 1.8. Therefore, subjects sensitized to pigeon antigen who have a chronic T lymphocyte alveolitis may have an expanded population of suppressor T cells. Costabel and colleagues[23] also found that among lymphocytes recovered from the lungs of patients with hypersensitivity pneumonitis there were relatively more OKT8-staining (suppressor) cells than there were among lymphocytes from controls or sarcoidosis patients; thus patients with hypersensitivity pneumonitis had a lower T4 cell/T8 cell ratio than did controls (1.1 and 1.6, respectively). More Ia antigen-bearing T cells (identified as activated cells) were present in hypersensitivity pneumonitis patients also. More evidence of this has been provided by Leatherman and colleagues.[24] They studied five asymptomatic pigeon breeders who had at least 10 years of regular exposure to pigeons and six subjects with chronic hypersensitivity, including two pigeon breeders and four patients with farmer's lung (all had appropriate serum antibodies). For controls, eight patients with sarcoidosis and eight healthy nonsmokers were used. Details of the cell counts (mean values) are given in TABLE 2. As shown, the percentage of OKT8-staining lymphocytes (T suppressor cells) was greater in the chronic hypersensitivity and pigeon breeder's groups; these groups had T4 cell/T8 cell ratios of less than 1. In contrast, T cells from sarcoidosis patients had an exaggerated proportion of T helper cells; this group had a high ratio of 4. This switch in the principal type of T lymphocyte in the alveoli of hypersensitivity patients, as compared to those found in normals and sarcoidosis patients, is fascinating, and may be a key finding to understanding more about immunoregulation in the lower respiratory tract.

The appearance of some alveolar macrophages is distinctive. Large cells with excessive cytoplasmic vacuoles (foamy macrophages) may constitute about 10% of the macrophage population, and clumps of macrophages may be found held together by epithelial junctions, as revealed by electron microscopy. Although eosinophils are not increased, as might be expected in an allergic form of lung disease, basophils (considered to be luminal mast cells) are definitely present in increased numbers (but constitute only 1% of respiratory cells).[1,10]

Total protein content in lavage fluid is increased but without a disproportionate increase in albumin, which might point to a significant leak of protein across the endothelial-alveolar barrier. Enhanced immunoglobulin content accounts for some of this because IgG and IgM levels are increased; special elevation of IgG4 was noted in pigeon breeders.[25] Specific antibody activity in IgG and IgA classes can be identified.[10,26] Apparently surfactant has an unusual composition in hypersensitivity pneumonitis, and specimens show increased levels of phosphatidylinositol compared to phosphatidylcholine; levels of phosphatidylethanolamine and glycerol are decreased.[27] The significance of these surfactant changes is uncertain.

EXPERIMENTAL MODELS

Having presented details of the alveolar and peripheral airway alterations that occur, as sampled by lung lavage, in acute and chronic stages of hypersensitivity

TABLE 2. Analysis of Lung Lavage Lymphocytes[a]

	Total Number of Cells ($\times 10^6$)	Lymphocytes (%)	T cells (% T3)	Helper/Inducer Cells (% T4)	Suppressor/Cytotoxic Cells (% T8)	T4:T8 Ratio
Nonsmoking controls	10	16	61	39	24	1.8
Chronic hypersensitivity patients	71	65	76	33	42	0.8
Asymptomatic pigeon breeder's disease patients	36	48	75	29	45	0.7
Sarcoidosis patients	18	38	80	61	19	4.0

[a] Adapted from Leatherman *et al.*[24] Saline solution lavages of 300 ml were used. Entries are mean values.

pneumonitis and reviewed lung biopsy histology from patients with chronic disease, it seems appropriate to examine experimental models that have attempted to create or mimic the human disease process. As the inciting antigens are known and available for immunizing animals, specific models should be possible to design. One tremendous advantage in studying this form of hypersensitivity lung disease is having the specific etiologic agents, which still presents a drawback in trying to create "sarcoidosis" in an animal model. Thus, one would have predicted that farmer's lung or pigeon breeder's disease could be created faithfully in a model, for the aerosol exposure pattern in terms of quantity of antigen deposition, frequency, and prolonged duration of exposure could be controlled (also, antigens could be administered to large numbers of animals). This has not turned out to be the case: the creation of satisfactory models, in general, has been disappointing, and they may not yet exist. The vagrancies of the animal models probably point out what is unknown and still puzzling about human susceptibility to disease from inhaled organic antigens—individual host resistance and the role of adjuvant-like substances to accentuate cellular hypersensitivity. Representative animal models will be reviewed.

Richerson and colleagues[28] sensitized New Zealand white rabbits in their footpads with ovalbumin emulsified in complete Freund's adjuvant (CFA). When the rabbits were challenged 3 weeks later with an aerosol of albumin, serum precipitins to ovalbumin developed. After the challenge, rabbits were killed at intervals, until 10 days had passed, so that changes in lung histology could be seen. No lung changes were apparent 5 hr after the challenge; alveolitis was maximal between 24 and 48 hr and had almost disappeared at 6 days. Only sensitized rabbits who were challenged developed a lung reaction which consisted of a patchy alveolitis of lymphocytes, large mononuclear cells, eosinophils, and plasma cells; peribronchiolitis was found, too, and some vasculitis. Sensitized but nonchallenged rabbits had a few scattered granulomas in lung thought to be due to oil in the adjuvant that escaped as emboli to the lungs. Rabbits only given aerosol antigen had no lung reaction. Thus, a transient acute inflammatory alveolitis was created that did not feature PMN influx and that was resolved in about a week; only with adjuvant was it possible to elicit a reaction. Repeated or prolonged airway sensitization was not attempted.

Moore and colleagues[29] used rabbits of the same species and sensitized them with a pigeon dropping extract by aerosol exposure, 5 days/week for 3-4 months, until serum precipitins to the extract had developed. Then the rabbits received a single intravenous dose of killed bacillus Calmette-Guérin (BCG) suspended in mineral oil and were again given aerosol antigen for another 3-4 weeks as before. Lung histology in this group was examined 6 and 24 hr after the last aerosol dose of extract, and changes were compared with controls given only IV BCG 3 weeks before and no aerosol antigen, and with normal control rabbits. Despite 3 months of exposure to repeated aerosol antigen and the development of specific serum-precipitating antibodies, rabbits had essentially normal lungs and no inflammatory reaction. But, if given a single dose of adjuvant and aerosol antigen challenge was continued another 3 weeks or so, a severe, exudative pneumonitis developed in 6 hr with PMN's in the vicinity of granulomas; however, in 24 hr after the last aerosol exposure, there was a noticeable clearing of the acute exudate and only an increased number of macrophages was apparent. This overall inflammatory reaction was brief considering the prolonged and extensive immunization these animals received. It is noteworthy that airway antigen exposure alone, even in the presence of specific serum antibody, did not produce a lung reaction or evidence of hypersensitivity pneumonitis; only after the introduction of an agent that induced cellular activation in some way (BCG in oil given IV, which probably was deposited almost quantitatively in the pulmonary vasculature) did an acute pneumonitis develop. PMN's were the principal inflammatory cells which responded. No evidence of hemorrhagic alveolitis was found as may be induced when complement fragments (C5a) or preformed immune complexes are instilled in the lungs,[30] for these models of acute lung injury appear to have reactions that are different from the hypersensitivity pneumonitis reactions.

The results of the work on rabbits by Moore *et al.*[29] were similar to the results of our work on monkeys (H. Y. Reynolds *et al.*, unpublished results). A group of five normal *Macaca mulatta* monkeys was given an aerosol exposure of *Micropolyspora faeni* cells. Five-milligram doses of 3-μ antigen particles (spores were not used) were given, during 15-30-min nebulization intervals, three times per week for 3 months. After a few weeks, antibody to the antigen preparation was detected in serum and in alveolar secretions, prepared as concentrated bronchoalveolar lavage fluid. Initial bronchoalveolar lavage fluid cell counts were normal, and about 6% of the cells present were lymphocytes.[31] Biweekly lavage cell analyses obtained during the immunization period, however, revealed no increased numbers of lymphocytes or inflammatory cells. Tissue histology of one lung sampled showed a virtually normal alveolar architecture. Thus, as Moore *et al.*[29] found in rabbits, prolonged aerosol exposure to an appropriate antigen elicited a humoral response, but, after this developed, no acute alveolitis would occur, suggesting that an antigen-antibody complex did not form or was not a sufficient stimulus in the sensitized airways to cause an inflammatory reaction or alveolitis. Only with an injection of a BCG adjuvant and continued aerosol antigen challenge did alveolitis develop that resembled human pathology. Our monkeys were not given a cellular adjuvant, as was done in the second phase of the Moore *et al.*[29] study. We were discouraged at this point, however, that months of arduous airway sensitization of normal subhuman primates would not produce a case of acute hypersensitivity pneumonitis, particularly after precipitating antibodies had formed. Perhaps the group of animals was too small, or perhaps the incorrect antigen was used (cell wall instead of spores). Perhaps unique susceptibility must be present (genetic predisposition) for the disease to result. The point for emphasis, as found in other animal models of this disease, is that it can be difficult to cause lung changes unless an adjuvant is added.

Harris and colleagues,[32] using New Zealand rabbits, inoculated the animals intratracheally with 50 mg of *Micropolyspora faeni* antigen in 3 ml of saline solution at 3-day intervals × 3. At 8 days and 2 and 3 weeks after this immunization, lungs were lavaged and studied histologically. Controls had received only saline injections. Maximal lung changes were observed in the samples taken after 8 days: a patchy pneumonitis was evident, and lung lavage cells reflected an increase in the number of macrophages and a 5% PMN component; the lymphocyte component increased from 2% (as in controls) to 7%. These modest inflammatory changes were no longer evident in the samples taken after 2 and 3 weeks. Although these rabbits did not receive adjuvant and received only three airway immunizations, they developed anti-*Micropolyspora faeni* precipitins in serum and lung secretions within 2 weeks, their skin test reactivity appeared (with both an acute Arthus and delayed component), and their alveolar macrophages displayed some evidence of cellular activation. It is interesting to compare the results of Moore *et al.*[29] and this present work[31] in which the same animal species but different antigen and immunization schedules were used. In both reports, without an adjuvant added, lung histologic changes were modest even with evidence that humoral immunity was stimulated. These findings are consistent with our results with a monkey model in which repeated aerosol antigen applications evoked humoral immunity but no alveolitis or obvious antigen-antibody immune complex injury in the lung.

Bernardo and colleagues[33] used outbred guinea pigs for their model and immunized them with ovalbumin and CFA parenterally. Ten days later, particulate ovalbumin

(2-6 μ in diameter) was instilled intratracheally; for specificity of the response, controls received a particulate human serum albumin or saline solution. Animals were studied immediately after challenge and after 1, 2, 4, and 10 days. Only guinea pigs immunized with CFA plus ovalbumin and given the homologous antigen in the airways developed a pulmonary reaction. This consisted of diffuse hemorrhage and a PMN pneumonitis that began at 4 hr, was maximal by 24 hr, and switched to a mononuclear cell response in 2-4 days; by 10 days the alveolitis had resolved and normal lung architecture was restored. The number of T lymphocytes in the lungs increased between 24 and 96 hr and then decreased, but a similar change in B lymphocytes did not parallel the T cell response. The antigen did cause lymphocyte-blast transformation in the adjuvant-immunized animals. In summary, an acute form of hemorrhagic, inflammatory cell (PMN) alveolitis resulted when guinea pigs were sensitized with adjuvant plus antigen which evolved through a mononuclear cell alveolitis phase and disappeared in 10 days. Similarities between the Richerson *et al.*[28] and Bernardo *et al.*[33] protocols are obvious, with the major difference being the use of rabbits instead of guinea pigs or perhaps the form of antigen used for airway challenge (aerosol of solubilized ovalbumin versus intratracheally instilled particulates). The guinea pigs had a hemorrhagic component of injury in the acute phase, but the rabbits did not. In another rabbit model[34] designed to create an Arthus lung reaction, rabbits were immunized with bovine IgG and incomplete Freund's adjuvant (to develop precipitating antibody without delayed hypersensitivity), then boosted 3 weeks later. One to 2 weeks later they were challenged with the IgG antigen, which was selectively instilled into a lower lobe bronchus. The lung lesions, developing after 6 hr had elapsed, were consistent with an Arthus-like reaction, featuring inflammatory cells (PMN's) and hemorrhage. Again, some form of adjuvant was required.

Fulmer and colleagues[35] used outbred guinea pigs and immunized them parenterally with pigeon serum (1:10 dilution) emulsified in CFA. After boosting the animals 2 weeks later, they allowed 2 more weeks to elapse before the first of four weekly 1-hr aerosol exposures to pigeon serum (1:2 dilution). Thus, the total period of sensitization and exposure challenge was up to 5 months. Animals were sacrificed at various times after the subsequent aerosol exposure intervals. Guinea pigs studied 4-6 hours after the first aerosol exposure had a hemorrhagic alveolitis that evolved, judging from the animals that were studied later, into a PMN alveolitis in 1-3 days. Animals studied after the second or third and fourth aerosol exposures, however, had an interstitial mononuclear alveolitis and some evidence of granuloma formation. This model seems particularly faithful for some of the characteristic lung lesions seen in chronic human hypersensitivity disease. But an adjuvant was required for the initial sensitization and booster injection, and a hemorrhagic phase of alveolitis occurred after the first airway exposure to antigen.

As mentioned, this review of hypersensitivity lung models is neither exhaustive nor inclusive, but these representative studies do underscore some differences between apparent human disease and experimental approaches to it. Animal species do not all react in the same way, and an adjuvant to boost cellular immunity seems to be a requisite for a successful and predictable model. Repeated airway exposure alone is sufficient to elicit humoral and respiratory antibodies but will not create impressive alveolitis. Intraairway administration of adjuvants has not been used because of the unsuitability of oily protein-containing substances which go into the lungs and themselves cause irritation and local inflammation. For humans, many periods of respiratory exposure may occur while the subject remains reasonably asymptomatic. No obvious cellular immunity from concomitant exposure to an adjuvant or infectious agent is known to occur. Antibodies develop. Thereafter, some people with continued exposure have episodic illness, but most others do not, although a few do have subclinical disease and more lymphocytes and antibodies recoverable from their airways (alveolitis?). Productive cough with expectoration that may contain erythrocytes or hemosiderin-containing macrophages, if intraalveolar hemorrhage has occurred, is unusual.

SUMMARY

It is surprising that forms of hypersensitivity pneumonitis do not occur more frequently, given the variety of biologic dusts and airborne antigens that have been found to cause disease. Exposure is almost universal in some occupations that involve handling animals or feed products, and development of humoral immunity occurs in most; however, overt respiratory illness is relatively infrequent or not easily recognized by the subject. What differs between symptomatic and asymptomatic subjects is not certain, but unique host resistance or susceptibility, as the case may be, appears to be a factor. This may have a genetic basis, but this has not been investigated vigorously. With repeated airborne exposure to appropriate antigens, a humoral and a local respiratory antibody response occur but perhaps with little disease consequence, as most subjects so immunized remain clinically asymptomatic. So far as is known, there is no other route of antigenic exposure except through the respiratory tract, but contact with the antigens could occur on the skin or on mucosal surfaces such as the conjunctiva, or antigens could be ingested by swallowing nasopharyngeal secretions. Except for serum antibodies, however, there is little documentation that other systemic organs are affected, as may occur with sarcoidosis. Of course there is great variability in the age of the subjects and the dosage of antigen to which the subject is exposed, and the frequency and duration of exposure can vary considerably. All of these would seem to be easily tested, however, in an animal model where most of the variables could be independently controlled and varied at will. Even the genetic and aging factors, which are the most difficult parameters to control in humans, could be investigated. Yet, it has been very difficult and perplexing not to have created a more faithful model of hypersensitivity pneumonitis in the laboratory. It is virtually impossible to cause predictable lung disease without the use of an adjuvant that will induce some measure of delayed or cellular hyperreactivity. The acute lung disease caused by antigen-antibody reactions seems too explosive and severe, for its acute disease counterpart of hypersensitivity pneumonitis in humans and the persistence of histologic changes in lung tissue is brief and is usually resolved within 1-2 weeks. A chronic model producing granulomas and fibrosis has been difficult to construct, although the work reported by Fulmer and colleagues[35] is very encouraging. For all models, systemic administration of adjuvants has been used, but not via the respiratory tract because suitable adjuvants for contact with mucosal surfaces do not exist or have not been tested in these lung models. Of course this is an ingredient or perhaps a prerequisite that has not been considered in determining susceptibility to disease in humans. Should an adjuvant be looked for? Has a concomitant exposure factor(s) been overlooked, perhaps one delivered in the airway along with the putative antigen? For example, pigeon droppings contain protein, and albumin is considered a probable sensitizing antigen, yet bacterial or fungal products in the droppings (or dust that develops from dried droppings) or an endotoxin-like substance may be respired with the same exposure and contribute to the stimulation of cellular hypersensitivity. There are two points for us to reflect upon: 1) Has the correct combination of airway antigens been determined? 2) Does cell-mediated immunity have to develop simultaneously with humoral immunity before lung disease (alveolitis) occurs?

Another confounding problem in the sensitized subject with humoral and local respiratory antibodies is that some subjects upon reexposure develop acute alveolitis attended by systemic symptoms, leukocytosis, and lung function impairment while others do not. Close inspection of the alveolar milieu, however, with lung lavage analysis of cells and proteins, shows that a low-grade alveolitis is often present[12] and that subclinical disease is present. Some or most of these asymptomatic subjects with continued exposure will convert to a more obvious form of disease, and will occasionally present the hallmarks of chronic disease. Is it simply persistent, recurrent antigen challenge and a culmination of exposure, or is aging, less effective host immunity, or, again, the effect of an unrecognized adjuvant the culprit?

With chronic disease, the lung architecture may have reversible damage, and fibrotic changes are fixed. This may not be true for the granulomatous response which is often prominent in subacute and chronic phases but has been noted to disappear and to resolve. Dynamic granulomas or the kinetics of this part of the inflammatory process need investigation. It could be that beryllium lung disease will provide insight into the resorbable granuloma process.

REFERENCES

1. REYNOLDS, H. Y. 1982. Hypersensitivity pneumonitis. *In* Clinics in Chest Medicine. Vol. **3:** 503-519. W. B. Saunders. Philadelphia, PA.
2. REYNOLDS, H. Y. 1984. Interstitial lung diseases: Classification, definition, and correlation between clinical and histologic staging. Semin. Respir. Med. **60:** 1-19.
3. REYNOLDS, H. Y. 1982. Immunologic lung disease. Chest **81:** 626-631, 745-751.
4. LACEY, J. & M. E. LACEY. 1964. Spore concentrations in the air of farm buildings. Trans. Br. Mycol. Soc. **47:** 547-552.
5. CAMPBELL, J. M. 1932. Acute symptoms following work with hay. Br. Med. J. **2:** 1143-1144.
6. SEAL, R. M. E., E. J. HAPKE & G. O. THOMAS. 1968. The pathology of the acute and chronic stages of farmer's lung. Thorax **23:** 469-489.
7. STUDDERT, T. C. 1953. Farmer's lung. Br. Med. J. **1:** 1305.
8. REED, C. E., A. SOSMAN & R. A. BARBEE. 1965. Pigeon breeder's lung. J. Am. Med. Assoc. **193:** 261-265.
9. HARGREAVE, F. E., J. PEPYS & J. L. LONGBOTTON. 1966. Bird breeder's (fancier's) lung. Lancet **i:** 445-449.
10. REYNOLDS, H. Y., J. D. FULMER, J. A. KAZMIEROWSKI, W. C. ROBERTS, M. M. FRANK & R. G. CRYSTAL. 1977. Analysis of cellular and protein components of bronchoalveolar lavage fluid from patients with idiopathic pulmonary fibrosis and hypersensitivity pneumonitis. J. Clin. Invest. **59:** 165-175.
11. DOPICO, G. A., W. G. REDDAN, F. CHMELIK, M. E. PETERS, C. E. REED & J. RANKIN. 1976. The value of precipitating antibodies in screening for hypersensitivity pneumonitis. Am. Rev. Respir. Dis. **113:** 451-455.
12. SOLAL-CÉLIGNY, P., M. LAVIOLETTE, J. HÉBERT & Y. CORMIER. 1982. Immune reactions in the lungs of asymptomatic dairy farmers. Am. Rev. Respir. Dis. **126:** 964-967.
13. VOISIN, C., A. B. TONNEL, C. LAHOUTE, H. ROBIN, J. LEBAS & C. AERTS. 1981. Bird fancier's lung: Studies of bronchoalveolar lavage and correlations with inhalation provocation tests. Lung **159:** 11-12.
14. FOURNIER, E. C., F. SANTORRO, C. AERTS, C. LAHOUTE & C. VOISIN. 1981. Study of bronchoalveolar lavage before and after the inhalation challenge test in bird fancier's disease: Deduction about immunological mechanism involved. *In* Sarcoidosis and Other Granulomatous Disorders. J. Chrétien, J. Marsac & J. C. Saltiel, Eds.: 578-583. Pergamon Press. Paris.

15. FOURNIER, E., P. GOSSET, A. B. TONNEL, B. WALLAERT, C. VOISIN & C. CAPRON. 1986. Early neutrophil alveolitis after inhalation challenge in bird fancier's disease contemporary of the appearance of a seric neutrophil chemotactic activity. Chest. In press.
16. CORMIER, Y., J. BÉLANGER, P. LEBLANC, J. HÉBERT & M. LAVIOLETTE. Ann. N.Y. Acad. Sci. This volume.
17. DICKIE, H. A. & J. RANKIN. 1958. Farmer's lung: An acute granulomatous interstitial pneumonitis occurring in agricultural workers. J. Am. Med. Assoc. **167:** 1069.
18. TOTTEN, R. S., D. H. S. REID & H. O. DAVIES. 1958. Farmer's lung: Report of two cases in which lung biopsies were performed. Am. J. Med. **25:** 803.
19. REYES, C. N., F. J. WENZEL & B. R. LAWTON. 1982. The pulmonary pathology of farmer's lung disease. Chest **81:** 142-146.
20. PACHECO, Y., G. CORDIER, M. PERRIN-FAYOLLE & J. P. REVILLARD. 1982. Flow cytometry analysis of T lymphocytes in sarcoidosis. Am. J. Med. **73:** 82-88.
21. MOORE, V. L., G. M. PEDERSEN & W. C. AUSER. 1980. A study of lung lavage materials in patients with hypersensitivity pneumonitis: *In vitro* response to mitogen and antigen in pigeon breeder's disease. J. Allergy Clin. Immunol. **65:** 365-370.
22. MORTIZ, E. D., J. M. SMIEJAN, B. A. KEOGH & R. G. CRYSTAL. 1982. Nonfibrotic pigeon breeder's syndrome: A disorder characterized by a chronic suppressor T cell alveolitis. Clin. Res. **30:** 453A.
23. COSTABEL, U., K. J. BROSS, H. MATTHYS & G. N. LOHR. 1982. Cell surface antigens of lung lymphocyte subpopulations in sarcoidosis and hypersensitivity pneumonitis. Bull. Eur. Physiol. Respir. **18:** 143A.
24. LEATHERMAN, J. W., A. F. MICHAEL, B. A. SCHWARTZ & J. R. HOIDAL. 1984. Lung T cells in hypersensitivity pneumonitis. Ann. Intern. Med. **100:** 390-392.
25. CALVANICO, N. J., S. P. AMBEGAONKAR, D. P. SCHLUETER & J. N. FINK. 1980. Immunoglobulin levels in bronchoalveolar lavage fluid from pigeon breeders. J. Lab. Clin. Med. **96:** 129-140.
26. PATTERSON, R., J. L. F. WANG, J. N. FINK, N. J. CALVANICO & M. ROBERTS. 1979. IgA and IgG antibody activities of serum and bronchoalveolar fluid from symptomatic pigeon breeders. Am. Rev. Respir. Dis. **120:** 113-118.
27. JOUANEL, P., C. MOTTA, J. BRUN, C. MOLINA & B. DASTUGUE. 1981. Phospholipids and microviscosity study in bronchoalveolar lavage fluids from control subjects and from patients with extrinsic allergic alveolitis. Clin. Chim. Acta **115:** 211-221.
28. RICHERSON, H. B., F. H. F. CHENG & S. C. BAUSERMAN. 1971. Acute experimental hypersensitivity pneumonitis in rabbits. Am. Rev. Respir. Dis. **104:** 568-575.
29. MOORE, V. L., G. T. HENSLEY & J. N. FINK. 1975. An animal model of hypersensitivity pneumonitis in the rabbit. J. Clin. Invest. **56:** 934-944.
30. JOHNSON, K. J. & P. A. WARD. 1974. Acute immunologic pulmonary alveolitis. J. Clin. Invest. **54:** 349-357.
31. KAZMIEROWSKI, J. A., A. S. FAUCI & H. Y. REYNOLDS. 1976. Characterization of lymphocytes in bronchial lavage fluid from monkeys. J. Immunol. **116:** 615-618.
32. HARRIS, J. O., D. BICE & J. E. SALVAGGIO. 1976. Experimental granulomatous pneumonitis: Bronchopulmonary response to *Micropolyspora faeni* in the rabbit. Chest **61**(Suppl. 1): 287-288.
33. BERNARDO, J., G. W. HUNNINGHAKE, J. E. GADEK, V. J. FERRANS & R. G. CRYSTAL. 1979. Acute hypersensitivity pneumonitis: Serial changes in lung lymphocyte subpopulations after exposure to antigen. Am. Rev. Respir. Dis. **120:** 985-994.
34. ZAVALA, D. C., M. L. RHODES, H. B. RICHERSON & R. OSKVIG. 1975. Light and immunofluorescent study of the Arthus reaction in the rabbit lung. J. Allergy Clin. Immunol. **56:** 450-463.
35. FULMER, J. D., A. FLINT & D. E. LAW. 1983. Experimental granulomatous lung disease in guinea pigs. Lung **161:** 337-348.

Report of the Commission on Granulomatous Diseases

D. GERAINT JAMES[a]

Royal Northern Hospital
London, England

W. JONES WILLIAMS

Llandough Hospital
Cardiff, Wales

INTRODUCTION

This commission was initiated in 1981 by Jacques Chrétien in Paris in order to define those granulomatous disorders which mimic sarcoidosis. They have similar sarcoid granulomas with circumscribed lesions showing aggregates of epithelioid cells, with or without necrosis, that are surrounded by varying numbers of lymphocytes, plasma cells, and fibroblasts (TABLE 1). The disorders under scrutiny may have many such lesions scattered through several organs or may be confined to a single organ or system. It is important to distinguish multisystem granulomatous disease from localized granulomatous reactions (TABLE 2).

CLASSIFICATION

Granuloma-forming disorders are classified under the following headings: infections, reactions to chemicals, immunological abberrations, enzyme defects, neoplasia, extrinsic allergic alveolitis, and miscellaneous disorders. Each of these headings is subclassified.

Infections

Infections remain the commonest contributor to granulomatous disorders worldwide, and for this reason all biopsy specimens must be scrutinized thoroughly for the

[a]Address for correspondence: Royal Northern Hospital, Holloway Road, London N7 6LD, England.

TABLE 1. A Histological Comparison of Various Granulomatous Disorders

Disorder	Features						
	Sarcoid Granulomas	Necrosis	Schaumann's Bodies	Interstitial Cellular Inflammation	Cavities	Vasculitis	Mediastinal Adenopathy
Sarcoidosis	+	–	+++	±	$\underline{\pm}$	±	++
Tuberculosis	+	++ (caseation)	$\underline{\pm}$	±	+	±	+ (primary)
Extrinsic allergic alveolitis	+ (acute stage)	–	±	++	–	++	–
Chronic beryllium disease	+	±	++	++	–	–	–
Wegener's granulomatosis	±	++ (infarction)	–	++ (giant cell)	++	+++	(rare)
Lymphomatoid granulomatosis	±	++	–	++ (immature)	++	++	(rare)
Bronchocentric granulomatosis	+	+	–	(eosinophil)	±	±	(rare)
Necrotic sarcoidal granulomatosis	+	++	–	++ (mature)	+	++	±
Churg-Strauss granulomatosis	+	++	–	++ (mature)	–	++	(rare)

TABLE 2. Differences between Multisystemic Sarcoidosis and a Nonspecific Local Sarcoid Tissue Reaction

Feature	Multisystemic Sarcoidosis	Local Sarcoid Tissue Reaction
Number of organs or systems involved	Several	Usually one
Ages of patients with the disease (years)	20-50	Any
Skin lesions	Frequent	
Chest radiograph	Abnormal (88%)	Normal
Slit lamp examination of eyes	Abnormal (15%)	Normal
Tuberculin skin test	Negative (66%)	Variable
Kveim test	Positive (80%)	Negative
Serum angiotensin-converting enzyme level	Elevated (60%)	Normal
Calcium metabolism	Abnormal (20%)	Normal
Response to corticosteroids	Good	Variable

NOTE: The percentages are those of patients in whom the given conditions applied.

causative organisms (TABLE 3). Tuberculosis, schistosomiasis, and leprosy are still common granulomatous infections in some parts of the world. The local histologist will be well acquainted with indigenous infections, but the speed of travel across the world now makes it imperative that we should all be aware of this wide range of causative agents.[1]

Reactions to Chemicals

Chronic beryllium disease contiunues to be a hazard because of its wide use in various industries, including metallurgy, ceramics, and atomic energy. The diagnosis is based on a history of exposure, compatible clinicoradiographic features in lungs and skin, widespread granulomas, the presence of beryllium in tissues and urine, and the beryllium lymphocyte transformation test.[2]

Other chemicals liable to produce granulomas are zirconium, which causes axillary deodorant granulomas; talc; and silicon. Pulmonary talc granulomatosis is due to inhalation or intravenous administration of talc or intravenous pentazocine which is 75% talc. Patients thus exposed had positive gallium scans, raised serum angiotensin-converting enzyme levels, and bronchoalveolar lymphocytosis. Measurement of talc crystals is of value in distinguishing injected (average size: 14 μm) from inhaled crystals (average size: 3.5 μm).[3,4] Polydimethylsiloxane fluid, or, silicone fluid, is widely used in breast augmentation and other cosmetic purposes. Injections and implants may give rise to granulomatous pulmonary infiltration and to granulomatous hepatitis.[5]

Immunological Aberrations

There is an immunological background or basis for a diverse number of granulomatous disorders. Some primarily affect the lung or alimentary tract, others are multisystemic. The defect may be associated with disordered cell-mediated immunity, humoral immunity, or immune complexes, or characterized by a prominent vasculitis. Some disorders are associated with more than one of these defects (TABLE 4). Their differentiation from sarcoidosis is made by a distinctive clinical picture, as in Crohn's regional enteritis, acquired immune deficiency syndrome (AIDS), giant cell arteritis, Peyronie's disease, and the Melkerrson-Rosenthal syndrome; serological tests, as in systemic lupus and hypogammaglobulinemia; histology; and electron microscopy, as in histiocytosis X.

Enzyme Defects

Chronic granulomatous disease of children (CGDC) is due to a leucocyte oxidase defect.

Killing of bacteria depends on a burst of respiratory enzyme activity, which leads to the production of hydrogen peroxide and superoxide in phagocytes. Neutrophils in CGDC, because they are deficient in enzymes needed for this superoxide respiratory burst, are unable to kill some ingested bacteria. Enzymes that may not be present in adequate amounts include nicotinamide adenine dinucleotide phosphate (NADPH) oxidase, myeloperoxidase, cytochrome *b,* pyruvate kinase, glucose-6-phosphate dehydrogenase, lysozyme, and lactoferrin. Each deficiency could contribute to a different clinical profile.

The classical X-linked disorder occurs in boys aged about 5 years, presenting with hepatosplenomegaly, generalized lymphadenopathy, weeping granulomatous skin lesions, and diffuse miliary lung infiltration. The histology is of multisystemic sarcoid granulomas. There may be more than one X-linked form and also more than one autosomal recessive variety. The group is heterogenous because there are now reports

TABLE 3. Causative Organisms of Granulomatous Disorders[a]

Bacteria	Fungi
Brucella	*Blastomyces dermatidis*
Francisella tularensis	*Coccidioides immitis*
Proprioni	*Histoplasma capsulatum*
Yersinia	*Sporthrix schenckii*
Mycobacteria tuberculosis	Aspergillus
M. leprae	*Cryptococcus neoformans*
M. kansasii	
M. intracellulare	Other
M. marinum	Chlamydia[c]
M. bovis[b]	Spirochaetes
	Treponema
	Leishmania
	Toxoplasma gondii
	Schistosoma
	Toxocara

[a] The organisms listed below constitute the infectious causes of granulomatous disorders, as described in the text.
[b] Bacille Calmette-Guérin.
[c] Associated with cat-scratch disease and lymphogranuloma.

of defective oxidative metabolism with phagocytic stimuli such as bacteria but not with nonphagocytic, soluble metabolic stimuli such as sodium fluoride or concanavalin A. There is certainly more than one mechanism for initiating oxidative metabolism.

Patients with CGDC only suffer from catalase-producing staphylococci and enterobacteria. Organisms that lack catalase supply the neutrophil with the hydrogen peroxide for their own destruction. Thus catalase-negative organisms, such as pneumococci or streptococci, present no problem to these patients.

Neutrophil leucocytes of normal patients with bacterial infections reduce colorless nitroblue tetrazolium to form blue-black formazan granules in the cytoplasm. This fails to occur in the leucocytes of children with CGDC or of mothers of children with the X-linked disorder.

Neoplasia

Granuloma formation is observed in reticuloses and in lymph nodes draining carcinomas. It is a well-recognized feature of pinealoma, dysgerminoma, seminoma, and malignant nasal granuloma. Sarcoid granulomas may be seen in lymph nodes draining carcinomas of the breast, stomach, thyroid, and ovaries and may sometimes be seen within these tumors. The granulomas of Hodgkin's disease commonly have eosinophils, which are absent in those of sarcoidosis.

There have been many claims of an association between neoplasia and sarcoidosis whereas others feel that the association is fortuitous rather than established.[1]

TABLE 4. Granulomatous Disorders Associated with Immunological Aberrations

T Cell Defects[a]	Vasculitis
Sarcoidosis	Giant cell arteritis
Crohn's regional enteritis	Wegener's granulomatosis
Primary billiary cirrhosis	Churg-Strauss granulomatosis
AIDS	Necrotizing sarcoidal granulomatosis
	Lymphomatoid granulomatosis
B Cell Defects	Unclassified Disorders
Hypogammaglobulinemia	Peyronie's disease
Immune Complex Disorders	Histiocytosis X
Systemic lupus erythematosus	Rosenthal-Melkerrson Syndrome (granulomatous cheilitis)
Circulating immune complex diseases	
Hepatic granulomatous disease (granulomatous hepatitis)	

[a] Disordered cellular immunity.

Extrinsic Allergic Alveolitis

A thorough occupational history should provide a pointer to extrinsic allergic alveolitis (hypersensitivity pneumonitis), which may be provoked by many different allergens (TABLE 5). The causative agent is not apparent by histology, but the presence

TABLE 5. Nature and Sources of Organic Dust Antigens in Extrinsic Allergic Alveolitis[a]

Disease	Dust Exposure	Antigen or Nature of Antigen with which Precipitin Is Formed
Farmer's lung	Moldy overheated hay	*Micropolyspora faeni* / *Thermoactinomyces vulgaris*
Bagassosis	Moldy overheated sugarcane bagasse	*Thermomycete sacchari*
Mushroom picker's lung	Mushroom compost dust	Thermophilic actinomycetes / mushroom spores
Maltworker's lung	Moldy barley or malt	*Aspergillus clavatus*
Bird fancier's lung	Pigeon and budgerigar droppings	Avian serum protein antigens
Pituitary snufftaker's lung	Powder of porcine and bovine posterior-pituitary extract	Serum protein and pituitary antigens
Wheat weevil disease	Infested wheat flour	*Sitophilus granarius*
Maple stripper's lung	Infected maple bark	*Cryptostroma corticale*
Sequoisis	Moldy redwood sawdust	*Aureobasidium pullulans* / *Graphium pullularia*
Suberosis	Cork dust	*Polyspora frequenta*
Woodworker's lung	Sawdusts of oak, cedar, etc.	Molds
Cheese washer's lung	Molds on cheese	*Penicillium* species
Paprika splitter's lung	Paprika	
Humidifier or air conditioner lung	Contaminated forced air system	Protozoa / Amoebae

[a] Revised by Dr. John Edwards.

of circulating precipitins is of diagnostic value. Granulomas are present in the acute stage but not in the chronic fibrotic stage of the disease, a distinctive contrast from chronic beryllium disease. The granulomas may be indistinguishable from those of sarcoidosis on light microscopy, electron microscopy, and histochemistry. The prominent alveolitis in this family of allergic disorders helps to segregate them from sarcoidosis (TABLE 6).

Miscellaneous Disorders

Granuloma formation may be prominent in several other clinical situations, but it should not be misconstrued as sarcoidosis. The conditions are unrelated to each other and are difficult to classify in earlier headings. They include chalazions, sebaceous cysts, dermoidal skin, annular granulomas, panniculitis, and Whipple's disease. Granuloma formation may also be noted after radiotherapy and cancer chemotherapy. Finally, its presence in patients with pyrexia of unknown origin and with allergic drug reactions may provide diagnostic pitfalls.

CONCLUSION

Sarcoidosis has many clinical and histological mimics. This joint clinicohistological classification of granulomatous disorders (TABLE 7) provides a modern differential

TABLE 6. Differences between Sarcoidosis and Extrinsic Allergic Alveolitis

Feature	Sarcoidosis	Extrinsic Allergic Alveolitis
Histology		
Granuloma distribution[a]	Widespread	Centrilobular
Interstitial pneumonitis	Mild	Prominent
Schaumann bodies	70%	5%
Occupational history	No	Yes
Systemic character	Always	Sometimes
Erythema nodosum	Common	Absent
Hilar adenopathy	Frequent	Very rare
Wheezing	Rare	Common
Uveitis	Frequent	Absent
Depression of delayed-type hypersensitivity	Yes	Yes
Circulating precipitins	Absent	Present
Raised or abnormal immunoglobulin levels	Yes	Yes
Kveim-Siltzbach test	Positive	Negative
Serum angiotensin-converting enzyme levels	Raised	Normal
Abnormal calcium metabolism	Frequent	Absent
Response to steroids	Good	Good
Prognosis	Good	Good, if removed from exposure to antigen

[a] The granulomas of sarcoidosis were identical to those of extrinsic allergic alveolitis.

TABLE 7. A Classification of Granulomatous Disorders

Infections (See TABLE 3)	
Reactions to Chemicals	
Immunological Aberrations (See TABLE 4)	
Enzyme Defects	
Neoplasias	
Reticulosis	Dysgerminoma formation
Reticulum cell sarcoma formation	Seminoma formation
Carcinoma formation	Malignant nasal granuloma formation
Pinealoma formation	
Extrinsic Allergic Alveolitis (See TABLES 5 & 6)	
Miscellaneous Disorders	
Chalazion formation	Granuloma annulare
Dermoidal skin	Reactions to radiotherapy
Sebaceous cyst formation	Reactions to cancer chemotherapy
Whipple's disease	Allergic reactions to drugs
Panniculitis	Pyrexia of unknown origin

diagnosis of sarcoidosis. It will, it is hoped, reduce the frequency with which the label sarcoidosis is mistakenly applied to clinical situations, to biopsy material, or to radiographic shadows. This analysis may also bring to light common denominators which may provide clues to the etiology of sarcoidosis.

FUTURE PROSPECTS

This commission was initiated during the conference held in Paris in 1981, and its subject, the classification of granulomatous diseases, will be a subject for future world congresses. It is hoped that the following questions will be addressed: 1) the geographic distribution and frequency of various granulomatous disorders throughout the world; 2) whether there are any granulomatoses that are mutually exclusive with sarcoidosis, such as tuberculosis in China or schistosomiasis in the Middle East or leprosy in Africa; 3) the reason why there is an increased recognition of sarcoidosis in India and Africa (Is it possible that sarcoidosis emerges in the wake of tuberculosis and leprosy?); and 4) whether the local environment in any part of the world contributes to any particular granulomatous disorders.

REFERENCES

1. JAMES, D. G. & W. JONES WILLIAMS. 1985. Sarcoidosis and Other Granulomatous Disorders. W. B. Saunders. Philadelphia, PA.
2. JONES WILLIAMS, W. & W. R. WILLIAMS. 1983. The value of beryllium lymphocyte transformation tests in chronic beryllium disease and in potentially exposed workers. Thorax **38:** 41-44.

3. FARBER, H. W., R. P. FAIRMAN & F. L. GLAISER. 1982. Talc granulomatosis: Laboratory findings similar to sarcoidosis. Am. Rev. Respir. Dis. **125:** 258-261.
4. ABRAHAM, J. L. & C. BRAMBILLA. 1979. Particle size for differentiation between inhalation and injection pulmonary talcosis. Am. Rev. Respir. Dis. **119:** 196.
5. CHASTRE, J., F. BASSET, F. VIAN, P. DOURNOVO, A. BOUCHAMA, A. AKESBI & C. GILBERT. 1983. Acute pneumonitis after subcutaneous infections of silicone in transsexual men. N. Engl. J. Med. **308:** 764-767.

Immunoregulation of Granuloma Formation in Murine Schistosomiasis Mansoni[a]

DOV L. BOROS[b]

Department of Immunology and Microbiology
Wayne State University School of Medicine
Detroit, Michigan 48201

INTRODUCTION

Life Cycle

Schistosomiasis mansoni is a tropical disease that affects over 120 million people.[1] It is caused by a trematode worm that measures 1.5 cm in length and lives in the mesenteric veins of infected humans or animals. The worms live in pairs, and each adult female produces about 300 eggs daily. The eggs contain a live embryo: the miracidum, which has to hatch in fresh water and find its intermediate host, the snail, in order to continue its life cycle. Miracidia within the snail undergo a complicated metamorphosis and after several weeks emerge in a new form: the fork-tailed cercariae. The free-swimming cercariae infect their definitive hosts, humans, upon water contact (fishing, washing, swimming, etc.) by skin penetration. After penetration cercariae shed their tails and transform into schistosomula that are adapted to live in the salty environment of the body. The young schistosomula migrate from the skin to the lungs by way of blood vessels and lymphatics and reside there for several days. During this time they grow and become impervious to the humoral or cellular attack of the host. The schistosomula then descend to the liver where they finish their maturation process and eventually reach their final habitat, the mesenteric venules. Here the mating of the sexes takes place, and the worm pairs live in perpetual copulation. Their life span is 5–10 years. During their residence in the blood stream, the worms successfully evade the immune attacks of the host by a variety of means, one of them being the acquisition and binding of host antigen onto their outer body surface: the tegument.

Pathology of the Disease

As part of their nutrition the worms ingest host red blood cells. This causes only negligible blood loss. In previously exposed individuals, reexposure to cercariae may

[a]This work was supported by Grant AI-12913 from the National Institutes of Health.

[b]Address for correspondence: Wayne State University School of Medicine, 540 East Canfield Avenue, Detroit, Michigan 48201.

cause dermatitis. In heavily infected persons, reexposure to *Schistosoma mansoni* may elicit Katayama fever, which is manifested by fever, hepatosplenomegaly, lymphadenopathy, and eosinophilia. The syndrome is suggestive of a serum sickness type of immune reaction. The main pathology of the disease, however, is due to the antigenic secretions of the eggs[2] that lodge in the liver and intestines and the subsequent host granulomatous response. The severity of the disease is in direct proportion to the number of eggs present in the tissues. The liver sustains the most damage during the disease. Chronic granulomatous inflammations heal by fibrosis that is cumulative over the long period of the disease. The development of "clay pipestem" fibrosis in the livers of infected humans may be the result of granulomatous inflammations as well as other still undefined host- and parasite-derived factors. In a certain number of genetically predisposed individuals, hepatosplenic disease develops.[3] It is characterized by hepatosplenomegaly, portal hypertension, ascites, the formation of esophageal varices, hematemesis, and, occasionally, death. The development of collateral portasystemic circulation allows the dissemination of eggs into the lungs, where granuloma formation, arteritis, and cor pulmonale develop.

MURINE MODEL OF SCHISTOSOMIASIS MANSONI

Our understanding of the pathology of the disease was greatly advanced by the development of the murine model. Mice infected with *S. mansoni* develop granulomas in the liver and intestines and elicit the clinical syndrome of hepatosplenomegaly tissue fibrosis, portal hypertension, ascites formation, and bleeding.[4] Injection of schistosome eggs alone also evokes granulomas at the site of embolization. This model is advantageous in that it utilizes synchronously growing granulomas, delineates the dynamics of the evolution and involution of the lesions, and excludes the histopathologic changes that obscure the granulomatous process in the infected animals. This model demonstrated that pulmonary granuloma formation was evoked by soluble egg antigens (SEA)[5] secreted by the glands of the mature miracidium. The antigens are a mixture of proteins, glycoproteins, and polysaccharides. The antigenic principle(s) are most probably glycoproteins[6,7] that sensitize the host to a T lymphocyte-mediated immune reaction. The T cell-mediated nature of the schistosome egg-induced granuloma has been confirmed by various experimental means. Granuloma formation was adoptively transferred by T lymphocytes but not by antiserum;[8] it could be suppressed by applying drugs (azathioprine or corticosteroids) and antilymphocyte or antithymocyte sera—means that eliminate T lymphocytes or suppress their activity.[9] Granuloma formation was greatly diminished in thymus-deprived normal mice or in athymic nude mice.[10–12] Finally, granuloma formation was correlated with the development of other parameters of T cell-mediated immune responses such as delayed skin reaction, lymphokine production, and antigen-induced lymphoproliferation.[13]

MODULATION OF THE GRANULOMATOUS INFLAMMATORY RESPONSE

An important early observation established that mice displayed diminished granulomatous reactions around freshly deposited eggs during the chronic stage of a light infection of *S. mansoni.*[14] Concurrent with the formation of smaller granulomas, an improvement in the pathophysiology of the disease was also recorded. This spontaneously modulated granulomatous response was then examined in great detail. As the disease reached the chronic stage, dynamic changes took place in the lymphocyte populations of the infected mice. A shift in the ratio of T lymphocytes to B lymphocytes favoring the latter was observed in the circulation, lymph nodes, spleen, and granulomas of the chronically infected mice.[15] Moreover, the number of anti-SEA antibody-producing plasma cells within the hepatic granulomas significantly increased.[16] A detailed immunological analysis has shown that chronically infected mice not only displayed down-modulated granulomatous responses, but also showed a lack of delayed skin responses to SEA, without exhibiting generalized anergy to other unrelated antigens. Whereas lymphokine production was maximal at the acute stage of the infection, at the chronic stage the splenic and lymph node lymphocytes ceased to produce macrophage migration-inhibitory factor (MIF)[17] and eosinophil-stimulation promoter (ESP) lymphokines.[18] The latter observations strongly indicate a link between diminished granuloma formation and impaired inflammatory lymphokine production.[19] With the progress of the infection an almost exponential rise was recorded in the level of circulating anti-SEA antibodies. Taken together, the changes in lymphocyte dynamics and function clearly indicate that certain regulatory mechanisms are active in the chronically infected mice. This assumption was corroborated by the adoptive transfer of lymphocytes of chronically infected mice to acutely infected mice (mice with 6-week-old infections) that resulted in diminished liver granulomas.[20] An analysis of the lymphocytes that adoptively transferred liver and lung granuloma suppression revealed that they are T cells that display I-associated (Ia) membrane antigens (FIG. 1). Significantly, following cell transfer, the numbers of Ia antigen-positive T lymphocytes also increased in the adoptively suppressed liver granulomas. The question of specificity was settled by showing that the transferred T lymphocytes did not suppress pulmonary granulomas that formed around artificial beads coated with unrelated antigens.[21] By the use of alloantisera that recognized membrane markers on the surface of T lymphocytes, a further delineation of the regulatory T cells was possible. Thus, the T lymphocytes that exerted suppression over the acutely infected animals' cells between 6 and 8 weeks after infection were further identified as belonging to the Lyt-1^+ subset of cells.[22] More light was shed on the complexity of regulatory mechanisms by adoptive transfer studies which utilized admixtures of splenic cells, which were taken from acutely or chronically infected mice and given to normal mice. Baseline observations established that when 4×10^7 splenic cells of acutely infected mice (mice with 8-week-old infections) were injected, along with eggs, into normal animals, a significantly more enhanced pulmonary granulomatous response was transferred than when splenic cells derived from chronically infected donors were injected. Admixture of 2×10^7 purified T lymphocytes obtained from the spleens of acutely or chronically infected donors resulted in a significant suppression of granulomas as measured 2 days after cell transfer. Alloantisera and complement treatments that selectively eliminated certain subsets of lymphocytes provided further information. Thus, the lymphocytes that transferred enhanced granulomatous responses in the recipients were identified as Lyt-1^+ T inflammatory cells that participate in delayed hypersensitivity reactions (T_{DH} cells). In contrast, the lymphocytes from chronically infected donors that suppressed the granuloma induction by T_{DH} cells were classified as Lyt-2.3^+ T suppressor (T_S) cells (FIG. 2).[23]

It is to be emphasized that mice which exhibit modulated responses still possess the capacity for granuloma formation, albeit at a diminished level. Moreover, their splenic lymphocytes are capable of transferring subdued granuloma formation in normal recipients. It was inferred from this that the state of modulation is to be

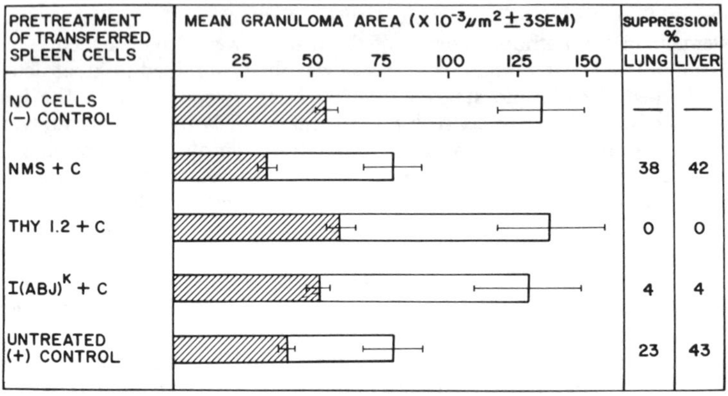

FIGURE 1. Abrogation of adoptive suppression by treatment of spleen cells with Thy-1 and Ia antisera. Spleen cells of donors with 32-week-old infections were treated with the indicated antisera or normal serum. Twenty million viable cells were transferred to each recipient. There were six mice in each group. Mean areas of lung (hatched bars) and liver (open bars) granulomas are shown. Reproduced from Chensue and Boros[21] by copyright permission of the American Association of Immunologists.

regarded as a dynamic process in which the inflammatory and regulatory lymphocytes interact in a way that favors the suppressor mode. This was corroborated by experiments in which chronically infected mice were injected with cyclophosphamide, a drug known to kill the rapidly dividing T_S cells or their precursors. Drug treatment indeed shifted the equilibrium. Because T_S cells were eliminated, the anticipated reversal of the modulated granulomatous response occurred. Restoration of vigorous granuloma formation was accompanied by the reappearance of MIF-active lymphokine production in the splenic cells of the majority of treated mice.[22] Similarly, injections of antiserum directed against the I-J subregion of the major histocompatibility complex (MHC) of CBA^k strain mice given to chronically infected animals also reversed granuloma modulation. This indicated that the T_S lymphocyte(s) that participate in the regulatory process display I-J subregion membrane markers, that is, are I-J^+.[24]

A central but as yet unanswered question concerns the signal(s) that trigger T_S cell activity. A large amount of an antigen that directly interacts with T lymphocytes may be one of the signals.[25] A changed mode of antigen presentation that specifically triggers T_S rather than T_{DH} cell activity has also been postulated.[26] Whereas no clues are available as yet in the schistosome model, evidence exists for the very early presence of T_S cells in the infected animals. When mice that have 8-week-old infections and are at the peak of their granulomatous response are splenectomized[27] or treated with cimetidine, a further enhancement of the granulomatous response is observed.[28] Apparently the removal of a low number of T_S cells (or their precursors) or the inhibition of their function by blockading H_2 receptors with cimetidine mitigated the incipient suppressor effect and allowed the full expression of the inflammatory activity of T_{DH} cells. Thus, an equilibrium between inflammatory and regulatory cells is present even at the early phase of the infection, but it is maintained in the inflammatory mode.

Over the years one major tenet was the relationship between inflammatory lymphokine production and granuloma formation.[29] Liver granulomas isolated from acutely infected mice produced,[30] whereas those obtained from animals that underwent modulation did not produce,[19] lymphokines. As mentioned previously, elimination of T_S cells restored both enhanced granuloma formation and lymphokine production.[22] Thus, analyzing the regulation of lymphokine production seemed a profitable approach for understanding the process of modulation. By means of alloantisera, we characterized the MIF lymphokine-producing cells in the spleens of mice with 8-week-old infections as non-Ia, Lyt-1^+ T_{DH} lymphocytes. These cells, in all probability, are identical with those that adoptively transfer the granulomatous response to normal recipients. Next, it was established that splenic lymphocytes of mice with 8-week-old infections produced MIF-active lymphokine, whereas cells derived from mice with 20-week-old infections did not. Admixture of the two cell populations in equal numbers resulted in the abrogation of lymphokine production (FIG. 3). Abrogation was specific because lymphokine production by an unrelated antigen was unhindered. By alloantisera, the suppressor population in the spleens of mice with 20-week-old infections was identified as belonging to the Lyt-2.3^+ T cells that also displayed I-C and I-J subregion membrane markers, that is, as a Lyt-2.3^+ I-C^+ I-J^+ T_S cell.[31] These studies delineated the interaction between an inflammatory and regulatory subset of lymphocytes in which the latter prevailed. The interaction must have occurred rapidly because *in vitro* lymphokine production occurs within hours of antigen stimulation, and the whole test is concluded within 20 hr. The rapidity of interaction indicated the involvement of soluble factor(s) that mediated the suppressor signal(s). Indeed, the existence of such suppressor factors (SF's) was proven by harvesting supernatant fluids

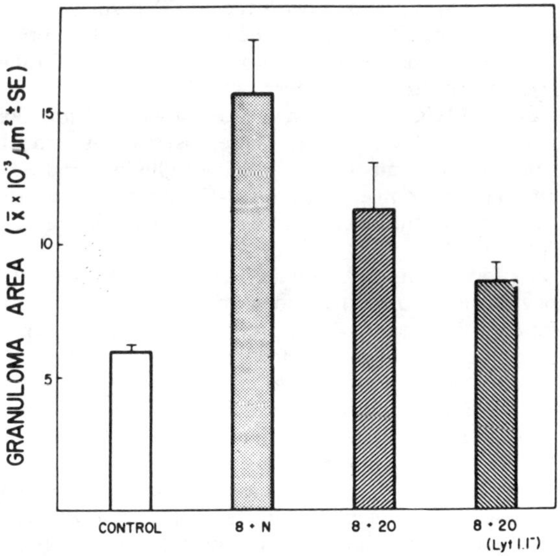

FIGURE 2. Suppression of adoptive granulomatous hypersensitivity in normal recipients with splenic suppressor T cells of mice with 20-week-old infections. Twenty million nylon wool-purified splenic T cells from mice with 8-week-old infections were mixed with an equal number of splenic T cells from normal mice (N) or cells purified by plate bonding from mice with 20-week-old infections before transfer into recipients. Spleen cells from mice with 20-week-old infections were depleted of Lyt-1.1-bearing cells with alloantiserum and complement prior to mixing. Reproduced from Wellhausen *et al.*[23] by copyright permission of the Elsevier Science Publishing Company.

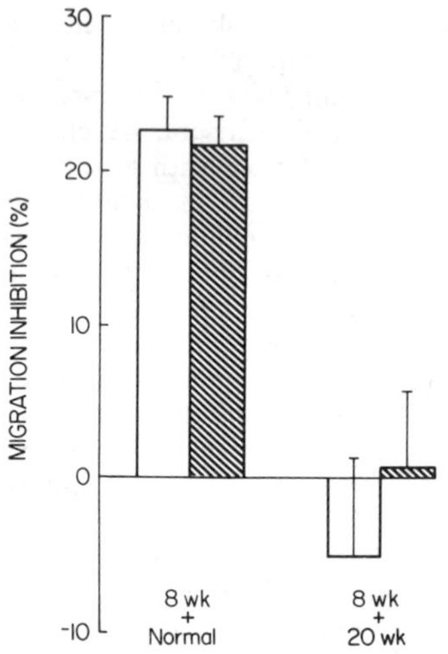

FIGURE 3. Suppression of MIF activity of splenic cells from mice with 8-week-old infections and from mice with 20-week-old infections. Equal numbers of spleen cells from mice with 8- and 20-week-old infections were mixed and added to 10^6 normal peritoneal exudate cells in graded doses (open bars: 5×10^4; hatched bars: 1×10^5) and then assayed for MIF activity. Bars represent means, and error bars SEM's, of three separate experiments. Reproduced from Chensue *et al.*[31] by copyright permission of the Rockefeller University Press.

from antigen-pulsed and cultured splenic cells of chronically infected mice. Supernatant fluid even in diluted form suppressed the *in vitro* production of lymphokine by splenic cells from mice with 8-week-old infections or SEA adjuvant-sensitized mice. The cell that produced the factor was identical with the one that suppressed T_{DH} cell activity and lymphokine production. SF acted specifically only on SEA-primed lymphocytes, and showed genetic restriction because it was ineffective on histoincompatible lymphocytes. Suppression was strong, however, with lymphocytes that shared the genes of the H-2 locus of the MHC, and was narrowed down to compatibility at the I-AB and I-C subregions of the H-2 complex. These observations strongly indicated that SF is composed in part of Ia membrane antigens. This was indeed corroborated by immunoadsorbant columns coupled with anti-I-C subregion antiserum that removed suppressor activity, and by the demonstration of suppression using I-C$^+$ substance eluted from the columns (FIG. 4).[32]

That granuloma formation and regulation depend on subsets of functionally different T lymphocytes has also been demonstrated in an *in vitro* model. *S. mansoni* worm pairs maintained in tissue culture produce embryonated eggs. Following the addition of splenic lymphocytes of infected mice, mononuclear cells adhere to the surface of the deposited eggs. In a few days, eggs show a variety of cellular reactions that range from a few adherent cells to complete circumoval aggregates. The cells that surround the eggs are lymphocytes, macrophages, and eosinophils—the actual components of the *in vivo* granuloma. The circumoval reaction is T lymphocyte dependent, and the effector cell is identified as an Lyt-1$^+$ cell.[33] Closely following the *in vivo* model, splenic cells of acutely infected mice formed larger, and those of chronically infected animals smaller, lesions around cultured eggs. Admixture of the two populations diminished the intensity of the cellular reaction. Alloantisera and complement treatment of splenic cells of chronically infected mice showed that the cell that exerted the suppression was an Lyt-2.3$^+$ T lymphocyte. When splenic cell populations of chronically infected mice became enriched with Lyt-1$^+$ T cells and such cells were mixed with splenic cell populations from acutely infected mice, or with cell populations from normal mice, a suppression of the granuloma was observed. From the foregoing it was concluded that splenic lymphocytes contain both inflammatory T_{DH} lymphocytes and at least two kinds of regulatory T_S cells: one that directly suppresses inflammatory T_{DH} cell activity (Lyt-2.3$^+$ cell) and another that can induce suppressor cell production in a normal splenic population (Lyt-1$^+$ suppressor/inducer cell).[34]

The experiments carried out *in vivo* and *in vitro* shed light on the complex interactions that take place during the process of regulation of the granulomatous response. Moreover, strong indications were obtained for the activity of soluble suppressor factors that convey suppressor signals among cells. Attempts to prove the relevance of SF in *in vivo* suppression, however, remained unsuccessful. In our laboratory, repeated injections of crude or affinity column-purified SF (I-C$^+$ SF) into vigorous granuloma-bearing mice failed to modulate the granulomatous response. It is possible that the relatively minute amounts of SF that were obtained from the immunoaffinity columns were simply inadequate to carry out the effect. Another laboratory, which used a different cell preparation, successfully demonstrated granuloma suppression. Cell-free sonicates obtained from the spleens or thymus cells of chronically infected mice and administered repeatedly over a period of 2 weeks to mice with 6-week-old infections suppressed both liver and lung granulomas. The extracts also suppressed the SEA-elicited delayed skin reactivity of infected mice. The suppression was specific because it did not affect an antigenically unrelated system.[35]

In order to gain further insight into the initial phase of the process of modulation, we examined the ability of SF in the recruitment of a suppressor population. To this end, splenic lymphocytes from mice with 8-week-old infections were used. Despite the vigorous granuloma-forming capacity of the mice it was previously shown that they possess a low contingent of suppressor lymphocytes. Splenic cells were incubated for 2 days with crude SF or I-C and I-J subregion-specific substances purified on immunoaffinity columns. At the end of the incubation period, washed cells were mixed with equal numbers of freshly harvested splenocytes from mice with 8-week-old infections, and the cell mixture was injected along with schistosome eggs into normal recipients. A significant suppression was achieved with crude as well as I-J$^+$ SF (FIG. 5). Again, the factor acted specifically, not influencing granuloma formation in an unrelated artificial granulomatous system. Because the number of I-J$^+$ cells increased over the period of incubation, and suppression was eliminated with anti-Thy-1.2 antiserum and complement, we concluded that the recruited suppressor lymphocyte was an I-J$^+$ T_S cell.

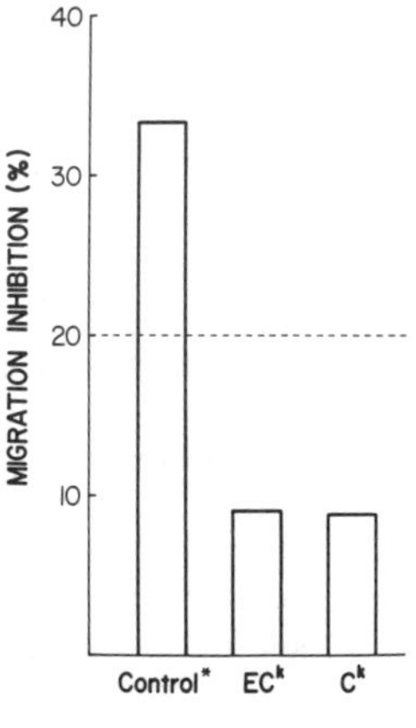

FIGURE 4. Suppressive effect of acid eluates from anti-I subregion immunoadsorbants. Immunoadsorbants that had bound MIF suppressor factor were treated with glycine buffer (pH 2.8) to elute bound material. Eluent material was dialyzed against fresh medium, reconstituted with antibiotics and serum, and then tested for suppressive activity. The control migration inhibition was considered to be that in the presence of eluate from a normal mouse serum column which did not remove suppressor activity. The dotted line shows baseline inhibition in a 1:2 dilution of normal spleen cell supernatant. Bars represent means of two separate experiments. Reproduced from Chensue *et al.*[32] by copyright permission of the Rockefeller University Press.

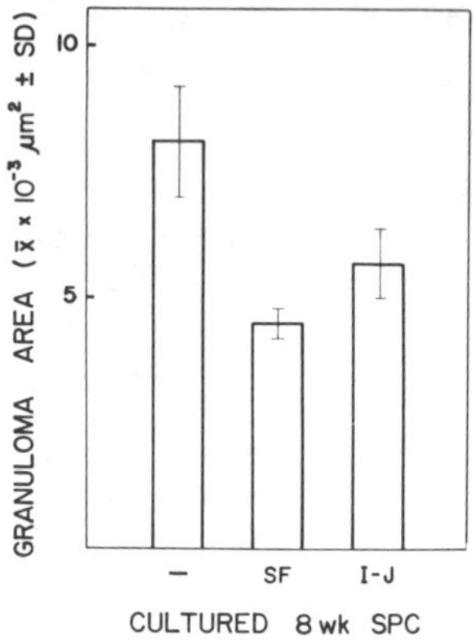

FIGURE 5. Recruitment of suppressor lymphocytes by soluble suppressor factor. Splenic lymphocytes from mice with 8-week-old infections were cultured for 48 hr with crude suppressor factor or I-J^+ factor eluted from an immunoadsorbant column. Then lymphocytes were washed and mixed with an equal number of freshly harvested splenic lymphocytes from mice with 8-week-old infections. The cell mixture along with eggs was injected IV into normal recipients. Granulomas were measured 2 days later.

So far it has been shown that SF's not only differ in their molecular composition, but also carry out different, direct suppressor or suppressor recruitment functions. Though these molecules seem to arise from the membranes or cytoplasm of suppressor lymphocytes, their exact composition still remains to be elucidated. Because the factors were specifically absorbed by affinity columns there is no doubt that part of their functional moiety is composed of I-C and I-J subregion membrane antigens. These antigens are known to promote cell-cell interactions in the murine immune system. The component that lends antigenic specificity to the system is still unknown. Among the substances that can specifically select T cells, one can enumerate the antigen and idiotypic or anti-idiotypic T cell determinants. According to a recent report, the partial characterization of SF that suppresses schistosome granuloma formation was achieved. Crude SF obtained from the thymus gland extracts of chronically infected mice exerted *in vivo* suppression of the granuloma only when homology existed at the I-J^k subregion of the H-2 complex between donor and recipient. Columns that carried bound SEA's did not remove suppressor activity, indicating that SF apparently did not comprise a T cell receptor with antigen-specific idiotype. Suppressor activity was absorbed, however, by immunoaffinity columns with bound anti-SEA IgG antibody. The inference from these experiments was that the suppressor molecule expressed anti-idiotypic reactivity and carried I-J subregion membrane determinants.[36] Whether the various receptors and determinants constitute one complex is still to be confirmed.

SUMMARY AND CONCLUSIONS

Schistosomiasis mansoni is a chronic, T lymphocyte-mediated granulomatous disease that affects mainly the liver and intestines of the infected host. The chronic inflammatory process and subsequent fibrous repair are the major factors in the pathology of the disease. In the murine model of schistosomiasis at the onset of the chronic stage of the infection, the granulomatous response undergoes spontaneous modulation with concomitant alleviation of the pathologic disturbance. Analysis of the process of modulation revealed that it results from the interaction between inflammatory and regulatory subpopulations of T lymphocytes. At the acute phase of the infection, the granulomatous response is initiated and maintained by inflammatory

T_{DH} cells that release lymphokines which mobilize and recruit the macrophages, eosinophils, etc. for the generation of the lesion. Already at this stage, while the inflammatory influence prevails, a low number of suppressor T lymphocytes are present. With the progress of the infection, the overheated inflammatory response is curbed by regulatory processes. At least two, but perhaps more, T suppressor lymphocytes are involved in the maintenance of the modulation of the granulomatous response. Modulation is an active process that needs constant maintenance, probably by recruitment of fresh suppressor cells. Removal of the suppressor population causes an immediate elevation of the granulomatous response. During modulation, T suppressor lymphocytes either abrogate or greatly diminish inflammatory lymphokine production. This in turn may be the cause for decreased cell recruitment and diminution in newly formed granuloma size. Apparently a total abrogation of the granulomatous response is not desirable because released egg antigens can be harmful to liver parenchyma cells. This has been demonstrated both in thymus-deprived and in nude, infected mice.[37,38] Thus, a smaller inflammatory response has the double advantage of not only being less destructive, but also shielding the underlying tissue from damage by parasite products. The various subpopulations of T lymphocytes communicate with one another by means of soluble suppressor factors that arise from the suppressor T cells. The factors may have different functions. One factor may regulate lymphokine production whereas another may recruit fresh suppressor cells from a pool of precursors. The factors act in an antigen-specific manner. Tentatively, one may assume that these factors are composed of two units: one is the I subregion membrane marker and the other is the specific recognition receptor. The nature of this receptor is still unclear, but it may be an anti-idiotypic determinant. Thus, for successful cell-cell interaction, a receptor for the I subregion membrane antigens as well as one for the proper idiotype-bearing T lymphocytes are necessary (TABLE 1).

In the foregoing, T cell circuitry that functions in the spleens of schistosome-infected mice has been characterized. It is inferred that the regulatory mechanisms that modulate inflammation are expressed at the level of the granuloma. Thus, future research is concentrated on the dynamics of the interacting T lymphocyte populations found within the granulomas.

Though research described in this review pertains to the murine model of schistosomiasis mansoni, an increasing number of clinical observations indicate that similar regulatory processes may also take place in infected humans. Suppressor T lymphocytes that regulate the specific proliferative responses of peripheral blood lymphocytes have been found in the circulation and spleen of infected humans.[39] Patients with hepatosplenic schistosomiasis had decreased numbers of $T4^+$ lymphocytes in the circulation and showed a decreased $T4^+$:$T8^+$ cell ratio.[40] Though it awaits confirmation, it is

TABLE 1. Summary of T Lymphocyte Interactions That Occur during the Modulation of the Granulomatous Response

1. The granulomatous response is mediated by T_{DH} lymphocytes that secrete inflammatory lymphokines.
2. The modulated granulomatous response results from the dynamic interaction between T_{DH} and T_S cells with decreased or abrogated lymphokine production.
3. Modulation is maintained by T_S cell-T_S cell interaction in which T_S precursor/helper lymphocytes generate T_S effector cells that exert suppression over T_{DH} cells.
4. T_S cells interact by means of I subregion-encoded, antigen-specific suppressor factors.
5. I-C^+ suppressor/effector factor acts on T_{DH} cells. I-J^+ suppressor/recruiter factor acts on T_S precursor cells.

likely that humans during the chronic phase of the infection also modulate their granulomatous responses.[41]

There is still much to learn about the mode of interactions among the inflammatory and regulatory subsets of T lymphocytes. At least experimentally, the manipulation of the granulomatous response has become feasible. Whereas the modulated inflammatory response appears to be advantageous to the infected host, it is still to be elucidated how the suppressed state influences tissue damage and repair. As the role of soluble suppressor factors becomes clearer, it will not be a farfetched belief that such natural regulatory substances may one day find clincial application in the modulation of the granulomatous response.

REFERENCES

1. WARREN, K. S. 1982. Immunol. Rev. **61:** 189-213.
2. HANG, L. M., K. S. WARREN & D. L. BOROS. 1974. Exp. Parasitol. **35:** 288-298.
3. ABDEL-SALAM, E., S. ISHAAC & A. A. F. MAHMOUD. 1979. J. Immunol. **123:** 1829-1831.
4. DEWITT, W. B. & K. S. WARREN. 1959. Am. J. Trop. Med. Hyg. **8:** 440-446.
5. BOROS, D. L. & K. S. WARREN. 1970. J. Exp. Med. **132:** 488-507.
6. PELLEY, R. P., R. J. PELLEY, J. HAMBURGER, P. A. PETERS & K. S. WARREN. 1976. J. Immunol. **117:** 1553-1560.
7. BOROS, D. L., R. TOMFORD & K. S. WARREN. 1977. J. Immunol. **118:** 373-376.
8. WARREN, K. S., E. O. DOMINGO & R. B. T. COWAN. 1967. Am. J. Pathol. **51:** 735-756.
9. WARREN, K. S. & D. L. BOROS. 1975. *In* Mononuclear Phagocytes in Immunity, Infection and Pathology. R. van Furth, Ed.: 1015-1028. Blackwell. Oxford.
10. BUCHANAN, R. D., D. P. FINE & D. G. COLLEY. 1973. Am. J. Pathol. **71:** 207-214.
11. PHILLIPS, S. M., J. J. DI CONZA, J. A. GOLD & W. A. REID. 1977. J. Immunol. **118:** 594-599.
12. AMSDEN, A. F., D. L. BOROS & A. T. HOOD. 1980. Infect. Immun. **27:** 75-80.
13. BOROS, D. L., H. J. SCHWARTZ, A. POWELL & K. S. WARREN. 1973. J. Immunol. **110:** 1118-1125.
14. DOMINGO, E. O. & K. S. WARREN. 1968. Am. J. Pathol. **52:** 369-380.
15. CHENSUE, S. W. & D. L. BOROS. 1979. Am. J. Trop. Med. Hyg. **28:** 291-299.
16. BOROS, D. L, A. F. AMSDEN & A. T. HOOD. 1982. J. Immunol. **128:** 1050-1053.
17. BOROS, D. L., R. P. PELLEY & K. S. WARREN. 1975. J. Immunol. **114:** 1437-1441.
18. COLLEY, D. G. 1975. J. Immunol. **115:** 150-156.
19. JAMES, S. L. & D. G. COLLEY. 1975. J. Reticuloendothel. Soc. **18:** 283-293.
20. COLLEY, D. G. 1976. J. Exp. Med. **143:** 696-700.
21. CHENSUE, S. W. & D. L. BOROS. 1979. J. Immunol. **123:** 1409-1414.
22. CHENSUE, S. W., S. R. WELLHAUSEN & D. L. BOROS. 1981. J. Immunol. **127:** 363-367.
23. WELLHAUSEN, S. R., S. W. CHENSUE & D. L. BOROS. 1980. *In* Basic and Clinical Aspects of Granulomatous Diseases. D. L. Boros & T. Yoshida, Eds.: 219-234. Elsevier/North-Holland. New York, NY.
24. GREEN, W. F. & D. G. COLLEY. 1981. Proc. Natl. Acad. Sci. USA **78:** 1151-1156.
25. DORF, M. E. & B. BENACERRAF. 1984. Annu. Rev. Immunol. **2:** 127-158.
26. SHERR, D. H., K. M. HEGHINIAN, B. BENACERRAF & M. E. DORF. 1980. J. Immunol. **124:** 1389-1395.
27. HOOD, A. T. & D. L. BOROS. 1980. Am. J. Trop. Med. Hyg. **29:** 586-591.
28. WEINSTOCK, J. V., S. W. CHENSUE & D. L. BOROS. 1983. J. Immunol. **130:** 423-427.
29. BOROS, D. L. 1981. Lymphokines **3:** 257-281.
30. BOROS, D. L., K. S. WARREN & R. P. PELLEY. 1973. Nature **246:** 224-226.
31. CHENSUE, S. W., D. L. BOROS & C. S. DAVID. 1980. J. Exp. Med. **151:** 1398-1412.
32. CHENSUE, S. W., D. L. BOROS & C. S. DAVID. 1983. J. Exp. Med. **157:** 219-230.
33. DOUGHTY, B. L. & S. M. PHILLIPS. 1982. J. Immunol. **128:** 30-36.
34. DOUGHTY, B. L. & S. M. PHILLIPS. 1982. J. Immunol. **128:** 37-42.

35. El Naggar, A. & D. G. Colley. 1982. Cell. Immunol. **72:** 151-156.
36. Abe, T. & D. G. Colley. 1984. J. Immunol. **132:** 2084-2088.
37. Buchanan, R. D., D. P. Fine & D. G. Colley. 1973. Am. J. Pathol. **71:** 207-214.
38. Byram, J. R., M. J. Doenhoff, R. Musallam, L. H. Brink & F. Von Lichtenberg. 1979. Am. J. Trop. Med. Hyg. **28:** 274-285.
39. Ellner, J. J., G. R. Olds, R. Kamel, G. S. Osman, A. El Kholy & A. A. F. Mahmoud. 1980. J. Immunol. **125:** 308-312.
40. Colley, D. G., N. Katz, R. S. Rocha, W. Abrantes, A. L. da Silva & G. Gazzinelli. 1983. Scand. J. Immunol. **17:** 297-302.
41. Rocklin, R. E., A. P. Brown, K. S. Warren, R. P. Pelley, V. Houba, T. K. A. Siongok, J. Ouma, R. F. Sturrock & A. E. Butterworth. 1980. J. Immunol. **125:** 1916-1923.

The Langerhans' Cell in Human Pathology

F. BASSET,[a] P. SOLER, AND A. J. HANCE

Institut National de la Santé
et de la Recherche Médicale Unité 82
Faculté Xavier Bichat
Paris, France

INTRODUCTION

The Langerhans' cell (LC) is a normal cellular component of the epidermis of mammals and appears to play an essential role in protecting the skin against foreign antigens which have penetrated the epithelial surface.[1,2] Under pathological situations, however, LC's may also be found in extraepidermal sites and may therefore play a role in the pathogenesis of a variety of diseases. It is useful to divide the pathological conditions in which LC's are found in abnormal locations into two broad groups. The first of these groups is the family of diseases assembled under the name histiocytosis X (HX). In HX, LC's are usually present in large numbers, and they probably play a fundamental role in the pathogenesis of these diseases. The second general group of disorders in which LC's are found in abnormal locations, referred to here as the "non-HX disorders," represents a heterogeneous group of diseases unrelated to HX, in which LC's may be found in small numbers in the involved tissues. Although they probably do not have primary pathogenetic significance in these disorders, LC's may play some role in non-HX disorders as well.

Better understanding of the disease-associated abnormalities of the LC may provide insight into the normal biology of this important cell. In this context, the purpose of this paper is fourfold: First, to describe briefly the origin, distribution, and function of the normal LC. Second, to describe the two types of circumstances in which LC's are found in extraepidermal sites. Third, to compare normal LC's with those in pathological situations with respect to their tissue distribution, morphology, and topographical arrangements within the lesions. Fourth, this information will be used to formulate hypotheses explaining the abnormal location and/or the activation of LC's in HX and the non-HX disorders.

[a] Address for correspondence: Institut National de la Santé et de la Recherche Médicale Unité 82, Faculté Xavier Bichat, 16 rue Henri Huchard, 75018 Paris, France.

NORMAL LC's

Four main cell populations are present in the epidermis: the keratinocytes, melanocytes, Merkel cells, and LC's. Because melanocytes and LC's have a dendritic shape, for many years there was considerable uncertainty concerning the relationship of these cells.[3] It is now recognized, however, that the origin and function of the LC is independent of the melanocyte.[1,2,4] It is now known that LC's are of mesenchymal origin[1,2,4] and are derived from a pool of precursor cells found in the bone marrow.[5] The immature LC's migrate, probably via the peripheral circulation, to the epidermis where they take their fully differentiated form.[6] LC's have also been demonstrated in the thymus and lymph nodes of humans and in those of normal experimental animals,[7–10] and therefore it is probable that the precursor cells can also migrate directly to these tissues. Within the tissue, the LC's are mobile cells. Following activation, they are able to migrate from the epidermis to the dermis and regional lymph nodes.[11,12]

The primary role of the LC is now thought to be immunologic in nature. In this context, LC's have been described as a "reticuloepithelial trap for internal contact antigens"[2] and therefore to serve as "a critical link between the extracutaneous environment and the organism."[13] LC's have been demonstrated to take up specifically a wide variety of antigens known to produce contact dermatitis.[11,12] Furthermore, LC's are able to present these and other antigens to thymus-derived (T) lymphocytes, and therefore initiate immune responses against such antigens.[14,15] In addition, it has been suggested that LC's may play a role in attracting T lymphocytes to the epidermis and dermis, may serve as a target in the rejection of skin grafts, and may play a role in the development of immature T lymphocytes within the thymus.[15]

An area of recent interest has been relationship between LC's, macrophages, and dendritic cells.[a] These cells share in common a number of important characteristics, and all can play an important role in initiating immune responses.[17,18] Each kind of cell can be distinguished, however, on the basis of its tissue distribution, its morphology, the nature of the surface glycoproteins it expresses, and/or its functional capabilities. Although all three cell types may be derived from the same, or closely related, bone marrow precursors, current evidence suggests that the development of the cells of monocyte/macrophage lineage is distinct from that of LC's and dendritic cells. It remains unestablished whether dendritic cells and LC's are products of distinct cell lineages or whether the LC represents a "differentiated" dendritic cell.[16,19]

CIRCUMSTANCES IN WHICH LC'S ARE FOUND IN EXTRAEPIDERMAL SITES

Under normal conditions the distribution of LC's is quite circumscribed, since these cells are apparently restricted to bone marrow (when they are in an immature form),[5] squamous epithelia (in the epidermis, cervix, or gingiva, for example),[1,20–24] and some lymphoid tissues.[7–10] In the non-HX disorders and in HX, LC's are found in additional sites. The sites in which LC's are found in these two groups of disorders are summarized below.

[a] The term dendritic cells encompasses a group of more or less similar cells identified in a variety of tissues and periphral blood which are characterized by a dendritic shape and appear to be important members of the immune system.[16]

Non-HX Disorders

Although the non-HX disorders encompass a wide variety of pathological conditions, certain common features may explain the presence of LC's in these diseases.

Squamous Metaplasia

A variety of pathological conditions are associated with squamous metaplasia of the epithelium. It is not uncommon to find LC's associated with such areas of abnormal epithelium. Vitamin A deficiency results in squamous metaplasia of the trachea and bladder, and LC's have been demonstrated in these abnormal locations.[25] Similarly, a variety of interstitial lung diseases, including idiopathic pulmonary fibrosis, pulmonary fibrosis associated with collagen-vascular diseases, and hypersensitivity pneumonitis, result in squamous metaplasia of the bronchiolar or alveolar epithelium, and LC's have been demonstrated to be in close proximity to these reactive epithelial changes.[26,27]

Tumors

Cell infiltrates associated with certain tumors may contain LC's.[28,29] In some cases the LC's are present in small numbers, but in some tumors, especially bronchiolo-alveolar tumors, LC's may be present in large numbers.[30] The fact that these tumors frequently arise from cells of epithelial origin raises the possibility that they produce chemotactic factors for LC's, factors ordinarily produced only by squamous epithelium.

Viral Reactions

A few LC's have been identified in a liver biopsy from a patient with viral hepatitis antigen.[31] LC's are also found in association with viral particles in vaccine pustules.[32] Furthermore, LC's may be present in increased numbers in lymph nodes of patients with a variety of viral diseases.[10]

Dermal Infiltrates

Increased numbers of LC's are observed in a variety of cutaneous disorders involving not only epidermis but also dermis. Some are reactive or inflammatory, such as lichen planus,[33] lichen aureus,[34] or actinic reticuloid.[35] Others are considered to represent T cell malignancies such as Sezary's syndrome and mycosis fungoides.[1] In addition to being present in an abnormal location (the dermis, for example), LC's in these disorders may show morphological alterations (see below).[1]

HX Disorders

In contrast to the non-HX disorders, in which LC's are occasionally found, HX represents a group of disorders characterized, in their active stages, by the constant presence of large numbers of LC's.[36–38] This observation, which is in agreement with the unifying concept, originally proposed by Farber[39] and Lichtenstein,[40] served two important functions. First, it focused attention on the fact that abnormalities of the LC were likely to be of importance in the pathogenesis of a group of diseases which may appear clinically heterogeneous (Letterer-Siwe disease, Hand-Schüller-Christian disease, and eosinophilic granuloma of bone, for example). Second, it permitted the distinction of the HX disorders from other clinically similar diseases in which the LC plays no pathogenetic role (malignant histiocytosis, familial lymphohistiocytosis, lipid storage diseases, and some histiocytic cutaneous disorders, for example).[36–38,41]

Currently, the HX disorders are divided into two groups: the disseminated forms (in which several different tissues are involved simultaneously or successively) and the localized forms (in which usually only one tissue is involved).

The disseminated form is usually subdivided into the acute forms (corresponding to Letterer-Siwe disease) and the subacute or chronic forms (corresponding to Hand-Schüller-Christian disease or multifocal eosinophilic granulomatosis). Although the acute form is more likely to occur in younger patients, to be associated with more widespread lesions, and to carry a worse prognosis than the more chronic forms, the tissues involved are usually similar. The tissues most commonly affected by disseminated HX are the skin (including the oral mucosa), bone and bone marrow, lymph nodes and spleen, liver, and lung. Less common sites of involvement include the pituitary, the thyroid, and the nervous system.[42]

In the localized forms of HX, the tissue distribution is more limited. Lesions are usually found in bone or lung, but localized HX of the skin has recently been described.[43,44]

It is apparent that tissue distribution of LC's is similar in the non-HX disorders and in HX. Bone is the only tissue in which LC's are found only in the context of HX lesions. One must remember that LC's are derived from a bone marrow precursor; this could mean that the disease induces an early maturation of this precursor, leading to the appearance of fully differentiated LC's in marrow and in bone. In fact, bone lesions in HX involve predominantly flat bones, which are the main producers of bone marrow.[45]

HISTOPATHOLOGICAL FEATURES OF LC's

Both HX and the non-HX disorders may be associated with alterations in the histopathological features of LC's. In this section, the topographical arrangement, cellular morphology, and immunohistochemical properties of normal LC's and of LC's present in HX and the non-HX disorders will be reviewed.

Normal LC's

In the skin, LC's are regularly dispersed throughout the suprabasal region of the spinous layer. The cellular processes of adjacent LC's are in close proximity, and thus the cells appear to form the meshwork of a net located below the stratum granulosum of the epidermis. LC's are seldom, if ever, present in the dermis of normal skin.[1,3]

The morphology of the LC (FIG. 1) is characterized by the presence of specific cytoplasmic inclusions: the LC granules. These granules, visible only with the electron microscope, have a very distinctive appearance. They consist of elongated structures of constant thickness formed by two bilaminar membranes surrounding a central core. Serial reconstructions have shown that the granules have a plate- or cup-like shape.[46] When a granule is sectioned perpendicular to its long axis, periodic striations are visible in the central core and the inner layer of the membranes.

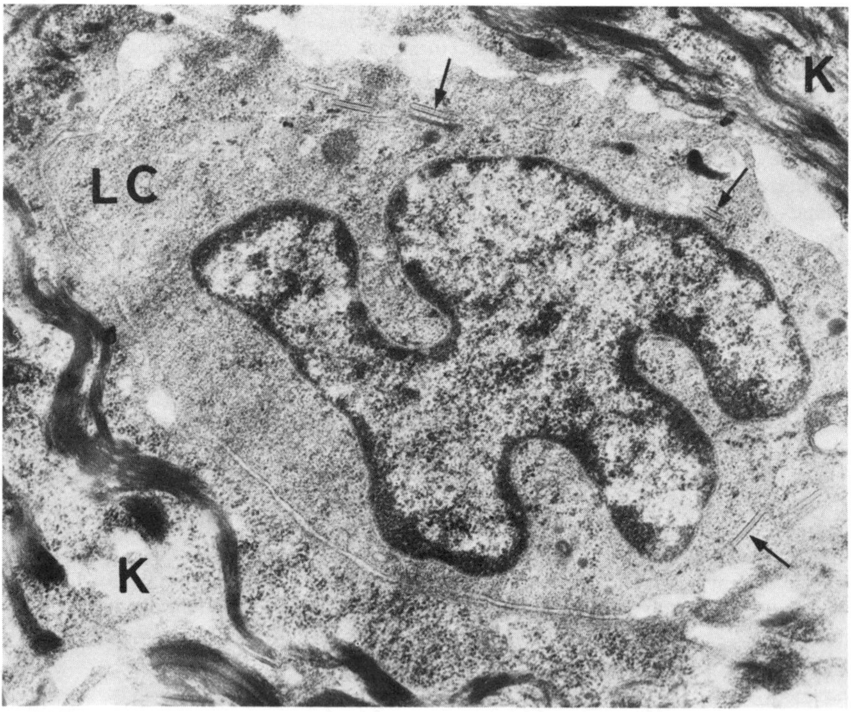

FIGURE 1. Electron micrograph of a normal epidermal Langerhans' cell (LC) with typical granules (arrows) between keratinocytes (K). Original magnification: × 18 000; enlarged to 108% of original size.

Most granules are located centrally in the cell, especially in the Golgi region, but occasionally these granules are in continuity with the plasma membrane.[3]

LC's normally have a dendritic shape,[16] one which results in long, irregular cytoplasmic extensions that may contain LC granules. Other morphological features of these cells include the presence of normal amounts of all usual cell organelles, such as mitochondria, Golgi apparatus, rough and smooth endoplasmic reticulum, intermediate-sized microfilaments, and lysosomes. Usually, few or no phagolysosomes are present, although some lipid droplets can be seen in the cytoplasm.[1] The nucleus is often indented or convoluted, and has little condensed chromatin. Mitotic figures are rarely observed in normal LC's.[1]

Normal LC's express, on their cell surfaces, a variety of glycoproteins characteristic of cells subserving an immune function. Like other cells capable of presenting antigens to T lymphocytes,[17,18] LC's display HLA-D surface antigens.[47,48] Furthermore, LC's display receptors for the Fc region of immunoglobulin G and the C3 fragment of complement[49] and therefore can interact with a variety of immune complexes. Recently, it has been demonstrated that LC's also express surface antigens detected by monoclonal antibody T4.[50] It has been suggested that this surface antigen, which is also present on helper T lymphocytes and monocytes,[51] may be important in the interaction of $T4^+$ cells with other cells expressing HLA-D surface antigens.[52,53] Thus, this surface glycoprotein may facilitate interaction between LC's and other $HLA\text{-}D^+$ cells, such as other LC's and activated T lymphocytes. Finally, the plasma membrane of the LC and, at least in some cases, the membranes of the LC granules strongly express the glycoprotein detected by the monoclonal antibody T6.[54,55] The function of this antigen, which is also expressed by immature but not by mature T lymphocytes, is unknown. Its structure is very similar, however, to that of HLA-A/B antigens.[56] Thus it is possible that this T6 antigen, like HLA-A/B antigens,[52] facilitates the ability of the LC to initiate immune responses against certain types of antigens.

LC's in the Non-HX Disorders

Although LC's are found in abnormal locations in the non-HX disorders, their distribution within the tissues is reminiscent of their normal distribution in the skin (FIG. 2). When found in areas of squamous metaplasia,[25–27] the cells are usually scattered within or below the abnormal epithelium; similarly, when found in association with tumors, the cells form a meshwork within the stroma of the tumor that surrounds the neoplastic cells.[29,30] Clumps of LC's are rarely encountered in the non-HX disorders except in the cutaneous reactions[32–35] and, rarely, in some tumors.[28]

Similarly, the shape of the cell is usually dendritic, whatever tissue is involved (metaplasia, tumor, or chronically inflamed connective tissue) (FIGS. 3 & 4). Furthermore, the cellular morphology of LC's in the non-HX disorders is usually normal. In non-HX LC's the organelles present are similar, and the surface glycoproteins are identical to those found in normal LC's. Mitotic activity is low in both non-HX and normal LC's, and the number of LC granules found in non-HX disorders is similar to that found in normal skin. Thus, the LC in the non-HX disorders usually appears to be an unusually located normal cell.

LC's in HX

The topographical arrangement of LC's in HX is markedly abnormal. Although some cells can be independent, most are clumped or arranged in irregular groups and therefore contribute, to a variable extent, to the development of granulomas. In this context, the eponym "Langerhans' cell granulomatosis" has been introduced by Lieberman *et al.*[57] as a substitute for "HX," to emphasize this characteristic organization of LC's into granulomas. Within the granulomas the LC's may be closely or

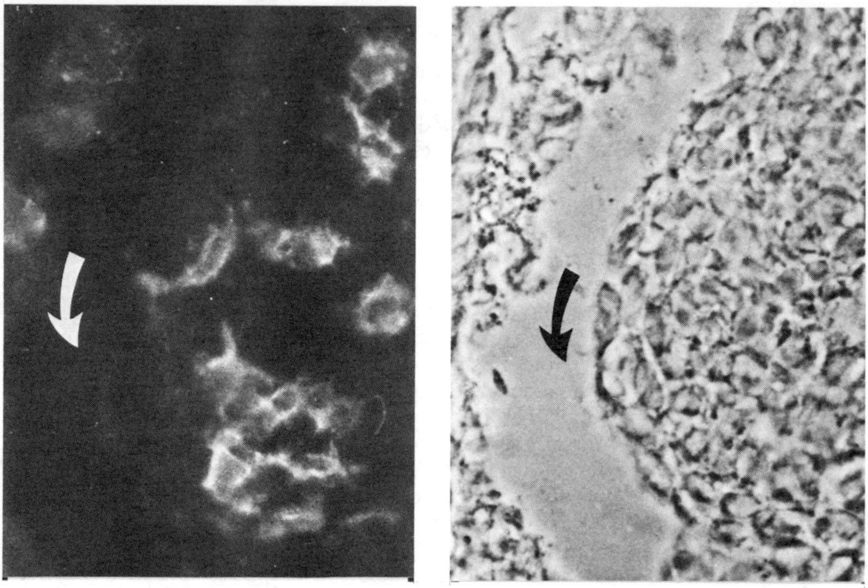

FIGURE 2. Fluorescence photomicrograph of OKT6 labeling (left) and phase-contrast microscopy (right) of the same field. LC's in an area of squamous metaplasia of the alveolar epithelium. Open lung biopsy in a patient with idiopathic pulmonary fibrosis. Arrows: residual alveolar lumen. Magnification: × 250.

loosely juxtaposed. No true junctional complexes appear to exist between them, however, and loose arrangements are most frequently observed.

The granulomas of HX are lesions which evolve in successive phases. Both the cell populations and the matrix elements composing these granulomas vary depending on the stage of the lesion. Early granulomas consist of cell infiltrates of variable size that destroy the preexisting structures. They may be compact, have a loose center, or be unmistakably cavitary (FIGS. 5 & 6). These early granulomas have little or no connective tissue framework and variable vascular supply. LC's often predominate in the central part of compact granulomas or in the walls of cavitary ones; neutrophils, eosinophils, and mast cells are associated in different proportions from place to place. Lymphocytes usually are more numerous in peripheral parts of the lesions, lesions which usually have poorly defined limits. In more advanced lesions, LC's decrease in number, and other cell types, especially macrophages and eosinophils, may become predominant; the connective tissue framework is much more developed, and fibrotic changes appear. In the final stage, the granulomas of the lesions are replaced by stellate areas of scar tissue surrounding clumps of macrophages laden with pigment and lipids. Lymphoid follicles may be present in the periphery of these lesions, but, not uncommonly, LC's are completely absent.

Although the arrangement of LC's in granulomas which evolve over time is common to all clinical forms of HX and all sites of tissue involvement, there are some pecularities in this process that depend on which tissue is affected.

In bone the lesions are usually bulky, poorly vascularized, and frequently undergo massive necrosis.[45] LC's can be identified with electron microscopy, even in necrotic areas, by the presence of numerous LC granules which are entangled in complicated clusters and which sometimes persist even when other cell structures have disappeared. The increase in the lipid content of macrophages is often very marked in late stages, and xanthomatous changes may result.

In the skin the lesions are usually small and are centered in the dermis, although the adjacent epidermis is often involved. Hemorrhagic areas are frequently present in their vicinity, and eosinophils are rarely observed within skin lesions.[58]

In the lung the lesions consist of multiple granulomas, which are often miliary, dispersed throughout both lungs.[59–61] They are located mainly in the subpleural region and frequently involve terminal or respiratory bronchioles. In general, granulomas with different appearances, which correspond to different evolutionary stages, are present simultaneously. Early lesions can be compact or cavitary, and are mainly composed of LC's. Necrosis is usually absent, even in cavitary lesions. The limits of lesions are usually poorly defined, and cell infiltrates expand into adjacent alveolar walls. In the more advanced lesions cavitation often becomes prominent, and the lesions consist of thick, partly fibrotic walls containing irregularly distributed cells (small nests of LC's, eosinophils, and macrophages laden with lipids and/or pigment, for example). In late lesions, remodeling of lung tissue, which is probably independent from the HX process itself, may become predominant.

When examined individually with the electron microscope, LC's in the lesions of HX do not differ greatly from normal LC's. The LC's in HX, however, usually have several features which serve to distinguish them from normal LC's. First, they have a more rounded shape with filopodia but few or no dendrites, especially when recovered

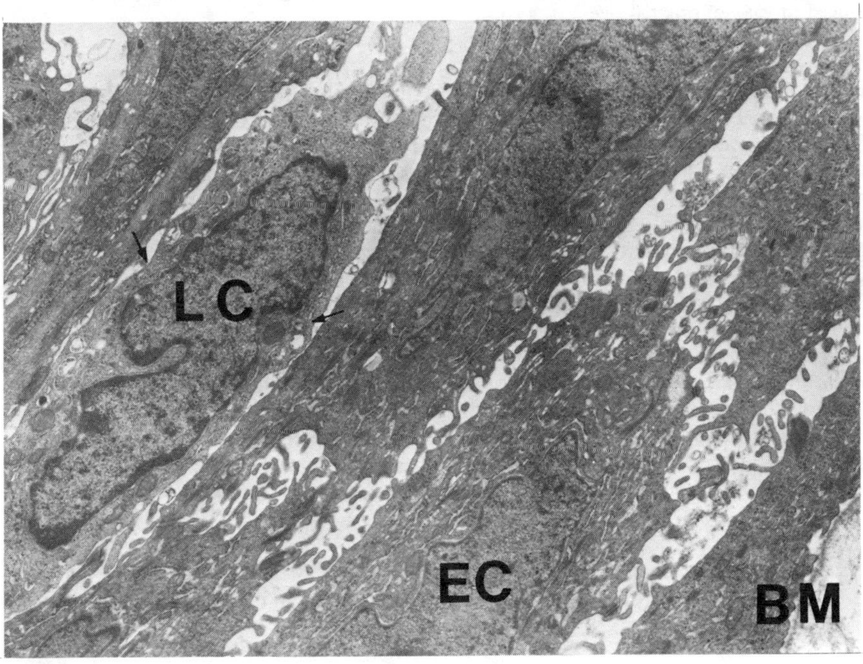

FIGURE 3. Electron micrograph of a Langerhans' cell (LC) in an area of squamous metaplasia of the alveolar epithelium. Open lung biopsy in a patient with idiopathic pulmonary fibrosis. EC = epithelial cell; BM = basement membrane. The arrows point to the LC granules. Original magnification: × 5000; reduced to 91% of original size.

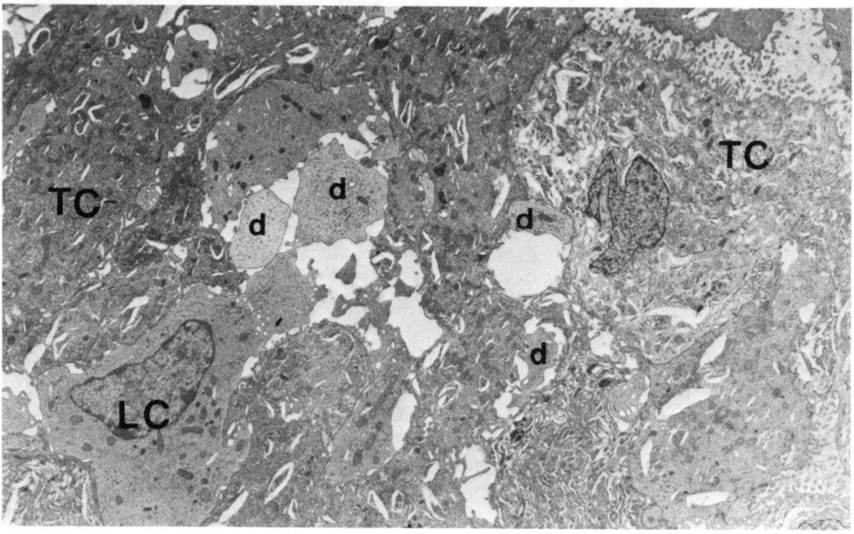

FIGURE 4. Electron micrograph of a Langerhans' cell (LC) in a bronchiolo-alveolar carcinoma, with dendrites (d) interspersed between tumor cells (TC). Original magnification: × 3600; reduced to 95% of original size.

by bronchoalveolar lavage.[62] In addition, LC's in HX have extremely convoluted and clear nuclei. Furthermore, they contain larger numbers of LC granules, which are often peripherally located and are much more often in continuity with the plasma membrane (FIG. 7). Similarly, usual cytoplasmic organelles often appear more developed in LC's from HX than in epidermal LC's, and some additional peculiar structures (serpentines or crystals in mitochondria) are sometimes present.[59,63] Finally, mitotic figures are not infrequent in lesions of HX, and this increased mitotic activity may explain the occasional presence of intranuclear LC granules observed in LC's from HX lesions.[64,65] Although the mitotic activity of LC's is increased in HX, changes typical of neoplastic cells are not seen (heteroploid and dedifferentiated cells, for example). In general, changes in the cellular morphology of LC's in HX are very similar to those observed in dermal LC's in actinic reticuloid[35] and various other cutaneous disorders.[1,32,34] As previously discussed, the LC's in these conditions appear to be normal cells which have been activated by the presence of a chronic inflammatory process in the skin. Thus, the morphologic changes observed in LC's of HX support the concept that the cells are activated but not neoplastic.

PATHOGENESIS OF ABNORMALITIES OF THE LC

From the preceding description, it is apparent that two general types of abnormalities of the LC are found in human pathological conditions. First, these may be abnormalities in the distribution of LC's. Second, there are disorders in which the fundamental abnormality is the appearance of increased numbers of LC's which are abnormally activated. In some cases, the abnormalities of tissue distribution and activation occur independently (abnormal tissue distribution of normal LC's in the non-HX disorders and abnormal activation of LC's without abnormal tissue distribution in HX of the skin, for example). In other conditions, however, these two abnormalities coexist, such as in pulmonary HX. Thus, in order to explain the pathogenesis of abnormalities of the LC, it is necessary to understand the factors which influence the tissue distribution of LC's, the factors which serve to "activate" LC's, and the relationship between the distribution and activation of LC's. Each of these topics is discussed below.

Factors Which May Influence the Distribution of LC's

Although it has been suggested that the process of keratinization is related to the appearance of LC's in the skin,[14,15] little specific information is available concerning the factors which normally regulate the distribution of LC's. The distribution of LC's observed in the non-HX disorders, however, suggests that two factors may be important in regulating LC distribution.

First, the appearance of LC's at sites of squamous metaplasia[25,27] and in association with certain tumors of epithelial origin[28–30] suggests that epithelial cells may play an important role in regulating LC distribution. The fact that LC's are restricted to certain layers of the normal epidermis and the fact that bronchiolo-alveolar tumors,[30] but not other lung carcinomas, are associated with LC accumulation suggest that only

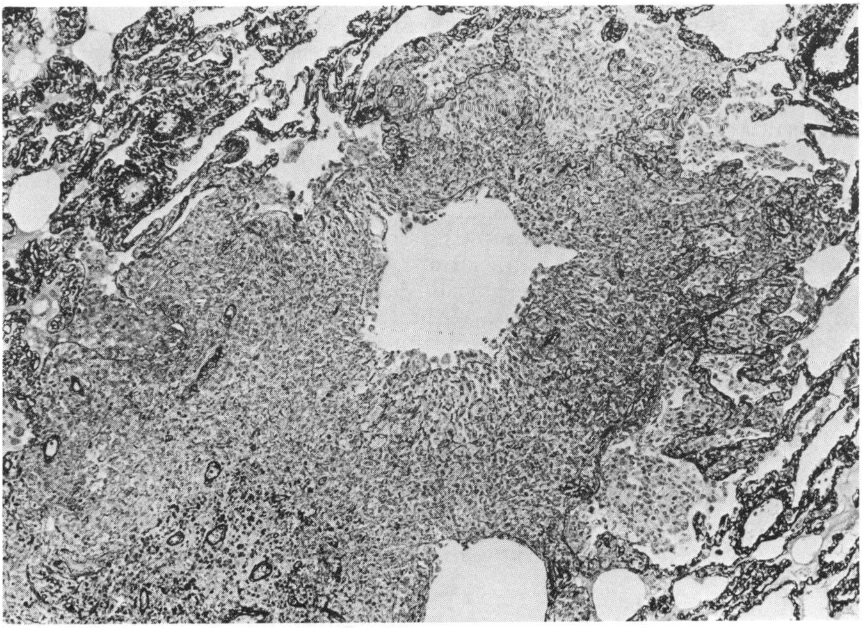

FIGURE 5. Histology section of an early granuloma in pulmonary HX. Periodic acid-silver methenamine stain. Original magnification: × 40; reduced to 81% of original size.

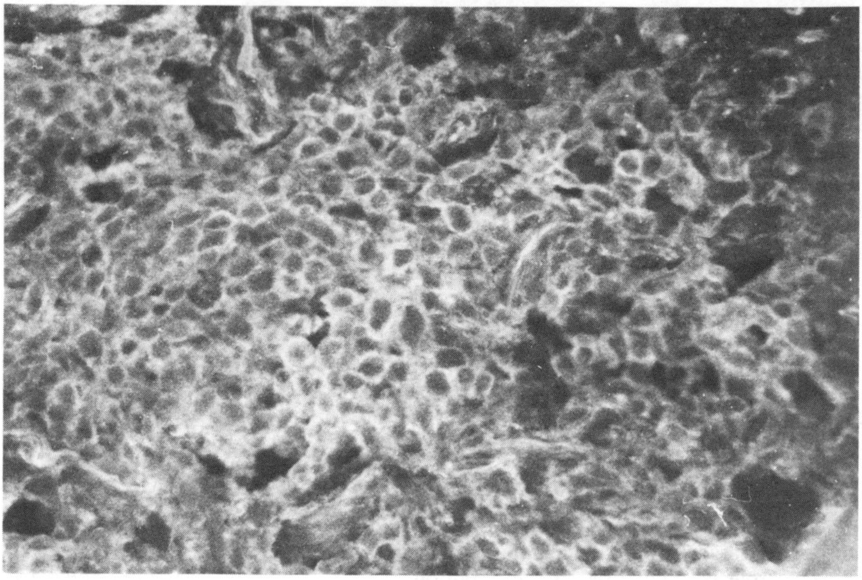

FIGURE 6. Fluorescence photomicrograph of OKT6 labeling. The LC's are densely packed in a granulomatous area of pulmonary HX. Original magnification: × 250; reduced to 93% of original size.

certain stages of epithelial cell differentiation may be associated with the ability to attract LC's. Presumably the influence of epithelial cells on LC distribution could result from either direct cell-cell interactions or the release by epithelial cells of chemotactic factors specific for LC's.

Second, a factor which also appears to influence LC distribution appears to be produced in the course of some viral infections. After viral vaccinations, LC's migrate from their usual location in the epidermis toward the dermis and regional nodes.[32] In other cases, viral infections are associated with the appearance of LC's ectopic locations, such as the liver.[31] The mechanism(s) responsible for the effect of viral infections remain unknown. Because the migration of LC's observed in viral vaccinations is similar to that observed in contact dermatitis and the Sezary syndrome,[1] it appears that products of the immune response are likely to play a role. On the other hand, LC's were recently reported to act as potent activators of human T cells to herpes simplex virus.[66] Better characterization of the stimuli associated with epithelial dysplasia and viral infections may provide insight into the factors which govern the normal distribution of LC's, in addition to explaining the abnormal distribution of LC's found in the non-HX disorders and in some forms of HX.

Factors Which Influence the Activation of LC's

The HX disorders are characterized by marked changes in the distribution of LC's within the tissues and a marked increase in the number of LC's present. Analysis of the morphology of the cells indicates that they are "activated." Although it has been suggested that these changes result from the neoplastic transformation of LC's, several findings argue against this concept.[37,38,40,42,45]

First, the ultrastructure of the LC in HX indicates that it remains a highly differentiated cell, and cellular abnormalities usually associated with malignancy are not present.

Second, the lesions of HX are usually localized to sites where LC's or their precursors are normally present (bone containing marrow, skin, and lymph nodes, for example) or to sites where normal LC's may be found in non-HX disorders (lung and liver, for example). They usually do not have a diffuse, metastasis-like dissemination.

Third, the granulomatous lesions of HX undergo a characteristic evolutionary process which in many respects resembles that of granulomatous reactions to infectious agents or foreign antigens. Finally, most clinical forms of HX,[39,40,45,57,60,61] including the fulminant forms such as Letterer-Siwe disease, may in at least 50% of the cases either evolve into a more chronic disease process, follow a relapsing course, or remit spontaneously or after treatment.[67] Mortality associated with pulmonary HX is usually the result of sequelae of the destructive granulomatous process (respiratory failure, for example) and not a result of progressive infiltration of tissues by LC's.[68]

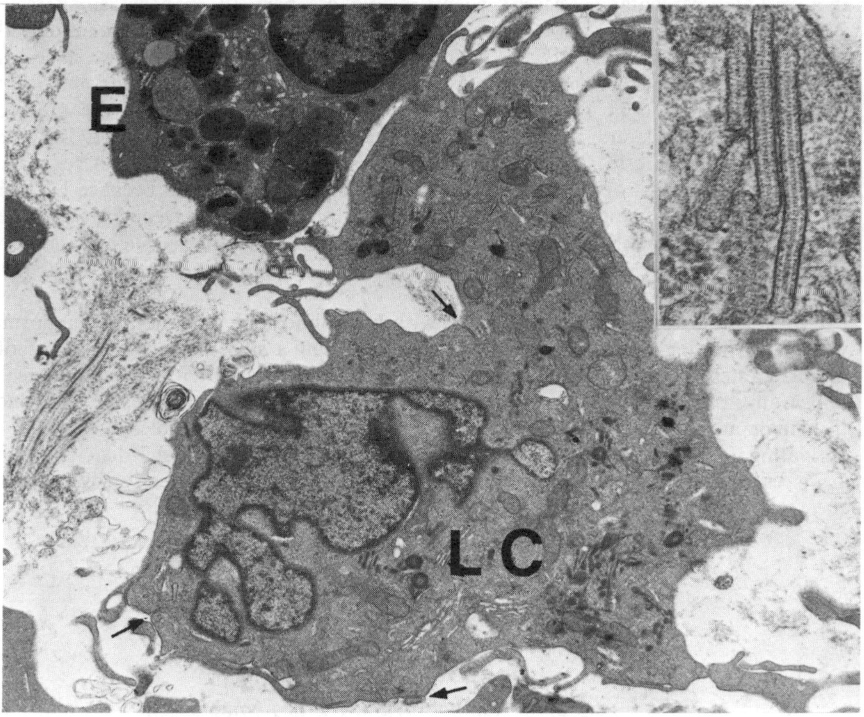

FIGURE 7. Electron micrograph of a Langerhans' cell (LC) in a granuloma of pulmonary HX. The arrows point to two granules in continuity with the plasma membrane. E = eosinophil. Insert: a higher magnification of the granules. Original magnification: × 7500 (that for the insert was × 60 000); enlarged to 104% of original size.

These findings suggest that the activation of LC's in HX is not a neoplastic process, but rather results from a reactive process which is immunologic in nature. Although mitotic figures are present in the granulomas of HX, the level of mitotic activity seen in these tissues appears insufficient to account for the large numbers of LC's present. Thus, this reactive process probably must also result in stimulation of the production of precursor cells in the bone marrow. The nature of the factors responsible for the activation of LC's and their precursors (viral infection and neo-antigens produced by the interaction of toxic substances with normal cells, for example), however, remains unknown.

The Relationship between Stimuli Influencing Distribution and Activation of LC's

As previously discussed, abnormal distribution and abnormal activation of LC's can occur independently. Thus, the presence of abnormally activated LC's in unusual locations may be contingent on distinct stimuli. The adult form of pulmonary HX may represent an example of such a process. A striking feature of this disease is that in a very high percentage of cases it occurs in smokers, particularly heavy smokers.[59–61] As discussed elsewhere,[69] however, it appears unlikely that cigarette smoking is directly responsible for pulmonary HX. In order to explain these observations, we have suggested that the adult form of HX may require the presence of two independent stimuli. One stimulus would be required to activate the LC's as discussed in the previous section. The second, independent stimulus would be required to attract LC's to the lung. Because cigarette smoking (particularly heavy smoking) is known to induce squamous metaplasia of the bronchial and alveolar epithelium, and because LC's are attracted to areas of squamous metaplasia, this stimulus could be frequently provided by smoking. Presumably less common causes of squamous metaplasia, such as radiation therapy[70,71] or environmental[60] exposure, could also provide this stimulus in the non-smoking patients with pulmonary HX.

In the other forms of HX associated with both abnormal activation and abnormal tissue distribution of LC's, it seems more likely that a single agent results in both abnormalities. For example, the acute forms of HX associated with the simultaneous appearance of granulomas in a variety of abnormal sites can be more easily explained if a single agent, such as a disseminated viral infection, is responsible. In addition to activating LC's, such an agent could also stimulate abnormal tissue distribution of LC's, either directly (viral-induced squamous metaplasia) or indirectly (by inducing the release of immune mediators).

CONCLUSION

Recent progress in the understanding of the LC has emphasized the importance of this cell in the normal immune defense system. In part, this knowledge has resulted from the study of diseases in which abnormalities of LC's play a role. Additional study of these disorders appear to offer an opportunity to better understand the factors which regulate the maturation, localization, and activation of LC's. The presence of large numbers of LC's in the lesions of HX suggests that involved tissue may be a convenient source from which to purify LC for *in vitro* studies. It is to be hoped that such studies will not only provide further insight into the normal LC, but also aid in the development of specific therapies for these unusual but debilitating diseases.

ACKNOWLEDGMENTS

We wish to thank S.I. Katz and V.J. Ferrans for their valuable insights and F. Miklovic for her editorial assistance.

REFERENCES

1. Rowden, G. 1981. The Langerhans cell. CRC Crit. Rev. Immunol. **3:** 95-180.
2. Shelley, W. B. & L. Juhlin. 1976. Langerhans cells form a reticuloepithelial trap for external contact antigens. Nature (London) **261:** 46-47.
3. Breathnach, A. S. 1965. The cell of Langerhans. Int. Rev. Cytol. **18:** 1-28.
4. Wolff, K. 1972. The Langerhans cell. Curr. Probl. Dermatol. **4:** 80-145.
5. Katz, S. I., K. Tamaki & D. H. Sachs. 1979. Epidermal Langerhans cells are derived from cells originating in bone marrow. Nature **282:** 324-326.
6. Shelley, W. B. & L. Juhlin. 1978. The Langerhans cell. Its origin, nature and function. Acta Derm. Venereol. Suppl. (Stockholm) **79:** 7-22.
7. Hoshino, T., A. Kukita & S. Sato. 1970. Cells containing Birbeck granules (Langerhans cell granules) in human thymus. J. Electron Microsc. **19:** 271-274.
8. Kondo, Y. 1969. Macrophages containing Langerhans cell granules in normal lymph nodes of the rabbit. Z. Zellforsch. Mikrosk. Anat. **98:** 506-511.
9. Shamoto, M., C. Kaplan & A. K. Katoh. 1971. Langerhans cell granules in human hyperplastic lymph nodes. Arch. Pathol. **92:** 46-52.
10. Vernon, M. L., L. Fountain, H. M. Krebs, L. Horta-Barbosa, D. A. Fuccillo & J. L. Sever. 1973. Birbeck granules (Langerhans cell granules) in human lymph nodes. Am. J. Clin. Pathol. **60:** 771-779.
11. Silberberg-Sinakin, I., R. L. Baer & G. J. Thorbecke. 1978. Langerhans cells. A review of their nature with emphasis on their immunologic functions. Prog. Allergy **24:** 268-294.
12. Thorbecke, G. J., I. Silberberg-Sinakin & T. J. Flotte. 1980. Langerhans cells as macrophages in skin and lymphoid organs. J. Invest. Dermatol. **75:** 32-43.
13. Wolff, K. & G. Stingl. 1983. The Langerhans cell. J. Invest. Dermatol. **80:** 17S-21S.
14. Stingl, G., S. I. Katz, E. M. Shevach, A. S. Rosenthal & I. Green. 1978. Analogous functions of macrophages and Langerhans cells in the initiation of the immune response. J. Invest. Dermatol. **71:** 59-64.
15. Friedmann, P. S. 1981. The immunology of Langerhans cells. Immunol. Today **2:** 124-128.
16. Tew, J. G., J. Thorbecke & R. M. Steinman. 1982. Dendritic cells in the immune response. Characteristics and recommended nomenclature. A Report from the Reticuloendothelial Society Committee on Nomenclature. J. Reticuloendothel. Soc. **31:** 371-380.
17. Unanue, E. R. 1981. The regulatory role of macrophages in antigenic stimulation. Part two: Symbiotic relationship between lymphocytes and macrophages. Adv. Immunol. **31:** 1-136.
18. Unanue, E. R., D. I. Beller, C. Y. Lu & P. M. Allen. 1984. Antigen presentation. Comments on its regulation and mechanism. J. Immunol. **132:** 1-5.
19. Hoefsmit, E. L. M., A. M. Duijvestijn & E. W. A. Kamperdijk. 1982. Relation between Langerhans cells, veiled cells and interdigitating cells. Immunobiology **161:** 255-265.

20. Younes, M. S., E. M. Robertson & S. A. Bencosme. 1968. Electron microscope observations on Langerhans cells in the cervix. Am. J. Obstet. Gynecol. **102:** 397-403.
21. Figueroa, C. D. & I. Caorsi. 1980. Ultrastructural and morphometric study of the Langerhans cell in the normal human exocervix. J. Anat. **131:** 669-682.
22. Waterhouse, J. P. & C. A. Squier. 1967. The Langerhans cell in human gingival epithelium. Arch. Oral. Biol. **12:** 341-348.
23. Mausle, E., W. Mootz & J. Schondorf. 1971. Evidence of Langerhans cells in the epithelium of the human tonsil. Cytobiologie **3:** 359-366.
24. Bock, P. 1974. Fine structure of Langerhans cells in the stratified epithelia of the esophagus and stomach of mice. Z. Zellforsch. Microsk. Anat. **147:** 237-247.
25. Wong, Y. C. & R. C. Buck. 1971. Langerhans cells in epidermoid metaplasia. J. Invest. Dermatol. **56:** 10-17.
26. Basset, F., P. Soler, L. Wyllie, F. Mazin & J. Turiaf. 1976. Langerhans cells and lung interstitium. Ann. N.Y. Acad. Sci. **278:** 599-611.
27. Kawanami, O., F. Basset, V. J. Ferrans, P. Soler & R. Crystal. 1980. Pulmonary Langerhans cells in patients with fibrotic lung disorders. Lab. Invest. **44:** 227-233.
28. Porfiri, B., M. Nigro & A. Garcovich. 1979. Sur la présence d'agrégats constitués de cellules de Langerhans et cellules lymphoides dans l'infiltrat péritumoral dans un cas de naevomatose baso cellulaire. Etude ultrastructurale. Ann. Dermatol. Venerol. (Paris) **106:** 237-240.
29. Palacios, J. J. N., M. A. M. Gonzalez & R. D. Gonzalez. 1984. Langerhans cells in a renal carcinoma. Ultrastruct. Pathol. **6:** 109-114.
30. Basset, F., P. Soler, L. Wyllie, R. Abelanet, M. Le Charpentier, B. Kreis & A. S. Breathnach. 1974. Langerhans cells in a bronchiolar alveolar tumour of lung. Virchows Arch. A **362:** 315-330.
31. Scotto, J. 1977. Cellules de Langerhans dans le foie humain. Nouv. Presse Med. **6:** 3864.
32. Nagao, S., S. Inaba & S. Iijima. 1976. Langerhans cells at the sites of vaccinia virus inoculation. Arch. Dermatol. Res. **256:** 23-31.
33. Bhan, A. K., T. J. Harrist, G. F. Murphy & M. C. Mihm. 1981. T cell subsets and Langerhans cells in lichen planus. *In situ* characterization using monoclonal antibodies. Br. J. Dermatol. **105:** 617-622.
34. Schitzler, L., J. L. Verret, B. Schubert, S. Belaich & P. Belperron. 1977. Lichen aureus ou lichen purpuricus. A propos de 5 cas. Intérêt de l'étude ultrastructurale. Ann. Dermatol. Venerol. (Paris) **104:** 731-736.
35. Schnitzler, L., J. L. Verrett, B. Schubert & M. D. Picard. 1975. Langerhans cells in actinic reticuloid. J. Cutan. Pathol. **2:** 170-178.
36. Basset, F., C. Nezelof & V. J. Ferrans. 1983. The histiocytoses. Pathol. Annu. **18**(2): 27-78.
37. Favara, B. E., R. C. McCarthy & G. W. Mierau. 1983. Histiocytosis X. Hum. Pathol. **14:** 663-676.
38. Risdall, R. J., L. R. Dehner, P. Duray, N. Kobrinky, L. Robison & M. E. Nesbit. 1983. Histiocytosis X (Langerhans cell histiocytosis). Prognostic role of histopathology. Arch. Pathol. Lab. Med. **107:** 59-63.
39. Farber, S. 1941. The nature of "solitary eosinophilic granuloma" of bone. Am. J. Pathol. **17:** 625-629.
40. Lichtenstein, L. 1964. Histiocytosis X (eosinophilic granuloma of bone, Letterer-Siwe disease and Schüller-Christian disease). Further observations of pathological and clinical importance. J. Bone J. Surg. **46**(A): 76-90.
41. Winkelmann, R. K. 1981. Cutaneous syndromes of non-X histiocytosis. A review of the macrophage-histiocyte diseases of the skin. Arch. Dermatol. **117:** 667-672.
42. Kepes, J. J. 1979. Histiocytosis X. *In* Handbook of Clinical Neurology. P. J. Vinken & G. W. Bruyn, Eds. Vol. **38:** 93-117. Elsevier/North-Holland. Amsterdam.
43. Hashimoto, K. & M. S. Pritzker. 1973. Electron microscopic study of retuculohistiocytoma. An unusual case of congenital, self-healing reticulohistiocytosis. Arch. Dermatol. **107:** 263-270.
44. Bonifazi, E., R. Caputo, A. Ceci & C. Meneghini. 1982. Congenital self-healing histiocytosis. Clinical, histologic and ultrastructural study. Arch. Dermatol. **118:** 267-272.
45. Nezelof, C. 1966. L'histiocytose X. Rev. Fr. Etud. Clin. Biol. **11:** 22-39.

46. SAGEBIEL, R. W. & T. H. REED. 1968. Serial reconstruction of the characteristic granule of the Langerhans cell. J. Cell Biol. **36:** 595-602.
47. KLARESKOG, L., U. M. TJERNLUND, U. FORSUM & P. A. PETERSON. 1977. Epidermal Langerhans cells express Ia antigens. Nature **268:** 248-250.
48. ROWDEN, G., M. G. LEWIS & A. K. SULLIVAN. 1977. Ia antigen expression of human epidermal Langerhans cells. Nature **268:** 247-248.
49. SILBERBERG, I., R. L. BAER & S. A. ROSENTHAL. 1974. The role of Langerhans cells in contact allergy. I. An ultrastructural study in actively induced contact dermatitis in guinea pigs. Acta Derm. Venereol. **54:** 321-331.
50. WOOD, G. S., N. L. WARNER & R. A. WARNKE. 1983. Anti-Leu 3/T4 antibodies react with cells of monocyte/macrophage and Langerhans lineage. J. Immunol. **131:** 212-216.
51. MOSCICKI, R. A., E. P. AMENTO, S. M. KRANE, J. T. KURNICK & R. B. CALVIN. 1983. Modulation of surface antigens of a human monocyte cell line, U937, during incubation with T lymphocyte-conditioned medium. Detection of T4 antigen and its presence on normal blood monocytes. J. Immunol. **131:** 743-748.
52. REINHERZ, E. L., S. C. MENER & S. F. SCHLOSSMAN. 1983. The delineation of antigen receptors on human T lymphocytes. Immunol. Today **4:** 5-8.
53. BLUESTONE, J. A. & R. J. HODES. 1983. Cell-surface molecules involved in T cell functions. Immunol. Today **4:** 256-259.
54. FITHIAN, E., P. C. KUNG, G. GOLDSTEIN, A. RUBENFELD, C. FENOGLIO & R. EDELSON. 1981. Reactivity of Langerhans cells with hybridoma antibody. Proc. Natl. Acad. Sci. USA **78:** 2541-2544.
55. MURPHY, G. F., A. K. BHAN, S. SATO, T. J. HARRIST & M. C. MIHM. 1981. Characterization of Langerhans cells by the use of monoclonal antibodies. Lab. Invest. **45:** 465-468.
56. KEFFORD, R. F., F. CALABI, I. M. FEARNLEY, O. R. BURRONE & C. MILSTEIN. 1984. Serum β_2-microglobulin binds to a T cell differentiation antigen and increases its expression. Nature (London) **308:** 641-642.
57. LIEBERMAN, P. H., C. R. JONES & D. A. FILIPPA. 1980. Langerhans cell (eosinophilic) granulomatosis. J. Invest. Dermatol. **75:** 71-72.
58. WINKELMANN, R. K. 1969. The skin in histiocytosis X. Mayo Clin. Proc. **44:** 535-548.
59. BASSET, F., B. CORRIN, H. SPENCER, J. LACRONIQUE, C. ROTH, P. SOLER, J.-P. BATTESTI, R. GEORGES & J. CHRÉTIEN. 1978. Pulmonary histiocytosis X. Am. Rev. Respir. Dis. **118:** 811-820.
60. FRIEDMAN, J. P., A. A. LIEBOW & J. SOKOLOFF. 1981. Eosinophilic granuloma of lung. Clinical aspects of primary pulmonary histiocytosis in the adult. Medicine **60:** 385-396.
61. COLBY, T. V. & C. LOMBARD. 1983. Histiocytosis X in the lung. Hum. Pathol. **14:** 847-856.
62. BASSET, F., P. SOLER, M. C. JAURAND & J. BIGNON. 1977. Ultrastructural examination of bronchoalveolar lavage for diagnosis of pulmonary histiocytosis X. Preliminary report on four cases. Thorax **32:** 303-306.
63. BASSET, F., J. ESCAIG & M. LE CROM. 1972. A cytoplasmic membranous complex in histiocytosis X cells. Cancer **29:** 1380-1386.
64. MORALES, A. R., G. FINE, R. C. HORN & J. H. L. WATSON. 1969. Langerhans cells in a localized lesion of the eosinophilic granuloma type. Lab. Invest. **20:** 412-423.
65. SHAMOTO, M. 1977. Mitotic histiocytes and intranuclear Langerhans cell granules in histiocytosis X. Virchows Arch. B **24:** 87-90.
66. BRAATHEN, L. R., E. BERLE, U. MOBECH-HANSSEN & E. THORSBY. 1980. Studies on human epidermal Langerhans cells. II. Activation of human T lymphocytes to herpes simplex virus. Acta Derm. Venereol. **60:** 381-387.
67. NEZELOF, C., F. FRILEUX-HERBET & J. CORNIER-SACHOT. 1979. Disseminated histiocytosis X. Analysis of prognostic factors based on a retrospective study of 50 cases. Cancer **44:** 1824-1838.
68. POWERS, M. A., F. B. ASKIN & D. H. CRESSON. 1984. Pulmonary eosinophilic granuloma. Am. Rev. Respir. Dis. **129:** 503-507.
69. HANCE, A. J., F. BASSET, G. SAUMON, C. DANEL, D. VALEYRE, J.-P. BATTESTI, J. CHRÉTIEN & R. GEORGES. Ann. N.Y. Acad. Sci. This volume.
70. SAJJAD, S. M. & M. A. LUNA. 1982. Primary pulmonary histiocytosis X in two patients with Hodgkin's disease. Thorax **37:** 110-113.
71. BURNS, B. F., T. V. COLBY & R. F. DORFMAN. 1983. Langerhans cell granulomatosis (histiocytosis X) associated with malignant lymphomas. Am. J. Surg. Pathol. **7:** 529-533.

In Vitro Granuloma Formation Using Defined Antigenic Nidi[a]

PATRICK J. LAMMIE, S. MICHAEL PHILLIPS, GERALD P. LINETTE, AMAL I. MICHAEL, AND ANNA G. BENTLEY

Department of Medicine
Section of Allergy and Immunology
University of Pennsylvania
School of Medicine
Philadelphia, Pennsylvania 19104

INTRODUCTION

The immobilization of certain infectious agents or foreign antigens in host tissues elicits a characteristic delayed-type hypersensitivity response which becomes manifest with the formation of a granuloma around the offending material. This reaction is critically dependent upon the presence of sensitized thymus-derived (T) cells and is apparently correlated with the production by T cells of lymphokines which both activate and recruit cells (see Boros[1] for a review). Chronic tissue exposure to antigenic stimuli can lead to fibrosis and its attendant sequelae through as yet undefined mechanisms.

In vivo experimental studies have contributed much to our understanding of the evolution of granulomatous responses, their cellular constituents, and the T cell subsets responsible for their immunoregulation.[1,2] Many questions, however, remain with regard to the nature of antigen recognition, the cellular signals responsible for the generation and regulation of the granulomatous response, and the relationship between immunologic reactivity and end-stage fibrosis. These questions are particularly compelling as they apply to idiopathic granulomatous diseases such as sarcoidosis and Crohn's disease for which appropriate experimental models do not exist.

The development of an *in vitro* model to analyze granuloma formation has been a long-term goal of our laboratory. These studies have focused initially on granulomas induced by eggs of the helminthic parasite, *Schistosoma mansoni,* a cause of significant morbidity in the developing world.[3-9] *In vitro* granuloma formation represents a useful and readily exploited model of *in vivo* granulomatous hypersensitivity. The assay offers a number of advantages for the study of mechanisms of granuloma formation at the cellular and molecular level. In the present report, we will briefly review the model and our recent work analyzing granuloma formation by cloned T cells and discuss new data relating to lymphokine-mediated regulation of granuloma formation. Our major goal in presenting this work is not to report specifics of the data, however, but

[a]This work was supported by Grant AI-15193 from the National Institutes of Health.

to convince other investigators of the utility of this model and its potential applicability to many granulomatous diseases.

MATERIALS AND METHODS

Infection

C_{57}Bl/6 mice (Jackson Laboratories, Bar Harbor, ME) were maintained according to established conditions of humane animal care. Mice were infected with 30 cercariae of the Puerto Rican strain of *S. mansoni* as previously described.[3]

Antigen and Bead Preparation

Soluble egg antigen (SEA) was generously provided by the UNDP/World Bank/WHO Program for Research and Training in Tropical Diseases. Antigen-bound Biogel P4 polyacrylamide beads (Biorad, Richmond, CA) were prepared by a carbodiimide coupling procedure as previously described.[8]

In Vitro *Granuloma Formation*

Single cell suspensions were prepared from the spleens of normal and infected animals in RPMI 1640 supplemented with antibiotics, 5×10^{-5} M 2-mercaptoethanol, 10 mM HEPES buffer, and 10% fetal calf serum. To generate *in vitro* granulomas, 2×10^6 spleen cells were incubated in 1 ml of medium per well of a 24-well plate with 200 antigen-coated beads. Cultures were set up in triplicate and were incubated at 37° C in a 5% CO_2-in-air atmosphere. After 6-9 days, cultures were observed with an inverted phase-contrast microscope equipped with a constant temperature stage heater set at 37° C. Cell-bead reactions were scored in a coded fashion according to the following set of criteria: 1) no cells attached to the bead; 2) 1-5 lymphoid cells; 3) 6-20 cells; 4) >20 cells; 5) a complete monolayer of cells; 6) multiple monolayers of cells. Evidence of mononuclear cell migration toward an individual bead adds 1 unit (U) to the score for that bead. Fifty or more reactions per well were scored, and then a mean reaction score or granuloma index (GI) was computed for each well. Data are reported as the mean of triplicate determinations.

The validity of the granuloma index as a quantitative means of determining the size of the reactions has been assessed by quantitative fluorometry. A significant correlation ($r = .71$; $p < .01$) was obtained between the granuloma score assigned to individual granulomas and their fluorescence following staining with acridine orange, a nonspecific stain for viable cells.

Antibodies

Monoclonal antibodies BP107 (directed against Ia antigens)[10] and GK1.5 (directed against L3T4 antigens)[11] were generously provided as ascites by Drs. Jonathan Sprent (University of Pennsylvania, Philadelphia, PA) and Frank Fitch (University of Chicago, Chicago, IL) respectively. Monoclonal antibody DMS2 (directed against interleukin-2 (IL-2))[12] was provided by Dr. Kendall Smith (Dartmouth Medical School, Hanover, NH). A rabbit antimurine immune interferon (IFN-γ) antibody, of high titer, was supplied by Genentech (San Francisco, CA). Anti-Ly-2.2 was purchased from New England Nuclear (Boston, MA).

Lymphokines

Recombinant murine immune interferon was supplied by Genentech (San Francisco, CA). Affinity-purified IL-2 (Jurkat) was generously provided by Dr. Kendall Smith.

RESULTS AND DISCUSSION

Definition of the Model

In initial studies, *in vitro* granulomas were generated by incubating cell populations from *S. mansoni*-infected hosts with eggs of the parasite.[3] Comparable reactions have also been demonstrated using antigens derived from the egg (SEA) covalently bound to polyacrylamide beads.[6] Morphological studies at the light and ultrastructural levels have established the sequence of reactions around these antigenic nidi.[3,5,6] Initial binding by the macrophage to the egg or bead is closely followed by T cell contact with the macrophage and the formation of macrophage-lymphocyte clusters (FIG. 1A). The active recruitment of additional mononuclear cells eventually leads to complete encapsulization of the egg or bead (FIG. 1B) and terminal stages of matrix protein deposition.

Granuloma formation *in vitro* recapitulates *in vivo* events. A significant correlation exists between the ability of spleen cells from infected animals to form *in vitro* granulomas and the size of hepatic granulomas at various times after infection (TABLE 1). Parallel experiments with PPD-immunized animals have also demonstrated a corre-

FIGURE 1. **(A)** A 4-day-old SEA bead granuloma to which macrophages have adhered. Macrophage processes have extended over the bead's surface. Note especially the formation of macrophage-lymphocyte clusters. These lymphocytes have been shown to be T cells by indirect immunofluorescence. **(B)** Side-by-side comparison of developmental stages of *in vitro* granuloma formation. Following initial T cell-macrophage contact and activation, a pronounced migration toward the bead occurs. Macrophages have coated the bead on the left. A complete monolayer of macrophages and lymphocytes has encapsulated the bead on the right. Original magnifications for **A** and **B**: × 1000; the figure has been reduced to 78% of its original size.

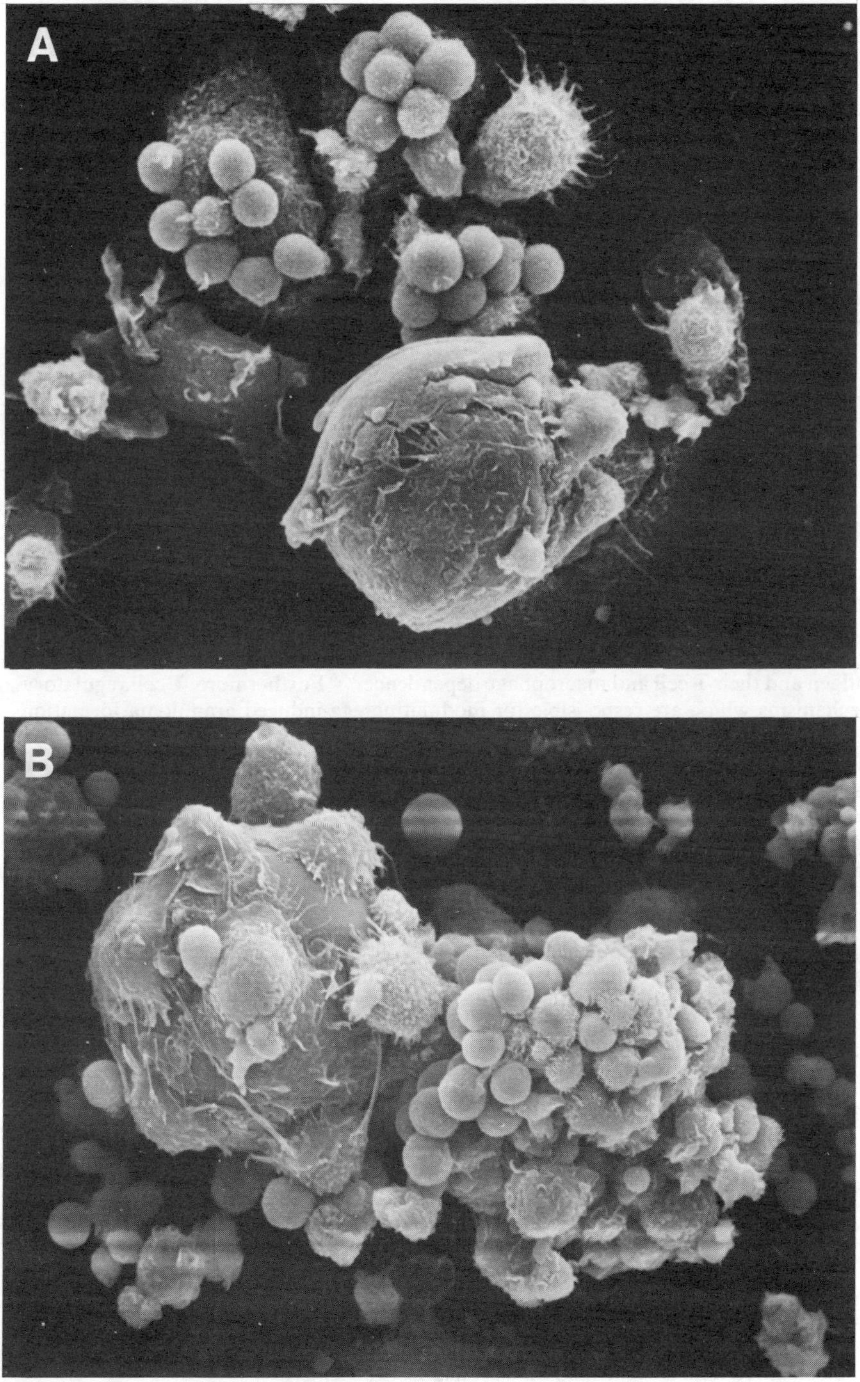
A
B

TABLE 1. Comparison of *in Vitro* Granuloma Formation and *in Vivo* Granuloma Formation or Delayed-type Hypersensitivity[a]

SEA[b]			PPD[c]		
Time[d]	GI	Diameter of Granuloma (μm)	Time[d]	GI	Delayed-type Hypersensitivity[e]
0	1.18		0	1.41	0.03
5	1.87	127	2	1.73	0.69
10	2.57	284	4	3.22	1.13
20	1.81	152	6	1.59	0.58
40	1.52	76	8	1.61	0.40

NOTE: GI versus granuloma size: $r = .78$; $p < .01$. GI versus delayed-type hypersensitivity: $r = .72$; $p < .05$.

[a] Summarized from Bentley *et al.*[6]

[b] Animals exposed to 125 *S. mansoni* cercariae.

[c] Animals sensitized with 0.5 ml of CFA.

[d] Interval in weeks between exposure and assay.

[e] Induration in mm at 36 hr.

spondence between *in vitro* and *in vivo* delayed-type hypersensitivity responses. These studies also illustrate the potential applicability of the *in vitro* granuloma model to other antigen systems.

In vitro reactions are like *in vivo* responses in their specificity for the sensitizing antigen and their T cell and macrophage dependence.[3,5,6] Furthermore, T cell regulatory mechanisms which are responsible for modulating egg-induced granuloma formation in the livers of chronically infected mice operate *in vitro* as well.[2,3] Comparable studies employing peripheral blood lymphocytes (PBL) of patients with schistosomiasis have also been undertaken.[7,9] These studies have shown that *in vitro* granuloma formation by human PBL is also under the regulatory control of T cell subsets and suggest that analogies exist between results obtained with human and murine cells (see TABLE 2 for a summary). Thus, an analytic approach to the mechanisms of immunoregulatory alterations in both human and experimental models of the disease is feasible.

We have recently initiated additional studies to characterize 1) *in vitro* granuloma formation in response to purified antigens (not discussed in this report); 2) essential elements of T cell-macrophage cooperation in granuloma formation (discussed below); 3) effector functions of cloned T cells (discussed in the next part of this section); and 4) the potential regulatory role of lymphokines in granuloma formation (discussed in

TABLE 2. Comparison of the Contributions of Human and Murine T Cell Subsets to *in Vitro* Granuloma Formation[a]

Cell Surface Marker			
Human	Murine	T Cell Subset	Effect of Cell Depletion on Granuloma Size
OKT3	Thy-1	All mature T cells	↓
OKT4	Ly-1	Helper/inducer T cells	↓
OKT8	Ly-2	Suppressor/cytotoxic T cells	↑↓

[a] Summarized from Doughty and Phillips[3] and Doughty *et al.*[7]

the last part of this section). Clearly these questions do not represent independent issues, but are interrelated aspects of the same cellular cascade. Our preliminary attempts to understand the events involved in the activation of granuloma formation have focused on the role of macrophage and T cell surface antigens in this process using the schistosomiasis model. Expression of Ia antigens by macrophages is a prerequisite for antigen presentation[13] whereas L3T4 antigen expression by T cells is required for class II MHC antigen-specific binding and lymphokine release.[14] The two molecules are thus intimately involved with the process of antigen recognition and initial T cell activation. Not surprisingly, antibodies directed against Ia and L3T4 antigens were both able to cause significant inhibition of the *in vitro* granulomatous response of immune spleen cells to SEA beads, even when added as late as day 4 of culture (TABLE 3). *In vitro* granuloma formation is, therefore, a dynamic process, involving ongoing cooperation between Ia antigen-positive macrophages and class II MHC-restricted T cells. Regulation of Ia antigen expression by IFN-γ may play a key role in determining the magnitude of the elicited response.[15,16] Experiments employing defined populations of macrophages and T cells (see below) are in progress to answer this question.

TABLE 3. Effect of Antibodies Directed against Ia and L3T4 Antigens on *in Vitro* Granuloma Formation

Antibody[a]	Day Added	Normal Spleen GI[c]	Normal Spleen Significance	Immune Spleen[b] GI[c]	Immune Spleen[b] Significance
None		2.75		3.84	
Anti-Ia	0	2.75	NS	3.29	$p < .05$
	2			3.04	$p < .01$
	4			3.33	$p < .01$
Anti-L3T4	0	2.84	NS	3.00	$p < .01$
	2			3.29	$p < .05$
	4			3.40	$p < .05$

[a] The anti-Ia antibody was diluted 1:100; the anti-L3T4 antibody was diluted 1:1000.
[b] Immune spleen cells were obtained from animals 8 weeks after infection.
[c] GI was determined 7 days after culture initiation.

In Vitro *Granuloma Formation by T Cell Clones*

T cell cloning technology has led to significant advances in our understanding of the nature of antigen recognition by T cells, genetic restrictions on immune responses, and the effector functions mediated by specific subpopulations of cells.[17] We applied this technology to our study of the *in vitro* granuloma model in order to begin to analyze the capabilities of the T cells responsible for granuloma formation and the cellular and molecular signals which regulate the process.[8] The clones we studied were derived from the spleens of acutely infected animals by cloning in the presence of IL-2 according to published procedures.[18] Sixteen clones were selected for expansion on the basis of their specificity for SEA in antigen-induced blastogenesis assays (representative data for four clones are shown in TABLE 4). SEA-specific clones were then

TABLE 4. Characteristics of T Cell Clones[a]

Clone	Response to SEA				Con A-induced FSA[f]
	Proliferation[b]	Delayed-type Hypersensitivity[c]	GI[d]	IL-2[e]	
Control	<200	3.4	2.56	0	1.6
A2	8869	11.5	3.46	2.48	4.4
A5	7492	9.0	3.67	7.75	4.7
G4	25 946	12.3	3.88	0.57	10.7
G6	1917	7.2	3.26	3.88	1.5

[a] Summarized from unpublished data and from Lammie *et al.*[8,19]

[b] Response in counts per minute of T cells + irradiated spleen cells (APC) + 50 μg/ml SEA; control = SEA + APC.

[c] Response in mm × 10^{-2} of footpad swelling elicited by 5 × 10^5 T cells + 10 μg SEA; control = normal spleen cells + SEA.

[d] *In vitro* GI of 1 × 10^5 T cells + 2 × 10^6 normal spleen cells; control = normal spleen cells alone.

[e] Units of IL-2 activity in supernatant of 1 × 10^6 T cells stimulated with 5 × 10^6 APC + SEA in CTLL proliferation assay; control = supernatant of APC + SEA.

[f] Ratio of fibroblast stimulatory activity (FSA) induced by serum-free supernatant of 1 × 10^6 T cells pulsed with con A; control = 5 × 10^6 normal spleen cells pulsed with con A.

tested for their ability to generate *in vitro* granulomas in response to SEA- or PPD-coated beads. In the absence of a source of antigen-presenting cells, T cells were unable to respond to the beads (GI <2). When 1 × 10^5 cells were supplemented with 2 × 10^6 normal spleen cells, however, significant responses were directed against SEA, but not PPD beads (GI = 3.69 and 2.67, respectively; means of data from 6 clones). Control cultures containing normal spleen cells alone were not responsive to either bead (GI = 2.60). T cell clone-generated granulomas were morphologically indistinguishable from those obtained with cultures of immune cells. Thus monoclonal T cells are capable of providing all the necessary signals to generate the *in vitro* response. Interestingly, the response of individual clones in the *in vitro* granuloma assay was significantly correlated with their ability to mediate local delayed-type hypersensitivity reactions, suggesting that T cell function *in vitro* and *in vivo* is analogous.

To provide a better understanding of how mediator production by T cells can contribute to granuloma formation, we also undertook an analysis of the lymphokines produced by the cloned cells. Individual clones were capable of producing a number of lymphokines in response to concanavalin A (con A) or SEA stimulation, including IL-2; IFN-γ, or macrophage-activating factor (MAF); macrophage migration-inhibitory factor (MIF); eosinophil-stimulation factor (ESP); and a T cell-derived fibroblast-stimulation factor (FSF-T).[19] While no obvious relationships exist between the production of specific mediators by individual clones and their capacity to induce *in vitro* granulomas, each of these lymphokines probably represents a significant component of the cascade of cellular activation and recruitment. The modulated granuloma of chronic schistosomiasis has, in fact, been attributed to suppressed production of MIF and ESP.[2,20,21] The experiments discussed below also support an autoregulatory role for T cell-produced IFN-γ and IL-2.

Developing a clearer understanding of the range of mediators produced by or in response to T cells is also crucial to efforts directed toward controlling granuloma formation and its associated fibrosis. The ability of T cells to produce fibroblast-stimulatory activity in response to con A in the complete absence of macrophages or other accessory cells (TABLE 4) suggests a direct molecular link between T cells and fibrosis.[19] The additional macrophage-mediated component of fibroblast stimulation, which exists[22] when accessory cells are present, may also be subject to T cell control via production of MAF. Further study of cloned T cells in the *in vitro* model may provide additional insights into the immunoregulatory aspects of fibroblast proliferation and collagen synthesis.

Lymphokine-mediated Regulation of Granuloma Formation

The demonstration of IFN-γ and IL-2 production by cloned T cells as well as the availability of purified lymphokines and antibodies directed against these mediators led us to investigate the effects of these two lymphokines on *in vitro* granuloma formation. Inclusion of polyclonal antimurine immune interferon or monoclonal anti-IL-2 consistently augmented responses (TABLE 5). Presumably, complete inhibition of IFN-γ or IL-2 would have suppressed the response because IFN-γ and IL-2 are required for induction of Ia expression and T cell growth, respectively. These antibodies do not block 100% of the lymphokine activity, however, and suppressive concentrations of either antibody were not reached in repeated experiments. In addition, no evidence of direct binding to SEA by either antibody was obtained. Thus, Fc receptor-mediated augmentation of bead binding was not the mechanism of enhanced responsiveness. While immune complex-mediated activation of macrophages may contribute to this effect, it is also possible that endogenous production of IFN-γ and IL-2 may achieve immunoregulatory levels. Confirmatory evidence has been obtained in experiments utilizing recombinant murine IFN-γ and affinity-purified IL-2. Both lymphokines suppressed *in vitro* granuloma formation by immune spleen cells in a dose-dependent fashion (data not shown). Consistent suppression was obtained with 10 U/ml IFN-γ and 0.5 U/ml IL-2, and these concentrations were utilized in subsequent experiments. It should be emphasized that no deleterious effects on cell viability were observed at these concentrations.

The ability of IL-2 to cause suppression may appear surprising given its requirement for T cell proliferation and its deficiency in immunosuppressed states.[23–25] The suppressive capacity of IL-2 may reflect an autoregulatory mechanism comparable to previously described feedback inhibition loops.[26] Because IL-2 is a required signal for IFN-γ release in both human and murine systems,[27–29] conceivably IL-2-induced

TABLE 5. Anti-IFN-γ and Anti-IL-2 Augment *in Vitro* Granuloma Formation

	Normal Spleen		Immune Spleen[b]	
Antibody[a]	GI	Significance	GI	Significance
	2.28		3.37	
Anti-IFN-γ	2.29	NS	4.01	$p < .01$
Anti-IL-2	2.84	$p < .05$	3.97	$p < .01$

[a] The anti-IFN-γ antibody was diluted 1:500; the anti-IL-2 antibody was diluted 1:25.
[b] Immune spleen cells were obtained from animals 8 weeks after infection.

suppression is also mediated via IFN-γ, which has well-characterized immunoregulatory effects.[30,31] Alternatively, exposure of cloned T cells to high levels of IL-2 is known to induce a transient state in which antigens do not provoke a response, a state which may result from a down regulation of IL-2 receptors.[23,32] Studies are in progress to resolve the issue by quantifying IL-2 receptor expression and IFN-γ production in this system.

Preliminary insight into a possible cellular mechanism of suppression was provided by cell-depletion experiments. Immune spleen cells treated with anti-Ly-2 plus complement were inhibited less by IL-2 and IFN-γ than untreated control cells were (TABLE 6). Addition of exogenous IFN-γ and IL-2 may, therefore, induce an Ly-2$^+$ suppressor cell population. IFN induction of suppressor cells has been previously reported, although the exact mechanism of the effect is undefined.[33] Some analogies may exist between suppressive effects induced by IL-2 and IFN-γ and previously described mitogen-induced nonspecific regulatory mechanisms.[34,35]

The physiological relevance of these observations is conjectural at present. Perhaps endogenous IL-2 and IFN-γ production *in vivo* control minimum and maximum rates of granuloma formation, preventing inadequate as well as overly aggressive responses. In any event, these experiments do point out the complexity of the lymphokine cascade as it applies to granuloma formation. Additional layers of complexity are no doubt imposed by IL-1 and other macrophage-associated factors. Obviously, years of study are required before we can understand mechanisms of granuloma formation at this level.

TABLE 6. Effect of IFN-γ and IL-2 on *in Vitro* Granuloma Formation

	GI of Culture		
Cell Population	Untreated	IL-2 (0.5 U/ml)	IFN-γ (10 U/ml)
Normal spleen	2.38	2.29[a]	2.30[a]
Immune spleen	3.67	2.19[b]	2.95[c]
Immune spleen (anti-Ly-2 depleted)	3.65	3.42[b]	3.59[a]

[a] Not significantly different from the control value.
[b] Significantly different from the control value: $p < .001$.
[c] Significantly different from the control value: $p < .01$.

SUMMARY

The *in vitro* granuloma model provides an excellent tool to study granulomatous hypersensitivity. In our studies of granuloma formation in schistosomiasis, we have demonstrated the utility of the model with respect to analysis of human PBL responses, cloned T cells, purified antigens of the parasite, and regulatory mechanisms. We have also presented data which demonstrate the applicability of this model to other antigenic systems. While the suggestion that this model may be suitable for the study of sarcoidosis may be premature, we would propose that the system may be adapted to screen potentially causative antigens. Furthermore, with the identification of the critical antigen(s), the *in vitro* granuloma model will facilitate studies at the clinical level.

ACKNOWLEDGMENT

The authors thank Anne Barr for her expert secretarial assistance.

REFERENCES

1. BOROS, D. L. 1978. Prog. Allergy **24:** 183-267.
2. COLLEY, D. G. 1981. *In* The Immunology of Parasitic Diseases. J. Mansfield, Ed. Vol. **1:** 1-83. Marcel Dekker. New York, NY.
3. DOUGHTY, B. L. & S. M. PHILLIPS. 1982. J. Immunol. **128:** 30-36.
4. DOUGHTY, B. L. & S. M. PHILLIPS. 1982. J. Immunol. **128:** 37-42.
5. BENTLEY, A. G., B. L. DOUGHTY & S. M. PHILLIPS. 1982. Am. J. Trop. Med. Hyg. **31:** 1168-1180.
6. BENTLEY, A. G., S. M. PHILLIPS, R. J. KANER, V. J. THEODORIDES, G. P. LINETTE & B. L. DOUGHTY. 1985. J. Immunol. **134:** 4163-4169.
7. DOUGHTY, B. L., E. A. OTTESEN, T. E. NASH & S. M. PHILLIPS. 1984. J. Immunol. **133:** 993-997.
8. LAMMIE, P. J., G. P. LINETTE & S. M. PHILLIPS. 1985. J. Immunol. **134:** 4170-4175.
9. DOUGHTY, B. L., D. M. ZODDA, A. EL KHOLY & S. M. PHILLIPS. 1984. Am. J. Trop. Med. Hyg. **33:** 1173-1177.
10. SYMINGTON, F. W. & J. SPRENT. 1981. Immunogenetics **14:** 53-61.
11. DIALYNAS, D. P., Z. S. QUAN, K. A. WALL, A. PIERRES, J. QUINTANS, M. R. LOKAN, M. PIERRES & F. W. FITCH. 1983. J. Immunol. **131:** 2445.
12. SMITH, K. A., M. F. FAVATA & S. OROSZLAN. 1983. J. Immunol. **131:** 1808-1815.
13. UNANUE, E. R., D. I. BELLER, C. Y. LU & P. M. ALLEN. 1984. J. Immunol. **132:** 1-5.
14. DIALYNAS, D. P., D. B. WILDE, P. MARRACK, A. PIERRES, K. A. WALL, W. HAVRAN, M. R. LOKEN, M. PIERRES, J. KAPPLER & F. W. FITCH. 1983. Immunol. Rev. **74:** 29-56.
15. STEEG, P. S., R. N. MOORE & J. J. OPPENHEIM. 1980. J. Exp. Med. **152:** 1734-1744.
16. ZLOTNIK, A., W. K. ROBERTS, A. VASIL, E. BLUMENTHAL, F. LAROSA, H. J. LEIBSON, R. O. ENDRES, S. D. GRAHAM, J. WHITE, J. HILL, P. HENSON, J. R. KLEIN, M. J. BEVAN, P. MARRACK & J. W. KAPPLER. 1983. J. Immunol. **131:** 794-800.
17. FATHMAN, C. G. & F. W. FITCH. 1982. Isolation, Characterization and Utilization of T Lymphocyte Clones. Academic Press. New York, NY.
18. SREDNI, B., H. Y. TSE, C. CHEN & R. H. SCWARTZ. 1981. J. Immunol. **126:** 341-347.
19. LAMMIE, P. J., A. I. MICHAEL, G. P. LINETTE & S. M. PHILLIPS. 1985. J. Immunol. In press.
20. CHENSUE, S. W., D. L. BOROS & C. S. DAVID. 1983. J. Exp. Med. **157:** 219-230.
21. JAMES, S. L. & D. G. COLLEY. 1975. J. Reticuloendothel. Soc. **18:** 283-291.
22. WYLER, D. J. 1983. *In* Cytopathology of Parasitic Disease. Ciba Foundation Symposium. Vol. **99:** 190-206. Pitman Books. London.
23. ROBB, R. J. 1984. Immunol. Today. **5:** 203-209.
24. PALACIOS, R. & G. MOLLER. 1981. J. Exp. Med. **153:** 1360-1365.
25. HAREL-BELLAN, M., M. SOSKOWICZ, D. FRADELIZI & H. EISEN. 1983. Proc. Natl. Acad. Sci. USA **80:** 3466-3469.
26. EARDLEY, D. D., J. HUGENBERGER, L. C. MCVAY-BOUDREAU, F. W. SHEN, R. K. GERSHON & H. CANTOR. 1978. J. Exp. Med. **147:** 1106-1115.
27. REEM, G. H. & N.-H. YEH. 1984. Science **225:** 429-430.
28. TORRES, B. A., W. L. FARRAR & H. M. JOHNSON. 1982. J. Immunol. **128:** 2217-2219.
29. KASAHARA, T., J. J. HOOKS, S. F. DOUGHERTY & J. J. OPPENHEIM. 1983. J. Immunol. **130:** 1784-1789.
30. HERON, I., K. BERG & K. CANTELL. 1976. J. Immunol. **117:** 1370-1373.

31. Kadish, A. S., F. A. Tansey, G. S. M. Yu, A. T. Doyle & B. R. Bloom. 1980. J. Exp. Med. **151:** 637-650.
32. Wilde, D. B., M. B. Prystowshy, J. M. Ely, S. N. Vogel, D. P. Dialynas & F. W. Fitch. 1984. J. Immunol. **133:** 636-641.
33. Vose, B. M., C. Riccardi, G. O. Bonnard & R. B. Herberman. 1983. J. Immunol. **130:** 768-772.
34. Tadakuma, T. & C. W. Pierce. 1978. J. Immunol. **120:** 481-486.
35. Aune, T. M. & C. W. Pierce. 1981. J. Immunol. **127:** 368-372.

Inhibition by Cyclosporin A of Streptococcal Cell Wall-induced Hepatic Granulomas in LEW/N Rats

JANICE B. ALLEN,[a] DAVID E. YOCUM, AND RONALD L. WILDER

Arthritis and Rheumatism Branch
National Institute of Arthritis, Diabetes, and Digestive and Kidney Diseases
National Institutes of Health
Bethesda, Maryland 20205

SHARON M. WAHL

Cellular Immunology Section
Laboratory of Microbiology and Immunology
National Institute of Dental Research
National Institutes of Health
Bethesda, Maryland 20205

INTRODUCTION

Noncaseating hepatic granulomas can be produced in susceptible female rats by a single intraperitoneal injection of group A streptococcal cell wall fragments.[1,2] Within 24 hr after injection, the liver becomes edematous with diffuse, polymorphonuclear leukocyte infiltration and fibrin deposition.[3] This reaction reaches maximum intensity by day 3 and gradually subsides. This acute reaction develops coincident with the deposition of cell wall fragments in the liver.[4] After about 2-3 weeks, the liver is infiltrated with inflammatory mononuclear cells. By 3-6 weeks, noncaseating granulomas primarily composed of macrophages, lymphocytes, and fibroblasts develop as an apparent consequence of the persistence of the cell walls in the liver.

Since lymphocytic infiltration is a prominent component of this granulomatous process and since bacterial cell walls are known modulators of mononuclear cell

[a] Address for correspondence: Arthritis and Rheumatism Branch, National Institute of Arthritis, Diabetes, and Digestive and Kidney Diseases, Building 10, Room 9N240, National Institutes of Health, Bethesda, Maryland 20205.

function,[4,5] we have hypothesized that the lesion reflects a cell-mediated immunologic reaction driven by the persistence of the cell walls in the mononuclear phagocytic cells in the liver.[6] To further address this hypothesis we have studied the effect of daily intramuscular injections of cyclosporin A (CS-A), a modulator of thymus-derived (T) lymphocyte function, on granuloma formation. CS-A is a hydrophobic oligopeptide with potent inhibitory effects on T cell-mediated immune responses.[7-10] Accumulating evidence suggests that CS-A interferes with the early stages of T lymphocyte activation.[11,12] We have demonstrated that CS-A significantly inhibits the development of the group A streptococcal cell wall-induced hepatic granulomas, without measurably affecting the dissemination of the cell wall antigens to the liver. These results provide evidence that T lymphocytes play a key role in the pathogenesis of this granulomatous process.

MATERIALS AND METHODS

Animals

Female, specific pathogen-free inbred LEW/N rats were obtained from the Small Animal Section of the National Institutes of Health. The animals weighed approximately 100 g at the beginning of each experiment.

Injection of Streptococcal Cell Walls

Group A streptococcal cell wall fragments (SCW) were prepared as previously described.[1] Briefly, a sterile suspension of sonicated streptococcal cell walls in phosphate-buffered saline (PBS), pH 7.4, was injected intraperitoneally into LEW/N females at a dose equivalent to 18 μg of cell wall rhamnose/g body weight.[13] Control animals were injected with an equal volume of PBS.

Treatment with CS-A

CS-A (gift of Sandoz Pharmaceuticals, East Hanover, NJ) was provided in powder form and dissolved initially in absolute ethanol. It was then diluted in sterile olive oil in a boiling water bath to final concentration. The final ethanol concentration was always 5% or less. It was prepared fresh every 4 days, stored at room temperature, and protected from light. CS-A was injected intramuscularly in the thigh on day -1 and daily thereafter. The dose, either 10 or 25 mg/kg, was adjusted according to body weight. Control rats included those injected with only SCW, PBS, olive oil and ethanol, or CS-A. CS-A-treated and control rats were handled identically for the duration of the experiment.

Histologic Evaluation

Specimens of liver were fixed in 10% buffered formalin, embedded in paraffin, sectioned, and stained with hematoxylin and eosin. The slides were coded and analyzed for evidence of an inflammatory reaction and/or other tissue abnormalities.

Immunoperoxidase Technique for Antigen Detection

Liver specimens were formalin fixed, paraffin embedded, sectioned, and stained for streptococcal cell wall antigens using an immunoperoxidase technique (ABC Vecta Stain Kit, Vector Laboratories, Burlington, CA) as previously described.[6,14] Controls included sections from saline-injected rats and/or CS-A-treated rats stained as above as well as sections from SCW-injected and/or CS-A-treated rats stained with normal rabbit globulin and no primary antibody. Specificity was verified by determining whether the antibody was absorbed onto the streptococcal cell walls, a process which completely eliminated positive staining. The black precipitate reaction product was an indication that the streptococcal cell wall antigen was present.

RESULTS

Streptococcal Cell Wall-induced Hepatic Granuloma Development

Previously published histopathologic analyses of LEW/N rats after intraperitoneal injections of group A streptococcal cell walls document the development of noncaseating, hepatic granulomas.[1,2] Within 24-72 hr after injection a predominantly polymorphonuclear leukocytic infiltrate with an intense fibrinous exudate is observed. This reaction gradually subsides. Two weeks after injection the predominant infiltrating cells are mononuclear leukocytes. This loose infiltrate of cells develops into organized aggregates of mature macrophages and lymphocytes, along with extensive fibroblast-like proliferation. These granulomas are present in the portal areas and in the parenchyma. Plasma cells, multinucleated giant cells, and eosinophils are also present. There is little evidence of hepatic cell death. We monitored the effects of CS-A on the granulomas 6 weeks after injection, by which time the granulomas were already well developed.

Effect of CS-A on Granuloma Development

Thirty-five female LEW/N rats, each weighing approximately 100 g, were divided into seven groups. Each rat in four of the groups was injected intraperitoneally with an aqueous suspension of group A streptococcal cell wall fragments at a dose of 18

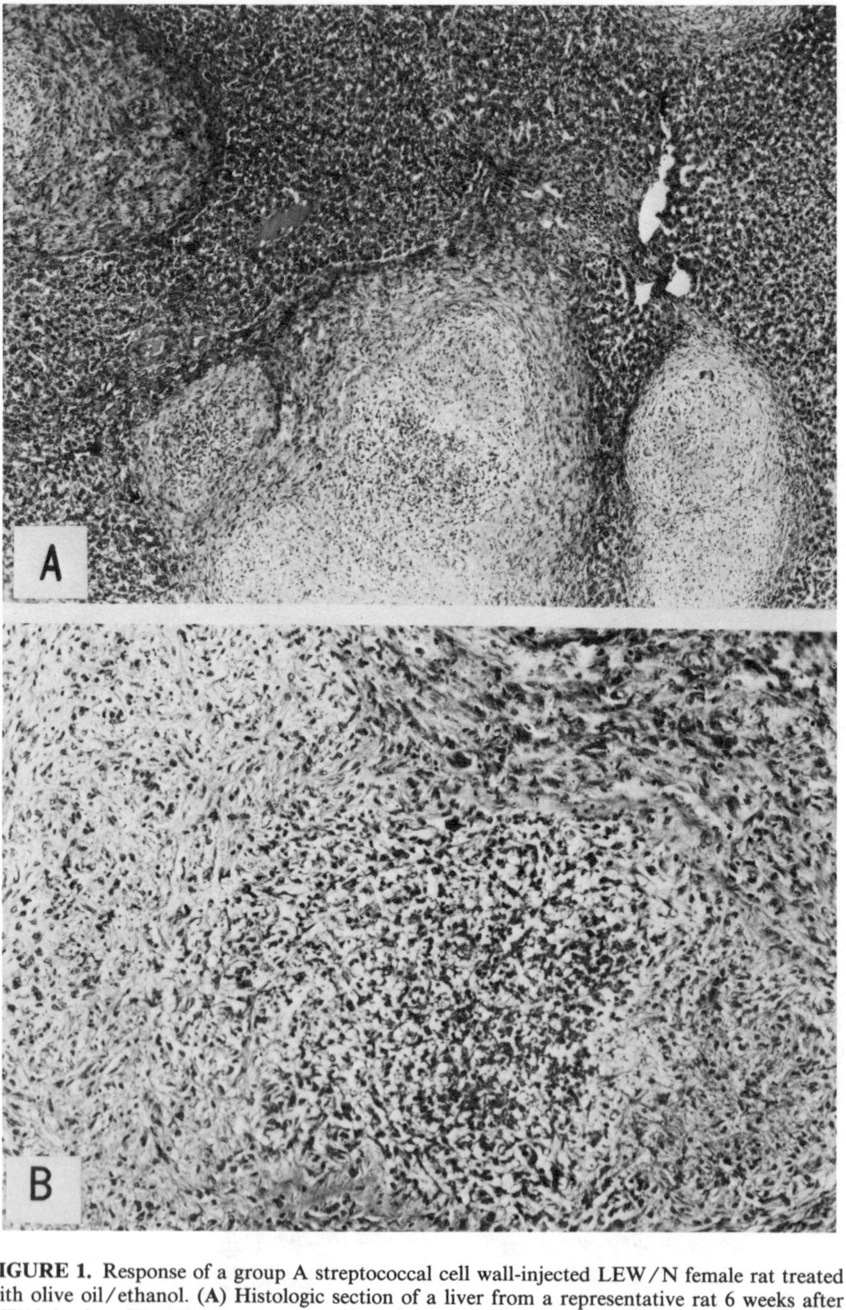

FIGURE 1. Response of a group A streptococcal cell wall-injected LEW/N female rat treated with olive oil/ethanol. (**A**) Histologic section of a liver from a representative rat 6 weeks after SCW injection. (**B**) A higher magnification of the section shown in **A**. The original magnifications for **A** and **B** were $\times$ 54 and $\times$ 220, respectively; the figure was enlarged to 111% of its original size.

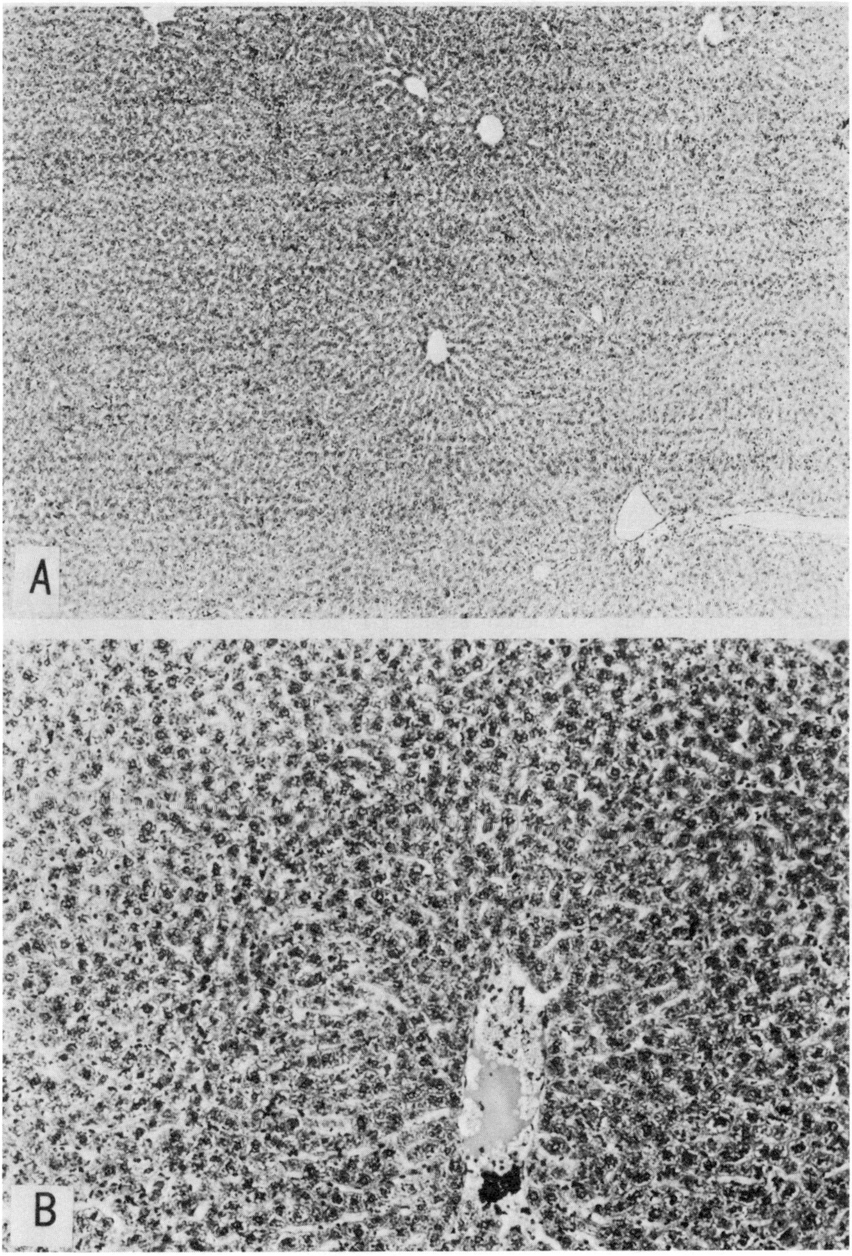

FIGURE 2. Response of a group A streptococcal cell wall-injected LEW/N female rat treated with CS-A at a dose of 25 mg/kg/day. (**A**) Histologic section of a liver from a representative rat 6 weeks after SCW injection. (**B**) A higher magnification of the section shown in **A**. The original magnifications for **A** and **B** were × 54 and × 200, respectively; the figure was enlarged to 111% of its original size.

μg rhamnose/g body weight. The remaining three groups (controls) were injected with an equal volume of PBS. Rats in these four groups received an intramuscular injection of olive oil/ethanol, CS-A at 25 mg/kg, CS-A at 10 mg/kg, or PBS 24 hr before the SCW injections and daily thereafter for the duration of the experiment. Rats in the other three groups were injected with PBS and received olive oil/ethanol, CS-A at 10 mg/kg/day, or CS-A at 25 mg/kg/day. After 6 weeks the rats were sacrificed, and the livers excised and analyzed for granuloma formation. Profound differences were observed among the SCW-injected groups. As demonstrated histologically in FIGURE 1, the liver from a representative rat in the olive oil-treated, SCW-injected group developed large noncaseating granulomas. The granulomas were extensive and consisted of macrophages, lymphocytes, plasma cells, and fibroblasts. In contrast, SCW-injected rats treated daily with CS-A at a dose of 25 mg/kg had an almost normal liver histology (FIGS. 2A & 2B). The only apparent abnormalities were the minimally increased lymphocytic cellularity, the slight dilation of hepatic sinusoids (around central veins), and the occasional mild periportal focal necrosis. There was no evidence of organized mononuclear cell foci or granuloma development throughout the liver. Livers from cell wall-injected rats treated with CS-A at a dose of 10 mg/kg/day were similar to those that received the higher dose (data not shown). Sections of livers from representative PBS-injected rats which received daily intramuscular injections of CS-A at 25 or 10 mg/kg, or no CS-A, showed no evidence of abnormal histology, as shown in FIGURES 3A & 3B. SCW-induced granulomas, as shown in FIGURE 3C, were identical to those in cell wall-injected rats who received the vehicle only. Thus, daily treatment of SCW-injected rats with 25 or 10 mg/kg of CS-A significantly inhibited the formation of hepatic granulomas.

Cell Wall Distribution

The persistence in tissues of the SCW antigens after intraperitoneal injection was demonstrated by immunoperoxidase staining. FIGURE 4 shows the localization of antigens in the cytoplasm of mononuclear phagocytic cells in the liver. Streptococcal cell wall antigens were detected in the livers of all cell wall-injected rats, with or without CS-A treatment. FIGURE 4A shows a section of liver from a representative rat in the SCW-injected group treated with olive oil/ethanol. The cell wall antigen was distributed throughout the tissue, but concentrated primarily in the granuloma. As depicted in FIGURE 4B, the section of liver from a representative rat in the CS-A-treated (25 mg/kg), SCW-injected group shows the antigen uniformly distributed throughout the entire tissue. Livers from cell wall-injected rats treated with CS-A at a dose of 10 mg/kg were similar to those that received the higher dose (data not shown). FIGURE 4C shows the absence of staining in a liver section from a PBS-injected rat stained with the anti-group A streptococci globulin.

FIGURE 3. Responses of LEW/N females 6 weeks after injection of PBS or streptococcal cell walls. **(A)** Histologic section of a liver from a representative rat injected with PBS and treated with CS-A at 25 mg/kg/day. **(B)** Section of liver from a representative rat injected with PBS only. **(C)** Section of a liver from a representative rat injected with streptococcal cell walls only. Original magnifications: × 130; figure enlarged to 127% of its original size.

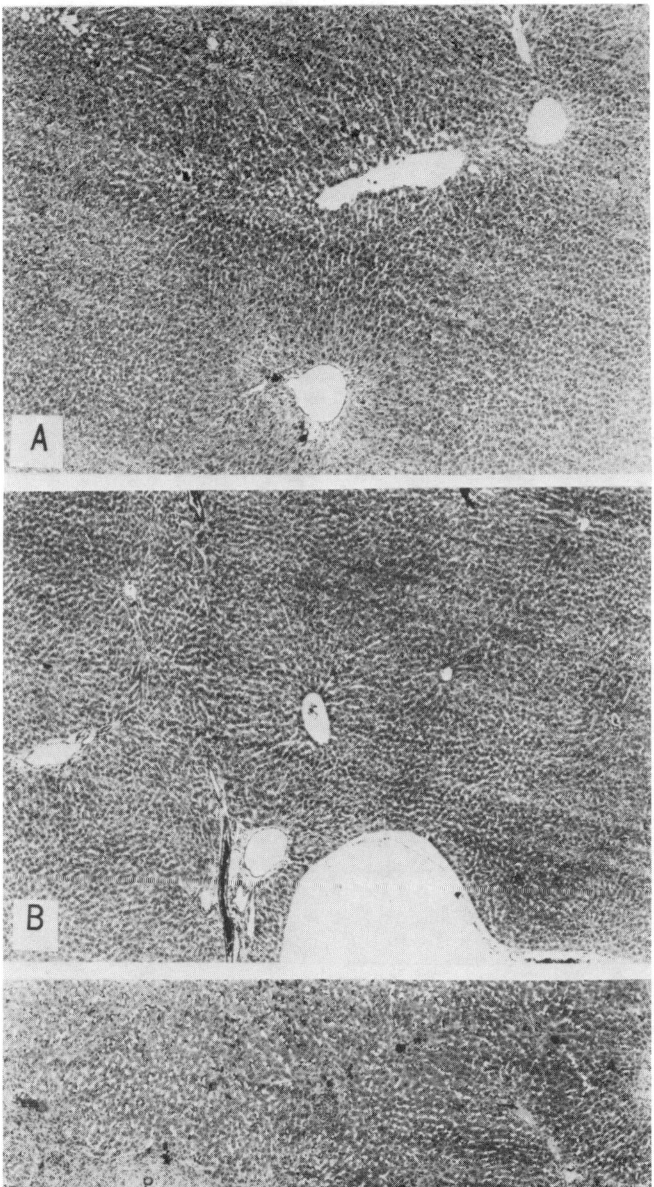
A
B
C

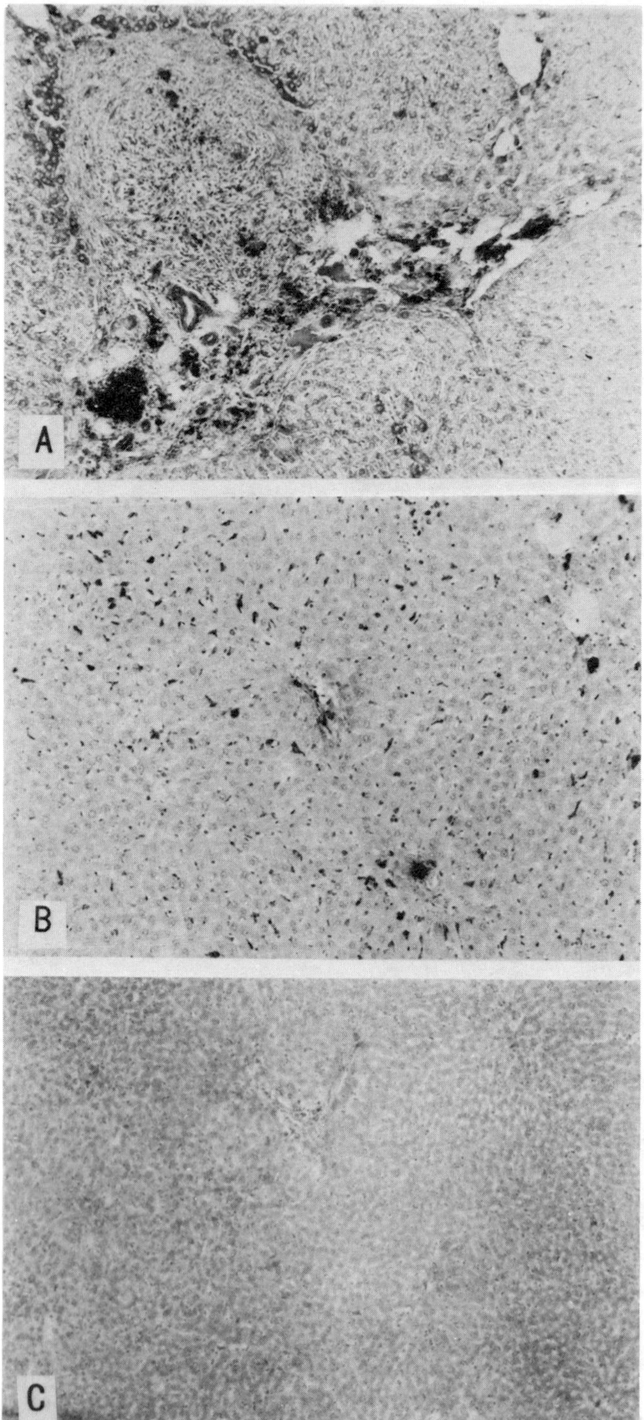
A
B
C

DISCUSSION

The formation of streptococcal cell wall-induced hepatic granulomas has been well documented.[1,2] The cellular mechanisms involved in the formation of these granulomas, however, are less well understood. The presence of large numbers of lymphocytes and monocyte-macrophages identified within the SCW-induced granuloma suggests that the following sequence of events may lead to the formation of discrete granulomas.[15,16] The hepatic Kupffer cells appear to phagocytize the poorly degradable cell walls, and following this uptake the cells may present the processed walls to T lymphocytes. The activated lymphocytes produce various lymphokines which may induce differentiation, proliferation, and mobilization of additional cells of the monocytic and lymphocytic series. The monocytes transform into tissue macrophages, enlarge, and display enhanced biochemical activity. This immobilization of blood monocytes around the focus of cell walls and their conversion into activated macrophages probably occur under the influence of T lymphocyte-derived lymphokines. The granuloma increases in size and is organized such that macrophages are arranged in a concentric structure surrounded by lymphocytes. This tight organization sequesters the cell walls from the surrounding tissues. Various cytokines may induce giant cell formation by promoting fusion between macrophages and may stimulate local fibroblast growth leading to fibrosis. Through the influx, local multiplication, and death of the macrophages and lymphocytes, the granuloma appears to be maintained as long as the cell walls persist in the site. Evidence that the T cells do indeed play a key role in the sequence of events leading to granuloma formation is provided by the CS-A studies reported here.

While the precise mechanisms of action of CS-A are not completely understood, data exist demonstrating that it exerts its effects by interfering with the early stages of T lymphocyte activation.[11,12] Thus, the drug is a very useful probe in determining the role of T lymphocytes in immunologically mediated disease. In our studies we observed that CS-A significantly inhibited the development of group A streptococcal cell wall-induced hepatic granulomas in LEW/N rats. Moreover, as determined by an immunoperoxidase technique, the cell wall antigen was deposited in phagocytic cells of the liver in both treated and untreated animals. Because the streptococcal cell walls were not eliminated in the CS-A-treated rats, and granuloma formation was still markedly inhibited, we conclude that T lymphocyte activation is a critical element in the development of these hepatic granulomas.

This conclusion is consistent with another relevant observation. We have completed studies in the nude rat that provide strong evidence that T lymphocyte-mediated immunological processes are necessary for the development of granulomas.[6] In addition, we have preliminary data which demonstrate by immunoperoxidase staining (unpublished data) that T cells, particularly of the T helper/inducer subset, are present in the granulomas and dispersed throughout the liver tissue. Although the livers of CS-A-treated animals are also sparsely infiltrated with lymphocytes, primarily of the helper/inducer subset, throughout the parenchyma, no aggregates of T lymphocytes can be demonstrated. While it is clear that the cell walls disseminate into the liver where they persist and that T lymphocytes migrate into the liver, even following CS-

FIGURE 4. Demonstration of group A streptococcal cell wall antigen in LEW/N female rat livers. **(A)** Section of liver from a representative rat treated with olive oil/ethanol in the cell wall-injected group. **(B)** Section of liver from a representative rat in the CS-A (25 mg/kg/day)-treated, cell wall-injected group. **(C)** Section of liver from a representative rat in the untreated, PBS-injected group. Original magnifications: × 80; figure enlarged to 126% of its original size.

A treatment, the T lymphocytes apparently do not become activated; therefore, granulomas do not develop.

Our findings may provide invaluable insights into the understanding of the pathogenesis of comparable human diseases and may also provide information on potential mechanisms of therapeutic intervention.

SUMMARY

A single intraperitoneal injection of an aqueous suspension of group A streptococcal cell wall fragments into susceptible LEW/N female rats results in the development of noncaseating hepatic granulomas as a consequence of deposition and persistence of the cell walls in the liver. We have studied the effect of daily intramuscular injections of CS-A, an inhibitor of T lymphocyte activation, on granuloma formation.

CS-A-treatment resulted in the pronounced inhibition of granuloma formation, although no appreciable differences in quantity of streptococcal cell wall antigens, which were deposited in the liver, could be demonstrated. These data suggest that activated T lymphocytes play a key role in the pathogenesis of this granulomatous process.

ACKNOWLEDGMENTS

We would like to thank Ms. Toni Vaughn for her assistance in preparing the manuscript, Dr. Marion Peters for her assistance in analyzing the liver histopathology, and Sandoz Pharmaceuticals for supplying the CS-A.

REFERENCES

1. WILDER, R. L., G. B. CALANDRA, A. J. GARVIN, K. D. WRIGHT & C. T. HANSEN. 1982. Strain and sex variation in the susceptibility to streptococcal cell wall-induced polyarthritis in the rat. Arthritis Rheum. **25:** 1064-1072.
2. HEYMER, B., H. SCHAFER, W. SCHACHENMAYR, D. HAFERKAMP & W. C. SCHMIDT. 1971. Streptococcal cell wall structure-induced hepatic granuloma. Arch. Pathol. **92:** 84-92.
3. ULEVITCH, R. J., P. S. TOBIAS & S. C. MATHISON. 1984. Regulation of the host response to bacterial lipopolysaccharides. Fed. Proc. **43:** 2755-2759.
4. WILDER, R. L., J. B. ALLEN, L. M. WAHL, G. B. CALANDRA & S. M. WAHL. 1983. The pathogenesis of group A streptococcal cell wall-induced polyarthritis in the rat: Comparative studies in arthritis-resistant and -susceptible inbred rat strains. Arthritis Rheum. **26:** 1442-1451.
5. GROSS, W. L. & M. SCHLAAK. 1984. Modulation of human lymphocyte functions by group A streptococci. Clin. Immunol. Immunopathol. **32:** 234-247.
6. ALLEN, J. B., D. G. MALONE, S. M. WAHL, G. B. CALANDRA & R. L. WILDER. 1985. The role of thymus-dependent lymphocytes in streptococcal cell wall-induced arthritis and hepatic granuloma formation: Comparative studies of pathology and cell wall distribution in athymic and euthymic rats. J. Clin. Invest. **76:** 1042-1056.

7. BOREL, J. G., C. FEURER, H. U. GUBLER & H. STAHELIN. 1976. Biological effects of cyclosporin A, a new antilymphocytic agent. Agents Actions **6:** 468-475.
8. KLAUS, G. G. B. 1981. The effects of cyclosporin A on the immune system. Immunol. Today **2:** 83-87.
9. BOREL, J. G., C. FEURER, C. MAGNEE & H. STAHELIN. 1977. Effects of the new anti-lymphocyte peptide cyclosporin A in animals. Immunology **32:** 1017-1025.
10. BRITTON, S. & R. PALACIOS. 1982. Cyclosporin A—Usefulness, risks and mechanism of action. Immunol. Rev. **65:** 5-22.
11. LILLEHOJ, H. S., T. R. MALEK & E. M. SHEVACH. 1984. Differential effect of cyclosporin A on the expression of T and B lymphocyte activation antigens. J. Immunol. **133:** 244-250.
12. KRONKE, M., W. J. LEONARD, J. M. DEPPER, S. K. ARYA, F. WONG-STAAL, R. C. GALLO, T. A. WALDMANN & W. C. GREENE. 1984. Cyclosporin A inhibits T cell growth factor gene expression at the level of mRNA transcription. Proc. Natl. Acad. Sci. USA **81:** 5214-5218.
13. DISCHE, Z. & L. B. SHETTLES. 1948. A specific color reaction of methylpentoses and a spectrophotometric micromethod for their determination. J. Biol. Chem. **175:** 595-603.
14. HSU, S. M. & H. J. REE. 1980. An improved immunoperoxidase technic for the detection of small amounts of antigens. Am. J. Clin. Pathol. **74:** 32-40.
15. BOROS, D. L. 1978. Granulomatous inflammations. Prog. Allergy **24:** 183-267.
16. ADAMS, D. O. 1976. The granulomatous inflammatory response. Am. J. Pathol. **84:** 164-191.

Flow Cytometry Assessment of Local T Cell Activation in Hypersensitivity Pneumonitis[a]

G. CORDIER,[b,c] J. F. MORNEX,[c,d] J. BRUNE,[c,d] AND J. P. REVILLARD[c]

[c]*Centre de Cytofluorométrie*
Unité d'Enseignement et de Recherche de Biologie Humaine
Institut National de la Santé et de la Recherche Médicale Unité 80
and
Equipe de Recherche Associée 782
du Centre National de la Recherche Scientifique
Hôpital E. Herriot
Lyons, France

[d]*Service de Pneumologie*
Hôpital L. Pradel
Lyons, France

INTRODUCTION

Repeated inhalation of organic antigens is known to induce, in a few susceptible individuals, an inflammatory disorder of the lower respiratory tract referred to as hypersensitivity pneumonitis (HP).[1-3] The major advantage of this clinical model, as opposed to most other cases of alveolitis, is that the etiological agent can be identified on the basis of clinical history, and the time course of exposure to specific antigen is usually known. Despite strong indirect evidence that suggests tissue damage is immunologically mediated, however, the relative contribution of an Arthus-like reaction, as suggested by the demonstration of precipitating specific antibodies[4-6] and that of a delayed-type hypersensitivity, thymus-derived (T) cell-mediated reaction[3,4] are still matters of controversy. Indirect evidence in support of the latter mechanism includes the presence of lymphocytes in the interstitial and alveolar cell infiltrates[7,8] and among the cells collected by bronchoalveolar lavage (BAL),[9-11] cells which constitute a high percentage of T cells.[10,11] Memory T cells which can undergo blast transformation, cell division, and/or lymphokine release upon exposure to a specific antigen have been demonstrated in the blood[12-14] and in the lung[13,14] of patients with breeder's disease or farmer's lung. Because T lymphocyte interaction with exogenous epitopes in the context of self-histocompatibility antigens results in a multistep activation process controlled by several helper or suppressor signals, the endpoint of any acti-

[a]This work was supported by Contrat de Recherche Libre INSERM 82.5.033.

[b]Address for correspondence: Institut National de la Santé et de la Recherche Médicale Unité 80, Hôpital E. Herriot, Pavillon P, 69374 Lyon Cédex 08, France.

vation signal cannot be ascertained from the sole demonstration of memory T cells by *in vitro* assays. Hence one may speculate that, depending on the efficiency of the suppressor cell circuits, the presence of antigen-sensitive T cells may be associated with a broad range of local immune responses, from the accumulation of resting T lymphocytes at one extreme to the presence of actively dividing cells which release lymphokines at the other. In the present study we collected alveolar lymphocytes by BAL from four patients with HP, and we studied changes in DNA and RNA content as well as the expression of T cell activation antigens. We confirmed the presence of dividing T lymphocytes, as already reported by our group in four other HP patients,[15] and we showed that T cell division occurred while other indications of T cell activation were apparent.

PATIENTS AND METHODS

Patients

Four female patients (range in ages: 41-61 years) with a diagnosis of hypersensitivity pneumonitis were studied. The diagnosis relied on the association of the following criteria:[1-3,9] chronic or acute onset of dyspnea; exposure to an antigen source known to be associated with hypersensitivity pneumonitis, that is, moldy hay, chicken feathers, isocyanate, or air conditioners (each patient had been exposed to a different source); a chest roentgenogram showing a diffuse reticular or reticulonodular pattern (three patients); a restrictive syndrome with decreased diffusing capacity and resting hypoxemia (three patients); and precipitating antibodies (three patients). Isocyanate hypersensitivity pneumonitis[16] was demonstrated by a positive challenge inhalation test.

BAL Cells

A flexible fiberoptic bronchoscope (Olympus BF2T or BFB2) was passed transnasally after local anesthesia and wedged into the middle lobe bronchus. The BAL began with the infusion of 0.9% sterile saline solution; after discarding the first 20 ml, 65-110 ml were recovered from each patient. The cell suspensions were filtered through sterile gauze, and the cells were counted on a hemocytometer. A differential count was performed on cytocentrifuge smears. The cells were washed twice in Ca^{2+}- and Mg^{2+}-free phosphate-buffered saline solution. No further separation was performed.

Peripheral Blood Cells

Blood leukocytes were obtained from heparinized blood after lysis of red cells.[17] Peripheral blood leukocytes from 34 healthy controls were used for immunofluorescence studies, and those from 15 of these healthy controls were used for lymphocyte cell cycle analysis.

Antigenic Membrane Expression

Antigenic membrane markers were identified by flow cytometry analysis after labeling with monoclonal antibodies. T lymphocytes and T cell subsets were identified with OKT3, OKT4, and OKT8 (Ortho Diagnostic Systems).[18] Monoclonal antibodies that were directed against HLA-DR, "Ia-like" antigens included OKIal (Ortho Diagnostic Systems),[19] I_2 (Coultronics),[20] rhodamine-conjugated anti-DR (Beckton-Dickinson),[21] and BL2 (raised by J. Brochier in our laboratory).[22] Monocytes were identified using MO2 (Coultronics)[23] and lymphocytes using BL16 (raised by J. Brochier in our laboratory). Membrane markers of lymphocyte activation were detected using MLR1, MLR2, and MLR3 (kindly provided by G. Corte and L. Moretta).[24]

Immunofluorescence staining and flow cytometry analysis were performed as detailed in another report.[25] Cell suspensions were run in a Cytofluorograf 50H (Ortho Instruments). Blood and alveolar lymphocytes were identified according to their light-scattering properties defining a lymphocyte cluster. In addition, more than 90% of the cells within the lymphocyte cluster were stained with BL16, a lymphocyte-specific antibody; less than 5% were stained with MO2. Fluorescence profiles were determined for each monoclonal antibody within this lymphocyte cluster. Ten thousand cells were analyzed for each sample.

Cell Cycle Analysis

Simultaneous measurement of the amounts of DNA and RNA contained in the cells was done after acridine orange staining as previously described.[15,25] The distribution of lymphocytes within the phases of the cell cycle was determined. For each sample 10 000 cells were analyzed.

Statistical Analysis

Data were analyzed using either the two-tailed *t* test or the Wilcoxon *t* test. Significance was determined at the $p < .05$ level.

RESULTS

T Lymphocyte Subsets

Patients' peripheral blood lymphocytes are characterized by slight but significantly decreased percentages of $OKT4^+$ and $OKT8^+$ cells as compared to normal blood lymphocytes (TABLE 1). An imbalance in the blood T lymphocyte subsets was observed in one case among three as shown by the OKT4:OKT8 ratio. Changes in the relative distribution of T cell subsets were observed between BAL fluid and blood in individual patients.

Expression of Class II Histocompatibility Antigens by T Cells

Expression of HLA-DR antigen by T cells was demonstrated by the added percentages of $OKT3^+$ cells and DR^+ cells (detected by OKIal, I_2, or BL2) exceeding 100% (FIG. 1). This situation was encountered in the BAL fluid of each patient but never in the blood of the patients and controls. In order to demonstrate the presence of lymphocytes simultaneously expressing OKT3 and DR, we performed in one of the patients an additional labeling with rhodamine-conjugated anti-DR. $OKT3^+$ lymphocytes were then sorted, using the sorting capabilities of the Cytofluorograf, and examined under a fluorescence microscope. Of the $OKT3^+$ cells, 15% were labeled with anti-DR.

TABLE 1. Blood and Lung T Cell Subsets in HP Patients

	Patient	Percentage of T Cells[a]			
		CD3	CD4	CD8	CD4/CD8
Controls[b]					
Blood		73	55	31	1.9
Patients					
Blood	1	65	41	28	1.5
	2	60	49	11	4.5
	3	72	43	30	1.4
	4	70	54	19	2.8
BAL fluid	1	75	45	22	2.0
	2	58	45	20	2.3
	3	94	22	57	0.4
	4	80	53	31	1.7

[a] Each T cell subset was defined according to its cluster of differentiation (CD). CD3 was recognized by OKT3, CD4 by OKT4, and CD8 by OKT8, as described in the text.
[b] $N = 34$

Expression of MLR Antigens

A marked increase in the number of $MLR1^+$ cells was found among lung lymphocytes from patients, as compared to normal peripheral blood lymphocytes (FIG. 2). The percentage of $MLR3^+$ cells was slightly increased whereas that of $MLR2^+$ cells was not.

Cell Cycle Analysis

Only one of the patients showed an increased percentage of blood lymphocytes in the S + (G2 + M) phases of the cell cycle as compared to normal blood lymphocytes. In marked contrast, lung lymphocytes from all the patients showed an increased

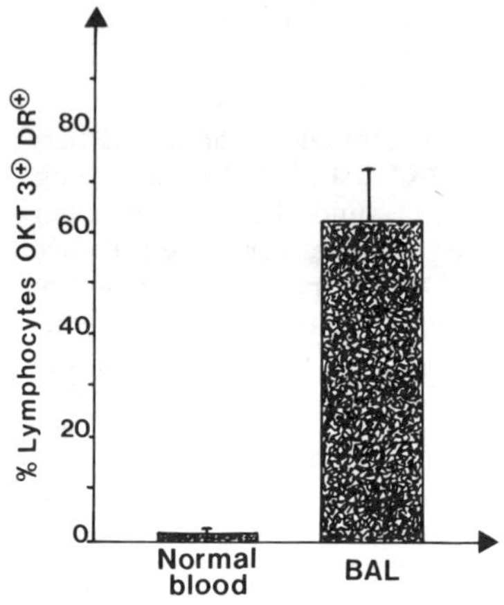

FIGURE 1. Expression of HLA-DR antigen by alveolar T lymphocytes. The percentage of OKT3$^+$ DR$^+$ lymphocytes in the BAL fluid of four patients is calculated as the sum of OKT3$^+$ and DR$^+$ lymphocytes minus 100%. Lymphocytes are identified by their light-scattering properties and labeling with BL16. Normal blood values are from Reinherz *et al.*[19]

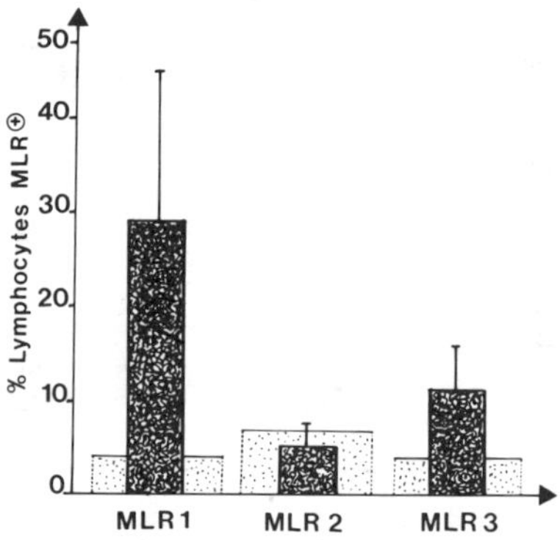

FIGURE 2. Expression of MLR antigens by alveolar lymphocytes. The BAL fluid values (from the four patients) are indicated by the dark bars. The blood values (from the normal subjects) are indicated by the light, dotted areas. The blood values were obtained from Corte *et al.*[24] and from Moretta (personal communication).

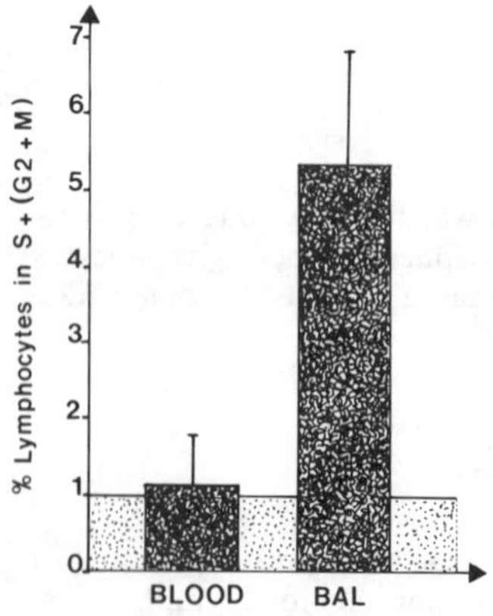

FIGURE 3. Cell cycle analysis of blood and alveolar lymphocytes. Lymphocytes in the S + (G2 + M) phases of the cell cycle in the blood and in the BAL fluid of the four patients contain more DNA and RNA. The light, dotted area represents normal blood lymphocyte values from 15 normal controls.

percentage of cells in S + (G2 + M) phases: 5.4 ± 1.4% of lung lymphocytes were in the S + (G2 + M) phases (FIG. 3).

DISCUSSION

In the present study lung lymphocyte activation was demonstrated in HP by flow cytometry analysis, a technique which provides a direct quantification of the number of activated cells. The same technique was used to assess the distribution of lymphocyte subsets identified by monoclonal antibodies. Among the patients we have investigated, T lymphocytes in BAL fluid showed only a minor imbalance between T cell subsets with an OKT4:OKT8 ratio that was slightly elevated when compared with that of blood lymphocytes. So far, decreased alveolar OKT4:OKT8 ratios have been reported in HP,[26–29] but the interpretation of this ratio in HP must take into account the time course of the disease and the time interval between the BAL and the last exposure to the antigen. Withdrawal from antigen exposure was reported to result in a reversal of the OKT4:OKT8 ratio.[29] One may therefore expect sequential variations in the T cell populations infiltrating the lung after *in vivo* antigen exposure similar to those after *in vitro* activation.[30]

The present study documents the presence of activated T lymphocytes in HP BAL fluid. As shown by *in vitro* models using mitogens, allogenic cells, or specific antigens, T cell activation can be regarded as a multistep phenomenon controlled by sequential signals (for a review see Mornex *et al.*[31]). A variety of surface structures identified by monoclonal antibodies are expressed by T cells only after activation. We studied the expression of two groups of antigens expressed late in the cell cycle: HLA-DR and MLR. Histocompatibility class II antigens (or, HLA-DR, "Ia-like" antigens) are expressed by T cells only after *in vivo* or *in vitro* activation.[19] Antigens identified by MLR1 and MLR2 antibodies are detectable on T cells after *in vitro* activation but not in resting T cells.[24,32] DR^+ T cells and/or $MLR1^+$ lymphocytes were found in the BAL fluid but not in the blood of the patients. Therefore the pathogenesis of HP appears to be characterized by local T cell activation. Since asymptomatic individuals exposed to specific antigens do disclose a lymphocytic alveolitis,[33] one may speculate that lung lymphocyte activation is associated with symptomatic HP.

The percentage of blood lymphocytes with increased DNA content (that is, in the S + (G2 + M) phases of the cell cycle) does not differ between patients and controls. Conversely, such dividing cells are present in the BAL fluid of all the patients under investigation. We have already reported such increased numbers of dividing lymphocytes within the T lymphocytes in the BAL fluid of four other patients with HP.[15] Further studies are needed to investigate the origin of activated T cells: they may be activated locally, within the mural alveolitis, or they may migrate from lymph nodes through the blood.[34]

The activation of T lymphocytes within the alveolar structure may be of critical importance in the pathogenesis of HP in recruiting and activating blood inflammatory cells, and thus inducing irreversible lung damage leading to fibrosis. The evidence of T lymphocyte activation emphasizes the role of a type IV immune reaction triggered by antigen exposure in the mechanism of HP. Measurement of T cell activation can be used to monitor the activity of the alveolitis.

ACKNOWLEDGMENTS

We wish to thank C. Molina for the precipitating antibody determinations; J. Brochier, G. Corte, and L. Moretta for kindly providing the monoclonal antibodies; and S. Alfano for the secretarial assistance.

REFERENCES

1. SALVAGGIO, J. E. & R. M. KARR. 1979. Chest **75**(Suppl.): 270-274.
2. WINTERBAUER, R. H. & S. P. HAMMAR. 1982. *In* Update: Pulmonary Diseases and Disorders. A. P. Fishman, Ed.: 225-230. McGraw Hill. New York, NY.
3. REED, C. E. & R. DE SHAZO. 1982. J. Am. Med. Assoc. **248:** 2683.
4. SCHATZ, M., R. PATTERSON & J. FIND. 1977. J. Allergy Clin. Immunol. **66:** 27-37.
5. BURRELL, R. & R. RYLANDEV. 1981. Eur. J. Respir. Dis. **62:** 332-343.
6. TERHO, E. O., P. LINDSTROM, R. MANTYJARVI, H. TUKIAINEN & O. WAGER. 1983. Allergy **38:** 347-352.
7. REYER, C. N., F. V. WENZEL, B. R. LAWTON & D. A. EMANUEL. 1982. Chest **81:** 142-148.
8. KAWANAMI, O., F. BASSET, R. BARRIOS, J. G. LACRONIQUE, V. J. FERRANS & R. G. CRYSTAL. 1983. Am. J. Pathol. **110:** 275-289.
9. REYNOLDS, H. Y., J. D. FULMER, J. A. KAZNIEROWSKI, W. C. ROBERTS, M. M. FRANK & R. G. CRYSTAL. 1977. J. Clin. Invest. **59:** 165-175.
10. HUNNINGHAKE, G. W., J. E. GADEK, O. KAWANAMI, V. J. FERRANS & R. G. CRYSTAL. 1979. Am. J. Pathol. **97:** 149-206.
11. GODART, P., J. CLOT, O. JONQUET, J. BOUSQUET & F. B. MICHEL. 1981. Chest **80:** 447-452.
12. CALDWELL, J. R., D. E. PEARCE, G. SPENCER, R. LEDER & R. H. WALDMAN. 1973. J. Allergy Clin. Immunol. **52:** 225-230.
13. SHUYLER, M. R., T. P. THIGPEN & J. E. SALVAGGIO. 1978. Ann. Intern. Med. **88:** 355-358.
14. MOORE, V. L., G. M. PEDERSEN, W. C. HAUSER & J. N. FINK. 1980. J. Allergy Clin. Immunol. **65:** 365-370.
15. PACHECO, Y., G. CORDIER, M. PERRIN-FAYOLLE & J. P. REVILLARD. 1982. Am. J. Med. **73:** 82-88.
16. CHARLES, J., A. BERNSTEIN, B. JONES, D. J. JONES, J. H. EDWARDS, R. M. F. SEARL & A. SEATON. 1976. Thorax **31:** 127-131.
17. HOFFMAN, R. A., P. C. KUNG, W. P. HANSEN & G. GOLDSTEIN. 1980. Proc. Natl. Acad. Sci. USA **77:** 4914-4917.
18. KUNG, P. C., F. GOLDSTEIN, E. L. REINHERZ & S. F. SCHLOSSMAN. 1979. Science **206:** 347-349.
19. REINHERZ, E. L., P. C. KUNG, J. M. PESANDO, J. RITZ, F. GOLDSTEIN & S. F. SCHLOSSMAN. 1979. J. Exp. Med. **150:** 1472-1482.
20. PESANDO, J. M., L. M. NADLER, H. LAZARUS, K. J. TOMASELLI, P. STASHENKO, J. RITZ, H. LEVINE, E. J. YUNIS & S. F. SCHLOSSMAN. 1981. Hum. Immunol. **3:** 67-69.
21. LAMPSON, L. A. & R. LEVY. 1980. J. Immunol. **125:** 293-299.
22. YONISH-ROUACH, E., G. CORDIER, J. COHEN, C. VINCENT & J. BROCHIER. 1983. *In* Protides of the Biological Fluids. H. Peeters, Ed. Vol. **30:** 487-490. Pergamon Press. Oxford.
23. TODD, R. F., L. M. NADLER & S. F. SCHLOSSMAN. 1981. J. Immunol. **126:** 1435-1442.
24. CORTE, G., L. MORETTA, F. DAMIANI, M. C. MINGARI & A. BARGELLESI. 1981. Eur. J. Immunol. **11:** 162-164.
25. MORNEX, J. F., G. CORDIER, J. PAGES, J. M. VERGNON, R. LEFEBVRE, J. BRUNE & J. P. REVILLARD. 1984. J. Allergy Clin. Immunol. **74:** 719-728.

26. Hirata, T., S. Nagai, S. Oshima & T. Izuni. 1982. Chest **82:** 232.
27. Moritz, E. D., J. M. Smiejean, B. A. Keogh & R. G. Crystal. 1982. Clin. Res. **30:** 435A.
28. Leatherman, J. W., A. F. Michael, B. A. Schwartz & J. R. Hoidal. 1984. Ann. Intern. Med. **100:** 390-392.
29. Costabel, U., K. J. Bross, J. Marxen & H. Matthys. 1984. Chest **85:** 514-518.
30. Burns, G. F. B., F. L. Battye & G. Goldstein. 1982. Cell. Immunol. **71:** 12-26.
31. Mornex, J. F., G. Cordier & J. P. Revillard. 1983. Rev. Fr. Mal. Respir. **11:** 787-812.
32. Canonica, G. W., M. Bagnasco, G. Corte, S. Ferrini, O. Ferrini & G. Giordano. 1982. Clin. Immunol. Immunopathol. **23:** 616-625.
33. Beaudoin, R., J. Beaudoin & M. Laviolette. 1983. Am. Rev. Respir. Dis. **127:** 64.
34. Beacham, C. H. & R. P. Daniele. 1982. Cell. Immunol. **74:** 284.

Lymphocyte Subpopulations in Extrinsic Allergic Alveolitis[a]

Y. CORMIER,[b,c] J. BÉLANGER, P. LEBLANC, J. HÉBERT, AND M. LAVIOLETTE

Centre de Pneumologie
Hôpital Laval
Sainte-Foy, Quebec, Canada

INTRODUCTION

Although the precise role of lymphocytes in the pathogenesis of extrinsic allergic alveolitis (EAA) is unknown, it is well recognized that the number of these cells is markedly increased in the bronchoalveolar lavage (BAL) fluid of these patients.[1] We have recently shown that the number of BAL lymphocytes is also increased in many asymptomatic dairy farmers[2] and in subjects with previously documented farmer's lung disease (FLD).[3] In another granulomatous disease, sarcoidosis, it has been demonstrated that most BAL lymphocytes were thymus-derived (T) cells with a high helper/suppressor subpopulation ratio.[4] Few studies have looked at lymphocyte subpopulations in allergic alveolitis. Recently Leatherman *et al.* reported an increase in the number of T cells, most of which were suppressor cells, in chronic EAA.[5] In the present study, we looked at BAL and peripheral blood (PB) lymphocyte subpopulations in a group of farmers who previously had acute disease. Although 26 out of 41 of these subjects were still in daily contact with the farm environment, all were in clinical remission at the time of the study. PB lymphocyte subpopulations were normal while overall BAL lymphocytes showed an increased proportion of T cells and a normal ratio of OKT4$^+$ cells to OKT8$^+$ cells (the OKT4/OKT8 ratio). This ratio, however, decreased when the number of BAL lymphocytes increased. These results were similar for subjects who had stayed on their farms and for those who had ceased all antigenic exposure.

MATERIALS AND METHODS

Forty-one farmers who had had at least one episode of acute FLD between 1 and 11 years previously were studied. The initial diagnoses were based on patient histories,

[a] This work was supported by the Medical Research Council of Canada, the Fondation J. D. Bégin de l'Université Laval, and the Quebec Lung Association.

[b] Address for correspondence and reprint requests: Centre de Pneumologie, Hôpital Laval, 2725 Chemin Sainte-Foy, Québec, Canada.

[c] A scholar of the Fonds de Recherche en Santé du Québec.

physical examinations, chest roentgenograms, pulmonary function tests, and serum precipitin analyses.[6] Further procedures, including BAL, transbronchial biopsy, and open lung biopsy were done when required to confirm each diagnosis. All subjects were free of acute episodes for at least 1 year, and none had taken corticosteroids for at least 6 months before the study. Twenty-six farmers were still on their farms (group I) while 15 had ceased all contact with the farm environment between 2 and 10 years before the study (group II).

After having signed a consent form, each subject had pulmonary function tests (of helium lung volumes, single-breath DL_{CO}, and forced expiratory flows). Serum precipitins to *Micropolyspora faeni* and *Thermoactinomyces vulgaris* (antigens from Greer Diagnostic) and to *Aspergillus fumigatus* (strains 3 and 5 from Greer Diagnostic and strain 6 from Bencard) were measured according to Ouchterlony's double-diffusion technique.[7] A range of concentrations from a 1/32 dilution to a fourfold concentration were tested; if no precipitins were detected at the highest concentration, the test was negative.

PB lymphocytes were separated by Ficoll-Hypaque gradient centrifugation as in previous experiments.[2] Eighteen normal volunteers also had blood samples drawn for PB lymphocyte analysis to provide control values.

All 41 of the subjects who once had FLD underwent fiberoptic bronchoscopy and BAL. Lavages were performed in a segmental or a subsegmental bronchus of the right middle lobe. Ten 30-ml boli of 0.9% sterile saline solution were instilled and withdrawn by syringe. The lavage fluid was centrifuged (500 $\times$ g for 10 min at 4° C), and the cell pellets were resuspended in RPMI 1640 (Flow Labs). Total cell counts were performed on a hemocytometer, and differential counts were performed on Wright-Giemsa- and nonspecific esterase-stained cytocentrifuged preparations. Cell viability, measured by trypan blue exclusion, was always greater than 90%. Lymphocytes were separated from macrophages by passage through a Sephadex G10 column.[8]

BAL and PB T lymphocytes and $OKT4^+$ and $OKT8^+$ T lymphocyte subpopulations were identified using specific monoclonal antibodies: Orthoclone OKT3 for T lymphocytes, OKT4 for the helper subpopulation, and OKT8 for the suppressor subpopulation (Ortho Pharmaceutical). Briefly, 5 μl of reconstituted monoclonal antibody solution were added to 200 μl of a lymphocyte suspension (4 $\times$ 10^6 cells/ml), and cells were incubated for 30 min at 4° C. Then the lymphocytes were washed twice, and 100 μl of fluorescein-labeled goat antimouse immunoglobulin (Tago and Immunodiagnostic Reagents) were added over 30 min at 4° C. The cells were then washed twice, resuspended in one or two drops of phosphate-buffered saline solution containing 30% (v/v) glycerol, and examined by fluorescence microscopy. A minimum of 100 cells was counted.

Statistics were done using the nonpaired Student's *t* test, except where specified. Correlations were calculated using a linear regression test.

RESULTS

There were 17 precipitin-positive subjects: 14 in group I and 3 in group II ($p > .2$, Fisher's exact test). Twenty-nine subjects had alveolitis, and more than 22% of the cells in their BAL samples were lymphocytes. Twenty-three of these patients were in group I ($p < .005$, Fisher's exact test). The total number of cells recovered by BAL was not different between the two groups (57.5 ± 36.4 and 37.1 ± 34.3 × 10^6 for groups I and II, respectively; $p > .05$) (FIG. 1A), but the percentage of lymphocytes was higher in group I (52.5 ± 21.2 and 26.3 ± 18.7, respectively; $p < .001$) (FIG. 1B).

Blood OKT

The numbers and percentages of $OKT3^+$, $OKT4^+$, and $OKT8^+$ cells in PB were measured in all 41 subjects. Values were similar to those of normal controls and were not different between groups I and II (FIG. 2), and no differences were apparent when subjects were regrouped according to serum precipitins or the presence of lymphocytic alveolitis ($p > .1$, all comparisons). Linear regression tests comparing PB variables (the OKT3, OKT4, and OKT8 values and the OKT4/OKT8 ratio) to BAL variables (the number of cells and the number and percentage of lymphocytes), failed to show any significant correlation. When PB OKT subpopulation values were plotted against pulmonary function test values, only a small correlation ($r = .36$; $p < .05$) between the OKT3 values and the forced expiratory volume (FEV_1)/forced vital capacity (FVC) ratio was found.

BAL OKT

BAL OKT3 values were measured in 26 out of 41 farmers (19 in group I and 7 in group II), and OKT4 and OKT8 values were measured in 24 subjects (19 in group

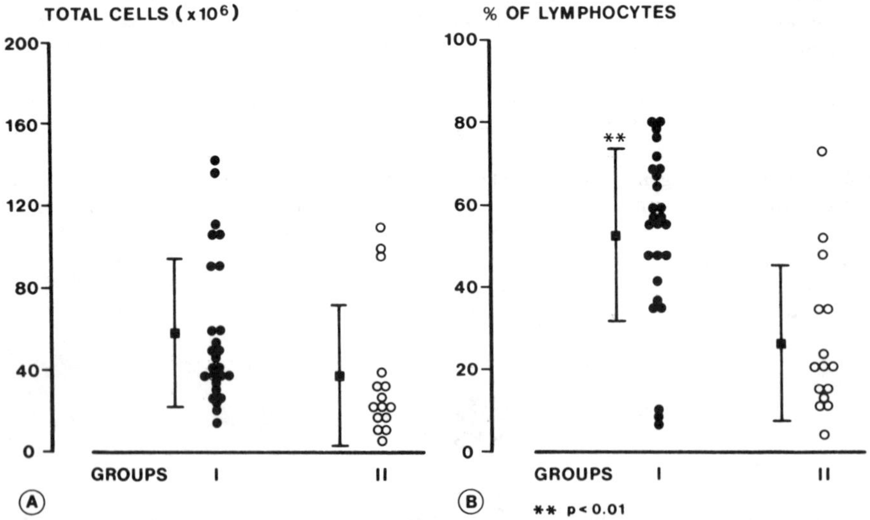

FIGURE 1. **(A)** The total number of cells recovered from group I (closed circles) and group II patients (open circles). Means ± SD's are indicated. **(B)** The percentages of lymphocytes in groups I and II (symbols as above).

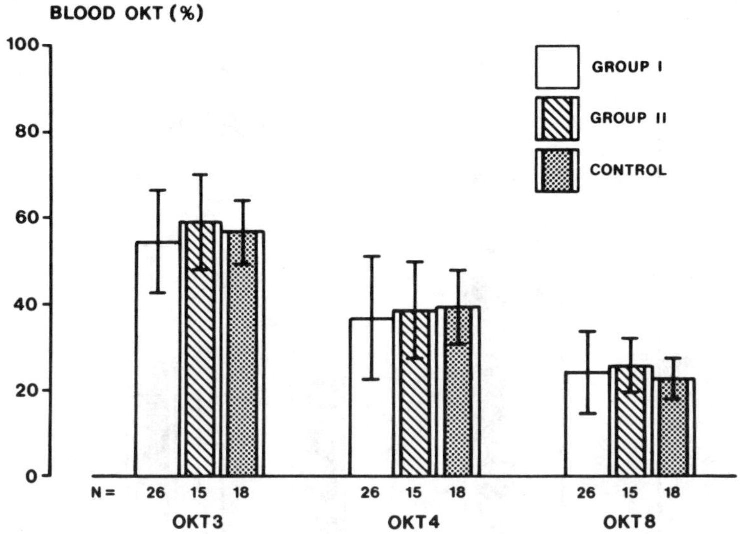

FIGURE 2. The blood OKT values for group I, group II, and controls (means ± SD's). The numbers below the bars represent the number of subjects in each group.

I and 5 in group II). Values for OKT3$^+$, OKT3$^+$, OKT8$^+$ lymphocytes were higher in BAL than in PB ($p < .001$, $p < .05$, and $p < .001$, respectively, Student's paired *t* test) (FIG. 3). The OKT4/OKT8 ratio was similar ($p > .2$) in both PB and BAL.

Groups I and II did not have significantly different BAL T cell populations (FIG. 4). Precipitin-positive and -negative subjects also had similar results ($p > .2$). As with PB OKT, there were no correlations with pulmonary function tests. Since only two subjects without alveolitis had a sufficient number of lymphocytes for our OKT technique, no statistical comparison could be made between OKT results for subjects with alveolitis and subjects with normal BAL. The percentage of cells in BAL fluid that were OKT4$^+$, however, was negatively correlated with the number of cells recovered ($r = .653$; $p < .001$) and the number of lymphocytes ($r = -.66$; $p < .001$) (FIG. 5A). The OKT8 values were positively correlated with both the number of BAL cells ($r = .546$; $p < .01$) and the number of lymphocytes ($r = .524$; $p < .01$) (FIG. 5B). The OKT4/OKT8 ratio was negatively correlated with both the number of cells ($r = -.436$; $p < .05$) and the number of lymphocytes ($r = -.416$; $p < .05$) (FIG. 6).

DISCUSSION

Our data show that PB lymphocyte subpopulations are normal in subjects that have had FLD. This result is consistent with that found for lymphocyte subpopulations in patients with chronic FLD.[5] In another study, Flaherty *et al.* have shown a decrease in the total number and percentage of T lymphocytes in PB in a group of patients

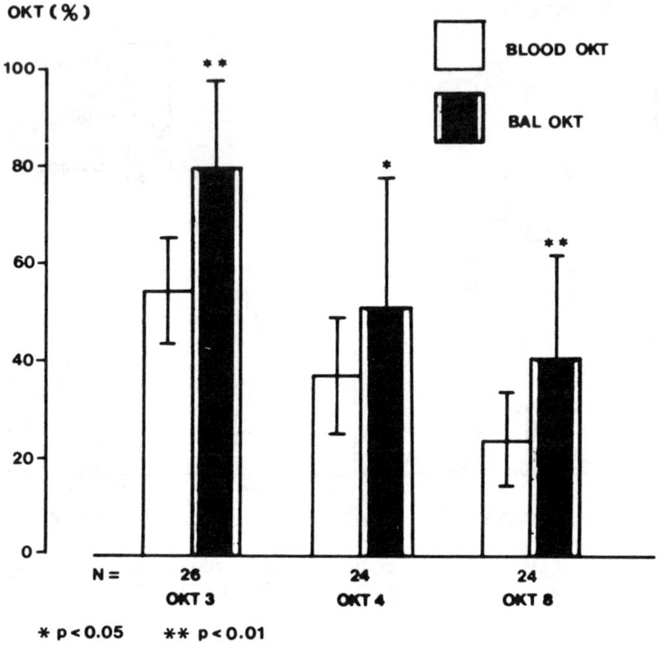

FIGURE 3. A comparison of blood and BAL OKT values. BAL OKT values were significantly higher than blood OKT values for the three antibodies. The numbers below the bars represent the number of subjects in each group.

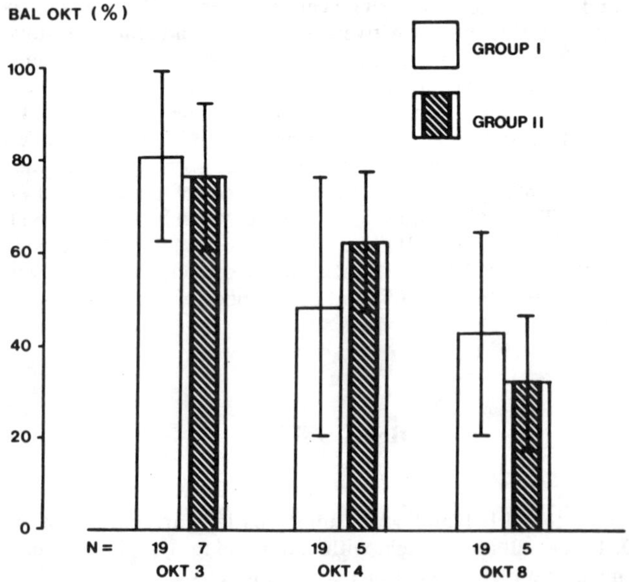

FIGURE 4. The BAL OKT values in groups I and II. The numbers below the bars represent the number of subjects in each group.

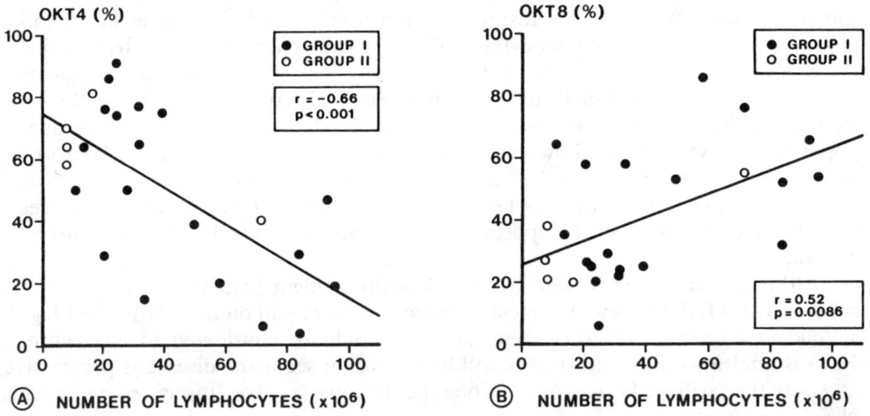

FIGURE 5. Correlations between the number of BAL lymphocytes and the numbers of $OKT4^+$ cells (**A**) and $OKT8^+$ cells (**B**). Closed circles represent subjects of group I; open circles, subjects of group II.

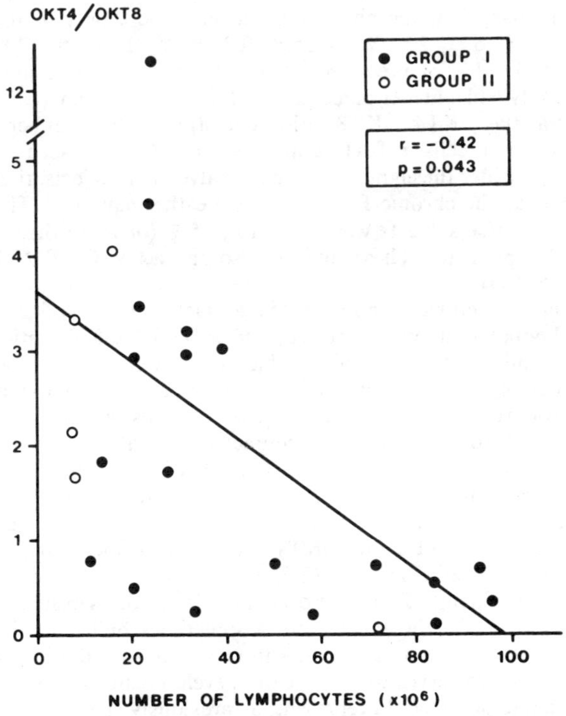

FIGURE 6. The negative correlation between the number of lymphocytes recovered by BAL and the OKT4/OKT8 ratio. Closed circles represent subjects of group I; open circles, subjects of group II.

similar to ours.[9] We did not measure the total number of lymphocytes but found a normal percentage of T lymphocytes in PB. The difference could be a technical one because our T cell populations were analyzed by indirect fluorescence microscopy, using the OKT3 monoclonal antibody, whereas Flaherty *et al.* used the E-rosette technique. We have no data, and are not aware of any, on the PB lymphocyte population in acute FLD; however, in severe chronic cases, results similar to ours were found.[5] In an animal model[10] it has been shown that a decreasing number of T suppressor cells rendered the monkeys more susceptible to EAA. Whether a decrease in number or function of T suppressor cells occurs in acute FLD is not currently known.

Although our patients were free of clinically evident disease at the time of the study, our BAL data show that most of those who were still on their farms had highly significant alveolitis. Whether these patients should be considered to have chronic FLD is unclear. Follow-up studies will be needed to see if the disease is progressive, and only then will we be able to see if one should consider alveolitis as being indicative of active disease.

The findings for the T cell subpopulations in BAL are interesting in that, for the group as a whole, the numbers of $OKT3^+$, $OKT4^+$, and $OKT8^+$ lymphocytes were increased whereas the OKT4/OKT8 ratio was normal. This increase in the number of BAL T cells is similar to that described in chronic FLD; however, our normal values for the OKT4/OKT8 ratio in patients who have had FLD are different from Leatherman's ratio. This can be explained by the fact that not all subjects tested here had high-intensity alveolitis, a condition seen in chronic EAA. Leatherman's subjects had severe pulmonary function alterations; in our group, only mild anomalies were present (DL_{CO} = 80.6 ± 26.4%, of predicted; FEV_1/FVC = 77.8 ± 9.2%; and TLC = 92.0 ± 13.1%, of predicted). Even the asymptomatic pigeon breeders in Leatherman's study had a higher percentage of lymphocytes than many of our subjects. When we look at the OKT4/OKT8 ratio in relation to the number of lymphocytes or the total number of cells in BAL, a negative correlation is seen.

We can also consider the eight high-intensity alveolitis subjects, that is, the subjects that were similar to the chronic EAA cases of Leatherman *et al.* The mean number of lavage cells for these subjects was 71×10^6, 65% (or more than 45×10^6 cells) of which were lymphocytes. These subjects also had a low OKT4/OKT8 ratio: 0.44 ± 0.28 (mean ± SD).

The five subjects who where no longer in contact with the antigen, in whom BAL lymphocyte subpopulations were assessed, had a OKT4/OKT8 ratio and a $OKT3^+$ cell percentage similar to those found in subjects who were in continued contact. This demonstrates that ongoing antigenic challenge may not be needed to maintain alveolitis with a high proportion of $OKT8^+$ cells, and that this situation can persist for a prolonged period (2-10 years) after the contact is ceased.

Little information is available on OKT3, OKT4, and OKT8 findings in acute FLD. We have performed tests for $OKT3^+$ cells and for $OKT4^+$ and $OKT8^+$ cells in only three and four cases, respectively. All three of the former had more $OKT3^+$ cells; three of the latter had a low OKT4/OKT8 ratio (mean: 0.4), and one of the latter had a high OKT4/OKT8 ratio (8.6).

The significance of a high T suppressor/cytotoxic alveolitis in subjects that formerly had FLD is unknown. In the presence of a sometimes high-intensity alveolitis and continued antigen challenge it is tempting to speculate that the increased number of suppressor lymphocytes serves to control the development of acute disease. The appearance of an acute phase could represent, as previously suggested, either a decrease in the suppressor activity (fewer or less active cells)[10,11] or a situation where the amount of antigen inhaled would overwhelm the suppressor capacity. EAA, however, does not appear to be an antibody-related disorder,[12] so it seems unlikely that the regulatory activity of $OKT8^+$ cells on bone marrow-derived (B) lymphocytes could play a role in protection against disease. By what mechanism T suppressor cells could protect against disease as suggested by Keller *et al.*[10,11] is unclear at the present; further knowledge on suppressor lymphocyte fractions and functions in various states of EAA is needed before one can understand the meaning of the present findings.

REFERENCES

1. REYNOLDS, H. Y., J. D. FULMER, J. A. KAZMIEROWSKI, W. C. ROBERTS, M. M. FRANK & R. G. CRYSTAL. 1977. Analysis of cellular and protein content of bronchoalveolar lavage fluid from patients with idiopathic pulmonary fibrosis and chronic hypersensitivity pneumonitis. J. Clin. Invest. **59:** 165-175.
2. SOLAL, P., M. LAVIOLETTE, J. HÉBERT & Y. CORMIER. 1982. Immune reactions in the lungs of asymptomatic dairy farmers. Am. Rev. Respir. Dis. **126:** 964-967.
3. LEBLANC, P., J. BÉLANGER, M. LAVIOLETTE & Y. CORMIER. 1983. Relationship between continued exposure, alveolitis, and the clinical state in farmer's lung disease (FLD). Chest **84:** 323.
4. HUNNINGHAKE, G. W. & R. G. CRYSTAL. 1981. Pulmonary sarcoidosis: A disorder mediated by excess helper T-lymphocyte activity at sites of disease activity. N. Engl. J. Med. **305:** 429-434.
5. LEATHERMAN, J. W., A. F. MICHAEL, B. A. SCHWARTZ & J. R. HOIDAL. 1984. Lung T cells in hypersensitivity pneumonitis. Ann. Intern. Med. **100:** 390-392.
6. CHMELIK, F., G. DO PICO, C. E. REED & H. DICKIE. 1974. Farmer's lung. J. Allergy Clin. Immunol. **54:** 180-188.
7. OUCHTERLONY, O. 1958. Diffusion-in-gel method for immunological analysis. *In* Progress in Allergy. P. Kallos, Ed. Vol. **5:** 1-78. Karger. Basel.
8. MARTINEZ, C., R. R. BERNABE, E. MORENO & F. DIAZ DE ESPADA. 1978. Depletion of monocytes from human peripheral blood leucocytes by passage through Sephadex G10 columns. J. Immunol. Methods **22:** 361-368.
9. FLAHERTY, D. K., J. E. SURFUS, F. CHMELIK, A. BRYANT, H. DICKIE, C. E. REED & J. RANKIN. 1976. Lymphocyte subpopulations in the peripheral blood of patients with farmer's lung. Am. Rev. Respir. Dis. **114:** 1093-1098.
10. KELLER, R. H., N. J. CALVANICO & J. O. STEVENS. 1982. Hypersensitivity pneumonitis in nonhuman primates. I. Studies on the relationship of immunoregulation and disease activity. J. Immunol. **128:** 116-122.
11. KELLER, R. H., J. N. FINK, S. LYMAN & G. PEDERSEN. 1982. Immunoregulation in hypersensitivity pneumonitis. I. Differences in T-cell and macrophage suppressor activity in symptomatic and asymptomatic pigeon breeders. J. Clin. Immunol. **2:** 46-54.
12. BURRELL, R. & R. RYLANDER. 1981. A critical review of the role of precipitins in hypersensitivity pneumonitis. Eur. J. Respir. Dis. **62:** 332-343.

Primary Biliary Cirrhosis

The Present Position

SHEILA SHERLOCK AND OWEN EPSTEIN

Department of Surgery and Medicine
Royal Free Hospital School of Medicine
London NW3 2QG, England

Primary biliary cirrhosis is a disease with progressive granulomatous destruction of small intrahepatic bile ducts. It is of unknown etiology. The disease is associated with a profound immunological disturbance, and this has been related to the bile duct destruction (TABLE 1). The final event seems to be an attack by cytotoxic lymphocytes on biliary epithelium. The antigen might be the individual's own human leukocyte antigens (HLA's), antigens also known as avidin-biotin complex (ABC), which are present in high concentrations on biliary epithelium. It is unclear why the reaction should be to normal rather than foreign proteins. Perhaps the patient's own lymphoid system is at fault so that self and self antigens are not recognized. This could be due to failure of schooling by cytotoxic T cells in the thymus. These cells are regulated by suppressor cells which have been shown to be diminished both in number and function in primary biliary cirrhosis.[1] Alternatively, and perhaps more likely, the HLA proteins may have become foreign due to an extrinsic environmental factor. The identification of such a factor is an ongoing challenge to all those investigating primary biliary cirrhosis.

In many respects, primary biliary cirrhosis is analogous to the graft-versus-host syndrome as seen, for instance, after bone marrow transplants and where the immune system has become sensitized to foreign HLA proteins.[2] Structural changes in the bile ducts are similar. Other ducts, such as the lacrimal and pancreatic ducts,[3] with high concentrations of HLA's on their epithelia are involved. The condition can be viewed as a dry gland syndrome.[2] Ultrastructural changes in the bile ducts are similar.

The granulomas might be related to immune complexes. Indeed, complement has been identified within them. They predominantly consist of cytotoxic T cells, monocytes, and macrophages, however, and such compositions are indicative of cell-mediated tissue injury. Patients with many granulomas are usually seen early in the disease where bile duct destruction is not prominent and the prognosis better. Such patients have normal or only slightly decreased concentrations of suppressor cells in the peripheral blood. This might be related to the rarity of diffuse bile duct destruction and the good prognosis.[4]

Copper is retained in the liver, but in a nonhepatotoxic form.[5]

EPIDEMIOLOGY AND GENETICS

The disease has been reported from all parts of the world. Asians, Caucasians, Jews, Negroes, and Orientals are affected. There is family clustering, and the prevalance of circulating mitochondrial antibodies is increased in relatives of patients. There is no excess of any particular ABO blood group, HLA antigen, or rhesus negativity.[6]

PRESENTATION

The patient is usually female, only 10% of the patients being male. Presentation is usually between 40 and 60 years old. The usual onset is as pruritus. Jaundice may appear at the same time or later. The patient is usually pigmented. The liver is variably enlarged. The spleen is often palpable.

TABLE 1. Immunological Changes in Primary Biliary Cirrhosis

Depressed skin energy
Granuloma formation
Circulating immune complexes
Complement activation
Fewer regulator/suppressor cells

THE ASYMPTOMATIC PATIENT

The widespread use of automated biochemical screening has resulted in an increasing number of patients being diagnosed when asymptomatic.[7] Similarly, the diagnosis may be made in patients under investigation for a condition known to be associated with primary biliary cirrhosis such as thyroid or collagen disease or in the course of family surveys. Such patients tend to be younger, and abnormal physical signs may be absent. Mitochondrial antibody is always positive. Serum alkaline phosphatase and bilirubin may be normal or only minimally increased. Serum cholesterol and transaminases can also be normal.

ASSOCIATED DISEASES

Nonhepatic disorders, especially the collagenoses, are found in about two-thirds of the patients, and autoimmune thyroiditis is also frequent. Primary biliary cirrhosis may be associated with scleroderma and with the whole CREST syndrome. Such patients usually have a nuclear centromere antibody.[8] A sicca complex of dry eyes and mouth with or without the arthritis which completes Sjögren's syndrome is found in about 75% of the patients.[2] Associated skin lesions include immune complex capillaritis and lichen planus, which is also a feature of graft-versus-host disease.[9] Primary biliary cirrhosis and jejunal villous atrophy, which together resemble celiac disease, have been reported.[10] Other complications include immunoglobulin M (IgM)-associated membranous glomerulonephritis and renal tubular acidosis.[11] Bacteriuria develops in 35% of the patients and may be asymptomatic.[12] It is unexplained, but it has been postulated that urinary organisms might be invoked in the pathogenesis of primary biliary cirrhosis. Finger clubbing is common and hypertrophic osteoarthropathy is occasionally evident.[13] Gallstones, usually the pigmented type, are present in a third of the patients.

BIOCHEMICAL TESTS

At the time of diagnosis, serum bilirubin values are rarely very high at the onset, usually less than 2 mg/100 ml in asymptomatic patients. Serum alkaline phosphatase (γ-glutamyl transpeptidase) levels are raised. The total serum cholesterol level is increased but not constantly. The serum albumin level is usually normal at presentation and the total serum globulin level only moderately increased. The serum IgM level is usually raised, and this estimation has been suggested for diagnosis. These increases are not constant, however, and this method is not reliable for diagnosis although an increase may add some diagnostic weight.

SERUM MITOCHONDRIAL TEST

Circulating antibodies against mitochondria are found in virtually all the patients with primary biliary cirrhosis, provided undiluted serum samples are used in a standard immunofluorescence test. They probably play no role in pathogenesis. Mitochondrial antibodies are not confined to primary biliary cirrhosis, being detected in 30% of the patients with chronic active hepatitis (HBsAg negative) and in 3% of the patients with connective tissue diseases. They are absent in patients with mechanical obstruction to the bile ducts, including that caused by primary sclerosing cholangitis.

The antigen(s) concerned is a component of the mitochondrial inner membrane. These antigens are heterogenous. The adenosine triphosphatase-associated antigen, termed M2, is said to be specific for primary biliary cirrhosis. A positive immunoassay for M2 may be specific for primary biliary cirrhosis.[14] Another antigen found on the outer mitochondrial membrane, termed M4, is associated with chronic active hepatitis, granulomas, and bile duct proliferation and must be distinguished from that found with classical primary biliary cirrhosis.

LIVER BIOPSY

The only hepatic lesion diagnostic of primary biliary cirrhosis is the injured septal or interlobular bile duct. The disease begins with damage to the epithelium of small bile ducts. Histometric examinations show that bile ducts less than 70-80 μm in diameter are destroyed, particularly in the early stages. Surrounding the damaged duct is a cellular reaction which includes lymphocytes, plasma cells, eosinophils, and histiocytes. Granulomas commonly form. Bile ducts become destroyed and are replaced by aggregates of lymphoid cells, and bile ducts begin to proliferate. Hepatic arterial branches can be identified in the portal zones but without accompanying bile ducts. Fibrosis extends from the portal tracts, and there is a variable degree of piecemeal necrosis. Substantial amounts of copper and copper-associated protein can be demonstrated histochemically. The fibrous septa gradually come to distort the architecture of the liver, and regeneration nodules form. These are often irregular in distribution, and cirrhosis may be seen in one part of a biopsy but not in another.

The histological appearances have been divided into four stages: stage I, florid bile duct lesions; stage II, ductular proliferation; stage III, scarring (septal fibrosis and bridging); and stage IV, cirrhosis.[15] Such staging is of limited value as the changes in the liver are focal and evolve at different speeds in different parts. Stages overlap. It is particularly difficult to separate stages II and III. The disease has a very variable course, and advanced stage III lesions may be seen in the asymptomatic patient. Moreover, serial biopsies have shown that the same stage may persist.

COURSE AND PROGNOSIS

Earlier diagnosis in the asymptomatic patient makes the duration seem much longer, and these patients usually survive at least 10 years.[16] In those with symptomatic disease and jaundice the survival is about 7 years.

The course of asymptomatic patients is variable and unpredictable, and counseling the patient and her family is very difficult. Overall, the life expectancy of these patients does not differ from that of the general population.[16,17] Only 6 out of 36 asymptomatic patients studied over 6 to 11.4 years died from liver disease.[16] Serum bilirubin values are the best indicators of prognosis.[18] When values are consistently greater than 6 mg/dl, the patient is unlikely to survive more than 2 years (FIG. 1).[19]

Other features at diagnosis predicting decreased survival include symptoms, advanced age, hepatosplenomegaly, ascites, and hypoalbuminemia (less than 3 g/dl).[20] Histologically, piecemeal necrosis, cholestasis, bridging fibrosis, and cirrhosis correlate with the worst prognosis. On the other hand, granulomas seen on an initial biopsy predict a longer survival,[4] perhaps because they indicate a less aggressive immune response. Autoimmune diseases such as thyroiditis, sicca syndrome, or Raynaud's phenomenon correlate with decreased survival.[16]

TREATMENTS

These apply to all patients with cholestasis. They include the control of pruritus and the management of steatorrhea. Fat-soluble vitamins A, D, and K must be given parenterally to all cholestatic patients. Oral calcium supplements are indicated. The patient should be encouraged to sunbathe: an ultraviolet lamp may be useful in northern climates. Medium-chain triglycerides may be helpful. The patient is encouraged to lead as normal a life as possible because the condition is compatible with a full domestic and professional life for many years.

Intractable pruritus and painful xanthomatous neuropathy can be treated by plasmaphersis. This is a specialized and costly treatment but may be considered in the exceptional patient. Corticosteroids might be expected to be beneficial, but they accentuate the bone thinning of cholestasis. Indeed, some of the most disastrous examples of skeletal crumbling that we have seen have been in patients with late-stage primary biliary cirrhosis treated with prednisolone. Corticosteroids might be useful in the early, anicteric patient, where bone thinning is not a problem, but this has never been subjected to controlled trials. Azathioprine was said to be of benefit in treatment, but these good results were not confirmed in prospective controlled clinical trials.[21,22]

D-Penicillamine would be expected to reduce hepatic copper levels, act immunologically by depressing the inflammatory response, and, conceivably, to reduce

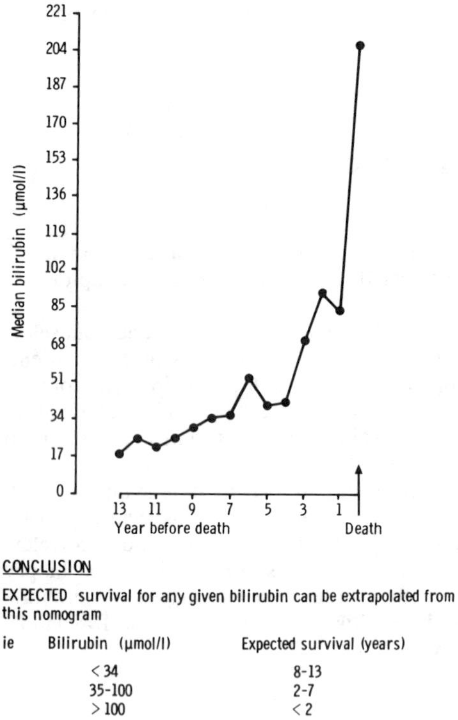

FIGURE 1. The evolution of liver failure in primary biliary cirrhosis. This nomogram is derived from the medians of pooled serum bilirubin results in patients followed serially from diagnosis to death.

hepatic fibrosis. Randomized, controlled trials have shown that D-penicillamine increases survival in primary biliary cirrhosis (FIG. 2).[23,24] Improvement in survival became apparent only after 18 months of treatment. Those dying early probably have irreversible liver disease. In surviving patients D-penicillamine treatment was associated with improved biochemical tests and decreases in copper levels in the liver. D-Penicillamine often reduces hepatic inflammation and piecemeal necrosis, but hepatic fibrosis continues to progress.

Side effects of D-penicillamine unfortunately lead to noncompliance and withdrawal of therapy. The most frequent is dyspepsia with nausea and vomiting. Taste may be lost, but this returns whether or not the drug is discontinued. Serious reactions include

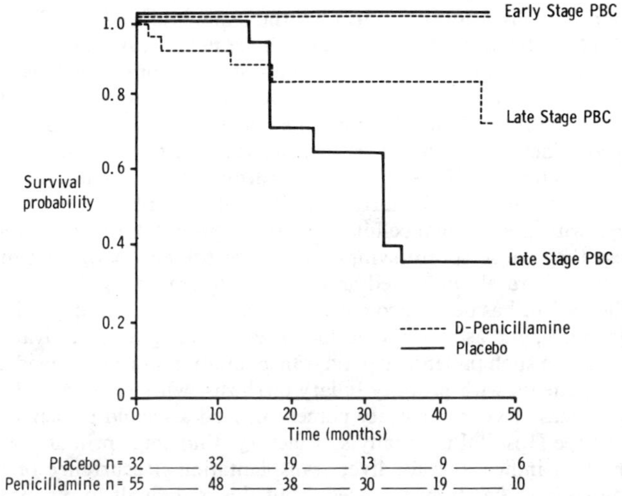

FIGURE 2. Survival probability in early and late histological stages of primary biliary cirrhosis (early stages: I and II; late stages: III and IV).

skin rashes, proteinuria, and blood dyscrasias such as thrombocytopenia and neutropenia. These usually lead to permanent withdrawal of therapy. Various autoimmune syndromes, including myasthenia, polymyositis, systemic lupus, and a Goodpasture-like picture are other complications.[25]

Other trials have shown less satisfactory results with D-penicillamine, recording a higher incidence of serious side effects.[26] Others have found no improvement in survival in those with fibrosis/cirrhosis on initial biopsy.[24] On small numbers of patients, statistical analysis is difficult.[19] D-Penicillamine is worth a trial in those who are symptomatic with a rising serum bilirubin level and who are unsuitable or have not reached the stage of consideration for liver transplantation (FIG. 3). There is little else to offer. D-Penicillamine should not be given to the asymptomatic.

D-Penicillamine treatment commences with a daily dose of 125 mg which is increased by 125 mg every 2 weeks until a daily dose of 500 mg is reached. Hemoglobin and white cell counts are measured, and proteinuria sought every week for the first 4 weeks, and then every month. The administration of the drug should be continued unless there is a serious complication or are manifestations of the late stages of primary biliary cirrhosis such as hematemesis, ascites, or the development of precoma.

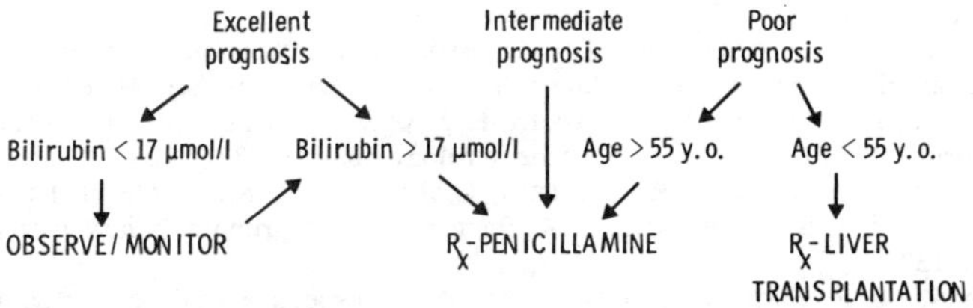

FIGURE 3. A rational approach to the treatment of primary biliary cirrhosis in 1984.

Cyclosporin A has a marked effect on the suppressor-inducer T lymphocytes in primary biliary cirrhosis.[27] The drug, however, is nephrotoxic and difficult to justify for long-term use. Less toxic derivatives are awaited. Chlorambucil and colchicine are under trial, but preliminary results suggest that the improvement is not dramatic.

Hemorrhage from esophageal varices may be early before a true nodular cirrhosis has developed. Therefore it is not surprising that porta-caval shunting gives good results in these patients.[28] Hepatic encephalopathy is an unusual complication. These encouraging results apply particularly to patients at little risk (grades A and B), rather than to those with poor hepatocellular function (grade C). Gallstones should be left *in situ* unless they cause severe symptoms or are present in the common bile duct. Cholecystectomy is rarely indicated and is badly tolerated.

When the patient has developed chronic hepatocellular failure, particularly rapidly deepening jaundice, and ascites, the outlook is extremely grave, survival being unlikely to exceed 1 year. In such patients hepatic transplantation must be considered.[29] Seventy percent of 40 patients with primary biliary cirrhosis, who were treated in Pittsburgh, survived for at least 1 year.[30] Twenty percent needed a second transplant. Experience at the Royal Free Hospital is equally satisfactory. End-stage primary biliary cirrhosis is one of the best indications for liver transplantation. Recurrence of the disease in the transplanted liver has been reported,[31] but this is difficult to distinguish from the graft-versus-host reaction of chronic rejection.[32]

REFERENCES

1. THOMAS, H. C. Potential pathogenic mechanisms in primary biliary cirrhosis. Semin. Liver Dis. **1:** 338-344.
2. EPSTEIN, O., H. C. THOMAS & S. SHERLOCK. 1980. Primary biliary cirrhosis is a dry gland syndrome with features of chronic graft-versus-host disease. Lancet **i:** 1166-1168.
3. EPSTEIN, O., R. G. W. CHAPMAN, G. LAKE-BAKAAR, A. V. FOO, S. B. ROSALKI & S. SHERLOCK. 1982. The pancreas in primary biliary cirrhosis and primary sclerosing cholangitis. Gastroenterology **83:** 1177-1182.
4. LEE, R. G., O. EPSTEIN, H. JAUREGUI, S. SHERLOCK & P. J. SCHEUER. 1981. Granulomas in primary biliary cirrhosis: A prognostic feature. Gastroenterology **81:** 983-986.
5. EPSTEIN, O., B. A. M. ARBORGH, M. SAGIV, R. WROBLEWSKI, P. J. SCHEUER & S. SHERLOCK. 1981. Is copper hepatotoxic in primary biliary cirrhosis? J. Clin. Pathol. **34:** 1071-1075.
6. HAMLYN, A. N. & S. SHERLOCK. 1974. The epidemiology of primary biliary cirrhosis: A survey of mortality in England and Wales. Gut **15:** 473-479.
7. LONG, R. G., P. J. SCHEUER & S. SHERLOCK. 1977. Presentation and course of asymptomatic primary biliary cirrhosis. Gastroenterology **72:** 1204-1207.
8. MAKINEN, D., M. FRITZER, P. DAVIS & S. SHERLOCK. 1983. Anticentromere antibody in primary biliary cirrhosis. Arthritis Rheum. **26:** 1914-1916.
9. GRAHAM-BROWN, R. A. C., I. SARKANY & S. SHERLOCK. 1982. Lichen planus and primary biliary cirrhosis. Br. J. Dermatol. **106:** 699-703.
10. ILIFFE, G. D. & D. A. OWEN. 1979. An association between primary biliary cirrhosis and jejunal villous atrophy resembling celiac disease. Dig. Dis. Sci. **24:** 802-806.
11. PARES, A., A. RIMOLA, M. BRUGUERA, E. MAS & J. RODÉS. 1981. Renal tubular acidosis in primary biliary cirrhosis. Gastroenterology **80:** 681-686.
12. BURROUGHS, A. K., I. J. ROSENSTEIN, O. EPSTEIN, J. M. T. HAMILTON-MILLER, W. BRUMFITT & S. SHERLOCK. 1984. Bacteriuria and primary biliary cirrhosis. Gut **25:** 133-137.
13. EPSTEIN, O., R. DICK & S. SHERLOCK. 1981. Prospective study of periostitis and finger clubbing in primary biliary cirrhosis and other forms of chronic liver disease. Gut **22:** 203-206.

14. BERG, P. A., R. KLEIN & J. LINDENBORN-FOTINOS. 1982. ATPase-associated antigen (M2): Marker antigen for serological diagnosis of primary biliary cirrhosis. Lancet **ii:** 1423-1425.
15. SCHEUER, P. J. 1980. Primary biliary cirrhosis. *In* Liver Biopsy Interpretation. 3rd edit.: 47-56. Williams and Wilkins. Baltimore, MD.
16. BESWICK, D. R., G. KLATSKIN & J. L. BOYER. Asymptomatic primary biliary cirrhosis: Long-term follow-up and natural history. Gastroenterology. In press.
17. JAMES, O., A. F. MACKLON & A. J. WATSON. 1981. Primary biliary cirrhosis: A revised clinical spectrum. Lancet **i:** 1278-1281.
18. SHAPIRO, J. M., H. SMITH & F. SCHAFFNER. 1979. Serum bilirubin: A prognostic factor in primary biliary cirrhosis. Gut **20:** 137-146.
19. EPSTEIN, O., D. G. COOK & S. JAIN. 1984. D-Penicillamine in PBC: An untested (and unstable?) treatment. Gut. In press.
20. ROLL, J., J. L. BOYER, D. BARRY & G. KLATSKIN. 1983. The prognostic importance of clinical and histologic features in asymptomatic and symptomatic primary biliary cirrhosis. N. Engl. J. Med. **308:** 1-7.
21. HEATHCOTE, J., A. ROSS & S. SHERLOCK. 1976. A prospective controlled trial of azathioprine in primary biliary cirrhosis. Gastroenterology **70:** 656-660.
22. CROWE, J., E. CHRISTENSEN & M. SMITH. 1980. Azathioprine in primary biliary cirrhosis: A preliminary report of an international trial. Gastroenterology **78:** 1005-1010.
23. EPSTEIN, O., S. JAIN, R. G. LEE, D. G. COOK, A. M. BOSS, P. J. SCHEUER & S. SHERLOCK. 1981. D-Penicillamine improves survival in primary biliary cirrhosis. Lancet **i:** 1275-1277.
24. DICKSON, E. R., R. H. WIESNER & W. P. BALDUS. 1984. D-Penicillamine trial for primary biliary cirrhosis. Gastroenterology **86:** 1062A.
25. MATLOFF, D. S. & M. M. KAPLAN. 1980. D-Penicillamine-induced Goodpasture-like syndrome in primary biliary cirrhosis: Successful treatment with plasmapheresis and immunosuppressives. Gastroenterology **78:** 1046-1049.
26. MATLOFF, D. S., E. ALPERT, R. H. RESNICK & M. M. KAPLAN. 1982. A prospective trial of D-PCA in primary biliary cirrhosis. N. Engl. J. Med. **306:** 319-326.
27. ROUTHIER, G., O. EPSTEIN, G. JANOSSY, H. C. THOMAS, S. SHERLOCK, P. C. KUNG & G. GOLDSTEIN. 1980. Effects of cyclosporin A on suppressor and inducer T lymphocytes in primary biliary cirrhosis. Lancet **ii:** 1223-1226.
28. SPISNI, R., G. SMITH-LAING, O. EPSTEIN & S. SHERLOCK. 1981. Results of portal decompression in patients with primary biliary cirrhosis. Gut **22:** 345-349.
29. SHERLOCK, S. 1983. Hepatic transplantation: The state of play. Lancet **ii:** 778-779.
30. VAN THIEL, D. H. 1984. The present results for liver transplantation. Gastroenterology. In press.
31. NEUBERGER, J., B. PORTMANN & B. R. D. MACDOUGALL. 1982. Recurrence of primary biliary cirrhosis after liver transplantation. N. Engl. J. Med. **306:** 1-4.
32. SNOVER, D. C., S. A. WEISDORF & N. K. RAMSAY. 1984. Hepatic graft-versus-host disease: A study of the predictive value of liver biopsy in diagnosis. Hepatology **4:** 123-130.

Introduction to the Sven Löfgren Memorial Lecture

ÅKE HANNGREN

Karolinska Institute
Stockholm, Sweden

It was more than 25 years ago that Sven Löfgren made his greatest contribution to the field of sarcoidosis and described what has come to be known as Löfgren's syndrome. Some of you may remember him from the third sarcoidosis conference, in Stockholm, when he could be found in his office, behind the desk that once belonged to Jörgen Schaumann, surrounded by Schaumann's paintings. He was at that time head of the tuberculosis clinic at St. Göran's Hospital.

The emphasis in sarcoidosis research at present is on the basic mechanisms of the disease, but it may well be worthwhile to remember that Sven Löfgren in his daily life was a clinician and was outstanding in diagnostics, even though he had very few tools in his hands. The next presentation, by Professor Turner-Warwick, Dean of the Cardiothoracic Institute of London, describes the tools available today in the management of sarcoidosis patients.

SVEN LÖFGREN MEMORIAL LECTURE

Do Measurements of Bronchoalveolar Lymphocytes and Neutrophils, Serum Angiotensin-converting Enzyme, and Gallium Uptake Help the Clinician to Treat Patients with Sarcoidosis?

M. TURNER-WARWICK,[a] P. L. HASLAM,
W. McALLISTER, A. BRITTON, AND R. LAWRENCE

Cardiothoracic Institute
Brompton and Royal Marsden Hospitals
London, England

INTRODUCTION

Opinions amongst physicians differ about if and when patients with pulmonary sarcoidosis should be treated with corticosteroids. Few would withhold treatment when the patient has obvious respiratory symptoms, particularly breathlessness. At the other extreme, many, but not all, physicians withhold treatment in asymptomatic patients with apparently newly developed radiographic changes because a substantial proportion of these patients (perhaps 60 to 70%) show spontaneous resolution within about 2 years. The main divergence of opinion in the United Kingdom concerns the middle group of patients who are asymptomatic but have known persisting radiographic parenchymal shadows. Some physicians commence treatment in an attempt to prevent irreversible changes, even when a patient's lung function is normal; others wait until there is deterioration of lung function measurements. Even when treatment has been started (on whatever basis) the problems are not over. Differences of opinion also exist about which corticosteroid doses should be used over time; about which measurements should be used in the titrations of the doses; about when corticosteroid treatment should be stopped; and about which indicator of relapse should be used to determine when corticosteroids should be reintroduced.

Against this background of well-defined and important clinical problems, efforts have been made to find more sensitive means of measuring "activity" than appraisals of a patient's symptoms, radiographs, or physiology. Such means include lymphocyte counts in bronchoalveolar lavage (BAL) samples and serum angiotensin-converting

[a] Address for correspondence: Department of Medicine, Cardiothoracic Institute, Brompton Hospital, Fulham Road, London SW3 6HP, England.

enzyme (ACE) level and gallium uptake determinations. In this paper these three measurements will be referred to as "WAG" (lung *W*ash, *A*ce level, and *G*allium uptake) measurements. Many physicians are already using these measurements of "activity" in preference to classical clinical measurements in making their therapeutic decisions. We need to consider how much evidence there is to justify this practice. The question is important because lavage causes the patient discomfort and is expensive in some countries, and gallium scans, which may be very expensive, contribute to the total radiation burden of the body. The problem is a difficult one because definite answers, which would require studies with long follow-up periods, are not easily obtained.

AIMS OF THE PRESENT STUDY

The present study was designed to answer certain specific questions despite the realization that the answers to these questions, which are outlined below, could only help solve part of the problem: 1) Do initial WAG measurements relate to the radiographic outcome following treatment? For this we studied patients before and at the time of maximum radiographic resolution. 2) Are WAG measurements consistently more sensitive indicators of "activity" than the chest radiograph? For this we analyzed WAG measurements at times when the chest radiograph had either returned to normal or had remained unchanged and stable over several months. 3) How well does the change, favorable or unfavorable, in a given WAG measurement correlate with the changes in the other two and with the change in clinical measurements? For this we considered the concordance between pairs of different clinical and WAG measurements. The details of this study will be published elsewhere. The purpose of this paper is to present an overall perspective of the problems, the study design, and the general conclusions.

METHODS

BAL was undertaken as described previously.[1] The cytospin method used for counting lavage lymphocytes was validated against cells prepared in suspension for electron microscopy and counted on 1-μm sections (Haslam, unpublished). The upper limit of normal for our laboratory was 15% for lymphocytes and 4% for neutrophils. A standard fluorimetric method was used to measure serum ACE levels.[2] The upper limit of normal for our laboratory was 52 nmol/ml/min. Quantitation of gallium scans was undertaken using absolute counts having defined areas of interest outlining the lung parenchyma and excluding the hilar regions. Standardization was achieved using counts/pixel/75 MBq/500 sec.

The chest radiographs were analyzed semiquantitatively using a modification of the International Labor Office (ILO) system where a profusion score of 0/0 to 3/3 was given to each lung providing a total score of abnormality of 18 for the whole chest radiograph. Linear shadows and upper lobe contraction was noted. Serial changes in the radiographs were also assessed using the side-by-side comparisons over a five-point scale ranging from much better, better, no change, worse, and much worse.

There was in fact good agreement between the ILO scores and side-by-side comparisons.

Lung function tests, including measurements of the transfer factor corrected for accessible lung volume (KCO), were undertaken using standard methods. The vital capacity and DL_{CO} have been selected for inclusion in the present analyses. All results have been expressed as percentages of those values that would have been predicted for normals.

The Population

Thirty-two patients who fulfilled our criteria for inclusion in this treatment program, that is, patients who continued to have abnormal radiographs for at least 1 year with or without breathlessness, were studied before and during corticosteroid treatment. All but five patients were Caucasian (one patient was black; four were Asian).

The Treatment Plan

The dose of corticosteroids was adjusted on clinical criteria only. A standard regimen was used beginning with 40 mg of corticosteroids for 4 weeks, titrating thereafter to 10 mg on alternate days over 3 months—so long as maximum radiographic improvement was maintained. In the few cases that had particularly severe abnormalities on their radiographs, 40 mg was maintained for 8 to 12 weeks to ensure maximum clearing. If radiographic relapse occurred the dose was increased to that achieving optimal clearing.[a] Lung volumes and transfer factors were monitored before treatment, at reviews 1 and 3 months after treatment, and at reviews every 6 months after treatment. They could not be used to titrate the dose because the lung volumes were frequently normal initially, and the transfer factors, although more often initially abnormal, often changed little during treatment.

WAG measurements were planned before treatment and at reviews 1, 3, and 12 months after treatment, so long as they were acceptable to the patients, all of whom gave their consent. The study was accepted by our ethics committee. The results of WAG measurements were not available to the clinicians at the times of review and were not used to change treatment. Thus the study design allowed changes in WAG measurements to be evaluated against the independent yardsticks of the chest radiograph and lung function measurements.

For practical reasons, not every patient had a complete set of measurements on every occasion. This was mainly due to technical factors relating to lack of availability of lavage or scanning time and the nonavailability of a small number of gallium scans for recounting by our improved technique. These deficiencies do not appear to have resulted in any consistent bias. They do, however, explain why different numbers are included in the various analyses.

[a] The radiograph showing optimal clearing was marked with a green "sticker" to facilitate and standardize later film comparisons in the detection of even slight changes.

RESULTS

Initial WAG Measurements and Radiographic Outcome

The patients were divided into three groups: group I, those showing complete radiographic clearing ($N = 12$); group II, those showing incomplete clearing ($N = 7$); and group III, those with incomplete clearing and with persistent linear shadows or evidence of contraction suggesting "fibrosis" ($N = 13$). Following treatment all but two patients showed marked radiographic clearing. Only 11 out of 32 patients had an initial abnormal vital capacity (that is, $< 80\%$ predicted for normals), and this remained abnormal following treatment in 5 of the 11 patients. The numbers of lavage lymphocytes were initially raised in all three groups (mean values: 27, 32, and 25%, respectively) and eventually fell in every group, although they all remained raised (means: 19, 23, and 16%, respectively). No difference was noted between the groups. In particular, 7 out of 12 patients had persistent abnormal lymphocyte levels even when their chest radiographs were normal. The mean lavage neutrophil level was raised in groups II and III (14 and 13%, respectively) but was normal in group I (2%) ($p < .05$). Neutrophil levels remained raised in groups II and III when restudied at the point of maximum radiographic clearing. The mean initial serum ACE levels were raised in all three groups initially (92, 76, and 93 units, respectively) and were within normal limits at maximum radiographic clearing (means: 44, 31, and 45 units, respectively). There was no difference between the groups. The initial gallium data were, unfortunately, incomplete (some records had become deleted) but showed raised mean values in all three groups with the greatest elevation being in group III (means: 60, 69, and 82 counts/pixel/75 MBq/500 sec, respectively). All fell substantially at the point of maximum radiographic clearing (means: 47, 56, and 53 counts/pixel/75 MBq/500 sec, respectively). There was no difference between the groups.

Incomplete clearing on the radiograph related to higher initial neutrophils, higher initial gallium scans, higher initial radiographic scores, and greater initial impairment of lung function.

WAG Measurements and Radiographs in Follow-up Trials

There were 15 incidences during follow-up examinations when the radiographs were normal and where complete simultaneous WAG data were available. BAL lymphocyte, ACE, and gallium uptake levels were also normal in only three patients (20%). BAL lymphocyte levels remained abnormal in 10 patients (67%); ACE levels in 7 (47%); and gallium scans in 6 (40%). Similar findings were seen in 18 instances when radiographs were stable but unchanged over several months (mean: 7 months). In these instances, the gallium scans were abnormal in 11 patients (61%); BAL lymphocyte levels in 10 (56%); and ACE levels in 7 (29%).

These studies might suggest that WAG measurements are more sensitive than the chest radiograph.

Analysis of the 31 occasions during follow-up when the BAL lymphocyte levels were normal, however, gave a different picture. The radiographs, ACE levels, and gallium scans were also normal in only six patients (19%). The radiographs were abnormal in 22 of the patients (71%); DL_{CO} values in 20 (65%); gallium uptake values in 14 (45%); vital capacity values in 13 (42%); and ACE levels in 8 (26%). Furthermore, the abnormal radiographs were not simply reflecting residual irreversible scarring because, in two-thirds of the patients, further radiographic improvement was seen even after the lymphocyte counts were observed as being normal. Similar analyses showed that when the gallium uptake or ACE level was normal, other measurements, including the chest radiograph and lung function, were frequently abnormal. Thus in this study no measurement appeared consistently more sensitive than the others.

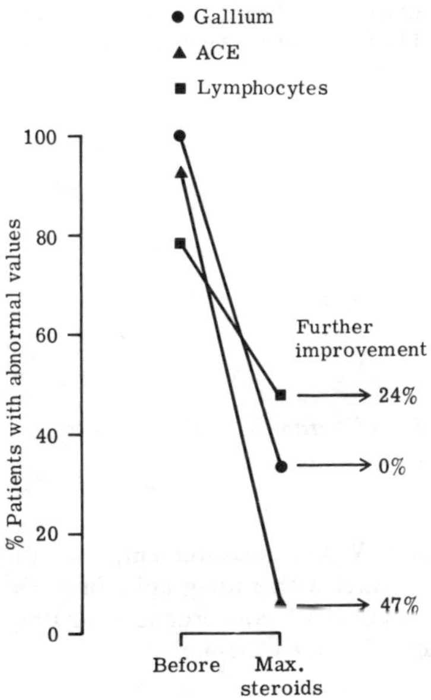

FIGURE 1. The percentage of patients ($N = 19$) with greater than normal values for gallium uptake, serum ACE, and BAL lymphocytes, before and after 1-3 months of treatment with the maximum dose of corticosteroids (usually 40 mg daily). This figure also shows the percentages of those patients with abnormal values at the end of treatment with high doses of steroids who showed further improvement in each parameter during the follow-up examinations.

The Relationship between WAG and Clinical Measurements and Corticosteroid Doses

To consider this question, the results before treatment and at the end of 4 weeks on 40 mg of corticosteroids were studied. The results are shown in FIGURES 1 & 2. The return towards normal was much greater for gallium and ACE values than for the radiograph, the lung function measurements, or the BAL lymphocyte counts. Persisting abnormal values after 1 month did not reflect maximum improvement in that further improvement was seen in 24% of those with raised lymphocyte counts and in 59% of those with persistently abnormal radiographs. Thus, overall, the chest radiograph returns to normal more slowly than other measurements; gallium and ACE values return to normal most rapidly; and BAL lymphocyte counts hold an intermediate position (FIG. 3).

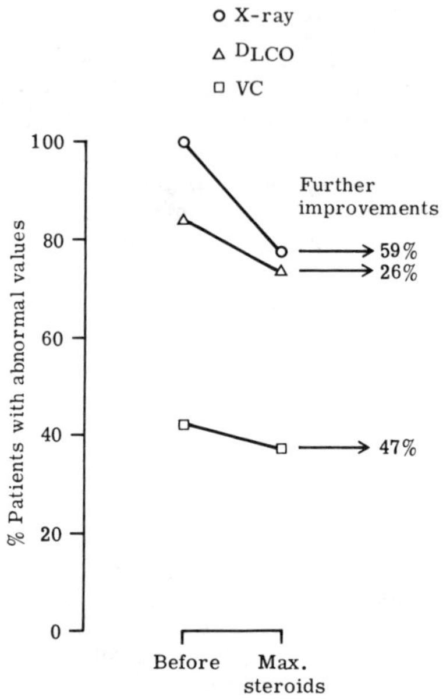

FIGURE 2. The percentage of patients ($N = 19$) with abnormal radiographs (parenchymal shadows) and abnormal DL_{CO} and vital capacity values before and after treatment with the maximum dose of corticosteroids. The format of the figure is the same as that in FIGURE 1.

Serial Changes in WAG Measurements and Radiographic and Lung Function Changes

The results of concordance studies between each WAG measurement, that is, lavage lymphocyte count, ACE level, or gallium uptake, with radiographs or with DL_{CO} and vital capacity values showed very similar results with concordances ranging from 41 to 57%. There were no significant differences between them.

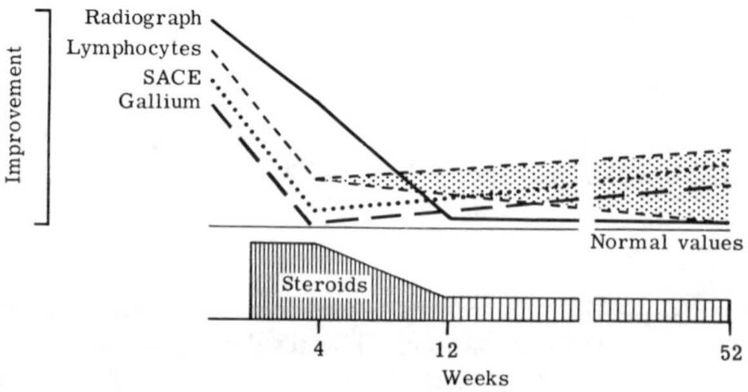

FIGURE 3. A general scheme representing the overall rates of return towards normal of the clinical and WAG measurements against time and steroid dosage. In particular it emphasizes the overall slower rate of return towards normal of the radiograph compared to WAG measurements. It also emphasizes that the radiograph may remain maximally clear while some of the WAG measurements become abnormal. In particular it emphasizes the great variability in BAL lymphocyte counts during the follow-up period which do not necessarily precede relapse of clinical parameters, nor parallel ACE or gallium measurements.

DISCUSSION AND CONCLUSIONS

In this short paper no attempt has been made to review the very substantial literature. It must be recognized that different conclusions will be made depending on the precise criteria and design of individual studies. In this study, irreversible radiographic and transfer factor changes were often seen in patients who had no respiratory symptoms. Thus, waiting for the development of symptoms before treatment does not appear logical if prevention of irreversible changes in structure and function is the objective.

During treatment, continued improvement, judging from radiographs and lung function tests, often occurred even on a reducing dose of steroids, when WAG components had already returned to normal. Therefore normal WAG values cannot be used to indicate an optimal improvement in the lung and cannot logically be used to dictate treatment. Moreover, some patients had persistently normal lymphocyte counts when the radiograph as well as ACE and gallium counts showed evidence of "activity" (FIG. 4).

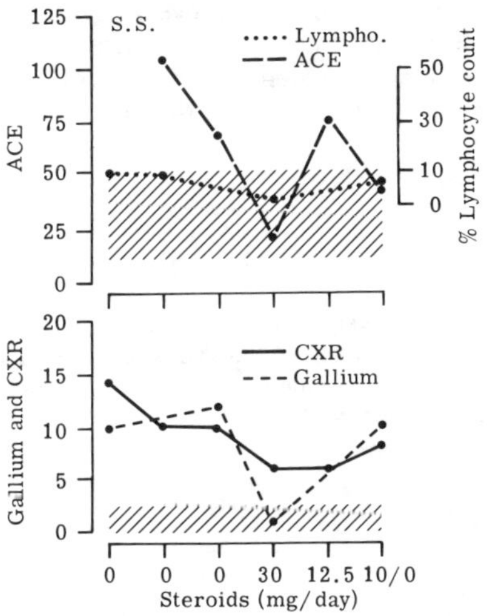

FIGURE 4. Serial ACE level measurements (in units) from a single patient. Lavage percent lymphocyte counts and gallium uptake and chest radiograph values are also shown (profusion scores using a modified ILO scheme). The range of normal values is shown by hatched lines. In this example the lymphocyte count remained consistently normal while the other measurements demonstrated fairly consistent changes before and during treatment on varying doses of steroids.

On the other hand, WAG components may be abnormal after the radiographs have returned to normal. This raises the possibility that WAG measurements might be an early indication of relapsing disease. This appeared to be the case in a small number of instances. Follow-up studies, however, showed that radiographs and lung function values frequently remained optimally normalized without change in the dose of steroids over many months of follow-up. In other words, abnormalities in WAG measurements did not consistently precede deterioration in the radiographs or lung function values over the time scale of our study. Whether these abnormal WAG values reflect subclinical activity of course remains a possibility, but they do not appear to be of clinical importance within the time scale of the present study. A determination of whether better long-term results would be obtained by using doses of steroids to maintain all WAG measurements (especially the lavage lymphocyte counts) normal, as well as optimal improvement of the radiographs and lung function values, would need a control trial lasting many years. The maintenance dose of steroids would certainly need to be higher than that used to maintain optimal improvement of the radiographs alone, and the side effects from such higher doses might well outweigh any possible benefits.

While we have not been able to identify any consistent advantage of WAG measurements over monitored radiographs in the titration of steroid dosage in our study, these measurements may be useful as additional tools in difficult individual cases where, for various reasons, the clinical measurements are discordant. For example, an increasingly breathless patient with stable radiographs and lung function values.

If the chest radiograph is to be used as the mainstay for clinical evaluation, rigorous and systematic comparisons of all radiographs during planned follow-up studies conducted over long periods with careful titration of steroids to maintain optimal improvement is at least logical, if irreversible changes are to be avoided.

This study does not answer completely all the questions concerning clinical management. It does, however, attempt to put in some perspective the relative values of clinical and new (WAG) measurements of activity and, in particular, suggests that the new measurements are not consistently more sensitive measurements against which corticosteroids can be titrated.

REFERENCES

1. Haslam, P. L., C. W. G. Turton, A. Lukoszek, A. J. Salsbury, A. Dewar, J. V. Collins & M. Turner-Warwick. 1980. Bronchoalveolar lavage fluid cell counts in cryptogenic fibrosing alveolitis and their relation to therapy. Thorax **35:** 328-339.
2. Friedland, J. & E. Silverstein. 1976. A sensitive fluorimetric assay for serum angiotensin-converting enzyme. Am. J. Clin. Pathol. **66:** 416-424.

Persistent High Alveolar Lymphocytosis as a Predictive Criterion of Chronic Pulmonary Sarcoidosis[a]

DOMINIQUE ISRAEL-BIET,[b] ALAIN VENET, AND JACQUES CHRÉTIEN

Institut National de la Santé et de la Recherche Médicale Unité 214
Hôpital Laennec
75007 Paris, France

INTRODUCTION

Sarcoidosis is a systemic granulomatous disorder of unknown origin and is characterized by the presence of noncaseating granulomas at sites of the disease.[1] If the vital prognosis can be threatened by some extrathoracic localizations, the central nervous system or heart, for instance, this disease is nonctheless generally benign in terms of overall mortality. Various degrees of lung structure derangement, however, can develop during the course of sarcoidosis, which can ultimately lead to pulmonary fibrosis. Thus, the morbidity rate of the disease is quite appreciable. These complications usually arise during the chronic stages of sarcoidosis, that is, after more than 2 years of evolution. The major problem is to predict the final outcome of the disease early enough to be able to treat the patients before any irreversible lung structure derangement has occurred. Early predictive criteria of final outcome have always been sought after, but contradictory data have been reported so far. Since the last international conference on sarcoidosis, several studies have indeed focused on the predictive value of bronchoalveolar lavage (BAL), either to help foresee the functional evolution[2] and the short-term outcome of the disease[3,4] or to get a more accurate assessment of the disease activity.[5–7] The results of these studies are rather conflicting, which is understandable considering the differences existing between the series concerning the criteria for the selection of patients, the durations of the follow-up studies, and, finally, the ultimate goals of these studies. The point is that the short-term evolution is not

[a] This work was supported in part by Contrat de Fonds Special des Comités Départementaux contre les Maladies Respiratoires et la Tuberculose 83 MR-12.

[b] To whom correspondence should be addressed.

always indicative of the final outcome, and that being able to predict the final outcome does not necessarily make the advantages of a particular therapeutic decision evident. We focused our interest on the outcome of the disease at 2 years, the threshold of the chronic phase, where some complications are more likely to occur, in order to be able to define among our population of sarcoidosis patients which ones were more likely to develop pulmonary complications. On the other hand, we were interested in clarifying the usefulness of BAL among the routine assessments of sarcoidosis and in determining the value of BAL assessments in predicting the outcome of the disease at 2 years. We thus designed a study taking into account all nonsmoking, untreated sarcoidosis patients referred to the department since 1977, provided that their disease was of recent onset, in order to really characterize the spontaneous evolutive features of the early stages of the disease.

METHODS

Patient Population

Among the patients with biopsy-proven pulmonary sarcoidosis referred to the department between 1977 and 1981, we selected 73 patients on the basis of nonsmoking habits, no previous treatment, and recent onset of the disease. This could be assessed by two different means. First of all, some patients presented Löfgren's syndrome, which has been described as the hallmark of recently developed sarcoidosis.[8] Otherwise, patients were referred to the department because of chest radiograph abnormalities detected through a routine roentgenographic screening program. We selected for our study those who had normal chest radiographs within the 6 months prior to the appearance of the recently detected abnormalities.

There were 37 females and 36 males, and the mean age of the patients was 32.3 ± 8.5 years. The follow-up for all patients lasted at least 2 years: the usual time of spontaneous recovery. None of the patients received any treatment during this 2-year follow-up period. We evaluated the likelihood of such a recovery among untreated patients with disease of recent onset and thus investigated the natural history of their disease.

Evaluation of Sarcoidosis

All patients underwent a complete evaluation of their disease at the time of diagnosis as well as at times throughout the follow-up period. This evaluation was clinical, biological, roentgenographic, and functional, and also comprised bronchoalveolar lavages.

General Evaluation of the Disease

The clinical examination focused on all respiratory and extrathoracic symptoms that could be related to the disease. Serum angiotensin-converting enzyme (SACE) was assayed by the spectrophotometric method of Cushman and Cheung,[9] as modified by Lieberman.[10] The SACE value of all patients was compared to that of 46 healthy volunteers, and was considered abnormal if it was higher than the mean plus two standard deviations (SD's) of the control value. The upper limit of the normal value was thus 35 U/ml. In order to assess the roentgenographic aspect as accurately as possible, three different observers, in each case, classified the patients according to the following categories: type I, patients with hilar adenopathy only; type II, patients with adenopathy and parenchymal involvement; and type III, patients with parenchymal involvement only. Each patient underwent a complete pulmonary function test (PFT). Because sarcoidosis is known to induce an essentially restrictive syndrome, however, our evaluation focused mostly on total lung capacity (TLC) and carbon monoxide diffusing capacity (DC). This last value was corrected for the alveolar volume. Both values, TLC and DC, were expressed as the percentage of the predicted values from the European Coal and Steel Community Survey.[11] They were considered abnormal if they were less than 80% of the predicted values.

BAL and Cell Analysis

The detailed technique of the lavage has already been published.[12] Briefly, it was performed with a total of 300 ml of sterile, warm (37° C) saline solution. A cell count was done on native fluid with a hemocytometer, and the cell differential was determined on May-Grünwald-Giemsa-stained cytocentrifuged smears.[13] The thymus-derived (T) lymphocytes were identified by their ability to spontaneously form rosettes with neuraminidase-treated sheep red blood cells at 4° C, using the same technique as with blood T lymphocytes.[14] The lymphocytosis was either expressed as a percentage of the total cell count or as being abnormal, if the percentage of lymphocytes was higher than the mean plus two SD's of the percentage of lymphocytes in the lavage of normal controls. In order to determine this normal value, 20 healthy nonsmoking volunteers underwent BAL. Their mean lymphocyte percentage in BAL, ± SD, was 6.1 ± 4.2. Therefore the upper limit for the normal percentage of lymphocytes in BAL was 15%.

Follow-up Assessments

Patients were assessed every 6 months by clinical, biological, roentgenographic, and functional evaluation. They also underwent serial BAL. We were particularly interested in the first evaluation, that at the entry into the study (t_0), and in the subsequent evaluations 12 months (t_{12}) and 24 months (t_{24}) after the beginning of the study. BAL was performed at t_0 in 73 patients, at t_{12} in 44 patients, and at t_{24} in 18 patients. Patients were considered cured if all clinical, biological, roentgenographic, functional, and lavage data were normal at t_{24}. They were considered uncured if at least one of these criteria was still abnormal at t_{24}.

Statistical Analysis

We used the two-tailed Student's *t* test, the chi-square test, and the Fisher exact probability test.[15] All results are expressed as means ± SD's.

RESULTS

General Presentation of Patients at the First Evaluation

A summary of the general presentation of patients at t_0 is given in TABLE 1.

Clinical Data

None of the patients complained of any respiratory symptoms, and their physical pulmonary examinations were utterly normal. Extrathoracic localizations (ETL's) of sarcoidosis were found in 21 patients (27%), and included skin, lymph nodes, liver, spleen, and parotids. No ETL's were found in 57 patients (73%).

Chest Radiographs

Interestingly, the majority of patients were classified as type I. Indeed, 39 patients (53%) presented a type I chest radiograph, and 34 patients (47%) presented a type II radiograph. No patient presented a type III radiograph.

TABLE 1. Presentation of Patients at the First Evaluation

Aspect of Presentation	Percentage of Patients[a]
Clinical Data	
Clinical pulmonary symptoms	0
ETL's	28
Radiographic Staging[b]	
Type I	53
Type II	47
Type III	0
PFT Values[c]	
Abnormal DC	12
Abnormal TLC	14
Abnormal DC and TLC	7
SACE Levels[d]	
Elevated	67

[a] Percentage of patients exhibiting a given aspect of the general presentation.

[b] Type I: hilar involvement only; type II: hilar and parenchymal involvement; type III: parenchymal involvement only.

[c] PFT values were considered abnormal if they were less than 80% of the predicted values.

[d] SACE levels were considered elevated if they were greater than 35 U/ml (the mean ± 2 SD's for the normal controls).

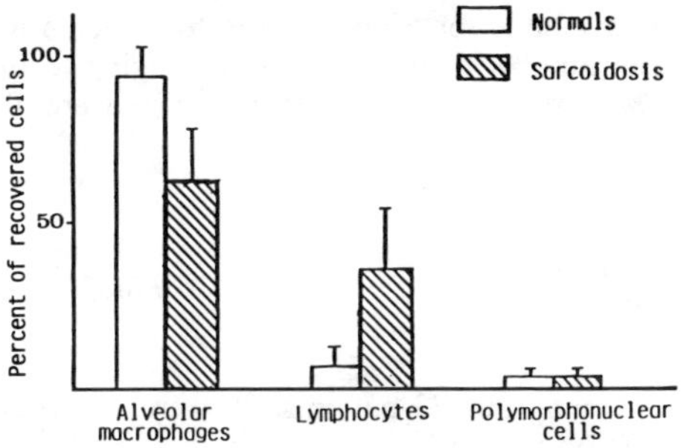

FIGURE 1. Cell differentials in controls ($N = 20$) and sarcoidosis patients ($N = 73$). The total cell numbers were 29 ± 16 × 10^6 in controls and 59 ± 37 × 10^6 in sarcoidosis patients, respectively.

PFT Values

As a whole, the patients had both TLC and DC within the normal range at t_0: these values reached 93.2 ± 13.2% and 95.9 ± 19.5% of their respective predicted values. Forty-nine patients (67%), however, did have normal PFT values; 9 others (12%) had abnormal TLC values (72.8 ± 6.1%); 10 (14%) had abnormal DC values (68.7 ± 8.4); and 5 (7%) had both PFT values abnormal.

SACE Levels

SACE determinations at t_0 were available in 43 patients. The mean value for all patients was 44.1 ± 22.9 U/ml. It was abnormal in 29 patients (67%) and was normal in 14 others (33%).

BAL Analyses

The fluid recovery was 57 ± 15% of the instilled saline solution, and was quite similar to that of normal controls ($p > .5$). The total cell count of our patients was 59.5 ± 36.8 × 10^6 and was significantly higher ($p < .01$) than that of controls (26.9 ± 13.7 × 10^6). As expected, the BAL cell analysis showed an important increase ($p < .01$) of the lymphocyte percentage in our patients compared to controls (34.9 ± 18.5% and 6.1 ± 4.2%, respectively). Concurrently, there was a decrease of the macrophage percentage (63.0 ± 18.9%), but because of the high cellularity observed in the BAL fluid of sarcoidosis patients, the population of alveolar macrophages was indeed expanded. Finally, polymorphonuclear leukocytes accounted for 1.3 ± 1.3% of the total cell count, a percentage quite similar to that for controls (2 ± 2%) (FIG. 1).

It is noteworthy that as many as 61 patients (84%) had an abnormal lymphocytosis at the time of diagnosis. Their values of lymphocytosis were homogeneously distributed all along a wide range (5 to 77%). Twenty-one patients disclosed a lymphocyte count between 15 and 30%; 24 between 30 and 50%; and 16 over 50%. A T cell determination was available for 50 out of the 61 patients with a high lymphocytosis at t_0, and the mean number of lymphocytes belonging to the T type was 83.5 ± 8.1%. More than 30% of the cells recovered by lavage were T lymphocytes in 48% of our patients.

Final Outcome

Among our 73 patients, 39 were eventually cured at t_{24} (53%) whereas 34 were not (47%).

All of the uncured patients still had abnormal chest radiographs, whether they were stable or deteriorated compared to their initial radiographic evaluations. As a matter of fact, 11 of the uncured patients (30%) had developed type III chest radiographs by t_{24}. All the uncured patients still had abnormal chest radiographs.

On the other hand, SACE was assayed in 28 uncured patients at t_{24} and was shown to have remained elevated in 14 of them (50%).

About the same proportion (47%) of uncured patients still had abnormal PFT values at 2 years, whether the values were of TLC alone (16%), of DC alone (25%), or of both TLC and DC (6%).

Finally, BAL was performed at t_{24} in 18 uncured patients. Eleven of them (61%) still had an abnormal lymphocytosis in BAL at 2 years, with a lymphocyte percentage of 21 ± 12%.

Predictive Value of Alveolar Lymphocytosis

We have tried to determine the predictive value of initial lymphocytosis in BAL by looking at it in different ways. First, we defined the cured and the uncured groups at t_{24} using all the recovery criteria already described and calculated for each group the mean initial lymphocytosis value at t_0. We did not find any significant difference ($p > .5$, Student's t test) between these two values, which were 34.8 ± 19.3% and 34.9 ± 17.8%, respectively. Besides, all the individual values were equally dispersed in both groups, ranging from 5 to 77% (FIG. 2). Second, we calculated within each range of initial values of lymphocytosis the number of eventually cured and uncured patients at t_{24}. Again, we found no difference between the recovery and the nonrecovery rates of the patients within each initial range of lymphocyte counts. It is therefore obvious that one cannot expect any help from the initial BAL data to foresee what the outcome will be 2 years later. It is important to underline the fact that the intensity of the lymphocytic alveolitis is devoid of any predictive value if evaluated during the very early stages of sarcoidosis, not only on a statistical basis, but also on an individual one.

Because we were also interested in the spontaneous evolution of the alveolitis among early stages of sarcoidosis, and since iterative lavages had been performed on our patients during the follow-up period, we observed the evolution of all these iterative BAL data and formed some interesting notions. First, the patients presenting a normal alveolar lymphocytosis at t_0 never disclosed an abnormal lymphocytosis at any subsequent time during the follow-up period. Second, patients who had an initially abnormal lymphocyte count, but a normalized one by t_{12}, never disclosed again any increase of their lymphocytosis. Third, each patient who did eventually have a normalized alveolar lymphocytosis developed it before the end of the first year after diagnosis.

We then wanted to see whether this evolutive feature of the alveolitis could be correlated in any way to the prognosis, and we did find a strong correlation between the persistence of an abnormal lymphocytosis at t_{12} and final nonrecovery. As a matter of fact, among the 44 patients who underwent a BAL at t_{12}, 23 disclosed a normal lymphocyte count at that time, and 21 a high one. Among these 23 patients 11 had lymphocyte counts within the normal range at t_0 which remained normal throughout the follow-up period; 12 had an abnormal lymphocytosis at t_0 which became normal by t_{12}. Altogether, this group of patients with a normal lymphocyte percentage at t_{12} reached a recovery rate of 81% at t_{24}. In marked contrast, the patients who still had an abnormal lymphocytosis at t_{12} only reached a recovery rate of 13% at t_{24} (FIG. 3).

We conclude from these results that the persistence of an abnormal alveolar lymphocytosis within the first year after diagnosis of an early stage sarcoidosis strongly argues for a nonrecovery at 2 years, and therefore for a chronic evolution.

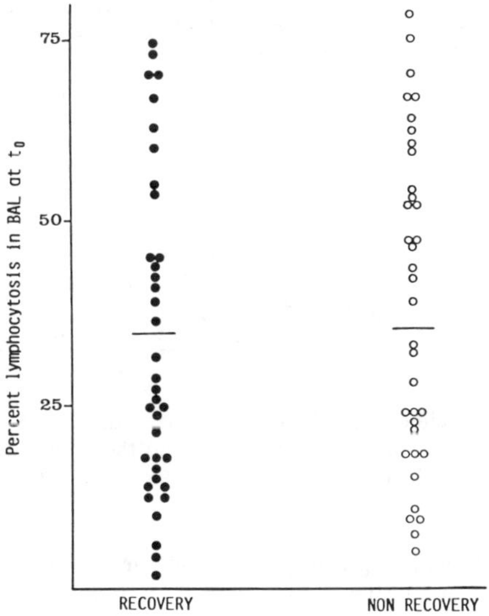

FIGURE 2. Individual values of initial alveolar lymphocytosis of all patients, whether they were classified in the recovery or the nonrecovery group after the 2-year follow-up period. Mean value of initial lymphocytosis in the recovery group: 34.8 ± 19.3%; in the nonrecovery group: 34.9 ± 17.8% ($p > .5$).

DISCUSSION

A major problem in sarcoidosis is to predict its natural outcome. Although a benign disease in terms of overall mortality, sarcoidosis has an appreciable morbidity rate. When treatment becomes necessary because of a compromised respiratory status, the histological changes in the lung structures are usually irreversible, and the treatment is not successful. Several studies so far have aimed at establishing reliable criteria to predict the evolution of sarcoidosis. Among these studies, several have focused on BAL, evaluating its predictive value for the overall evolution of the disease.[2-4] The results reported so far are rather conflicting, possibly because of the extreme variability of clinical presentation of sarcoidosis, making the series and the patients in the series nonhomogeneous, and hardly comparable to one another. This is due to large differences in the time of prior disease before entry into the study, in the duration of the follow-up studies, in smoking habits, or in previous treatments. To better study the natural history of sarcoidosis, we selected patients with sarcoidosis of confirmed recent onset, and followed the spontaneous course of their disease for at least 2 years. To further eliminate any factor which could possibly modify this course, we excluded all smokers and all previously treated patients. Moreover, no patients were ever treated throughout the follow-up period. We thus came up with a very homogeneous population of recent onset sarcoidosis patients.

Our study population was found to be quite representative of the usual sarcoidosis, as far as sex ratio, age, and existence of ETL's were concerned. The spontaneous outcome is also quite comparable to that of other series[16,17] with a 53% rate of recovery at 2 years. It must be stressed, however, that none of our patients initially had any

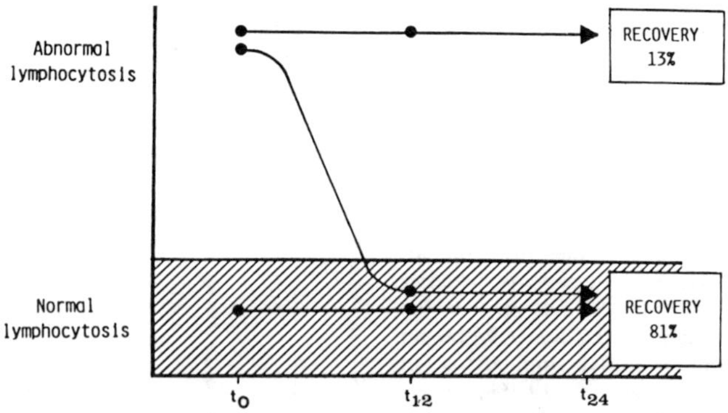

FIGURE 3. Evolution of alveolar lymphocytosis and final outcome of the disease in the patients with a normal lymphocytosis and those with an abnormal lymphocytosis at t_{12}. Recovery rate in the first group: 81%; in the second group: 13% ($p < .001$).

clinical respiratory symptoms or presented a type III chest radiograph, and that 67% of our patients had normal PFT values at t_0. Not only that, but 39 patients (53%) had a type I chest radiograph. This may be rather different from other series, which generally comprise fewer type I and more type II or type III patients, and where clinical or functional symptoms are more frequent at time of presentation. Once again, this should not be too surprising, since we deal here with sarcoidosis of very recent onset. Such a selection of patients has been possible because of the routine chest X-ray screening program that exists in France. In addition, because Laennec Hospital is a reference center for interstitial lung diseases, patients are referred to our department with chest radiograph abnormalities detected before the development of any clinical or functional symptoms.

Because all our patients had a pulmonary localization of their disease, and because BAL is a reliable means of assessing the alveolitis, we thought it would be interesting to characterize the evolution of the alveolitis all along the natural course of recent onset sarcoidosis. In addition, a high lymphocyte count in BAL seems to be a very common feature of early stage sarcoidosis, in our series (84% of our patients presented an abnormal lymphocytosis) as well as in others.[18] Because the recovery rate was 53% at 2 years, it was obvious that some patients with a high initial lymphocytosis were nonetheless eventually cured. We thus tried to determine the time it took for the alveolar lymphocyte count to return to normal during the course of the disease, and found it to be approximately 12 months after diagnosis. We then focused on the subsequent evolution of the patients who did have a normal lymphocytosis at that time compared to that of patients who did not. In other words, we looked for a possible correlation between the lymphocytosis, whether initial or persistent, and the final outcome of the disease.

We showed that assessments of initial lymphocytosis could not enable us to predict the final outcome of a recent onset sarcoidosis. As a matter of fact, no statistical correlation could be established between initial values of lymphocytosis and outcome. Moreover, on an individual basis it was impossible, in front of a patient presenting any lymphocytosis at t_0, whether high or low, to predict whether or not he would be cured at t_{24}. More specifically, an abnormal lymphocyte count at t_0, even a very high one, by no means implied an evolution towards a chronic phase. This is quite consistent with the study by Valeyre *et al.*[18] Their study showed that all their patients with Löfgren's syndrome had an abnormal lymphocytosis detected by BAL at presentation, and 92% of them recovered within a year.

Conversely, we found a strong correlation between the persistence of a high lymphocytosis detected by BAL at t_{12} and final nonrecovery ($p < .001$, chi-square test). Indeed, 87% of the patients with a high lymphocytosis at t_{12} were not cured at 2 years. On the other hand, 81% of the patients with a normal lymphocyte count at t_{12} were cured at t_{24}. It is noteworthy that among the latter one can find patients with a lymphocytosis which had always been normal as well as patients with an abnormal lymphocyte count at t_0 that had returned to normal by t_{12}. There was no difference, however, between the recovery rates of these two subgroups of patients (data not shown). Thus, it is striking that, no matter what the initial lymphocytosis is, a normal BAL lymphocyte count at t_{12} is indicative of an evolution towards recovery, whereas its persistence argues for an evolution towards a chronic phase. It has to be stressed that we deal here with a statistical likelihood, and that a persistent abnormal lymphocytosis is not always predictive on an individual basis. As a matter of fact, 13% of such patients were actually cured at t_{24}.

Although these results might look different from those previously published, we think that they do not express any conflicting ideas. Most of the previous studies dealing with BAL had not focused on long-term outcome. They either studied the reliability of BAL in assessing the cellular changes occurring in interstitial structures during sarcoidosis,[19] the importance of the site of lavage or more reproducibility,[20] the nature of the immune phenomenon occurring within the lung,[21–27] or the predictive value of alveolitis for the respiratory status during an ensuing 6-month interval.[2] In the last study, Keogh *et al.* showed that patients with a high-intensity alveolitis (that is, one in which more than 28% of the cells recovered by BAL are T lymphocytes and in which gallium lung scans are positive) were likely to show some deterioration in at least one of their PFT values within 6 months whereas patients with a low-intensity alveolitis (one in which fewer than 28% of the cells recovered by BAL are T lymphocytes and/or in which gallium lung scans are negative) would remain stable. We think that these results are quite complementary with ours. Indeed, a high-intensity alveolitis, even if it suggests a functional deterioration within the 6 months following its assessment, does not imply any undesirable long-term evolution, provided that it is found in an early stage of the disease. Conversely, the persistence of such a high-intensity alveolitis not only suggests a functional deterioration, but also an overall chronic evolution, one possibly leading to some irreversible lung structure derangements and permanently altered PFT values.

We found that a nonrecovery of sarcoidosis at 2 years was likely if the alveolar lymphocytosis was persistently abnormal 1 year after the onset of the disease. It must, however, be kept in mind that some of these patients will nonetheless be cured at 2 years, which is the threshold of the chronic phase of sarcoidosis, and that some more patients will spontaneously recover during this chronic phase. In other words, we do not advocate any systematic treatment of patients that have a high lymphocytosis detected by BAL at t_{12}, but we suggest that such patients should be watched more closely than any others, because *some* of them are at a greater risk for complications.

Finally, the belief that lymphocytes are implicated in the pathogenesis of the disease has been proved correct: evidence of their activation at sites of the disease has been found, and the role of some lymphokines in the different steps of the pathological events that characterize sarcoidosis is now known.[21–27] Our study points out another important characteristic of the lymphocytes in this disease, a characteristic which is relevant to clinical studies, particularly studies designed to determine prognoses. BAL has long proved to be the most reliable, the safest, and the most repeatable way to recover the constitutive elements of the sarcoidosis alveolitis, and this argues for its importance within the routine assessment of sarcoidosis patients and in obtaining more information about the pathogenesis and clinical course of sarcoidosis.

SUMMARY

A homogeneous population of 73 sarcoidosis patients with recent onset sarcoidosis, no smoking habits, and no previous treatments was serially evaluated in a study of the spontaneous evolution of sarcoidosis. This evaluation comprised clinical, radiographic, biological, and functional assessments as well as assessments of fluids recovered by BAL. We determined the natural history of alveolar lymphocytosis in early stage sarcoidosis and the predictive value of such lymphocytosis for the outcome of the disease. We focused on the outcome at 2 years because it is the usual time of spontaneous recovery; after 2 years the disease enters the chronic phase, and more complications are likely to occur. We found that the initial lymphocytosis observed during the very early stages of the disease had no predictive value for the outcome. Conversely, the persistence of a high alveolar lymphocytosis within the first year of evolution is strongly correlated to a nonrecovery at 2 years, and thus to a chronic phase of sarcoidosis.

ACKNOWLEDGMENTS

We would like to thank A. M. Laval for technical assistance in processing the BAL fluids and D. Guillemot for secretarial assistance.

REFERENCES

1. MITCHELL, A. & J. SCADDING. 1974. State of the art: Sarcoidosis. Am. Rev. Respir. Dis. **110:** 774-800.
2. KEOGH, B. A., G. W. HUNNINGHAKE, B. R. LINE & R. G. CRYSTAL. 1983. The alveolitis of pulmonary sarcoidosis: Evaluation of natural history and alveolitis-dependent changes in lung function. Am. Rev. Respir. Dis. **128:** 256-265.
3. BRAMBILLA, G., L. CHAVEZ, E. BRAMBILLA, F. MOREL, P. GROSLAMBERT, D. MAINSONNEUVE, A. VINCENT, A. DAMAK, D. RIGAUD & B. PARAMELLE. 1981. Prognostic value of bronchoalveolar lavage and angiotensin-converting enzyme in sarcoidosis. *In* Sarcoidosis and Other Granulomatous Disorders. J. Chrétien, J. Marsac & J. C. Saltiel, Eds.: 419-423. Pergamon Press. Paris.
4. STANISLAS-LEGUERN, G., D. CHOUDAT, A. ARNOUX, P. DURIEUX, J. LACRONIQUE, C. BAUMANN, G. J. HUCHON, J. H. MARSAC & J. CHRÉTIEN. 1981. Prognostic value of angiotensin-converting enzyme and alveolar lymphocytes in sarcoidosis. *In* Sarcoidosis and Other Granulomatous Disorders. J. Chrétien, J. Marsac & J. C. Saltiel, Eds. 424-429. Pergamon Press. Paris.
5. ROSSI, G. A., O. SACCO, E. COSULICH, G. DAMIANI, G. CORTE, A. BARGELLESI & C. RAVAZZONI. 1984. Pulmonary sarcoidosis: Excess of helper T lymphocytes and T cell subset imbalance at sites of disease activity. Thorax **39:** 143-149.
6. RAZMA, G., J. P. LYNCH III, B. S. WILSON, P. A. WARD & S. L. KUNKEL 1984. Expression of Ia-like (DR) antigen on human alveolar macrophages isolated by bronchoalveolar lavage. Am. Rev. Respir. Dis. **129:** 419-424.
7. CEUPPENS, J. L., L. M. LACQUET, G. MARIEN, M. DEMEDTS, A. VAN DEN EECKHOUT & E. STEVENS. 1984. Alveolar T-cell subsets in pulmonary sarcoidosis: Correlation with disease activity and effect of steroid treatment. Am. Rev. Respir. Dis. **129:** 563-568.
8. SILTZBACH, L. E., D. G. JAMES, E. NEVILLE, J. TURIAF, J. P. BATTESTI, O. P. SHARMA, Y. HOSODA, R. MIKAMI & M. ODAKA. 1974. Course and prognosis of sarcoidosis around the world. Am. J. Med. **57:** 847-852.
9. CUSHMAN, D. W. & H. S. CHEUNG. 1971. Spectrophotometric assay and properties of the angiotensin-converting enzyme of rabbit lung. Biochem. Pharmacol. **250:** 262-265.
10. LIEBERMAN, J. 1975. Elevation of the serum angiotensin-converting enzyme level in sarcoidosis. Am. J. Med. **59:** 365-372.
11. Commission des Communautés Européennes. 1967. Tables de références pour les examens spirographiques: 13-818-2-67. Service des Publications des Communautés Européennes. Luxembourg.
12. ROTH, C., G. J. HUCHON, A. ARNOUX, G. STANISLAS-LEGUERN, J. H. MARSAC & J. CHRÉTIEN. 1981. Bronchoalveolar cells in advanced pulmonary sarcoidosis. Am. Rev. Respir. Dis. **124:** 9-12.
13. MORDELET-DAMBRINE, M., A. ARNOUX, G. STANISLAS-LEGUERN, D. SANDRON, J. CHRÉTIEN & G. HUCHON. 1984. Processing of lung lavage fluid causes variability in bronchoalveolar cell counts. Am. Rev. Respir. Dis. **130:** 305-306.
14. WEINER, M. S., C. BIANCO & V. NUSSENZWEIG. 1973. Enhanced binding of neuraminidase-treated sheep erythrocytes to human T lymphocytes. Blood **42:** 939-946.
15. COLQUHOUN, D. 1971. Lectures on Biostatistics: An Introduction to Statistics with Applications in Biology and Medicine. Clarendon Press. Oxford.
16. BACHARACH, T. 1961. Sarcoidosis: A clinical review of 111 cases. Am. Rev. Respir. Dis. **84:** 12-16.
17. CHRÉTIEN, J., G. STANISLAS-LEGUERN & J. C. SALTIEL. 1981. Course and treatment of sarcoidosis in 350 patients: A follow-up study for ten years. *In* Proceedings of the International Symposium on Sarcoidosis. R. Mikami & Y. Hosoda, Eds.: 301-314. University of Tokyo Press. Tokyo.
18. VALEYRE, D., G. SAUMON, R. GEORGES, J. L. KEMENY, D. BLADIER, J. AMOUROUX, J. PRE & J. P. BATTESTI. 1984. The relationship between disease duration and noninvasive pulmonary explorations in sarcoidosis with erythema nodosum. Am. Rev. Respir. Dis. **129:** 938-943.

19. Hunninghake, G. W., O. Kawanami, V. J. Ferrans, R. C. Young, Jr., W. C. Roberts & R. G. Crystal. 1981. Characterization of the inflammatory and immune effector cells in the lung parenchyma of patients with interstitial lung disease. Am. Rev. Respir. Dis. **123:** 407-412.
20. Cantin, A., R. Begin, M. Rola-Pleszczynski & R. Boileau. 1983. Heterogeneity of bronchoalveolar lavage cellularity in stage III pulmonary sarcoidosis. Chest **83:** 485-486.
21. Crystal, R. G., W. C. Roberts, G. W. Hunninghake, J. E. Gadek, J. D. Fulmer & B. R. Line. 1981. Pulmonary sarcoidosis: A disease characterized and perpetuated by activated lung T-lymphocytes. Ann. Intern. Med. **94:** 73-94.
22. Hunninghake, G. W., J. D. Fulmer, R. C. Young, J. E. Gadek & R. G. Crystal. 1979. Localization of the immune response in sarcoidosis. Am. Rev. Respir. Dis. **120:** 49-57.
23. Hunninghake, G. W., J. E. Gadek, R. C. Young, Jr., O. Kawanami, V. J. Ferrans & R. G. Crystal. 1980. Maintenance of granuloma formation in pulmonary sarcoidosis by T-lymphocytes within the lung. N. Engl. J. Med. **302:** 594-598.
24. Hunninghake, G. W. & R. G. Crystal. 1981. Pulmonary sarcoidosis: A disorder mediated by excess helper T-lymphocytes at sites of disease activity. N. Engl. J. Med. **305:** 429-434.
25. Hunninghake, G. W. & R. G. Crystal. 1981. Mechanisms of hypergammaglobulinemia in pulmonary sarcoidosis: Site of increased antibody production and role of T-lymphocytes. J. Clin. Invest. **67:** 86-92.
26. Pinkston, P., P. B. Bitterman & R. G. Crystal. 1983. Spontaneous release of interleukin-2 by lung T-lymphocytes in active pulmonary sarcoidosis. N. Engl. J. Med. **308:** 793-800.
27. Daniele, R. P., J. H. Dauber & M. D. Rossman. 1980. Immunologic abnormalities in sarcoidosis. Ann. Intern. Med. **92:** 406-416.

Systemic and Lung Protein Changes in Sarcoidosis

Lymphocyte Counts, Gallium Uptake Values, and Serum Angiotensin-converting Enzyme Levels May Reflect Different Aspects of Disease Activity[a]

IRENE J. CHECK, MARYBETH R. KIDD, AND GERALD W. STATON, JR.[b]

Department of Pathology and Laboratory Medicine
and
Department of Medicine
Emory University School of Medicine
Atlanta, Georgia 30322

INTRODUCTION

Over the years a number of tests have been proposed for assessing disease activity in sarcoidosis.[1] Bronchoalveolar lavage (BAL) lymphocyte percentages (the number of lymphocytes counted expressed as a percentage of the total number of cells recovered by BAL), gallium-67 scans, and serum angiotensin-converting enzyme (SACE) level determinations have been proposed as useful clinical tests.[1-3] These tests, however, do not always correlate,[4,5] and seem to measure different aspects of the inflammatory process.

Because most inflammatory processes produce local and sometimes systemic protein changes, we evaluated paired sera and BAL fluids from normal subjects and sarcoidosis patients by high-resolution agarose gel electrophoresis to determine how protein patterns related to these clinical measures of disease activity.

[a] This work was supported by a grant from the Carlyle Fraser Heart Center.

[b] Address for correspondence and reprint requests: 35 Linden Avenue, N.E., Suite 5311, Atlanta, Georgia 30365.

MATERIALS AND METHODS

Patient Population, BAL, and Gallium-67 Studies

Twenty-one patients seen in the Emory University Affiliated Hospitals between January 1982 and October 1983 were studied. All had chest radiographs, pulmonary function tests, BAL's, gallium-67 lung scans, and SACE level determinations in routine initial and follow-up evaluations of biopsy-proven sarcoidosis. An additional tube of serum was frozen at −70° C for later analysis. Twelve patients had 1 evaluation, seven patients had 2, and two patients had 3, for a total of 32 evaluations. Each evaluation was considered a separate event for purposes of data analysis. The characteristics of the patients are summarized in TABLES 1 & 2.

BAL was performed through a fiberoptic bronchoscope wedged in the right middle lobe or lingula. Normal saline solution, in 35- to 50-ml aliquots, to a total volume of 100 to 200 ml, was instilled through the suction channel and gently aspirated into a sterile trap. Total and differential cell counts and percent viability (trypan blue exclusion) were determined.[9] Lavage fluid was centrifuged and the supernatant removed and frozen at −70° C until analysis.

Using computer-interfaced, wide-field scintillation cameras, gallium-67 lung scans were performed 48 hr after intravenous injection of 3 to 5 mCi gallium-67 citrate. Posterior images of chest and abdomen were obtained.

A computer-based technique was used to quantitate the deposition of gallium-67 in the lungs relative to a background area below the kidney, expressed as a total lung to background (TL/B) ratio.[10]

TABLE 1. Patient Characteristics

Characteristics	Number of Patients
Sex	
Male	6
Female	26
Smoking Status	
Nonsmokers	8
Former smokers	10
Smokers	14
Treatment Status	
Treated	12
Untreated	20
Chest Radiographic Type[a]	
Type 0	9
Type I	1
Type II	17
Type III	5

[a] Type 0: normal; type I: bilateral hilar adenopathy without pulmonary infiltrates; type II: bilateral hilar adenopathy with pulmonary infiltrates; and type III: pulmonary infiltrates alone.

TABLE 2. Pulmonary Function Tests[a]

Test	Mean ± SEM
FVC (%)	75 ± 2
TLC (%)	73 ± 2
DLVA (%)	78 ± 4
PaO_2 (torr)	85 ± 2

[a] Pulmonary function tests were performed on standard spirometry, lung volume, single breath diffusing capacity, and arterial blood gas equipment. Percent predicted values for forced vital capacity (FVC), total lung capacity (TLC), and single breath diffusing capacity (DLVA) were calculated using the regression equations of Crapo *et al.*[6-8]

BAL and Serum Analyses

Total protein contents in serum and BAL supernatant, respectively, were measured using a Coomassie blue binding assay (Biorad protein assay, Biorad Laboratories, Richmond, CA). BAL fluids were concentrated 100-fold using a Minicon-B15 filter (Amicon, Danvers, MA). The agarose gel electrophoresis procedure was modified from that of Jeppsson *et al.*[11] Gels 1-mm thick were cast onto 125 × 245 mm Gelbond film (FMC, Rockland, ME) using a 1% agarose solution (Seachem ME agarose, FMC, Marine Colloids Division, Rockland, ME) in barbital buffer (pH 8.6). Four-microliter samples of serum or 5 to 20 μl of concentrated BAL fluid were applied over an application foil (Worthington Diagnostics, Freehold, NJ) on an area preblotted with 4-cm wide chromatography paper (Whatman, Clifton, NJ). Electrophoresis was carried out at 10° C for 45 min on an LKB Multiphor unit (LKB Instruments, Rockville, MD) set at 20 V/cm. Gels were fixed in picric acid fixative (Worthington Diagnostics, Freehold, NJ), pressed, dried, and stained with 0.25% amido black for serum or with 0.5% Coomassie blue for BAL fluid.

The major protein fractions were quantitated using a Cliniscan densitometer (Helena Laboratories, Beaumont, TX). The gels were scanned at 595 nm, and six fractions were quantitated (albumin and the α_1-, α_2-, β_1-, β_2-, and γ-globulins). Visual interpretation scores of serum and BAL patterns for each patient were made by two pathologists who did not know the patient's name or diagnosis. Serum protein patterns were scored as normal, acute inflammatory (given two or more of the following changes: increased α_1- or α_2-globulin levels or decreased prealbumin or α-lipoprotein levels), or chronic inflammatory (given increased γ-globulin levels and decreased albumin and transferrin levels).[11]

Statistical Analysis

All data were stored in an ALTOS microcomputer (Altos Computer Systems, San Jose, CA) using the DBASE II database management program (Ashton-Tate, Culver City, CA). Correlation coefficients among the tests were calculated using linear regression analysis, and statistical significance of the difference between means was determined using two-tailed unpaired *t* tests using ABSTAT statistical software programs (Anderson-Bell, Denver, CO). All data are presented as means ± SEM.

RESULTS

Examination of the patient sera revealed 9 specimens with inflammatory changes and 23 specimens with normal protein patterns.

The patient BAL fluids showed a wide range of total protein values (0.037 to 0.878 mg/ml) compared to those shown by BAL fluids from normal subjects (0.028 to 0.135 mg/ml). Although some patients had normal agarose gel protein patterns (some albumin and, occasionally, minimal amounts of β_1-globulin would be found), others had abnormal patterns, with bands corresponding to most of the serum proteins including γ-globulin. Many patients with normal amounts of total protein in their BAL specimens had abnormal agarose patterns. Therefore, we grouped the BAL specimens on the basis of the γ-globulin concentrations and high-resolution agarose gel electrophoresis patterns. The first BAL specimen type ($N = 10$), labeled normal, was defined as having < 0.02 mg/ml of γ-globulin and only albumin and minimal amounts of β_1-globulin on electrophoresis. The total protein level ranged from 0.037 to 0.116 mg/ml. The second type ($N = 8$), labeled intermediate, was defined as having ≥ 0.02 mg/ml (0.02 to 0.07 mg/ml) of γ-globulin and more intense protein bands in the α_1-, α_2-, and γ-globulin regions. The total protein level ranged from 0.101 to 0.126 mg/ml. The third type ($N = 14$), labeled abnormal, was also defined as having > 0.02 mg/ml of γ-globulin (0.021 to 0.356 mg/ml), but with an electrophoretic pattern showing more intense bands for all proteins. The total protein level ranged from 0.09 to 0.878 mg/ml. Nine patients also had bands of restricted heterogeneity in the γ-globulin region suggestive of immune complexes.[12]

The patient population exhibited three of the four possible combinations of sera pattern (normal or inflammatory) and BAL specimen type (normal or abnormal). Each patient in group 1 ($N = 9$) had an inflammatory serum pattern and an abnormal BAL specimen (FIG. 1A); each patient in group 2 ($N = 13$) had normal serum and an intermediate to abnormal BAL specimen (FIG. 1B); and each patient in group 3 ($N = 10$) had normal serum and a normal BAL specimen (FIG. 1C). No patient with an inflammatory serum pattern had a normal BAL specimen. The concentrations of total protein and of each of the major protein fractions in the BAL specimens decreased from group 1 to group 3 (FIG. 2). The BAL specimens of patients in group 3 were very similar to normal BAL specimens.

To evaluate whether the amount of a given protein was disproportionately increased in the lung, the protein's concentration in a BAL specimen was compared to its concentration in serum. Because albumin is synthesized in negligible amounts within the lung, we corrected for increases in alveolar permeability by including serum and BAL albumin values to calculate a protein index similar to the immunoglobulin G (IgG) synthetic index for cerebrospinal fluid.[13]

FIGURE 3 illustrates the BAL protein indices for the α_1-globulins, (predominantly α_1-antitrypsin), the β_1-globulins (predominantly transferrin), and the γ-globulins for each of the three groups as compared to the normal indices. A BAL protein index of greater than 1.0 suggests there is a disproportionate amount of that protein in the BAL specimen relative to serum. The β_1-globulin and γ-globulin indices were > 1 in groups 1 and 2 but not in group 3 or in the normal individuals. The α_1-globulin index was < 1.0 in all the groups and in the normals.

On the basis of serum and BAL protein abnormalities, patients in group 1 appeared to have more active pulmonary and systemic disease than did those in groups 2 or 3. To evaluate how these results correlated with the other laboratory tests of disease activity, BAL lymphocyte percentages, gallium-67 lung uptake values (TL/B ratios), and SACE levels were related to the protein pattern groups. The BAL lymphocyte

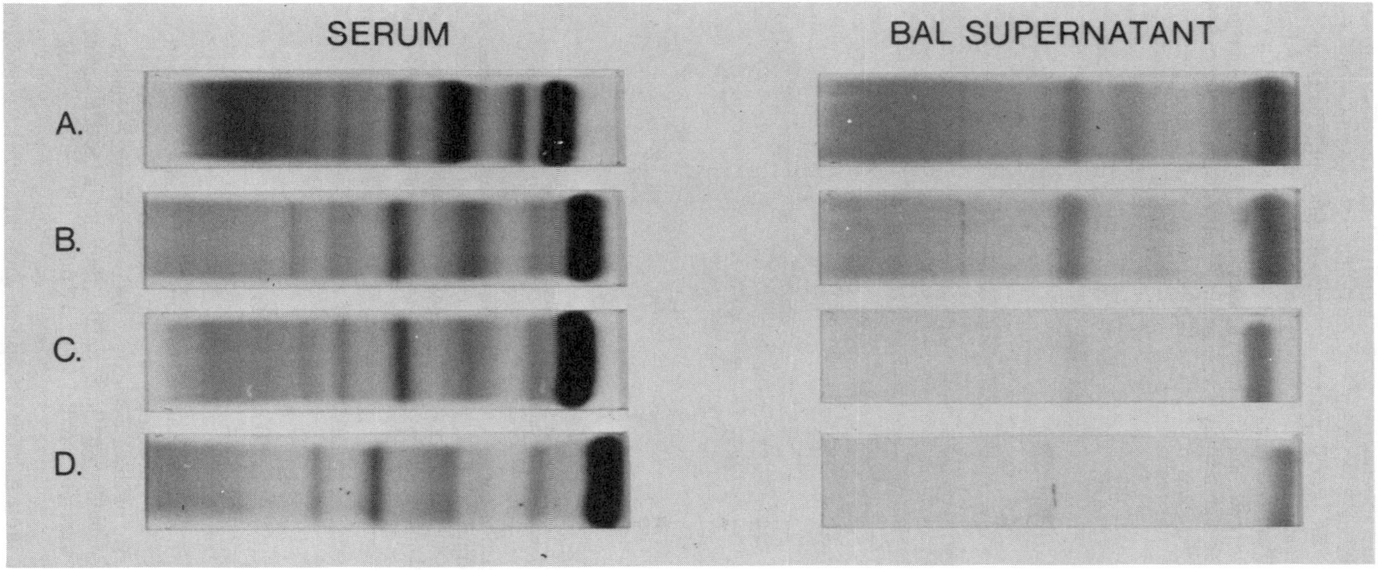

FIGURE 1. Representative paired sera and BAL fluid high-resolution agarose electrophoresis specimens. (**A**) Inflammatory serum and abnormal BAL supernatant patterns typical of group 1 patients ($N = 9$). (**B**) Normal serum and abnormal BAL supernatant patterns typical of group 2 patients ($N = 13$). (**C**) Normal serum and normal BAL supernatant patterns typical of group 3 patients ($N = 10$). (**D**) Normal serum and normal BAL supernatant patterns typical of normal subjects ($N = 10$).

percentages were highly abnormal in group 1 and fell markedly both from group 1 to group 2 and from group 2 to group 3 (FIG. 4). The relationship of the quantitated gallium-67 uptake and the protein pattern groups was different. The group 1 patients, the ones with inflammatory changes in serum proteins, had the most highly abnormal TL/B ratio. Although patients in groups 2 and 3 had slightly abnormal TL/B ratios, group 2 patients, who had abnormal BAL specimens but normal serum protein patterns, did not differ significantly from group 3 patients, who had normal BAL specimens (FIG. 5). There was no relationship between SACE level and the protein groups (FIG. 6).

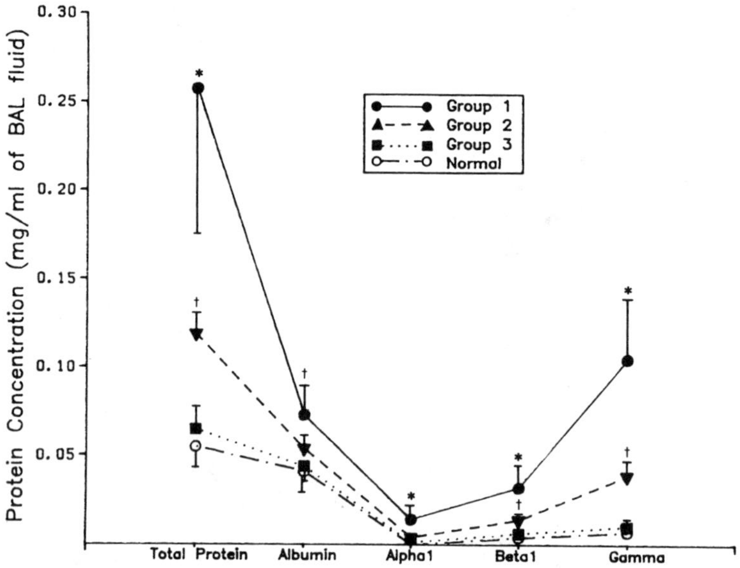

FIGURE 2. Protein fraction concentrations in BAL supernatants from sarcoidosis patients grouped according to serum and BAL protein patterns. Groups 1, 2, and 3 are as they were described in FIGURE 1. Normal values for protein analysis were determined from lavage fluid obtained from 10 normal nonsmoking subjects. * = $p < .05$ versus group 2, group 3, and normal values; † = $p < .05$ versus group 3 and normal values.

DISCUSSION

This study has shown that proteins in serum and BAL fluid are frequently abnormal in sarcoidosis. Patients with increasingly abnormal serum and BAL protein levels also had changes in two tests of disease activity, BAL lymphocyte percentage determinations and quantitated gallium-67 lung uptake, but not in SACE levels. The fact that the relationships were not parallel suggests that each test measures a different aspect of inflammation.

Changes in serum protein levels consistent with inflammation probably reflect systemic sarcoidosis, although they might also result from severe pulmonary disease.

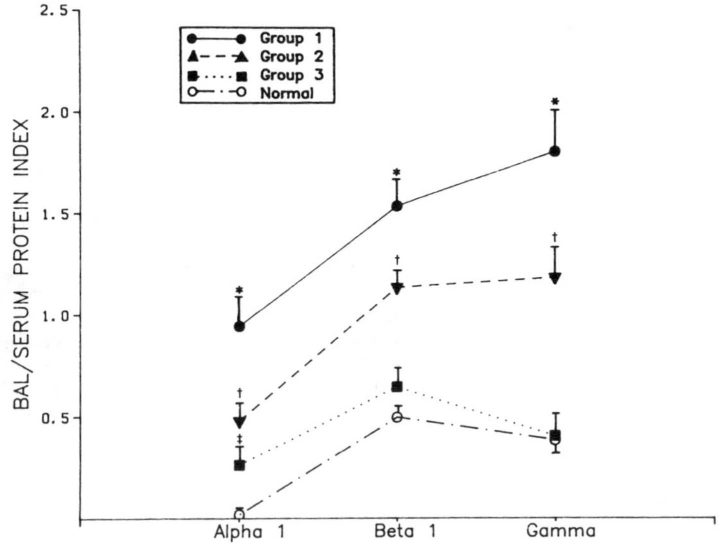

FIGURE 3. Protein indices for α_1-, β_1-, and γ-globulin fractions. The protein index relates the concentration of a protein in a band from a BAL fluid electrophoresis specimen to the protein's serum concentration and, to correct for alveolar permeability, to the albumin levels in serum and in BAL fluid. The index for γ-globulin, for example, is calculated as follows: (mg γ-globulin in BAL fluid) (mg albumin in BAL fluid)$^{-1}$/(mg γ-globulin in serum) (mg albumin in serum)$^{-1}$. Groups 1, 2, and 3 and normal subjects are as they were described in FIGURES 1 & 2. $*=p < .05$ versus group 2, group 3, and normal values; $\dagger=p < .05$ versus group 3 and normal values; and $\ddagger=p < .05$ versus normal values.

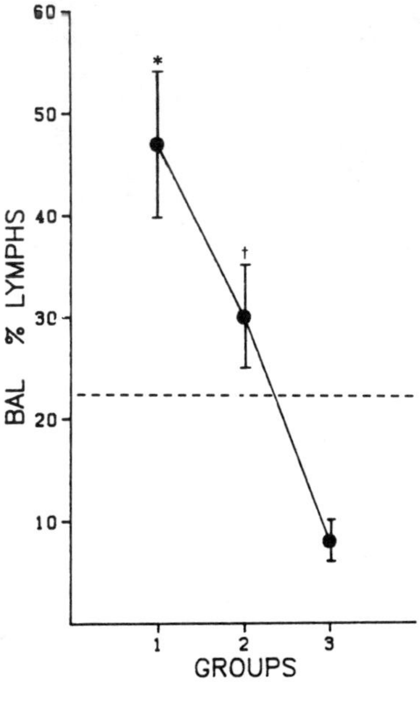

FIGURE 4. BAL lymphocyte percentages (BAL % lymphs) in the three groups of sarcoidosis patients described in FIGURE 1. Normal values for cell counts were obtained by performing BAL on 17 normal nonsmoking subjects. The upper limit for normal lymphocyte percentages (-----) was determined by adding two SD's to the means of the values from the normal subjects. $*=p < .05$ versus group 2 and group 3 values; $\dagger=p < .05$ versus group 3 values.

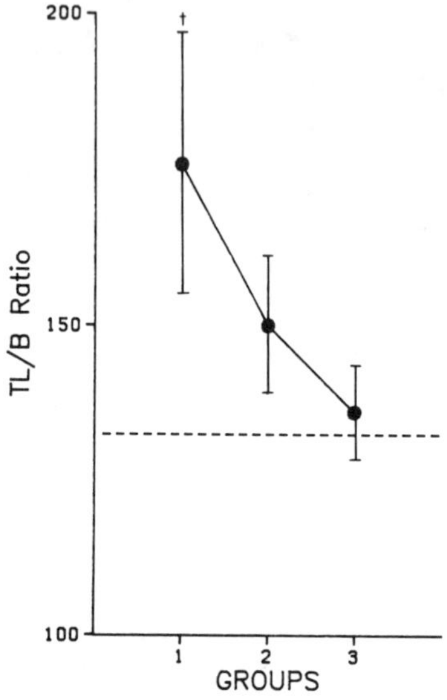

FIGURE 5. Quantitated gallium-67 uptake (TL/B ratios) in the three groups of sarcoid patients described in FIGURE 1. Normal values for the TL/B ratio were established by performing gallium lung scans in five patients who exhibited no clinical evidence of pulmonary disease and who were being scanned for nonpulmonary inflammatory lesions. The upper limit for normal TL/B ratios (----) was determined by adding two SD's to the means of the values of the normal subjects. †=$p < .05$ versus group 3 values.

The increased albumin levels in BAL fluid are due to increased permeability,[15] and the increased γ-globulin levels to synthesis of immunoglobulins by B lymphocytes and plasma cells in the lung.[16,17] Interestingly, none of the patients with inflammatory changes in serum protein had normal BAL protein patterns. Patients with abnormal serum and BAL specimens may have more severe disease than those with normal serum and abnormal BAL specimens or those with normal serum and normal BAL specimens.

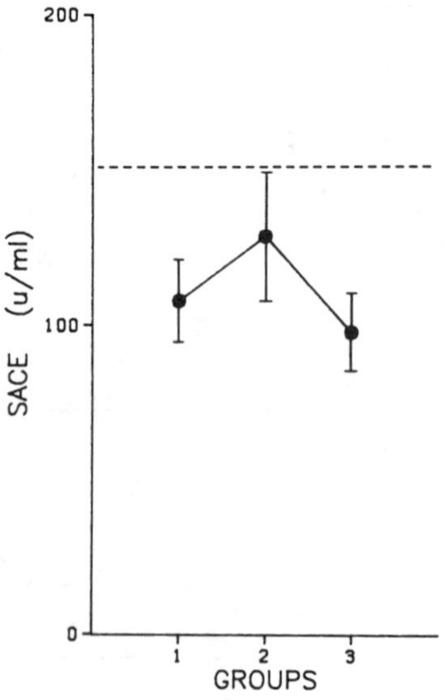

FIGURE 6. SACE levels in the three groups of sarcoidosis patients described in FIGURE 1. SACE levels were measured by radioassay using the method of Rohatgi and Ryan.[14] Normal values were established by testing 41 normal subjects. The upper limit for normal SACE values (----) was determined by adding two SD's to the means of the values of the normal subjects.

This suggestion is supported by the changes in BAL lymphocyte percentages and gallium-67 lung uptake values among these groups. The BAL lymphocyte percentages, thought to measure the degree of lymphocytic infiltrate in the lung parenchyma,[18] best paralleled the changes in BAL protein levels, including those of γ-globulin. Because T cells constitute the predominant class of lymphocytes in the BAL fluid of patients with sarcoidosis,[2,19] these data suggest that T cells play an immunoregulatory role in the local synthesis of immunoglobulin and the pathogenesis of increased alveolar permeability. Alternatively, increased numbers of T cells and higher BAL protein (albumin and γ-globulin) levels may reflect similar underlying disease mechanisms.

Values for gallium-67 uptake in the lung parenchyma also differed among the groups of patients with different patterns of serum and BAL protein. Interestingly, the patients with the highest gallium-67 uptake values were those with serum protein changes suggestive of systemic inflammation. We do not know the cause of this association. Quantitated gallium-67 lung uptake is thought to reflect the degree of activation of alveolar macrophages[20] and is likely to be mediated by transferrin receptors on cells.[21] These patients may have low iron saturation of transferrin, as seen in some patients with systemic inflammation. This might allow binding of more gallium to transferrin, resulting in more gallium uptake by activated cells (possibly activated monocytes/macrophages with transferrin receptors[22]). Our finding of a disproportionate increase in the β_1-globulin fraction, composed primarily of transferrin, in some patients with sarcoidosis may indicate increased transferrin synthesis by macrophages within the lung,[23] selective binding to transferrin receptors on pulmonary cells (a transferrin sink),[22] or increased transfer of cell-bound transferrin from the circulation.

In contrast to the BAL lymphocyte percentage and gallium-67 lung uptake studies, we found no relationship between the protein pattern groups and SACE levels. Other investigators have also failed to find correlations between serum IgG or BAL IgG/albumin and SACE levels.[24] Although SACE levels have been proposed to measure the mass of total body granulomas,[3] its relationship to disease activity is uncertain.[1,2] These data suggest that SACE levels are probably not related to the systemic or pulmonary inflammation process.

In summary, systemic and pulmonary proteins relate to other measures of disease activity, but not in parallel, suggesting that each measures a different aspect of inflammation. Further studies of serum and lung proteins may help elucidate the mechanisms of BAL cell changes and increased gallium-67 lung uptake in sarcoidosis.

SUMMARY

BAL lymphocyte percentages, quantitated gallium-67 lung uptake, and SACE levels have all been proposed as measures of disease activity in sarcoidosis. We analyzed 32 paired sera and BAL fluids from sarcoidosis patients by high-resolution agarose electrophoresis to look for protein changes characteristic of systemic or local inflammation and compared the results with those from the above tests.

Nine patients (group 1) had serum inflammatory protein changes and increased total protein, albumin, β_1-globulin (transferrin), and γ-globulin levels in fluid recovered by BAL. Thirteen patients (group 2) had normal protein levels in sera but abnormal protein levels in BAL specimens. Ten patients (group 3) had normal protein levels in sera and in BAL specimens. Patients in groups 1 and 2 had a disproportionate increase in β_1-globulin (transferrin) and γ-globulin levels in their BAL specimens. The BAL lymphocyte percentage changes paralleled the BAL protein level changes, suggesting relationships among the immunoregulatory role of these cells, increased local immunoglobulin synthesis, and the pathogenesis of altered alveolar permeability. Gallium-67 uptake was highest in patients with serum inflammatory protein changes. Thus, systemic inflammation may facilitate pulmonary gallium-67 uptake, possibly by changes in BAL fluid or serum transferrin saturation and/or kinetics. SACE levels showed no relationship to changes in the levels of serum or BAL proteins. These data suggest that the various proposed measures of disease activity reflect different aspects of inflammation in sarcoidosis.

ACKNOWLEDGMENTS

We thank Drs. E. Honig, M. Gilman, G. Grossman, M. Duffell, J. Pine, and A. Plummer for referring patients to the study; Ms. M. Brantley and Ms. C. Drwiega for performing the bronchoalveolar fluid analyses; Dr. D. Sgoutas for performing the SACE analyses; and Ms. J. Wyndham for preparing this manuscript for publication.

REFERENCES

1. Fanburg, B. L., Ed. 1983. Sarcoidosis and Other Granulomatous Diseases of the Lung. *In* Lung Biology in Health and Disease. Vol. **20.** Marcel Dekker. New York, NY.
2. Crystal, R. G., W. C. Roberts, G. W. Hunninghake, J. E. Gadek, J. D. Fulmer & B. R. Line. 1981. Pulmonary sarcoidosis: A disease characterized and perpetuated by activated lung T-lymphocytes. Ann. Intern. Med. **94:** 73-94.
3. Lieberman, J., L. A. Schleissner, A. Nosal, A. Sastre & F. S. Mishkin. 1983. Clinical correlations of serum angiotensin-converting enzyme (ACE) in sarcoidosis. Chest **84:** 522-528.
4. Staton, G., M. Gilman, J. Pine, L. Greenwald, W. Fajman & I. Check. 1983. Comparison of clinical evaluation, bronchoalveolar lavage, gallium-67 lung uptake, and serum angiotensin-converting enzyme in the assessment of pulmonary sarcoidosis. Am. Rev. Respir. Dis. **127**(Suppl.): 89.
5. Beaumont, D., J. Y. Herry, M. Sapene, P. Bourgret, J. J. Larzul & B. Delabarthe. 1982. Gallium-67 in the evaluation of sarcoidosis: Correlation with serum angiotensin-converting enzyme and bronchoalveolar lavage. Thorax **37:** 11-18.
6. Crapo, R. O., A. H. Morris & R. M. Gardner. 1981. Reference spirometric values using techniques and equipment that meet ATS requirements. Am. Rev. Respir. Dis. **123:** 659-664.
7. Crapo, R. O., A. H. Morris, P. D. Clayton & C. R. Nixon. 1982. Lung volumes in healthy nonsmoking adults. Bull. Eur. Physiopathol. Respir. **18:** 419-425.
8. Crapo, R. O. & A. H. Morris. 1981. Standardized single breath normal values for carbon monoxide diffusing capacity. Am. Rev. Respir. Dis. **123:** 185-189.
9. Hunninghake, G. W., J. E. Gadek, O. K. Kawanami, V. J. Ferrans & R. G. Crystal. 1979. Inflammatory and immune processes in the human in health and disease: Evaluation by bronchoalveolar lavage. Am. J. Pathol. **97:** 148-206.
10. Fajman, W. A., L. V. Greenwald, G. Staton, I. Check, J. Pine, M. Gilman, K. Scheidt & E. McClees. 1984. Quantitative 67-gallium citrate lung imaging in sarcoidosis: Comparison of three methods and correlation with bronchoalveolar lavage. Am. J. Roentgenol. **142:** 683-688.

11. JEPPSSON, J. O., C. B. LAURELL & B. FRANZEN. 1979. Agarose gel electrophoresis. Clin. Chem. **25:** 629-638.
12. KELLY, R. H., M. A. SCHOLL, V. S. HARVEY & A. G. DEVENYI. 1980. Qualitative test for circulating immune complexes by use of zone electrophoresis on agarose. Clin. Chem. **26:** 396-402.
13. LINK, H. & G. TIBBLING. 1977. Principles of albumin and IgG analyses in neurological disorders. II. Relationship of the concentration of the proteins in serum and cerebrospinal fluid. Scand. J. Clin. Lab. Invest. **37:** 396-397.
14. ROHATGI, P. & J. W. RYAN. 1980. Simple radioassay for measuring serum activity of angiotensin-converting enzyme in sarcoidosis. Chest **78:** 69-76.
15. BAUGHMAN, R. P., C. H. BOSKEN, P. HURTUBISE & R. G. LOUDON. 1982. Bronchoalveolar lavage in patients with sarcoidosis: Evidence for an albumin leak. Am. Rev. Respir. Dis. **125**(Suppl.): 54.
16. RANKIN, J. A., G. P. NAEGEL, C. E. SCHRADER, R. A. MATTHAY & H. Y. REYNOLDS. 1983. Air-space immunoglobulin production and levels in bronchoalveolar lavage fluid of normal subjects and patients with sarcoidosis. Am. Rev. Respir. Dis. **127:** 442-448.
17. HUNNINGHAKE, G. W. & R. G. CRYSTAL. 1981. Mechanisms of hyperglobulinemia in pulmonary sarcoidosis: Site of increased antibody production and role of T-lymphocytes. J. Clin. Invest. **67:** 86-92.
18. HUNNINGHAKE, G. W., O. KAWANAMI, V. J. FERRANS, R. C. YOUNG, W. C. ROBERTS & R. G. CRYSTAL. 1981. Characterization of the inflammatory and immune effector cells in the lung parenchyma of patients with interstitial lung disease. Am. Rev. Respir. Dis. **123:** 407-412.
19. HUNNINGHAKE, G. W., J. D. FULMER, R. C. YOUNG, J. E. GADEK & R. G. CRYSTAL. 1979. Localization of the immune response in sarcoidosis. Am. Rev. Respir. Dis. **120:** 49-57.
20. HUNNINGHAKE, G. W., B. R. LINE, S. V. SZAPIEL & R. G. CRYSTAL. 1981. Activation of inflammatory cells increases the localization of gallium-67 at sites of disease. Clin. Res. **49:** 171A.
21. LARSON, S. M., Z. GRUNBAUM & J. S. RASEY. 1981. The role of transferrins in gallium uptake. Int. J. Nucl. Med. Biol. **8:** 257-266.
22. HIRATA, T., P. PINKSTON, P. BITTERMAN, A. HANCE & R. CRYSTAL. 1984. Alveolar macrophage transferrin receptors in pulmonary sarcoidosis. Am. Rev. Respir. Dis. **129:** A20.
23. STECHER, V. J. & G. J. THORBECKE. 1967. Site of synthesis of serum proteins. I. Serum protein produced by macrophages *in vitro*. J. Immunol. **99:** 643-652.
24. VALEYRE, D., G. SAUMON, D. BLADIER, J. AMOUROUX, J. PRE, J. P. BATTESTI & R. GEORGES. 1982. The relationships between noninvasive explorations in pulmonary sarcoidosis of recent origin, as shown in bronchoalveolar lavage, serum, and pulmonary function tests. Am. Rev. Respir. Dis. **126:** 41-45.

Predictive Value of Bronchoalveolar T Cell Subsets for the Course of Pulmonary Sarcoidosis

U. COSTABEL,[a] K. J. BROSS, J. GUZMAN, A. NILLES,
K. H. RÜHLE, AND H. MATTHYS

Medizinische Universitätsklinik
Albert-Ludwigs-Universität
Freiburg, West Germany

INTRODUCTION

Pulmonary sarcoidosis is characterized by increased proportions and numbers of thymus-derived (T) lymphocytes in bronchoalveolar lavage (BAL) fluid.[1-6] In active disease, most of these T lymphocytes are OKT4-positive helper-inducer cells.[3-6] Compared to serum angiotensin-converting enzyme (SACE) level and gallium uptake measurements, we found that determinations of BAL helper cell proportions provided the best means of assessing activity in pulmonary sarcoidosis.[6] Recently the proportions and absolute numbers of I-associated (Ia) antigen-positive, activated T cells in BAL fluid have been found to be markedly increased in pulmonary sarcoidosis with elevated T4/T8 (helper/suppressor) ratios compared to those patients with normal ratios.[7]

It is not clear whether BAL lymphocyte subpopulations can be correlated to predictions of disease outcome in cases of sarcoidosis, or whether knowing these proportions can help us identify those patients who should be treated for progressive disease. Thus, the purpose of this study was to assess the predictive value of BAL helper and suppressor cell counts as well as of cell counts of Ia antigen-positive T cells for the course of pulmonary sarcoidosis.

METHODS

Patients

Thirty-one patients with pulmonary sarcoidosis, all of whom entered our department consecutively, were included in our study. All of these patients had undergone BAL since October 1981 and fulfilled the following criteria: histologically proven

[a] Address for correspondence: Medizinische Universitätsklinik, Hugstetterstrasse 55, D-7800 Freiburg, West Germany.

disease; no treatment with steroids for at least 3 months before the first BAL; and clinical, physiologic, and radiographic evaluations, with controls, over a follow-up period for at least 12 months after the first BAL. Twenty patients underwent a second BAL during the follow-up period.

According to the initial T4/T8 ratios in BAL fluid, two groups of patients were formed: one group included all patients with elevated T4/T8 ratios, that is, with ratios above 3.5 (the mean value plus two SD's for healthy control subjects), and the other group included all patients with normal T4/T8 ratios. Clinical and laboratory characteristics of the two groups are shown in TABLE 1. Data are given as mean values ± one SD.

BAL

Each BAL was performed by applying 100 ml of saline solution in five 20-ml aliquots. BAL cells were counted. Cell differentials were made from each smear after it was stained with May-Grünwald-Giemsa and 1000 cells were counted.

Lymphocyte subsets were identified by the peroxidase-antiperoxidase method performed on glass slides as previously described.[7–9] The following monoclonal antibodies were used: OKT3, to determine the total number of T cells; OKT4, to mark helper-inducer T cells; OKT8, to mark suppressor-cytotoxic T cells; and OKIa, to mark Ia antigen-positive (HLA-DR^+), activated T cells.

Pulmonary Function Tests

Lung volumes were measured by body plethysmography, and the CO diffusing capacity was measured using the single-breath method. Our values are reported as diffusing capacity/lung volume. Arterial blood gases were measured at rest and during exercise.

SACE Activity

SACE activity was measured using a spectrophotometric assay described by Lieberman.[10]

Gallium Index

To calculate the gallium index of ^{67}Ga lung scans, the uptake by the lung area was computed as a percentage of the uptake by the liver area.

TABLE 1. Clinical and Laboratory Characteristics of Patients with Elevated and of Patients with Normal T4/T8 Ratios[a]

	Patients with Elevated T4/T8 Ratios	Patients with Normal T4/T8 Ratios	Significance
Number of patients	16	15	
Number of males/females	5/11	9/6	NS
Number of smokers/nonsmokers	4/12	4/11	NS
Average age (years)	42 ± 17	35 ± 11	NS
Duration of disease before BAL (months)	21[b]	16[c]	NS
Length of follow-up period (months)	21 ± 7	18 ± 6	NS
Number of Patients in Each Radiographic Stage			
Type I	7	1	
Type II	4	10	
Type III	5	4	
Lung function Tests			
Vital capacity (%)	80 ± 12	91 ± 14	$p < .05$
DL_{CO}/VL (%)	78 ± 14	92 ± 13	$p < .01$
PaO_2 at exercise (%)	100 ± 12	107 ± 14	NS
SACE level (U/ml)	52 ± 26	43 ± 11	NS
Gallium index	38 ± 27	24 ± 20	NS
BAL Data			
Fluid recovered (%)	60 ± 13	59 ± 10	NS
Total number of cells recovered ($\times 10^6$)	25 ± 18	13 ± 8	$p < .05$
Percentage of lymphocytes among BAL cells	45 ± 21	32 ± 20	NS
Percentage of $T4^+$ cells among lymphocytes	81 ± 5	53 ± 15	$p < .0001$
Percentage of $T8^+$ cells among lymphocytes	13 ± 9	30 ± 9	$p < .0001$
T4/T8 ratio	8.7 ± 3.4	1.9 ± 0.8	$p < .0001$
Percentage of Ia antigen$^+$ cells among lymphocytes	20 ± 18	5 ± 8	$p < .01$

[a] T4/T8 ratios above 3.5 were considered elevated.
[b] Range: 0-108 months.
[c] Range: 0-60 months.

Signs of Deterioration: Criteria for the Decision to Treat Patients

The signs of deterioration were as follows: symptoms developed or were progressive (cough, dyspnea, or systemic symptoms), values for one lung function test fell to less than 10% of those recorded initially (IVC, TLC, CO diffusing capacity, or PaO_2 at exercise), and successive chest radiographs indicated the disease was progressive.

If, during the follow-up period, one of the conditions listed above occurred, the course was classified as having deteriorated; if one of these conditions began to clear, it was classified as having improved; if no change occurred, it was classified as being stable.

RESULTS

Course of Disease in Patients with Normal T4/T8 Ratios in Initial BAL

In this group of 15 patients, 10 patients improved during the follow-up period of 18 ± 6 months, 3 patients remained stable, and only 2 patients had to be treated with steroids because of persistent symptoms. Neither of these last two patients suffered a relapse after their withdrawal from therapy (FIG. 1).

Chest radiographs showed improvement in eight and lung function was improved in four patients of this group. Deterioration of these parameters occurred in none of these 15 patients.

Course of Disease in Patients with Elevated T4/T8 Ratios in Initial BAL

In this group of 16 patients, 6 patients deteriorated without therapy during the subsequent follow-up period of 21 ± 7 months, and 4 patients had to be treated with steroids because of severe symptoms and/or reduced lung function. Three of these four treated patients relapsed when treatment was stopped after 6 months.

Chest radiographs revealed deterioration in four patients that had elevated T4/T8 ratios (in three of these four patients the stage progressed from I to II), and improvement in only three patients. Lung function deteriorated in eight and improved in two patients of this group.

Interestingly, also in stage I disease, elevated T4/T8 ratios were found in about half of the cases associated with a deteriorating course (FIG. 2). In stage III disease, four out of five patients with elevated T4/T8 ratios had conditions which deteriorated whereas three out of four patients with normal ratios improved or were stable.

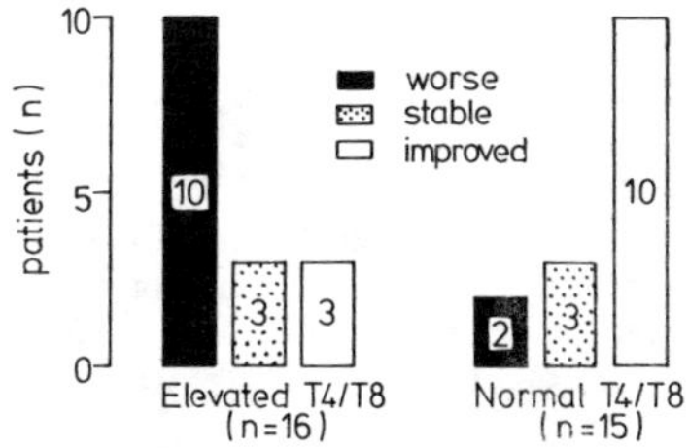

FIGURE 1. A comparison of the course of sarcoidosis in 16 patients with initially elevated T4/T8 ratios and in 15 patients with initially normal T4/T8 ratios in BAL fluid.

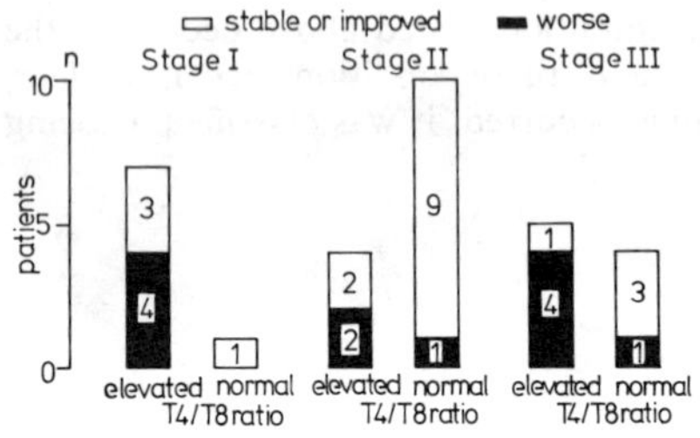

FIGURE 2. A comparison of the course of sarcoidosis in patients with initially elevated or normal BAL T4/T8 ratios in the different chest roentgenograph stages.

Predictive Value of BAL T Cell Subset Ratios

Information for assessing the value of T4/T8 ratios for predicting the course of sarcoidosis is shown in the left side of TABLE 2. A normal ratio is highly predictive for nondeterioration; 87% of the patients with normal ratios ultimately improved or remained stable. A high sensitivity value was calculated taking only T4/T8 ratios into account (83% of the patients whose conditions ultimately deteriorated had elevated ratios); however, the specificity value that resulted was low (68%), and the false-positive value (the percentage of patients whose conditions did not deteriorate even though they had elevated ratios) was relatively high (38%).

TABLE 2. The Value of Considering T Cell Subset Ratios and Activated T Cell Levels When Predicting the Course of Sarcoidosis

	Patients with Elevated and Normal T4/T8 Ratios		Patients with Elevated and Normal Activated T cell Levels[a]	
	Elevated ($N = 16$)	Normal ($N = 15$)	Elevated ($N = 11$)	Normal ($N = 19$)
Number of patients whose conditions deteriorated	10	2	9	3
Number of patients whose conditions improved or remained stable	6	13	2	16
	Evaluations of Predictions for Deterioration Based on the Single Criterion[b] (%)		Evaluations of Predictions for Deterioration Based on the Two Criteria[c] (%)	
Sensitivity	83		75	
Specificity	68		89	
False positive	38		18	
False negative	13		16	

[a] The former had elevated T4/T8 ratios; the latter had either elevated or normal T4/T8 ratios. Activated T cell levels were considered elevated if >25% of the lymphocytes in the lavage fluid were Ia antigen positive or if >9000 lymphocytes/ml of lavage fluid were Ia antigen positive.

[b] $p < .01$.

[c] $p < .001$.

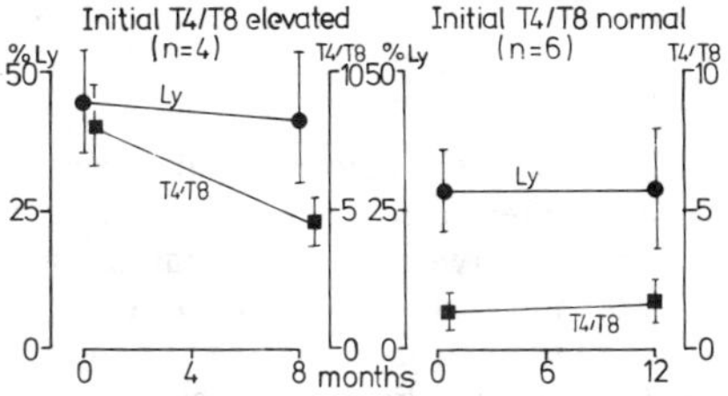

FIGURE 3. Changes in T4/T8 ratios and lymphocyte percentages in untreated sarcoidosis.

The specificity and false-positive values clearly improved when Ia antigen-positive, activated T cell levels were considered in the evaluation of alveolitis (TABLE 2, right side). The specificity value was 89%, and the false-positive value was reduced to 18%.

Changes in BAL Lymphocyte Percentages and T4/T8 Ratios during the Course of Sarcoidosis

FIGURE 3 shows that in stable cases of sarcoidosis in which therapy is withheld and initial T4/T8 ratios are elevated, the T4/T8 ratios decrease after 8 months whereas the lymphocyte percentages remain unchanged. In stable sarcoidosis with initially normal T4/T8 ratios, the T4/T8 ratios and lymphocyte percentages remain unchanged after 12 months. There is a large variation of the mean values of the lymphocyte percentages because the patient population did not behave uniformly; that is, some patients had increases in their percentages over the course of the study, and others had decreases. The patients reacted more uniformly with respect to their T4/T8 ratios.

FIGURE 4 shows the effect of steroids, as evaluated by serial lavages. BAL T4/T8 ratios and lymphocyte percentages continuously decreased during therapy.

Other Tests of Activity

Single lung function tests, SACE level determinations, gallium indices, and BAL fluid lymphocyte counts without subtyping were not of the same predictive value for the course of pulmonary sarcoidosis as BAL fluid T cell counts with subtyping (data not shown).

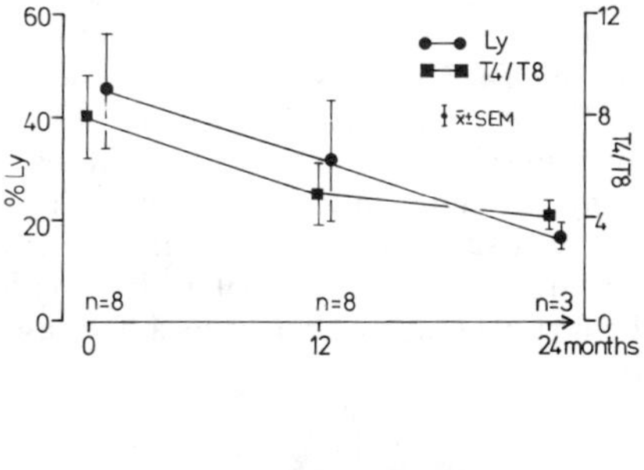

FIGURE 4. The effect of steroid therapy on T4/T8 ratios and lymphocyte percentages in sarcoidosis.

DISCUSSION

In sarcoidosis, conventional clinical, roentgenographic, and lung function parameters are often unreliable in predicting a patient's outcome[1,11-13] because they cannot distinguish between active inflammation and irreversible fibrosis.[1] The data of this study demonstrate that the proportions of lymphocyte subsets, which reflect the activity of the inflammatory processes in the lungs of sarcoidosis patients, are predictive of the subsequent clinical course of the disease. This study confirms our previous observations[14] and extends them by having used larger numbers of patients and a longer follow-up period.

Deterioration revealed by chest roentgenograms occurred only in patients with initially elevated T4/T8 ratios in BAL fluid. Even in stage I disease, where usually only 10-20% of patients will progress to stage II or III,[15] an elevated T4/T8 ratio was followed by deterioration in four out of seven patients.

A normal T4/T8 ratio was found to be highly predictive for nondeterioration. The specificity of an elevated T4/T8 ratio to predict deterioration correctly improved considerably when the levels of Ia antigen-positive T cells in BAL fluid were taken into account. Ia antigens are not expressed on normal T cells unless they are activated.[16] When we used both T4/T8 ratios and the levels of activated T cells in BAL fluid as

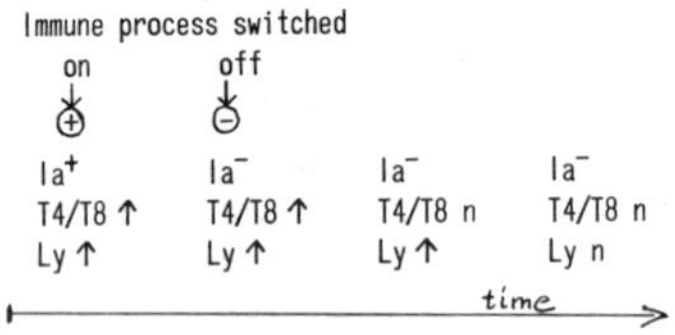

FIGURE 5. A hypothesis of the evolution of lymphocyte subpopulations in the alveolitis of sarcoidosis. See the text for more details.

criteria for predicting the outcome of sarcoidosis, our results were as good as those of Keogh *et al.*[13] who showed that the conditions of certain patients were likely to deteriorate: patients that have high proportions of BAL cells made up of T cells (> 28%) and positive gallium scans. Compared to T cell subset determinations, gallium scans have the disadvantage of a relatively high radiation burden to the patient[17] and of requiring 48 hr for completion.

In addition to these studies, Baughman *et al.*[18] reported that knowing the absolute gallium uptake as well as the absolute number of T4-positive cells in fluid was useful when predicting the response to therapy in sarcoidosis. This indicates that these parameters assess an alveolitis which is still active and thus susceptible to therapy.

Prednisone is known to induce a fall in the number of T4-positive cells and in the proportion of lymphocytes made up of T4-positive cells.[19] This was also observed in our study, where repeated lavages revealed a fall in the percentage of lymphocytes and the T4/T8 ratios after steroids were applied.

Finally, we would like to offer a hypothesis of the evolution of lymphocyte subpoulations in the alveolitis of sarcoidosis (FIG. 5). Once the immune process is switched on by an unknown triggering agent, T cells are activated and express Ia antigens on their cell surfaces, and T4-positive cells rapidly and uncontrollably proliferate. Once the immune process is switched off, either spontaneously or as a result of therapy, the first consequence might be a decrease in the number of Ia antigen-positive T cells, a decrease which could even occur before the gradual normalization of T4-positive cell levels (the proportion of BAL cells made up of lymphocytes ultimately becomes normalized as well). This hypothesis has yet to be tested; studies in which serial lavages are performed and in which larger numbers of patients and longer observation periods are used will probably be required.

In conclusion, this study demonstrated the usefulness of knowing lymphocyte subset proportions when predicting the outcome of pulmonary sarcoidosis.

SUMMARY

To study the value of knowing the proportions of bronchoalveolar T cell subsets when predicting the course of pulmonary sarcoidosis, we subjected 31 patients to clinical, physiologic, and radiographic evaluations, with controls, for at least 12 months. Initially, when all patients were untreated, BAL's were performed, and BAL lymphocyte subsets were marked by the following monoclonal antibodies: OKT3 (expressed by all T cells), OKT4 (to mark helper-inducer T cells), OKT8 (to mark suppressor-cytotoxic T cells), and OKIa (to mark Ia antigen-positive, activated T cells). A normal T4/T8 ratio was highly predictive of a favorable course: the conditions of 13 out of 15 patients with normal ratios remained stable or improved, and only 2 of these 15 patients had to be treated because of persistent symptoms. On the other hand, the conditions of 10 out of 16 patients with elevated T4/T8 ratios deteriorated during the follow-up period. The specificity of T cell subsets for predicting deterioration was improved by considering both the T4/T8 ratio and the number of Ia antigen-positive, activated T cells present. Deterioration occurred in 9 out of 11 patients with elevated T4/T8 ratios and elevated levels of activated T cells. These results suggest that the subtyping of BAL lymphocytes may be useful in determining prognosis in pulmonary sarcoidosis

REFERENCES

1. Crystal, R. G., W. C. Roberts, G. W. Hunninghake, J. E. Gadek, J. D. Fulmer & B. R. Line. 1981. Ann. Intern. Med. **94:** 73-94.
2. Rossman, M. D., J. H. Dauber, M. E. Cardillo & R. P. Daniele. 1982. Am. Rev. Respir. Dis. **125:** 366-369.
3. Hunninghake, G. W. & R. G. Crystal. 1981. N. Engl. J. Med. **305:** 429-434.
4. Costabel, U., K. J. Bross, H. Matthys & G. W. Löhr. 1982. Bull. Eur. Physiopathol. Respir. **18:** 142P.
5. Ginns, L. C., P. D. Goldenheim, R. C. Burton, R. B. Colvin, L. G. Miller, G. Goldstein, C. Hurwitz & H. Kazemi. 1982. Clin. Immunol. Immunopathol. **25:** 11-20.
6. Costabel, U., K. J. Bross & H. Matthys. 1983. Klin. Wochenschr. **61:** 349-356.
7. Costabel, U., K. J. Bross, K. H. Rühle, G. W. Löhr & H. Matthys. 1985. Am. Rev. Respir. Dis. **131:** 337-342.
8. Bross, K. J., G. A. Pangalis, C. G. Staatz & K. G. Blume. 1978. Transplantation **25:** 331-334.
9. Costabel, U., K. J. Bross & H. Matthys. 1985. Bull. Eur. Physiopathol. Respir. **21:** 381-387.

10. LIEBERMAN, J. 1975. Am. J. Med. **59:** 365-372.
11. WINTERBAUER, R. H. & J. F. HUTCHINSON. 1980. Chest **78:** 640-647.
12. DEREMEE, R. A. 1983. Chest **83:** 128-133.
13. KEOGH, B. A., G. W. HUNNINGHAKE, B. R. LINE & R. G. CRYSTAL. 1983. Am. Rev. Respir. Dis. **126:** 256-265.
14. COSTABEL, U., K. J. BROSS, D. BURGER, E. CARLGREN, J. GUZMAN & H. MATTHYS. 1983. Am. Rev. Respir. Dis. **127**(4,2): 62.
15. HILLERDAL, G., E. NÖU, K. OSTERMAN & B. SCHMEKEL. 1984. Am. Rev. Resir. Dis. **130:** 29-32.
16. WINCHESTER, R. J. & H. G. KUNKEL. 1979. Adv. Immunol. **28:** 221-229.
17. MIRD: Dose estimate report No. 2. 1973. J. Nucl. Med. **14:** 755-756.
18. BAUGHMAN, R. P., M. FERNANDEZ, C. H. BOSKEN, J. MANTIL & P. HURTUBISE. 1984. Am. Rev. Respir. Dis. **129:** 676-681.
19. SLADE, J. D. & B. HEPBURN. 1983. J. Lab. Clin. Med. **101:** 479-487.

Radionuclides in Detecting Active Granuloma Formation

Gallium-67 Scintigraphy and Histopathology with Autoradiographic Findings

A. VAN MAARSSEVEEN,[a] C. ALBERTS,[b]
J. VAN DER SCHOOT,[c] E. VAN ROYEN,[c] C. HENS,[a]
H. MULLINK,[a] AND J. DE GROOT[a]

[a] *Department of Pathology*
Free University Hospital
1007 MB Amsterdam, the Netherlands

[b] *Department of Pulmonology*
and
[c] *Department of Nuclear Medicine*
Academic Medical Center
1105 AZ Amsterdam, the Netherlands

INTRODUCTION

Pulmonary sarcoidosis is characterized by epithelioid cell granulomas in the alveolar interstitium.[1] These granulomas are composed of macrophages, epithelioid cells, multinucleated giant cells, and lymphocytes and of fibroblasts in the periphery. Macrophages are considered to be the basic cellular element.[2] Current concepts of the pathogenesis of pulmonary sarcoidosis suggest that granuloma formation is preceded by an alveolitis,[3] and activated thymus-derived (T) lymphocytes within the alveolar structures may have a role in establishing and maintaining granuloma formation.

The course of the disease is unpredictable. Most patients have a self-limited form, but in about 20% of the patients there is progression to interstitial fibrosis. Patients with persistent or progressive pulmonary involvement need special attention and become candidates for treatment with corticosteroids. The problem in managing pulmonary sarcoidosis is the identification of the activity of the disease.

Previous reports have focused attention on ^{67}Ga scintigraphy in staging the disease activity.[4-8] Gallium-67 scintigraphy has been found a valuable supplement to chest radiography.

The ^{67}Ga accumulation mechanism, however, remains poorly understood. Studies in neoplastic[9,10] and inflammatory disease[11] have been performed. Current ideas suggest that radionuclide activity is related to either transferrin-lactoferrin-binding cells[12,13] or lysosomal binding in tumor and inflammatory cells, such as macrophages, granulocytes, or lymphocytes.[14,15] In sarcoidosis, ^{67}Ga may accumulate in tissue structures[16] in association with the activated inflammatory and granulomatous reaction. It seems reasonable that positive ^{67}Ga scintigraphy results may be due to ^{67}Ga uptake by active granulomas.[4,8] There are data, however, that suggest a direct role for lymphocytes with respect to ^{67}Ga accumulation.[3,17,18]

The present study investigates granuloma formation in the lungs of guinea pigs. The granulomatous response was activated by administration of Freund's complete adjuvant (FCA). Autoradiography was performed in an attempt to elucidate the mechanism of ^{67}Ga accumulation in pulmonary sarcoidosis.

MATERIALS AND METHODS

Each guinea pig was sensitized with FCA by one 0.1-ml FCA injection into each of its footpads and two 0.3-ml FCA injections into its nuchal muscles. Pulmonary granulomatosis was activated by an intravenous booster injection of 0.25 ml of FCA at various times after sensitization.

Histopathology and autoradiography with [^{3}H]thymidine and ^{67}Ga citrate were performed. To prevent interference in the autoradiographic studies, these two radionuclides were used separately in two series of animals.

Guinea pigs that were sensitized or boosted with FCA were used in DNA synthesis studies. The animals were given two intravenous injections of 100 μCi of [^{3}H]thymidine, the second injection 30 min after the first, and were killed 30 min after the second injection. Lungs were removed, fixed in phosphate-buffered formalin, and embedded in paraffin. Tissue sections 5-μm thick were covered with an Ilford G-5 photographic emulsion which was diluted with an equal amount of distilled water. After 3 weeks of exposure at 4° C, the emulsion was developed in Kodak D-19, fixed in Kodak Unifix, and washed and stained with eosin hematoxylin.

FCA-sensitized guinea pigs were subjected to whole-body ^{67}Ga scintigraphy. Gallium-67 scintigraphy was performed 48 hr after an intravenous injection of 0.5 mCi of ^{67}Ga citrate. Images from anterior and posterior aspects were obtained by using a large-field gamma camera. Immediately after scintigraphy the animals were killed by ether anesthesia. Lungs were removed for activity counting in a gamma counter. The activity measured was expressed as counts/g of tissue.

Cell suspensions from the lung tissue were obtained by cutting in fresh Hanks' balanced salt solution (HBSS). Gallium-67 activity in cells, lung fragments, and washing fluid was determined after three washings with HBSS. Sedimentation centrifugation preparations were made from the cells. Autoradiography was performed by dipping these slides into Kodak NTB-3 nuclear track emulsion diluted with distilled water (1:7). After drying, the slides were exposed for 3 to 5 days at 4° C, developed in Kodak D-19, fixed in Kodak Unifix, and washed thoroughly before they were stained with eosin hematoxylin.

RESULTS

In untreated guinea pigs a normal pulmonary structure without any granulomatous reaction was shown. Sensitization with FCA revealed a gradual increase of pulmonary granulomatous tissue (TABLE 1). The intravenous injection of FCA enhanced granuloma formation in the lung. Autoradiographs of pulmonary tissue after the intravenous injection of [^{3}H]thymidine revealed substantial [^{3}H]thymidine incorporation in cells, an indication of DNA synthesis. No remarkable incorporation of [^{3}H]thymidine could be demonstrated in the pulmonary tissues of nonsensitized guinea pigs. Less than 5 days after an intravenous injection of FCA, however, synthesis was induced in pulmonary lymphocytes, macrophages, and some epithelioid cells in nonsensitized animals, as well as in animals sensitized 1 month previously (TABLE 2). Prolongation of the sensitization time did not result in an increase in the number of cells which synthesized DNA. Three months after sensitization, an intravenous booster with FCA was given 5 days before the experiment, and a dramatic increase in the number of macrophages and epithelioid cells which synthesized DNA was observed, as compared to animals that were not given a booster.

The results of ^{67}Ga scintigraphy in FCA-sensitized guinea pigs, whether or not they received intravenous boosters of FCA, are shown in TABLE 3. Gallium-67 scin-

TABLE 1. Pulmonary Granulomatosis in Guinea Pigs Evoked by FCA Sensitization

		Histopathological Quantification of Pulmonary Tissue			
Months after FCA Sensitization	FCA Booster[a]	Alveolitis	Mononuclear Cell Proliferation	Granuloma Formation	Necrosis
0	No	−	−	−	−
	Yes		+	+	−
3	No	+	±	±	−
	Yes		++	++	±
12	No	+	±	+	−
	Yes		+±	++	±
17	No	+	+	+±	−

[a] Note how the intravenous booster injection of FCA enhanced granuloma formation.

tigraphy was strongly positive for animals that had received boosters. Animals that had not received boosters had negative or slightly positive ^{67}Ga scans which seemed to be independent of the prolongation of the sensitization time. Cell suspensions prepared from lungs of guinea pigs that had received boosters contained more ^{67}Ga activity per cell than did those prepared from the lungs of animals that had not received boosters. Gallium-67 radioactivity was not only associated with cells, but could be detected, in small amounts, in the washing fluid.

Autoradiography of the cell sedimentation centrifugation preparations showed that ^{67}Ga activity was principally related to macrophages (FIG. 1). The ^{67}Ga experiments showed that ^{67}Ga bound almost exclusively to macrophages and that binding was greatly enhanced by the injection of boosters (TABLE 4).

DISCUSSION

As already mentioned, the localization of ^{67}Ga in different pathologic processes seems to vary.[9-11,14,15] Clinical experience suggests that ^{67}Ga uptake varies and that it

TABLE 2. *In Situ* Localization of DNA-synthesizing Mononuclear Cells in the Lungs of FCA-sensitized Guinea Pigs

Months after FCA Sensitization	FCA Booster[a]	[^{3}H]Thymidine Incorporation[b] (%) Lymphocytes	Macrophages	Epithelioid Cells
0	No[c]	0	0	0
	Yes	3.2 ± 0.1	4.8 ± 0.3	0.5 ± 0.7
1	Yes	3.9 ± 1.6	4.1 ± 0.3	2.1 ± 0.8
3	No	3.1 ± 0.8	3.4 ± 0.6	0
	Yes	3.8 ± 1.5	10.0 ± 0.5	2.6 ± 1.7
12	No	2.8 ± 0.8	3.8 ± 0.7	0

[a] The intravenous FCA booster injections were given 5 days before the experiments.

[b] [^{3}H]Thymidine incorporation is expressed as the percentage of mononuclear cells that were labeled.

[c] No granulomatous tissue formed, and no [^{3}H]thymidine incorporation was evident.

depends on the activity of the process.[4-8] In studies designed to elucidate why ^{67}Ga accumulation was found mostly in patients with an active granulomatous process, we used intravenous injections of FCA for 5 days in sensitized guinea pigs and thus provided a model of pulmonary granulomatosis.[19-21] In this way an accelerated gran-

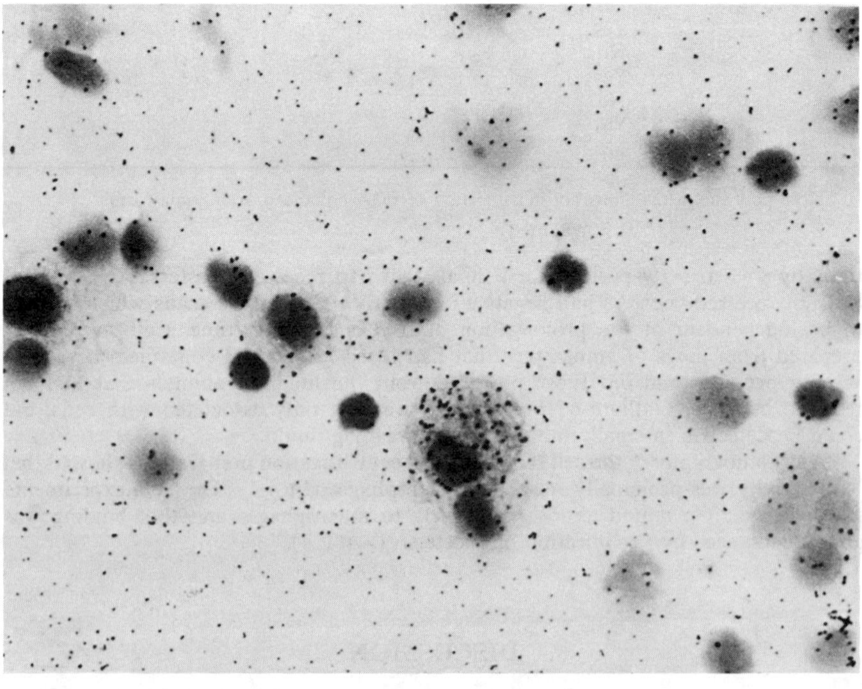

FIGURE 1. Autoradiograph of a cell suspension preparation showing the localization of ^{67}Ga in a pulmonary macrophage of an FCA-sensitized guinea pig.

TABLE 3. Gallium-67 Localization in Different Portions of Pulmonary Tissue Suspensions of FCA-sensitized Guinea Pigs

Months after FCA Sensitization	FCA Booster	Lung Tissue (g)	Radioactivity[a] (cpm $\times$ 10^3/g)	Activity[b] (%) Free	Cell Associated	Fragment Associated	cpm/ 10^4 Leukocytes
3	No	4.06	30.2	18	10	72	4
	No	3.38	26.8	12	18	69	4
	Yes	8.46	293	30	23	47	48
12	No	4.54	44.5	10	24	65	6
	No	6.06	21.0	8	24	68	2
	Yes	7.50	301	27	24	48	25

[a] The radioactivities of lung tissue samples were determined in counts per minute (cpm) $\times$ 10^3 and related to the weights of the samples.

[b] The activity distribution among the extracellular (free), intracellular (cell associated), and undisrupted fragment portions of each suspension is expressed in percentages.

ulomatous response was evoked as compared to that in animals that had not previously received boosters. Local DNA synthesis in such granulomatous tissue, a process of cell proliferation, can be measured by determining the extent of [^{3}H]thymidine incorporation. The very active lesions, which were present in our animals that had received boosters, contain many proliferating young mononuclear phagocytes (± 10% of the macrophage population). In this active granulomatosis, ^{67}Ga is taken up in the macrophages as shown by autoradiography.

Although ^{67}Ga uptake is related to the macrophages, this study gives no information about the ultimate sites of deposition. The processes which facilitate the transfer of protein-bound ^{67}Ga in the plasma to intra- or intercellular binding sites are not yet clearly understood.[12,14] Gallium-67-labeled glycoproteins may be bound to cells in other ways.

TABLE 4. Gallium-67 Accumulation in Cells Recovered in Suspensions from the Lungs of FCA-sensitized Guinea Pigs

Months after FCA Sensitization	FCA Booster[a]	cpm/ 10^4 Leukocytes	Cells with ^{67}Ga Activity[b] (%)		
			Lymphocytes	Macrophages	Neutrophils
3	No	4	0	2.5	0
	No	4	0	3.1	0
	Yes	48	0.5	6.3	0
	Yes	47	0	8.4	0
	Yes	42	1.4	12.2	0
12	No	6	0.5	1.8	0
	No	2	0	0.9	0
	Yes	25	0	9.1	0
	Yes	11	0	4.8	0
	Yes	13	ND	ND	ND
17	No	11	0	0	0
	No	3	0	0	0

[a] The intravenous FCA booster injections were given 5 days before the experiments.
[b] The percentage of cells with ^{67}Ga activity could be determined autoradiographically.

The present results are consistent with our experience with ^{67}Ga scintigraphy in patients with pulmonary sarcoidosis.[4,5] The data support, again, the usefulness of ^{67}Ga scintigraphy for the localization and grading of active granulomatous lesions. Gallium-67 scintigraphy results in pulmonary sarcoidosis may be comparable to those obtained in the abovementioned animal model of pulmonary granulomatosis. It seems reasonable, in view of the well-documented interaction between lymphocytes and macrophages,[3,17] that the activated T lymphocytes may mediate the ^{67}Ga uptake of macrophages in sarcoidosis.

We have recently started an additional study. Five patients suffering from pulmonary involvement and peripheral lymphadenopathy underwent lymph node biopsy to establish the diagnosis of sarcoidosis. In order to evaluate the ^{67}Ga accumulation in these patients, scintigraphy was performed 48 hr after intravenous injection of 2 mCi gallium-67 citrate. More or less ^{67}Ga uptake by the lymph nodes could be demonstrated in all patients. Thereafter lymph node biopsies were done. Cell suspensions of the lymph nodes showed only low ^{67}Ga activities, ones comparable to those found in sensitized guinea pigs that had not received boosters. Autoradiography of these lymph nodes was not conclusive.

In conclusion, pulmonary granulomatosis induced in guinea pigs by sensitization with FCA resulted in little or no uptake of ^{67}Ga. The ^{67}Ga scans were similar to the negative ^{67}Ga lung scans seen in inactive pulmonary sarcoidosis. Activation of the granulomatosis by a booster injection of FCA resulted in strongly positive ^{67}Ga lung scans, scans similar to those seen in active pulmonary sarcoidosis.

SUMMARY

Granuloma formation studies were performed on lungs of guinea pigs sensitized with FCA over 2 to 17 months. Prolonged time of sensitization revealed more granulomatous pulmonary tissue. An intravenous booster of FCA in the animals that had been sensitized for 3 months yielded enhanced granuloma formation within 5 days. The histopathology of these lungs was comparable with that seen in lungs of animals after 17 months of sensitization without booster. Enhanced local proliferation of macrophages, measured by [^{3}H]thymidine incorporation and autoradiography, was seen in the lungs of the animals that had received boosters. Moreover, ^{67}Ga scintigraphy was strongly positive in these animals. Scintigraphy of cell suspensions of pulmonary tissue from these animals showed that ^{67}Ga was predominantly taken up (quantitatively as well as qualitatively) by the alveolar macrophages.

Cell suspensions of sarcoidosis patients, prepared in the same way, showed only a low level of ^{67}Ga uptake, one comparable to that of the pulmonary cell suspensions of the sensitized animals that had not received boosters.

It is suggested that a negative scintigraphy in patients with chronic pulmonary granulomatous disorders could be (partly) explained by the absence of activated macrophages.

ACKNOWLEDGMENTS

We wish to thank Mrs. Kolk of the Antoni van Leeuwenhoek Hospital for the autoradiographic preparations, Mrs. Sokole-Busemann for correcting the English text, and Mr. Dolman for typing the manuscript.

REFERENCES

1. MITCHELL, D. N. & J. J. SCADDING. 1974. Sarcoidosis. Am. Rev. Respir. Dis. **110:** 774-802.
2. SPECTOR, W. G. 1976. Epithelioid cells, giant cells, and sarcoidosis. Ann. N.Y. Acad. Sci. **278:** 3-5.
3. CRYSTAL, R. G., G. W. HUNNINGHAKE, J. E. GADEK, B. A. KEOGH, S. I. RENNARD & P. B. BITTERMAN. 1981. State of the art: The pathogenesis of sarcoidosis. *In* Ninth International Conference on Sarcoidosis and Other Granulomatous Disorders. J. Chrétien, J. Marsac & J. C. Saltiel, Eds.: 13-35. Pergamon Press. Paris.

4. ALBERTS, C., J. B. VAN DER SCHOOT & A. S. GROEN. 1981. ^{67}Ga scintigraphy as an index of disease activity in pulmonary sarcoidosis. Eur. J. Nucl. Med. **6:** 205-212.
5. ALBERTS, C., J. B. VAN DER SCHOOT, J. J. DAATSELAAR, M. C. P. BRAAT & C. M. ROOS. 1983. ^{67}Ga scintigraphy, serum lysozyme, and angiotensin-converting enzyme in pulmonary sarcoidosis. Eur. J. Respir. Dis. **64:** 38-46.
6. BEAUMONT, D., J. Y. HERRY, M. SAPENE, P. BOURGET, P. LARZUI & B. DE LABARTHE. 1982. Gallium-67 in the evaluation of sarcoidosis: Correlations with serum angiotensin-converting enzyme and bronchoalveolar lavage. Thorax **37:** 11-18.
7. LINE, B. R., J. D. FULMER, H. Y. REYNOLDS, W. C. ROBERTS, A. E. JONES, E. K. HARRIS & R. G. CRYSTAL. 1978. Gallium-67 citrate scanning in the staging of idiopathic pulmonary fibrosis: Correlation with physiologic and morphologic features and bronchoalveolar lavage. Am. Rev. Respir. Dis. **118:** 355-365.
8. KLECH, H., H. KOHN, F. KUMMER & A. MOSTBECK. 1982. Assessment of activity in sarcoidosis: Sensitivity and specificity of ^{67}Ga scintigraphy, serum ACE levels, chest roentgenography, and blood lymphocyte subpopulations. Chest **82:** 732-738.
9. HAYES, R. L., B. NELSON, D. C. SWARTZENDRUBER, J. E. CARLTON & B. L. BYRD. 1970. Gallium-67 localization in rat and mouse tumours. Science **167:** 289-290.
10. LANGHAMMER, H., G. GLAUBIT, S. F. GREBE, J. F. HAMPE, U. HAUBOLD, J. HÖR, A. KAUL, P. KOEPPE, J. KOPENHAGE, H. D. ROEDLER & J. B. VAN DER SCHOOT. 1972. ^{67}Ga for tumour scanning. J. Nucl. Med. **13:** 25-30.
11. GELRUD, L. G., J. C. ARSENEAU, M. S. MILDER, R. J. KRAMER, S. J. SWANN, G. P. CANELLOS & G. S. JOHNSTON. 1974. The kinetics of ^{67}Ga incorporation into inflammatory lesions: Experimental and clinical studies. J. Lab. Clin. Med. **83:** 489-495.
12. HOFFER, P. B. 1978. Mechanisms of localization. *In* Gallium-67 Imaging. P. B. Hoffer, C. Bekerman & R. E. Henkin, Eds.: 4-8. Wiley. New York, NY.
13. SEPHTON, R. G. & A. W. HARRIS. 1981. Studies on the uptake of ^{67}Ga and ^{59}Fe and the binding of transferrin by cultured mouse tumour cells. Int. J. Nucl. Med. Biol. **8:** 333-339.
14. HAYES, R. L., B. NELSON, D. E. SWARTZENDRUBER, J. E. CARLTON & B. L. BYRD. 1971. Studies of intracellular deposition of ^{67}Ga. J. Nucl. Med. **12:** 364.
15. HAMMERSLEY, P. A. G. & D. M. TAYLOR. 1974. The role of lysosomal enzyme activity in the localization of ^{67}Ga citrate. Eur. J. Nucl. Med. **4:** 261-270.
16. LOPEZ-MAJANO, V. & P. SANSI. 1982. Gallium-67 uptake in cutaneous sarcoidosis. Eur. J. Nucl. Med. **7:** 95-96.
17. LINE, B. R., G. W. HUNNINGHAKE, B. A. KEOGH, A. E. JONES, G. S. JOHNSTON & R. G. CRYSTAL. 1981. Gallium-67 scanning to stage the alveolitis of sarcoidosis: Correlation with clinical studies, pulmonary function studies, and bronchoalveolar lavage. Am. Rev. Respir. Dis. **123:** 440-446.
18. MERZ, T., L. MALMUD, K. MCKUSICK & H. N. WAGNER. 1974. The mechanisms of ^{67}Ga association with lymphocytes. Cancer Res. **34:** 2495-2499.
19. MASIH, N., J. MAJESKA & T. YOSHIDA. 1979. Studies on experimental pulmonary granulomas. I. Detection of lymphokines in granulomatous lesions. Am. J. Pathol. **95:** 391-402.
20. BASSETT, F., P. SOLER, L. WYLIE & J. TURIAF. 1974. Pulmonary sarcoid-like granulomatosis provoked by injecting Freund's complete adjuvant intravenously in the rat. *In* Proceedings of the Sixth International Conference on Sarcoidosis. K. Iwai & Y. Hosoda, Eds.: 121-125. University Park Press. Tokyo.
21. LIEBERMAN, J., W. KANESHIRO, A. SASTRO, K. WEISSER & T. REA. 1980. Serum angiotensin-converting enzyme and lysozyme in rabbits with pulmonary granulomatosis induced by complete Freund's adjuvant and BCG. *In* Eighth International Conference on Sarcoidosis and Other Granulomatous Diseases. W. Jones Williams & B. H. Davies, Eds.: 111-117. Alpha Omega. Cardiff.

Prognostic Significance of Gallium Lung Scans in Sarcoidosis

ALBERT H. NIDEN,[a] FRED S. MISHKIN,[b]
FRANK SALEM,[c] ALVIN V. THOMAS, JR.,[a] AND
VIJAY KAMDAR[a]

[a]*Department of Medicine*
[b]*Department of Radiology*
and
[c]*Department of Pathology*
Charles R. Drew Medical School
University of California School of Medicine
Los Angeles, California

INTRODUCTION

Nonspecific adrenocorticosteroid therapy has been shown to ameliorate symptoms, induce remission, and improve the quality of life in patients with active pulmonary sarcoidosis.[1–8] The efficacy of such therapy to alter the ultimate course of the disease and prevent progressive pulmonary fibrosis, however, remains controversial.[1–27] Recent studies suggest that glucocorticoid therapy does not improve pulmonary function because similar changes, that is, spontaneous remissions and relapses, are noted in untreated patients with active pulmonary sarcoidosis.[15,17,20,21,23,26,27] A major problem with corticosteroid therapy is frequent relapses of disease activity as therapy is tapered. Suppression without elimination of disease activity may explain the failure of long-term corticosteroid therapy to prevent physiologic deterioration. Regulation of therapy has traditionally been by symptomatic, radiographic, and, to a lesser degree, physiologic responses. These parameters cannot distinguish pulmonary dysfunction resulting from an inflammatory reaction in the lung from those secondary to pulmonary fibrosis.[26,28–30] The former is potentially reversible whereas the latter is not. Use of a sensitive marker of pathologic disease activity to monitor response to therapy might permit better regulation of therapy and thus prevent progressive physiologic deterioration.

In recent years, gallium lung scans have been utilized to initially evaluate patients with sarcoidosis.[30–49] Gallium lung uptake has been correlated with the inflammatory cellular infiltrate associated with chronic diffuse pulmonary infiltrative processes.[30,32,49–51] In sarcoidosis, a disease associated with pulmonary infiltration of macrophages and activated T cell lymphocytes,[45,52–56] the degree of gallium uptake correlates with the numbers of these cells retrieved by bronchoalveolar lavage[29,40,41,44–46,49,53,55] and with histologic evidence for active disease.[32,49,51] Such studies have suggested that gallium accumulation is a sensitive indicator of pathologic activity and is helpful in clinical staging of the disease. There are no long-term studies, however, evaluating the usefulness of gallium imaging for predicting the course of the disease and for regulating therapy to prevent physiologic deterioration.

The present study was designed to test the following hypothesis: Failure of current therapy for sarcoidosis to alter the course of the disease results from therapy being regulated to control the clinical manifestations, that is, symptoms, chest roentgenogram, and pulmonary physiologic responses, rather than the pathologic activity of the disease. Because the gallium scan should more accurately reflect pathologic disease activity, physiologic deterioration might be prevented if therapy was adjusted to obtain and maintain a normal gallium scan.

MATERIALS AND METHODS

The conditions of patients with pulmonary sarcoidosis were followed for at least 1 year by the pulmonary division at a 300-bed, acute-care county hospital in this study. The diagnosis of sarcoidosis was established in all patients by the demonstration of noncaseating epithelioid granulomas in the appropriate clinical setting. The patient population consisted of 18 black women and 7 black men, 22 to 44 years of age with a mean age of 32.4 years. Duration of observation was 1 to 10 years with a mean follow-up period of 4 years and 4 months.

Conventional spirometry using a 13.5-l, water-sealed spirometer (Warren E. Collins, Baintree, MA) was performed on all patients. The best trial of duplicate or triplicate measurements was chosen. To evaluate long-term effects of therapy and the relationship of gallium scan activity to course of disease, the most recently measured pulmonary function studies were compared to the best recorded results obtained at or shortly after (within 3 months of) initiation of therapy.

Imaging from head to thigh was performed 72 hr after the intravenous injection of 4 mCi gallium-67 citrate following a 72-hr delay to minimize background activity. In the early years of the study, anterior and posterior scans were obtained with a dual-probe crystal rectilinear scanner, which was 20 cm in diameter and appropriately collimated; in more recent years a Siemens Pho-Con planar tomographic scanner was used to obtain 12 simultaneous images at 2-cm intervals. Gallium scans were interpreted by F.M., who had no knowledge of the clinical status of any of the patients. Gallium imaging of the lung was interpreted as being normal, 0, if accumulation in the lung did not exceed that of the soft tissues of the shoulder; 1+ if greater than that of thoracic soft tissue but less than that of the liver; 2+ if equal to hepatic uptake; and 3+ if greater than hepatic uptake.

Pathologic inflammatory tissue reactions were assessed by a pathologist, F.S., who did not know the clinical status of any of the patients. The degree of inflammation was arbitrarily graded without regard to the degree of fibrosis. A grade of 0 was applied to normal cases, cases where granulomas and inflammatory cells (lymphocytes, macrophages, and histiocytes) were absent. Pathologic activity was graded as being 1+ if granulomas were rare and/or a minimal number of inflammatory cells were present; 2+ if between two and four granulomas per low power field and/or a moderate number of inflammatory cells were present; 3+ if more than four granulomas per low power field and/or many inflammatory cells were present.

Therapy was necessary if at least one of the following was evident: disabling symptoms; a vital capacity less than 60% of that predicted for normal subjects; a decrease in vital capacity greater than 15% during the follow-up period; and/or a diffusing capacity less than 60% of that predicted for normal subjects and a vital capacity between 60% and 80% of that predicted for normal subjects. A gallium scan that revealed an abnormal uptake level in itself was not an indication to initiate therapy. Once therapy was started, however, gallium lung scan activity was used as an indicator to adjust or restart therapy if it had been discontinued. Therapy initially consisted of 40-60 mg prednisone daily. During the first 3 months patients were evaluated every 2 to 4 weeks by interviews; examinations; and spirometry, serum angiotensin-converting enzyme level, and diffusing capacity determinations. When clinically stable (usually after 3 to 4 months), patients were subjected to another gallium imaging. If a patient's gallium scan was normal, prednisone was slowly tapered over the next 6 to 8 months, and reevaluations were conducted each month until a maintenance dose of therapy was obtained (usually 10 to 15 mg prednisone). Once started on therapy, patients were maintained on prednisone for a minimum of 2 years. During the first year, gallium scans were repeated twice. Prednisone therapy was adjusted to obtain and maintain, if possible, a normal scan. After the first year all patients had a minimum of at least one gallium scan, chest roentgenogram, and complete pulmonary function study per year. More frequent examinations were obtained as clinically indicated. Four patients failed to respond to the above regimen and were treated with azathioprine (two patients) and cyclophosphamide (two patients).[2]

Informed consent was obtained after the nature of the procedures was fully explained.

RESULTS

Twenty-four of the 25 patients required therapy during the period of observation. Three patients died during the study period: a noncompliant patient died due to respiratory failure secondary to subacute active pulmonary sarcoidosis; another patient died due to cor pulmonale and inactive pulmonary sarcoidosis (confirmed at autopsy); and another patient died due to an unrelated cause (acute myocardial infarction). For the entire group of patients there was an average decline in vital capacity of 203 ml (range: +763 ml to −912 ml). The 24 patients who required treatment had a mean decrease of 212 ± 470 ml in vital capacity during or following therapy ($.01 < p < .025$ by paired t test analysis).

Relationship of Initial Gallium Scan with Response to Therapy

Three patients had an initial gallium scan grade of 0 while 10 patients had an initial grade of 1+ and 12 patients an initial grade of 2-3+ (FIG. 1). Of the 13 patients with a normal or 1+ accumulation of gallium in the lung when first seen, the average decline in vital capacity was −2.6% (range: +21% to −22%). The vital capacity improved more than 10% in three patients, was stable in five, and deteriorated more than 10% in five. The 12 patients who had initial gallium scan readings of 2+ or 3+ demonstrated a mean loss in vital capacity of −12.7% (range: +24% to −42%). The vital capacity improved in only one patient, was stable in four, and deteriorated in seven.

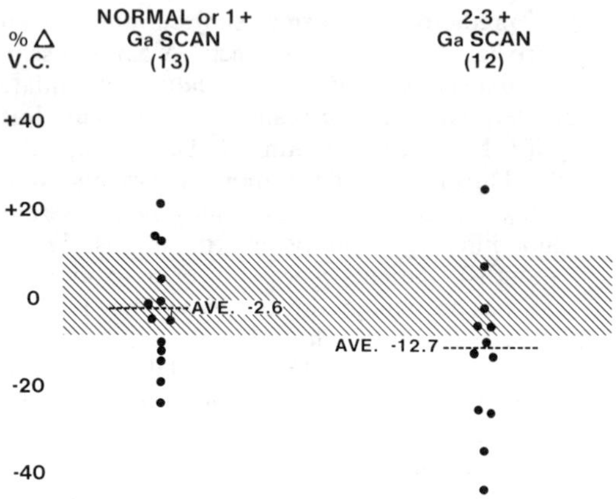

FIGURE 1. The relationship of initial gallium scan activity in the lung to the subsequent response to therapy as measured by vital capacity. In this and following figures, the shaded area represents a +10% to −10% change in vital capacity (stable vital capacity). Values above this area indicate improvement; values below indicate deterioration in physiologic function. Note that patients with normal and low-grade (1+) gallium scans had a better prognosis than those with more reactive (2-3+) scans.

Response of Gallium Scan and Lung Function to Therapy

With therapy, six patients' gallium lung scans returned to normal and remained normal throughout the study period (FIG. 2). In this group, there was a mean improvement in vital capacity of +16.5%. None in this group had a condition which deteriorated whereas three had conditions which improved and three others had conditions which remained stable. Of the conditions of 10 patients whose scans were never above 1+ while on therapy, only one was improved, two remained stable, and seven deteriorated, with an average decline in vital capacity of −11.5%. Eight patients had 2-3+ gallium scans some time during their course of therapy. The mean loss of vital capacity in this group was −15.3%. Five of these patients deteriorated physiologically, three of them remained stable, and none of them improved.

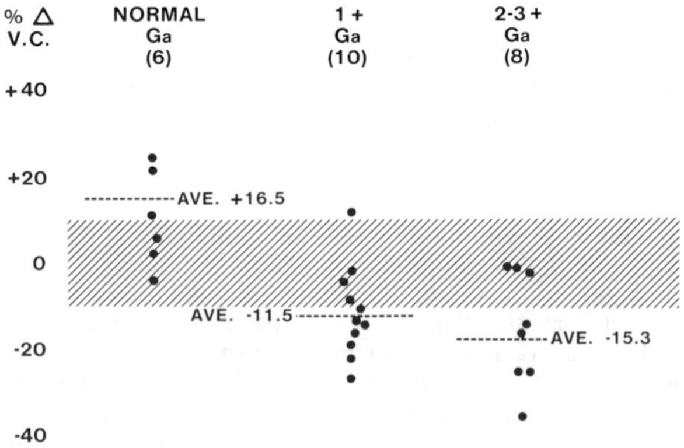

FIGURE 2. The relationship of gallium lung scan findings during therapy to the eventual changes in vital capacity. No physiologic deterioration occurred in patients whose gallium scans returned to and remained normal during follow-up whereas 7 out of 10 patients with low-grade activity (1+) had loss of function.

Thus 18 of the 24 patients treated had one or more relapses in gallium scan activity after scan activity had returned to normal in 13 patients or improved but failed to reach normal in 5 patients (FIG. 3). In this group of 18 patients there was a mean decline in vital capacity of −14% (range: +14% to −42%). Only 1 of these patients improved whereas 5 remained stable and 12 deteriorated physiologically.

Correlation between Gallium Scan and Tissue Pathologic Activities

Thirty-two patients with sarcoidosis had gallium imaging of the lung within 1 week of percutaneous needle biopsy (29 patients) or within 3 weeks of autopsy (3 patients). In 29 patients, a core of lung tissue measuring 2 to 3 mm in diameter and 1.5 to 2.5 cm in length was obtained using a Franklin-Vim-Silverman needle. There were no serious complications. Four of these cutting needle biopsies were repeat studies at a time patients were being treated.

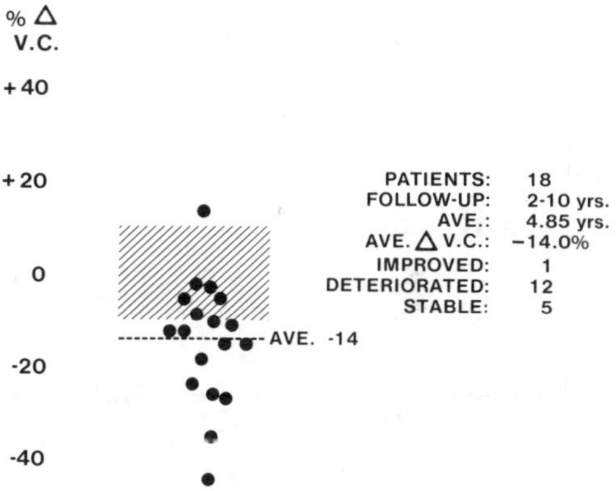

FIGURE 3. Vital capacity response of 18 patients whose gallium lung image abnormality relapsed after returning to normal or improved but failed to become normal with therapy. Twelve of the 18 patients had deterioration of physiologic function.

All 27 patients with an abnormal scan (1-3+) had evidence of pathologically active lung disease, and there was moderate agreement between gallium scan activity and pathologic activity (FIG. 4). In those patients with normal gallium scans (grade 0), however, there was disagreement with pathologic activity in three of the five patients: one patient with 1+ and two with 2+ inflammatory tissue reactions.

DISCUSSION

Effective therapy for pulmonary sarcoidosis remains elusive. Despite relatively aggressive, tightly controlled therapy, two-thirds of our study group failed to remain in remission but rather had one or more relapses of disease activity as determined by gallium lung scans. Moreover, 50% of our treated patients slowly deteriorated physiologically. The number of patients studied was too small to permit a control group.

Thus we cannot state with certainty whether or not we were able, with our protocol, to either reduce the number of patients who deteriorated physiologically or the extent of that deterioration. Most likely, we did not alter the course of their disease.

There are some conclusions that can be drawn from our study. First, although there was considerable individual variability, patients with normal or 1+ gallium lung scans when first seen had a better prognosis with regard to preservation of vital capacity than those patients with initial lung scans that were 2-3+. Second, return to and maintenance of a normal gallium scan with therapy is a good prognostic sign because none of these patients ultimately had a loss of physiologic function. When this group of patients was first seen, however, there was nothing to indicate they would respond well to therapy. Three of these six patients had initial gallium scans that were 2-3+. Third, continued or intermittent low-grade disease activity, as evidenced by 1+ gallium lung scans, in a patient on therapy was a poor prognostic sign (7 out of 10 patients deteriorated physiologically) even though disease inactivity was suggested by conventional measures. Fourth, an abnormal gallium scan is a good

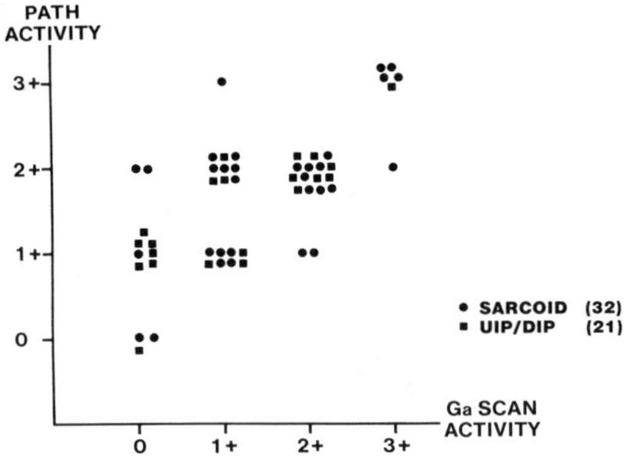

FIGURE 4. Correlation of independently graded pathologic activity and gallium scan activity in 32 patients with sarcoidosis (●) and 21 patients with idiopathic interstitial pneumonitis (■). All patients with abnormal accumulation of gallium had pathologically active lung disease. Three out of five sarcoidosis patients with normal scans had pathologically active disease.

indicator of pathologically active disease; all of our patients with an abnormal accumulation of gallium in the lung had pathologically active disease demonstrated on lung biopsy. Fifth, a normal gallium scan does not rule out pathologically active disease. This degree of pathologic activity, however, does not appear to be clinically significant because patients with normal scans showed no physiologic deterioration. Finally, despite its limitation, gallium imaging makes rough predictions of the course of disease possible.

Our patients may have relapsed following a reduction of prednisone therapy after complete pathologic remission of their disease. Alternatively, the patients who relapsed may represent those individuals who had continued low-grade pathologically active disease associated with a normal gallium scan. This latter possibility is consistent with our findings of biopsy-active disease with a normal gallium scan. The incidence of falsely negative scans is unknown because it was difficult to justify lung biopsy in patients who were clinically stable and had a normal gallium lung scan.

Treatment failure results from either the use of an ineffective drug (adrenocorticosteroid) or the inadequate use of an effective drug. Until we have a more sensitive marker of disease activity in patients with sarcoidosis, we cannot say whether prednisone is an ineffective drug for treating patients with sarcoidosis or that we are using an inadequate dose and/or too short a treatment period to induce and maintain pathologic remission.

In summary: 1) In general, the more reactive the gallium scan, the greater the loss of lung function. 2) No physiologic deterioration occurs if a normal scan is obtained and maintained. 3) Even low-grade gallium accumulation (1+) in the lung is likely to be associated with a loss in vital capacity. 4) The goal of therapy is the maintenance of a normal gallium scan. 5) An abnormal scan is a good indicator of pathologically active disease whereas a normal scan does not rule out disease activity. 6) Current therapy for sarcoidosis is inadequate to maintain suppression of disease activity and prevent functional deterioration. 7) Gallium imaging is a noninvasive test that adequately identifies patients with sarcoidosis who require more aggressive therapy but is limited in its ability to identify those patients who will lose function while on therapy or to guide therapy to prevent such loss of function. 8) Improvement or worsening of the gallium scan is an approximate predictor of the course of the disease. 9) In patients with sarcoidosis, a more sensitive marker of pathologic disease activity is needed to more effectively monitor response to and regulate therapy. Such a test, however, may not have a better predictive value.

REFERENCES

1. JAMES, D. G. & A. D. THOMPSON. 1959. The course of sarcoidosis and its modifications by treatment. Lancet **i:** 1057-1061.
2. SONES, M. & H. L. ISRAEL. 1960. The course and prognosis of sarcoidosis. Am. J. Med. **29:** 84-93.
3. SCADDING, J. G. 1961. Prognosis of intrathoracic sarcoidosis in England: A review of 136 cases after 5 years' observation. Br. Med. J. **2:** 1165-1172.
4. ELLIS, K. & G. RENTHAL. 1962. Pulmonary sarcoidosis: Roentgenographic observations on the course of the disease. 1962. Am. J. Roentgenol. **88:** 1070-1083.
5. RUGBERG-ROOS, I. 1962. The course and prognosis of sarcoidosis as observed in 296 cases. Acta Tuberc. Scand. **41:** 1-42.
6. JAMES, D. G., L. S. CARSTAIRS, J. TROWELL & O. P. SHARMA. 1967. Treatment of sarcoidosis: Report of a controlled therapeutic trial. Lancet **ii:** 526-528.
7. JOHNS, C. J., J. B. ZACHARY & W. C. BALL, JR. 1974. A ten-year study of corticosteroid treatment of pulmonary sarcoidosis. Johns Hopkins Med. J. **134:** 271-283.
8. JOHNS, C. J., M. I. MACGREGOR, J. B. ZACHARY & W. C. BALL. 1976. Extended experience in the long-term corticosteroid treatment of pulmonary sarcoidosis. Ann. N.Y. Acad. Sci. **278:** 722-731.
9. STONE, O. J., A. SCHWARTZ, J. A. FELLMAN & F. J. LOVELOCK. 1953. Pulmonary function in sarcoidosis: Results with cortisone therapy. Am. J. Med. **15:** 468-476.
10. SMELLIE, H., G. H. APTHORP & R. MARSHALL. 1961. The effect of corticosteroid treatment on pulmonary function in sarcoidosis. Thorax **16:** 87-90.
11. BOUSHY, S. F., R. S. KURTZMAN, N. D. MARTIN & G. M. LEWIS. 1965. The course of pulmonary function in sarcoidosis. Ann. Intern. Med. **62:** 939-955.
12. SHARMA, O. P., C. COLP & M. H. WILLIAMS. 1966. Course of pulmonary sarcoidosis with and without corticosteroid therapy as determined by pulmonary function studies. Am. J. Med. **41:** 541-551.
13. STONE, R. J. & A. SCHWARTZ. 1966. Long-term study of sarcoid and its modification by steroid therapy: Lung function and other factors in prognosis. Am. J. Med. **41:** 528-540.
14. EMIRGIL, C., B. J. SOBOL & M. H. WILLIAMS. 1969. Long-term study of pulmonary sarcoidosis: The effects of steroid therapy as evaluated by pulmonary function studies. J. Chronic Dis. **22:** 69-86.
15. YOUNG, R. L., L. E. HARKLEROAD, R. E. LORDON & J. G. WEG. 1970. Pulmonary sarcoidosis: A prospective evaluation of glucocorticoid therapy. Ann. Intern. Med. **73:** 207-212.

16. Block, A. J. & R. W. Light. 1973. Alternate day steroid therapy in diffuse pulmonary sarcoidosis. Chest **63:** 495-500.
17. Israel, H. L., D. W. Fouts & R. A. Beggs. 1973. A controlled trial of prednisone treatment of sarcoidosis. Am. Rev. Respir. Dis. **107:** 609-614.
18. Refvem, O. 1974. Long-term corticosteroid treatment of pulmonary sarcoidosis. *In* Proceedings of the Sixth International Conference on Sarcoidosis. K. Iwai & Y. Hosoda, Eds.: 533-538. University Park Press. Baltimore, MD.
19. Colp, C., S. S. Park & M. H. Williams, Jr. 1976. Pulmonary function follow-up of 120 patients with sarcoidosis. Ann. N.Y. Acad. Sci. **278:** 301-307.
20. DeRemee, R. A. 1977. The present status of treatment of pulmonary sarcoidosis: A house divided. Chest **71:** 388-393.
21. Selroos, O. & T. L. Sellergren. 1979. Corticosteroid therapy of pulmonary sarcoidosis: A prospective evaluation of alternate day and daily dosage in stage III disease. Scand. J. Respir. Dis. **60:** 215-221.
22. Bottger, D. 1980. Results of a controlled therapeutic trial of prednisolone in chronic non-fibrotic pulmonary sarcoidosis. *In* Eighth International Conference on Sarcoidosis and Other Granulomatous Diseases. W. Jones Williams & B. H. Davies, Eds.: 629-631. Alpha Omega. Cardiff.
23. Eule, H., I. Roth & W. Weide. 1980. Clinical and functional results of a controlled clinical trial of the value of prednisone therapy in sarcoidosis stage I and II. *In* Eighth International Conference on Sarcoidosis and Other Granulomatous Diseases. W. Jones Williams & B. H. Davies, Eds.: 624-628. Alpha Omega. Cardiff.
24. Middleton, W. G. & A. C. Douglas. 1980. Prolonged corticosteroid therapy in pulmonary sarcoidosis. *In* Eighth International Conference on Sarcoidosis and Other Granulomatous Diseases. W. Jones Williams & B. H. Davies, Eds.: 632-647. Alpha Omega. Cardiff.
25. Refvem, O. & O. K. Refvem. 1980. Long-term corticosteroid treatment of pulmonary sarcoidosis. *In* Eighth International Conference on Sarcoidosis and Other Granulomatous Diseases. W. Jones Williams and B. H. Davies, Eds.: 648-651. Alpha Omega. Cardiff.
26. Winterbauer, R. H. & J. F. Hutchinson. 1980. Clinical significance of pulmonary function tests on the management of sarcoidosis. Chest **78:** 640-647.
27. Harkleroad, L. E., R. L. Young, P. J. Savage, D. W. Jenkins & R. E. Lordon. 1982. Pulmonary sarcoidosis: Long-term follow-up of the effects of steroid therapy. Chest **82:** 84-87.
28. Keogh, B. A. & R. G. Crystal. 1980. Pulmonary function testing in interstitial pulmonary disease: What does it tell us? Chest **78:** 856-865.
29. Crystal, R. G., J. E. Gadek, V. J. Ferrans, J. D. Fulmer, B. R. Line & G. W. Hunninghake. 1981. Interstitial lung disease: Current concepts of pathogenesis, staging and therapy. Am. J. Med. **70:** 542-568.
30. Niden, A. H. & F. S. Mishkin. 1983. Role of gallium-67 citrate scanning in diffuse interstitial lung disease. Pract. Cardiol. **9:** 141-163.
31. McKusick, K. A., J. S. Soin, A. Ghiladi & H. N. Wagner. 1973. Gallium-67 accumulation in pulmonary sarcoidosis. J. Am. Med. Assoc. **223:** 688.
32. Niden, A. H., F. S. Mishkin & M. M. L. Khurana. 1976. ^{67}Gallium citrate lung scans in interstitial lung disease. Chest **69:** 266-288.
33. Siemsen, J. K., S. F. Grebe & A. D. Waxman. 1978. The use of gallium-67 in pulmonary disorders. Semin. Nucl. Med. **8:** 235-249.
34. Niden, A. H. & F. S. Mishkin. 1979. Clinical usefulness of gallium lung scans. Compr. Ther. **5:** 24-34.
35. Bekerman, C., P. B. Hoffer, J. D. Bitran & R. G. Gupta. 1980. Gallium-67 citrate imaging studies of the lung. Semin. Nucl. Med. **10:** 286-301.
36. Heshiki, A., S. Schatz, K. A. McKusick, D. W. Bowersox, J. S. Soin & H. N. Wagner. 1974. Gallium-67 citrate scanning in patients with pulmonary sarcoidosis. Am. J. Roentgenol. **122:** 744-749.
37. Siemsen, J. K., S. F. Grebe, E. N. Sargent & D. Wentz. 1976. Gallium-67 scintigraphy of pulmonary diseases as a complement to radiography. Radiology **118:** 371-375.
38. Nosal, A., L. A. Schleissner, F. S. Mishkin & J. Lieberman. 1979. Angiotensin I-

converting enzyme and gallium scan in noninvasive evaluation of sarcoidosis. Ann. Intern. Med. **9:** 328-331.

39. WILLIAMS, J. A., A. ANSARI, T. TANAKA, M. KHURANA, A. THOMAS, F. S. MISHKIN & A. H. NIDEN. 1979. Correlation between angiotensin converting enzyme and ^{67}gallium scan in sarcoidosis. Am. Rev. Resp. Dis. **119**(2): A86.
40. LINE, B. R., G. W. HUNNINGHAKE, B. A. KEOGH, A. E. JONES, G. S. JOHNSTON & R. G. CRYSTAL. 1981. Gallium-67 scanning to stage the alveolitis of sarcoidosis: Correlation with clinical studies, pulmonary function studies, and bronchoalveolar lavage. Am. Rev. Respir. Dis. **123:** 440-446.
41. BEAUMONT, D., J. Y. HERRY, M. SAPENE, P. BOURGUET, J. J. LARZUL & B. DELABARTHE. 1982. Gallium-67 in the evaluation of sarcoidosis: Correlations with serum angiotensin-converting enzyme and bronchoalveolar lavage. Thorax **37:** 11-18.
42. GUPTA, R. G., C. BEKERMAN, L. SICILIAN, S. OPARIL, S. M. PINSKY & J. P. SZIDON. 1982. Gallium-67 citrate scanning and serum angiotensin-converting enzyme levels in sarcoidosis. Radiology **144:** 895-899.
43. KLECH, H., H. KOHN, F. KUMMER & A. MOSTBECK. 1982. Assessment of activity in sarcoidosis: Sensitivity and specificity of ^{67}gallium scintigraphy, serum ACE levels, chest roentgenography, and blood lymphocyte subpopulations. Chest **82:** 732-738.
44. SCHOENBERGER, C. I., B. R. LINE, B. A. KEOGH, G. W. HUNNINGHAKE & R. G. CRYSTAL. 1982. Lung inflammation in sarcoidosis: Comparison of serum angiotensin-converting enzyme levels with bronchoalveolar lavage and gallium-67 scanning assessment of the T lymphocyte alveolitis. Thorax **37:** 19-25.
45. KEOGH, B. A., G. W. HUNNINGHAKE, B. R. LINE & R. G. CRYSTAL. 1983. The alveolitis of pulmonary sarcoidosis: Evaluation of natural history and alveolitis-dependent changes in lung function. Am. Rev. Respir. Dis. **128:** 256-265.
46. LAWRENCE, E. C., R. B. TEAGUE, M. S. GOTTLIEB, S. G. JHINGRAN & J. LIEBERMAN. 1983. Serial changes in markers of disease activity with corticosteroid treatment in sarcoidosis. Am. J. Med. **74:** 747-756.
47. LIEBERMAN, J., L. A. SCHLEISSNER, A. NOSAL, A. SASTRE & F. S. MISHKIN. 1983. Clinical correlations of serum angiotensin-converting enzyme (ACE) in sarcoidosis: A longitudinal study of serum ACE, ^{67}gallium scans, chest roentgenograms, and pulmonary function. Chest **84:** 522-528.
48. ROHATGI, P. K. & H. BAIER. 1983. Quantitative gallium scanning in pulmonary sarcoidosis. Respiration **44:** 304-313.
49. ABE, S., M. MUNAKATA, M. NISHIMURA, Y. TASUNETA, T. TERAI, I. NAKANO, Y. OHSAKI & Y. KAWAKAMI. 1984. Gallium-67 scintigraphy, bronchoalveolar lavage, and pathologic changes in patients with pulmonary sarcoidosis. Chest **85:** 650-655.
50. LINE, B. R., J. D. FULMER, H. Y. REYNOLDS, W. C. ROBERTS, A. E. JONES, E. K. HARRIS & R. G. CRYSTAL. 1978. Gallium-67 citrate scanning in the staging of idiopathic pulmonary fibrosis: Correlation with physiologic and morphologic features and bronchoalveolar lavage. Am. Rev. Respir. Dis. **118:** 355-365.
51. THOMAS, A., A. H. NIDEN, F. S. MISHKIN & V. J. KAMDAR. 1984. Correlation of gallium lung scan (GLS) and pathologic activity in sarcoidosis (S) and idiopathic interstitial pneumonitis (IIP). Am. Rev. Respir. Dis. **129**(2): A53.
52. DANIELE, R. P. & D. T. ROWLANDS. 1976. Lymphocyte subpopulations in sarcoidosis: Correlation with disease activity and duration. Ann. Intern. Med. **85:** 593-600.
53. HUNNINGHAKE, G. W., J. E. GADEK, R. C. YOUNG, JR., O. KAWANAMI, V. J. FERRANS & R. G. CRYSTAL. 1980. Maintenance of granuloma formation in pulmonary sarcoidosis by T-lymphocytes within the lung. N. Engl. J. Med. **302:** 594-598.
54. HUNNINGHAKE, G. W. & R. G. CRYSTAL. 1981. Pulmonary sarcoidosis: A disorder mediated by excess helper T-lymphocyte activity at sites of disease activity. N. Engl. J. Med. **305:** 429-434.
55. HUNNINGHAKE, G. W., O. KAWANAMI, V. J. FERRANS, R. C. YOUNG, JR., W. C. ROBERTS & R. G. CRYSTAL. 1981. Characterization of the inflammatory and immune effector cells in the lung parenchyma of patients with interstitial lung disease. Am. Rev. Respir. Dis. **123:** 407-412.
56. HUNNINGHAKE, G. W., G. N. BEDELL, D. C. ZAVALA, M. MONICK & M. BRADY. 1983. Role of interleukin-2 release by lung T-cells in active pulmonary sarcoidosis. Am. Rev. Respir. Dis. **128:** 634-638.

Gallium-67 Activity in Bronchoalveolar Lavage Fluid in Sarcoidosis

H. A. TRAUTH,[a] K. HEIMES,[b] R. SCHUBOTZ,[a] AND P. VON WICHERT[a]

[a]*Medizinische Poliklinik*
Zentrum Innere Medizin
and
[b]*Nuklearmedizinische Poliklinik*
Zentrum Radiologie
Philipps Universität
D-3550 Marburg, Federal Republic of Germany

INTRODUCTION

Sarcoidosis is a systemic granulomatous disease. The etiology is still unknown. The disease, through its natural history, is generally benign and needs no treatment; however, in nearly 20-30% of the cases permanent lung dysfunction develops. Assessment of the degree of lung involvement is a prerequisite for optimal management of the disease.[1-3] Studies about alveolar inflammation may also lead to a better understanding of the pathogenesis of the disease.

There are several well-established methods employed in assessing the staging of pulmonary sarcoidosis: clinical evaluation, pulmonary function testing, blood testing, and chest radiography.[4-8]

More recently, cytological analysis of fluid obtained by bronchoalveolar lavage (BAL) as well as gallium-67 imaging have been used and proved to be very sensitive tools to assess activity and to document spread of sarcoidosis.[9-14]

A characteristic finding in sarcoidosis is an increased number of mononuclear phagocytes and activated thymus-derived (T) lymphocytes in tissue.[15] Gallium-67 scans are usually positive in active sarcoidosis; however, the quantitation of activity with gallium-67 lung scans may be difficult. One current method of evaluating gallium-67 lung uptake is a semiquantitative approach, one which depends on rather subjective judgments provided by an individual examiner.[14-16] Another, more accurate procedure is the quantitative computer score, which is based on lung activity versus liver activity ratios.[17,18]

There are conflicting results about the correlation between gallium-67 uptake values and cell counts in BAL fluid.[13,19-22] Beaumont *et al.* and Gupta *et al.* could not find a correlation between gallium-67 uptake in the lung and the number of cells in BAL fluid,[21,22] but others did.[13,19,20]

We initiated this study to determine whether gallium-67 could be found in BAL fluid, whether gallium-67 levels in BAL fluid could be dependent on the activity of sarcoidosis, and whether the amount of gallium-67 found in BAL fluid could be related to other measures of disease activity.

PATIENTS AND METHODS

Patient Population

Sixteen patients with recently diagnosed, active, and untreated sarcoidosis were included in the study. Each patient had either stage I or stage II sarcoidosis; patients with stage III pulmonary sarcoidosis were excluded. All 16 patients were nonsmokers.

The control population consisted of nine patients that did not have sarcoidosis and had normal lungs, and five patients that had cryptogenic fibrosing alveolitis (CFA).

The diagnosis of noncaseating epithelioid cell granulomas of the type found in sarcoidosis was established by means of peribronchial lung biopsy and bronchial biopsy (14 cases); open lung (2 cases), skin (2 cases), lymph node (2 cases), conjunctiva (1 case), and liver (2 cases) biopsies were taken as well. All the patients had decreased tuberculin sensitivity. Eleven out of 16 patients had recently developed clinical signs of sarcoidosis activity, and 14 out of 16 patients had roentgenological findings typical of sarcoidosis.

Definition of Activity

Sarcoidosis was considered active if 1) epithelioid cell granulomas of the type associated with sarcoidosis were found in tissues obtained from recently performed biopsies; 2) clinical signs such as erythema nodosum, symmetrical arthralgia, fever, ocular involvement, skin lesions, a cough, and shortness of breath had appeared recently (and could not be attributed to any cause but sarcoidosis); and 3) roentgenographs and time course changes characteristic of active sarcoidosis were found.

Gallium-67 Scanning and Measurement of Gallium-67 Activity

About 48 hr after intravenous injection of 2-3.3 mCi of gallium-67 citrate, BAL and anterior, posterior, and lateral rectilinear whole-body scans were performed. The intensity and spread of gallium-67 uptake in the lungs and in lymph node and extrapulmonary regions was estimated. Gallium-67 activity was measured in a well counter in a cell-containing sample (1 ml of BAL fluid) immediately after centrifugation, and in a cell-free sample (1 ml NaCl). Gallium-67 activity was measured in counts per minute (cpm) and was expressed as cpm/mCi/10^6 cells.

BAL

BAL was performed about 3 hr before gallium-67 imaging using a modification of the method described by Hunninghake *et al.*[23] We instilled two 50-ml aliquots of 0.9% sterile saline solution into a segmental bronchus of the middle lobe. The recovered volume was centrifuged for at least 1 min at 2000 rpm and thus separated into cell-containing (1 ml) and cell-free fractions.

Cells in BAL

After gallium-67 activity was measured, cell pellets were resuspended in modified Hanks' salt solution. Cell smears were cytocentrifuged and then stained with May-Grünwald-Giemsa.[24] A differential count of 500 cells was performed. Cases in which erythrocytes were found and/or in which more than 1% of the cells in BAL fluid were granulocytes (typical conditions for smokers and patients with stage III pulmonary sarcoidosis[25]) were excluded, for erythrocytes and granulocytes may store gallium.[26]

Angiotensin-converting Enzyme

Serum angiotensin-converting enzyme (SACE) levels and lavage fluid ACE (LACE) levels (that is, cell-free fluid levels) were measured by direct *in vitro* radioassay. The normal range for SACE levels is 30–124 U/ml. SACE levels of about 125 U/ml were considered elevated.

α_1-Antitrypsin

The α_1-antitrypsin (α_1-AT) levels were measured in serum and in lavage fluid according to the colorimetric test. Normal α_1-AT levels ranged from 190 to 340 mg/dl.

Statistics

Statistics were done with the two-tailed *U* test (Wilcoxon, Mann, and Whitney) and with the rank correlation test (Spearmann).

RESULTS

Gallium-67 Activity in Lavage Fluid

Gallium-67 activity ranged from 16 to 6160 cpm/ml of injected gallium-67 citrate.

In active sarcoidosis gallium-67 activity in the cell-containing pool of BAL fluid ranged from 1096 to 6160 cpm/mCi of injected gallium-67 citrate. The difference between gallium-67 activity in lavage fluid in subjects with CFA (activity ranged from 601 to 1657 cpm/mCi) and that in healthy subjects, that is, in subjects with healthy lungs (activity ranged from 64 to 4558 cpm/mCi), is significant.

It is striking that two patients, with gallium-67 activities of 4558 and 2329 cpm/mCi, respectively (the latter patient was in the control population), had suffered from acute cases of sarcoidosis that had spontaneously regressed 20 and 12 years ago, respectively. They now have no signs of sarcoidosis activity evident by clinical, roentgenological, or seralogical means; by lung function tests; or by whole-body gallium-67 scans.

Gallium-67 activity does not strictly correlate with the total number of nucleated cells in BAL fluid. Also, we found that healthy individuals show low activity and low numbers of cells.

Gallium-67 activity in the cell-containing lavage fluid sample is significantly higher in patients with sarcoidosis than it is in patients with CFA ($\alpha = .01$) or in patients with healthy lungs ($\alpha = .01$) (FIG. 1).

Gallium-67 Activity and Lymphocyte Counts

A close correlation was found, using the Spearmann rank correlation test, between the number of lymphocytes in lavage fluid and gallium-67 activity in the cell-containing sample of lavage fluid in sarcoidosis ($r_s = .6979$; $\alpha = .005$). No correlation was seen in CFA patients ($r_s = .567$; NS), and poor correlation was seen in patients with normal lungs ($r_s = .6958$; $\alpha = .05$) (FIG. 2). In normal subjects we found low gallium-67 activity and low lymphocyte counts.

Two patients with serologically and bacteriologically proven acute yersiniosis, without histological signs of sarcoidosis, but with arthralgia and erythema nodosum showed a surprisingly elevated number of lymphocytes but low gallium-67 activity.

Gallium-67 Activity and Macrophage Counts

Only poor correlation ($r_s = .3628$; $\alpha = .1$) was found between the number of mononuclear phagocytes and the gallium-67 activity in lavage fluid in active sarcoidosis. No correlation was seen in individuals with healthy lungs or in patients with CFA.

Gallium-67 Activity in BAL Fluid and the Stage of Sarcoidosis

Whether gallium-67 scans showed lung uptake or only lymph node involvement, there was no significant difference in gallium-67 activity in BAL.

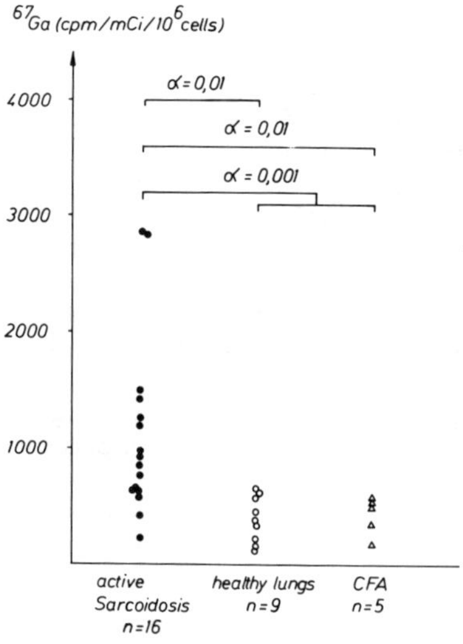

FIGURE 1. Gallium-67 activities in the cell-containing fractions of BAL specimens. Significantly higher activities were found among the specimens from patients with active sarcoidosis than among those from patients without sarcoidosis ($\alpha = .01$) or with CFA ($\alpha = .01$). The correlations were determined using the *U* test.

Gallium-67 Activity in BAL Fluid and Biochemical Parameters of Activity

We found no correlation between SACE levels and lavage gallium-67 activity, or between LACE levels and lavage gallium-67 activity. When SACE or serum α_1-AT levels (or both) are increased in active sarcoidosis, gallium-67 activity is significantly higher than in cases with normal SACE or serum α_1-AT levels ($\alpha = .05$). We found increased SACE or serum α_1-AT levels especially in cases with high gallium-67 activity in BAL fluid (TABLE 1).

Gallium-67 Activity in BAL Fluid and Clinical Signs

In cases with fully developed clinical signs of sarcoidosis activity, we found higher BAL fluid gallium-67 activities ($\alpha = .1$). Cases of acute sarcoidosis, or cases in which deterioration had become evident, had higher gallium-67 activities in their BAL specimens ($\alpha = .05$) (TABLE 2).

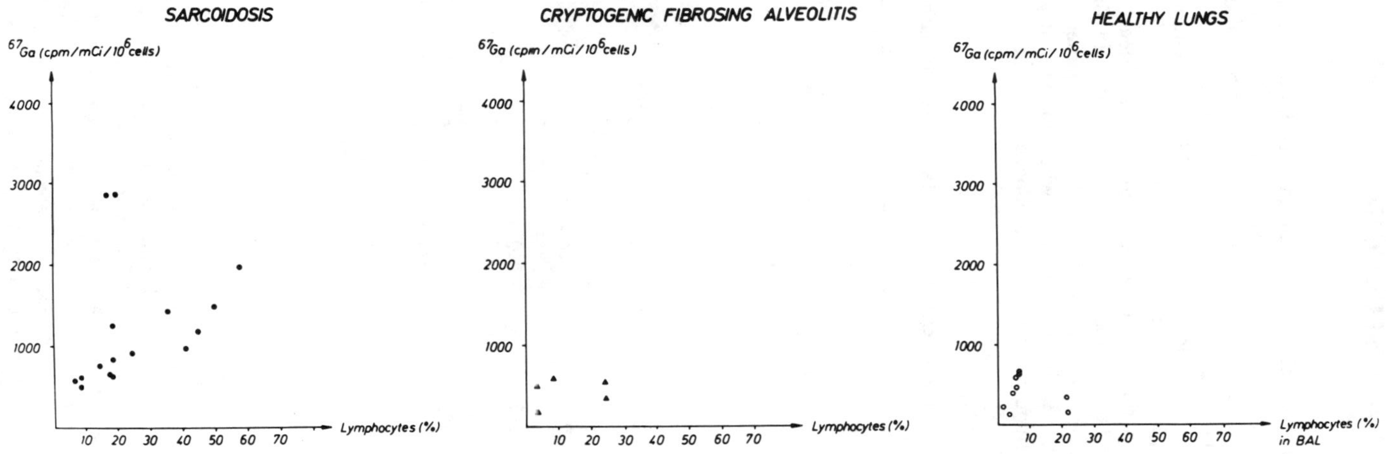

FIGURE 2. The correlations, as determined using the Spearmann rank correlation test, between gallium-67 activity and the percentage of lymphocytes in BAL fluid for patients with active sarcoidosis, CFA, and healthy lungs. The correlation was significant for patients with active sarcoidosis (r_s = .6979; α = .005); insignificant for patients with CFA (r_s = .567); and poor for patients without sarcoidosis (r_s = .6958; α = .05).

DISCUSSION

The study shows that gallium-67 can be found in BAL fluid. Gallium-67 activity is found in the cell-containing fraction of lavage fluid and may be correlated to the number of nucleated cells. Fluid devoid of cells is practically free of gallium-67. In patients with active sarcoidosis gallium-67 activity in lavage fluid is usually higher than it is in patients without sarcoidosis, in normal subjects, in sarcoidosis patients with healthy lungs, or in patients with CFA.

The most striking result of the study is that only in patients with active sarcoidosis may gallium-67 activity in lavage fluid be closely correlated with the number of lymphocytes in lavage fluid ($\alpha = .05$); it does not in CFA patients and healthy subjects. This result is supported by Merz *et al.*,[27] who showed that gallium-67 associates tenaciously to the thymus-dependent lymphocytes—to the activated as well as to the nonactivated cells.

TABLE 1. Gallium-67 Activities and Other Measures of Active Sarcoidosis in 16 Patients

Gallium-67 Activity[a] (cpm/mCi/10^6 cells)	Serum α_1-AT (U/ml)	SACE (U/ml)	LACE (U/ml)	Gallium-67 Scan
2.865	476	105	21	+
2.846	182	143	7.2	–
1.980	730	112	8	+
1.492	686	83	0.3	+
1.427	380	198	19	+
1.250	431	69	0	+
1.209	350	105	0	–
0.980	328	158	14	+
0.932	292	78	5	+
0.849	219	76	4	–
0.772	190	86	7	+
0.645	343	210	1.3	+
0.633	KA	KA	8	+
0.625	343	210	1.3	+
0.577	292	84	5	+
0.223	190	86	7	+

[a]Each value represents the activity found in the cell-containing fraction of the BAL fluid recovered from a single patient.

The poor correlation seen between the number of mononuclear phagocytes and gallium-67 activity in lavage fluid in active sarcoidosis does not agree with data shown by Rossi *et al.*,[28] who found gallium-67 in alveolar macrophages in lavage fluid samples. The reason for this difference may be that different stages of sarcoidosis were investigated in the two papers, and, different cell separation methods may have been used.

There is no difference in mean gallium-67 activity in BAL fluid between patients with hilar lymph node sarcoidosis only and with involvement in lung parenchyma. The reason is that there is probably an involvement of lung parenchyma in roentgenological stage I sarcoidosis as well, one not detectable by roentgenography but known to exist from data obtained by lung biopsies and gallium-67 scintigraphy.[29,30]

TABLE 2. Gallium-67 Activities in and Symptoms and Spontaneous Time Courses of 16 Patients with Active Sarcoidosis

	Symptoms[b]					
Gallium-67 Activity[a] (cpm/mCi/10^6 cells)	Arthralgia	Erythema Nodosum	Malaise	Cough and Dyspnea	Extrapulmonary Involvement	Spontaneous Time Course
2.865			++	++(+++)		Unknown[c]
2.846	+		++	+		+++
1.980	+++	+(++)	++			−
1.492	++	+				+
1.427			+		Eyes	Unknown[c]
1.250						− − −
1.209	+(++)		+(++)			++
0.980	+++	+	+++	+++	Skin	+++
0.932	++	+				−
0.849						Unchanged
0.772			++		Lymph nodes	Unchanged
0.645	+		++	++		Unknown[c]
0.633			+			0
0.625			+	+		Unknown[c]
0.577					Eyes	−
0.223			++	+	Cervical lymph nodes	−

[a]Each value represents the activity found in the BAL fluid recovered from a single patient. High activity was indicative of acute sarcoidosis and/or physiological deterioration; low activity indicated improvement was likely.

[b]Parentheses indicate which symptoms in a given case became more pronounced.

[c]The spontaneous time course could not be determined because the patient had been treated.

Lieberman[4] reported that SACE levels reflected the activity of sarcoidosis. Furthermore, LACE levels were assumed to be indicative of lung involvement in sarcoidosis.[31] The lack of correlation between LACE levels and both gallium-67 scans and gallium-67 activities in lavage fluid, and between SACE levels and gallium-67 activities in lavage fluid, limits the usefulness of the assumption that SACE levels or LACE levels reflect the degree of lung involvement. High gallium-67 activity in lavage fluid may be correlated to the acuteness of sarcoidosis and of its symptoms. High gallium-67 activity seems to be an indicator of the short-term time course. It is striking that low gallium-67 activity in lavage fluid seems to indicate that change for the better is imminent.

Measurement of gallium-67 activity in BAL fluid gives quantitative information about gallium-67 uptake in pulmonary sarcoidosis. The data shown here suggest that the number of gallium-67 counts in BAL cell pellets, together with lymphocyte counts in lavage fluid, reflect the activity of pulmonary sarcoidosis. Thus quantitation of gallium-67 activity in BAL cell pellets could be a further parameter to determine the activity and, perhaps, the short-term time course of pulmonary involvement in sarcoidosis.

SUMMARY

Roentgenograms and gallium-67 scans and gallium-67 counts of BAL fluid samples, together with differential cell counts, have proved to be useful in assessing activity and lung involvement in sarcoidosis. In active pulmonary sarcoidosis gallium-67 scans are usually positive. Quantitation of gallium-67 uptake in lung scans, however, may be difficult. Because gallium-67 uptake and cell counts in BAL fluid may be correlated, we set out to investigate gallium-67 activity in BAL fluid recovered from patient of different groups.

Sixteen patients with recently diagnosed and untreated sarcoidosis, nine patients with healthy lungs, and five patients with CFA were studied. Gallium-67 uptake of the lung, gallium-67 activity in the lavage fluid, SACE and LACE levels, and α_1-AT activity were measured.

Significantly more gallium-67 activity was found in BAL fluid from sarcoidosis patients than in that from CFA patients ($\alpha = .001$) or patients with healthy lungs ($\alpha = .001$). Gallium-67 activity in BAL fluid could be well correlated with the number of lymphocytes in BAL fluid, but poorly with the number of macrophages. Subjects with increased levels of SACE or serum α_1-AT showed higher lavage gallium-67 activity than did normals, but no correlation could be established. High gallium-67 activity in lavage fluid may be correlated with acute sarcoidosis or physiological deterioration; low activity denotes change for the better.

The results show that gallium-67 counts in BAL fluid reflects the intensity of gallium-67 uptake and thus of activity of pulmonary sarcoidosis.

ACKNOWLEDGMENTS

We wish to thank Miss G. Barth for her skillful technical assistance and Dr. H. Prinz for his advice on how to conduct the statistical analysis.

REFERENCES

1. CRYSTAL, R. G., G. W. HUNNINGHAKE, J. E. GADEK, B. A. KEOGH, S. J. RENNARD & J. B. BITTERMAN. 1983. State of the art: The Pathogenesis of sarcoidosis. *In* Sarcoidosis and Other Granulomatous Disorders. J. Chrétien, J. Marsac & J. C. Saltiel, Eds.: 13-35. Pergamon Press. Paris.
2. CRYSTAL, R. G., W. C. ROBERTS, G. W. HUNNINGHAKE, J. E. GADEK, J. D. FULMER & B. R. LINE. 1981. Pulmonary sarcoidosis: A disease characterized and perpetuated by activated lung T-lymphocytes. Ann. Intern. Med. **94:** 73-94.
3. HUNNINGHAKE, G. W., B. A. KEOGH, B. R. LINE, J. E. GADEK, O. KAWANAMI, V. J. FERRANS & R. G. CRYSTAL. 1980. Pulmonary sarcoidosis: Pathogenesis and therapy. *In* Basic and Clinical Aspects of Granulomatous Disorders. D. Boros & Yoshida, Eds.: 275-290. Elsevier/North-Holland. New York, NY.
4. LIEBERMAN, J. 1975. Evaluation of serum angiotensin-converting enzyme (ACE) levels in sarcoidosis. Am. J. Med. **59:** 365-372.
5. SCHMEKEL, B., R. HALLGREN, G. STALENHEIM & P. VENGE. 1983. Lactoferrin, β_2-microglobulin, lysozyme and ECP: Differential indices reflecting inflammatory cell activity in sarcoidosis. *In* Sarcoidosis and Other Granulomatous Disorders. J. Chrétien, J. Marsac & J. C. Saltiel, Eds.: 378-382. Pergamon Press. Paris.
6. VALEYRE, D., G. SAUMON & D. BLADIER. 1982. The relationships between noninvasive explorations in pulmonary sarcoidosis of recent origin, as shown in bronchoalveolar lavage, serum, and pulmonary function tests. Am. Rev. Respir. Dis. **126:** 41-45.
7. GUPTA, R. G., C. BEKERMAN, I. SICILIAN, S. OPARIL, S. M. PINSKY & J. P. SZIDON. 1982. Gallium-67 citrate scanning and serum angiotensin-converting enzyme levels in sarcoidosis. Radiology **144:** 895-899.
8. GUPTA, R. G., S. OPARIL & J. P. SZIDON. 1979. Clinical significance of serum angiotensin-converting enzyme levels in sarcoidosis. J. Lab. Clin. Med. **93:** 940-949.
9. HUNNINGHAKE, G. W., J. E. GADEK, O. KAWANAMI, V. J. FERRANS & R. G. CRYSTAL. 1979. Inflammatory and immune processes in the human lung in health and disease: Evaluation by bronchoalveolar lavage. Am. J. Pathol. **97:** 149-206.
10. COSTABEL, U., K. J. BROSS, J. FISCHER, J. GUZMAN & H. MATTHYS. 1983. Die Bedeutung der Helfer-T-Lymphocyten in der bronchoalveolaren Lavage für die Aktivitätsbeurteilung der Sarkoidose. Prax. Klin. Pneumol. **37:** 574-577.
11. ROTH, C., C. J. HUCHON, A. ARNOUX, G. STANISLAS-LEGUERN, J. H. MARSAC & J. CHRÉTIEN. 1981. Bronchoalveolar cells in advanced pulmonary sarcoidosis. Am. Rev. Respir. Dis. **124:** 9-12.
12. TRAUTH, H. A., R. SCHUBOTZ, & K. HERBERT. 1983. Die Galliumszintigraphie in der Aktivitätsdiagnostik der Sarkoidose. Dtsch. Med. Wochenschr. **108:** 1804-1806.
13. LINE, B. R., G. W. HUNNINGHAKE, B. A. KEOGH, A. E. JONES, G. S. JOHNSTON & R. G. CRYSTAL. 1981. Gallium-67 scanning to stage the alveolitis of sarcoidosis: Correlation with clinical studies, pulmonary function studies, and bronchoalveolar lavage. Am. Rev. Respir. Dis. **123:** 440-446.
14. ALBERTS, C., J. B. VAN DER SCHOOT & A. S. GROEN. 1981. ^{67}Ga scintigraphy as an index of disease activity in pulmonary sarcoidosis. Eur. J. Nucl. Med. **6:** 205-212.
15. SCHOENBERGER, C. I., B. R. LINE, B. A. KEOGH, G. W. HUNNINGHAKE & R. G. CRYSTAL. 1982. Lung inflammation in sarcoidosis: Comparison of serum angiotensin-converting enzyme levels with bronchoalveolar lavage and gallium-67 scanning assessments of the T-lymphocyte alveolitis. Thorax **37:** 19-25.
16. KLECH, H., H. KOHN, D. KUMMER & A. MOSTBECK. 1982. Assessment of activity in sarcoidosis. Chest **82:** 732-735.
17. JOHNSON, D. G., H. M. JOHNSON, C. C. HARRIS, C. A. PIANTADOSI, R. A. BLINDER & R. E. COLEMAN. 1984. Gallium-67 uptake in the lung in sarcoidosis. Radiology **150:** 551-555.
18. FAJMAN, W. A., L. V. GREENWALD & G. STATON. 1984. Assessing the activity of sarcoidosis: Quantitative ^{67}Ga citrate imaging. Am. J. Roentgenol. **142:** 683-688.
19. LAWRENCE, E. C., M. S. GOTTLIEB, R. B. TEAGUE, J. LIEBERMAN, S. G. JHINGRAN & B. F. ORMAN. 1983. Correlation of disease activity in sarcoidosis with serum angiotensin-

converting enzyme, ^{67}Ga lung scanning and bronchoalveolar lavage. *In* Sarcoidosis and Other Granulomatous Disorders. J. Chrétien, J. Marsac & J. C. Saltiel, Eds.: 430-433. Pergamon Press. Paris.

20. HUCHON, G. J., E. BERRISOUL, L. G. BARRITAULT, A. VENOT, J. MARSAC, J. C. ROUCAYROL & J. CHRÉTIEN. 1983. Comparison of bronchoalveolar lavage and gallium-67 lung scanning to assess the activity of pulmonary sarcoidosis. *In* Sarcoidosis and Other Granulomatous Disorders. J. Chrétien, J. Marsac & J. C. Saltiel, Eds.: 440-445. Pergamon Press. Paris.
21. BEAUMONT, D., J. J. LARZUL, J. Y. HERRY, M. SAPENE, J. KERNEC, P. DELAVAL & B. DE LABARTHE. 1983. Serum angiotensin-converting enzyme determination, gallium-67 scanning and bronchoalveolar lavage in the evaluation of sarcoidosis. *In* Sarcoidosis and Other Granulomatous Disorders. J. Chrétien, J. Marsac & J. C. Saltiel, Eds.: 434-439. Pergamon Press. Paris.
22. GUPTA, R. G., C. BEKERMAN, L. SKILIAN & J. P. SZIDON. 1979. Relationship between bronchoalveolar cellular and gallium-67 citrate uptake in sarcoidosis. Clin. Res. **27:** 662.
23. HUNNINGHAKE, G. W., J. E. GADEK, O. KAWANAMI, V. J. FERRANS & R. G. CRYSTAL. 1979. Inflammatory and immune processes in the human lung in health and disease: Evaluation of bronchoalveolar lavage. Am. J. Pathol. **97:** 149-206.
24. REYNOLDS, H. G., J. D. FULMER, J. A. KAZIEROWSKI, W. C. ROBERTS, M. M. FRANK & R. G. CRYSTAL. 1977. Analysis of cellular and protein content of bronchoalveolar lavage fluid from patients with idiopathic pulmonary fibrosis and chronic hypersensitivity pneumonitis. J. Clin. Invest. **59:** 165-175.
25. CANTIN, A., R. BEGIN, M. ROLA-PLESZYNSKI & R. BOILEAU. 1983. Heterogeneity of bronchoalveolar lavage cellularity in stage III pulmonary sarcoidosis. Chest **83:** 485-486.
26. GERUD, L. G. & J. C. ARSENEU. 1973. Metabolism. *In* Atlas of Gallium-67 Scintigraphy. G. S. Johnson & A. E. Jones, Eds.: 7-9. Plenum. New York, NY.
27. MERZ, T., L. MALMUD, K. MCKUSICK & H. N. WAGNER. 1974. The mechanism of ^{67}Ga association with lymphocytes. Cancer Res. **34:** 2495-2499.
28. ROSSI, G. A. 1983. Assessment of activity and extent of the granulomatous process: An appraisal. *In* Sarcoidosis and Other Granulomatous Disorders. J. Chrétien, J. Marsac & J. C. Saltiel, Eds. Pergamon Press. Paris.
29. STJERNBERG, N., H. BJÖRNSTAD-PETERSEN & H. TRUEDSON. 1980. Flexible fiberoptic bronchoscopy in sarcoidosis. Acta Med. Scand. **208:** 397-399.
30. LEUENBERGER, P., J. P. ZELLWEGER, R. VEJDOUSKY & G. FAVEZ. 1983. L'examen histologique et cytologique des biopsie bronchiques et pulmonaries transbronchique aux differents stades de la sarcoidose endothoracique. Schweiz. Med. Wochenschr. **111:** 98-101.
31. BRAMBILLA, C., L. CHAVEL, E. BRAMBILLA, F. MOREL, P. GROSLAMBERT, D. MAWONNENVE, A. VINCENT, A. DAMAK, D. RIGAUD & B. PARAMELLE. 1983. Prognostic value of bronchoalveolar lavage and angiotensin-converting enzyme in sarcoidosis. *In* Sarcoidosis and Other Granulomatous Disorders. J. Chrétien, J. Marsac & J. C. Saltiel, Eds.: 419-423. Pergamon Press. Paris.

Assessment of Gallium-67 Scanning in Pulmonary and Extrapulmonary Sarcoidosis

HAROLD L. ISRAEL,[a] GEORGE F. GUSHUE,[a]
AND CHAN H. PARK[b]

[a]*Division of Pulmonary Diseases*
Department of Medicine
and
[b]*Division of Nuclear Medicine*
Department of Radiation Therapy and Nuclear Medicine
Thomas Jefferson University Hospital
Philadelphia, Pennsylvania

INTRODUCTION

In the decade since abnormal uptake of gallium-67 was observed in patients with sarcoidosis,[1] scanning has received extensive investigation and wide clinical use in this disease. Early studies indicated poor correlation of gallium-67 uptake and clinical activity,[2-5] but Crystal *et al.*,[6] after studying gallium-67 scans in conjunction with bronchoalveolar lavage, concluded that scanning was the most convenient way of assessing the intensity of the alveolitis which, they considered, was the most reliable predictor of progressive sarcoidosis requiring corticosteroid therapy. Subsequent studies of the value of gallium-67 scans for determining the need for treatment have been carried out with varying results.[7-13] The duration of follow-up has been brief in most of these studies. The present study attempts to relate gallium-67 uptake to more prolonged observation, and to compare the value of scans and serum angiotensin-converting enzyme (ACE) levels in assessing persistent or recurrent clinical activity in long-standing cases of sarcoidosis.

MATERIALS AND METHODS

One hundred four gallium-67 scans, serum ACE determinations, and chest roentgenograms were performed in 97 patients and compared with evaluations of clinical activity based on symptoms, physical signs, serial roentgenograms, and pulmonary and hepatic function tests. All tests were performed before corticosteroid therapy or after it had been suspended for at least 3 weeks. Most, but not all, patients judged to be clinically active required corticosteroid therapy.

The patient population consisted of 33 whites (13 males and 20 females) and 64 blacks (13 males and 51 females) with biopsy-supported diagnoses of sarcoidosis. Gallium-67 scans were not performed in patients in whom the diagnosis was easily established by conventional methods and were not used to assess the need for treatment in cases of obviously active and symptomatic disease. Scanning was employed for the purposes of 1) detecting clinically inapparent involvement suitable for tissue biopsy, 2) detecting relapse in patients with chronic sarcoidosis after cessation of corticosteroid therapy, or 3) distinguishing inflammation and fibrosis as the cause of symptoms and impaired function in patients with disease of long duration. These problems were often encountered in patients with extrapulmonary sarcoidosis. The proportion of the patient population represented by extrapulmonary sarcoidosis patients in our study (40%) was greater than that in other gallium-67 scanning studies, which have largely been concerned with pulmonary sarcoidosis.

Fifty patients were scanned as an aid to diagnosis. Thirteen were referred for study because of uveitis; 27 because of neural, hepatic, articular, upper respiratory, glandular, cutaneous, or other extrapulmonary manifestations; and 10 because of atypical respiratory symptoms or chest roentgenographic abnormalities. The other 47 patients had known sarcoidosis and were scanned to assess persistent or recurrent clinical activity. In addition, we reviewed lung scans made between 1973 and 1976 of 20 patients with various types of sarcoidosis.[4]

Each anterior or posterior scan was performed 48-72 hr after an intravenous injection of 3 mCi of gallium-67 using a whole-body scanner, and spot images were made using an Anger camera. Scans were interpreted without knowledge of clinical and roentgenographic data. A numerical grade was assigned to each assessment of lung uptake according to the classification scheme of Lawrence *et al.*:[10] 0: normal; 1+: lung $<$ bone; 2+: lung $=$ bone; 3+: lung $>$ bone; and 4+: lung $\geq$ liver.[10] Abnormal uptake in mediastinal, hilar, and peripheral nodes as well as in lacrimal glands, parotids, liver, and spleen was noted, but not graded.

Serum ACE levels were measured in the Clinical Laboratories of Thomas Jefferson University Hospital employing a radioassay with reagents obtained from Ventrex Laboratories (Portland, ME). Values above 162 units in men and above 140 units in women were classified as elevated.

Chest roentgenograms were classified as follows: 0: normal; I: hilar/mediastinal adenopathy; and II/III: parenchymal disease.

RESULTS

Long-term Observation

Thirteen patients scanned between 1973 and 1976 remained under observation for 3 years or more (TABLE 1). Also included in TABLE 1 are observations on 19 patients who were subsequently scanned and who have been observed for 3 years or more.

There was no relationship between the initial gallium-67 scan findings and ultimate outcome of the disease in the 32 cases. Ten patients had pulmonary uptake: in two instances it was slight (grade I), but it was more pronounced in eight others (grades III or IV). All were treated with corticosteroids, but only three had progressive or persistent disease under treatment in 1984, and seven were inactive with minimal residuals at the time of the last evaluation.

Eighteen patients had mediastinal/hilar but no pulmonary uptake, and six of these patients had uptake that was predominantly extrathoracic. Eight of the 18 patients had clinically recovered at the time of the last study. The other 10 patients had progressive disease: 2 had persistent liver disease; 4, pulmonary disease; 2, severe upper respiratory tract involvement; 1, severe cerebral disease; and 2, disfiguring skin disease. Eight patients were still under treatment in 1984. Four patients with known sarcoidosis had completely normal scans: two continued in remission, but two had later progression.

Gallium-67 Scans and ACE Levels as Indicators of Clinical Activity

Serum ACE level determinations and gallium-67 scans were performed on 104 occasions in 97 patients. Sarcoidosis was clinically active at the time of the test in 80 instances, and inactive in 24 instances. Serum ACE levels were elevated in 54 of the 104 tests, were elevated in 45 patients with active and in 9 patients with inactive disease, and were normal in 35 patients with active and in 15 patients with inactive disease. Sensitivity was 56.3% and specificity 62.5%. The positive predictive value of ACE level elevation was 83.3%; the negative predictive value, 30.0%.

TABLE 1. Initial Gallium-67 Scan Findings Related to Outcome of Sarcoidosis

	Recovered Patients (N = 32)	Patients Followed > 3 Years (N = 17)
Number of patients with pulmonary uptake	10	7
Number of patients with no pulmonary uptake		
Predominantly mediastinal	12	7
Predominantly extrathoracic	6	1
Negative scan	4	2

NOTE: No significant differences were found using the chi-square test.

Marked elevation was misleading in one patient who had long-standing disease and whose gallium-67 scan was negative. At necropsy, 6 months later, only a few granulomatous residues were found, and the ACE level elevation was thought to be due to alcoholic cirrhosis. Although false-positive ACE level elevations were not a major problem in this series, normal values were obtained in 42.7% of patients with clinically active disease. In many instances the discrepancy was striking: patients with intense radiologic and scan evidence of fresh and extensive pulmonary sarcoidosis had normal ACE levels.

Gallium-67 scans were more sensitive and reliable than ACE levels as indicators of clinical activity. Abnormal uptake (in the lung, mediastinum, or elsewhere) was found in 96.3% of the 80 tests in patients with clinically active sarcoidosis (TABLE 2). In three patients, however, normal gallium-67 scans were obtained in patients who had active disease: one of these patients had myopathic disease, and two others had pulmonary disease. Gallium-67 uptake was increased in 15 patients with clinically inactive disease, in 12 instances in the mediastinum or in lacrimal glands. In three

TABLE 2. Gallium-67 Scans in Active and Inactive Sarcoidosis

	Patients with Positive Scans (N = 92)	Patients with Negative Scans (N = 12)
Number of patients with active disease	77	3
Number of patients with inactive disease	15	9
	Predictive Values (%)	
Sensitivity	96.3	
Specificity	37.5	
Positive predictive value	83.7	
Negative predictive value	75.0	

patients who recovered from extrapulmonary sarcoidosis and who had no clinical, radiologic, or physiologic evidence of pulmonary disease, abnormal lung uptake ranged from 1+ to 3+. The specificity of gallium-67 scans as an indicator of sarcoidal activity was 37.5%. The positive predictive value was 83.7%; the negative predictive value, 75.0%.

Gallium-67 Scans as an Aid to Diagnosis of Extrapulmonary Sarcoidosis

Forty patients were referred to us because they exhibited extrathoracic manifestations of sarcoidosis (TABLE 3). Thirteen had uveitis: 10 with mediastinal adenopathy, 2 with pulmonary nodulation, and 1 with a normal chest roentgenogram. Gallium-67 uptake was observed in lacrimal or nasal areas in each case: nine had mediastinal and two had pulmonary uptake. The scans were useful in selecting the biopsy site in three cases: a transbronchial biopsy, a nasal mucosal biopsy, and an inguinal node biopsy were taken.

Seven patients were examined because of hepatic disease. Six of these patients had normal chest roentgenograms. Mediastinal uptake of gallium-67 was noted in four patients and pulmonary uptake in three.

Six patients with central nervous system disease were studied. Two of these patients had normal chest roentgenograms. In one remarkable case of unexplained fever and meningitis, a gallium-67 scan showed diffuse pulmonary uptake even though the patient had a normal chest roentgenogram. Transbronchial biopsy revealed noncaseating granulomas, and the meningitis responded to corticosteroid therapy.

Gallium-67 scans were also useful in patients with cutaneous, muscular, and glandular disease. Mediastinal or other characteristic uptake was found in 5 out of 10 of these patients, who had normal chest roentgenograms.

In the total of 40 patients with extrathoracic presentations, 17 of whom had normal chest roentgenograms, increased mediastinal uptake of gallium-67 was noted in 25, increased lung uptake in 8, and abnormal extrathoracic uptake in 26 patients. Serum ACE levels were raised in 62.5% of the 40 cases, a percentage similar to that observed in patients with pulmonary sarcoidosis.

DISCUSSION

Following the report of Crystal *et al.*[6] that gallium-67 uptake in the lungs was the most accurate indicator of which patients would later develop physiologic deterioration, gallium-67 scanning has been widely applied in studies of the course of sarcoidosis.

Klech *et al.*[9] compared gallium-67 scan (mediastinal as well as pulmonary) uptake scores in 35 patients with active and in 25 patients with inactive sarcoidosis and noted abnormal uptake in 91% of the former but in only 32% of the latter; interestingly, the gallium-67 scan score was higher in patients with type I disease only than in those with type II/III disease or extrapulmonary sarcoidosis. They concluded that scanning was valuable in facilitating therapeutic decisions and dosage adjustment. They pointed out, however, that scanning is of doubtful reliability during steroid therapy, and they therefore interrupted therapy for 3 days before the gallium-67 injection.

Lawrence *et al.*[10] evaluated gallium-67 scans (measuring pulmonary uptake only) in 12 patients before and after treatment with prednisone for 6 weeks, and studied five patients 18-24 months after the start of a year of prednisone treatment. In most instances, gallium-67 uptake fell rapidly and remained low throughout the period of treatment. In two patients, gallium-67 uptake rose within a few months of cessation of treatment in a manner similar to that noted in patients in the series of Klech *et al.*[9]

McAllister *et al.*[11] assessed the value of scanning in 24 patients with pulmonary sarcoidosis treated 4-36 months. In this study, gallium-67 scanning proved to be no more consistent or sensitive a marker of change than chest roentgenograms.

Keough *et al.*[12] presented data on 10 patients with untreated pulmonary sarcoidosis observed for 12 months after gallium-67 scanning. Six patients had normal scans at outset. One of these six patients showed physiological deterioration at 12 months. Four patients had increased gallium-67 uptake: three had conditions which subsequently deteriorated, and one improved. The changes in ventilatory function, however, were slight, and there was no corresponding deterioration in diffusing capacity.

Robbins *et al.*[13] noted marked reductions in gallium-67 scores (measuring lung and hilar uptake) and ACE levels after approximately 5 months of prednisone treatment. No improvement was noted in pulmonary function, however, suggesting that neither ACE nor gallium-67 score reductions reflect significant effects of prednisone on the granulomatous inflammation.

A review of these studies indicates that investigations of untreated patients are by definition confined to mild cases in which the eventual outcome can be determined

TABLE 3. Increased Gallium-67 Uptake in Patients Studied for Extrathoracic Sarcoidosis

Reason for Referral	Number of Patients	Increased Gallium-67 Uptake		
		Mediastinal	Pulmonary	Extrathoracic
Ocular	13	9	2	10
Hepatic	7	4	3	3
CNS	6	3	2	3
Cutaneous	4	4	0	3
Myopathy	4	2	1	2
Other	6	3	0	5

only after many years of follow-up. On the other hand, studies of the course of disease in patients requiring steroids presumably include most of the cases who develop pulmonary fibrosis or irreparable extrapulmonary damage. Corticosteroid therapy diminishes both serum ACE levels[14] and gallium-67 uptake,[10,13] and hence these parameters are not reliable for monitoring disease activity in patients receiving treatment.

The use of gallium-67 scans to monitor the progress of sarcoidosis appears to be impractical because the radiation exposure (equivalent to that of an upper gastrointestinal X-ray study) makes repetition more often than twice yearly undesirable and because prednisone therapy inhibits gallium-67 uptake. Depression of serum ACE levels in nonsarcoid subjects given prednisone has been reported,[14] and the parallel behavior of gallium-67 scans and serum ACE levels in patients with sarcoidosis during treatment with prednisone[10,13] suggests that a similar nonspecific effect of gallium-67 uptake occurs. This possibility cannot be tested because of the impropriety of subjecting patients to repeated gallium-67 scans. It remains uncertain how long such depression lasts after discontinuation of prednisone therapy in patients with sarcoidosis. The observations of Lawrence *et al.*[10] suggest that some weeks or months are required for gallium-67 uptake scores to rise after prednisone therapy is ended. Thus the practice[9] of performing gallium-67 scans 72 hr after suspending treatment has given results of doubtful reliability. It is our belief that absence of gallium-67 uptake in the lungs or elsewhere should not be assumed to indicate absence of inflammatory activity unless the patient has been off prednisone for several months. This represents a major obstacle to use of gallium-67 scans as a guide to termination of corticosteroid therapy.

Although scepticism appears justified regarding the value of the gallium-67 scan for determining the need for corticosteroid therapy in fresh cases of sarcoidosis, a better case can be made for other uses of the gallium-67 scan. Weinreb *et al.*[15] called attention to the use of gallium-67 scans in patients with uveitis, reporting that abnormal uptake in the lacrimal glands was found in 87% of patients with sarcoidosis, as compared to 31% in patients with nonsarcoid ocular or systemic diseases. The difficulty in distinguishing normal and mildly abnormal uptake in lacrimal glands has proven to be a major impediment, and few ophthalmologic centers have adopted the policy of securing gallium-67 scans in patients with uveitis and no clinical or roentgenographic evidence of sarcoidosis. We performed gallium-67 scans in 16 patients with uveitis: abnormal lacrimal gland uptake was found in 8 patients with abnormal chest roentgenograms, but no increase in lacrimal uptake was observed in 8 patients with normal chest films.[16] Of the 13 patients in the present study referred to us because of uveitis and found to have sarcoidosis, 12 had roentgenographic mediastinal enlargement and 2 had pulmonary nodulation. The yield of gallium-67 scanning in patients with ocular disease and no other evidence of sarcoidosis is too small to warrant routine use of this procedure.

Gallium scans are more rewarding when noncaseating granulomas have been demonstrated in extrathoracic sites and when roentgenographic evidence of nodal or pulmonary involvement is absent. In cases of hepatic, cardiac, osseous, renal, and especially neural granulomatosis, the diagnosis of sarcoidosis is often best corroborated by a demonstration of granulomas in distant tissues characteristically involved in sarcoidosis. For this purpose, whole-body gallium-67 scanning may demonstrate uptake indicating systemic involvement. Three patients in the present series with hepatic granulomatosis and normal chest roentgenograms had abnormal pulmonary uptake of gallium-67, and one had lacrimal uptake which led to positive conjunctival biopsy.

The frequency with which gallium-67 scanning helped resolve these difficult diagnostic problems suggests that this procedure is worthwhile in cases of suspected sarcoidosis in which corroboration of the diagnosis by tissue analysis is not available by cutaneous, glandular, or pulmonary biopsies.

The value of gallium-67 scans in assessing persistent or recurrent activity in long-standing sarcoidosis is limited largely to patients with pulmonary disease.[17] Recurrence of cough, fatigue, and malaise, especially after recent cessation of corticosteroid therapy, is difficult to evaluate. Gallium-67 uptake may be demonstrable when there are no roentgenographic changes and may be regarded as fairly reliable evidence of activity. We have, however, encountered three instances in which such uptake was misleading. A completely normal gallium-67 scan provides reassuring evidence that recurrent symptoms are not the result of sarcoidosis. In many cases, however, the only abnormalities found will be mediastinal uptake, a finding not necessarily indicative of clinical activity. Patients with chronic hilar sarcoidosis and without any spreading of clinical manifestations of the disease will demonstrate abnormal mediastinal uptake for decades.[18]

Serum ACE levels proved to be far less sensitive indicators of clinical activity and far less reliable indicators of inactivity.

Sarcoidosis is a multifocal disease, and no single parameter—gallium-67 scans, ACE levels, or physiologic or biochemical markers—can be relied upon in evaluating its pathologic and clinical manifestations. Sarcoidosis is not just a pulmonary disease, and measurement of "alveolitis" is not a reliable predictor of outcome or the need for treatment. Sarcoidosis is extraordinary not only in the spectrum of tissues it may affect, but in its duration. Remarkably transient in some individuals, it is a life-long problem for others, and markers of prognosis and outcome of the disease cannot be determined by short-term studies.

SUMMARY

Gallium-67 scans have been widely employed in patients with sarcoidosis as a means of indicating alveolitis and the need for corticosteroid therapy. Observation of 32 patients followed 3 or more years after gallium scans showed no correlation between findings and later course: of 10 patients with pulmonary uptake, 7 recovered with minor residuals; of 18 patients with mediastinal of extrathoracic uptake, 10 had persistent or progressive disease; of 4 patients with negative initial scans, 2 had later progression. The value of gallium-67 scans as an aid to diagnosis was studied in 40 patients with extrapulmonary sarcoidosis. In 12 patients, abnormal lacrimal, nodal, or pulmonary uptake aided in selection of biopsy sites. Gallium-67 scans and serum ACE levels were compared in 97 patients as indices of clinical activity. Abnormal gallium-67 uptake was observed in 96.3% of the tests in active disease, and ACE level elevation occurred in 56.3%. In 24 patients with inactive or recovered disease, abnormal gallium-67 uptake occurred in 62.5% and ACE level elevation in 37.5%. Gallium-67 scans have a limited but valuable role in the diagnosis and management of sarcoidosis.

REFERENCES

1. McKusick, K. A. 1973. Gallium accumulation in pulmonary sarcoidosis. J. Am. Med. Assoc. **233:** 688.
2. Hershiki, A., S. L. Schatz, K. A. McKusick, D. W. Bowersox, J. S. Soin & N. N. Wagner. 1975. Gallium-67 citrate scanning in patients with pulmonary sarcoidosis. Am. J. Roentgenol. Radium Ther. Nucl. Med. **122:** 744-749.

3. Niden, A. H., F. S. Mishkin & M. Khurana. 1976. Use of gallium-67 lung scan to assess pathologic activity of pulmonary sarcoidosis. Am. Rev. Respir. Dis. **113:** 164.
4. Israel, H. L., C. H. Park & C. M. Mansfield. 1976. Gallium scanning in sarcoidosis. Ann. N.Y. Acad. Sci. **278:** 514-516.
5. Nosal, A., L. A. Schleissner, F. S. Mishkin & J. Lieberman. 1979. Angiotensin-converting enzyme and gallium scan in non-invasive evaluation of sarcoidosis. Ann. Intern. Med. **90:** 328-333.
6. Crystal, R. G., Moderator. 1981. Pulmonary sarcoidosis: A disease characterized and perpetuated by activated lung T-lymphocytes. Ann. Intern. Med. **94:** 73-94.
7. Alberts, C., J. B. van der Schoot & A. S. Groen. 1981. ^{67}Ga scintigraphy as an index of disease activity in pulmonary sarcoidosis. Eur. J. Nucl. Med. **6:** 205-212.
8. Beaumont, D., J. Y. Herry, M. Sapene, P. Bourquet, J. J. Larzul & B. De-Labarthe. 1982. Gallium-67 in the evaluation of sarcoidosis correlation with serum angiotensin-converting enzyme and bronchoalveolar lavage. Thorax **37:** 11-18.
9. Klech, H., H. Kohn, F. Kummer & A. Mostbeck. 1982. Assessment of activity in sarcoidosis: Sensitivity and specificity of ^{67}gallium scintigraphy, serum ACE levels, chest roentgenography and blood lymphocyte subpopulations. Chest **82:** 732-739.
10. Lawrence, E. C., R. B. Teague, M. S. Bottlieb, S. G. Jhingran & J. Lieberman. 1983. Serial changes in markers of disease activity with corticosteroid treatment of sarcoidosis. Am. J. Med. **74:** 747-756.
11. McAllister, W. A. C., P. Haslam, A. Davidson, A. Britten, J. Payne & M. Turner-Warwick. 1983. A longitudinal study of ^{67}Ga scan, alveolar lavage, and SACE in the assessment of pulmonary sarcoidosis during therapy. Am. Rev. Respir. Dis. **127** (Suppl.): 63.
12. Keough, B. A., G. W. Hunninghake, B. R. Line & R. G. Crystal. 1983. The alveolitis of pulmonary sarcoidosis: Evaluation of natural history and alveolitis-dependent changes in lung function. Am. Rev. Respir. Dis. **128:** 256-265.
13. Robbins, P. S., H. Patrick, H. H. Maurer & J. W. Fewell. 1983. Effect of corticosteroid therapy on objective gallium scoring of pulmonary sarcoidosis. Am. Rev. Respir. Dis. **127**(Suppl.): 76.
14. Baughman, R. R., V. Poly Song Sang, R. D. Roberts & L. Srivastava. 1983. Effects of sarcoidosis and steroids on angiotensin-converting enzyme. Am. Rev. Respir. Dis. **128:** 631-633.
15. Weinreb, R. N., E. Z. Yavitz, G. R. O'Connor & R. A. Barth. 1981. Lacrimal gland uptake of gallium citrate gallium-67. Am. J. Ophthalmol. **92:** 16-20.
16. Israel, H. L. & A. G. Desai. 1983. Gallium scans in diagnosis of ocular sarcoidosis. Presented at the Fourth European Conference on Sarcoidosis. Sorrento. Italy.
17. Wallaert, B., P. Ramon, E. Fournier, A. B. Tonnel & C. Voisin. 1982. Bronchoalveolar lavage, serum angiotensin-converting enzyme, and gallium-67 scanning in extrathoracic sarcoidosis. Chest **82:** 553-555.
18. Israel, H. L., M. Sperber & R. M. Steiner. 1983. Course of chronic hilar sarcoidosis in relation to markers of granulomatous activity. Invest. Radiol. 1-5.

A European Survey on the Usefulness of ^{67}Ga Lung Scans in Assessing Sarcoidosis

Experience in 14 Research Centers in Seven Different Countries[a]

G. RIZZATO[b]

Ambulatorio della Sarcoidosi
Divisione Medica Vergani
Ospedale Niguarda-Cà Granda
Milan, Italy

A. BLASI

Clinica Tisiologica
Facoltà di Medicina e Chirurgia
Ospedale Monaldi
Naples, Italy

INTRODUCTION

Many problems on the usefulness of the ^{67}Ga lung scan in sarcoidosis have not been definitely solved. With a view toward solving some of these questions, we have endeavored to put together the data of various research centers in Europe known for their studies on the ^{67}Ga lung scan in sarcoidosis. Each center received a questionnaire with 18 tables, and the centers which completed and returned their questionnaires are listed in TABLE 1. Only patients with histologically proven sarcoidosis were taken into consideration.

[a] See TABLE 1 in the text for more details and a list of all the participants.

[b] Address for correspondence: Via Juvara 9, 20129 Milan, Italy.

TABLE 1. Participating Centers

City	Hospital	Authors
Amsterdam	Vrije Universiteit Amsterdam	C. Alberts
Barcelona	Hospital de Bellvitge "Princeps d'Espanya"	F. Badrinas, M. Ramos, I. Ricart, L. Puchal, E. Buendia, M. Mestre, and F. Fernandez Nogués
Bruges	A.Z. Sint-Jan	R. Pannier
Genoa	Ospedale Civili di Genova	G. Rossi, B. Balbi, E. Balzano, D. Pelucco, E. Cerri, and C. Ravazzoni
Lyons	Hôpital Louis Pradel	J. Mornex, B. Lahneche, P. Chauvot, P. Mary, J. Vergnon, M. Vincent, J. Cordier, and J. Brune
Milan	Ospedale Niguarda-Cà Granda	G. Rizzato, F. Spinelli, and P. Fraioli
Naples	Ospedale Monaldi	A. Blasi, L. Carratù, E. Marangio, A. Cuomo, A. Pesci, and M. Sofia
New York	Mount Sinai Hospital	A. Teirstein
Paris	Hôpital Bichat	J. Smiejan, P. Dournovo, P. Thibault, and F. Basset
Philadelphia	Thomas Jefferson University Hospital	H. Israel, C. Park, and G. Gushue
Rennes	Centre Hospitalier Université	P. Delaval, P. Bourguet, J. Herry, D. Coetmeur, and L. Nicol
Rome	Ospedale Monteverde	F. Pigorini
St.-Genis-Laval	Hôpital Sainte-Eugénie	M. Perrin-Fayolle, D. Gindre, D. Azzard, P. Moret, R. Harf, B. Taviot, N. Biot, and Y. Pacheco
Vienna	Wilhelminenspital	H. Klech, H. Köhm, F. Kummer, and A. Mostbeck

QUESTIONS OF THE SURVEY

Question 1: Are There Correlations between Scoring Systems?

The centers in Barcelona, Bruges, Milan, Naples, New York, Paris, Rennes, Rome, and Vienna compared pulmonary (or mediastinal) uptake to hepatic uptake of ^{67}Ga using a subjective scoring method.[1] The center in Philadelphia used a similar subjective scoring system, which compared uptake in the lungs to that in the bones and liver.[2] The center in Saint-Genis-Laval used a ^{67}Ga index in which a subjective score (of 0, 1, 2, or 3) would be chosen based on comparisons to hepatic activity and multiplied by the percentage of the area of the lung that was involved. The center in Genoa used a semiquantitative index.[3] The center in Amsterdam used 1) a quantitative method, in which a gamma camera linked to a computer system was used to determine the number of counts per pixel for each of the regions of interest in the chest,[4] and 2) a subjective method, in which pulmonary lung uptake was compared to the activity in the liver, the spine, and the soft tissue of the neck and shoulders.[5] The center in Lyons used the semiquantitative index[3] and a totally quantitative index, in which a gamma camera associated with a computer processed digitalized data.[6] Thus the results of our survey must be interpreted taking into account these different techniques.

The only center where a correlation between two scoring systems was researched was that in Lyons. The researchers at Lyons were unable to find any correlation between the two methods of evaluation, which were applied on the same scans. The center in Amsterdam is currently investigating the same problem. The problem has also been studied by Fajman *et al.*[7] and by Patrick *et al.*[8] Both groups have found a good correlation between the visual index and the computer-assisted ^{67}Ga index.

Question 2: Which Method Gives the Most Reliable Score?

The methods based on digital evaluation seem better because they allow little bias. The center in Amsterdam has shown that in patients with stage 1 sarcoidosis increased lung activity may be found in 16% of all the patients by using subjective scoring methods, and in 58% of the first 12 patients studied by digital evaluation of ^{67}Ga scintigraphy.[4] Also, Fajman *et al.*,[7] Patrick *et al.*,[8] and Bourguet *et al.*[9] have found that the objective computer-assisted method is more sensitive than subjective scoring for detecting active disease and for separating patients with inactive and patients with active sarcoidosis. Bourguet *et al.*[9] have shown that for high ^{67}Ga uptake there is a strong correlation between the two methods; for lower uptake, the absolute quantitative method allows a better discrimination between patients with inactive sarcoidosis and controls.

Question 3: Is the ^{67}Ga Lung Scan or Radiography More Sensitive?

We have studied a group of 632 untreated patients. TABLES 2 & 3 show that in untreated patients the highest positivity is present in early sarcoidosis (stages 1 and

TABLE 2. Gallium-67 Uptake in Untreated Patients in Different Radiographic Stages

		Number of Patients with Elevated ^{67}Ga Uptake[a]		
Radiographic Stage	Total Number of Patients	Mediastinal and/or Pulmonary Uptake	Pulmonary Uptake	Number of Patients without Elevated ^{67}Ga Uptake[a]
0	82	36 (44.0)	10 (12.2)	46 (56.0)
1	190	164 (86.3)	40 (21.1)	26 (13.7)
2	248	213 (85.9)	160 (64.5)	35 (14.1)
3	112	71 (63.4)	65 (91.5)	41 (36.6)
	632	484 (76.6)	265 (41.9)[b]	148 (23.4)

[a]Percentages are shown in parentheses.

[b]The number of patients with elevated pulmonary uptake expressed as a percentage of patients with elevated mediastinal and/or pulmonary uptake is 54.7%.

2). In stage 1, lung uptake is detected in about 20% of patients in spite of clear lung fields on their X-ray pictures; this percentage increases with increasing stage and reaches 65% in stage 2 and exceeds 90% in stage 3. Nearly half (44%) of the stage 0 patients, that is, patients with normal X-ray pictures, have positive ^{67}Ga scans, and 12% of all stage 0 patients show some lung uptake. The new digital methods of ^{67}Ga scoring will probably show higher percentages.

We found that 183 of the above patients did not require therapy and could be studied 3 to 9 months later with a second simultaneous paired observation of ^{67}Ga scans and X-ray pictures. A worsened scan with an unchanged X-ray picture was observed in 24 of them, and an improved scan with an unchanged X-ray picture in 53: thus the ^{67}Ga lung scan was more sensitive than chest radiography in detecting changes in 77 patients (42.1%). By contrast, a worsened or an improved X-ray picture with an unchanged scan was seen in only 10 patients. In other words, the ^{67}Ga lung scan was far more sensitive than chest radiography in detecting changes. In 35 of the 53 patients with improved scans and unchanged X-ray pictures, further observations (up to nine) were available, and a late improvement on X-ray film could be observed in 24 of 35 patients (68.8%). Thus in a wide subset X-ray picture improvement occurs later than ^{67}Ga lung scan improvement.

Also, 199 of the above patients required therapy and could be studied similarly during the follow-up period (TABLE 4). At the time of the second study a worsened

TABLE 3. Discrepancies of Improvement in Serial Studies of Untreated Patients

		Unchanged X-Ray Picture		Unchanged Scan	
	Serial, Paired Observations[a]	Worsened Scan	Improved Scan	Worsened X-Ray Picture	Improved X-Ray Picture
Number of patients	183	24	53 (28.9)[b]	6	4

[a] The ^{67}Ga scan and the radiograph were taken no more than 5 days apart.
[b] Thirty-five of these 53 patients had a second X-ray picture taken of them, and 24 of these 35 patients (68.8%) showed improvement.

scan (in spite of therapy) with an unchanged X-ray picture was seen in 17 patients (8.5%), and an improved scan with an unchanged X-ray picture was seen in 74 patients (37.2%). Thus in a total of 91 patients (45.7%) the scan was more sensitive than chest radiography in detecting changes. One patient showed an improved X-ray picture with an unchanged scan; no patients showed a worsened X-ray picture with an unchanged scan. Late follow-up was available in 35 of the 74 patients with improved scans and unchanged X-ray pictures: a late improvement of the X-ray pictures of 9 out of these 35 patients was observed (25.7%). Thus also during therapy the ^{67}Ga lung scan is far more sensitive than chest radiography in evaluating the response to therapy, but the late improvement of chest X-ray pictures occurs in a narrower subset.

Question 4: Is the ^{67}Ga Lung Scan or Bronchoalveolar Lavage More Sensitive?

Lymphocyte percentages in bronchoalveolar lavage (BAL) fluid have been postulated to predict an active inflammatory process which is likely to progress, but what

TABLE 4. Serial Comparisons between ^{67}Ga Lung Scans and Chest X-Ray Pictures during Steroid Therapy[a]

		Unchanged X-Ray Picture		Unchanged Scan	
	Serial, Paired Observations	Worsened Scan	Improved Scan	Worsened X-Ray Picture	Improved X-Ray Picture
Number of Patients	199	17	74 (37.7)[b]	0	1

[a] Only patients that initially had elevated ^{67}Ga uptake were considered.
[b] Thirty-five of these 74 patients had a second X-ray picture taken of them, and 9 of these 35 (25.7%) showed improvement.

lymphocyte percentage predicts active disease has not been clearly defined. Crystal *et al.*[10] think that high-intensity alveolitis is that state in which both T lymphocytes and alveolar macrophage components are at a high level (that is, when >28% of the cells in BAL fluid are T cells) and in which elevated ^{67}Ga uptake is seen. Lawrence *et al.*,[11] however, have shown that lymphocyte percentages above 20% are associated with disease activity, and Huchon *et al.*[12] have shown that lymphocyte percentages above 15% are predictive of an active process. The T lymphocyte percentage in BAL fluid is a marker of clinical activity, but it is not clearly defined what lymphocyte percentage predicts active disease.

TABLE 5 shows our results. In a group of 39 untreated patients with negative scans, the T lymphocyte percentage was over 28% in 6 (15.4%) and over 15% in 11 (28.2%) patients. Thus lymphocyte alveolitis was present in 15 to 28% of the untreated patients with negative scans.

In a group of 136 untreated patients with positive scans, the T lymphocyte percentage was $\leq$ 15% in 16 (11.8%) and $\leq$ 28% in 35 (25.7%) patients. Thus the scan was positive in 12 to 26% of the patients without significant lymphocytosis.

On the basis of the above data we think that the ^{67}Ga lung scan appears more sensitive than BAL when using the 28% level, and less sensitive than BAL when using the 15% level. At present, however, comparing BAL results from different laboratories is difficult: according to Law *et al.*,[13] lymphocytes constitute 1 to 2% of the BAL cells of normal nonsmokers; according to Godard *et al.*,[14] the lymphocyte percentage reaches 18.6 ± 1.3% for normal nonsmokers.

TABLE 5. Comparison between ^{67}Ga Lung Scans and Lymphocyte Percentages for Untreated Patients

	Number of Patients with Lymphocytosis[a]		Number of Patients without Lymphocytosis[a]	
	15%	28%	15%	28%
Patients with elevated uptake (N=136)			16 (11.8)	35 (25.7)
Patients without elevated uptake (N=39)	11 (28.2)	6 (15.4)		

[a] Two threshold values were used to determine whether lymphocyte percentages were elevated: the value suggested by Crystal *et al.*,[10] 28%, and the value suggested by Huchon *et al.*,[12] 15%. Percentages above the threshold values were considered elevated; those equal to or below the threshold values were not considered elevated.

Question 5: Are There Correlations between ^{67}Ga Lung Scan Results and BAL Results?

Up till now the literature has given conflicting results: Beaumont *et al.*[15] found no correlation whereas Huchon *et al.*[12] and Line *et al.*[16] could show a good correlation between the ^{67}Ga index and BAL lymphocyte percentages. In our study, the centers in Lyons and Milan failed to find any correlation, and this could suggest that the two markers reflect different stages of the granulomatous process. The center in Saint-Genis-Laval failed to find any correlation between the ^{67}Ga index and various parameters of BAL (total protein levels, lymphocyte percentages, and alveolar ACE levels), but found good correlation between the intensity of ^{67}Ga uptake (a score of 0,1,2, or 3 upon subjective evaluation) and lymphocyte percentages, total protein levels, and alveolar ACE levels in each area lavaged: these results suggest that the generally applied blind method of BAL, always in the same previously determined area, could be a source of false-negative results, and that more positive results could be reached if the site of BAL could be guided by ^{67}Ga data. Finally, the center of Vienna found a positive correlation between the ^{67}Ga scan and BAL lymphocyte percentages (N = 14, $p < .05$).

Question 6: Is the ^{67}Ga Lung Scan or the ACE Level More Sensitive?

Many authors[15,17,18] have shown that the ^{67}Ga lung scan is more sensitive than the ACE level. In our survey, 810 untreated patients had simultaneous ^{67}Ga lung scans and serum ACE level determinations. In a total of 206 patients with negative scans, 60 had elevated ACE levels (TABLE 6). Thus 1) ACE levels were higher than normal in 29.1% of the patients with negative scans, and 2) the ACE level was more sensitive than the ^{67}Ga scan in 7.4% of all untreated patients.

On the other hand, in a total of 419 patients without elevated ACE levels, 243 had positive scans. Thus 1) the ^{67}Ga lung scan was positive in 58.0% of the patients without elevated ACE levels, and 2) the ^{67}Ga lung scan was more sensitive than the ACE level in 30% of the untreated patients.

On the basis of these data we confirm that the ^{67}Ga lung scan is more sensitive than the ACE level, but, in a small percentage of patients (7.4% in our survey), the ACE level is the superior indicator. This behavior could occur, and for the following reasons: 1) ^{67}Ga and ACE are markers of different phenomena that occur in different stages of the granulomatous process. 2) In patients with extrapulmonary sarcoidosis ACE levels are elevated more often than is ^{67}Ga uptake. 3) Many patients could present normal levels of ACE for the whole span of the disease; however, the possibility that patients with initially normal ACE levels could have rising ACE levels in a later phase of the disease is an open question that needs critical assessment. 4) In about 30% of patients an ACE inhibitor in the serum of patients could be the cause of normal ACE levels.[19]

Question 7: Are There Correlations between ^{67}Ga Lung Scan Results and ACE Results?

For ^{67}Ga scores and ACE determinations, Schoenberger *et al.*[17] have shown poor correlation; Alberts *et al.*,[20] weak correlation; and Beaumont *et al.*,[15] Rohatgi and

Baier,[21] and Klech *et al.*,[22] good correlation in untreated patients. Our results are also varied. Amsterdam and Vienna of course confirmed the weak correlations already published,[20,22] but the centers in Lyons and Saint-Genis-Laval found no correlations: these different results could have been caused by the use of different ^{67}Ga scoring methods.

Question 8: In What Percentage of Untreated Patients Is the ^{67}Ga Lung Scan the Only Noninvasive Means of Determining Clinical Activity?

We have assumed the presence of other signs of clinical activity when one or more of the six criteria listed in TABLE 7 were present. BAL was not taken into consideration because it is a somewhat invasive procedure. TABLE 7 shows that the ^{67}Ga lung scan appeared to be the only noninvasive method able to detect clinical activity in 20% of the 481 patients with positive scans.

TABLE 6. Comparison between ^{67}Ga Lung Scans and Serum ACE Levels for Untreated Patients

		Patients without Elevated ^{67}Ga Uptake		Patients with Normal ACE Levels	
Center	Total Number of Patients	Number	Number with Elevated ACE Levels	Number	Number with Elevated ^{67}Ga Uptake
Amsterdam	76	6	4	27	25
Barcelona	127	41	16	65	40
Bruges	9	1	0	8	4
Genoa	29	7	2	17	3
Lyons	23	1	0	4	4
Milan	132	45	12	86	53
New York	18	11	4	7	4
Paris	29	16	3	15	2
Philadelphia	97	12	4	49	30
Rennes	70	2	2	37	28
Rome	10	3	2	3	2
St.-Genis-Laval	48	12	5	21	15
Vienna	142	49	6	80	33
Total	810	206 (25.4)	60[a] (7.4)	419 (51.7)	243[b] (30.0)

[a]This number expressed as a percentage of the number of patients with elevated ^{67}Ga uptake is 29.1%.

[b]This number expressed as a percentage of the number of patients with normal ACE levels is 58.0%.

Some authors prefer to consider only the lungs, and not the mediastinum, when determining whether patients have elevated ^{67}Ga uptake. Taking lung uptake only into consideration, in TABLE 7 we show that lung uptake is present in about 40% of all untreated patients with positive scans and is the only marker of clinical activity in 15% of them. All the above percentages will probably rise with the new digital methods of ^{67}Ga scoring.

TABLE 7. Comparison between ^{67}Ga Lung Scans and Signs of Clinical Activity in Untreated Patients

	Patients with Elevated ^{67}Ga Uptake		
	Mediastinal and/or Pulmonary Uptake (N = 481)	Pulmonary Uptake (N = 205)[a]	Patients without Elevated ^{67}Ga Uptake (N = 179)
Number of patients with no other signs of clinical activity[b]	97 (20.1)	32 (15.6)	
Number of patients with other signs of clinical activity			51 (28.5)

[a]This number expressed as a percentage of the number of patients with mediastinal and/or pulmonary uptake is 42.6%.

[b]The purpose of this row was to find in what percentage of patients the ^{67}Ga scan was the only noninvasive procedure by which clinical activity could be determined. The signs of clinical activity that were assessed were as follows: 1) deteriorating sequential X-ray pictures; 2) progressive symptoms (dyspnea and cough); 3) elevated serum ACE levels; 4) systemic symptoms (fever, weight loss, and arthralgias); 5) clinical or laboratory evidence of prominent extrathoracic involvement; and 6) worsened pulmonary function test results (a 10% decrease or more in vital capacity, forced expiratory volume, or TL_{co}). Lymphocyte percentages were not assessed because BAL is considered an invasive procedure.

By contrast, in a group of 179 untreated patients with negative scans, other signs of clinical activity could be shown in 51. Thus in about 30% of patients with negative scans clinical activity may be detected by other means.

Question 9: In What Percentage of Patients Is a Negativization of ACE, the ^{67}Ga Lung Scan, or BAL Seen during Steroid Therapy?

In a group of 10 patients Beaumont *et al.*[15] showed frequent persistence of ^{67}Ga uptake during steroid therapy in spite of normal ACE levels, and the same result was confirmed by Rizzato *et al.*[23] in a group of 40 patients. By contrast, Lawrence *et al.*[2] think that the ACE test may be the preferred test for the follow-up if the ACE level is initially elevated.

In patients requiring, and receiving, steroid therapy, we studied markers of activity (ACE, ^{67}Ga, BAL lymphocytes) in three different situations: 1) in 108 patients (from Amsterdam, Barcelona, Bruges, Genoa, Lyons, Paris, and Rennes) during therapy; 2) in 138 patients (from Milan and Naples) after steroid therapy had been discontinued for 7 days; 3) in 17 patients (from Saint-Genis-Laval) after steroid therapy had been discontinued for 1 month.

TABLE 8 shows that in the seven centers where markers were studied during steroid therapy, ACE levels, ^{67}Ga uptake, and lymphocyte percentages were still elevated in 17, 38, and 72% of the patients studied, respectively. The questionnaire did not ask how many of these patients were nonresponders; how many were underdosed in an attempt to reduce steroid levels; or how many, on their own initiative, had taken a lower dose than that prescribed. Therapy, however, appears to suppress ACE levels more than ^{67}Ga uptake and ^{67}Ga uptake more than BAL lymphocyte percentages.

TABLE 7 also shows what happened to the markers of clinical activity after steroid therapy was discontinued (data on BAL, however, are insufficient to permit evaluation). The comparison of rebounds between different patients is surely liable to criticism; however, TABLE 8 suggests that the time course of the ACE level rebound seems quicker than that for the ^{67}Ga uptake rebound. To have more reliable data we would have to submit patients to an ACE level determination, BAL, and a ^{67}Ga lung scan three times in one month, but this cannot be done.

Question 10: What Is the Value of the ^{67}Ga Lung Scan during Concomitant Steroid Therapy?

In 1978 Waxman *et al.*[24] showed a reduced ^{67}Ga uptake by central nervous system tumors in patients on steroid therapy, a reduction which was probably due to biochemical reasons that could not be explained by that paper. Klech *et al.*[22] and Rizzato *et al.*[25] think that if ^{67}Ga is administered to sarcoidosis patients during concomitant steroid therapy, the value of scoring is doubtful because of possibly suppressed ^{67}Ga uptake in the granuloma tissue; thus they discontinue steroid therapy, respectively, 3 and 7 days before administering ^{67}Ga, to avoid the suppression of ^{67}Ga uptake. However, the difference between the positivities for the ^{67}Ga lung scans during therapy and 7 days after the discontinuation of therapy is not so high as to support this hypothesis (TABLE 8). Thus this remains at present an open question.

Question 11: In What Percentage of Patients Does the ^{67}Ga Lung Scan Return to Positivity, and What is the Time Course of This Return, after Steroid Therapy Has Been Reduced or Discontinued?

In many patients, due to the negativity of markers of activity, it was suggested that steroid therapy be discontinued or that steroid doses be reduced, after a mean period of steroid therapy lasting over 1 year. TABLE 9 shows that the rebound to

TABLE 8. Serum ACE Levels, ^{67}Ga Lung Scans, and Lymphocyte Percentages during Steroid Therapy

Status of Steroid Therapy	Total Number of Patients	Number of Patients with Elevated Serum ACE Levels	Number of Patients with Elevated ^{67}Ga Uptake	Number of Patients with Lymphocytosis[a]
Current	108	15/87 (17.2)	36/95 (37.9)	28/39 (71.8)
Discontinued for 7 days	138	23/100 (23.0)	63/124 (50.8)	3/6 (50.0)
Discontinued for 1 month	17	12/17 (70.6)	10/17 (58.8)	12/17 (70.6)

[a]A threshold value of 15% was used.

TABLE 9. The Rebound to Positivity of the ^{67}Ga Lung Scan after the Reduction or Discontinuation of Steroid Therapy

Status of Steroid Therapy	Mean Duration of Steroid Therapy (days)	Total Number of Patients	Number of Patients Not Showing Rebounds[a]	Number of Patients Showing Rebounds	Time before Rebound Was Observed (days)	
					Mean	Range
Reduced[b]	591	80	65 (81.2)	15 (19.0)	73	30–211
Discontinued	386	66	39 (59.0)	27 (41.0)	176	30–1005

[a] After at least 6 months.
[b] When steroid therapy was reduced to 10 mg or less of prednisone per day or equivalent doses of other steroids were used.

positivity for the ^{67}Ga lung scan occurred in about 40% of patients after discontinuation and in about 20% of patients after reduction of therapy. The time of discovery of rebounds ranged from 1 month to 3 years.

Question 12: What Is the Best Dose of ^{67}Ga?

We asked the centers what the cost of 1 mCi of ^{67}Ga was and which dose they used for each scan. Only seven centers replied to these two questions, and the data are shown in TABLE 10. It appears that we in Milan are using about half the dose that is used in the other centers. Thus we should have less positivities on the ^{67}Ga lung scan than do the other centers. TABLE 11 compares the results of our center in Milan to the results of all the other centers shown in TABLE 10. All the centers used the subjective score method. To our surprise it is clear that in all the situations studied

TABLE 10. Doses of ^{67}Ga and Costs of ^{67}Ga Scans in Different Research Centers

Center	Dose[a]	Cost per mCi[b]
Barcelona	2.5–3.0	16.5
Bruges	3–5[c]	20.0
Milan	1.5	15.0
Naples	35 μCi/kg	25.0
Philadelphia	3	5.0
Rennes	3	27.5
Rome	3	17.0

[a]Doses are expressed in mCi unless otherwise marked.
[b]Costs are expressed in U.S. dollars (December 1983)
[c]Doses varied according to weight.

in the present work and reported in TABLE 11 that the 1.5 mCi dose of ^{67}Ga seems as useful as the more usual dose (3 to 5 mCi) for clinical purposes, when evaluating ^{67}Ga lung scans with the subjective method. This reduces the cost and the radiation burden by half. Also, Abe *et al.*[26] have recently used a low dose of ^{67}Ga (2 mCi) and obtained good results on positivity.

Question 13: What Is the Cost?

Many think that ^{67}Ga is expensive. TABLE 10 shows that the mean cost (related to U.S. dollars in December 1983) was $18.00 per mCi. Of course the final cost is dose dependent. Giving the dose that we suggest in Milan for clinical purposes, the cost of ^{67}Ga would be $27.00 per scan.

TABLE 11. Comparison between ^{67}Ga Lung Scans Made Using Different Doses of ^{67}Ga[a]

	Milan (dose: 1.5 mCi)		Other Centers (dose: ≥3 mCi)	
	Number of Patients Found to Have Elevated ^{67}Ga Uptake			
	Mediastinal and/or Pulmonary Uptake	Pulmonary Uptake	Mediastinal and/or Pulmonary Uptake	Pulmonary Uptake
Patients in different radiographic stages				
Stage 1	34/40 (85.0)	10/40 (25.0)	130/150 (86.6)	30/150 (20.0)
Stage 2	22/25 (88.0)	13/25 (52.0)	191/223 (85.6)	147/223 (65.9)
Stage 3	12/28 (42.8)	11/28 (39.3)	59/84 (70.2)	54/84 (64.3)
Patients with no other signs of clinical activity	24/95 (25.3)	4/47 (8.5)	73/386 (18.9)	28/158 (17.7)
Patients with normal serum ACE levels	53/86 (61.6)	22/86 (25.6)	122/200 (61.0)	66/200 (33.0)
	Number of Patients Whose ^{67}Ga Scans Were More Sensitive Than Their X-Ray Pictures during the Follow-up			
Untreated patients	10/26 (38.5)		67/157 (42.6)	
Treated patients	32/78 (41.0)		59/121 (48.7)	
	Number of Patients Whose ^{67}Ga Scans Rebounded to Positivity			
Patients whose steroid therapy was discontinued	7/14 (50.0)		20/52 (38.4)	
Patients whose steroid therapy was reduced	4/27 (14.8)		11/53 (20.7)	

[a]The chi-square test was used for the statistical analysis ($p > .05$) for all differences between Milan and the other centers.

Question 14: Could the ^{67}Ga Lung Scan Be Used to Guide Lung Biopsy?

Up till now the literature has given few and disappointing results: Niden *et al.*[27] found good agreement between ^{67}Ga accumulation in the lung and the presence of active granulomatous inflammation in the lung tissue obtained at biopsy; however, Ackart *et al.*[28] showed that ^{67}Ga scanning is neither efficacious nor cost-effective in predicting the diagnostic yield of transbronchial lung biopsy in 19 patients with sarcoidosis.

In our survey, only the center in Barcelona correlated the lung biopsy data with the ^{67}Ga lung scan results in the same area: a positive biopsy was found in 7 out of 11 patients that had biopsies taken from areas that had positive scans; a negative biopsy was found in 3 out of 6 patients that had biopsies taken from areas that had negative scans. Moreover, a patient in Bruges underwent two lung biopsies, one before treatment and one 1 month after treatment began: the improvement detected with ^{67}Ga scans corresponded with a nearly complete regression of alveolitis and of fresh granulomas. Our data are inconclusive, and the lung scan-guided biopsy surely needs further studies.

Question 15: Could the ^{67}Ga Lung Scan Be Used to Guide BAL?

The usefulness of BAL is based on the assumption that a particular segmental lavage reflects the situation throughout both lungs. This assumption was based on studies on a few patients, studies which revealed only minor differences in BAL cellularity at different lavage sites of patients with sarcoidosis[29] or some other interstitial lung disease.[30] This assumption, however, is now subject to criticism, in the case of sarcoidosis. Cantin *et al.*[31] have shown conflicting results in different BAL sites. Consequently, the question arises if BAL could give better results when performed in segments which have positive scans. In our survey, only the centers in Bruges, Lyons, and Saint-Genis-Laval correlated the data of BAL with the positivity of the ^{67}Ga lung scan in the same areas. On a total of 119 BAL's in zones which had positive ^{67}Ga scans (in 72 patients), alveolitis could be shown in 99 zones (thus 20 patients had positive scans but had normal BAL fluid). On this basis, lung scan-guided BAL may be very interesting and surely needs further studies.

SUMMARY

Fifty-eight contributors from 12 European and 2 American sarcoidosis centers have collaborated in a survey to define many questions concerning the use of ^{67}Ga lung scan in sarcoidosis. The new quantitative scoring methods based on digital evaluation seem better in detecting lung activity. In 20.1% of untreated patients, the ^{67}Ga lung scan appeared to be the only noninvasive method with which clinical activity could be detected. ^{67}Ga scans may be useful in guiding lung biopsy and in choosing pulmonary segments for BAL. Of 382 patients studied during follow-up (154 patients with three to nine scans at intervals of 2 to 12 months), the ^{67}Ga scan was far more sensitive than chest radiography, both in detecting improvement and in foreseeing relapses. Steroid therapy appears to suppress ACE levels more than ^{67}Ga uptake, and ^{67}Ga uptake more than the alveolitis detectable by BAL. Gallium-67 uptake rebounds to positivity occur in about 40% of patients after steroid discontinuation and in about 20% of patients after steroid reduction to daily doses of 10 mg or less of prednisone. The ^{67}Ga dose of 1.5 mCi seems appropriate for clinical purposes and is recommended for the subjective scoring method in order to reduce the cost and the radiation burden.

ACKNOWLEDGMENTS

We wish to thank Drs. C. Alberts (Amsterdam), F. Badrinas (Barcelona), R. Pannier (Bruges), G. Rossi (Genoa), J. Mornex (Lyons), M. Perrin-Fayolle (Saint-Genis-Laval), L. Carratù (Naples), A. Teirstein (New York), J. Smiejan (Paris), H. Israel (Philadelphia), P. Delaval (Rennes), F. Pigorini (Rome), and H. Klech (Vienna) for sending us the data that permitted us to carry out this survey.

REFERENCES

1. NOSAL, A., L. A. SCHLEISSNER, F. S. MISHKIN & J. LIEBERMAN. 1979. Angiotensin I-converting enzyme and gallium scan in noninvasive evaluation of sarcoidosis. Ann. Intern. Med. **90:** 328-331.
2. LAWRENCE, E. C., R. B. TEAGUE, M. S. GOTTLIEB, S. G. JHINGRAN & J. LIEBERMAN. 1983. Serial changes in markers of disease activity with corticosteroid treatment in sarcoidosis. Am. J. Med. **74:** 747-756.
3. LINE, B. R., J. D. FULMER, H. Y. REYNOLDS, W. C. ROBERTS, A. E. JONES, E. K. HARRIS & R. G. CRYSTAL. 1978. Gallium-67 citrate scanning in the staging of idiopathic pulmonary fibrosis: Correlation with physiologic and morphologic features and bronchoalveolar lavage. Am. Rev. Respir. Dis. **118:** 355-365.
4. VAN UNNIK, J. G., E. A. VAN ROYEN, C. ALBERTS & J. B. VAN DER SCHOOT. 1983. A method of quantitative ^{67}Ga scintigraphy in the evaluation of pulmonary sarcoidosis. Eur. J. Nucl. Med. **8:** 351-353.
5. ALBERTS, C., J. B. VAN DER SCHOOT & A. S. GROEN. 1981. ^{67}Ga scintigraphy as an index of disease activity in pulmonary sarcoidosis. Eur. J. Nucl. Med. **6:** 205-212.
6. MARY, P., J. F. MORNEX, B. LAHNECHE, J. M. VERGNON, P. CHAUVOT, M. VINCENT & J. BRUNE. 1982. Quantitative evaluation of the pulmonary ^{67}Ga uptake in the staging of interstitial lung diseases. Eur. J. Respir. Dis. **63**(Suppl. 125): 128-129.
7. FAJMAN, W. A., L. V. GREENWALD, G. STATON, I. J. CHECK, J. PINE, M. GILMAN, K. A. SCHEIDT & E. C. MCCLEES. 1984. Assessing the activity of sarcoidosis: Quantitative ^{67}Ga citrate imaging. Am. J. Radiol. **142:** 683-688.
8. PATRICK, H., P. S. ROBBINS, R. A. VITTI, A. H. MAURER & J. W. FEWELL. 1985. Pulmonary gallium-67 activity in patients with sarcoidosis: Pitfalls in subjective and objective assessments. Sarcoidosis **2:** 73.
9. BOURGUET, P., P. DELAVAL, L. NICOL & J. Y. HERRY. 1985. Absolute quantitation of pulmonary gallium-67 uptake in sarcoidosis. Sarcoidosis **2:** 70.
10. CRYSTAL, R. G., G. W. HUNNINGHAKE, J. E. GADEK, B. A. KEOGH, S. I. RENNARD & P. B. BITTERMAN. 1983. State of the art: The pathogenesis of sarcoidosis. *In* Sarcoidosis and Other Granulomatous Disorders. J. Chrétien, J. Marsac & J. C. Saltiel, Eds.: 13-35. Pergamon Press. Paris.

11. LAWRENCE, E. C., M. S. GOTTLIEB, R. B. TEAGUE, J. LIEBERMAN, S. G. JHINGRAN & B. F. ORMAN. 1983. Correlation of disease activity in sarcoidosis with serum angiotensin-converting enzyme, ^{67}Ga lung scanning and bronchoalveolar lavage. *In* Sarcoidosis and Other Granulomatous Disorders. J. Chrétien, J. Marsac & J. C. Saltiel, Eds.: 430-433. Pergamon Press. Paris.
12. HUCHON, G. J., F. BERRISSOUL, L. G. BARRITAULT, A. VENOT, J. MARSAC, J. C. ROUCAYROL & J. CHRÉTIEN. 1983. Comparison of bronchoalveolar lavage and gallium-67 lung scanning to assess the activity of pulmonary sarcoidosis. *In* Sarcoidosis and Other Granulomatous Disorders. J. Chrétien, J. Marsac & J. C. Saltiel, Eds.: 440-445. Pergamon Press. Paris.
13. LAW, D., L. JACKSON & J. FULMER. 1982. Bronchoalveolar lavage analysis in the interstitial diseases. Am. Rev. Respir. Dis. **125:** 105.
14. GODARD, P., J. CLOT, T. O. JONQUE, J. BOUSQUET & F. B. MICHEL. 1981. Lymphocyte subpopulations in bronchoalveolar lavages of patients with sarcoidosis and hypersensitivity pneumonitis. Chest **80:** 447-452.
15. BEAUMONT, D., J. Y. HERRY, M. SAPENE, P. BOURGUET, J. J. LARZUL & B. DE LABARTHE. 1982. Gallium-67 in the evaluation of sarcoidosis: Correlations with serum angiotensin-converting enzyme and bronchoalveolar lavage. Thorax **37:** 11-18.
16. LINE, B. R., G. W. HUNNINGHAKE, B. A. KEOGH, A. E. JONES, G. S. JOHNSTON & R. G. CRYSTAL. 1981. Gallium-67 scanning to stage the alveolitis of sarcoidosis: Correlation with clinical studies, pulmonary function studies and bronchoalveolar lavage. Am. Rev. Respir. Dis. **123:** 440-446.
17. SCHOENBERGER, C. I., B. R. LINE, B. A. KEOGH, G. W. HUNNINGHAKE & R. G. CRYSTAL. 1982. Lung inflammation in sarcoidosis: Comparison of serum angiotensin-converting enzyme levels with bronchoalveolar lavage and gallium-67 scanning assessment of the T lymphocyte alveolitis. Thorax **37:** 19-25.
18. KLECH, H., H. KOHN, F. KUMMER & A. MOSTBECK. 1983. Value of different parameters for the assessment of activity in sarcoidosis: X-ray, ^{67}Ga scanning, serum ACE levels and blood lymphocyte subpopulations. *In* Sarcoidosis and Other Granulomatous Disorders. J. Chrétien, J. Marsac & J. C. Saltiel, Eds.: 389-397. Pergamon Press. Paris.
19. LIEBERMAN, J. & A. SASTRE. 1985. Presence of an ACE inhibitor in human serum. Sarcoidosis **2:** 73.
20. ALBERTS, C., J. B. VAN DER SCHOOT, J. J. VAN DAATSELAAR, M. C. P. BRAAT & C. M. ROOS. 1983. ^{67}Ga scintigraphy, serum lysozyme and angiotensin-converting enzyme in pulmonary sarcoidosis. *In* Sarcoidosis and Other Granulomatous Disorders. J. Chrétien, J. Marsac & J. C. Saltiel, Eds.: 398-403. Pergamon Press. Paris.
21. ROHATGI, P. K. & H. BAIER. 1983. Quantitative gallium scanning in pulmonary sarcoidosis. Respiration **44:** 304-313.
22. KLECH, H., H. KOHN, F. KUMMER & A. MOSTBECK. 1982. Assessment of activity in sarcoidosis. Chest **82:** 732-738.
23. RIZZATO, G., F. SPINELLI, M. VERCELLONI, M. MANTERO, S. LO CICERO & L. BERTOLI. 1983. Utilità della scintigrafia polmonare con gallio nella patologia del mediastino. *In* Atti della XXVIII Settimana Medica degli Ospedali. R. Celentano & M. Gregorj, Eds.: 223-227. Ente Pettimana Medica Ospedale. Rome.
24. WAXMAN, D., J. R. BELDON, W. RICHLI, D. E. TANASESCU & J. K. SIEMSEN. 1978. Steroid-induced suppression of gallium uptake in tumors of the central nervous system: Concise communication. J. Nucl. Med. **19:** 480-482.
25. RIZZATO, G., F. SPINELLI, G. TANSINI, M. VERCELLONI, S. LO CICERO, M. MANTERO & L. BERTOLI. 1983. Assessment of sarcoidosis activity by ^{67}Ga lung scan: A study with follow-up. Respiration **44:** 360-367.
26. ABE, S., M. MUNAKATA, M. NISHIMURA, Y. TSUNETA, T. TERAI, I. NAKANO, Y. OHSAKI & Y. KAWAKAMI. 1984. Gallium-67 scintigraphy, bronchoalveolar lavage, and pathologic changes in patients with pulmonary sarcoidosis. Chest **85:** 650-655.
27. NIDEN, A. H., F. S. MISHKIN & M. KHURANA. 1976. Use of gallium lung scan to assess pathologic activity of pulmonary sarcoidosis. Am. Rev. Respir. Dis. **113:** 164.
28. ACKART, R. S., T. L. MUNZEL, J. J. RODRIGUEZ, C. J. DONLAN, R. J. KLAYTON & D. R. FOREMAN. 1982. Efficacy of ^{67}Ga scintigraphy in predicting the diagnostic yield of transbronchial lung biopsy in pulmonary sarcoidosis. Chest **82:** 7-9.

29. Weinberger, S. E., J. A. Kelman, N. A. Elson, J. Fulmer & R. G. Crystal. 1978. Bronchoalveolar lavage in interstitial lung disease. Ann. Intern. Med. **89:** 459-466.
30. Tonnel, A. B., C. Voisin, J. J. Lafitte, P. Ramon & C. Aerts. 1979. Variations des populations cellulaires recueillies par lavage bronchoalvéolaire en fonction de la topographie des lésions et de l'etage exploré. INSERM **84:** 271-280.
31. Cantin, A., B. Raymond, M. Rola-Pleszczynski & R. Boileau. 1983. Heterogeneity of bronchoalveolar lavage cellularity in stage III pulmonary sarcoidosis. Chest **83:** 485-486.

Summary Statement on Disease Activity Assessment

J. CHRÉTIEN,[a] A. VENET, D. ISRAEL-BIET,
F. CLAVEL, AND D. SANDRON

*Institut National de la Santé
et de la Recherche Médicale Unité 214
75007 Paris, France*

The term activity is currently widely used in clinical descriptions of sarcoidosis. Nevertheless, as pointed out in several papers[1-5] and as discussed at the last meeting in Paris, there is still no real consensus as to its precise meaning.

In fact, its meaning differs between papers, and these differences lead to various means of assessment and to various interpretations of the data collected. Moreover, this lack of a precise and definite meaning may be misleading when forming prognoses and, hence, when making therapeutic recommendations.

Originally the term activity was probably developed in sarcoidosis in reference to infectious diseases and particularly to tuberculosis. In the latter, for instance, the term of activity as currently used implies that the disease is still evolving. In other words, the patient has not recovered, and, regardless of whether clinical symptoms are present at the time, if untreated, the disease may relapse at some time in the future. Thus an active disease requires specific treatment to prevent progression or relapse. In tuberculosis we possess a specific treatment, and we know that it is effective. In sarcoidosis, however, the persistence of the disease does not imply that it will get worse and must therefore be treated. The real problem in this disease is the uncertainty concerning both the evolution and the benefit of treatment.

In the light of this problem, the acceptance of the label of activity in sarcoidosis must not lead to mistakes as unfortunately it has in various papers. Some current misinterpretations must be underlined: 1) Activity should not be mistaken for the extent of the disease, which is reflected by the extent and the density of the granulomatous process, or for the stage of the granuloma (recent or ancient). The gallium scan, for instance, may indicate these two parameters and nothing more.[5] 2) Activity should not be mistaken for the evolution and the outcome of the disease. For instance, in Löfgren's syndrome, the disease is often known to be intense as assessed by a severe inflammatory syndrome, a high-intensity alveolitis, a marked increase in the serum angiotensin-converting enzyme level, and a high gallium scan index, and has been described as being "active" and, sometimes, as being "highly active." Nevertheless, most patients spontaneously recover and usually do so within a short time and without corticosteroids.[6] 3) Activity should be considered in the context that sarcoidosis is a multisystem disease. Great intensity of the granulomatous process within one organ (for instance, an intense involvement of the alveoli by inflammation, that is, a high-intensity alveolitis) does not necessarily imply serious general involvement. 4) Finally,

[a] President of the Ninth International Conference on Sarcoidosis and Other Granulomatous Disorders and a member of the International Committee on Sarcoidosis.

the notion of activity should not lead to unnecessary corticosteroid treatment.[2,5] The principal misleading aspect of the notion of activity is the implication that active disease should be treated with corticosteroids.

Taking all these possible pitfalls into account, it seems that we could, and should, define activity as "the maintenance of granuloma formation, or, of granuloma production."[5] Sarcoidosis is characterized by multisystem granuloma formation, but the mechanism of this granuloma formation is as yet unknown.

In accepting this definition of activity, however, we can identify many symptoms and signs of the disease itself, as can be seen, for instance, in the excellent and exhaustive list presented by D. G. James and W. Jones Williams.[7] This list includes clinical, biochemical, and immunological markers of "activity." Finally, and because of the imprecision of this concept of activity, almost all features of the disease (clinical, biological, and isotopic) have so far been considered (alone or combined) as possible criteria or markers of activity. In fact, the data given express only that the disease is going on and nothing more. They do not indicate that treatment is always necessary.

What we need in medical practice is to determine whether the disease is likely to worsen and whether treatment is required or not. Therapeutic decisions have to be built upon well-defined predictive criteria that are not merely activity criteria or markers.

Finally, it seems preferable to avoid the term activity, as well as the terms high or low activity, which are equivocal and sources of misinterpretation, and to use the terms *predictive criteria* and *therapeutic guidelines*. Among predictive criteria and therapeutic guidelines, one should distinguish between those referring to the functional integrity of one particular organ (for instance, the lungs, heart, or eyes) and those referring to the general outcome of the disease. The involvement of some organs, however, 1) determines the particular organ function and 2) might also determine the vital prognosis. Thus, these criteria should predict 1) the functional evolution of an affected organ or system[8,9] and 2) the possible spreading of the disease towards still unaffected organs or systems.

The criteria usually proposed can be separated into several groups. Clinical criteria include the development of fever, splenomegaly, and skin lesions (skin lesions may indicate severe and chronic disease); biochemical criteria include elevated serum calcium and serum angiotensin-converting enzyme levels; physiological criteria include increased gallium-67 uptake in the lung and elevated angiotensin-converting enzyme and immunoglobulin levels in bronchoalveolar lavage fluid; other, general criteria, some of which may be assessed using Kveim reaction and, possibly, Mantoux tests, include elevated serum immunoglobulin and lysozyme microglobulin levels and increased sedimentation rates.

The value of a given criterion in forming prognoses or making therapeutic decisions may be expressed in terms of the *specificity* and *sensitivity* of the criterion. To determine the specificity and sensitivity of a given criterion at only one examination, it is necessary to know the mechanism of the criterion. Furthermore, in other cases (in which the number of lymphocytes in bronchoalveolar fluid is increased, for example[10]), follow-up studies may be required to determine the predictive values of certain criteria.[10–12]

In this context, and in summary, we should propose for the next international conference and future works the following suggestions: 1) To use terms predictive criteria and therapeutic guidelines instead of the term activity, unless the term has been clearly defined. 2) To evaluate each biological or clinical criterion or marker of predictive value only on the basis of previous sequential studies with a sufficiently long follow-up. According to these sequential studies the sensitivity and the specificity of each criterion will be evaluated. 3) To use combined criteria leading to the determination of a "score" useful for therapeutic guidelines. 4) To assess the validity of each criterion in both treated and untreated groups of patients. 5) To look for new criteria, on the basis of either technological advances or new insights into the pathogenesis of the disease.

In this way, new aspects, such as the metabolic steps of vitamin D_3 in cell cultures or in human studies, may be developed.

REFERENCES

1. JAMES, D. G. 1981. Angiotensin-converting enzyme. *In* Sarcoidosis and Other Granulomatous Disorders. J. Chrétien, J. Marsac & J. C. Saltiel, Eds.: 362-365. Pergamon Press. Paris.
2. SHARMA, O. P. 1981. Treatment of sarcoidosis: What next? *In* Sarcoidosis and Other Granulomatous Disorders. J. Chrétien, J. Marsac & J. C. Saltiel, Eds.: 492-498. Pergamon Press. Paris.
3. TURNER-WARWICK, M. 1981. Assessment of the activity and extent of the granulomatous process. *In* Sarcoidosis and Other Granulomatous Disorders. J. Chrétien, J. Marsac & J. C. Saltiel, Eds.: 450-453. Pergamon Press. Paris.
4. JUNOD, A. 1981. Assessment of activity and extent of the granulomatous process. *In* Sarcoidosis and Other Granulomatous Disorders. J. Chrétien, J. Marsac & J. C. Saltiel, Eds.: 409-413. Pergamon Press. Paris.
5. DE LABARTHE, B. & J. CHRÉTIEN. 1981. Les indices d'activité de la sarcoidose: Signification et valeur. Ann. Med. Interne **132:** 221-224.
6. VALEYRE, D., G. SAUMON, R. GEORGES, J. L. KEMENY, D. BLADIER, J. AMOUROUX, J. PRE & J. P. BATTESTI. 1984. The relationship between disease duration and noninvasive pulmonary explorations in sarcoidosis with erythema nodosum. Am. Rev. Respir. Dis. **129:** 938-943.
7. JAMES, D. G. & W. JONES WILLIAMS. 1985. Sarcoidosis and Other Granulomatous Disorders. W. B. Saunders. Philadelphia, PA.
8. CRYSTAL, R. G., P. B. BITTERMAN, S. I. RENNARD, A. J. HANCE & B. A. KEOGH. 1984. Interstitial lung diseases of unknown cause: Disorders characterized by chronic inflammation of the lower respiratory tract. N. Engl. J. Med. **310:** 154-166, 235-244.
9. KEOGH, B. A., G. W. HUNNINGHAKE, B. R. LINE & R. G. CRYSTAL. 1983. The alveolitis of pulmonary sarcoidosis: Evaluation of natural history and alveolitis-dependent changes in lung function. Am. Rev. Respir. Dis. **128:** 256-265.
10. ISRAEL-BIET, D., G. STANISLAS-LEGUERN, A. VENET, A. ARNOUX, G. HUCHON & J. CHRÉTIEN. Persistent lymphocytosis in bronchoalveolar lavage is associated with chronic sarcoidosis. First International Conference on Bronchoalveolar Lavage. May 1984. Columbia, MD.
11. BEAUMONT, D., S. Y. HERRY, M. SAPENE, P. BOURGUET, J. J. LARZUL & B. DE LABARTHE. 1982. Gallium-67 scans in the evaluation of sarcoidosis: Correlation with serum angiotensin-converting enzyme and bronchoalveolar lavage. Thorax **37:** 11-18.
12. KLECH, T. H., H. KOHN, F. KUMMER & A. MOSTBECK. 1982. Assessment of activity in sarcoidosis: Sensitivity and specificity of 67-gallium scintigraphy, serum ACE levels, chest roentgenography, and blood lymphocyte subpopulations. Chest **82:** 732-738.

Breathing Pattern in Sarcoidosis and Idiopathic Pulmonary Fibrosis

G. RENZI,[a,b] J. MILIC-EMILI,[c] AND A. E. GRASSINO[b,c]

[b]*Notre Dame Hospital*
University of Montreal
Montreal, Quebec, Canada

[c]*Meakins-Christie Laboratory*
McGill University
Montreal, Quebec, Canada

INTRODUCTION

Interstitial lung disease (ILD) comprises a group of chronic disorders that involve the lung parenchyma and lead to pulmonary fibrosis.[1] Physiologically, patients with these disorders have a restrictive pattern characterized by decreased lung volumes, displacement of the lung's pressure-volume curve to the right, and variable abnormalities of ventilation perfusion.[2-4] The degree of lung impairment varies considerably from patients with ILD to patients suffering from idiopathic pulmonary fibrosis (IPF). The latter patients have a greater degree of restriction and poorer prognosis[5,6] than patients with sarcoidosis.[5] In fact, few of the patients affected with sarcoidosis will develop significant and severe pulmonary fibrosis.[7,8]

The physiological abnormalities of ILD lead to an abnormal breathing pattern with increased ventilation at rest. Tidal volume and frequency are related to the inspiratory neuromuscular drive, and this in turn is related to lung elastance.[9] The altered breathing pattern in ILF, however, can also be caused by various physiopathological mechanisms, with factors which may be described as being "inflammatory," "irritative," "mechanical," etc.[10-13]

The purpose of this paper is to compare the resting ventilatory pattern and drive in IPF and sarcoidosis and to discuss possible mechanisms involved in the resulting breathing pattern.

METHODS

Studies were performed on 25 patients (16 women and 9 men) with a histological diagnosis, obtained from open lung biopsy, of chronic interstitial lung fibrosis; 16 had a diagnosis of sarcoidosis and 9 of idiopathic lung fibrosis. Healthy subjects matched

[a]Address for correspondence: Notre Dame Hospital, 1560 Sherbrooke Street, Montreal, Quebec H2L 4M1, Canada.

for age, height, weight, and sex served as controls. The criteria for the inclusion of patients in this study were that each patient have a diagnosis, by both histologic and roentgenographic means, of diffuse lung fibrosis; that each patient be a nonsmoker; that each patient have a forced expired volume in 1 sec (FEV_1)/forced vital capacity (FVC) ratio not lower than that predicted for normal patients; and that each patient have a normal arterial Po_2. At the time of the study all patients were in a stable clinical state.

The test involved measuring the static pressure-volume characteristics of the lungs of patients while they sat and the volume and time components of the respiratory cycle and the mouth occlusion pressures of patients that were breathing air while at rest.

The static pressure-volume curve was measured in expiration over the vital capacity range. Transpulmonary pressure was measured via a 10-cm-long latex balloon placed in the middle of the esophagus, and the lung volume was determined by integrating mouth flow. Static lung compliance was measured in the tidal volume range from the average of five pressure-volume curves which were reproducible within 10%. The breathing cycle was studied in resting subjects. Each of these subjects breathed through a mouth piece and a Fleisch 3 pneumotachograph attached to a two-way valve that separated the inspiratory line from the expiratory line. The inspiratory line was provided with a silent, electrically operated valve which could be closed during expiration and opened automatically about 0.3 sec after the onset of the following occluded inspiration. The dead space of the valve and mouth piece was 80 ml. Mouth occlusion pressure (P.1) was measured with a Sanborn 267 B transducer; mouth flow with the pneumotachograph; and volume by integrating flow. The signals were recorded on a Hewlett Packard eight-channel recorder using a paper speed of 50 mm/sec.

After the patient had breathed room air in the circuit for 15 min, the inspiratory line was occluded 6 to 10 times at the rate of 1 occlusion/min. Care was taken that the subject had no warning of the occlusion by placing a screen between the subject and the operator. Music of the subject's choice was provided via earphones. After the last mouth occlusion pressure was measured, a sample of arterial blood was withdrawn from a previously anesthetized radial artery and analyzed for Po_2, Pco_2, and pH (IL 213 analyzer). End-tidal CO_2 was monitored throughout the test. Each control subject underwent a similar protocol except for the measurement of lung elastance and blood gas levels.

On a separate occasion, within a few days after the initial test, each patient had the following measured: total lung capacity (TLC) and its subdivisions, using the helium dilution method, and FEV_1/FVC. Dead space and %VD/VT were measured using the Bohr equation. In the control subjects only spirometry was measured.

Approval for this study was obtained from the Ethics Committee of Notre Dame Hospital.

RESULTS

A summary of the anthropometric characteristics and lung function data of 16 sarcoidosis and 9 IPF patients are shown in TABLE 1. The patients in the IPF group were significantly older ($p < .05$) and had the more severe restrictive abnormalities.

FIGURE 1 illustrates the ventilatory and drive parameters in the two groups, that is, the sarcoidosis (S) and IPF (F) groups, compared to those of the normal (N) group.

TABLE 1. Anthropometric Characteristics and Lung Function Values in 16 Sarcoidosis and 9 IPF Patients

	Sarcoidosis (mean ± SD)		IPF (mean ± SD)		Significance[a]
Age (years)	41.2	15.8	55.0	10.4	$p < .05$
Height (m)	1.64	0.1	1.60	0.1	NS
Weight (kg)	64.8	11.1	63.1	13	NS
TLC (% of predicted)	77.3	10.0	55.2	8.8	$p < .005$
VC (% of predicted)	80.3	12.8	50.9	11.2	$p < .005$
FEV_1/FVC (%)	83.6	7.2	81.7	9.1	NS
Lung elastance (cm H_2O/1)	11.3	5.2	23.1	10.3	$p < .005$
PaO_2 (mm Hg)	79.3	6.1	75.0	6.3	NS
$PaCO_2$ (mm Hg)	38.3	2.8	40.9	2.3	NS

[a] Significance was determined using Student's *t* test.

IPF patients have higher $\dot{V}_E$ values, while breathing, and smaller V_T and higher f values than sarcoidosis patients. IPF patients also have higher ventilatory drive valves; that is, they have higher V_T/inspiration time (TI) ratios and P.1 values.

FIGURE 2 shows the relationship of lung elastance with P.1 and TI. As noted, P.1 increases ($p < .001$) and TI decreases ($p < .01$) with elastance: both relationships are linear. IPF patients have higher P.1 and lower TI values than do sarcoidosis patients.

FIGURE 3 compares elastance with the breathing pattern. A significant positive relationship was found between f and elastance ($p < .01$), and an inverse relationship was found between V_T and elastance ($p < .05$). Note that IPF patients generally have higher f and smaller V_T values than sarcoidosis patients.

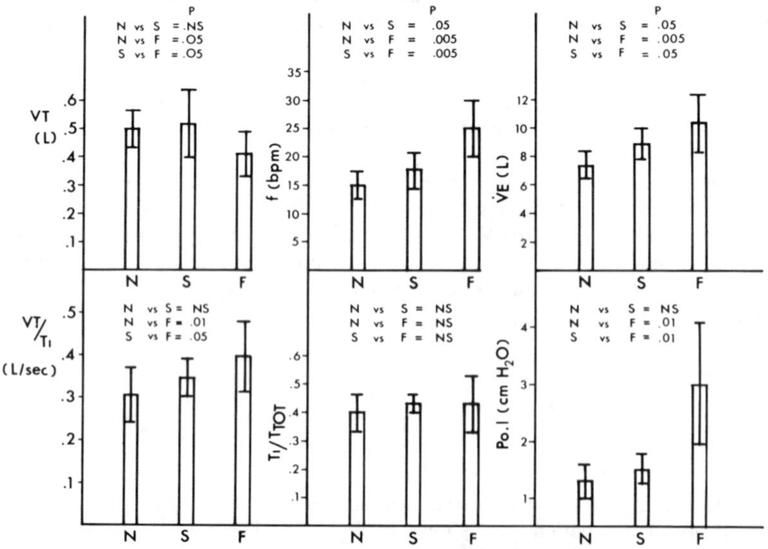

FIGURE 1. Relationship between the ventilatory and drive parameters in 16 sarcoidosis (S) and 9 IPF (F) patients when compared to each other and to those in normals (N) matched for age, height, and sex.

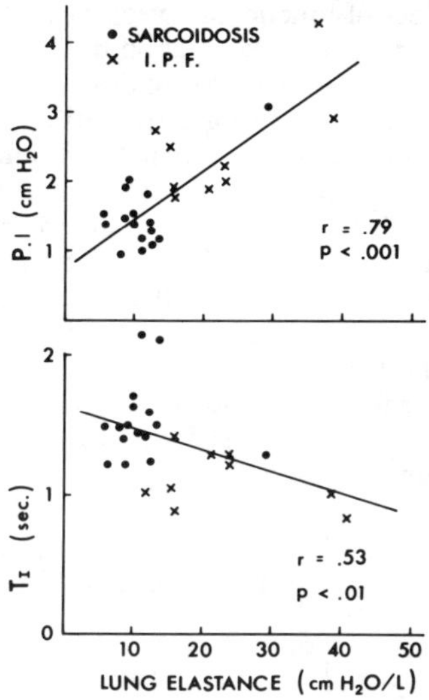

FIGURE 2. Relationship between P.1 and TI, respectively, and lung elastance in 16 sarcoidosis and 9 IPF patients.

FIGURE 4 compares lung elastance to the effective inspiratory impedance (P.1/VT/TI) and shows a significant positive relation ($p < .001$). In the same figure, the %VD/VT is related to elastance and shows a strong linear correlation.

DISCUSSION

ILD comprises a group of heterogeneous, often fatal diseases that involve the lung parenchyma and are characterized by derangement of the alveolar interstitium and

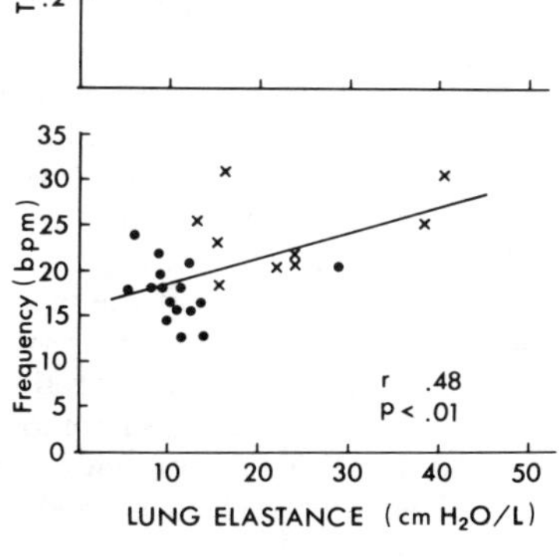

FIGURE 3. Tidal volume and frequency plotted as functions of lung elastance in 16 sarcoidosis and 9 IPF patients that were at rest and breathing room air.

loss of functional alveolar capillary units.[14] IPF and sarcoidosis patients both present a chronic inflammation in the lower respiratory tract; however, some differences have been observed. Sarcoidosis is characterized by a lymphocyte alveolitis whereas IPF shows a neutrophil alveolitis. The latter represents a high-intensity alveolitis and leads to more severe scarring and pulmonary fibrosis and deterioration of pulmonary function.[15] In addition, free collagenase is routinely detected in lavage fluid of patients with IPF and is not found in that of patients with sarcoidosis.[16] The presence of this enzyme within the alveolar structure may account in part for the disorganization of collagen fibers and the accumulation of type I collagen which is characteristic of IPF.

The effector function of inflammatory and immune cells constituting the alveolitis in IPF and that of cells constituting the alveolitis in sarcoidosis are different: the neutrophil component in IPF releases important mediators of inflammation.[17,18] This leads to increased fibrosis which represents an elastic load eliciting a small V_T and an increased f.

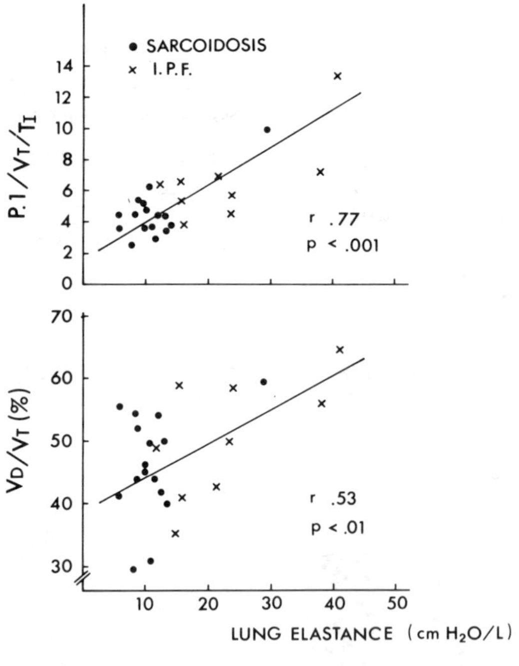

FIGURE 4. Comparison between effective inspiratory impedance (P.1/V_T/TI) and %V_D/V_T, respectively, and lung elastance in 16 sarcoidosis and 9 IPF patients.

The increased load and inspiratory neuromuscular output is inversely related to the pulmonary compliance. FIGURE 5 shows the relationship between P.1 and the static lung compliance in 16 sarcoidosis and 9 IPF patients. Even though the sarcoidosis patients had lower compliance values (mean: 0.089 1/cm H_2O), they did not attain the threshold value for increasing the output of the respiratory center (about 0.06 1/cm H_2O). Most IPF patients (mean static compliance: 0.043 1/cm H_2O) modified their breathing pattern because of the increased output of the respiratory center.

It has been shown[9] that the decrease in V_T is due to shortening of TI, and not a reduction in neuromuscular output or the inspiratory flow, and these findings are more accentuated in IPF than in sarcoidosis.

Our previous data[9] also shows that modifications of lung elastance caused by IPF or by external loads imposed on normal subjects elicit qualitatively similar modifi-

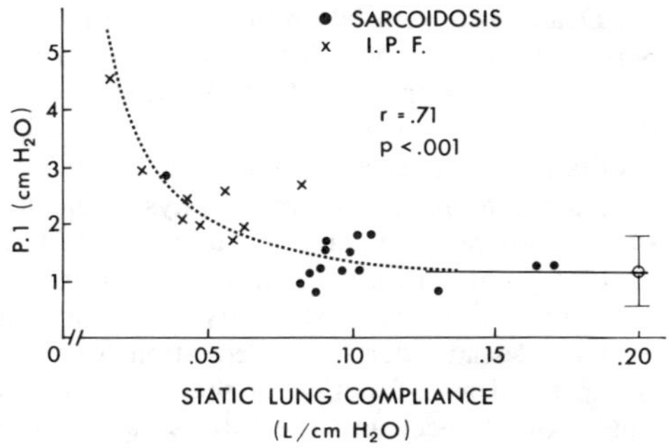

FIGURE 5. Relationship between P.1 and static lung compliance in 16 sarcoidosis and 9 IPF patients. Mean values of P.1 ± 2 SD's for normal subjects are included. The best fitting function is hyperbolic ($r = 71$; $p < .001$).

cations in the breathing pattern. These consist of reduced VT and increased frequency, and both variables change progressively as a function of increased elastance.

Disorders associated with ILD are characterized by alveolitis with inflammatory and immune cells as effectors.[15] In this stage, vagal airway and lung parenchymal receptors (stretch, irritant, and J receptors) may be activated by liberation of inflammatory mediators produced in the lung parenchyma leading to a further increase in f.[19–22]

In order to evaluate factors besides elastance that influence the pattern of breathing, we plotted f as a function of total elastance in 33 normal subjects breathing with inspiratory elastic loads,[10,23–26] in 16 sarcoidosis patients, and in 9 IPF patients (FIG. 6). The sarcoidosis and IPF patients tended to have higher f values than did the elastically loaded normal subjects. It is therefore possible to assume that factors besides elastance affect the breathing pattern.

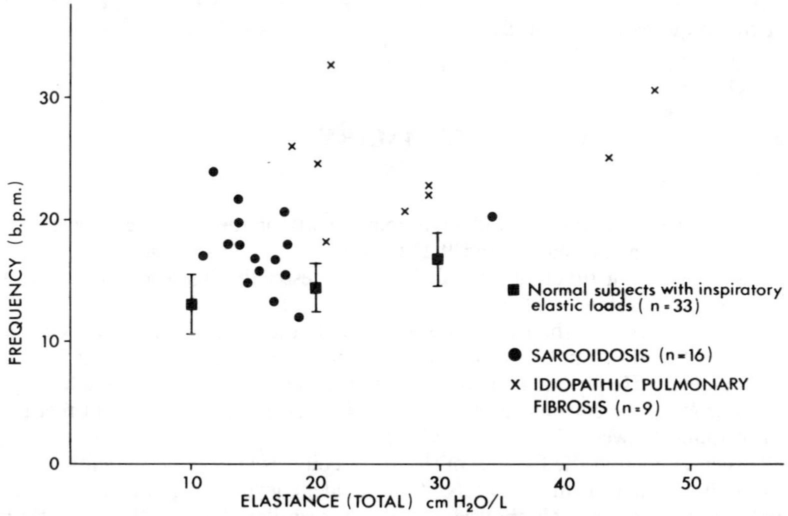

FIGURE 6. Breathing frequency at rest plotted as a function of total elastance in 16 sarcoidosis and 9 IPF patients and in normal subjects breathing against added elastic loads. The frequencies at elastances of 10, 20, and 30 cm $H_2O/1$ in loaded normal subjects are shown as averages ± SD's and were obtained from earlier studies.[10,23–26]

Dead-space ventilation may be another important factor influencing the breathing pattern because $\%V_D/V_T$ is increased in ILD secondary to the decrease of V_T or increase of V_D or both. Total ventilation is the sum of the alveolar ventilation and the dead-space ventilation, and any increase in anatomical or physiological dead space results in an increased requirement for inspiratory muscle force development.[27]

Furthermore, an increased physiological dead-space and V/Q imbalance necessitate an increased ventilation to eliminate CO_2. Patients with ILD frequently hyperventilate, which results in chronic hypocapnea.[28] Respiratory rate is set at a particular frequency which is least costly to the average force developed by the respiratory muscles. Mead[29] derived an equation for this optimal frequency in which frequency is expressed as a function of the time constant of the respiratory system (resistance times compliance) and the ratio of alveolar ventilation to dead space. Both factors are modified in ILD.

More recently, Dimarco *et al.*[30] showed that patients with ILD and small V_T have reduced rib cage expansion. This may add another mechanism by which respiratory drive and timing are altered.

CONCLUSION

We have compared the breathing patterns of patients with IPF to those of patients with sarcoidosis. We observed that the two groups of patients showed a significant correlation between V_T, f, P.1, and lung elastance. Hence the main factor affecting the breathing pattern in lung fibrosis is the influence of the elastic load on the control of breathing, with IPF having higher f and lower V_T values because of the increased elastance. Other factors influencing the breathing pattern are the decreased V_T and increased $\%V_D/V_T$ values. Inflammation may stimulate the vagal receptors to increase f, but this requires further study.

SUMMARY

We measured the volume and time components of the breathing cycle together with the P.1 in 16 sarcoidosis and 9 IPF patients. Patients in the IPF group were older, and their lung functions revealed a more restrictive pattern with small TLC, VC, and higher elastance values.

We observed that in the two groups of patients there was a significant correlation between V_T, f, and P.1 and lung elastance, and that the stiffer IPF patients had higher drive parameters. Hence, the main factor affecting the breathing pattern in both groups is the influence of the elastic load on the control of breathing. A significant relationship was also found between $\%V_D/V_T$ and elastance.

We then compared the f values of the 16 sarcoidosis and 9 IPF patients with those of elastically loaded normal subjects. At equivalent levels of elastance, even though the patients and the normals showed qualitatively similar changes, the patients tended to have higher frequencies for the equivalent elastic load.

In conclusion, ventilatory and drive parameters in interstitial lung diseases increased as a function of the elastic load, this load being greater in IPF than in sarcoidosis. Inflammation may stimulate the vagal receptors to increase the frequency of breathing, but this requires further study.

REFERENCES

1. SPENCER, H. 1977. Pathology of the Lung. W. B. Saunders. Philadelphia, PA.
2. BOUSHY, S. F. & L. B. NORTH. 1973. Pulmonary function in infiltrative lung disease. Chest **62:** 939-955.
3. FULMER, J. D., W. C. ROBERTS & E. R. VON GAL. 1979. Morphologic-physiologic correlates of the severity of fibrosis and degree of cellularity in idiopathic pulmonary fibrosis. J. Clin. Invest. **63:** 665-676.
4. GIBSON, G. J. & N. B. PRIDE. 1976. A reappraisal of lung mechanics in fibrosing alveolitis. Chest **69**(Suppl.): 256.
5. CARRINGTON, C. B., E. A. GAENSLER & R. E. COUTU. 1962. Natural history and treated course of usual and desquamative interstitial pneumonia. Am. Rev. Respir. Dis. **126:** 1005-1012.
6. RUDD, R. M., P. L. HASLAM & M. TURNER-WARWICK. 1981. Cryptogenic fibrosing alveolitis. Am. Rev. Respir. Dis. **124:** 1-8.
7. SMELLIE, H. & C. HOYLE. 1960. The natural history of pulmonary sarcoidosis. Q. J. Med. **29:** 539-558.
8. RENZI, P. & G. RENZI. 1983. La sarcoidose de type Québécois. Un. Med. Can. **II:** 1-5.
9. RENZI, G., J. MILIC-EMILI & A. E. GRASSINO. 1982. The pattern of breathing in diffuse lung fibrosis. Bull. Eur. Physiopathol. Respir. **18:** 461-472.
10. AGOSTONI, E., E. D'ANGELO, G. TORRI & L. RAVENNA. 1977. Effects of uneven elastic loads on the breathing pattern of anesthetized and conscious men. Respir. Physiol. **30:** 153-168.
11. TRENCHARD, D., D. GARDNER & A. GUZ. 1972. Role of pulmonary vagal afferent nerve fibers in the development of rapid shallow breathing in lung inflammation. Clin. Sci. **42:** 251-263.
12. CAMPBELL, E. J. M., O. P. DINNICK & J. B. L. HOWELL. 1961. The immediate effects of elastic loads on the breathing of man. J. Physiol. (London) **156:** 260-273.
13. TURINO, G. M., R. V. LOURENCO, L. A. DAVIDSON & A. D. FISHMAN. 1963. The control of ventilation in patients with reduced pulmonary distensibility. Ann. N.Y. Acad. Sci. **109:** 932-940.
14. FULMER, J. D. & R. G. CRYSTAL. 1979. Interstitial lung disease. *In* Current Pulmonology. D. H. Simmons, Ed. Vol **1:** 1-65. Houghton Mifflin. Boston, MA.
15. CRYSTAL, R. G., J. E. GADEK, V. J. FERRANS, J. D. FULMER, B. R. LINE & G. W. HUNNINGHAKE. 1981. Interstitial lung disease: Current concepts of pathogeneses, staging and therapy. Am. J. Med. **70:** 542-568.
16. GADEK, J. E., J. A. KELMAN & G. A. FELLS. 1979. Collagenase in the lower respiratory tract of patients with idiopathic pulmonary fibrosis. N. Engl. J. Med. **301:** 737-742.
17. HAVERMAN, K. & A. JANOFF, Eds. 1978. Neutral Proteases of Human Polymorphonuclear Leukocytes: Biochemistry, Physiology and Clinical Significance. Urban and Schwarzenberg. Baltimore, MD.
18. TILL, G. O., K. J. JOHNSON, R. KUNKEL & P. A. WARD. 1982. Intravascular activation of complement and acute lung injury: Dependency on neutrophils and toxic oxygen metabolites. J. Clin. Invest. **69:** 1126-1135.
19. BLEECKER, E. R., D. J. COTTON, S. P. FISHER, P. D. GRAF, W. M. GOLD & J. A. NADEL. 1976. The mechanism of rapid, shallow breathing after inhaling histamine aerosol in exercising dogs. Am. Rev. Respir. Dis. **114:** 909-916.
20. COTES, J. E., G. R. JOHNSON & A. MCDONALD. 1970. Breathing frequency and tidal volume: Relationship to breathlessness. *In* Breathing: Hering-Breuer Centenary Symposium. R. Porter, Ed.: 297-314. Churchill. London.
21. PHILLIPSON, E. A., E. MURPHY, L. F. KOZAR & R. K. SCHULTZE. 1975. Role of vagal

stimuli in exercise ventilation in dogs with experimental pneumonitis. J. Appl. Physiol. **39:** 76-85.

22. REMMERS, J. E. 1973. Extrasegmental reflexes derived from intercostal afferents: Phrenic and laryngeal responses. J. Physiol. (London) **233:** 45-62.
23. POPE, H., R. HOLLOWEY & E. J. M. CAMPBELL. 1968. The effects of elastic and resistive loading of inspiration on the breathing of conscious man. Respir. Physiol. **4:** 363-372.
24. CHERNIACK, R. & C. GUENTER. 1961. The efficiency of the respiratory muscles in obesity. Can. J. Biochem. Physiol. **39:** 1215-1222.
25. McILROY, M. B., F. L. ELDRIDGE, J. THOMAS & R. V. CHRISTIE. 1956. The effect of added elastic and nonelastic resistances on the pattern of breathing in normal subjects. Clin. Sci. **15:** 337-344.
26. BLAND, S., L. LAZEROU, G. DYCK & R. M. CHERNIACK. 1967. The influence of the chest wall on respiratory rate and depth. Respir. Physiol. **3:** 47-54.
27. KILLIAN, K. J. & E. J. M. CAMPBELL. 1963. Dyspnea and exercise. Annu. Rev. Physiol. **45:** 465-477.
28. KORNBLUTH, R. & G. M. TURINO. 1980. Respiratory control in diffuse interstitial lung disease and diseases of the pulmonary vasculature. Clin. Med. **1:** 91-102.
29. MEAD, J. 1960. Control of respiratory frequency. J. Appl. Physiol. **15:** 325-336.
30. DIMARCO, A. F., S. G. KELSEN, N. S. CHERNIACK & B. GOTHE. 1983. Occlusion pressure and breathing pattern in patients with interstitial lung disease. Am. Rev. Respir. Dis. **127:** 425-430.

Exercise Testing in the Physiologic Assessment of Sarcoidosis

LAURENCE ATHOS, JOHN G. MOHLER,
AND OM P. SHARMA

Los Angeles County-University of Southern California Medical Center
Los Angeles, California 90033

INTRODUCTION

Discrepancies between subjective, radiologic, and physiologic assessments of sarcoidosis severity, although previously demonstrated, have not been evaluated in conjunction with invasive symptom-limited maximum exercise testing. Exercise testing may provide unique observations into the integrated response of the cardiopulmonary systems to physiologic stress.[1] The present study, therefore, examined 39 patients with sarcoidosis who underwent multiple pulmonary physiologic studies including incremental exercise to determine maximum oxygen consumption (Vo_2).

MATERIALS AND METHODS

Thirty-nine patients with proven sarcoidosis underwent an exercise study after their informed consent was obtained. Almost all subjects underwent spirometry and lung volume and Dco determinations. The race, sex, and age distributions are shown in TABLE 1. Seven subjects had normal chest radiographs (stage 0); 9 had bilateral hilar adenopathy (stage 1); 15 had bilateral adenopathy and parenchymal densities (stage 2); and 8 had limited parenchymal infiltrates only (stage 3). None had evidence of markedly intense fibrosis or honeycombing (stage 4).

Thirty-nine patients met the criteria for adequately motivated exercise to maximum Vo_2, as defined below. Data from these 39 subjects were correlated with our modified health questionnaire. We also reviewed the medical chart for reports of symptoms of cough and dyspnea.

Forced vital capacity (FVC), forced expiratory volume in 1 sec (FEV_1), and maximal voluntary ventilation (MVV) were measured with a 13-liter Stead-Wells spirometer. Lung volumes were determined by whole-body volume phlethysmography (Mead-Leath) in 25 subjects and by a 7-min helium dilution (McMichael) in 12 subjects. A modification of the single-breath method (Forster) was used to measure Dco. Increment symptom-limited exercise was accomplished on a motor-driven treadmill by methods described previously.[2] The symptoms that limited exercise were most often dyspnea, weakness or pain in the legs, or general fatigue of a vague nature (for example, a patient might remark, "I don't feel well").

Reference values for spirometry were those of Morris *et al.*,[3] and a 13% reduction factor was used for those patients of African ancestory.[4] Reference values for lung volume determinations were those of Goldman and Becklake,[5] and a correction for race similar to the one described above was used. DCO and KCO reference values were obtained from Van Ganse and Cotes[6] (no correction for race). Resting arterial blood gas reference values were obtained from Mellemgaard.[7]

All subjects were graded for the severity of the symptoms of dyspnea and cough on a 0-4 scale: dyspnea grades were as outlined in the British Medical Research Council questionnaire,[8] and cough grades included those for no (0), occasional (1), frequent but not daily (2), daily/exertional but not troublesome (3), or always troublesome (4) coughing. The standard statistical method of comparing data to reference values was used in this report; that is, the Z statistic, where Z = (observed value-reference value)/SD of the reference, was used. A single-tailed value representing 95% confidence limits is $Z < -1.64$. We do not use ratios such as percentages of predicted values, which admittedly are popular but nonetheless erroneous.

TABLE 1. Subject Demographics

Race	
Black	37
Caucasian	1
Hispanic	1
Sex	
Male	12
Female	27
Age (years)	
Mean	39
Range	21-75

During exercise, subjects were scored on a 0-4 scale for five physiologic parameters: mouth breathing, supraclavicular retraction, sternocleidomastoid muscle retraction, length of spoken word string, and stressed quality to the voice. The sum score of these parameters, the dyspnea sum index (DSI), was then calculated. In previously published studies we have demonstrated a high correlation between the DSI and $\dot{V}O_2$ as $\dot{V}O_2$ increases to maximum $\dot{V}O_2$ on graded exercise; healthy subjects always reached a DSI score of 18 or higher at maximal exercise as did 25 of 27 patients with chronically obstructed airways.[2] For this study, a maximum DSI score of 17 or higher was accepted as evidence of satisfactory exercise motivation. Also accepted as objective evidence of maximum $\dot{V}O_2$ and symptom-limited exercise were a heart rate 0.9 or more times the calculated reference value, $210 - (.65 \times \text{age})$, or a dyspnea index above 90 (based on measured MVV which was equal to or greater than 30 times the FEV_1). Abnormal ventilatory mechanics (defined below), or an exercise PaO_2 of 60 mm Hg or less without elevating the PCO_2 compared to resting, may reduce exercise capacity and were also accepted as evidence for achieving true maximal exercise.

Subjects were categorized as being limited by pulmonary impairment in their ability to achieve their expected maximum $\dot{V}O_2$ values if they demonstrated one or more of the following abnormalities of ventilation, lung mechanics, or gas exchange: a dyspnea index (DI = $\dot{V}E/MVV$) of 90 or above, a breathing rate of 60 or more breaths/min at a V_T/FVC ratio of less than .46, a maximal exercise V_D/V_T greater than 30, a $\dot{V}E/\dot{V}O_2$ at maximal exercise above 53, a $\dot{V}E/\dot{V}CO_2$ at maximal exercise above 42, or an exercise PaO_2 of 60 mm Hg or lower while sustaining a resting level of PCO_2.

RESULTS

Twenty-five of 39 subjects satisfied one or more of the preceding criteria and were thus characterized as having pulmonary impairment which would be expected to limit exercise. Fourteen of the 25, in fact, had a maximum $\dot{V}O_2$/kg body weight which was below the 95% confidence level determined using the data of Bruce *et al.*[9]

Four other subjects failed to achieve the 95% confidence band for maximum $\dot{V}O_2$/kg body weight. These subjects, of which one was in stage 0, two in stage 1, and one in stage 2, had no demonstrable pulmonary limitations to exercise. Their exercise limitation was ascribed to a lack of muscle fitness secondary to general inactivity or cardiovascular disorders. At maximum $\dot{V}O_2$, one of these subjects had a low heart rate, which suggested he had heart disease; another one had an unusually high heart rate, which suggested he had poor conditioning. Two had systolic and diastolic hypertensive responses. The data from these subjects were excluded from analysis, except where noted. The remaining 10 subjects attained a maximum $\dot{V}O_2$/kg body weight within the 95% confidence band of Bruce *et al.*,[9] and did not demonstrate gas exchange or ventilatory mechanical abnormalities to such a degree where one would categorize them as being limited by their pulmonary abnormalities.

The data was dichotomized into an "abnormal" group and a "no demonstrated abnormality" group. For this analysis, symptom scores of 2 or greater for dyspnea or cough were labeled "abnormal," as were Z scores of -1.65 or less for FVC, FEV_1, total lung capacity (TLC), residual volume (RV), DCO, KCO, resting PaO_2, and $P(A\text{-}a)O_2$ (that is, outside the 95% confidence level for normality, as determined using one-tailed tests); in addition, three subjects with high RV and high RV/TLC were labeled as "abnormal."

When patients were divided into two groups (those with, and those without, pulmonary limitation to exercise), abnormal resting $P(A\text{-}a)O_2$, DCO, TLC, and FVC were found to be the most sensitive indicators of whether patients had such limitations. Pulmonary symptoms were present in less than half of the subjects with pulmonary limitation to exercise (TABLE 2). Separating subjects into those without parenchymal infiltration evident on chest X-rays (CXR's) (group A: subjects in stages 0 and 1), and those with parenchymal infiltration evident on CXR's (group B: subjects in stages 2 and 3), demonstrated a significant dichotomy. Four of 14 (29%) group A subjects had demonstrated pulmonary exercise limitation as compared to 21 of 22 (95%) group B subjects. Pulmonary symptoms were present in only one group A subject as compared to 50% of the group B subjects. Approximately 33% of the group A subjects had significant abnormalities of resting physiologic measurements as contrasted to approximately 66% of the group B patients (TABLE 3).

The chest radiograph proved to be the best overall predictor of exercise performance in this study. Twenty-one of the 25 subjects with pulmonary limitation to exercise were in radiographic stages 2 and 3. When these subjects were labeled as "likely abnormal exercise" subjects and those in stages 0 and 1 as "likely normal exercise" subjects, a sensitivity of 84%, a specificity of 90%, a positive predictive value of 95%,

TABLE 2. Abnormal Pulmonary Symptoms and Resting Physiologic Parameters as Indicators of Pulmonary Exercise Limitation.

Indicator	Pulmonary Exercise Limitation[a] Correctly Identified	Not Identified
Cough	9	15(1)
Dyspnea	12	13
PaO_2	14	11
$P(A\text{-}a)O_2$	17	8
FVC	16	9
FEV_1	14	10(1)
TLC	15	9(1)
RV	10	14(1)
DCO	16	5(4)
KCO	7	14(4)

[a]Twenty-five subjects had demonstrated pulmonary exercise limitation. Numbers in parentheses indicate the numbers of missing observations.

TABLE 3. Frequency of Abnormalities of Pulmonary Symptoms, Resting Physiologic Parameters, and Exercise Parameters with Relation to Radiographic Stage

	Number of Patients Displaying Abnormality			
	Group A[b]		Group B	
Abnormality[a]	Stage 0 (N=6)	Stage 1 (N=7)	Stage 2 (N=14)	Stage 3 (N=8)
Rest				
Cough	0	1	6	3
Dyspnea	0	0	10	3
PaO_2	0	3	5	7
$P(A\text{-}a)O_2$	3	5	11	3
FVC	2	0	11	4
FEV_1	0	1	10	3
TLC	1	2	9	6
RV	2	3	6	4
DCO	1	3	8	6
KCO	0	3	3	3
Exercise				
Dyspnea Index (>90)	0	1	3	2
Abnormal f at low V_T	0	1	1	0
V_E/VO_2 (>53)	0	1	1	1
V_E/VCO_2 (>42)	0	3	3	5
V_D/V_T (>30)	0	1	4	5
PaO_2 (<60 mm Hg)	1	0	9	6
Low maximum VO_2/kg body weight	1	1	8	4
Pulmonary exercise limitation (total)	1	3	14	7

[a] Numbers in parentheses indicate threshold values.
[b] Radiographic classification (see text).

a negative predictive value of 69%, and an overall accuracy (test efficiency) of 86% were found (FIG. 1).

We also compared the Z statistic of the physiologic data to the that of the maximum $\dot{V}O_2$ data to determine relationships (TABLE 4). Resting $P(A-a)O_2$ had a low specificity (38%) which reduced its test efficiency to 63% overall. DCO had a high specificity (78%) and, except for CXR staging, had the best overall test efficiency (77%), followed by TLC, FVC, and FEV_1 at 71% and resting PaO_2 at 66%. Pulmonary symptoms of cough and dyspnea were highly specific (90% and 89%, respectively) but had low sensitivities (38% and 48%, respectively). Making the criteria more strict by altering the definitions of abnormality, or limiting the Z values to 1.0, 1.5, or 2.0 SD's from reference values failed to improve upon these test efficiencies, and the accuracy worsened.

We then combined those physiologic tests with the highest test accuracy, DCO, TLC, FVC, and FEV_1, into a "predictive battery." Each test was scored as 0 if normal and 1 if abnormal, and these scores were summed. Scores of 0 to 4 are possible, where 0 meant no abnormalities and 4 meant all four tests were abnormal. We found that

		Pulmonary Disease Limitation	
		Demonstrated	Not Demonstrated
Test Parameter	Abnormal	True Positive (a)	(b) False Positive
	Not Abnormal	False Negative (c)	(d) True Negative

Stable properties:
$a/(a+c)$ = sensitivity
$d/(b+d)$ = specificity

Frequency - dependent properties:
$a/(a+b)$ = positive predictive value
$d/(c+d)$ = negative predictive value
$(a+d)/(a+b+c+d)$ = accuracy: "test efficiency"

FIGURE 1. Schema for defining statistical terminology.

a majority of the patients with pulmonary exercise limitation had high battery scores whereas those subjects without pulmonary exercise limitation had low battery scores (TABLE 5).

Not identified by this screening, however, would have been a 46-year-old black woman with radiographic stage 3 sarcoidosis who desaturated to a PaO_2 of 60 mm Hg on exercise; her only significant abnormality on pre-exercise screening was a complaint of an annoying cough (her resting PaO_2 was 84; her $P(A-a)O_2$, 25). A 50-year-old black male with radiographic stage 2 sarcoidosis complained of a troublesome cough and dyspnea on exertion; his resting physiologic studies failed to demonstrate abnormality apart from a resting $P(A-a)O_2$ of 34 (−2.9 SD's below referent values; PaO_2 was 87). This subject deoxygenated to a PaO_2 of 48 mm Hg with maximal exercise, and he had a respiratory rate of 64 breaths/min with a $\dot{V}E/\dot{V}O_2$ of 52 and a V_D/V_T of 33. Three of five subjects with only one abnormality on routine physiologic screening who had demonstrated pulmonary limitation to exercise also had abnormalities of resting arterial blood gases, that is, of $P(A-a)O_2$ and PaO_2.

$P(A-a)O_2$ usually widens moderately with heavy exercise, possibly due to a lower mixed venous O_2 content or to rapid pulmonary transit or both; however, a $P(A-a)O_2$ greater than 33 is distinctly abnormal.[10,11] Conversely, PaO_2 generally rises with exercise (attributed to decreased $PaCO_2$, increased R, and improved ventilation-perfusion

TABLE 4. Predicting Exercise Limitation due to Pulmonary Disorder

	Sensitivity (%)			Specificity (%)			Positive Predictive Value (%)			Negative Predictive Value (%)			Test Efficiency (Accuracy)		
	All	Group		All	Group		All	Group		All	Group		All	Group	
Parameter	Subjects	A	B	Subjects	A	B	Subjects	A	B	Subjects	A	B	Subjects	A	B
Cough	38	—	43	90	89	—	90	—	100	38	67	—	53	62	43
Dyspnea	48	—	62	89	100	—	92	—	93	38	67	—	59	62	59
Z $P(A\text{-}a)O_2$	68	75	67	38	44	100	77	38	100	38	80	13	63	54	68
Z PaO_2	56	50	57	90	89	100	93	75	100	45	80	10	66	77	59
Z FVC	64	25	71	90	89	100	94	50	100	50	73	14	71	69	73
Z FEV_1	58	33	62	100	100	100	100	100	100	50	82	11	71	83	64
Z TLC	67	25	70	80	78	—	89	33	93	50	70	—	71	62	67
Z RV	42	25	50	50	56	—	67	20	91	26	63	—	44	46	48
Z DL_{CO}	76	100	70	78	75	—	89	50	100	58	100	—	77	80	70
Z KCO	33	50	30	78	75	—	78	33	100	33	86	—	47	70	30
CXR[a]	84			90			95			69			86		

[a] Subjects in stages 0 and 1 (group A) were considered normal; subjects in stages 2 and 3 (group B) were considered abnormal. Abnormality is defined in the text.

matching). Thus a Pa_{O_2} below 75 mm Hg at moderate exercise has been suggested as a marker for disease.[10] In this study, $P(A-a)_{O_2}$ widened to above 33 mm Hg in 29 subjects, to an average of 56 mm Hg. Pa_{O_2} fell in all but five subjects, all of whom had stage 0 and stage 1 radiographic findings. In 16 subjects, the Pa_{O_2} fell to 60 mm Hg or less. The most striking deoxygenation occurred in patients with stage 2 and stage 3 sarcoidosis and in one patient with stage 0 sarcoidosis who had previously had parenchymal infiltrate evident on chest radiography (TABLE 6).

DISCUSSION

Uncertainty as to the natural history of untreated sarcoidosis, and disparities between subjective, radiologic, and physiologic assessments of disease severity (with or without treatment), have frustrated attempts to rigidly assess disease activity. In addition, these problems make it difficult to judge severity and formulate indications for therapeutic intervention.[12] The consensus is that drugs should be administered only to symptomatic patients.[13] The observation has been frequently made, however, that many patients with poor physiologic function do not have significant pulmonary

TABLE 5. The DCO, TLC, FVC, and FEV_1 Predictive Battery

Pulmonary Limitation to Exercise	Total Points[a]					
	0	1	2	3	4	Sum
Yes	2	5	7	2	9	25
No	4	4	2	0	0	10

[a] One point was assigned for each test which evidenced an abnormality.

symptoms and, conversely, that some patients with good function are symptomatic.[14] Winterbauer and Hutchinson[15] urged caution in attaching significance to pulmonary function tests and outlined a scheme utilizing chest radiographs and FVC and DCO values, initially and in follow-up, to guide therapy. They found no evidence that pulmonary compliance or arterial blood gas measurements aided the clinician, but they did not address exercise testing.

It has long been recognized that impairment of gas exchange as demonstrated in widening of the $P(A-a)_{O_2}$ with exercise can be present in sarcoidosis,[16] but only modest widening of the $P(A-a)_{O_2}$ has generally been demonstrated in nonfibrotic sarcoidosis patients.[17–21] These investigators uniformly investigated subjects at submaximal exercise levels, such as 2-5 min of bicycling, or stopped exercise when a level of 1 1/min V_{O_2} or a pulse rate of 120-160/min was reached. Jones and Campbell have addressed the hazards of extrapolating maximal exercise behavior from submaximal exercise testing.[22] We have noted similar difficulty in using pulse rate to determine maximum V_{O_2}, especially in patients with interstitial fibrosis and abnormality of gas exchange.[23] In this study all subjects were exercised to symptom-limited maximum V_{O_2}. Twenty-nine of our 39 patients fell outside the 95% confidence interval for maximum V_{O_2}/kg body weight; 25 of these demonstrated distinctly abnormal responses to exercise.

It is uncommon for exercising subjects to reach a maximal ventilation more than two-thirds their measured MVV.[10,24] Six of our subjects reached a maximum ventilation greater than 90% of their measured MVV. The most common ventilatory pattern with exercise is to increase V_T more than respiratory frequency up to a V_T/VC of 55 ± 8.7.[10] Thereafter, respiratory frequency increases, but rarely above 60 breaths/min. This pattern minimizes work of breathing in patients free of marked restriction

TABLE 6. Change in Arterial Blood Gas Values with Exercise[a]

Radiographic Stage	Rest[b]		Exercise	
	PaO_2	$P(A-a)O_2$	PaO_2	$P(A-a)O_2$
0	79	(26)	57	66
	94	13	76	42
	101	11	96	27
	82	21	75	41
	89	(23)	93	31
	92	16	91	34
	99	(21)	91	34
1	(68)	(22)	85	43
	(84)	(38)	85	43
	87	21	73	53
	88	21	91	35
	98	17	101	25
	100	21	85	44
Mean ± SD	89.93 ± 9.2	20.8 ± 6.4	84.5 ± 11.3	39.8 ± 10.6
2	(62)	(44)	39	82
	(66)	(56)	42	87
	(70)	(32)	60	58
	(77)	(34)	52	72
	(80)	(34)	77	49
	(81)	(26)	55	66
	84	17	66	50
	87	(34)	48	81
	89	(33)	57	72
	89	19	58	64
	89	(28)	77	50
	97	20	50	68
3	(61)	(53)	50	79
	(71)	20	54	67
	(72)	(33)	47	76
	(72)	(36)	54	65
	82	20	47	73
	84	25	60	56
	109	22	76	55
Mean ± SD	80.1 ± 11.8	30.9 ± 10.5	56.3 ± 10.8	66.8 ± 11.2

[a] Data could be obtained from 32 of 39 patients tested. This table incorporates data from all 32 of these patients.

[b] Numbers in parentheses indicate abnormal values. Experimental values were considered abnormal if Z was > −1.65 when compared to reference values for seated, resting patients.

of lung volume. Five of our subjects had a maximal respiratory frequency of 60 breaths/min or higher; two of these were breathing at an abnormally low V_T/VC.

The ventilatory equivalent for V_{O_2} (V_E/V_{O_2}) will normally increase to 35 or 40 with vigorous incremental exercise, especially above about 60 to 70% of maximal

$\dot{V}O_2$. A ratio greater than 53, however, would clearly be abnormal.[10] Three of our patients had a ventilatory equivalent for oxygen above 53, which was associated, in all cases, with other exercise abnormalities. The ventilatory equivalent for CO_2 ($\dot{V}E/\dot{V}CO_2$) normally falls with progressive exercise; an index of greater than 42 would fall outside the 95% confidence limits.[10] Eleven sarcoidosis patients had ventilatory equivalents for CO_2 above this level which were associated with other exercise abnormalities in nine cases. V_D/V_T also normally falls with progressive exercise.[10,25] Ten of our tested sarcoidosis subjects had an abnormally high V_D/V_T at maximal exercise, suggesting worsening matching of perfusion to ventilation and increased dead space.

Significantly abnormal gas exchange in this population was best demonstrated by the marked increases in $P(A-a)O_2$ and marked decreases in PaO_2 which occurred at maximal exercise. Overall, the mean PaO_2 fell from 83.8 to 67.8 and $P(A-a)O_2$ increased from 26.8 to 55.9. Subjects with stage 0 and stage 1 sarcoidosis had less marked changes; their mean PaO_2 decreased from 89.3 to 84.5 and their $P(A-a)O_2$ increased from 20.8 to 39.8. Subjects with stage 2 and stage 3 sarcoidosis had marked changes, with their mean PaO_2 falling from 80.1 to 56.3 and their mean $P(A-a)O_2$ increasing from 30.8 to 66.8.

This frequency and severity of abnormality in gas exchange is more marked than those reported by Miller *et al.*,[26] probably reflecting the more strenuous exercise imposed on our subjects. Our findings are also more abnormal than those reported by Matthews and Hooper,[27] who studied their sarcoidosis subjects with an ear oximeter-monitored bicycle exercise to maximal incremental exercise, but sampled blood gases only at 75% of maximum work load. We demonstrated pulmonary limitation to exercise to occur in 29% of our subjects with stage 0 and stage 1 sarcoidosis, and in 95% of our subjects with stage 2 and stage 3 disease. This compares to an 11% incidence of pulmonary exercise limitation in stage 1, 50% in stage 2, and 75% in stage 3 sarcoidosis subjects reported by Matthews and Hooper.

Colp has reported that a detailed questionnaire or exercise tolerance testing or both improves the correlation between spirometry and DCO studies and the evaluation of respiratory disability in sarcoidosis patients; noteworthy is the fact that she reported some marked discrepancies.[28] We likewise found a high positive predictive value but a low sensitivity for symptoms of cough or dyspnea. Highest test efficiencies in this study occurred with spirometry and DCO and lung volume determinations. Some patients with no spirometric, lung volume, or DCO abnormalities (to the 95% confidence level), however, had significant derangements of exercise performance. Overall, with a preponderance of exercise abnormalities in sarcoidosis patients stages 2 and 3, we could not improve upon the chest radiograph as a predictor of exercise limitation. A finding of multiple abnormal pulmonary function tests strongly suggests, however, that exercise will similarly be abnormal.[27]

Despite the failure of many to correlate pathologic features of sarcoidosis with radiographic parenchymal changes,[17,18,29] our data clearly shows that the radiographic staging of sarcoidosis is associated with significant differences in physiology, as seen in the preponderance of disordered pulmonary function tests and exercise studies among our patients with stage 2 and stage 3 sarcoidosis. In this we agree with the findings of others.[19,30]

In summary, we have demonstrated that severe abnormalities of gas exchange occur more frequently in sarcoidosis than previously reported from submaximal exercise studies. No single test or combination of pulmonary function, arterial blood gas, or pulmonary symptom tests could precisely predict pulmonary limitation to exercise in patients with sarcoidosis. Grading the chest radiograph or scoring the volume-dependent tests (TLC, FVC, FEV_1, and DCO) are the best means of predicting limitation of exercise activity.

ACKNOWLEDGMENT

We wish to thank Mary Wasserman for her patient and dedicated assistance in the typing of this manuscript.

REFERENCES

1. WASSERMAN, K. & B. J. WHIPP. 1975. Exercise physiology in health and disease. Am. Rev. Respir. Dis. **112:** 219-249.
2. MOHLER, J. G. 1982. Quantification of dyspnea confirmed by voice pitch analysis. Bull. Eur. Physiopathol. Respir. **18:** 837-850.
3. MORRIS, J. F., A. KOSKI & L. C. JOHNSON. 1971. Spirometric standards for healthy nonsmoking adults. Am. Rev. Respir. Dis. **103:** 57-67.
4. SELTZER, C., A. B. SIEGELAUB & G. D. FRIEDMAN. 1974. Differences in pulmonary function related to smoking habits and race. Am. Rev. Respir. Dis. **110:** 598-608.
5. GOLDMAN, H. I. & M. R. BECKLAKE. 1959. Respiratory function tests: Normal values at medium altitude and the prediction of normal results. Am. Rev. Tuber. **79:** 457-467.
6. VAN GANSE, W. F. & J. E. COTES. 1972. Cigarette smoking and pulmonary diffusing capacity (transfer factor). Am. Rev. Respir. Dis. **105:** 30-41.
7. MELLEMGAARD, K. 1966. The alveolar-arterial oxygen difference: Its size and components in normal man. Acta Physiol. Scand. **67:** 10-20.
8. FAIRBAIRN, A. S., C. H. WOOD & C. M. FLETCHER. 1959. Variability in answer to questionnaire on respiratory symptoms. Br. J. Prev. Soc. Med. **13:** 175-193.
9. BRUCE, R. A., F. KUSUMI & D. HOSMER. 1973. Maximal oxygen intake and nomographic assessment of functional aerobic impairment in cardiovascular disease. Am. Heart J. **85**(4): 546-562.
10. HANSEN, J. E., D. I. SUE & K. WASSERMAN. 1984. Predicted values for clinical exercise testing. Am. Rev. Respir. Dis. **129**(Suppl.): S49-S55.
11. MOHSENIFAR, Z., D. P. TASHKIN, S. E. LEVY, R. D. BJERKE, P. J. CLEMENTS & D. FURST. 1981. Lack of sensitivity of measurements of V_D/V_T at rest and during exercise in detection of hemodynamically significant pulmonary vascular abnormalities in collagen vascular disease. Am. Rev. Respir. Dis. **123:** 508-512.
12. WILLIAMS, M. H., JR. 1983. Pulmonary function in sarcoidosis. *In* Sarcoidosis and Other Granulomatous Diseases of the Lung. B. L. Fanburg, Ed.: 77-98. Marcel Dekker. New York, NY.
13. SHARMA, O. P. 1984. Sarcoidosis: Clinical Management. Bulterworths. London.
14. COLP, C., S. S. PARK & M. H. WILLIAMS, JR. 1976. Pulmonary function follow-up of 120 patients with sarcoidosis. Ann. N.Y. Acad. Sci. **278:** 301-307.
15. WINTERBAUER, R. H. & J. F. HUTCHINSON. 1980. Clinical significance of pulmonary function tests: Uses of pulmonary function tests in the management of sarcoidosis. Chest **78**(4): 640-647.
16. SVANBORG, N. 1961. Studies on the cardiopulmonary function in sarcoidosis. Acta Med. Scand. Suppl. **170:** 366.
17. YOUNG, R. L., R. E. LORDEN, R. A. KRUMHOLZ, L. E. HARKLEROAD, G. E. BRANAM & J. G. WEG. 1968. Pulmonary sarcoidosis: Pathophysiologic correlations. Am. Rev. Respir. Dis. **97:** 997-1008.
18. CARRINGTON, C. B., E. A. GAENSLER, J. P. MIKUS, A. W. SCHACHTER, G. W. BURKE & A. M. GOFF. 1976. Structure and function in sarcoidosis. Ann. N.Y. Acad. Sci. **278:** 265-283.
19. MILLER, A., A. S. TEIRSTEIN & M. T. CHUANG. 1977. The sequence of physiologic changes in pulmonary sarcoidosis: Correlation with radiographic stages and response to therapy. Mt. Sinai J. Med. N.Y. **44**(6): 852-865.

20. RISK, C., G. R. EPLER & E. A. GAESNER. 1984. Exercise alveolar-arterial oxygen pressure difference in interstitial lung diseases. Chest **85**(1): 69-74.
21. KEOGH, B. A., E. LAKATOS, D. PRICE & R. G. CRYSTAL. 1984. Importance of the lower respiratory tract in oxygen transfer: Exercise testing in patients with interstitial and destructive lung diseases. Am. Rev. Respir. Dis. **129**(Suppl.): S76-S80.
22. JONES, N. L. & E. S. M. CAMPBELL. 1982. Clinical Exercise Testing. W. B. Saunders. Philadelphia, PA.
23. MOHLER, J., L. ATHOS & O. SHARMA. 1983. Dyspnea and voice stress analysis in health, obstructive airways disease and sarcoidosis. Chest **84:** 327.
24. COTES, J. E. 1963. Exercise limitation in health and disease. Br. Med. Bull. **19**(1): 31-36.
25. JONES, N. L., G. J. R. MCHARDY, A. NAIMARK & E. J. M. CAMPBELL. 1966. Physiological dead space and alveolar-arterial gas pressure differences during exercise. Clin. Sci. **31:** 19-29.
26. MILLER, A., M. CHUANG, A. S. TEIRSTEIN & L. E. SILTZBACH. 1976. Pulmonary function in stage I and II pulmonary sarcoidosis. Ann. N.Y. Acad. Sci. **278:** 292-300.
27. MATTHEWS, J. & R. G. HOOPER. 1983. Exercise testing in pulmonary sarcoidosis. Chest **83**(1): 75-81.
28. COLP, C. 1981. Communication to the editor. Chest **80**(2): 245.
29. YOUNG, R. C., J. G. CARR, M. SHELTON, M. MANN, A. FERRIN, J. R. LAUREY & K. A. HARDEN. 1967. Sarcoidosis: Relationship between changes in lung structure and function. Am. Rev. Respir. Dis. **95:** 224-238.
30. HUANG, C. T., A. E. HEUNCH, Y. ROSEN, S. MOON & H. A. LYONS. 1979. Pulmonary sarcoidosis: Roentgenographic, functional and pathologic correlations. Respiration **37:** 337-345.

Total and Regional Lung Function in Sarcoidosis

Smokers versus Nonsmokers[a]

ROBERT E. DUTTON,[b,c] PAOLO M. RENZI,[d,e]
VINCENT LOPEZ-MAJANO,[f] AND GILDO D. RENZI[e]

[c]Albany Medical College
Albany, New York

[e]Notre Dame Hospital
Montreal, Quebec, Canada

[f]Cook County Hospital
Chicago, Illinois

INTRODUCTION

Sarcoidosis is a generalized disease that frequently involves lung parenchyma. Histologically, granulomata are typically deposited in peribronchial and perivascular tissue. They occur in relation to lymphatics, subpleurally, and along lobular septa; they also occur scattered throughout alveolar walls and encroach upon airway epithelium. Subsequent fibrosis can occur and result in widespread interstitial fibrosis, bronchiolectasis, and distortion of airways and lung parenchyma.[1]

The correlation between total pulmonary function tests such as lung volume, diffusion of the lung, and static compliance compared to chest radiographs is poor in early sarcoidosis, and lung volumes, diffusion, and compliance are decreased in advanced fibrosis.[2,3] Most authors ascribe the decreased diffusion to an alveolar-capillary block.[4] An uneven ventilation-perfusion ratio is present in sarcoidosis, however, and this contributes to a decreased diffusion at rest.[5]

Smoking in the absence of other known causes for pulmonary disease has been shown to affect the small airways.[6] Airways normally smaller than 2 mm in diameter are narrowed or obliterated either reversibly by inflammation and mucus or irreversibly by fibrosis. Regional abnormalities consisting of hyperinflation of the lower lobes have been identified in young smokers by the xenon-133 method for determination of

[a]This research was supported by Notre Dame Foundation Grant 6315 and by U.S. Public Health Service–National Institutes of Health Grants HL-12564 and GM-15426.

[b]Address for correspondence: Department of Physiology, Albany Medical College, Albany, New York 12208.

[d]Present address: Pulmonary Unit, Massachusetts General Hospital, Boston, Massachusetts 02181.

regional residual volume.[7] Small airway disease also occurs in nonsmokers with sarcoidosis.[8] The incidence of small airway disease in smokers with sarcoidosis appears to be significantly higher than in smokers without pulmonary disease.[8,9] The combination of smoking and sarcoidosis is apparently synergistic, thus causing small airway obstruction earlier in the course of these diseases.

The objective of the present study was to evaluate the site and severity of pulmonary involvement by means of total and regional lung function tests in order to compare the pathophysiological changes of sarcoidosis alone in nonsmokers with the pathophysiological changes of sarcoidosis in smokers who have an added danger of developing obstructive pulmonary disease due to smoking.

METHODS

Twenty patients, 13 nonsmokers and 7 smokers, with sarcoidosis proven by lymph node or lung biopsy were studied. These studies included previously reported patients who subsequently underwent regional lung function tests,[8] plus other patients not previously reported. The choice of patients was oriented to interstitial and fibrotic lesions of the lung. None of the patients had a history of chronic bronchitis, a history of asthma or repeated respiratory infection, or clinical evidence of pulmonary hypertension or cor pulmonale. Each patient had a negative intradermal tuberculin reaction, a negative sputum cytology, and an absence of pathogenic fungi and bacteria in sputum cultures. Inspiratory posteroanterior and lateral chest radiographs were obtained on each patient. The chest radiographs were graded according to the following classification: stage 0: normal chest radiograph; stage I: bilateral hilar lymphadenopathy; stage II: slight infiltration or fibrosis; stage III: moderate to heavy infiltration or fibrosis. The radiographs were then subdivided into upper, middle, and lower zones and subsequently interpreted by an independent observer for the presence or absence of pulmonary infiltration. Total lung capacity (TLC) and its subdivisions were determined while patients remained seated. Residual volume (RV) was obtained by the helium dilution method.[10] Forced expiratory volume in 1 sec (FEV_1)/forced vital capacity (FVC) was measured as well as maximum midexpiratory flow rate, that is, forced expiratory flow from 25% to 75% of FVC ($FEF_{25-75\%}$). The diffusing capacity of the lung for carbon monoxide was measured by the steady-state end-tidal method.[11] Transpulmonary pressure was measured following the method of Milic-Emilie *et al.*[12] with the use of a Sanborn 267 B transducer. Flow was measured through a Fleisch pneumotachograph connected to a Sanborn 270 transducer. Volume was obtained by electrical flow integration. After previous inspiration to TLC, static pressure-volume curves were constructed by having the patient inspire in a stepwise fashion from functional residual capacity (FRC) to TLC and exhale in the same way. Static compliance (Cs) was obtained on the deflation curve 0.5 to 1.0 l above FRC. Airway resistance (Raw) was obtained by the method of von Neergaard and Wirz.[13]

The regional distribution of ventilation and perfusion as well as the regional distribution of lung volumes were studied with the subject seated in front of 12 scintillation counters, 6 of which were on each side. (Regional lung function studies were performed at the Meakins–Christie Institute, Montreal, Quebec.) Regional count rates were converted to regional concentration.[14] The subject rebreathed xenon-133 from a closed circuit, until the gas was equilibrated, and made a series of breathholds at TLC while regional count rates were recorded. These count rates represented a known, equilibrated xenon-133 concentration and allowed regional count rates resulting from bolus administration to be converted into regional concentration and thence to be reported as an index of ventilation per unit volume.[15] Distribution of regional perfusion in the subject, who remained in the same position, was measured through injection in the antecubital vein of a 2 mCi bolus of xenon-133 and then by a full inspiration to TLC where, again, regional count rates were measured and thence reported as index of perfusion per unit volume. Regional volume at RV or FRC was measured where the subject would inhale from any one of these two volumes, all the way to TLC, a known concentration of xenon-133-enriched air.[15] Regional counts

TABLE 1. Clinical Characteristics of 20 Patients with Sarcoidosis

Patient Number	Age (years)	Sex	Approximate Duration of Disease (years)	Stage of Disease on Chest X-ray
		Nonsmokers		
1	46	F	14	II
2	34	F	6	III
3	66	F	7	II
4	40	M	6	III
5	29	M	1	III
6	35	F	4	III
7	38	F	6	III
8	53	M	4	III
9	47	F	3	III
10	56	F	2	II
11	34	M	4	I
12	47	F	5	II
13	34	F	1	II
Mean ± SEM	43.0 ± 2.4		4.8 ± 0.8	
		Smokers		
14	26	M	5	0
15	43	F	3	III
16	30	F	4	0
17	40	M	1	II
18	25	M	2	II
19	49	F	19	II
20	24	M	1	II
Mean ± SEM	33.9 ± 2.2		5.0 ± 1.4	
Significance[a]	NS		NS	

[a]A difference was not considered significant if p was greater than .05.

would then be measured and related to the regional distribution at TLC during equilibration. Closing volume was obtained by the xenon-133 bolus technique.[9]

RESULTS

TABLE 1 shows the clinical characteristics of 20 patients, 13 nonsmokers and 7 smokers, with sarcoidosis. Their mean age was 39.8 years, and their mean duration of disease was 4.9 years. Although the mean age of smokers was lower than that of nonsmokers, this difference was not statistically significant. The mean duration of disease was also not significantly different between the two groups. Chest radiographs showed parenchymal infiltration in 17 out of 20 patients.

Pulmonary function values for both groups are illustrated in TABLES 2 & 3; some of these values are expressed as percentages of those that would have been predicted for healthy controls (% predicted). There was no significant difference between nonsmokers and smokers in vital capacity, but TLC was increased in the smokers ($p <$ .02), as well as RV ($p < .01$). The RV/TLC ratio remained comparable between the groups. DL_{co} and Cs were moderately decreased in both groups and were not significantly different. TABLE 3 compares the airway function in nonsmokers and smokers. Total tests for airway function did not reveal any differences between groups. The most important abnormalities were found in the $FEF_{25-75\%}$, Raw at 60 breaths/min (Raw_{60}), and closing volume (CV/VC). The test for CV/VC is a regional one due to the effect of gravity on the lung in the upright position. CV/VC is expressed in TABLE 3 as a ratio of absolute determinations and as a percentage of the value that would have been predicted for healthy controls.

TABLE 4 shows regional lung function data obtained by the xenon-133 techniques. There was no difference between nonsmokers and smokers in the regional distribution of ventilation, that is, their respective ventilation indices, but the incidence of abnormal regional lung volumes was significantly higher in the smokers ($p < .05$). FIGURE 1 compares the number of abnormal regions on chest radiographs versus static compliance (Cs) for all patients ($r = -.45$, $p < .05$). The correlation of Cs with the number of these regions is much higher when smokers are excluded ($r = -.63$, $p < .01$).

Pulmonary function tests were compared statistically for significant correlations. A low, but significant correlation was found between CV/VC (% predicted) and $FEF_{25-75\%}$ ($r = -.45$, $p < .05$) (FIG. 2). The dashed lines in the figure indicate the lower limit of normal $FEF_{25-75\%}$ (% predicted) at 80% and the upper limit of normal CV/VC (% predicted) at 120%. Both of these tests are indicative of the presence of small airway disease if large airway disease has been excluded by normal FEV_1/FVC ($\geq$ 70%) plus an airway resistance during spontaneous breathing of 4 cm $H_2O/1/$sec or less. All smokers had a CV/VC (% predicted) greater than 120%.[8] Only four subjects, all nonsmokers, had no evidence of airway disease in these tests (right lower quadrant of the figure). Five of the seven smokers were abnormal on both tests, but three of the five had evidence of large airway disease, thus rendering a diagnosis of small airway disease invalid on the basis of CV/VC or $FEF_{25-75\%}$. Small airway disease, however, has not been excluded in those three patients.

There was also a significant correlation between Raw during spontaneous breathing and FEV_1/FVC ($r = -.58$, $p < .01$). The correlation is much reduced if the one patient (number 3) with severe airway disease, as reflected by a $Raw_{SP\ BR}$ of 12 cm $H_2O/1/sec$, is excluded from the analysis ($r = -.42$, $p < .05$).

The xenon-133 RV ventilation index obtained during an inspiration from RV showed abnormal regions that correlated with the degree of abnormality of dynamic compliance measured at 60 breaths/min (Cd_{60}). As the number of zones of $\dot{V}$ index abnormalities increases, the Cd_{60} decreases ($r = -.64$, $p < .01$) (FIG. 3).

FIGURE 4 shows the number of abnormal regions determined by the xenon-133 RV ventilation index in 13 nonsmokers and 7 smokers. The highest proportion of abnormalities was in the upper lobes. There was no significant difference between nonsmokers and smokers by chi-square analysis, and 51 of 58 abnormalities were due to decreases in the ventilation index (TABLE 4). All seven increases, however, were in smokers.

TABLE 2. Pulmonary Function Data in 20 Patients with Sarcoidosis

Patient Number	VC[a]	TLC[a]	RV[a]	RV/TLC (× 100)	DL_{CO}	Cs[b] (l/cm H_2O)
			Nonsmokers			
1	102	94	77	28	111	0.147
2	65	85	122	44	70	0.058
3	72	79	90	43	55	0.125
4	73	78	81	29	52	0.161
5	58	74	123	40	76	0.066
6	89	89	91	30	89	0.120
7	84	98	112	36	75	0.080
8	64	85	113	44	78	0.123
9	83	88	85	32	87	0.107
10	114	115	105	32	65	0.162
11	109	111	101	24	77	0.232
12	90	103	124	41	84	0.178
13	80	80	81	33	73	0.068
Mean ± SEM	83.3 ± 3.9	90.7 ± 2.9	100.4 ± 3.9	35.1 ± 1.5	76.3 ± 3.8	0.125 ± 0.010
			Smokers			
14	91	97	109	24	69	0.118
15	74	82	88	35	69	0.096
16	104	116	138	37	63	0.131
17	101	125	161	37	84	0.296
18	103	114	133	29	118	0.095
19	93	125	181	50	60	0.200
20	83	103	166	38	—	0.145
Mean ± SEM	92.7 ± 2.5	108.9 ± 3.5	139.4 ± 7.4	36.4 ± 1.6	77.2 ± 5.0	0.154 ± 0.020
Significance[c]	NS	$p < .02$	$p < .01$	NS	NS	NS

[a]Each of these values is expressed as a percentage of the value that would have been predicted for healthy controls.
[b]Normal Cs = 0.200.
[c]A difference was not considered significant if p was greater than .05.

TABLE 3. Airway Function Data in 20 Patients with Sarcoidosis

Patient Number	FEV_1/FVC (× 100)	$FEF_{25-75\%}$ [a]	$Raw_{SP\ BR}$ (cm H_2O/1/sec)	Raw_{60} (cm H_2O/1/sec)	Cd_{60}/Cs (× 100)	CV/VC (× 100)	CV/VC[a]
			Nonsmokers				
1	71	51	3.3	4.3	79	20	110
2	59	16	12.0	25.0	—	40	350
3	92	145	2.1	2.6	—	16	106
4	66	69	2.0	3.4	67	14	88
5	83	49	3.6	3.0	53	18	150
6	88	98	3.6	3.6	70	19	130
7	91	90	3.8	3.3	92	16	100
8	73	44	3.1	2.6	79	28	133
9	63	34	6.0	6.1	44	28	155
10	77	96	2.3	2.1	96	25	114
11	85	136	1.0	1.3	100	26	186
12	82	93	1.9	2.2	114	34	190
13	93	105	—	—	—	12	90
Mean ± SEM	78.7 ± 2.6	78.9 ± 8.7	3.73 ± 0.67	4.96 ± 1.48	79.4 ± 5.3	22.8 ± 2.8	146.3 ± 15.6
			Smokers				
14	73	51	2.1	3.7	86	16	140
15	80	69	3.4	3.8	72	20	128
16	68	42	6.7	9.6	106	20	170
17	80	100	4.0	2.6	95	25	156
18	61	41	4.7	7.5	109	32	290
19	78	93	1.3	1.7	73	14	127
20	79	62	4.4	3.4	102	25	132
Mean ± SEM	74.1 ± 1.6	65.4 ± 5.3	3.80 ± 0.41	4.61 ± 0.65	91.9 ± 3.7	21.7 ± 1.4	163.3 ± 13.0
Significance[b]	NS	NS	NS	NS	NS	NS	NS

[a] Each of these values is expressed as a percentage of the value that would have been predicted for healthy controls.
[b] A difference was not considered significant if p was greater than .05.

TABLE 4. Regional Abnormalities Detected Using Radiography and Xenon-133 RV Indices

Patient Number	Regional Abnormalities[a]					
	Radiography		Ventilation Index		Volume Index	
	Location[b]	Number	Location[c]	Number	Location[c]	Number
Nonsmokers						
1[d]	RU,LU	2	↓RU,↓LU	2	Normal	0
2	RU,RM,RL,LU,LM,LL	6	↓RU,↓LM,↓LL	3	↓RU,↑RL,↓LU,↑LL	4
3[d]	RU,LU	2	↓RU,↓LU,↓RL	3	Normal	0
4[d]	RU,RM,RL,LU,LM,LL	6	↓RU,↓LU,↓LM	3	↓RU,↓LU	2
5[d]	RU,RM,RL,LU,LM,LL	6	↓RU	1	↓RU	1
6	RU,RM,RL,LU,LM,LL	6	↓RM,↓RL,↓LM,↓LL	4	Normal	0
7[d]	RU,RM,RL,LU,LM	5	↓RU,↓RL,↓LU,↓LM,↓LL	5	Normal	0
8[d]	RU,RM,RL,LU,LM,LL	6	↓RU,↓RM,↓RL,↓LU,↓LM,↓LL	6	—	—
9	RU,RM,RL,LU,LM	5	↓RU,↓RM,↓RL,↓LU,↓LM	5	↓RU,↓LU	2
10[d]	RU	1	↓RU,↓LU,↓LL	3	↓RU	1
11	Normal	0	Normal	0	Normal	0
12[d]	LL	1	↓RL	1	Normal	0
13	RU,LU	2	↓RU,↓LU	2	↓RU	1
Mean ± SEM		3.8 ± 0.5		2.9 ± 0.4		0.6 ± 0.2
Smokers						
14	Normal	0	↓RU,↓LU	2	↓LU,↑LL	2
15[e]	RU,RM,RL,LU,LM,LL	6	↑RU,↓RL,↑LU,↓LL	4	↓LU,↑LL,↑RL	3
16[e]	Normal	0	↓RU,↓LU	2	↓LU,↑LL,↑RL	3
17[d]	RU,RM,LU	3	Normal	0	↓LU,↓RU,↑RL	3
18	RU,RM,LU	3	↑RU,↑RM,↓RL,↓LM,↓LL	5	↓LU,↑LL,↓RU,↓RM	4
19[e]	LL	1	↑RU,↓RL,↑LU,↓LL	4	↑RL	1
20[e]	RU,LU	2	↑RU,↓RL,↓LL	3	↓RU,↑RL,↑LL	3
Mean ± SEM		2.1 ± 0.5		2.9 ± 0.4		2.7 ± 0.4
Significance[f]		NS		NS		$p < .05$

[a] R: right; L: left; U: upper; M: middle; L: lower.
[b] The regions below were abnormal because of increased density.
[c] The regions below were abnormal because of increased (↑) or decreased (↓) density.
[d] Patients that were normal according to xenon-133 regional perfusion studies.
[e] Patients that were abnormal according to xenon-133 regional perfusion studies (15: ↓RL; 16: ↑RU,↓RL; 19: ↓RL,↓LL; 20: ↓RL,↓LL).
[f] A difference was not considered significant if p was greater than .05.

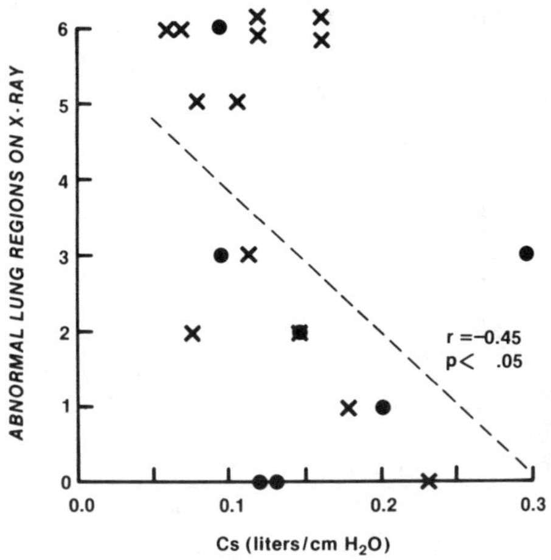

FIGURE 1. The number of abnormal regions of increased density evident in chest radiographs plotted against Cs of the lungs for individual nonsmokers (×) and smokers (●) with sarcoidosis ($r = -.45$, $p < .05$). The dashed line, obtained by linear regression analysis, yields the following equation: number of abnormal regions evident in radiographs = -17.88 Cs + 5.62 ($p < .05$).

FIGURE 5 shows the number of abnormal regions determined by xenon-133 volume index as measured from RV in 12 nonsmokers and 7 smokers. In contrast to the results of the ventilation index, there was a significantly higher incidence, determined by Student's t test and chi-square analysis, of regional volume abnormalities as measured by the volume index in smokers (TABLE 4). This was due to the presence of hyperinflation of the lower lobes in smokers as compared to nonsmokers (note the asterisks and solid bars in FIG. 5). The remaining abnormalities, predominantly in the upper lobes, were all reductions in volume index. The difference between nonsmokers and smokers yielded a chi-square of 8.3 using Yates' correction ($p < .001$). This combination of reduced volume in the upper lobes and hyperinflation of the lower lobes resulted in a loss of the normal gradient of volume index from apex to base in one or both lungs in six of the seven smokers with sarcoidosis.

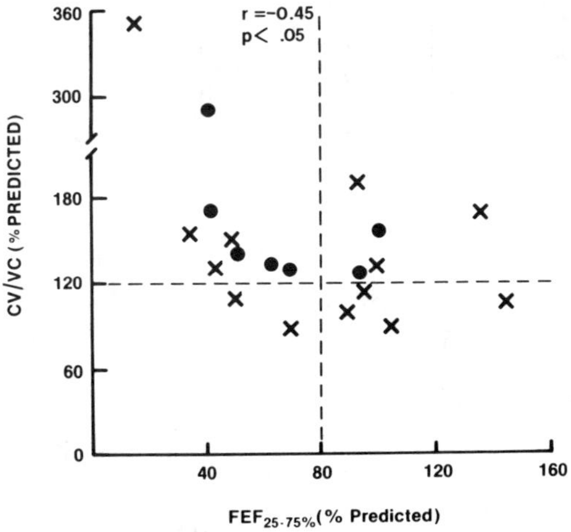

FIGURE 2. The xenon-133 CV/VC (% predicted) plotted against the $FEF_{25-75\%}$ (% predicted) for individual nonsmokers (×) and smokers (●) ($r = -.45$, $p < .05$). The dashed lines indicate the lower limit of normal $FEF_{25-75\%}$ (% predicted) and upper limit of normal CV/VC (% predicted). Linear regression analysis yields the following equation: CV/VC (% predicted) = -0.85 $FEF_{25-75\%}$ (% predicted) + 215.5 ($p < .05$).

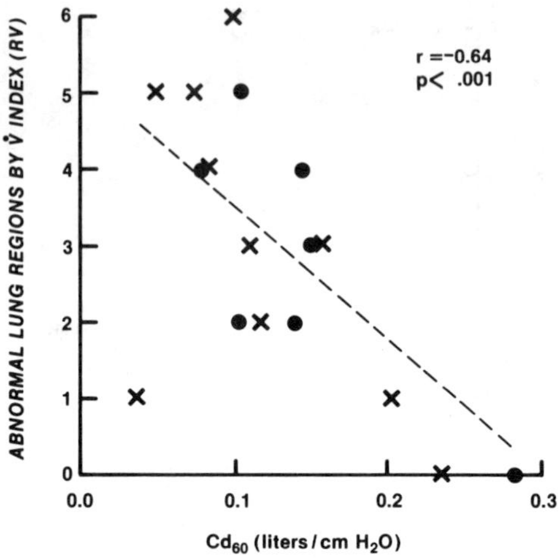

FIGURE 3. The number of abnormal lung regions found using the xenon-133 RV ventilation index plotted against Cd_{60} for individual nonsmokers (×) and smokers (●) ($r = -.64$, $p < .05$). The dashed line, obtained by linear regression analysis, yields the following equation: number of abnormal regions found using the xenon-133 RV ventilation index $= -16.6\ Cd_{60} + 4.7$.

FIGURE 6 shows the distribution of abnormal regions determined by radiography. The number of abnormalities is greater than those found with either the xenon-133 $\dot{V}$ or volume indices, and the abnormalities are predominantly in the upper lobes. This greater frequency of abnormalities is due to the high incidence in nonsmokers, as smokers had a reduced number of abnormalities apparent on radiographs when compared to either the $\dot{V}$ index or the volume index. The perfusion index was normal in the eight nonsmokers tested. There was a decrease in the perfusion index in one or both bases of four of five smokers tested (TABLE 4). This is significant by Fisher's exact test ($p < .05$).

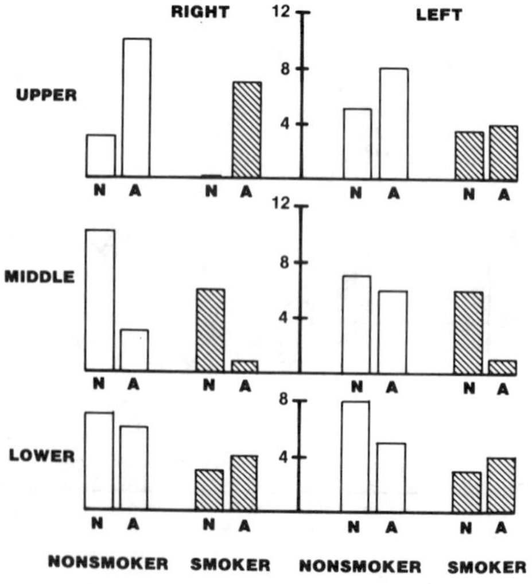

FIGURE 4. The number of abnormal lung regions (A), in each of the three zones of the lung, found using the xenon-133 RV ventilation index compared to the number of normal regions (N) for 13 nonsmokers and 7 smokers with sarcoidosis. All but 7 of 58 abnormal regions were decreases in the RV ventilation index. The seven increases in the RV ventilation index were in smokers (see TABLE 4).

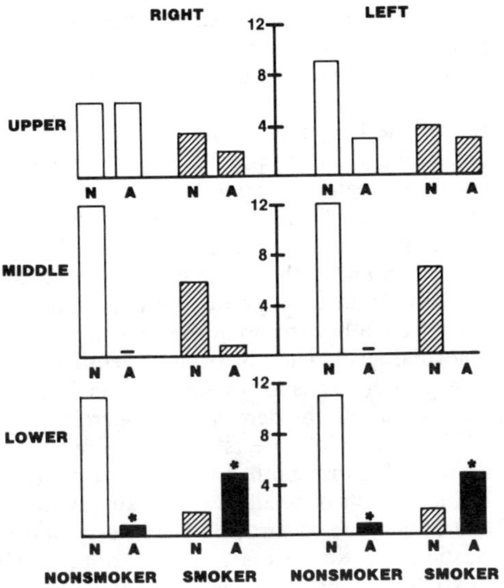

FIGURE 5. The number of abnormal lung regions (A), in each of the three zones of the lung, found using the xenon-133 RV volume index compared to the number of normal regions (N) for 12 nonsmokers and 7 smokers with sarcoidosis. All lower zone abnormalities were increases in the RV volume index (solid bars). All middle and upper zone abnormalities were decreases in the RV volume index.

DISCUSSION

Sarcoidosis has been classically described as a disease that creates physiological abnormalities of a restrictive nature, which in turn lead to losses of lung volume, reduced pulmonary compliance, and abnormalities in gas exchange.[16–20] Sarcoidosis also frequently affects airway function in both nonsmokers and smokers.[3,8,21–24] Smoking is a well-recognized cause of small airway obstruction.[9,25,26] A significantly higher

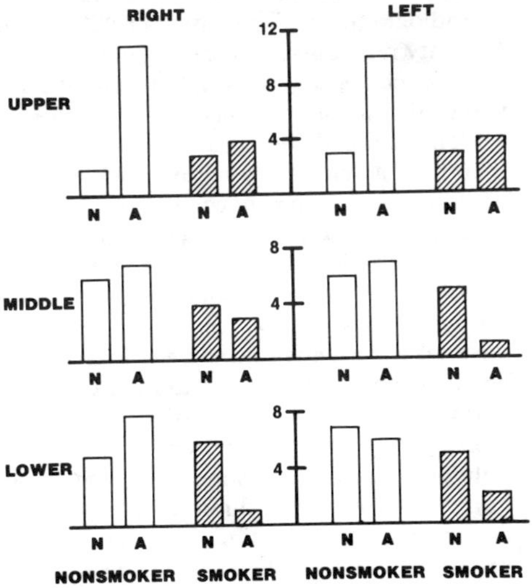

FIGURE 6. The number of abnormal lung regions (A), that is, regions showing parenchymal infiltration, in each of the three zones of the lung, evident in chest radiographs compared to the number of normal lung regions (N) for 13 nonsmokers and 7 smokers with sarcoidosis.

occurrence of airway obstruction in smokers with sarcoidosis led Dutton *et al.*[8] to propose that smoking and sarcoidosis have a detrimental synergism that induces a high incidence of hyperinflation of the lungs in smokers with sarcoidosis as compared to smokers with otherwise normal lungs. Coates and Comroe[16] observed an increased RV of the lung in patients with sarcoidosis, but did not differentiate smokers from nonsmokers. In the present study, significantly higher RV and TLC were found in smokers. Regional lung volumes determined by the xenon-133 method have identified the location of this hyperinflation to be at the lung bases in smokers. Only one nonsmoker had hyperinflation of lower lobes by this test, thus making a compensatory hyperinflation of the lower lobes in response to restrictive disease in the upper lobes unlikely as an eitology for the hyperinflation. Restrictive disease in the upper lobes does place a burden upon the remainder of the lung to sustain alveolar ventilation at a normal level. The diversion of ventilation to the lower lobes in smokers may result in a greater exposure to smoke than in smokers with otherwise normal lungs, thus accounting for the detrimental synergism of smoking and sarcoidosis.

Total or global tests of airway function did not differentiate nonsmokers from smokers because both groups had important deviations from normal in each test, including tests of small and large airway function. This confirms the presence of airway alterations due to sarcoidosis alone in nonsmokers. In lung diseases leading to high elastic recoil, such as sarcoidosis, both reversible and irreversible (fibrotic) lesions tend to stiffen the parenchyma and hold airways open during dynamic maneuvers, thus masking the severity of airway involvement. Powell *et al.*[24] have recommended maximal expiratory flow-pressure measurements as an additional precise method of defining airway abnormalities in the presence of high elastic recoil, but these were not obtained in the present patients.

Inherent to any study of regional ventilation are flow rates. Xenon-133 ventilation studies were done using flow rates less than 0.3 1/sec or in quasi-static conditions. Regional distribution of ventilation under these conditions is determined by regional compliance. Thus, one can assume that regional stiffness rather than small airway alterations is the cause of an abnormal xenon-133 ventilation index. This may account for the finding of a normal xenon-133 ventilation index in lower lung zones when both an increased xenon-133 volume index and an elevated CV are present. The negative correlation between Cs and the incidence of regional abnormalities evident on radiographs is also consistent with the presence of regional stiffness. There is less certainty regarding the meaning of a negative correlation between dynamic compliance and the incidence of xenon-133 ventilation abnormalities because dynamic compliance is sensitive to the presence of airway obstruction as well as regional stiffness.

The regional abnormalities in nonsmokers with sarcoidosis appear to be predominantly of a ventilatory nature, mostly diminished in the upper lobes, while perfusion is maintained within normal limits. The perfusion index was found to be normal in all the nonsmokers tested. This is in sharp contrast to the findings of McCarthy and Cherniak,[26] who studied regional ventilation-perfusion ratios in cryptogenic fibrosing alveolitis. While they found the distribution of ventilation to be normal, perfusion at the lung bases was decreased and was redistributed to the upper and middle zones. Arterial hypoxemia and increased alveolar-arterial gradients of oxygen tension could be correlated with the distribution of pulmonary blood flow, but not with the distribution of pulmonary ventilation. This was accompanied by marked hypoxemia, pulmonary hypertension, and cor pulmonale. West[27] has predicted that with increasing pulmonary artery pressure, perfusion of the lung in a seated patient would become more uniform, with a diminution of the top to bottom gradient normally present. An abnormal pattern of diminished perfusion at one or both lower zones was observed in four of five smokers in the present study, but perfusion appeared to be well maintained in the remainder of the lungs. In our series no patients with pulmonary infiltration had clinical, radiological, or electrocardiographic evidence of pulmonary hypertension or cor pulmonale. The well-maintained perfusion of the lung may be responsible for the favorable prognosis in sarcoidosis as reported by Hoyle.[28]

Regional abnormalities evident in chest radiographs were more frequent than regional abnormalities during any xenon-133 test. This indicates a greater sensitivity of the radiographic method to the presence of disease. A relative lack of sensitivity of the xenon-133 methods occurs in the presence of diffuse lung disease. If regional abnormalities are distributed equally in all zones, xenon-133 methods will fail to detect any abnormality. For example, in the present study patient number 5 had six abnormal regions evident in radiographs, and his pulmonary function tests were compatible with lung fibrosis. Regional xenon-133 studies showed only one territorial abnormality for ventilation and lung volume. Despite this limitation, xenon-133 studies are useful in defining regional inequalities of lung function when they exist. There was a good correlation between the number of abnormal regions evident in radiographs and the xenon-133 ventilation index ($r = .61$). This would have been even higher if the above limitation did not exist.

In summary, total pulmonary function tests, regional interpretation of the chest radiograph, and regional pulmonary function tests by means of xenon-133 methods are complementary and provide information that expands our understanding of the physiopathology of the lung in patients with sarcoidosis whether they are nonsmokers or smokers. A dominant feature in smokers with sarcoidosis is hyperinflation of the lower lobes and loss of the normal regional volume gradient from top to bottom in the lungs. The hyperinflation is accompanied by a high incidence of impaired blood flow to these lobes, requiring redistribution of blood flow to the middle and upper zones of the lungs.

REFERENCES

1. Longcope, W. T. & D. H. Freiman. 1952. A study of sarcoidosis based on a combined investigation of 160 cases including 30 autopsies from the Johns Hopkins Hospital and Massachusetts General Hospital. Medicine **31:** 1-32.
2. Snider, G. L. & L. R. Doctor. 1964. The mechanics of ventilation in sarcoidosis. Am. Rev. Respir. Dis. **89:** 897-908.
3. Renzi, G. & R. E. Dutton. 1974. Pulmonary function in diffuse sarcoidosis. Respiration **31:** 124-136.
4. Hamer, N. A. J. 1963. Changes in the components of the diffusing capacity in pulmonary sarcoidosis. Thorax **18:** 275-287.
5. Renzi, G., N. R. Antonisen, A. Grassino, L. Knight & R. R. Martin. 1974. Regional lung function in sarcoidosis. Scand. J. Respir. Dis. Suppl. **85:** 64.
6. Hogg, J. C., P. T. Macklem & W. M. Thurlbeck. 1968. Site and nature of airway obstruction in chronic obstructive lung disease. N. Engl. J. Med. **278:** 1355-1360.
7. York, L. E. & R. L. Jones. 1981. Effect of smoking on regional residual volume in young adults. Chest **79:** 12-15.
8. Dutton, R. E., P. M. Renzi, V. Lopez-Majano & G. D. Renzi. 1982. Airway function in sarcoidosis: Smokers versus nonsmokers. Respiration **43:** 164-173.
9. McCarthy, D. S., R. Spencer, R. Greene & J. Milic-Emili. 1972. Measurement of "closing volume" as a simple and sensitive test for early detection of small airway disease. Am. J. Med. **52:** 747-753.
10. Meneely, G. R., C. O. T. Ball, R. C. Kary, J. J. Gallaway, J. M. Merrill, R. E. Mabe, D. C. Roehm & N. L. Kaltreider. 1960. A simplified closed circuit helium

dilution method for the determination of the residual volume of the lungs. Am. J. Med. **28:** 824-831.

11. Bates, D. V., C. R. Woolf & S. D. Paul. 1962. Chronic bronchitis: A report on the first two stages of the coordinated study of chronic bronchitis in the Department of Veterans Affairs, Canada. Med. Serv. J. Can. **18:** 211-279.
12. Milic-Emilie, J., J. Mead, J. M. Turner & E. M. Glauser. 1964. Improved technique for estimating pleural pressure from esophageal balloons. J. Appl. Physiol. **19:** 207-211.
13. von Neergaard, K. & K. Wirz. 1927. Über eine Methode zur Messung der Lungen-elastizät am lebenden Menschen insbesondere beim Emphysem. Z. Klin. Med. **105:** 35-82.
14. Ball, W. C., Jr., P. B. Stewart, L. G. S. Newsham & D. V. Bates. 1962. Regional pulmonary function with xenon-133. J. Clin. Invest. **41:** 519-531.
15. Milic-Emili, J., J. A. M. Henderson, M. B. Dolovich, D. Trop & K. Kaneko. 1966. Regional distribution of inspired gas in the lung. J. Appl. Physiol. **21:** 749-759.
16. Coates, E. O. & J. H. Comroe, Jr. 1951. Pulmonary function studies in sarcoidosis. J. Clin. Invest. **30:** 848-852.
17. Austrian, R., J. McClement & A. D. Renzetti. 1951. Clinical and physiologic features of some types of pulmonary disease with impairment of alveolar-capillary diffusion. Am. J. Med. **11:** 667-685.
18. Riley, R. L., M. C. Riley & H. McD. Hill. 1952. Diffuse pulmonary sarcoidosis: Diffusing capacity during exercise and other lung function studies in relation to ACTH therapy. Bull. Johns Hopkins Hosp. **91:** 345-370.
19. Sellers, R. D. & A. A. Siebens. 1965. The effects of sarcoidosis on pulmonary function with particular reference to changes in pulmonary compliance. Am. Rev. Respir. Dis. **91:** 660-664.
20. Young, R. C., Jr., C. Carr, T. G. Shelton, M. Marin, A. Ferrin, J. R. Laurey & K. A. Harden. 1967. Sarcoidosis: Relationship between changes in lung structure and function. Am. Rev. Respir. Dis. **98:** 224-238.
21. Levinson, R. S., L. F. Metzger, S. N. Nigel, S. G. Kelsen, M. D. Altose, N. S. Cherniack & J. S. Brody. 1977. Airway function in sarcoidosis. Am. J. Med. **62:** 51-59.
22. Kaneko, K. & O. P. Sharma. 1977. Airway obstruction in pulmonary sarcoidosis. Bull. Eur. Physiopathol. Respir. **13:** 231-240.
23. Renzi, G., P. M. Renzi, V. Lopez-Majano & R. E. Dutton. 1981. Airway function in sarcoidosis: Effect of short-term steroid therapy. Respiration **42:** 98-104.
24. Powell, E., G. Renzi & P. T. Macklem. 1980. Severity and site of airflow obstruction in sarcoidosis. Am. Rev. Respir. Dis. **121**(Suppl.): 178.
25. McFadden, E. R., R. Kiker, B. Holmes & W. J. DeGroot. 1974. Small airway disease: An assessment of the tests of peripheral airway disease. Am. J. Med. **57:** 171-182.
26. McCarthy, D. & R. M. Cherniak. 1973. Regional ventilation-perfusion and hypoxia in cryptogenic fibrosing alveolitis. Am. Rev. Respir. Dis. **107:** 200-208.
27. West, J. B. 1969. Ventilation-perfusion inequality and overall gas exchange in computer models of the lung. Respir. Physiol. **7:** 88-110.
28. Hoyle, C. 1961. Prognosis of pulmonary sarcoidosis. Lancet **ii:** 611-615.

The Long-term Course of Airflow Obstruction in Obstructive Variants of the Fibrotic Stage of Sarcoidosis and of Idiopathic Pulmonary Fibrosis

J. MEIER-SYDOW, M. G. RUST, A. KAPPOS,
H. KRONENBERGER, K. NERGER, AND
G. SCHULTZE-WERNINGHAUS

Division of Pneumology
Department of Internal Medicine
Hospital of the Johann Wolfgang Goethe University
Frankfurt, Federal Republic of Germany

INTRODUCTION

Pulmonary fibrosis is, in functional terms, a restrictive disorder. But it is an old clinical experience that in addition to restriction, an airflow obstruction (AO) may occur. This experience refers to extrinsic diseases like tuberculosis with a diffuse cicatrization, the fibrotic stage of coal worker's pneumoconiosis, and many others. It also refers to cryptogenic entities.

Recently we gave a review[1] on clinical entities showing the association of diffuse pulmonary fibrosis and AO. We proposed a classification and mentioned some elements of the pathogenesis.

TABLE 1 gives examples of the incidence of AO in two cryptogenic conditions, the fibrotic stage of sarcoidosis (FSS) and idiopathic pulmonary fibrosis (IPF), with a remarkable agreement between different authors.[1–6] Another example[7] is histiocytosis X with the same incidence of obstructive variants (21%).

In previous studies[4,8,9] we presented comparative data of nonobstructive versus obstructive variants of these two conditions. The results are summarized in TABLE 2. Two remarkable aspects should be emphasized: 1) the degree and the constancy of the parameters indicating AO, and 2) the experience that the additional load of AO generally makes the patient suffer more but does not essentially influence the prognosis.

The topic of this presentation is restricted to the phenomenon of AO. Therefore our study deals exclusively with the obstructive variants of the two conditions. Moreover, only the parameters of AO, their progression or nonprogression in the course of the disease, will be presented. It has to be emphasized that only cases with definite airflow obstruction are dealt with, not, for instance, small airway disease.

The study has to answer two questions: 1) What is the long-term course of AO

TABLE 1. Reported Incidence of AO in patients with an FSS and IPF

Disorder	Number of Patients with AO[a]	FEV_1/VC (%)	Raw ($cm\ H_2O \cdot sec \cdot l^{-1}$)	Reference Number
FSS	7/19 (37)	<70		2
	6/16 (38)	<70		3
	8/14 (57)	<70	>3.5	4
IPF	4/19 (21)	<70		5
	13/53 (24)	<70		6
	7/37 (19)	<70	>3.5	4

[a] The fraction shows the number of patients out of the study population that had AO. The corresponding percentage is indicated in parentheses.

in FSS and IPF? 2) Do the two parameters of AO, forced expiratory volume in 1 sec related to vital capacity (FEV_1/VC) and airway resistance (Raw), run parallel or do they divert?

MATERIALS AND METHODS

For this study we selected patients who had a fibrotic lung disease—synonymous with pulmonary fibrosis—in association with definite AO. A fibrotic lung disease was considered to be present in a patient if his history was compatible with an interstitial lung disease, his radiographs showed signs of fibrotic lung disease, his biopsy was positive, and his lung function parameters showed a restrictive pattern. A definite AO was assumed with $FEV_1/VC < 65\%$. The minimum follow-up period was 4 years.

Depending on the course of the two parameters, FEV_1/VC and Raw, both calculated between the initial and the last determination, we assigned our patients to three groups. Group 1 did not have a significant change of either parameter, group 2 had a significant concordant change of both parameters, and group 3 had a significant divergent change of at least one of the two parameters.

Two patients who died during the first 2 years of the follow-up period had to be excluded from the evaluation because an assignment to one of the three groups after such a short follow-up period did not seem reasonable.

A change was considered to be significant if FEV_1/VC changed $\geq 20\%$. The

TABLE 2. Nonobstructive versus Obstructive Variants of FSS and IPF[a]

Degree of restriction	Considerable (VC about 2 l); no difference between FSS and IPF; no difference between nonobstructive and obstructive variants of the disease.
Degree of AO	Considerable (FEV_1/VC about 60%, Raw about 3.5 $cm\ H_2O \cdot sec \cdot l^{-1}$); no difference between FSS and IPF.
Course	Restriction and airway obstruction essentially constant over 3 to 4 years.
Prognosis	No significant difference between nonobstructive and obstructive variants of FSS and IPF.

[a] This table incorporates results from experiments conducted between 1980 and 1983.

change of Raw was considered to be significant if the difference was $\geq 25\%$ and at least 2 cm $H_2O \cdot sec \cdot l^{-1}$.

FEV_1 and VC were measured using a pneumotachograph; Raw was measured using a volume-constant body plethysmograph (E. Jaeger, Würzburg).

RESULTS

TABLE 3 shows the distribution we found for our 19 patients. About half of them had no significant change of both parameters (group 1). Only three patients showed a concordant change (group 2): all of them deteriorated. Of special interest were the remaining seven patients with a divergency of the two parameters: five of them had no change of FEV_1/VC, but a significant increase of Raw. Two patients showed different patterns.

TABLE 4 describes our patients. As far as sex and age distribution are concerned, there was no significant difference between the groups. FSS was found mainly in group

TABLE 3. Assignment of Patients According to the Course of FEV_1/VC and Raw[a]

	FEV_1/VC	Raw	*N*
Group 1	Stable	Stable	9
Group 2	Deteriorated	Deteriorated	3
	Improved	Improved	0
Group 3	Stable	Deteriorated	5
	Stable	Improved	1
	Deteriorated	Stable	1
	Improved	Stable	0

[a] Patients with stable FEV_1/VC values were assigned to group 1; patients with concordant changes in these values, to group 2; patients with divergent changes in these values, to group 3.

1 whereas IPF was distributed evenly. There was a considerable proportion of patients with a smoking history in all three groups. TABLE 5 compiles the lung function at the time of the initial evaluation. It is apparent that the restriction and the AO are both considerable in all groups. The parameters did not differ significantly between group 1 and group 3. Group 2 could not be compared because it comprised only three patients.

FIGURE 1 shows the course of FEV_1/VC and of Raw in group 1. It was astonishing to find that about half of our patients were assigned to this group with stable parameters of AO. Moreover, this constancy was maintained for long follow-up periods.

FIGURE 2 shows the course of the two parameters in group 2, which comprised only a minority of our patients. In these three patients FEV_1/VC and Raw both deteriorated.

FIGURE 3 shows group 3 comprising patients in whom we found a divergency as far as the course of both parameters is concerned. In the majority of patients (five out of seven) FEV_1/VC did not change while Raw increased. From the remaining two patients one improved concerning the Raw, and the other deteriorated concerning the FEV_1/VC, keeping the other parameter constant (TABLE 3).

TABLE 4. Study Population[a]

	Group		
	1	2	3
Total number of patients	9	3	7
Number of females	5	2	4
Number of males	4	1	3
Average age of patients (years)	48.3 ± 9.4	56.3	46.8 ± 18.1
Number of patients with FSS	5	2	2
Number of patients with IPF	4	1	6
Number of smokers or exsmokers	6	3	4

[a] Two patients could not be assigned to a group because they died during the first 2 years of follow-up.

DISCUSSION

The phenomenon of AO in diffuse pulmonary fibrosis has been thoroughly discussed recently.[1] Therefore in this context we will restrict ourselves to the findings presented.

The remarkable constancy, that is, nonprogression of AO observed by us in our previous short-term investigations (TABLE 2),[4,8,9] could be corroborated by the long-term results presented in this paper.

Another point is worth discussing: What is the significance of the surprising result that in one-third of all patients the two parameters of AO drifted apart, a phenomenon we called "divergency"?

We herein propose an explanation. In TABLE 6 the mechanical components influencing the two parameters of AO are listed. Let us first consider the "ordinary" AO, in which there is a decrease of bronchial diameter, centrilobular emphysema, and ventilatory inhomogeneity: all three features have the uniform effect of decreasing FEV_1/VC and increasing Raw. The mechanical components of parenchymal and peribronchial fibrosis, however, do not have such a uniform influence. Whereas the

TABLE 5. Pulmonary Function at the Time of the Initial Evaluation

	Group		
	1	2	3
VC (l)	2.3 ± 0.68	2.0	2.6 ± 0.92
FEV_1 (l)	1.2 ± 0.53	1.2	1.5 ± 0.58
FEV_1/VC (%)	50.4 ± 9.6	58.0	60.6 ± 11.3
Raw (cm $H_2O \cdot sec \cdot l^{-1}$)	6.8 ± 5.7	6.2	4.3 ± 3.8
TGV (l)	3.4 ± 0.72	2.8	3.5 ± 1.23
Cstat (l/cm H_2O)	0.16 ± 0.08	0.17	0.17 ± 0.08
pO_2 (mm Hg)	70.0 ± 10.6	57.5	65.4 ± 11.9

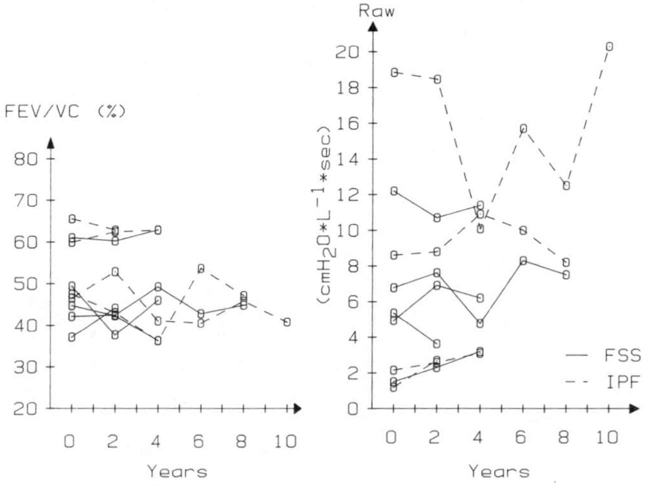

FIGURE 1. Course of FEV_1/VC and Raw in patients with stable parameters of AO (group 1).

distortion of bronchi and the irregular or bullous emphysema have the same effect as "ordinary" AO, the remaining two components diverge from the former: The elevation of the elastic recoil, which does not influence Raw, has a clear positive effect on FEV_1/VC. In nonobstructive cases this ratio is about 80%, which is abnormally high, and this abnormality can "mask" an AO.[10] Finally, the ventilatory inhomogeneity has to be discussed. It is due to the patchy distribution of fibrotic areas so typical for a diffuse pulmonary fibrosis. This inhomogeneity can induce an elevated alveolar resistance by producing a phase displacement of flow and alveolar pressure[11] simulating an AO. The phase displacement found by the plethysmographic method has been

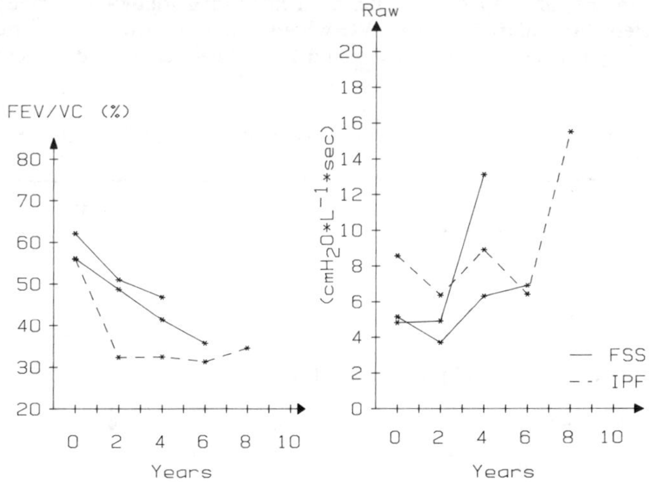

FIGURE 2. Course of FEV_1/VC and Raw in patients with a concordant change of both parameters (group 2).

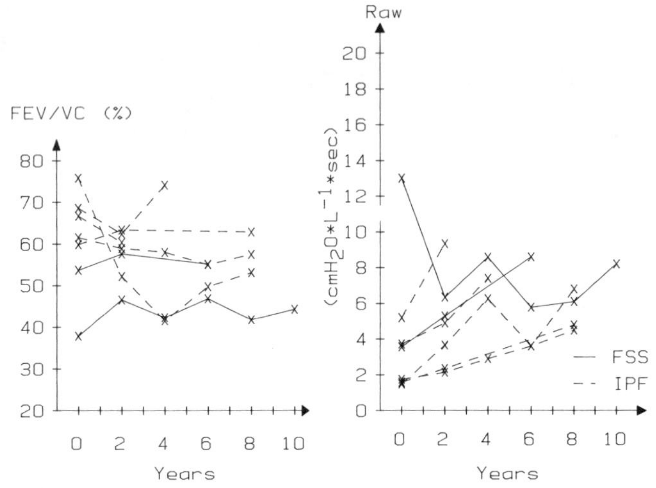

FIGURE 3. Course of FEV_1/VC and Raw in patients with a divergent change of both parameters (group 3).

confirmed by oscillation technique measurements of airway resistance in fibrotic disorders.[12] So in diffuse pulmonary fibrosis FEV_1/VC has a tendency to give falsely negative results, and thus "mask" the AO while Raw may give falsely elevated values.

The above-mentioned remarks refer to the scheme presented in TABLE 6. It is important to remember that our study concerns only patients with considerable AO because we excluded patients with an $FEV_1/VC \geq 65\%$. Under these assumptions only a potential false result of Raw is conceivable and not of FEV_1/VC.

Our conclusions are as follows: 1) Investigating the obstructive variants of FSS and IPF we found a remarkable constancy (nonprogression) of lung function parameters of AO in the majority of patients, even after long follow-up periods. 2) This constancy refers particularly to FEV_1/VC whereas in one-third of the patients there was a divergency between this parameter and Raw. These cases of divergency do not

TABLE 6. AO and Diffuse Pulmonary Fibrosis: A Concept of Divergency of FEV_1/VC and Raw

	FEV_1/VC	Raw
Consequences of airflow obstruction		
Decrease of bronchial diameter Centrilobular emphysema Ventilatory inhomogeneity	↓	↑
Consequences of parenchymal and peribronchial fibrosis		
Distortion of bronchi Irregular, bullous emphysema	↓	↑
Elevation of elastic recoil	↑	→
Ventilatory inhomogeneity	→	→ or ↑

with certainty reflect a deterioration of the functional status of the patient if FEV_1/VC remains constant. 3) There is strong evidence that the prognosis of the obstructive variants is not inferior to that of the nonobstructive groups. 4) Obstructive variants of FSS, IPF, and other cryptogenic interstitial entities merit more observation.

SUMMARY

We investigated patients with obstructive variants ($FEV_1/VC < 65\%$) of FSS ($N = 9$) and IPF ($N = 12$) and assessed the course of the lung function parameters of AO during observation times of 2 to 10 years. Three groups of patients could be formed: group 1 ($N = 9$), no significant change of FEV_1/VC and Raw; group 2 ($N = 3$), significant decrease of FEV_1/VC and significant increase of Raw; group 3 ($N = 7$), divergent changes of FEV_1/VC and Raw. Two patients died before they could be assigned to a group. The definite constancy of FEV_1/VC (group 1 and the majority of group 3) assessed in this long-term study corroborated our previous results. Thus the great majority of our patients showed no deterioration of AO. "Divergency" of Raw (group 3) can at least partially be interpreted as "false positive." The prognosis of the obstructive variants is essentially not inferior to that of the nonobstructive groups in these two conditions.

REFERENCES

1. MEIER-SYDOW, J., T. GEBHARDT, H. KRONENBERGER, K. NERGER, H. RIEMANN, M. RUST, M. SCHNEIDER, L. SCHMIDTS, G. SCHULTZE-WERNINGHAUS & S. TUENGERTHAL. 1983. Diffuse pulmonary fibrosis with airflow obstruction: Clinical entities and classification. Prax. Klin. Pneumol. **37:** 335-341.
2. DOLL, E. & K. KRÖPELIN. 1972. Atemmechanische Untersuchungen bei der Lungensarkoidose. Pneumonologie **148:** 7-23.
3. MILLER, A., A. S. TEIRSTEIN, I. JACKLER, M. CHUANG & L. E. SILTZBACH. 1974. Airway function in chronic pulmonary sarcoidosis with fibrosis. Am. Rev. Respir. Dis. **109:** 179-189.
4. MEIER-SYDOW, J. & M. RUST. 1983. Obstruktive Ventilationsstörung und Emphysem bei interstitiellen Lungenerkrankungen. Atemwegs Lungenkrankh **9:** 8-15.
5. YERNAULT, J. C., M. DE JONGHE, A. DE COSTER & M. ENGLERT. 1975. Pulmonary mechanics in diffuse fibrosing alveolitis. Bull. Eur. Physiopathol. Respir. **11:** 231-244.
6. CARRINGTON, C. B., E. A. GAENSLER, R. E. COUTU, M. X. FITZGERALD & R. G. GUPTA. 1978. Natural history and treated course of usual and desquamative interstitial pneumonia. N. Engl. J. Med. **298:** 801-809.
7. BASSET, F., B. CORRIN, H. SPENCER, J. LACRONIQUE, C. ROTH, P. SOLER, J. P. BATTESTI, R. GEORGES & J. CHRÉTIEN. 1978. Pulmonary histiocytosis X. Am. Rev. Respir. Dis. **118:** 811-820.
8. MEIER-SYDOW, J., M. RUST, H. KRONENBERGER & K. NERGER. 1982. Über die Kombination von diffuser Lungenfibrose mit Bronchialobstruktion. *In* Third European Conference on Sarcoidosis and Other Granulomatous Diseases. B. Djuric, Ed.: 339-348. Sremska Kamenica. Novi Sad.
9. RUST, M., A. D. KAPPOS & J. MEIER-SYDOW. 1981. Obstructive lung function pattern in patients with fibrotic stage of sarcoidosis. Bull. Eur. Physiopathol. Respir. **17:** 74P.
10. MACKLEM, P. T. 1983. Airway involvement in sarcoidosis. *In* Sarcoidosis and Other

Granulomatous Disorders. J. Chrétien, J. Marsac & J. C. Saltiel, Eds.: 310-311. Pergamon Press. Paris.

11. RODENSTEIN, D. O., D. C. STANESCU & C. FRANCIS. 1982. Demonstration of failure of body plethysmography in airway obstruction. J. Appl. Physiol.: Respir. Environ. Exercise Physiol. **52:** 949-954.

12. KAPPOS, A., E. GONSIOR, G. SCHULTZE-WERNINGHAUS & D. GIESE. 1981. Zur Interpretation der Unterschiede bei plethysmographischer und oszillatorischer Bestimmung des Atemwegswiderstandes. Prax. Pneumol. **35:** 772-775.

Bronchial Hyperreactivity in Fresh Stage I Sarcoidosis

F. MANRESA PRESAS, P. ROMERO COLOMER, AND
B. RODRIGUEZ SANCHÓN

Seccion de Fisiopatologia Respiratoria
Servicio de Aparato Respiratorio
Hospital de Bellvitge "Princeps d'Espanya"
Hospitalet de Llobregat
Barcelona, Spain

INTRODUCTION

In a significant number of patients with sarcoidosis there is an alteration of lung mechanics, and although the restriction in volume is classically considered the most prevalent alteration, the presence of airways obstruction is more frequent than is generally accepted.

This obstructive pattern was initially observed in advanced forms of the disease, but recent studies have shown an involvement of large and small airways even in the early forms.[1–3]

In our laboratory we have found that among 48 nonsmoking stage I sarcoidosis patients, the incidence of involvement was 23% in large airways and 66% in small airways.[4]

In 1981, Olafsson and Simonsson[5] reported the presence of airways hyperreactivity in some patients with stage I or stage II sarcoidosis. We have investigated the prevalence of bronchial hyperreactivity in a selected group of nonsmokers with stage I sarcoidosis.

MATERIALS AND METHODS

We have studied nine female and three male nonsmokers, between 24 and 63 years of age, with stage I sarcoidosis, 15 to 65 days after the onset of their initial symptoms.

None of the patients had a previous history of atopy, bronchial asthma, or recent pulmonary disease. All patients were diagnosed on clinical and radiological criteria, and the diagnoses were confirmed by findings of noncaseating granulomas in different tissues (lymph node, skin, muscle, and bronchial mucosa).

Five males of appropriate ages and heights were selected to form a control group. The response of the control group to nonspecific stimuli was compared to that of the experimental group.

A protocol was carried out on all the subjects, consisting in the analysis of different pulmonary mechanical parameters before and 5 min after the inhalation of saline, the inhalation of progressively increasing doses of methacholine, and the inhalation of ipratropium bromide (IB).

The inhalation of methacholine was performed according to the protocol of Irwin *et al.*,[6] and the procedure was as follows: a solution of 5 or 25 mg/ml of methacholine diluted in 10% isotonic phosphate-buffered saline was inhaled by means of a Bird nebulizer which delivered particles of less than 5 μ in size at a flow rate of 5 l/min with a pressure of 20 psi.

All the inhalations of methacholine were initiated at functional residual capacity (FRC), ended at total lung capacity (TLC), and were done regularly and slowly by the subject. The initial dose was one inhalation from a 5 mg/ml methacholine solution. This concentration was equivalent to 5 dose units (DU's), a DU being equal to the concentration of the methacholine solution in mg/ml times the number of inhalations from FRC to TLC.

Solutions of increasing DU's were given until a cumulative total dose of 180 DU's had been reached. The DU sequence was as follows: 5 (one inhalation from a 5 mg/ml solution), 25 (one inhalation from a 25 mg/ml solution), 50 (two inhalations from a 25 mg/ml solution), and 100 (four inhalations from a 25 mg/ml solution) DU's, for a total cumulative dose of 180 DU's.

The IB was inhaled at a dose of 240 μg by means of a metered-dose inhaler.

Prior to the inhalation provocation, pulmonary function was evaluated by spirometry and maximal expiratory flow-volume curves. Airway resistance, specific conductance of the airways (SGaw), and FRC as well as the TLC and residual volume (RV) were determined by body plethysmography. The transfer factor for CO (TCO) was obtained by the single-breath method and analyzed with an HP 47305 A analyzer.

After the inhalation of saline, each cumulative dose of methacholine, and of IB, plethysmography, spirometry, and flow-volume curve analyses were repeated three times (5 min after methacholine and 20 min after IB inhalations). The following parameters were obtained: SGaw, FRC, TLC, RV, forced vital capacity (FVC), forced expiratory volume in 1 sec (FEV_1), and maximal expiratory flows at 25 and 50% of the forced expiratory capacity (MEF_{25} and MEF_{50}, respectively). This sequence was maintained throughout the study.

We considered a fall in the SGaw of more than 35% its basal value a positive response.

The analysis of the changes in the aforementioned parameters during the methacholine inhalation was done comparing the evolution of the mean values of the control group. For FVC, FEV_1, FRC, and MEF_{50}, variations above one SD were considered. For MEF_{25} a change over two SD's was taken as positive.

Statistical analysis was done using Student's *t* test for comparisons between means.

RESULTS

TABLE 1 shows the results of the lung function tests of all the patients and the comparison between the groups. No differences were observed in any of the tests between the groups of patients: between responders and nonresponders and between both experimental groups and the normal control one.

FIGURE 1 shows the variations of SGaw as a percentage of its basal value in the 12 patients in comparison to the normal group. We observe that the dose-response

TABLE 1. Baseline Lung Function Data for the Patient Groups and the Control Group[a]

Subject	Age (years)	TLC (%)	FVC (%)	FEV_1 (%)	FEV_1/FVC (%)	MEF_{50} ($1 \cdot sec^{-1}$)	MEF_{25} ($1 \cdot sec^{-1}$)	SGaw ($1 \cdot sec^{-1} \cdot cm\ H_2O^{-1}$)	RV (%)	TCO (%)
Nonresponders										
1	47	99	92	94	76	2.70	0.70	0.16	120	140
2	37	107	93	98	77	3.80	1.40	0.22	151	127
3	32	90	95	87	71	3.00	0.75	0.22	156	100
4	29	98	92	88	80	3.00	1.00	0.20	116	81
5	37	109	104	103	77	2.60	0.80	0.24	113	84
6	63	109	106	108	71	1.80	0.50	0.21	121	80
Mean ± SD	40.8 ± 12.4	102.0 ± 7.6	97.0 ± 6.3	96.3 ± 8.3	75.3 ± 3.6	2.91 ± 0.65	0.56 ± 0.31	0.21 ± 0.027	129.5 ± 18.8	102.0 ± 25.7
Responders										
7	32	101	110	105	75	3.00	1.13	0.18	72	94
8	48	117	79	79	74			0.17	91	101
9	43	109	90	73	61	1.65	0.50	0.08	149	85
10	38	117	99	104	81	3.70	1.10	0.16	172	80
11	24	88	88	85	87	3.40	3.00	0.33	85	77
12	34	92	81	85	82	2.90	1.05	0.22	145	115
Mean ± SD	36.5 ± 8.5	104.0 ± 12.4	102.1 ± 11.7	88.5 ± 13.2	75.0 ± 7.5	2.93 ± 0.78	1.35 ± 0.95	0.18 ± 0.08	119.1 ± 41.2	92.0 ± 14.3
Controls										
Mean ± SD	32.5 ± 4.8	92.0 ± 17.5	94.2 ± 15.1	86.5 ± 8.7	4.24 ± 0.90	1.55 ± 0.44	0.36 ± 0.21			

[a] Individual results are shown for the patients. Comparisons are made between the means of the patient groups and the mean of the control group.

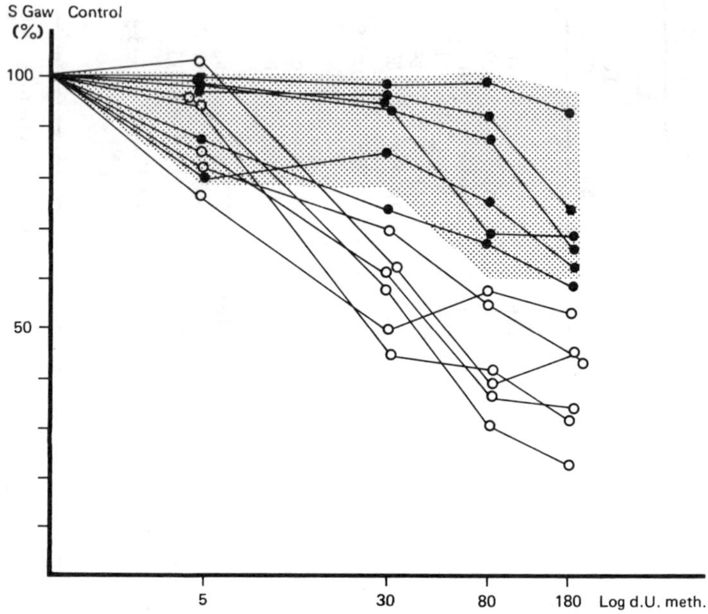

FIGURE 1. Dose-response curves in logarithmic scale for all the individuals in the two groups of patients. The curves describe the changes in SGaw during the progressive inhalation of methacholine. The shaded area shows the limits of the normal, control group response. ●——●: non responders; ○——○: responders. See the text for details.

TABLE 2. Global Analysis of the Modifications of the Flow and Volume Responses after the Inhalation of 30 DU's of Methacholine[a]

Subjects	Flow Response Modification[b]	Volume Response Modification[c]
Nonresponders		
1	−	+
2	−	+
3	−	+
4	+	−
5	−	+
6	−	+
Responders		
7	+	−
8	+	−
9	+	−
10	+	−
11	+	−
12	+	−

[a] The plus and minus signs indicate changes greater and less than, respectively, one SD for FEV_1, MEF_{50}, FVC, and RV, and changes greater and less than, respectively, two SD's for MEF_{25}.

[b] FEV_1, MEF_{50}, and MEF_{25}.

[c] FVC and RV.

curve of the nonresponders falls in the normal area. The dose of methacholine that induced a fall of 35% of the basal SGaw value for the responders was similar to that for the asthmatic patients, and the responders and the asthmatic patients had similar, steep-sloped dose-response curves.

Although the SGaw of most of the responders falls at low DU's of methacholine, we continued the protocol until a total of 180 DU's was reached in order to obtain a satisfactory dose-response curve.

We have compared the changes in SGaw after the inhalation from 30 DU's of methacholine, a dose above the one causing a fall in 35% in the SGaw in the responders, to those of the other parameters studied (FEV_1, FVC, RV, MEF_{25}, and MEF_{50}) to evaluate the possibility of a different site of action of the drug. TABLE 2 shows the behavior of the volume and flow response. FVC and RV were taken as volume parameters and FEV_1, MEF_{25}, and MEF_{50} as flow parameters.

In the group of nonresponders, defined as those patients whose SGaw values fell within normal limits after the inhalation from 30 DU's of methacholine, we could find that the methacholine induced a change in lung volumes in five out of six patients; on the other hand, in the group of responders we obtained a flow response in all of the six patients.

DISCUSSION

Bechtel *et al.*[7] pointed out in their article that "those patients with an abnormal response to the inhaled methacholine had a greater degree of baseline airways obstruction." At the same time, they concluded that "other factors apart from the basal airways geometry could be responsible for the modification in the response to the methacholine."

These authors separated the responders from the nonresponders on the basis of three functional criteria: 1) a higher degree of baseline airways obstruction, 2) a smaller FVC, and 3) a lower TCO. Clinically, they found that the responders were more symptomatic (coughing and wheezing) and had a longer duration of the disease.[7]

In our study we have not been able to confirm these findings: no differences were observed in the degree of baseline airways obstruction, FVC, clinical symptoms, or the duration of the disease; only a tendency for a smaller TCO was seen in the group of responders.

The selection of the patients in the early stages of the disease and the shortness of the symptomatic period could explain the differences between our results and those of Bechtel *et al.*[7]

The results of the methacholine test indicate two types of airways reactivity in a similar group of 12 patients. Why do some of them react as if they were asthmatics?

The degree of basal bronchial caliber has already been mentioned as a factor determining a different response to inhaled bronchoactive agents: those bronchi with small caliber react more intensively that those with normal lumen.[8] This may sometimes, however rarely, be the only explanation for this response, as Bechtel *et al.*[7] have already proposed in their article.

Turner-Warwick and Haslam[9] found an increase in histamine content in the bronchoalveolar lavage fluid of some patients with sarcoidosis, particularly in that of patients in advanced stages, but also in that of some patients in earlier stages. It may be hypothesized that the release of some bronchoactive mediators by the cells present in the alveoli is responsible for this abnormal reaction to methacholine.

Most of the patients in early stages of sarcoidosis present granulomas in their bronchial walls. The granulomatous inflammation by inducing changes in the anatomical and functional structures of the bronchial wall may alter its compliance and determine an abnormal response to some drugs or nonspecific stimuli.

Finally, a modification in the threshold of the cholinergic receptors of the bronchial tree may account in part for the response to the inhaled methacholine.

The significance of the flow, or volume, response has been examined before.[10,11] If we consider that the changes in different mechanical parameters that occur after the inhalation of a bronchoactive drug may reflect the predominant site of action of the drug (central or peripheral airways), as has been shown in asthmatics after bronchodilatation,[10–12] our results would suggest a different site of action of methacholine was more likely than a true absence of reactivity in the nonresponders group.

In fact, in this group, the change in lung volumes (RV and FVC) was clearly different than that in a similar normal population. If this is so, the hyperreactivity in sarcoidosis would be a more general phenomenon than has been accepted up till now, although its pathogenesis remains unclear.

Other interpretations of this fact are possible but would require measurements that have not been made in our study to substantiate them. If our considerations are confirmed, the choice of a single parameter (SGaw or FEV_1) to analyze the hyperreactivity in sarcoidosis and, perhaps, other related diseases may be unreliable.

In conclusion, we have shown that the prevalence of airways hyperreactivity is frequent in early sarcoidosis and that this may explain the high incidence of airways obstruction seen in this disease. The mechanism by which this abnormal response takes place is a matter of conjecture.

SUMMARY

In order to analyze the mechanism of airways obstruction seen in patients with early sarcoidosis, we have studied the bronchial reactivity in 12 patients with stage I sarcoidosis.

The patients were given progressively increasing doses of methacholine to inhale. A fall of more than 35% of the SGaw was taken as the index of response.

In 6 out of 12 patients (responders), we observed a dose-response curve similar to that seen in subjects with highly reactive airways.

We could not find any difference between responders and nonresponders that could explain the diverse responses to the methacholine. Nevertheless, the modifications in different mechanical parameters showed that the inhaled methacholine induced two types of changes: 1) a change in lung volumes (RV and FVC), observed mainly in the nonresponders, and 2) a change in forced expiratory flows (FEV_1, MEF_{25}, and MEF_{50}), observed in the responders. These types of response may suggest a different site of action of the inhaled agent.

We conclude that the presence of airways hyperreactivity is frequent in early sarcoidosis and could perhaps explain the incidence of airways obstruction seen in this disease.

REFERENCES

1. DINES, D. E., J. E. STUBBS & J. C. MCDOUGALL. 1978. Obstructive disease of the airways associated with stage I sarcoidosis. Mayo Clin. Proc. **53:** 788-791.
2. KANEKO, K. & O. P. SHARMA. 1977. Airway obstruction in pulmonary sarcoidosis. Bull. Eur. Physiopathol. Respir. **13:** 231-240.
3. OLSSON, T., H. BJORNSTAD-PETERSON & N. L. STJENBERG. 1979. Bronchostenosis due to sarcoidosis. Chest **75:** 663-670.
4. MANRESA PRESAS, F., M. J. FERNANDEZ SAMMAMED, B. RODRIGUEZ SANCHÓN, P. ROMERO COLOMER & F. BADRINAS. 1981. Función pulmonar en la sarcoidosis: Estudio prospectivo. Med. Clin. (Barcelona) **76:** 433-438.
5. OLAFSSON, M. & B. G. SIMONSSON. 1983. Nonspecific bronchial hyperreactivity as a sign of activity in fresh cases of pulmonary sarcoidosis: A pilot study. *In* Sarcoidosis and Other Granulomatous Disorders. J. Chrétien, J. Marsac & J. C. Saltiel, Eds.: 651-652. Pergamon Press, Paris.
6. IRWIN, R. S., W. M. CORRAO & M. R. PRATTER. 1981. Chronic persistent cough in the adult: The spectrum, frequency, and causes and the successful outcome of specific therapy. Am. Rev. Respir. Dis. **123:** 27-32.
7. BECHTEL, J. L., T. STARR III, D. R. DANTZKER & T. S. BOWER. 1981. Airway hyperreactivity in patients with sarcoidosis. Am. Rev. Respir. Dis. **124:** 759-761.
8. BOUSHEY, H. A., M. H. HOLTZMAN, J. R. SHELLER & J. A. NADEL. 1980. Bronchial hyperreactivity. Am. Rev. Respir. Dis. **122:** 383-413.
9. TURNER-WARWICK, M. & P. HASLAM. 1982. Personal communication. Course on Advanced Thoracic Medicine. London.
10. PARÉ, P. D., L. M. LAWSON & L. D. BROOKS. 1983. Patterns of response to inhaled bronchodilators in asthmatics. Am. Rev. Respir. Dis. **127:** 680-685.
11. RAMSDELL, J. W. & G. M. TISI. 1979. Determination of bronchodilation in the clinical pulmonary function laboratory. Chest **76:** 622-628.
12. FAIRSHTER, R. D. & A. F. WILSON. 1980. Relationship between the site of airflow limitation and localization of the bronchodilators response in asthma. Am. Rev. Respir. Dis. **122:** 27-32.

Clinical Study on Cardiac Sarcoidosis

T. TACHIBANA,[a,b] F. OHMORI,[c] AND E. UEDA[d]

[b] *Osaka Prefectural Hospital*
[c] *National Cardiovascular Center*
and
[d] *National Toneyama Hospital*
Osaka, Japan

INTRODUCTION

Cardiac involvement is the main cause of death by sarcoidosis in Japan. By the end of 1980 the Japan Sarcoidosis Committee had considered the autopsies of 73 cases from all over Japan. All of the cases had died of sarcoidosis: 53 of them (approximately 72.6%) had died of myocardial sarcoidosis; 12, of pulmonary sarcoidosis; and 8, of central nervous system sarcoidosis. Therefore, the early detection and treatment of cardiac lesions is of the utmost importance, and should be the subject of clinical studies of sarcoidosis.

Matsui *et al.*[1] have published a clinicopathological study on fatal myocardial sarcoidosis in Japan. Roberts *et al.*[2] and Silverman *et al.*[3] have published clinicopathological studies on cardiac sarcoidosis, and have considered cases that did not have cardiac dysfunction due to sarcoid heart disease.

Numao *et al.*[4] have used electrocardiograms (ECG's) and endomyocardial biopsies in clinical studies on cardiac involvement in sarcoidosis; Sekiguchi *et al.*[5] have conducted a clinical study on the prognosis of cardiac sarcoidosis; and Fleming[6] has conducted a clinical study in the United Kingdom on 200 patients with cardiac sarcoidosis, 65 of whom had necropsy confirmation.

We have studied cardiac involvement in sarcoidosis by using thallium-201 myocardial scans, gated blood pool scans, 24-hr ECG recording, two-dimensional and M-mode echocardiography, and serum angiotensin-converting enzyme (SACE) activity estimates. Examinations were serially performed over a 3-year period in most cases. In this study we demonstrate the clinical significance of the combination of these examinations in detecting cardiac involvement in sarcoidosis.

MATERIALS AND METHODS

Forty-one unselected patients with sarcoidosis (12 males and 29 females) with and without normal ECG's were studied. Only six of them showed cardiac symptoms with

[a] Address for correspondence: Osaka Prefectural Hospital, 3-Chrome, Bandai-higashi, Sumiyoshi-ku, Osaka, Japan.

abnormal ECG's. The mean age of the patients was 45 years, and ages ranged from 27 to 73 years. Radiographic staging was as follows: stage 0: 7 patients; stage 1: 25 patients; stage 2: 7 patients; and stage 3: 2 patients.

Thallium-201 myocardial perfusion scans were performed in a routine manner, after intravenous injection of 4 mCi of ionic thallium-201 chloride, with anterior views; 30°-, 45°-, and 60°-left anterior oblique views; and left lateral views. Myocardial images, containing 300 000 counts each, were recorded with a high-resolution scintillation camera (Ohio Nuclear Σ410S) and a high-resolution, low-energy collimator (Shimazu-Searle LFOB).

Gated blood pool scans were performed using radiolabeled red blood cells. The cells were labeled *in vivo* by intravenously injecting 20-25 mCi of technetium-99m pertechnetate. Data were recorded, in a multiple-gated mode on a magnetic disc, with a digital computer (DEC γ-11). A computer-based procedure gated to the ECG was used to collect and organize data into a series of images, and the left ventricular ejection fraction was determined using validated system software.

Each two-dimensional echocardiogram was obtained with one of two ultrasonoscopes: a Toshiba SSH 11A with a 2.4 MHz transducer, or a Toshiba 40A with a 3.5 MHz transducer. During the examinations, patients were supine or in various left-lateral decubitus positions to optimize image quality. Sector scans were recorded on Polaroid film and videotape for analysis. Each echocardiographic study included standard views from parasternal, apical, and subcostal transducer positions. Conventional M-mode echocardiograms were recorded simultaneously with an ECG and a phonocardiogram on the Honeywell strip-chart recorder attached to the main equipment with the same transducer used for the two-dimensional recordings. The beam direction for obtaining the M-mode echocardiogram was confirmed by the cursor in the real-time, two-dimensional image.

The pulsed Doppler echocardiograms were obtained with a bidirectional ultrasonic-pulsed Doppler flowmeter (Toshiba SDS 10A or SDS 12A) in combination with a cross-sectional echocardiograph (Toshiba SSH 11A or 40A). The frequency of the pulsed Dopper flowmeter was 2.5 MHz, and the pulsed repetition rate was 4.5 KHz. The Dopper signal was recorded simultaneously with the M-mode echocardiogram, phonocardiogram, and ECG using a strip-chart recorder.

ECG's were also recorded after patients had exercised and over 24-hr periods (Holter ECG).

Measurement of SACE activity was performed with a modified method of Cushman and Cheung as already described.[7] Serum was incubated with 3.5 mM Hip-His-Leu, 300 mM sodium chloride, and 100 mM borate/carbonate buffer (pH 8.3) instead of the phosphate buffer used in the original method. Assays were done in duplicate with a concurrent control serum.

RESULTS

Thallium-201 Myocardial Perfusion Scans

Thallium-201 myocardial perfusion scans (TMPS's) revealed the focal left ventricular defects in 5 out of 41 patients with sarcoidosis. TABLE 1 shows a summary of the results for these five patients.

In case 1, a patient who had no cardiac symptoms, inferior and apical left ventricular perfusion defects were found (FIG. 1, upper panels). These defects disappeared

TABLE 1. Patients with the Left Ventricular Perfusion Defect

	Case Number				
	1	2	3	4	5
Age	46Y	60Y	27Y	60Y	60Y
Sex	Male	Male	Male	Female	Female
ECG abnormalities	None	Complete AV block; pacing	CRBBB; VT	CRBBB	None
Left ventricular perfusion defect	Inferoapical ⊕ → ⊖ → ⊕ → ⊖ (2Y, 1Y, 6M)	Inferior ⊕ ——→ ⊖ (3Y)	Extensive (anterior and posterior)	Anteroseptal ⊕ ——→ ⊖ (3Y)	Anteroseptal ⊕ ——→ ⊖ (2Y)
Radiographic stage	BHL ⊕ → ⊖ ——→ ⊖	BHL ⊕ ——→ ⊖	Stage 0	BHL ⊕ → ⊖ ——→ ⊖	BHL ⊕ → ⊖ ——→ ⊖
SACE activity	(↑) → (→) → (↑) → (→)	(→)		(↑) ——→ (↑)	(↑) ——→ (↑)
Steroid treatment	3.5Y	3Y	None	None	None
Histological confirmation	Liver biopsy	Lymph node biopsy	Autopsy[a]	Lymph node biopsy	Lymph node biopsy

NOTE: Y: years; M: months; ⊕: present; ⊖: absent; (↑): elevated; (→): normal.
[a]The autopsy confirmed that the patient had fatal myocardial sarcoidosis.

(FIG. 1, middle panels) concomitant with normalization of chest radiograph findings and SACE activity after the patient was treated with steroids (60 mg of prednisolone every other day). The defects reappeared, however, concomitant with the reelevation of SACE levels after the steroid dose was decreased to 15 mg of prednisolone every other day (FIG. 1, lower panels). The perfusion defects disappeared again, concomitant with the normalization of SACE levels, after the steroid dose was increased. (The dose was increased to 60 mg of prednisolone every other day.)

In case 2, a patient who had Adams-Stokes disease, complete atrioventricular (AV) block on ECG and inferior left ventricular perfusion defect on TMPS were found. In this case a permanent pacemaker was implanted and a biopsy taken from the mediastinal lymph node to show granulomas. After long-term steroid treatment

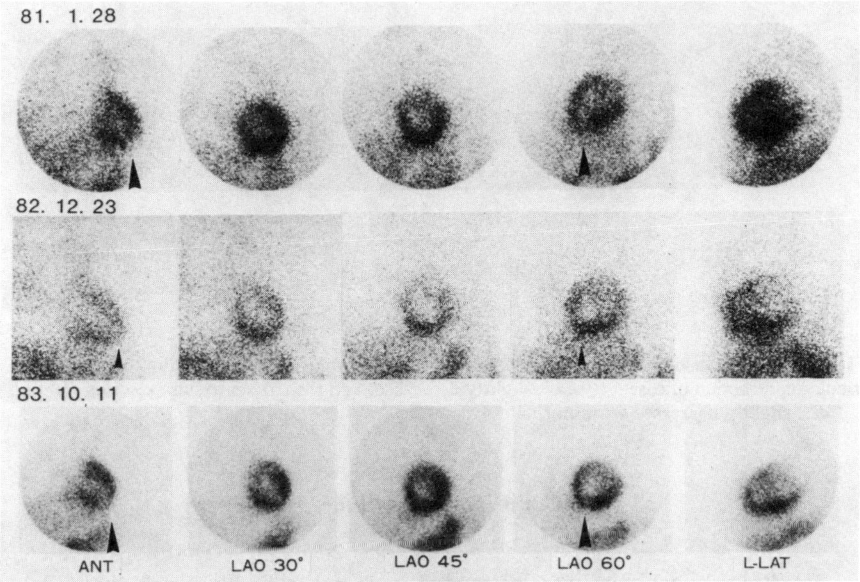

FIGURE 1. TMPS's before and after steroid therapy. Upper panels: The focal left ventricular perfusion defects in the inferior and apical regions (large arrowheads), which were probably due to sarcoid infiltration, were found before steroid treatment. Middle and lower panels: The defects shown in the upper panels disappeared (small arrowheads) in the 3 years after treatment with steroids began, but reappeared (large arrowheads) after the doses of the steroid were decreased.

the left ventricular perfusion defect disappeared concomitant with the normalization of SACE activity, and successive chest radiographs became clearer. The left ventricular perfusion defect also disappeared in cases 4 and 5.

In case 3, fatal myocardial sarcoidosis was found. The patient complained of various cardiac symptoms such as orthopnea and palpitation with syncopal attack. His ECG showed complete right bundle branch block (CRBBB) and occasional ventricular tachycardia. The thallium-201 uptake was found only at the inferior wall of the left ventricle, and broad anterior and posterior perfusion defects were found on the TMPS. This suggested the patient had an extensive ventricular myocardial lesion, the presence of which was confirmed later at autopsy. An extensive fibrotic lesion was found macroscopically in the left ventricular wall, where extensive lesions with many giant cells, including typical asteroid bodies, were found microscopically.

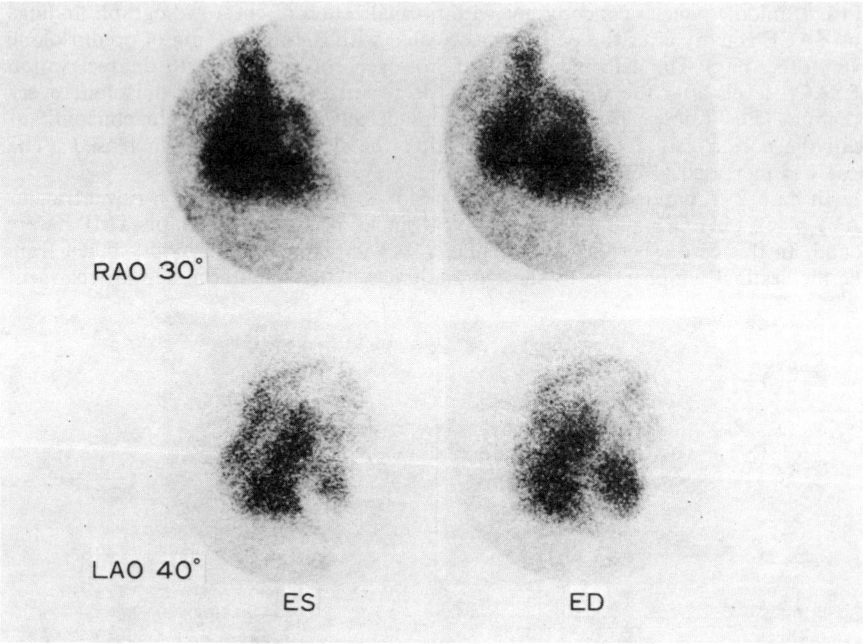

FIGURE 2. Gated blood pool scans with decreased left ventricular contraction. The left ventricular contraction of case 1 appears slightly decreased, and the left ventricular ejection fraction is 48%, slightly decreased from normal.

Gated Blood Pool Scans

Gated blood pool scans were performed in 41 patients with sarcoidosis, and 14 of them showed a decreased left ventricular ejection fraction (LVEF). FIGURE 2 shows the gated blood pool scan for case 1. The value for the LVEF was 48%, slightly decreased from normal. The LVEF was decreased in 3 out of 5 patients with left ventricular perfusion defect and in 11 out of 36 patients without left ventricular perfusion defect (TABLE 2).

TABLE 2. Correlation between the Left Ventricular Perfusion Defect and the LVEF

	Decreased LVEF		
	Present	Absent	Total
Left ventricular perfusion defect			
Present	3	2	5
Absent	11	25	36
Total	14	27	41

Echocardiograms

Two-dimensional and M-mode echocardiography was performed in 41 patients that had sarcoidosis. No marked abnormalities were found, but one patient did have fatal myocardial sarcoidosis. The two-dimensional echocardiogram for this patient showed generalized hypokinesis of the left ventricular, thin anterior, and posterior walls (FIG. 3A); the M-mode echocardiogram showed that the motion of these walls was poor (FIG. 3B). Pulsed Doppler echocardiography did not show any remarkable change.

ECG Findings

CRBBB's, heart blocks, and premature contractions were found in 4, 3, and 4 patients, respectively, out of 41 patients subjected to routine electrocardiography (TABLE 3). Exercise ECG's showed premature contractions in 7 out of the 27 patients that were examined. Holter ECG's showed premature contractions in 13 out of the 32 patients that were examined.

Change in ECG Findings with Steroid Treatment

ECG abnormalities such as frequent premature ventricular contraction (PVC), premature supraventricular contraction (PSC), and incomplete and complete AV blocks disappeared following steroid therapy in five patients (TABLE 4). In two of them (cases 7 and 9), ECG abnormalities such as frequent PVC and complete AV block reappeared after the steroid dose was reduced to 15 mg of prednisolone every other day, and disappeared again after the steroid dose was increased to 60 mg of prednisolone every other day.

SACE Activity

SACE activity correlated well with the appearance and disappearance of the left ventricular perfusion defect on the TMPS of case 1. The sequence of events in this patient is shown in detail in FIGURE 4.

The SACE level was elevated in all three patients examined (cases 1, 4, and 5) when the left ventricular perfusion defect on the TMPS was found. Furthermore, it was normal in two patients (cases 1 and 2) when the left ventricular perfusion defect disappeared after long-term steroid treatment. On the other hand, it was still elevated in two other patients (cases 4 and 5) when the left ventricular perfusion defect disappeared without steroids having been applied.

The SACE level was elevated in all 3 patients that had the left ventricular perfusion defect and in 16 out of the 36 patients that did not have the left ventricular perfusion defect (TABLE 5). The SACE activity of patients that did not have sarcoidosis but

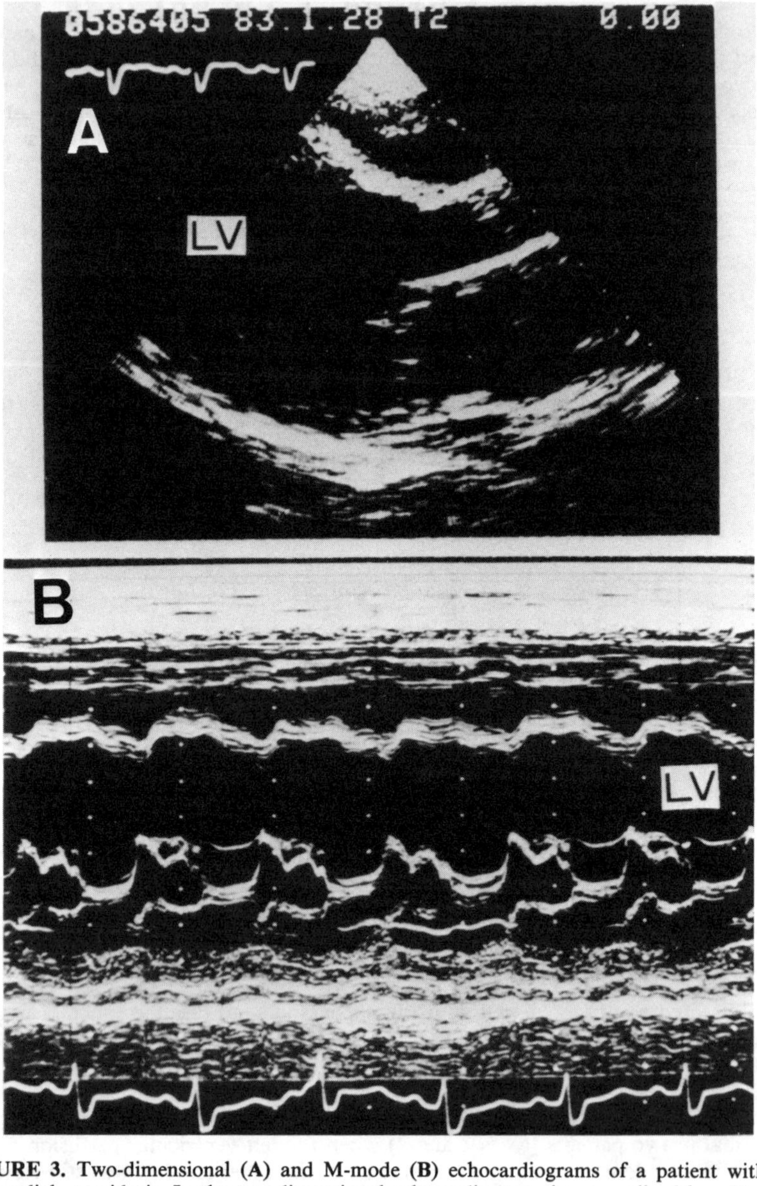

FIGURE 3. Two-dimensional (**A**) and M-mode (**B**) echocardiograms of a patient with fatal myocardial sarcoidosis. In the two-dimensional echocardiogram the generalized hypokinesis of the motion of the left ventricular, thin anterior, and posterior walls is shown. The M-mode echocardiogram also shows that the mobility of these walls was abnormally decreased.

TABLE 3. ECG Findings

	Routine ECG	Exercise ECG	Holter ECG
CRBBB	4	—	—
Heart block	3	—	—
PVC	2	3	6
PVC and PSC	1	2	5
PSC	1	2	2

did have the left ventricular perfusion defect was also investigated. It was normal in three patients that had acute myocardial infarction and in two patients that had dilated cardiomyopathy.

The correlation between LVEF and SACE was not significant (TABLE 6).

DISCUSSION

The paper by Bulkley *et al.*[8] was the first of several reports[9–11] on the left ventricular perfusion defect and on how this defect could be detected in patients with sarcoid heart lesions by performing a TMPS. All five patients in Bulkley's series had both marked cardiac symptoms and extensive myocardial sarcoid lesions. An autopsy confirmed the presence of these lesions in one case. An autopsy performed on a case in our series also confirmed the presence of extensive myocardial sarcoid lesions, lesions which had been detected as a left ventricular perfusion defect in a TMPS. In Kinney's series,[9] 14 out of 44 patients with sarcoidosis showed a left ventricular perfusion defect

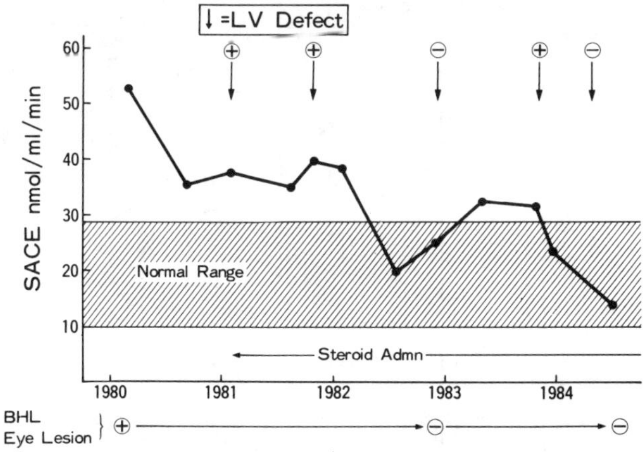

FIGURE 4. Correlation between SACE levels and the left ventricular perfusion defect in patients that received treatment. SACE activity was elevated when the left ventricular perfusion defect was first found. SACE activity was normalized after steroid treatment began, but became elevated again after the doses of the steroid were reduced: these changes parallel the disappearance and reappearance of the left ventricular perfusion defect.

TABLE 4. Improvements in Patients with ECG Abnormalities after Steroid Therapy

Case Number	Age (years)	Sex	ECG Abnormalities	Steroid Treatment (years)	SACE Activity at Present
6	53	Male	CRBBB → CRBBB PVC, PSC → CRBBB	4	Normal
7	61	Male	Frequent PVC → ⊖[a]	4	Normal
8	51	Female	Incomplete AV Block → ⊖	1	Normal
9	53	Female	CRBBB → Complete AV Block PVC → ⊖[a]	8	Normal
10	26	Male	Complete AV Block → ⊖	3	Normal

[a]The ECG abnormalities reappeared after the steroid doses were decreased; they disappeared again after the doses were increased.

TABLE 5. Correlation between the Left Ventricular Perfusion Defect and SACE Activity in Patients with Sarcoidosis

	SACE Activity		
	Elevated	Normal	Total
Left ventricular perfusion defect			
Present	3	0	3
Absent	16	20	36
Total	19	20	39

on TMPS although none of these 14 patients showed clinical cardiac dysfunction. In our series, only 6 out of 41 patients showed cardiac symptoms. Three out of five patients with left ventricular perfusion defects detected in TMPS's showed cardiac symptoms; one patient complained of Stokes-Adams syncopal attack and had to have a permanent pacemaker implanted to resolve a complete AV block.

In contrast to Kinney's series, all the patients in Haywood's series[10] had subjective or objective cardiac symptoms. Four out of 30 patients in this series showed the left ventricular perfusion defect in TMPS's, and the frequency of the appearance of this defect resembles that of our series. Moreover, the left ventricular perfusion defect disappeared after the steroid treatment in one case, a result identical to one in our series. After the steroid dose was decreased, however, the left ventricular perfusion defect reappeared and persisted in this case. In one patient of our series, the left ventricular perfusion defect reappeared after the steroid dose was decreased, but disappeared again after the dose was increased. From these observations, it is suggested that long-term therapy with steroids is very important in preventing the recurrence of sarcoid heart disease.

In the Japanese literature, the left ventricular perfusion defect was revealed in TMPS's in nine patients with cardiac sarcoidosis who had both cardiac symptoms and ECG abnormalities. Two of them had fatal myocardial sarcoidosis, in four of them endomyocardial biopsy was positive, and in two of them the SACE level was elevated. After steroid treatment the left ventricular perfusion defect disappeared in one case and was ameliorated in another one. Moreover, the SACE level, which had been elevated, became normal in the latter case. The left ventricular perfusion defect became more pronounced, however, in another case after 1 year without steroid therapy.

TABLE 6. Correlation between the LVEF and SACE Activity in Patients with Sarcoidosis

	SACE Activity		
	Elevated	Normal	Total
Decreased LVEF			
Present	6	7	13
Absent	13	13	26
Total	19	20	39

In Kinney's series the left ventricular perfusion defect could be correlated with echocardiographic evidence of left ventricular dysfunction. The latter was not prominent in our series, however, except in the case with fatal myocardial sarcoidosis.

In the Japanese literature, echocardiographic abnormalities were revealed in 16 patients with cardiac sarcoidosis who showed both cardiac symptoms and ECG abnormalities. In five of them left ventricular hypoperfusion was revealed in TMPS's, and the motion of this segment of the wall was revealed as being consistent with hypokinesis or dyskinesis by echocardiography.

Numao *et al.*[4] have reported that the incidence of ECG abnormalities such as PVC, PSC, CRBBB, and AV block in patients with sarcoidosis was more frequent than in controls. Our data is shown in TABLE 5. Stein *et al.*[12] have reported that seven out of eight patients with cardiac sarcoidosis displayed ventricular arrhythmia after exercising. Among our unselected patients with sarcoidosis, only a few displayed PVC and/or PSC after exercising. Kinney *et al.*[9] have reported that PVC, as detected in Holter ECG's, did not occur more frequently in patients with sarcoidosis than in the controls. In contrast to this finding, 13 out of 32 patients with sarcoidosis in our study showed PVC and/or PSC. Three of these 13 cases had the left ventricular perfusion defect; 1, complete AV block; and 2, frequent PVC. The abnormalities in the three latter cases disappeared after steroid treatment.

There are some reports that steroid treatment is effective in causing the disappearance of ECG abnormalities in patients with cardiac sarcoidosis.[13–17] In Japan, Hashida, as our co-worker, reported in 1964 that CRBBB and bilateral hilar lymphadenopathy (BHL) both disappeared after 4 months of steroid treatment. Since then, it has been reported in Japan that such ECG abnormalities as AV block, frequent PVC, CRBBB, and QS patterns disappeared after steroid treatment in nine patients with cardiac sarcoidosis. In our series, ECG abnormalities such as frequent PVC, PSC, and AV block disappeared after steroid treatment in five patients, when SACE activity was normal. Furthermore, after decreasing the dose of the steroid, the ECG abnormalities reappeared. These abnormalities disappeared again in two of our patients, the patients that had their dose of steroid increased. From these ECG observations, it is clear that long-term steroid treatment is necessary to prevent cardiac sarcoidosis.

The SACE level was elevated in most of the patients with the left ventricular perfusion defect in Haywood's series,[10] a finding identical to one in our series. The SACE level was elevated in all three patients examined with the left ventricular perfusion defect in our series. In one of them, the elevation and normalization of the SACE level correlated well with the appearance and disappearance of the left ventricular perfusion defect. The SACE level was not elevated in five patients without sarcoidosis but with the left ventricular perfusion defect. Although the SACE level reflects the summation of all the epithelioid cell granulomas in the body of a patient with sarcoidosis, determining whether the SACE level was elevated in a patient suspected of having cardiac sarcoidosis seemed to help the diagnosis.

FIGURE 5 demonstrates the correlation between SACE activity and clinical course in a case of fatal myocardial sarcoidosis (a case other than the one already discussed).

Her ECG at first showed CRBBB. It showed complete AV block 2 years later, when she complained of Adams-Stokes attack. A permanent pacemaker was subsequently implanted. After 6 years she died of congestive heart failure, at the age of 56. She had received low doses of a steroid and had markedly elevated SACE activity before her death. An autopsy confirmed the presence of systemic lesions of epithelioid cell granulomas, some of which were found in the myocardium. This is a typical case in that elevated SACE activity reflected the presence of systemic sarcoid granulomas, including those in the myocardium.

SUMMARY

Forty-one patients with sarcoidosis were investigated for cardiac involvement. The results are summarized as follows: 1) The focal left ventricular perfusion defect was found on the TMPS's of 5 out of 41 patients with sarcoidosis. The defect disappeared in four of these five patients over a 3-year period, but remained in the patient with fatal myocardial sarcoidosis. 2) A decreased left ventricular ejection fraction was found in 14 out of 41 patients with sarcoidosis, and in 3 out of 5 patients with the left ventricular perfusion defect. 3) Echocardiographic examination did not reveal left ventricular wall dysfunction at the site of the left ventricular perfusion defect, except in one patient with fatal myocardial sarcoidosis. 4) Holter ECG's showed such abnormalities as CRBBB, heart blocks, PVC, and PSC in 13 out of 32 patients with sarcoidosis. 5) SACE activity was elevated in all three patients with the left ventricular perfusion defect that were examined, and it could be correlated with changes in the left ventricular perfusion defect in one of them.

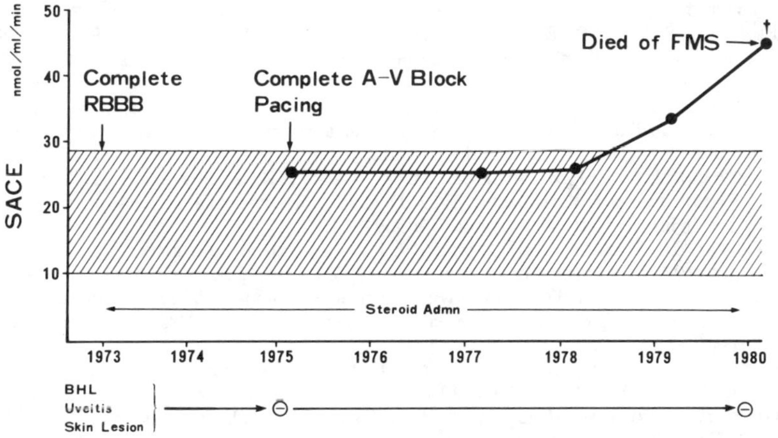

FIGURE 5. Changes in the SACE level of a female patient with fatal myocardial sarcoidosis (FMS). SACE activity was elevated before death in a pacing female patient with FMS. An autopsy confirmed the presence of systemic lesions of epithelioid cell granulomas, including some in the myocardium.

Combining the results of TMPS's, myocardial perfusion scans, gated blood pool scans, echocardiograms, Holter ECG's, and SACE activity estimates is useful in detecting and in monitoring the steroid treatment of sarcoid heart disease.

REFERENCES

1. Matsui, Y., K. Iwai, T. Tachibana, T. Fruie, N. Shigematsu, T. Izumi, H. Homma, R. Mikami, O. Hongo, Y. Hiraga & M. Yamamoto. 1976. Clinicopathological study on fatal myocardial sarcoidosis. Ann. N. Y. Acad. Sci. **278:** 455-469.
2. Roberts, W. C., H. A. McAllister, Jr. & V. J. Ferrans. 1977. Sarcoidosis of the

heart: A clinicopathologic study of 35 necropsy patients (group I) and review of 78 previously described necropsy patients (group II). Am. J. Med. **63:** 86-108.
3. Silverman, K. J., M. H. Hutchins & B. H. Bulkley. 1978. Cardiac sarcoid: A clinicopathologic study of 84 unselected patients with systemic sarcoidosis. Circulation **58:** 1204-1211.
4. Numao, Y., M. Sekiguchi, T. Fruie, Y. Matsui, T. Izumi & R. Mikami. 1980. A study of cardiac involvement in 963 cases of sarcoidosis by ECG and endomyocardial biopsy. *In* Eighth International Conference on Sarcoidosis and Other Granulomatous Diseases. W. Jones Williams & B. H. Davies, Eds.: 607-614. Alpha Omega. Cardiff.
5. Sekiguchi, M., T. Suda, T. Fruie, Y. Matsui, Y. Numao, H. Osada, T. Tachibana, M. Yamamoto & R. Mikami. 1983. Long-term prognosis of cardiac sarcoidosis patients with permanent pacemaker implantation: A Japanese study. *In* Sarcoidosis and Other Granulomatous Disorders. J. Chrétien, J. Marsac & J. C. Saltiel, Eds.: 658. Pergamon Press. Paris.
6. Fleming, H. A. 1983. Sarcoid heart disease in the United Kingdom (1971-1981): Report of 200 cases with necropsy comfirmation in 65. *In* Sarcoidosis and Other Granulomatous Disorders. J. Chrétien, J. Marsac & J. C. Saltiel, Eds.: 616. Pergamon Press. Paris.
7. Ueda, E., T. Kawabe, T. Tachibana & T. Kokubu. 1980. Serum angiotensin-converting enzyme activity as an indicator of prognosis in sarcoidosis. Am. Rev. Respir. Dis. **121:** 667-671.
8. Bulkley, B. H., J. R. Rouleau, J. Q. Whitaker, H. W. Strauss & B. Pitt. 1977. The use of ^{201}thallium for myocardial perfusion imaging in sarcoid heart disease. Chest **72:** 27-32.
9. Kinney, E. L., G. L. Jackson, W. C. Reeves, R. Zelis & E. Beers. 1980. Thallium-scan myocardial defects and echocardiographic abnormalities in patients with sarcoidosis without clinical cardiac dysfunction: An analysis of 44 patients. Am. J. Med. **68:** 497-503.
10. Haywood, L. J., O. P. Sharma, M. E. Siegel, R. J. Siegel, S. L. Gottlieb, J. Caldwell & J. K. Siemsen. 1982. Detection of myocardial sarcoidosis by thallium-201 imaging. J. Natl. Med. Assoc. **74:** 959-964.
11. Valeyre, D., J. Marsac, G. Gambini, J. Lanfranchi, N. Baubion, D. Palsky, J. C. Saltiel, J.-P. Battesti & J. Chrétien. 1983. Clinical assessment of sarcoidosis heart disease: A study of 37 patients with thoracic sarcoidosis. *In* Sarcoidosis and Other Granulomatous Disorders. J. Chrétien, J. Marsac & J. C. Saltiel, Eds.: 296-300. Pergamon Press. Paris.
12. Stein, E., B. Stimmel & L. E. Siltzbach. 1976. Clinical course of cardiac sarcoidosis. Ann. N. Y. Acad. Sci. **278:** 470-474.
13. Gozo, E., I. Cosnow, H. C. Cohen & L. Okun. 1971. The heart in sarcoidosis. Chest **60:** 379-388.
14. Fleming, H. A. 1974. Sarcoid heart disease. Br. Heart J. **36:** 54-68.
15. Friedman, H. S., N. H. Parikh, N. Chander & J. Calderon. 1976. Sarcoidosis with incomplete bilateral bundle branch block pattern disappearing following steroid therapy: An electrophysiological study. Eur. J. Cardiol. **4:** 141-150.
16. Lash, R., J. Coker & B. Y. S. Wong. 1979. Treatment of heart block due to sarcoid heart disease. J. Electrocardiol. **12:** 325-329.
17. Serwer, G. A., S. B. Edwards, D. W. Benson, P. A. W. Anderson & M. Spach. 1978. Ventricular tachyarrhythmia due to cardiac sarcoidosis in a child. Pediatrics **62:** 322-325.

The Prognosis of Sarcoid Heart Disease in the United Kingdom

HUGH A. FLEMING AND SHEILA M. BAILEY

East Anglian Regional Cardiac Unit
Papworth Hospital
Cambridge, England

Until recently sarcoid heart disease has been considered uncommon or even rare. The first case found in the United Kingdom was reported by Forbes and Usher in 1962.[1] This remained the only case reported in the United Kingdom until 1972, when we published a paper on six necropsy proven cases.[2] This led to our establishing the present study to identify and follow-up as many cases as possible in the United Kingdom.

By 1974 we were able to report our findings on 50 cases, 20 of which had necropsy confirmation, and we emphasized that sarcoid heart disease is not rare.[3] Sarcoid heart disease is commonly overlooked in life, and, in cases of sudden death, even at necropsy. We made a further report in 1981.[4] Presentation is most frequently accompanied by cardiac symptoms. Other manifestations of sarcoidosis may not be obvious and should be carefully sought. Many important studies of sarcoid heart disease have been reported from Japan.[5]

Since 1971 we have gathered and retained in the series a total of 250 cases, and we have recorded details annually. The present analysis takes us up to November 1983. All the data of the series will soon be entered into a computer, and modified, up-to-date figures will be available.

Criteria for inclusion in the series must be strict. They are as follows: 1) a cardiac condition compatible with sarcoidosis, 2) a clinical diagnosis of sarcoidosis, and/or 3) histological evidence of sarcoidosis.

Obviously necropsy is the only way of making the etiological diagnosis certain. In the vast majority of surviving patients, indeed, in 80% of them, there is histological confirmation of sarcoidosis in some system.

Using these criteria, a large number of submitted cases have been rejected because of inadequate evidence of sarcoidosis.

Sarcoid heart disease does have a high mortality, but there are few significant reports on survival. In 1977 Roberts *et al.*[6] reported that 73% of their patients with cardiac dysfunction died within 1 year. In 1982 Koide *et al.*[7] reported on a case that survived 12 years, and claimed that this case had the longest survival time ever reported. The oldest case we know of died at the age of 88 years.[8] Our series puts these reports in perspective: long survival is not rare.

We have looked at our series from the point of view of survival and present some of the results. The general composition of the 250 is shown in TABLE 1.

It should be noted that there is no particular sex preponderance, that only 21 cases are non-white, and that there is necropsy confirmation in 88 cases. Most of the patients presented with cardiac problems, sometimes many years after the other manifestations of sarcoidosis (ocular, bilateral hilar lymphadenopathy, and erythema no-

TABLE 1. Composition of the Series

	Number of Patients
Male	137
Female	113
Caucasian	229
Black	21
Deceased	107
Subjected to necropsy	88

dosum) had apparently cleared, and sometimes years *before* other manifestions had appeared. The cardiac problems were varied, and, indeed, sarcoidosis should be considered in any case of difficult heart disease, particularly those involving intractable and varied rhythm problems, complete heart block at an early age, or unexplained heart failure.

The predominant cardiac features at time of presentation are shown in TABLE 2. The valve lesion is commonly mitral incompetence. This can be transient and is probably due to papillary muscle dysfunction. It can be permanent, and in two cases has necessitated mitral valve replacement. Pericarditis is not uncommon, and pericardial involvement is extremely frequent at necropsy.

The age and sex distribution of patients presenting with sudden death is shown in FIGURE 1. The incidence in relatively young males is noteworthy.

The distribution of all deaths is similiarly shown in FIGURE 2. Again, the earlier peak in males is noted, as is the increased number of deaths recorded in males. The age distribution is wide.

The age at cardiac presentation in the whole series is shown in FIGURE 3. The age range is wide in both sexes, and the greatest incidence is between the ages of 25 and 65, emphasizing that this is a disease which affects relatively young people.

The cause of death in those who did not present with sudden death is shown in TABLE 3. Sudden death is common in all groups. Progressive heart failure is particularly common in those presenting as cardiomyopathy.

Of the 101 patients that have survived longer than 5 years, 74 are alive, 36 have survived for more than 10 years, and 7 have survived for more than 20 years. Analysis

TABLE 2. Predominant Cardiac Features

Cardiac Feature	Number of Patients
Complete heart block	49
Ventral ectopics or ventricular tachycardia	48
Myocardial disease	43
Sudden death	37
First-degree heart block or bundle branch block	33
Supraventricular arrhythmia	23
Valve lesion	21
Simulating myocardial infarction	15
Pericarditis	6
Accidental death	4

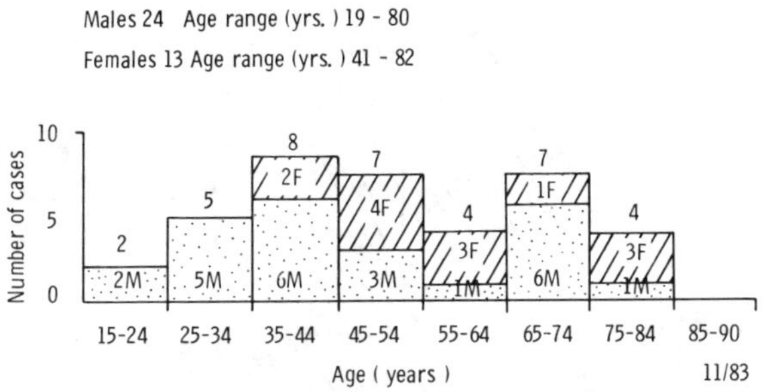

FIGURE 1. Age and sex distribution of patients presenting with sudden death.

of those patients that died after surviving more than 5 years after diagnosis yielded the figures shown in TABLE 4. Again the age range is wide, and there is no particular sex difference.

The mode of clinical presentation of the 36 cases which survived more than 10 years is shown in TABLE 5. There was often a mixed presentation. Congestive cardiac failure, heart block, ventricular arrhythmias, and supraventricular tachycardias are the common forms of presentation. All clinical types of patient are capable of survival.

The average age of presentation for each of several groups of patients among the 36 cases which survived more than 10 years is shown in TABLE 6. Note the wide age range, the similarity between the sexes, and the fact that steroids have been used in 24 and pacing in 5 patients.

Treatment has naturally been extremely varied. All possible cardiac drugs for heart failure and rhythm problems have been used. Pacing has frequently, but by no means invariably, been used for heart block. Steroids have been used commonly. The data are unsuitable for more detailed analysis.

Scrutiny of cases who have died usually showed that more energetic treatment would have been unlikely to alter the outcome in many, but we do feel that emphasis

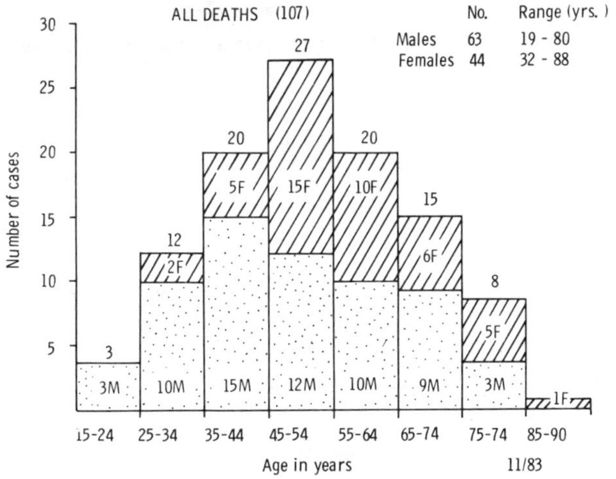

FIGURE 2. Age and sex distribution of all patients that died.

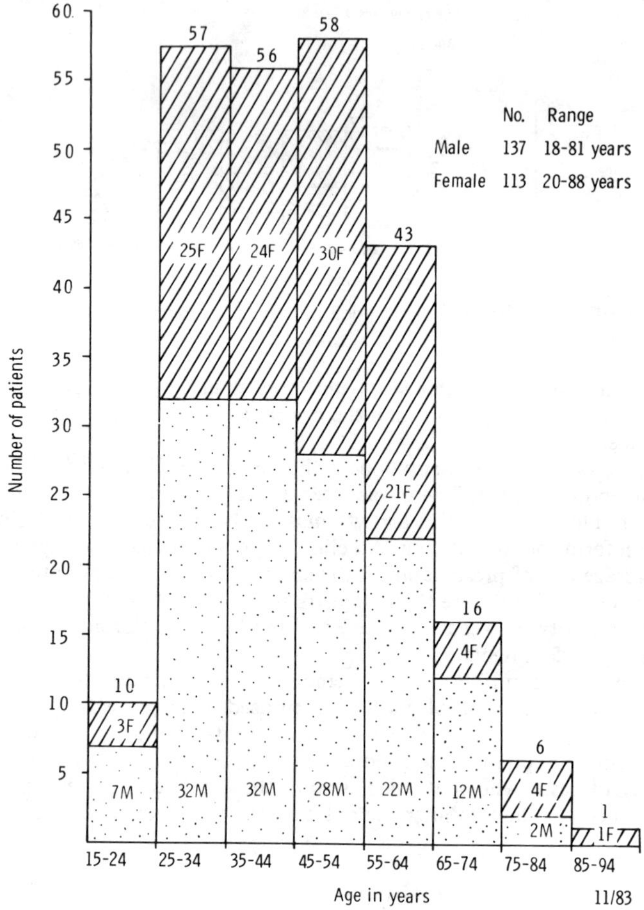

FIGURE 3. Age and sex distribution at the time of cardiac presentation, in a series with a total of 250 cases.

TABLE 3. Deaths Other than Those by Sudden Presentation

	Mode of Death		
Presentation	Congestive Heart Failure	Sudden	Other
Cardiomyopathy	19	9	2
Heart block	5	12	3
Arrhythmia	5	9	3

TABLE 4. Data for Patients That Survived at Least 5 Years after Diagnosis

	Number of Patients	Age at Death (years)		Survival Time (years)	
		Range	Average	Range	Average
Male	14	38-76	58.9	5-20	8.4
Female	13	43-73	59.3	5-28	11.3

should be placed on early diagnosis, earlier and more energetic treatment, and the more frequent and prolonged use of steroids, even in patients who are being paced. Successful steroid treatment has been reported in many papers.[9,10]

We have the impression that those patients which present with ventricular arrhythmia do less well than the others, and we have hopes that amiodarone (Cordarone) may benefit this group. The occasional severe side effects of this drug must be remembered.

We also have the impression that patients who have obvious lung or hilar node involvement fare better, perhaps because the etiological diagnosis is more apparent.

There are many interesting examples of long survival in severe cases, and we would like to quote one which has been particularly well managed. The essential elements of this patient's history are as follows.

In 1969, at the age of 38, she presented with progressive dyspnoea, cough, palpitations, central chest pain, peripheral circulatory failure, very rapid tachycardia, and a pericardial rub. She was defibrillated and treated with many necessary drugs for rhythm problems and heart failure. She had gross cardiomegaly, pericardial effusion, bilateral hilar lymphadenopathy, and erythema nodosum. She had a skin lesion which was biopsied and was positive for sarcoidosis, and a firm diagnosis of sarcoid heart disease was made. The disease was energetically treated through many difficult illnesses. She made a rapid response to treatment with steroids, and over the years she has been given digoxin, frusemide (Lasix), potassium, propranolol (Inderal), and more steroids. In 1984 she remains well (without treatment) and is working. FIGURE 4 shows a radiograph taken of her chest in 1969; FIGURE 5, one taken of her chest in 1970. A great improvement in the cardiomegaly is evident in the latter film.

FIGURE 6 shows samples of some of her rhythm problems. In 1968 she had ventricular tachycardia, which was followed by first-degree heart block. In 1971 there were marked Q wave and ST changes consistent with transmural myocardial infarction, and there were multifocal ventricular ectopics. In 1969 there were additional T wave

TABLE 5. Modes of Clinical Presentation for Patients that Survived at Least 10 Years after Diagnosis

Cardiac Feature	Number of Patients
Congestive heart failure	12
Heart block	9
Ventral ectopics	7
Tachycardia	7
Simulating myocardial infarction	2
Pericarditis	1

TABLE 6. Ages of Presentation for Patients That Survived at Least 10 Years after Diagnosis

	Age of Presentation (years)	
	Range	Average
Male	18-55	36
Female	20-59	42
Steroid treated		24
Paced		5

changes. In 1978 there was atrial flutter and later ventricular tachycardia. In 1981 she still had partial heart block and ventricular ectopic beats. This is a 15-year history of continuing problems that required energetic management, but a good clinical result was ultimately obtained.

In conclusion, recognition of sarcoid heart disease is important. Adequate treatment cannot be given unless the correct diagnosis is made. Presentation with sudden death is common, and there is little that can be done about this. Clinical sarcoidosis of other organs may be inconspicuous and must be diligently sought. When the diagnosis of sarcoid heart disease has been made the prognosis is not necessarily bad,

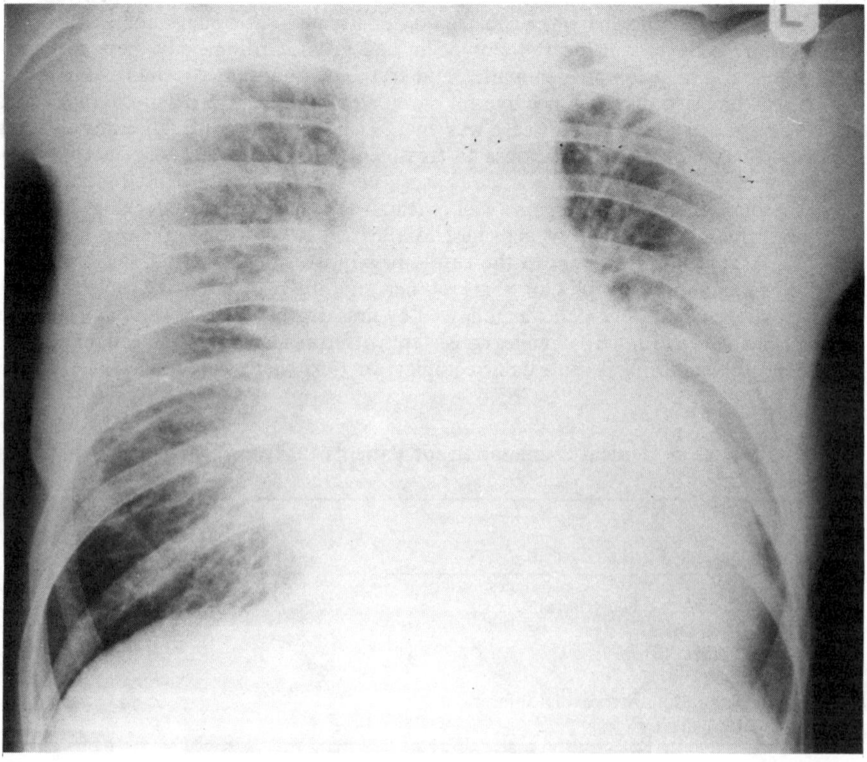

FIGURE 4. A chest radiograph taken in 1969. Cardiomegaly, pericardial effusion, pulmonary infiltration, and pulmonary edema are evident.

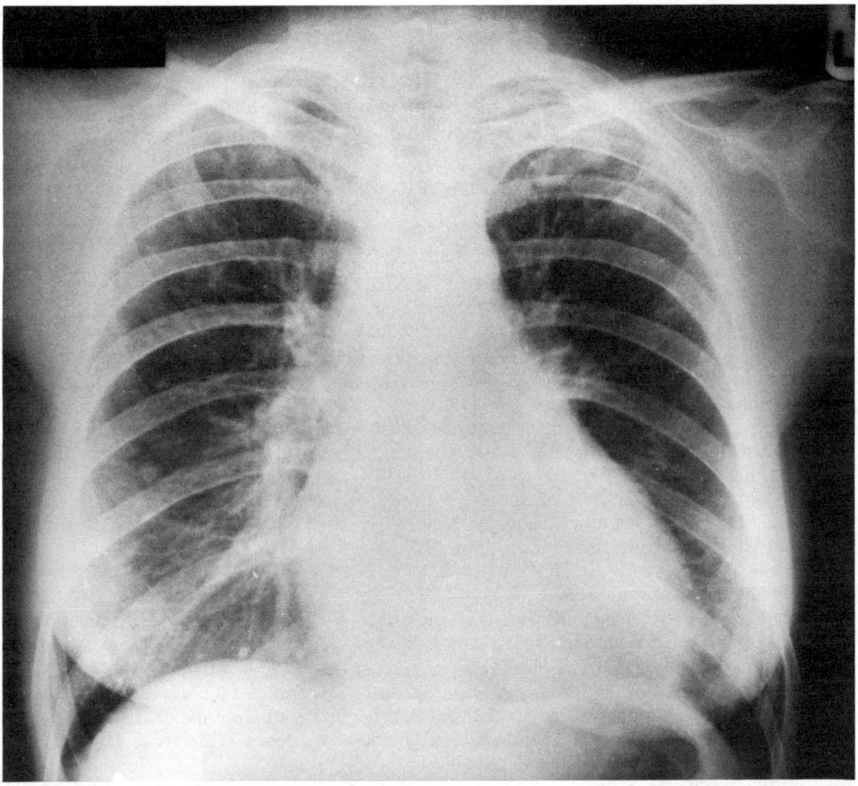

FIGURE 5. A chest radiograph taken in 1970. A considerable improvement in all details may be seen compared to the chest radiograph taken in 1969.

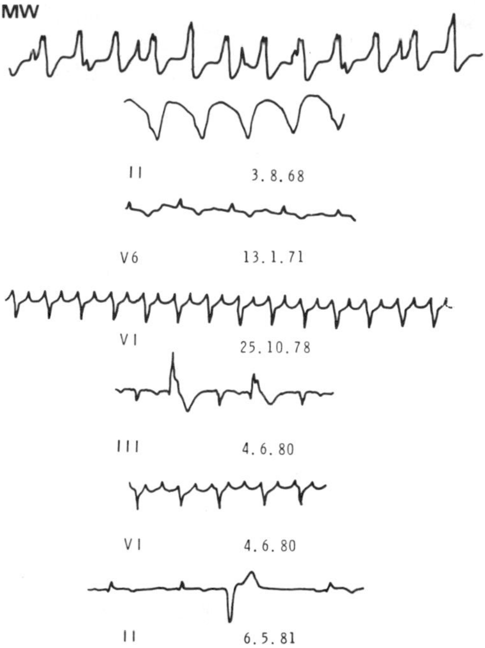

FIGURE 6. Sample electrocardiographs recorded over a 13-year period. See the text for details.

and energetic treatment with all cardiac drugs and pacing is indicated. The progress of patients must be followed carefully, clinically, and with chest radiographs, sufficiently frequent 24-hour electrocardiographic tapes, and echocardiography. Nuclear studies are of less proven value.

Steroids should be used more energetically, earlier, and for sufficiently long periods.

REFERENCES

1. FORBES, G. & A. USHER. 1962. Fatal myocardial sarcoidosis. Br. Med. J. **2:** 771-773.
2. GHOSH, P., H. A. FLEMING, G. A. GRESHAM & P. G. I. STOVIN. 1972. Myocardial sarcoidosis. Br. Heart J. **34:** 769-773.
3. FLEMING, H. A. 1974. Sarcoid heart disease. Br. Heart J. **35:** 54-68.
4. FLEMING, H. A. & S. M. BAILEY. 1981. Sarcoid heart disease: Report of 107 UK cases with necropsy confirmation in 62. J. R. Coll. Physicians London **15:** 245-253.
5. MATSUI, Y., K. IWAI, T. TACHIBANA, T. FRUIE, N. SHIGEMTSU, T. IZUMI, A. H. HOMMA, R. MIKAMI, O. HONGO, Y. HIRAGA & M. YAMAMOTO. 1976. Clinicopathological studies of fatal myocardial sarcoidosis. Ann. N.Y. Acad. Sci. **278:** 455-469.
6. ROBERTS, W. C., H. A. MCALISTER & V. J. FERRANS. 1977. Sarcoidosis of the heart. Am. J. Med. **63:** 86-108.
7. KOIDE, T., S. ITOYAMA, K. KATO, A. KATO & O. MURAO. 1982. Cardiac sarcoidosis with twelve-year survival. Jpn. Heart J. **23:** 263-270.
8. FLEMING, H. A. 1981. The oldest case of sarcoidosis in the world. Br. Med. J. **283:** 502.
9. YAMAMOTO, M., M. MURAMATSU & T. SUZUKI. 1980. Successful corticosteroid treatment of 7 cases of probable myocardial sarcoidosis. *In* Eighth International Conference on Sarcoidosis and Other Granulomatous Diseases. W. Jones Williams & B. H. Davies, Eds.: 615-623. Alpha Omega. Cardiff.
10. ISHIKAWA, T., H. KONDOH, S. NAKAGAWA, Y. KOIWAYA & K. TANAKA. 1984. Steroid therapy in cardiac sarcoidosis. Chest **85:** 445-447.

Ocular Sarcoidosis[a]

D. GERAINT JAMES

Royal Northern Hospital
London N7 6LD, England

BACKGROUND

The earliest descriptions of sarcoidosis drew attention to the cutaneous manifestations of the disease. Nearly 60 years were to elapse before it became accepted that the eye could be involved in a similar process. Jonathan Hutchinson was an able ophthalmologist as well as an observant dermatologist. He was, therefore, well qualified to note any possible association between inflammatory disease of the eye and the purple plaques which he had described. His voluminous writings do not suggest that he had perceived such a link, although he does accurately record examples of subacute relapsing iridocyclitis with postcorneal precipitates, which may well have been due to sarcoidosis.[1]

Schumacher[2] (1909) and Bering[3] (1910) first drew attention to iritis accompanying sarcoidosis. They independently noted, in addition to lesions of the eye, simultaneous involvement of the parotid and submaxillary glands. In view of positive tuberculin skin reactions, they concluded that their patients had tuberculous iritis.

The Danish ophthalmologist Heerfordt[4] (1909) drew attention to "febris uveoparotidea subchronica" characterized by uveitis and enlargement of the parotid glands. The condition ran a chronic and usually febrile course; was frequently complicated by cranial nerve palsies, especially of the seventh cranial nerve; and was associated with pleocytosis of the cerebrospinal fluid. Heerfordt described three cases and referred to others in the literature. Because the latter had been ascribed to mumps, Heerfordt believed that his examples were due to the same cause.

During the following quarter-century the etiology of Heerfordt's syndrome was fiercely debated. Two main schools of thought favored either mumps or tuberculosis. Garland and Thompson[5] (1933) favored a tuberculosis etiology on the basis of their observations of one case and a review of 46 examples from the literature. They recommended that the syndrome be termed "uveoparotid tuberculosis."

Controversy ended when Bruins-Slot[6] (1936), Longcope and Pierson[7] (1937), Pautrier[8] (1937), and Waldenstrom[9] (1937) identified uveoparotid fever as but another manifestation of sarcoidosis. Waldenstrom[9] described five patients with uveoparotitis attending the medical, surgical, and ophthalmic clinics in Uppsala. They had bilateral parotid gland enlargement and bilateral uveitis. The disease was clearly multisystemic, for one or other of these patients had evidence of involvement of the neurological system, lungs, lymph nodes, or skin, as well as fever or hyperglobulinemia. Waldenstrom drew particular attention to bizarre neurological manifestations which included

[a]This work would not have been possible but for generous financial support from the Roger Gibbs Research Foundation and the E. B. Hutchinson Trust. I am also grateful to the Friends of the Royal Northern Hospital for their help.

right facial or hypoglossal nerve palsy and bilateral neuritis; and at the same time indicated meningeal involvement with cerebrospinal fluid pleocytosis. A decade later, Colover[10] (1948) uncovered papilloedema in 16 out of 118 cases of neurosarcoidosis. The cerebrospinal fluid was abnormal in 23 of these 118 patients.

Ocular sarcoidosis involving both anterior and posterior segments is now universally well recognized.[11–24]

Apart from seeing papilloedema,[11] we see choroidoretinitis,[12] periphlebitis retinae,[14,17] retinal hemorrhage,[15,19] and, rarely, neovascularization.[20]

There is a variable incidence of ocular involvement detected in different world series,[24,25] depending partly on whether slit lamp examination is routinely done to uncover silent latent uveitis (TABLE 1). It is hoped that this technique will be universally adopted in the investigation of sarcoidosis.

TABLE 1. Incidence of Ocular Sarcoidosis in a Worldwide Survey[a]

City	Number of Patients	Patients with Ocular Sarcoidosis	
		Number	Percentage
London	537	147	27
New York	311	62	20
Paris	350	37	11
Los Angeles	150	17	11
Tokyo	282	91	32
Reading	425	69	16
Lisbon	89	5	6
Edinburgh	502	53	11
Novi Sad	285	43	15
Naples	624	0	0
Geneva	121	15	12
Western total	3676	539	15
Eastern total	2066	33	1.6
Worldwide total	5742	572	10

[a] The survey included 3676 patients from 11 cities[13] and 2066 patients from Eastern Europe.[24]

PRESENT SERIES

In a personal series of 818 patients with histological confirmation of sarcoidosis, 224 patients (27%) had ocular involvement. Most of these patients were between 20 and 40 years old, and two-thirds of them were female (TABLE 2). Ocular involvement is but one feature of a multisystemic disorder, and it is most commonly associated with intrathoracic disease, skin lesions, and positive Kveim and negative tuberculin skin tests, and hypercalcemia is often observed.

In the series of 224 patients, 66% had anterior uveitis, 14% had posterior uveitis, and another 13% had both. The conjunctiva was involved in 19% and the sclera in only 2% (TABLE 3). The relative infrequency of posterior uveitis is artificial because it is difficult to detect retinitis in the presence of acute inflammation in the anterior

TABLE 2. Clinical and Other Features in a Series of Patients with Ocular Sarcoidosis Compared to Those in a Series of Patients with Sarcoidosis Overall[a]

Feature	Percentage of Patients with the Feature	
	Patients with Ocular Sarcoidosis	Patients with Sarcoidosis Overall
Female	68	61
Age between 20 and 50 years at presentation	76	74
Intrathoracic involvement	75	88
Reticuloendothelial involvement (lymph nodes and spleen)	44	39
Skin lesions	36	21
Erythema nodosum	26	31
Central nervous system involvement	15	9
Facial palsy	12	5
Enlarged parotids	10	6
Bone cysts	8	3
Enlarged lachrymal glands	7	3
Positive Kviem test	80	84
Negative tuberculin skin test	87	70
Hypercalcemia	20	18

[a] The former series included 224 patients; the latter, 818 patients.

chamber. Now that anterior uveitis is rapidly controlled by corticosteroids, posterior uveitis is less likely to be overlooked in the future.

Anterior Uveitis

Anterior uveitis is the most frequent manifestation of ocular sarcoidosis. Populations of patients with anterior uveitis can be divided into subpopulations, of patients

TABLE 3. Frequency of Anatomical Involvement in a Series of Patients with Ocular Sarcoidosis[a]

Type of Ocular Involvement	Percentage of Patients Affected
Anterior uveitis	66
Posterior uveitis	14
Generalized uveitis (anterior and posterior)	13
Conjunctiva	19
Sclera	2
Enlarged lachrymal glands	7

[a]The series included 224 patients.

with acute or chronic iridocyclitis, depending on the onset, course, duration, and clinical associations (TABLE 4). Acute sarcoid iridocyclitis has an abrupt onset and causes pain, photophobia, blurred vision, and red eyes. It occurs most often in women that are between 20 and 30 years old, and is sometimes associated with circumcorneal ciliary congestion; a turbid aqueous humor; keratic precipitates in the anterior chamber; and other acute manifestations such as erythema nodosum and bilateral hilar lymphadenopathy. It responds well to corticosteroid therapy, and the whole course usually subsides uneventfully in a matter of weeks or months. Vitreous aggregations of cytotoxic white cells resemble snowballs. By way of contrast, chronic sarcoid iridocyclitis has an insidious onset in an older age group. There is no ciliary congestion, but gray "mutton fat" keratic precipitates may be seen in the anterior chamber. Ocular fibrosis leads to secondary glaucoma and cataract formation, so the prolonged course is often measured in terms of years or a lifetime. Lesions in other systems—lupus pernio, bone cysts, and pulmonary fibrosis—also reflect irreversible tissue fibrosis.

TABLE 4. Differences between Acute and Chronic Iridocyclitis due to Sarcoidosis

	Iridocyclitis	
	Acute	Chronic
Onset	Abrupt	Insidious
Age in years of patients during onset	20-35	35-50
Course	Transient	Persistent
Signs	Ciliary congestion; turbid aqueous humor; keratic precipitates	Fatty nodules; synechiae
Sequelae	Rare	Lens opacities; glaucoma; cataracts; blindness
Chest radiograph	Hilar adenopathy	Pulmonary fibrosis
Skin lesions	Erythema nodosum	Lupus pernio
Bone cysts	No	Yes
Response to corticosteroids	Good	Poor
Alternative treatment	Indomethacin	Chloroquine; methotrexate

Posterior Uveitis

Posterior uveitis was evident in 14% of the patients in this series without anterior involvement and in another 13% with anterior segment involvement (TABLE 3).

There is always a vitreous cellular infiltrate, and periphlebitis is present in three-quarters of patients, followed in frequency by disc edema and changes in the subretinal pigment epithelium. The disease has a low visual morbidity unless neovascularization develops.[20]

Choroidal nodules are usually scattered discrete off-white waxy exudates, and sometimes cause retinal venous constriction and periphlebitis. These lesions were first described by Walsh.[21] Franceschetti and Babel[23] (1949) used the term choroidoretinitis, "en tache de bougie," to describe their appearance. They may be so numerous as to merit the term birdshot chorioretinopathy. Peripheral choroiditis is symptomless. Involvement of the macula will cause blurring and loss of vision. Fundal lesions are painless, but an associated anterior lesion may cause pain. The more severe the posterior lesion, the greater the probability that it will be associated with some anterior manifestation of the disease.

Fluorescein angiography has brought a fresh dimension to the assessment of sarcoid uveitis, for the leakage of dye displays with clarity the retinal vasculitis. There is a close relationship between granuloma formation and blood vessels; in the central nervous system this is particularly evident in the walls of veins and capillaries, where granulomatous periphlebitis may be produced. This is shown most elegantly by venous leakage with fluorescein angiography in retinal sarcoidosis.

Periphlebitis retinae and peripheral vein occlusion may, though rarely, lead to distinct new vessels and retinal neovascularization.

Papilloedema

Papilloedema occurs more frequently in women and is commonly associated with facial palsy, as well as with pain and hyperalgesia of bizarre distribution on the trunk mimicking pleurisy, appendicitis, or spinal arthritis.[25,26] One of our patients, so afflicted, endeavored to claim compensation for a minor chest injury which he felt was the cause of his condition.[27] The cerebrospinal fluid and pressure may be normal; in one-half of the patients there may be increased protein levels and greater numbers of cells.

In patients with papilloedema, the diagnosis of neurological sarcoidosis should be entertained when it develops rapidly in adults, particularly women, and also especially if there is facial weakness or other cranial nerve palsies or unusual sensory symptoms over the trunk.

In our reported series of patients with papilloedema due to sarcoidosis,[11] evidence of multisystemic involvement, histological evidence of sarcoid tissue, a positive Kveim-Siltzbach test, a gratifying response to corticosteroids, and a subsequent benign course all served to differentiate neurosarcoidosis from the alternative diagnosis of a cerebral tumor. We may now add the value of computerized axial tomography (CAT) scans in making such a differentiation.

Conjunctival Involvement

Phlyctenular or nonspecific conjunctivitis is more commonly bilateral and often coincides with erythema nodosum and bilateral hilar lymphadenopathy as a manifestation of acute, transient sarcoidosis. We have observed it in 28 patients, and granulomas were obtained by biopsy from obvious phlyctenules when the latter were readily seen.

Conjunctival follicles have been noted in only nine patients in our series. Granulomas were readily obtained on biopsy of these follicles, which appear as nodular collections in the conjunctival folds of the lower eyelids.

Keratoconjunctivitis Sicca

Keratoconjunctivitis sicca is bilateral in women nearing menopause. It is a manifestation of chronic fibrotic sarcoidosis. The dry eyes show corneal staining and degenerative changes, but corneal ulceration is not a feature of sarcoidosis. It is accompanied by other chronic, persistent features including enlarged lacrimal and parotid glands, splenomegaly, lymphadenopathy, and pulmonary fibrosis.

Scleritis

Scleritis is a manifestation of acute sarcoidosis and is associated with erythema nodosum and bilateral hilar lymphadenopathy, which suggests that it is one component of a circulating immune complex disorder.

Lachrymal Gland Involvement

Lachrymal gland involvement has been noted in 22 patients, almost all of whom were black women from the West Indies. Biopsy evidence will help to distinguish enlargement due to sarcoidosis, tuberculosis, lymphoma, and Sjögren's and Mikulicz's syndromes.

OCULAR SYNDROMES

The literature abounds with descriptive syndromes, some of them eponymous and all of them emphasizing the multisystemic character of sarcoidosis (TABLE 5).

Heerfordt's Syndrome

This could equally well have been termed Waldenstom's syndrome.[9] It is characterized by uveitis and parotid gland enlargement, runs a chronic and usually febrile course, and is frequently complicated by cranial nerve palsies, especially of the seventh cranial nerve. Other components include bizarre neurological manifestations, lethargy, hyperalgesia, meningism, papilloedema, and cerebrospinal fluid pleocytosis.

We observed parotid gland enlargement in 6% and uveitis in 27% of the 818 patients with sarcoidosis in our series. Conversely, parotid gland enlargement occurred in 10% and facial palsy in 12% of the 147 patients with ocular sarcoidosis in another series.[27,28]

Löfgren's Syndrome

The late Sven Löfgren of Stockholm delineated the association of erythema nodosum and bilateral hilar lymphadenopathy due to sarcoidosis.[29] Uveitis occurred in 13 of 212 patients (6%), and roughly the same incidence was found in cases with and without erythema nodosum. Eight of the 13 patients with uveitis had concurrent parotitis. Löfgren's syndrome is associated with acute iritis. The syndrome is self-limiting and carries a good prognosis, with ultimate complete resolution of sarcoidosis.

Sjögren-like Syndrome

Keratoconjunctivitis sicca with or without parotid and lacrimal gland involvement mimics Sjögren's syndrome with its distressing symptoms of dry eyes and dry mouth, but there is no arthritis, which is such a prominent feature of Sjögren's syndrome.

TABLE 5. Clinical Patterns of Ocular Sarcoidosis

Disease	Features
Heerfordt's or Waldenstrom's syndrome	Uveitis; parotitis; fever; facial palsy
Löfgren's syndrome	Acute iritis; erythema nodosum; bilateral hilar lymphadenopathy; polyarthralgia
Sjögren-like syndrome	Keratoconjunctivitis sicca; parotid dysfunction; lachrymal dysfunction
Chronic fibrotic sarcoidosis	Chronic uveitis; lupus pernio; bone cysts; pulmonary fibrosis; secondary cataract; secondary glaucoma; cor pulmonale

Chronic Uveitis

Chronic fibrotic sarcoidosis may present itself insidiously, with long-standing subacute or chronic uveitis, lupus pernio (FIG. 1), bone cysts, and pulmonary fibrosis. Irreversible fibrosis has occurred in all systems, so ultimate resolution is unlikely to occur. Systemic steroids may provide symptomatic relief but do not quell the underlying fibrosis.

HISTOLOGICAL CONFIRMATION

When confronted with suspected ocular sarcoidosis, histological confirmation should be sought without delay. The differential diagnosis of uveitis is so wide that

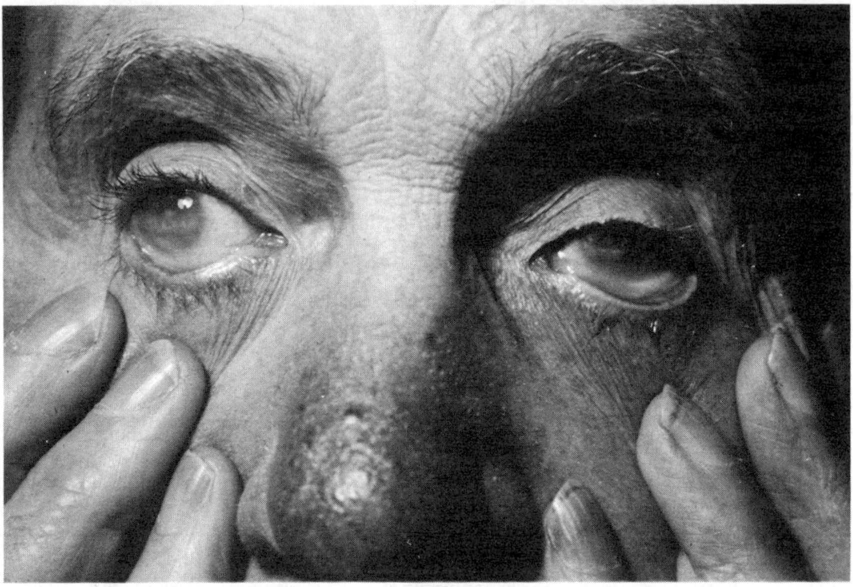

FIGURE 1. The woman pictured above is blind because of chronic fibrotic ocular fibrosis with secondary cataract formation following long-standing chronic relapsing iridocyclitis, which occurred in the days before steroid therapy. Also note the well-developed lupus pernio of the nose due to sarcoidosis.

histology becomes essential. It must be distinguished from Behçet's disease (TABLE 6). This may be obtained by biopsy of a conjunctival follicle or phlyctenule, or of skin, lymph node, lung, bronchus, liver, minor salivary gland, gum, or muscle tissue. Fiberoptic bronchoscopy is now a popular technique for yielding both bronchial mucosa and lung tissue.

Minor salivary gland biopsy is helpful not only for confirming sarcoidosis[30] but also in the investigation of Sjögren's disease with which sarcoidosis may be confused (TABLE 7).

The Kveim-Siltzbach skin test provides histological confirmation and is also a helpful marker of activity of sarcoidosis.

The Usefulness of Blind Conjuctival Biopsy

Sarcoid granulomas are readily obtained from obvious conjunctival follicles and phlyctenules, but blind biopsy is unrewarding. This means that it is of little value in unraveling the riddle of uveitis, whether the uveitis due to sarcoidosis or its many other causes; blind biopsy of the normal-looking conjunctiva is rarely helpful.

Now that I have painted this gloomy picture of the place of conjuctival biopsy in the investigation of sarcoidosis, allow me to restore some optimism. Karma[22] analyzed 79 patients with ocular sarcoidosis in a series of 218 patients and obtained histological evidence of conjunctival granulomas in 37 of them: thus an incidence of 17% among the 218 patients was found. A pitfall that must be emphasized is that conjunctival biopsy may produce nonspecific, foreign-body, giant-cell granulomas, and these must not be misconstrued as the granulomas of sarcoidosis.

MANAGEMENT: A 13-POINT PLAN

1. A full general medical examination should include ophthalmoscopy.
2. Slit lamp examination of the eyes should be used, for otherwise silent lesions may be overlooked.
3. Fluorescein angiography should be used if posterior uveitis is suspected.
4. Chest radiography should be used, for intrathoracic disease occurs in three-quarters of patients with ocular sarcoidosis (TABLE 2).
5. Histological confirmation may be obtained by fiberoptic bronchoscopy, or by biopsy of conjunctival follicle, or of lacrimal gland, lymph node, skin, liver, minor salivary gland, gum, or muscle tissue.

TABLE 6. Comparison of Ocular Sarcoidosis and Behçet's Disease

Features	Ocular Sarcoidosis	Behçet's Disease
Age range in years	20-40	20-40
Ratio of males to females	Equal	Predominantly male
Uveitis		
Anterior	+	+
Posterior	+	+
Oro-genital ulceration	−	+
Erythema nodosum	+	+
Neurologic disease	+	+
Thrombophlebitis	−	+
Cardiac involvement	+	+
Dermatographia	−	+
Fluorescein angiography	Leaking vasculitis	Leaking vasculitis
Chest radiography	Characteristic	Pleural effusion
Serum angiotensin-converting enzyme level	Raised	Normal
Kveim test	+	−
Tuberculin test	−	+
Human leukocyte antigens	B8; A1	B5
Response to treatment		
Steroids	+	+
Azathioprine	±	+
Cyclosporin	±	+
Colchicine	−	+

TABLE 7. Differential Diagnosis of Combined Ocular and Thoracic Disease

	Features				
	Ocular				
Disorder	Anterior Uveitis	Posterior Uveitis	Other	Radiographic	Other
Sarcoidosis	+	+	Enlarged lachrymal glands	Adenopathy; infiltration	Erythema nodosum; other skin lesions
Still's juvenile rheumatoid arthritris	+			Interstitial fibrosis; pleural effusion	Polyarthritis
Histoplasmosis		+		Disseminated opacities	Erythema nodosum
Wegener's granulamatosis	+	+		Migrating infiltrates; cavities	Nasopharyngeal and renal involvement
Ankylosing spondylitis	+			Apical fibrosis	Sacroiliitis; spondylitis
Behçet's disease	+	+	Hypopion	Pleural effusion	Erythema nodosum; oro-genital ulceration
Sjögren's disease			Enlarged lachrymal glands; kerato-junctivitis sicca	Diffuse infiltration	Plasma cell involvement of parotids
Stevens-Johnson syndrome	+		Conjunctivitis; keratitis; corneal ulceration	Pneumonia	Erythema multiforme; cold agglutinins

6. The Kveim-Siltzbach skin test is a safe, simple, and specific out-patient technique. It is positive in 80% of patients with ocular sarcoidosis (TABLE 2), but it takes 1 month to read the result. Fiberoptic bronchoscopy has reduced its popularity but not its specificity. Moreover, a positive Kveim test underlines activity of the disease. Although used less often in investigations of pulmonary disease, it is still widely used in investigations of uveitis, erythema nodosum, idiopathic hypercalciuria, and hepatic granulomatous disease.

7. One should make sure that the disorder is multisystemic.

8. The tuberculin skin test is negative in most patients with ocular sarcoidosis, and only faintly positive in the remainder. A strongly positive tuberculin skin test rules out active sarcoidosis. A negative tuberculin skin test in a patient who has had a BCG vaccination points to impaired cellular immunity and to the impaired memory of T lymphocytes.

9. Determining the serum angiotensin-converting enzyme level is not a good diagnostic test, for it has too many false-positives, but it is invaluable in long-term management. It provides a handy monitor of progress of the disease.

10. Serum calcium levels are elevated in up to 20% of patients with ocular sarcoidosis. Urine calcium levels, however, which may be monitored over 24 hr, are even better indicators, for hypercalciuria may occur with normal serum calcium levels (but never the reverse).

11. Special situations may include radioactive gallium as a monitor of progress of pulmonary and salivary gland disease; radioactive thallium to delineate myocardial sarcoidosis; and CAT scans for neurosarcoidosis.

12. One should determine whether the disease is acute or chronic (TABLE 4).

13. Patients should be treated vigorously with steroids to prevent the complication of ocular fibrosis.

TREATMENT

The mainstays of treatment comprise topical and oral corticosteroids together with local atropine eye drops. The latter is most important to maintain a dilated pupil and to prevent the inflamed iris from adhering to the lens and to the back of the cornea.

For anterior uveitis, steroid eye drops are applied frequently during the day, reinforced with a steroid eye ointment at night. If there is no substantial and continuing improvement after 1 week, then the concentration of corticosteroid in the anterior segment of the eye may be increased by cortisone from a local subconjunctival depot. Oral steroid therapy is indicated if local treatment does not lead to a rapid response or if ophthalmoscopy reveals posterior uveitis. Very often, of course, oral steroids are also indicated for extraocular involvement, particularly intrathoracic disease, neurosarcoidosis, cardiac disorder, disfiguring skin lesions, and lacrimal-parotid or reticuloendothelial involvement.

Local steroid therapy needs to be monitored carefully by intraocular pressure levels, for topical steroids may provoke rises or even precipitate secondary glaucoma. This is not a particular complication of oral steroids. High intraocular pressure indicates that a switch from topical to oral steroids is desirable, and that timolol eye drops (Timoptol) should be given to reduce the pressure to normal.

Other Drugs

Treatment may be necessary when there are contraindications to steroid therapy. Under compelling circumstances the alternatives listed below should be considered.

Indomethacin

Indomethacin may prove helpful in acute uveitis, a situation in which prostaglandins are present in large amounts in the aqueous humor.

Cyclosporin

Cyclosporin is an effective immunosuppressive drug which is of proven value in organ transplantation, and may be sight-saving in posterior uveitis due to Behçet's disease. It has not yet been adequately tested in ocular sarcoidosis.

Azathioprine

The immunosuppressive azathioprine has a steroid-sparing effect that permits a significant (up to 50%) reduction in the steroid dose needed.

REFERENCES

1. HUTCHINSON, J. 1900. Mabey's malady and lupus pernio. Arch. Surg. **11:** 205-211.
2. SCHUMACHER, G. 1909. Fall von beiderseitiger Iridougclitis Chronica bei Boeckshem multiplem benignem Sarkoid. Münch. Med. Wochenschr. **56:** 2664.
3. BERING, F. 1910. Zur Kentnis des Boeckshen Sarcoids. Dermatol. Z. **17:** 404-412.
4. HEERFORDT, C. F. 1909. Uber Eine 'Febris uveo-parotidea subchronica' an der glandula parotis under der uvea des anges lokalisiert und haufig mit pareden Cerebrospinaler neuen Kompliaiert. V. Graefes. Arch. Ophthalmol. **70:** 254-273.
5. GARLAND, H. G. & J. G. THOMPSON. 1933. Uveo-parotid tuberculosis (febris uveo-parotidea of Heerfordt). Q. J. Med. **26:** 157-177.
6. BRUINS-SLOT, W. J. 1936. Ziekte von Besnier-Boeck en febris uveoparotidea (Heerfordt). Ned. Tijdschr. Geneeskd. **80:** 2859-2863.
7. LONGCOPE, W. T. & J. W. PIERSON. 1937. Boeck's sarcoidosis. Bull. Johns Hopkins Hosp. **60:** 223-296.
8. PAUTRIER, L. M. 1937. Syndrome de Heerfordt et maladie de Besnier-Boeck-Schaumann. Bull. Soc. Hop. Paris **53:** 1608-1620.
9. WALDENSTROM, J. 1937. Some observations on uveoparotitis and allied conditions with special reference to symptoms from the nervous system. Acta Med. Scand. **91:** 53-68.
10. COLOVER, J. 1948. Sarcoidosis of the nervous system. Brain **71:** 451-473.

11. JAMES, D. G., M. A. ZATOUROFF, J. TROWELL & F. C. ROSE. 1967. Papilloedema in sarcoidosis. Br. J. Ophthalmol. **51:** 526-529.
12. JAMES, D. G., E. NEVILLE & D. A. LANGLEY. 1976. Ocular sarcoidosis. Trans. Ophthalmol. Soc. U.K. **96:** 133-139.
13. JAMES, D. G., E. NEVILLE, L. E. SILTZBACH, J. TURIAF, J. P. BATTESTI, O. P. SHARMA, Y. HOSODA, R. MIKAMI, M. ODAKA, T. G. VILLAR, B. DJURIČ, A. C. DOUGLAS, W. MIDDLETON, A. KARLISH, A. BLASI, D. OLIVIERI & P. PRESS. 1976. A worldwide review of sarcoidosis. Ann. N.Y. Acad. Sci. **278:** 321-334.
14. AINSLIE, D. & D. G. JAMES. 1953. Sarcoidosis with ocular involvement. Arch. Middlesex Hosp. **3:** 71-83.
15. GOULD, H. & H. E. KAUFMAN. 1961. Sarcoid of the fundus. Arch. Ophthalmol. **65:** 453-456.
16. JAMES, D. G. 1964. The diagnosis and treatment of ocular sarcoidosis. Acta Med. Scand. Suppl. **425:** 203-206.
17. AINSLIE, D. & D. G. JAMES. 1956. Ocular sarcoidosis. Br. Med. J. **1:** 954-964.
18. DOW, D. S. 1965. Ocular sarcoidosis: Report of a case characterized by vitreous and retinal hemorrhage, extensive phlebitis, anterior uveitis and secondary glaucoma and with extensive multiple and system involvement. Am. J. Opthalmol. **59:** 93-97.
19. QUOCK, G. P. & R. F. DONOHUE. 1967. Flame-shaped retinal hemorrhage in sarcoidosis. J. Am. Med. Assoc. **202:** 230-234.
20. SPALTON, D. J. & M. D. SANDERS. 1981. Fundus changes in histologically confirmed sarcoidosis. Br. J. Opthalmol. **65:** 348-358.
21. WALSH, F. E. 1939. Ocular importance of sarcoidosis. Arch. Ophthalmol. (Chicago) **21:** 421-438.
22. KARMA, A. 1979. Ophthalmic changes in sarcoidosis. Acta Ophthalmol. **141**(Suppl.): 1-94.
23. FRANCESCHETTI, A. & J. BABEL. 1949. La chorionretinite "en tache de bougie" manifestation de la maladie Besnier-Boeck. Ophthalmologica **118:** 701-710.
24. DJURIČ, B., L. MANDI, S. YEZENDI & CELIKOGLY. 1980. Sarcoidosis in six European cities. *In* Eighth International Conference on Sarcoidosis and Other Granulomatous Diseases. W. Jones Williams and B. H. Davies, Eds.: 527-531. Alpha Omega. Cardiff.
25. MATTHEWS, W. B. 1965. Sarcoidosis of the nervous system. J. Neurol. Neurosurg. Psychiatry **28:** 23-29.
26. SILVERSTEIN, A., M. M. FEUER & L. E. SILTZBACK. 1965. Neurologic sarcoidosis. Arch. Neurol. (Chicago) **12:** 1-11.
27. JAMES, D. G. & O. P. SHARMA. 1967. Neurological complications of sarcoidosis. Proc. Roy. Soc. Med. **60:** 1169-1172.
28. GREENBERG, G., R. ANDERSON, P. SHARPSTONE & D. G. JAMES. 1964. Enlargement of the parotid gland due to sarcoidosis. Br. Med. J. **2:** 861-862.
29. LÖFGREN, S. 1946. Erythema nodosum: Studies on etiology and pathogenesis in 185 adult cases. Acta Med. Scand. **124**(Suppl. 174): 1-197.
30. NESSAN, V. J. & J. R. JACOWAY. 1979. Biopsy of minor salivary glands in diagnosis of sarcoidosis. N. Engl. J. Med. **301:** 922-924.

Treatment of Intraocular Complications of Sarcoidosis

ALAN G. PALESTINE,[a] ROBERT B. NUSSENBLATT, AND CHI-CHAO CHAN

Clinical Ophthalmic Immunology Section
Clinical Branch
National Eye Institute
National Institutes of Health
Bethesda, Maryland 20205

INTRODUCTION

Sarcoidosis may affect the ocular structures in numerous ways. The percentage of patients reported to have ocular sarcoidosis varies considerably among different studies. Thirty-eight percent of patients in one study from the Southeast United States with systemic sarcoidosis have ocular involvement,[1] and 52.5% of those patients with ocular disease had intraocular inflammation and 25.3% had posterior segment inflammation (chorioretinal lesions, retinal periphlebitis, and vitritis). A second study found 27% of patients with systemic sarcoidosis had ocular involvement.[2] Although many of the forms of intraocular sarcoidosis respond to corticosteroid therapy,[3] other therapeutic modalities may be utilized. This paper will illustrate several forms of surgical therapy in the treatment of selected complications of intraocular sarcoidosis and the use of systemic cyclosporin A (CsA) in steroid nonresponders.

MATERIALS AND METHODS

CsA Therapy

Five patients with anterior and posterior ocular inflammation related to sarcoidosis were treated. The diagnosis of sarcoidosis was biopsy proven in three of the patients and presumed in the fourth and fifth on the basis of an abnormal gallium scan of the lung and abnormal pulmonary function testing compatible with the diagnosis of sarcoidosis. The ocular and systemic findings for these five patients are summarized in TABLE 1, and one of these patients, number 1, is discussed in detail as case A

[a] Address for correspondence: National Institutes of Health, National Eye Institute, Building 10, Room 10N 222, Bethesda, Maryland 20205.

TABLE 1. CsA Therapy in Ocular Sarcoidosis

Patient Number	Age (years)/Sex/Race	Systemic Involvement	Maintenance CsA Dose (mg/kg)	Maintenance Prednisone Dose (mg daily)	Duration of Therapy (months)
1	35/F/B	Liver; lung; parotid glands	5	None	9
2	39/F/B	Mediastinum	3.3	15	18
3	23/M/B	Bone marrow	15[a]	60[a]	3[a]
4	36/F/W	Lung; central nervous system	15[a]	10[a]	2[a]
5	57/M/W	Lung; axillary nodes; central nervous system?	5	15	16

[a]Not controlled.

below. All patients had been poorly controlled on systemic corticosteroids or had developed severe side effects.

Treatment began with a daily dose of 10 mg/kg CsA taken orally. If there was no response of the ocular inflammation in 2 weeks, the dose was increased to 15 mg/kg. The dose was lowered in response to decreased renal function or hypertension, or if the patient experienced severe subjective side effects.

In general, decreased renal function of up to 50% (as indicated by a doubling of the pretreatment creatinine) was tolerated without alteration of the CsA dose. If adequate control of the intraocular inflammation could not be achieved with CsA alone, 15 mg of prednisone was added daily. Serum chemistries and hematology profiles were followed monthly.

Case Illustrations

Three case histories will be presented to illustrate a variety of surgical techniques as well as to illustrate the use of CsA.

Case A

A 34-year-old black female was diagnosed in 1977 as having hepatic sarcoidosis on liver biopsy following evaluation for fever. She developed recurrent bilateral anterior and posterior granulomatous uveitis beginning in 1977 which could be controlled with daily doses of 10-30 mg of systemic prednisone. She had several inflammatory episodes in both eyes and, by 1980, had developed a low-grade chronic granulomatous inflammation with mutton-fat keratic precipitates, white vitreoretinal nodules, and white retinal punctate lesions. She developed elevated intraocular pressure in 1980 related to steroid therapy. Topical prednisolone or systemic prednisone caused a marked rise in intraocular pressure. She was placed on topical timolol 0.5% and oral acetazolamide 500 mg twice daily so that steroid therapy of the ocular inflammation could be continued. For the next 2 years her vision remained in the 20/30 range in both eyes, and her uveitis was controlled with topical fluorometholone (FML) with the careful addition of oral prednisone as needed. In September 1982 she had an abrupt decrease in acuity in the left eye to counting fingers at 1 foot. There was a moderate posterior vitritis, and a subretinal neovascular membrane was present temporal to the optic disc with retinal edema extending into the left macula (FIG. 1A). Argon-laser photocoagulation was performed which led to resolution of this membrane (FIG. 1B). The laser power was 300 to 400 mW, and sixty-five burns 50 μ in diameter were made. The patient's vision improved to 20/200 over the next month.

She continued to have recurrent episodes of uveitis in both eyes during the next year. When these episodes occurred, the dose of oral prednisone was increased to 15 to 30 mg each day for 2 to 3 weeks, after which time the dose was returned to 10 mg every other day. Topical FML, timolol, and oral neptazine (50 mg three times a day) were continuously utilized. The increases in oral prednisone were accompanied by a marked increase, to between 40 and 50 mm Hg, in intraocular pressure. In September 1982 an early Bjerrum's scotoma was noted in the right eye compatible with early glaucomatous damage. Oral steroid administrations were discontinued. The patient's intraocular inflammation increased in the right eye, and her vision decreased from

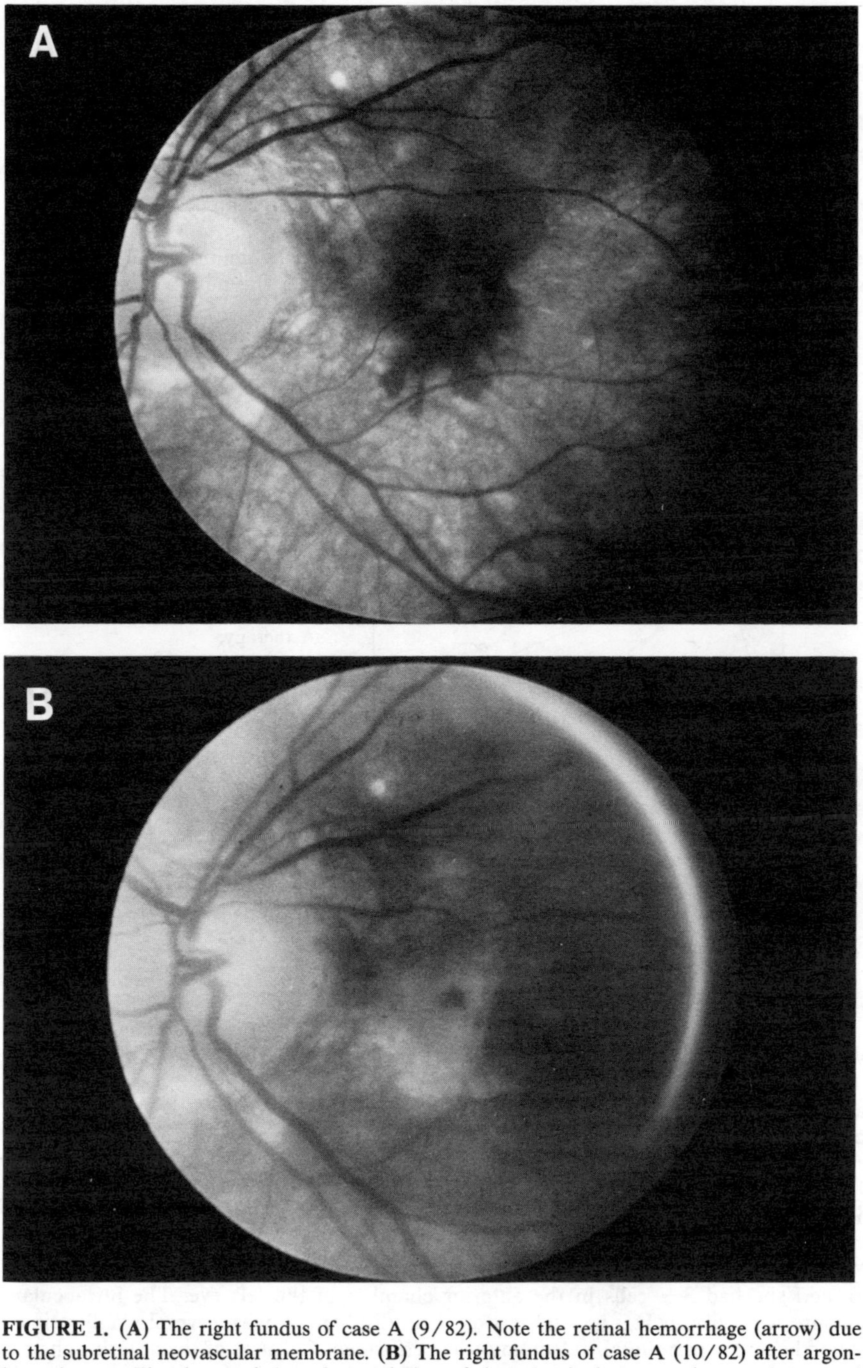

FIGURE 1. (**A**) The right fundus of case A (9/82). Note the retinal hemorrhage (arrow) due to the subretinal neovascular membrane. (**B**) The right fundus of case A (10/82) after argon-laser therapy. The therapy led to the resolution of the subretinal neovascular membrane and left residual scarring.

20/20 to 20/40. Her alkaline phosphatase and γ-glutamyl transpeptidase levels increased as shown in FIGURE 2. Her gallium scan was abnormal and showed parotid (FIG. 3A) and lacrimal gland involvement. Because of the increased ocular and hepatic inflammation and the steroid-related glaucoma, the patient was begun on 10 mg/kg of CsA (TABLES 1 & 2). Her serum chemistries improved (FIG. 2), and her vision improved to 20/20 in the right eye and remained 20/200 in the left. The ocular inflammation became quiet. The CsA doses were gradually decreased because of nausea and decreased renal function over the next 2 months. In December 1983 the patient was using 5 mg/kg of CsA daily and continued using topical FML and timolol. Serum chemistries (FIG. 2) continued to improve as did the gallium scan (FIG. 3B), and the patient's ocular inflammation remained quiet over the next 6 months.

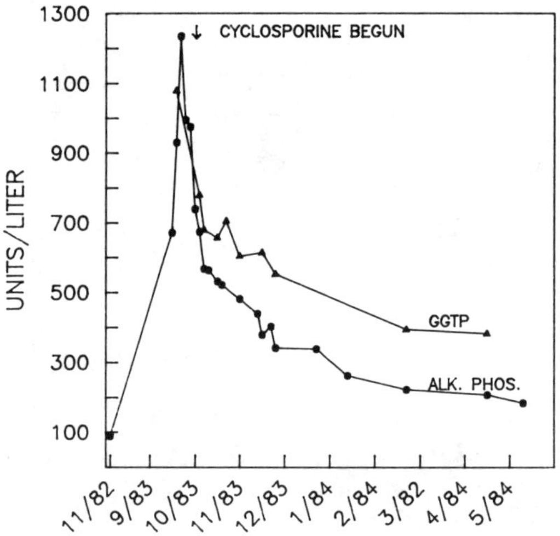

FIGURE 2. Serum alkaline phosphatase and γ-glutamyl transpeptidase levels in case A as related to CsA therapy.

Case B

A 6-year-old white female developed acute iritis with corneal edema, posterior synechiae, iris nodules, and elevated intraocular pressure in the left eye in June 1982. The antinuclear antibody and rheumatoid factor levels were normal; the sedimentation rate was 10 mm/hr; the serum angiotensin-converting enzyme level was 31.5 units (normal level: less than 25 units); the PPD skin test was positive; and the sputum and gastric cultures were negative. She was placed on topical prednisolone, isoniazid (10 mg/kg), and rifampin (15 mg/kg). Her inflammation continued over the next 2 months, and iris nodules were again noted in August 1982. There was an increase in anterior segment inflammation. She continued to have elevated intraocular pressure. When examined at the National Eye Institute in September 1982 her vision was 20/40, and she had 3+ cells in the anterior chamber of the left eye. The intraocular pressure was 36 mm Hg, and there was optic disc edema with several small retinal hemorrhages. A peripheral iridectomy was performed. Cultures of the anterior chamber fluid were negative for microorganisms. Pathology of the iris specimen showed

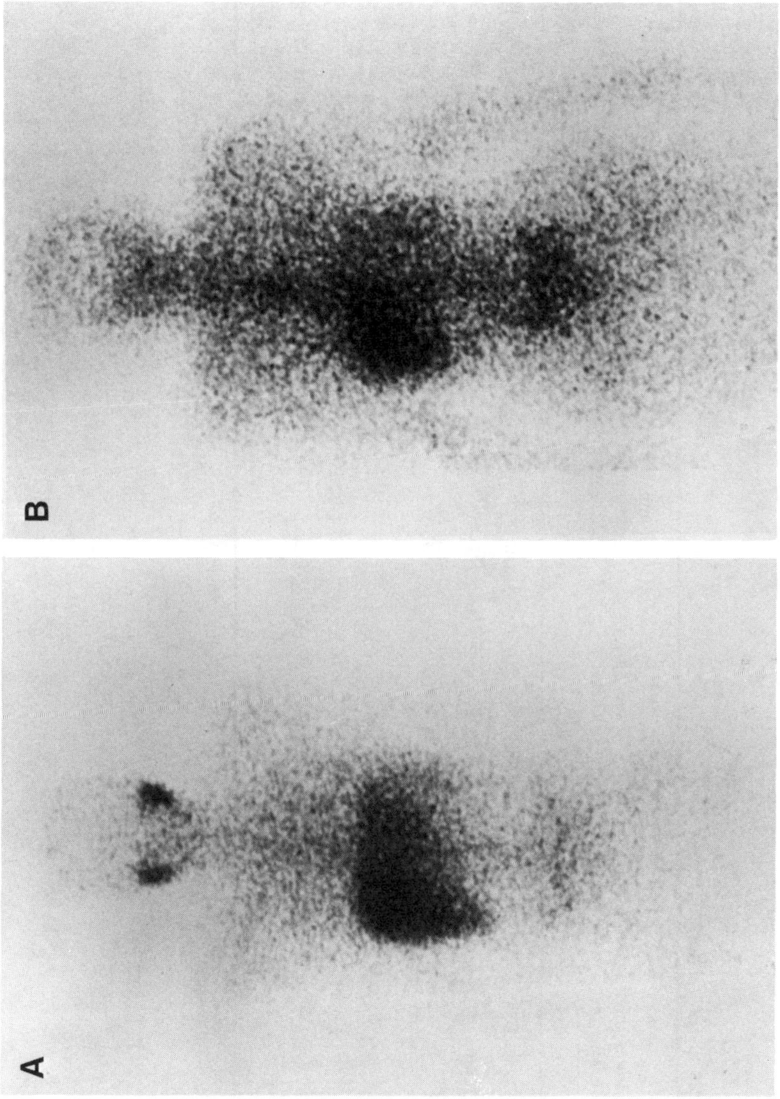

FIGURE 3. **(A)** Gallium scan of case A (9/83) showing increased gallium uptake in the parotid glands before CsA therapy. **(B)** Another gallium scan of case A (5/84), showing the abnormal uptake of gallium in the parotid glands to be resolved.

TABLE 2. Effects of CsA Therapy

Patient	Ocular Inflammation before Therapy		Vision before Therapy		Vision during Therapy		Inflammation during Therapy			
Number	OD	OS	OD	OS	OD	OS	OD	OS	Comments	Side Effects
1	2+	2+	20/40	20/200	20/20	20/200	0	0	Liver function improved	Nausea on 10 mg/kg CsA
2	3+	3+	20/160	20/200	20/30	20/40	Trace	Trace	Preexisting chronic pyelonephritis; pretreatment creatinine clearance: 70	Decreased renal function requiring a decrease in CsA
3	–	3+	Blind	20/200	Blind	CF[a]	–	4+		None
4	2+	2+	20/200	20/200	CF[a]	CF[a]	1+	1+		Tremor; hyperesthesia
5	2+	2+	20/200	20/70	20/50	20/30	Trace	Trace	Aseptic meningitis while on CsA; stopped CsA after 16 months; vision stable.	Renal toxicity; epigastric discomfort; tremor

[a]The patient could count fingers held 1 foot away.

noncaseating granulomatous inflammation (FIG. 4). Stains for acid-fast organisms were negative. The patient was given 25 mg of oral prednisone each day, and significant improvement in the inflammation was evident over the next week. Vision returned to 20/20 in the left eye, and the optic disc edema resolved. She was tapered off oral steroids over 6 weeks.

Case C

A 22-year-old black female had a 7-year history of granulomatous uveitis involving the anterior and posterior segments of both eyes. In January 1982 she had a marked increase in inflammatory activity with a decrease in vision. Chest radiographs had

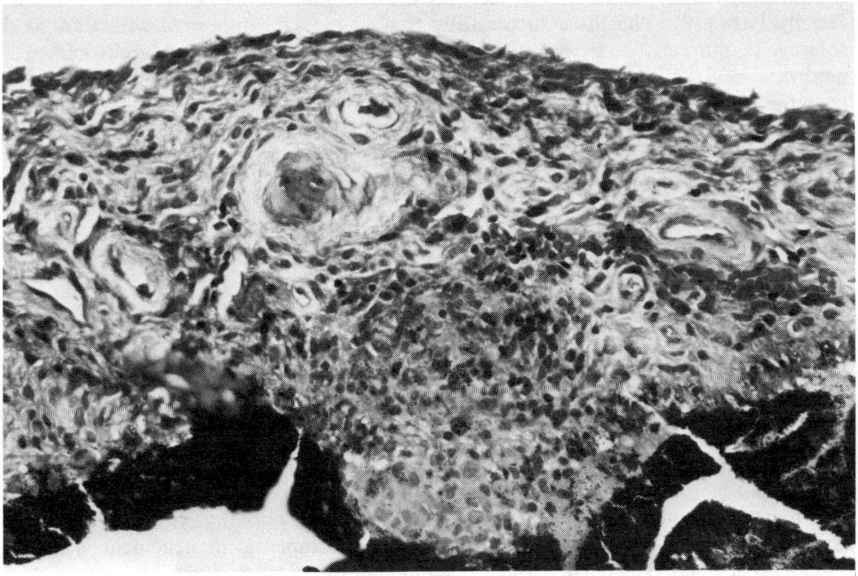

FIGURE 4. Iris specimen from case B showing noncaseating granulomatous inflammation.

shown hilar adenopathy, and the patient was anergic to skin testing. The patient had been treated with topical prednisolone every 2 hr and 20-40 mg of oral prednisone daily to control the inflammation. In June 1982 her vision was 20/50 and 20/400 in her left and right eyes, respectively. Intraocular pressure was 3 and 0 mm Hg in her left and right eyes, respectively. The anterior chambers were quiet, there were early posterior subcapsular cataracts, and 1+ vitreous cells were present in each eye. Macular edema and optic disc edema were present bilaterally. She underwent argon-laser therapy to 270° of trabecular meshwork in the left eye in an attempt to occlude the meshwork. The pressure increased to 4 mm Hg. The cataracts progressed in both eyes, and she required 20 mg of prednisone daily to control the uveitis. In January

1983 she underwent extracapsular cataract removal in the left eye via a limbal incision. The vitreous fluid was observed to be hazy, and an anterior vitrectomy was also performed. Vision improved from 20/400 to 20/25. She continued to require 20-30 mg of prednisone every other day for the uveitis. An attempt to taper the prednisone resulted in a severe flare-up of inflammation, and her vision was reduced to 20/50 in the left eye. In July 1983 she underwent pars plana lensectomy and vitrectomy in the right eye. The vision improved from counting fingers at 1 foot to 20/25. She was continued on 20 mg of prednisone every other day.

RESULTS OF CsA THERAPY

Three of the five patients treated with systemic CsA for sarcoid uveitis had significantly improved vision and decreased inflammation; two of the five were unaffected (TABLE 2). The three successfully treated patients improved with CsA as the sole agent, but renal toxicity in patient 2 (exacerbated by preexisting chronic pyelonephritis) and patient 5 required the addition of low doses of prednisone. This represented a marked lowering of their prednisone dosage in that 60 mg each day failed to control the inflammation. Patient number 5 had fever and aseptic meningitis while on CsA. This may represent a failure to control sarcoidosis of the central nervous system in this patient.

DISCUSSION

The majority of ophthalmic publications dealing with sarcoidosis emphasize the multitude of varied ocular manifestations which may occur in sarcoidosis. These include conjunctival nodules, anterior uveitis, vitritis, chorioretinitis, retinal periphlebitis, optic nerve inflammation, and lacrimal gland and orbital involvement.[1,2,4] Complications secondary to the chronic inflammation often include cataracts, glaucoma, and macular edema, and infrequently include band keratopathy, vitreous hemorrhaging, and subretinal neovascular membranes.[1,2,4] Therapeutic management is less frequently discussed. The cornerstone of ocular therapy of sarcoidosis is corticosteroids.[2] These may be used in topical, periocular, or systemic form. Some patients with severe anterior and posterior uveitis fail to respond to systemic steroids or cannot tolerate this therapy. It is these patients in whom we have utilized CsA as an alternate therapy. In addition, complications such as glaucoma, cataracts, vitreous opacities, and subretinal neovascular membranes do not respond to medical therapy, but are amenable to surgical therapy.

CsA is a cyclic endecapeptide which has a marked suppressive effect on helper T cell function. It prevents the production of interleukin-2 and will block the response of lymphocytes to this lymphokine under certain conditions. CsA has been primarily utilized for the prevention of graft rejection in kidney, liver, and heart transplantation.[5] We have treated 70 patients with systemic CsA for uveitis of presumed autoimmune etiology who had failed on systemic prednisone.[6,7] These include patients with Behçet's syndrome, Vogt-Koyanagi-Harada syndrome, pars planitis, and idiopathic intermediate uveitis as well as sarcoidosis. Approximately 90% of patients have had a favorable initial response, but only 60% can tolerate the toxicity of the treatment over the long term.[7] Side effects have included nephrotoxicity, hypertension, hirsutism, gingivitis, hyperesthesias, and epigastric distress.[8] Approximately 50% can be controlled with CsA as the sole agent. No lymphoma or opportunistic infections have occurred, in contrast to the organ transplant patients in whom the rate of these complications is no lower than with conventional immunosuppressive therapy.[5]

The size of the population we studied, five patients, prevents us from making broad generalizations about the effectiveness of CsA in sarcoidosis. Three of the five patients had significant, favorable responses, but patients 3 and 4 clearly worsened in spite of high doses of CsA and prednisone.

The serum chemistry abnormalities in patient 1 (Case A) became much less pronounced, indicating a possible effect by CsA on systemic disease, but patient 5 had fever and aseptic meningitis, symptoms that may have represented sarcoidosis of the central nervous system, while being treated with CsA. Only one of the three CsA responders could be treated with this drug as the only systemic therapy. CsA did significantly reduce the steroid requirement and provided improved control of inflammation as compared to prednisone alone. CsA, however, may alter the metabolism and therefore the effect of prednisone by increasing its half-life.[9] It is therefore difficult to assess the contribution of CsA in reducing the steroid requirement. CsA may have a role in the therapy of sarcoidosis, and further studies are needed to define the correct usage of this agent.

Several types of surgical intervention are illustrated in the case examples in this paper. Case C illustrates cataract removal with vitrectomy to remove lens and vitreous opacities. Cataracts occur in uveitis as a result of the inflammation and steroid therapy. One study found these in 8.4% of patients, but this may understate the incidence because cataracts evolve slowly with time.[1] With current vitrectomy instrumentation, lens and vitreous opacities may be removed through small incisions, thereby minimizing the trauma to the eye. Any surgical procedure may induce increased inflammatory activity, and it is advisable to begin with a quiet eye when possible. Although cataracts may be removed by intracapsular extraction, extracapsular extraction, or pars plana lensectomy, we prefer the latter technique because it permits a smaller incision and the removal of pathological vitreous tissue, and because it does not cause trauma to the trabecular meshwork.

Glaucoma in sarcoidosis may result from trabecular meshwork inflammation, trabecular meshwork occlusion from synechiae, pupillary block from synechiae (case B), steroid therapy, or a combination of factors (case A). The acute glaucoma from pupillary block is best treated with iridectomy as in case B. This may be done surgically or with an argon laser; however, laser iridectomies are small and tend to close if the inflammation persists. Chronic glaucoma (case A) requires medical therapy and may require filtering surgery. Filtering surgery was avoided in this patient by discontinuing oral steroid and using systemic CsA.

Ocular hypotension (case C) is an uncommon complication of sarcoidosis for which there is no accepted therapy. It results from inflammatory ciliary body damage and a subsequent decrease in aqueous humor secretion. Laser therapy was utilized in this case in an attempt to decrease aqueous outflow by damaging the trabecular meshwork, and was accompanied by a small, but sustained increase in intraocular pressure. Pars plana vitrectomy may also be used to treat ocular hypotension if a cyclitic membrane is present.

Subretinal neovascular membrane formation (case A) is another uncommon occurrence in sarcoidosis,[10,11] but it is very common in other ocular disorders such as senile macular degeneration. The new vessels grow beneath the retina and cause edema and hemorrhaging. Argon-laser photocoagulation can lead to resolution of the membrane,[11] but permanent retinal damage can occur from both the membrane and the laser therapy. The natural course of these membranes in sarcoidosis is not well documented, but they do not appear to resolve with systemic steroid therapy, in contrast to the optic disc and epiretinal neovascular proliferation that may also occur in sarcoidosis.

We have illustrated a number of therapeutic modalities for the treatment of the intraocular complications of sarcoidosis. In addition to steroid therapy for inflammation, cataract removal, vitrectomy, glaucoma surgery, and laser photocoagulation have a role in the management of these patients. The role of systemic CsA in ocular sarcoidosis is still not well defined, but CsA may be useful in selected patients in whom steroid therapy is ineffective or is producing undesirable complications.

ACKNOWLEDGMENTS

We would like to thank Dr. Merlyn Rodrigues for her assistance with case B and Dr. Douglas Gaasterland for his assistance in the laser treatment of case C.

REFERENCES

1. Obenauf, C. D., E. S. Harold, C. F. Sydnor & G. K. Klintworth. 1978. Sarcoidosis and its ophthalmic manifestations. Am. J. Ophthalmol. **86:** 648-655.
2. James, D. G., E. Neville & D. A. Langley. 1976. Ocular sarcoidosis. Trans. Ophthalmol. Soc. U.K. **96:** 133-145.
3. Spalton, D. J. & M. D. Sanders. 1981. Fundus changes in histologically confirmed sarcoidosis. Br. J. Ophthalmol. **65:** 348-358.
4. Henkind, P. 1982. Sarcoidosis: An expanding ophthalmic horizon. J. Roy. Soc. Med. **85:** 153-159.
5. Ho, M., C. P. Wajszczuk, A. Haryd, J. S. Dummer, T. E. Starzi, T. R. Hakala & H. T. Bahnson. 1983. Infections in kidney, heart, and liver transplant recipients on cyclosporine. Transplant. Proc. **15**(Suppl. 1): 2768-2772.
6. Nussenblatt, R. B., A. G. Palestine & C. C. Chan. 1983. Cyclosporin A therapy in the treatment of intraocular inflammatory disease resistant to systemic corticosteroids and cytotoxic agents. Am. J. Ophthalmol. **96:** 275-282.
7. Nussenblatt, R. B., A. G. Palestine & C. C. Chan. Ocular Pharmacol. In press.
8. Palestine, A. G., R. B. Nussenblatt & C. C. Chan. Side effects of cyclosporine in nontransplant patients. Am. J. Med. **77:** 652-656.
9. Ost, L. 1984. Effects of cyclosporin on prednisolone metabolism. Lancet **i:** 451.
10. Frank, K. W. & H. Weiss. 1983. Unusual clinical and histopathological findings in ocular sarcoidosis. Br. J. Ophthalmol. **67:** 8-16.
11. Gragoudas, E. S. & C. D. J. Regan. 1981. Peripapillary subretinal neovascularization in presumed sarcoidosis. Arch. Ophthalmol. **99:** 1194-1197.

Different Mechanisms of Hypercalciuria in Sarcoidosis

Correlations with Disease Extension and Activity

ALAIN MEYRIER,[a,b] DOMINIQUE VALEYRE,[c]
ROGER BOUILLON,[d] FRANÇOISE PAILLARD,[e]
JEAN-PAUL BATTESTI,[c] AND ROBERT GEORGES[f]

[b]*Service de Néphrologie*
and
[c]*Service de Pneumologie*
Hôpital Avicenne
93000 Bobigny, France

[d]*Laboratorium voor Experimentelle Geneeskunde*
Rega Instituut
3000 Louvain, Belgium

[e]*Laboratoire d'Explorations Fonctionnelles*
Hôpital Tenon
75970 Paris, France

[f]*Institut National de la Santé*
et de la Recherche Médicale Unité 82
Faculté Xavier-Bichat
75018 Paris, France.

INTRODUCTION

Hypercalcemia has long been recognized a complication of sarcoidosis.[1] Its frequency has been diversely appreciated.[2] The prevalence of hypercalciuria has less often been evaluated, although it seems much higher than that of hypercalcemia.[3] These disorders of calcium metabolism have been the subject of extensive research since it was shown that patients with sarcoidosis exhibit an acquired disorder of vitamin D_3 metabolism.[4–9] This interest was stimulated by recent observations which disclosed high serum levels of 1,25-dihydroxyvitamin D_3 (1,25-$(OH)_2$-D_3) in this disease,[10–16] and culminated when a coherent body of clinical and experimental data demonstrated that, in patients with sarcoidosis, the production of this dihydroxylated metabolite of vitamin D_3 can be extrarenal.[17–20] In spite of this growing knowledge, the mechanism(s)

[a]To whom correspondence should be addressed.

of hypercalciuria of sarcoidosis has rarely been investigated. Moreover, in spite of a few studies that showed the hypercalciuria of sarcoidosis could be either of intestinal or of skeletal origin,[21–23] no attempts were made to make correlations between the type of hypercalciuria and the course of sarcoidosis. The present study was undertaken in an effort to gain further insight in these issues.

METHODS

Patients

Thirty-nine untreated patients, all suffering from confirmed thoracic sarcoidosis, were investigated between October 1980 and May 1981. Renal function was normal in all. The demographic characteristics of the patients are shown in TABLE 1. The patients were evaluated on the basis of 1) the radiological staging, evaluated according

TABLE 1. Demographic Features of the Patients

	Group 1 (N = 12)	Group 2 (N = 14)	Group 3 (N = 13)
Number of males	8	8	10
Number of females	4	6	3
Number of whites	10	7	10
Number of blacks	2	7	3
Average age (years)	34.0 ± 7.4	34.0 ± 8.2	35.0 ± 11.0

to the method described by Siltzbach *et al.*;[24] 2) extrathoracic dissemination, evaluated according to clinical criteria; and 3) the evolutive trend of sarcoidosis, evaluated by clinical and radiological surveillance (over the ensuing year in 23 patients in whom no treatment was judged necessary and over the 6 months preceding the study in 12 patients who were treated with corticosteroids after the completion of this study). The patients fell into two groups: those with stable or regressive signs and symptoms and those with aggravated signs and symptoms, that is, patients with nonevolutive and evolutive disease, respectively. The biological markers of activity that were considered were the serum angiotensin-converting enzyme (SACE) level and the lymphocyte percentage, that is, the percentage of cells in fluid recovered by bronchoalveolar lavage (BAL) that were lymphocytes.

Laboratory Methods

Calcium levels were determined by atomic absorption flame photometry (Perkin-Elmer); creatinine and phosphate levels, by the usual colorimetric methods, using an autoanalyzer (Technicon); cyclic AMP (cAMP) levels, by radiocompetition assay (Amersham). Parathyroid hormone (PTH) radioimmunoassay was conducted with an antibody recognizing the COOH-terminal end of the molecule (IRE). Serum 25-OH-D_3 was determined by competitive protein-binding assay. Serum 1,25-$(OH)_2$-D_3 was determined by radioimmunoassay as described elsewhere.[25,26] In 30 patients BAL was performed as described elsewhere.[27] Counts of lymphocytes in lavage fluid were expressed as lymphocyte percentages (the number of lymphocytes per ml/the total number of cells per ml). SACE was assayed with hippuryl-histidine-leucine as substrate.[28]

Conduct of the Study

The study was conducted in two periods. During an observation period of several days the patients had an unrestricted diet. In the mornings, before the patients ate, blood samples were taken for calcium and phosphate determinations, and urine was collected over a 24-hr period for calcium determinations. During the same period of time lung investigations were carried out, and blood samples were taken in order that SACE, 25-OH-D_3, and 1,25-$(OH)_2$-D_3 levels be determined. Hypercalciuria was diagnosed if calcium excretion over 24 hr was greater than 0.1 mmol/kg body weight; hypercalcemia, if serum calcium levels were equal to or greater than the mean of the control values plus three SD's, that is, 2.60 mmol/1.

The calcium absorption test was conducted as described by Pak *et al.*,[29,30] after 3 days during which the patient had a diet containing less than 400 mg of calcium per day and drank only softened water. Blood (B1) and urine (Ul) samples were drawn at 9:30 AM. The patient was then given a standard breakfast and absorbed 1000 mg of calcium (Sandoz Forte). Blood (B2) and urine (U2) samples were collected again at 1:30 PM.

The following determinations were made: B1: the calcium, phosphate, PTH, 25-OH-D_3, and 1,25-$(OH)_2$-D_3 levels; U1: the value for the tubular reabsorption of phosphate (TRP), the calcium/creatinine ratio, and the secreted nephrogenous cAMP level; B2: the calcium, phosphate, and PTH levels; and U2: the calcium/creatinine ratio and the nephrogenous cAMP level. The means and SD's of the control values for these items are shown in the tables and/or in the test.

Means and SD's are used throughout. Means were compared using Student's *t* test. Correlations were made when a linear relationship between parameters could be found using the least-squares method.

RESULTS

Results of the Calcium Absorption Test

Three groups of patients were distinguished when the calcium/creatinine ratios corresponding to the fasting and post-calcium load periods were analyzed (TABLES 1-3). The control values for the ratios corresponding to these periods were 0.150 ± 0.079 and 0.369 ± 0.098, respectively. Experimental values within two SD's were

TABLE 2. Calcium Absorption Test Results

	Serum Calcium (mmol/l)	Serum Phosphorus (mmol/l)	Urinary Calcium (mmol/kg body weight)	Secreted cAMP (pmol/ml GFR)	PTH (ng/ml)	25-OH-D_3 (ng/ml)	1,25-$(OH)_2$-D_3 (pg/ml)
Controls	2.310 ± 0.095 (50)	1.05 ± 0.08 (50)	< 0.100 (50)	17.40 ± 2.60 (30)	1.00 ± 0.30 (50)	13.4 ± 9.0 (31)	42.0 ± 13.0 (78)
Group 1	2.390 ± 0.137 C^a (12)	0.97 ± 0.16 (12)	0.078 ± 0.031 (12)	11.00 ± 7.84 C^d (11)	0.59 ± 0.20 C^d (11)	7.5 ± 3.5 (9)	39.0 ± 15.1 (11)
Group 2	2.450 ± 0.145 C^d (14)	1.15 ± 0.11 $G1^a$ (14)	0.113 ± 0.046 $G1^a$ (14)	15.50 ± 4.67 (13)	0.64 ± 0.39 C^d (13)	9.6 ± 3.2 (6)	59.0 ± 14.2 C^dG1^b (12)
Group 3	2.560 ± 0.254 C^d (13)	1.12 ± 0.17 $G1^a$ (13)	0.146 ± 0.071 $G1^b$ (13)	9.00 ± 4.46 C^dG2^c (12)	0.53 ± 0.10 C^d (13)	8.5 ± 3.0 (7)	57.0 ± 22.1 C^b (9)

NOTE: The abbreviations C, G1, and G2 indicate where comparisons had been made with the corresponding values for the control group, group 1, and group 2, respectively. The number of patients for each determination is shown in parentheses.

[a] $p < .05$.

[b] $p < .01$.

[c] $p < .002$.

[d] $p < .001$.

TABLE 3. Relationships between Calcium Absorption Test Results and the Status of Sarcoidosis

	Radiographic Stage			Patients with Extrathoracic Extension (%)	Patients with Evolutive Disease (%)	SACE[a] (U/ml)	Lymphocyte Percentage[b]
	1	2	3				
Group 1 (Normal)	6	4	2	17	22	42.0 ± 24.1[c]	46.0 ± 22.9[c]
Group 2 (Absorptive)	4	7	3	36	57	62.0 ± 20.1[c]	51.0 ± 22.7[c]
Group 3 (Resorptive)	3	7	3	85	82	65.0 ± 32.1[c]	46.0 ± 19.5[c]

[a] Normal values of SACE: 22.00 ± 4.38 U/ml.
[b] Normal values for the lymphocyte percentage: 9.10 ± 3.91.
[c] $p < .001$ compared to controls.

considered normal. The PTH and nephrogenous cAMP levels were low in all three groups. The serum phosphorous levels and the TRP values were normal. The serum 25-OH-D_3 and 1,25-$(OH)_2$-D_3 levels were low (TABLE 2).

Group 1

In 12 patients the fasting and post-calcium load urinary calcium/creatinine ratios were normal (0.120 ± 0.067 and 0.354 ± 0.107, respectively).

In this group extrathoracic localizations were rare. Sarcoidosis was evolutive in two out of nine patients in whom aggravation could be established. SACE levels were lower than those in groups 2 and 3, but these differences were not statistically significant. Mean serum calcium levels were slightly but significantly higher than the level in controls. Urinary calcium excretion over a 24-hr period was normal, and the 1,25-$(OH)_2$-D_3 levels were normal.

Group 2

In 14 patients the fasting urinary calcium/creatinine ratio was normal (0.19 ± 0.07) whereas the post-load calcium/creatinine ratio was high (0.84 ± 0.27). These patients were considered to have absorptive hypercalciuria.

In this group extrathoracic localizations were present in one-third of the patients. Sarcoidosis was evolutive in most of the patients. SACE levels were higher than those in group 1, but these differences were not statistically significant. Serum calcium levels were significantly higher than those in controls, two patients being unmistakably hypercalcemic (2.85 and 2.67 mmol/1, respectively). In this group, the patients had higher urinary calcium excretion per 24 hr than did patients of group 1, but this difference between the two groups was not statistically significant. The 1,25-$(OH)_2$-D_3 levels in patients of group 2 were significantly higher than those in patients of group 3.

Group 3

In 13 patients both the fasting and the post-calcium load urinary calcium/creatinine ratios were elevated (0.43 ± 0.15 and 0.94 ± 0.31, respectively). These patients were considered to have resorptive hypercalciuria.

In this group extrathoracic localizations were present, and sarcoidosis was evolutive in most of the patients. SACE levels were elevated in the same proportion of patients as that in group 2. Four patients were unmistakably hypercalcemic (3.15, 2.75, 2.66, and 2.91 mmol/1, respectively). This was correlated with the degree of hypercalciuria, which was higher than that in the absorptive group. Serum 1,25-$(OH)_2$-D_3 levels were significantly higher than those in controls and in group 1, but there was no difference with the absorptive group.

Relationships between the Calcium Absorption Test and Vitamin D Metabolites

A significant correlation was made between the serum 1,25-$(OH)_2$-D_3 level and the post-calcium load urinary calcium/creatinine ratio ($N=32$, $r=.36$, $p<.05$). The 1,25-$(OH)_2$-D_3 level was also correlated with the serum calcium level, but only for Caucasians ($N=19$, $r=.53$, $p<.02$).

Relationships between Sarcoidosis and Calcium Metabolism

Fasting and post-load calcium/creatinine ratios and the amount of calcium excreted over 24-hr periods varied significantly according to the degree of extension and whether the disease was evolutive. SACE levels were higher in the patients with

TABLE 4. Predictive Value of the Calcium Absorption Test on Sarcoidosis Extension and Aggravation

	Extension			Aggravation		
	Yes ($N=18$)	Significance[a]	No ($N=21$)	Yes ($N=15$)	Significance[a]	No ($N=19$)
Urinary calcium (mmol/kg body weight)	0.14	$p < .01$	0.09	0.14	$p < .01$	0.08
Calcium/creatinine ratio						
Fasting	0.34	$p < .001$	0.16	0.31	$p < .05$	0.17
Post-calcium load	0.86	$p < .05$	0.63	0.88	$p < .001$	0.59
SACE (U/ml)	76.6	$p < .001$	44.4	62.0	NS	51.0

[a] Comparisons with controls by Student's *t* test.

extrathoracic localizations ($N=18$, 76.6 ± 38.0 U/ml versus $N=21$, 44.4 ± 18.5 U/ml) ($p<.003$), and could be correlated with the amount of calcium excreted over 24-hr periods ($N=39$, $r=.37$, $p<.02$). No significant relationship was found between calcium metabolism and the markers of activity, particularly lymphocyte percentages. Serum 1,25-$(OH)_2$-D_3 and 25-OH-D_3 levels did not seem to depend on the degree of extension or on whether the disease was evolutive.

DISCUSSION

The knowledge that sarcoidosis can be attended by hypercalcemia dates back to 1939.[1] In 1954, Henneman *et al.*[4] and Anderson *et al.*[6] demonstrated that patients with sarcoidosis have an acquired metabolic disorder characterized by an abnormal sensitivity to, or excessive endogenous production of, vitamin D_3, and that this disorder was reversible with corticosteroid treatment. Several epidemiological studies have shown that the prevalence of hypercalcemia is on the order of 11%.[2] The frequency of hypercalciuria has been less thoroughly studied. It appears to be higher, and seems to reach 60% of the cases.[3,31] Few studies have so far been dedicated to the mechanism of the hypercalciuria of sarcoidosis. In fact, the bulk of calcium studies in sarcoidosis was essentially dedicated to the derangement of vitamin D_3 metabolism. In this respect, two major steps were the demonstration that the serum 1,25-$(OH)_2$-D_3 level is elevated in sarcoidosis,[10–16] and the demonstration that this increase can be observed in the absence of renal 1,α-hydroxylase.[17] There is more evidence that sarcoid granulomas (or macrophages) are able to elaborate 1,25-$(OH)_2$-D_3 or 1,α-hydroxylase.[32] In spite of this growing knowledge, few attempts have been made to examine the relationships between calcium and vitamin D_3 disorders on the one hand, and the clinical extension and the development of sarcoidosis on the other.

In 1980, we had the opportunity to study some patients with sarcoidosis that had hypercalcemia and hypercalciuria. We realized that in some of them both disorders persisted with a calcium-poor diet, and found that in such cases hypercalciuria was apparently due to bone resorption rather than solely explained by intestinal calcium hyperabsorption. These cases prompted us to investigate a large number of consecutive sarcoidosis patients, in order to evaluate the respective frequencies of absorptive and of resorptive hypercalciuria and their relationships with vitamin D_3 metabolism, and to specify their links with the clinical course of the disease. The results of this study have been presented in detail elsewhere.[33] They showed that excessive calcium excretion in sarcoidosis is not a simple disorder, as one-third of our sarcoidosis patients exhibited an absorptive type of hypercalciuria whereas another third seemed to have both intestinal hyperabsorption and bone resorption. In all, parathyroid secretion was reduced, as shown by low serum levels of PTH and by subnormal secretion of nephrogenic cAMP. This ruled out the possible coincidence with a parathyroid adenoma.

The mechanism or mechanisms of hypercalciuria deserve discussion. High serum levels of 1,25-$(OH)_2$-D_3 certainly play a major role in this disorder as patients with normal serum levels of 1,25-$(OH)_2$-D_3 were normocalciuric. It is well established that this metabolite of vitamin D_3 stimulates the intestinal absorption of calcium. This is in agreement with the correlation made in our study between 1,25-$(OH)_2$-D_3 and the abnormal rise of the urinary calcium/creatinine ratio after an oral load, and suffices to explain the hypercalciuria of the absorptive group. Nevertheless, the fact that half of the hypercalciuric patients had a pattern of bone resorption calls for further explanation.

Our data confirm previous works that, using different methodology, had already shown that in some cases the hypercalciuria of sarcoidosis was not merely explained by high intestinal calcium absorption but could also be ascribed to osteolysis.[21–23] Our subgroup of patients with resorptive hypercalciuria is of particular interest, and the mechanism of resorptive hypercalciuria is not evident. The role of excess 1,25-$(OH)_2$-D_3 must be considered, as this metabolite exerts a bone-resorbing effect, an effect that has been demonstrated in bone tissue cultures *in vitro*[34–37] as well as in human experiments.[38] Nevertheless, some other factor must be involved in bone resorption because the serum levels of 1,25-$(OH)_2$-D_3 were similarly elevated in both the absorptive and resorptive subsets. The patients with resorptive hypercalciuria were those with the largest clinical extrathoracic dissemination of the disease. They also exhibited higher SACE activity, although this trend did not reach statistical significance due to dispersion of the data points in this small sample. Thus, bone resorption seemed to be related to the extent of the granulomatous process.

A first explanation would be direct bone resorption by sarcoid granulomas. There are numerous data in the literature on this classical localization, a localization that has been correlated with sarcoid dissemination, especially in the skin.[39–42] Its frequency is diversely estimated: from 3-4% in France and Belgium to 14-30% in the United States and Scandinavia.[40] In fact, most of the studies are radiological, and there appears to be an underestimation of bone involvement in the absence of bone biopsies. One can imagine that osseous granulomas could be responsible for a resorptive type of hypercalciuria. Osteopenia due to diffuse skeletal granulomatosis has been described by Fallon *et al.*[43] In their observation, hypercalciuria was probably resorptive as it persisted on a calcium-poor diet, and bone photon-absorption densitometry showed low density of the skeleton. Bone biopsy disclosed peritrabecular granulomas and osteoclastic resorption. We did not perform systematic bone biopsies in our patients, and we cannot exclude the possibility of bone granulomas in the resorptive group. Yet we did not observe bone rarefaction on skeletal surveys, and, when performed in three patients of the resorptive group, gallium scans did not disclose skeletal fixation of the isotope.

The role of a bone-resorbing substance adding its own effect to that of 1,25-$(OH)_2$-D_3 should therefore be considered. A likely candidate is the osteoclast-activating factor (OAF)[44] which is produced by normal, activated lymphocytes or by phytohemagglutinin-activated mononuclear cells, especially when macrophages are added to the lymphocytes.[45–47] The interaction between macrophages and T lymphocytes fits with the nature of sarcoid lesions.[48] It is therefore tempting to postulate that granulomas could be the source of OAF, thereby inducing bone resorption. The rapid response of hypercalcemia to corticosteroid therapy would also find here a logical explanation. This would also explain why our patients in group 1 had a tendency to be slightly hypercalcemic and had low parathyroid secretion in spite of normal 1,25-$(OH)_2$-D_3 serum concentrations. It is highly probable that ACE is produced by sarcoid granulomas, and that its serum concentration reflects the amount of granulomatous tissue in the body.[49] This would be relevant to the higher SACE levels in patients with resorptive hypercalciuria in our cases.

In conclusion, analyzing the type of hypercalciuria in sarcoidosis provides a sensitive approach to the calcium and vitamin D_3 disorders of this disease. Hypercalciuria and especially the post-calcium load urinary calcium/creatinine ratio may be well correlated with serum 1,25-$(OH)_2$-D_3 levels. There is a significant relationship between the urinary calcium/creatinine ratio for fasting patients and indices of disease activity, making this simple determination one of the best tests of sarcoid dissemination and of whether sarcoidosis is evolutive. Two types of hypercalciuria can be distinguished. In one, intestinal hyperabsorption of calcium can be explained by high 1,25-$(OH)_2$-D_3 serum levels. In the other, we speculate that superimposed bone resorption could be due to bone granulomas and/or to the cumulative effects on osteoclasts of 1,25-$(OH)_2$-D_3 and of an OAF produced by sarcoid granulomas (both agents being equally sensitive to corticosteroids). It is hoped that this hypothesis could be demonstrated by further studies of sarcoid granulomas in culture and determinations of bone-resorbing and of 1,α-hydroxylase activities in the cell culture medium.

REFERENCES

1. HARREL, G. T. & S. FISHER. 1939. Blood chemical changes in Boeck's sarcoid with particular reference to protein, calcium and phosphatase values. J. Clin. Invest. **18:** 687-693.

2. STUDDY, P. R., R. BIRD, E. NEVILLE & D. G. JAMES. 1980. Biochemical findings in sarcoidosis. J. Clin. Pathol. **33:** 528-533.
3. LEBACQ, E., H. VERHAEGEN & V. DESMET. 1970. Renal involvement in sarcoidosis. Postgrad. Med. J. **46:** 526-529.
4. HENNEMAN, P. H., E. F. DEMPSEY, E. L. CARROLL & F. ALBRIGHT. 1956. The cause of hypercalcuria in sarcoid and its treatment with cortisone and sodium phytate. J. Clin. Invest. **53:** 1229-1242.
5. GLECKLER, W. J. 1956. Hypercalcemia and renal insufficiency due to sarcoidosis: Treatment with cortisone. Ann. Intern. Med. **44:** 174.
6. ANDERSON, J., C. HARPER, C. E. DENT & G. R. PHILPOT. 1954. Effect of cortisone on calcium metabolism in sarcoidosis with hypercalcaemia: Possibly antagonistic actions of cortisone and vitamin D. Lancet **ii:** 720-724.
7. DANOWSKI, T. S. 1962. Calcium, phosphorus, parathyroids, and bone. *In* Clinical Endocrinology. R. Hoover, Ed.: 270. Williams & Wilkins. Baltimore, MD.
8. BELL, N. H., J. R. GILL, JR. & F. C. BARTTER. 1964. On the abnormal calcium absorption in sarcoidosis. Am. J. Med. **36:** 500-513.
9. BELL, N. H. & F. C. BARTTER. 1964. Transient reversal of hyperabsorption of calcium and of abnormal sensitivity to vitamin D in a patient with sarcoidosis during an episode of nephritis. Ann. Intern. Med. **61:** 702-710.
10. PAPAPOULOS, S. E., L. J. FRAHER, L. M. SANDLER, T. L. CLEMENS, I. G. LEWIN & J. L. H. O'RIORDAN. 1979. 1,25-Dihydroxycholecalciferol in the pathogenesis of the hypercalcaemia of sarcoidosis. Lancet **i:** 627-630.
11. BELL, N. H., P. H. STERN, E. PANTZER, T. K. SINHA & H. F. DELUCA. 1979. Evidence that increased circulating 1,25-dihydroxyvitamin D is the probable cause for abnormal calcium metabolism in sarcoidosis. J. Clin. Invest. **64:** 218-225.
12. STERN, P. H., J. DE OLAZABAL & N. H. BELL. 1980. Evidence for abnormal regulation of circulating 1,25-dihydroxyvitamin D in patients with sarcoidosis and normal calcium metabolism. J. Clin. Invest. **66:** 852-855.
13. ZERWEKH, J. E., C. Y. C. PAK, R. A. KAPLAN, J. L. MCGUIRE, K. UPCHURCH, N. BRESLAN & R. JOHNSON, JR. 1980. Pathogenetic role of 1,25-dihydroxyvitamin D in sarcoidosis and absorptive hypercalciuria: Different response to prednisolone therapy. J. Clin. Endocrinol. Metab. **51:** 381-386.
14. CHESNEY, R. W., A. J. HAMSTRA, H. F. DELUCA, S. HOROWITZ, E. F. GILBERT, R. HONG & W. BORCHERDING. 1981. Elevated serum 1,25-dihydroxyvitamin D concentrations in the hypercalcemia of sarcoidosis: Correction by glucocorticoid therapy. J. Pediatr. **98:** 919-922.
15. KOIDE, Y., N. KUGAI, S. KIMURA, T. FUJITA, N. YAMASHITA, T. HIRAMOTO, J. SUKEGAWA, E. OGATA & K. KAMASHITA. 1981. Increased 1,25-dihydroxycholecalciferol as a cause of abnormal calcium metabolism in sarcoidosis. J. Clin. Endocrinol. Metab. **52:** 494-498.
16. LEMAIRE, V., L. CANIELA, H. DUREPAIRE, S. LAFOREST, L. MIRAVET & A. RYCKEWAERT. 1982. Hypercalcémie isolée révélatrice d'une sarcoidose: Un cas avec élévation du 1,25-dihydroxycholecalciferol. Nouv. Presse Med. **11:** 1143-1144.
17. BARBOUR, G. L., J. W. COBURN, E. SLATOPOLSKY, A. W. NORMAN & R. L. HORST. 1981. Hypercalcemia in an anephric patient with sarcoidosis: Evidence for extrarenal generation of 1,25-dihydroxyvitamin D. N. Engl. J. Med. **305:** 440-443.
18. MAESAKA, J. K., V. BATUMAN, N. C. PABLO & S. SHAKAMURI. 1982. Elevated 1,25-dihydroxyvitamin D levels: Occurrence with sarcoidosis with end-stage renal disease. Arch. Intern. Med. **142:** 1206-1207.
19. ZIMMERMAN, J., M. F. HOLICK & J. SILVER. 1983. Normocalcemia in a hypoparathyroid patient with sarcoidosis: Evidence for parathyroid hormone-independent synthesis of 1,25-dihydroxyvitamin D. Ann. Intern. Med. **98:** 338.
20. MITCHELL, T. H., T. C. B. STAMP, M. V. JENKINS, E. B. MAWER & J. L. BERRY. 1983. Hypercalcaemic sarcoidosis in hypoparathyroidism. Br. Med. J. **286:** 764-765.
21. HENDRIX, J. Z. 1966. Abnormal skeletal mineral metabolism in sarcoidosis. Ann. Intern. Med. **64:** 797-803.
22. KUHLMANN, U., F. FINKEL, U. BINSWANGER & W. SIEGENTHALER. 1980. Calciumstoffwechselstorungen bei Sarkoidose. Inzidenz, Ausmass, Pathogenese und renal Folgeerkrankungen. Klin. Wochenschr. **58:** 17-23.

23. REINER, M., G. SIGURDSSON, V. NUNZIATA, M. A. MALIK, G. W. POOLE & G. F. JOPLIN. 1976. Abnormal calcium metabolism in normocalcaemic sarcoidosis. Br. Med. J. **2:** 1473-1476.
24. SILTZBACH, L. E., D. G. JAMES, E. NEVILLE, J. TURIAF, J. P. BATTESTI, O. P. SHARMA, Y. HOSODA, R. MIKAMI & M. ODAKA. 1974. Course and prognosis of sarcoidosis around the world. Am. J. Med. **57:** 847-852.
25. BOUILLON, R., P. DE MOOR, E. G. BAGGIOLINI & R. USKOKOVIC. 1980. A radioimmunoassay for 1,25-dihydroxycholecalciferol. Clin. Chem. **26:** 562-567.
26. BOUILLON, R., F. A. VAN ASSCHE, H. VAN BAELEN, W. HEYNS & P. DE MOOR. 1981. Influence of the vitamin D-binding protein on the serum concentration of 1,25-dihydroxyvitamin D_3. J. Clin. Invest. **67:** 589-596.
27. VALEYRE, D., G. SAUMON, D. BLADIER, J. AMOUROUX, J. PRÉ, J. P. BATTESTI & R. GEORGES. 1982. The relationships between noninvasive explorations in pulmonary sarcoidosis of recent origin, as shown in bronchoalveolar lavage, serum, and pulmonary function tests. Am. Rev. Respir. Dis. **126:** 41-45.
28. SANDRON, D., D. LECOSSIER, F. MOREAU, A. GRODET, G. BASSET & J. P. BATTESTI. 1979. Angiotensin-converting enzyme in sarcoidosis and other pulmonary diseases: A comparison of two methods of determination. Lung **157:** 31-38.
29. PAK, C. Y. C., R. KAPLAN, H. BONE, J. TOWNSEND & O. WATERS. 1975. A simple test for the diagnosis of absorptive, resorptive and renal hypercalciurias. N. Engl. J. Med. **292:** 497-500.
30. PAK, C. Y. C. 1979. Physiological basis for absorptive and renal hypercalciurias. Am. J. Physiol. **237**(6): F415-F423.
31. GOLDSTEIN, R. A., H. L. ISRAEL, K. L. BECKER & C. F. MOORE. 1971. The infrequency of hypercalcemia in sarcoidosis. Am. J. Med. **51:** 21-30.
32. ADAMS, J. S., O. P. SHARMA, M. A. GACAD & F. R. SINGER. 1983. Metabolism of 25-hydroxyvitamin D_3 by cultured pulmonary alveolar macrophages in sarcoidosis. J. Clin. Invest. **72:** 1856-1860.
33. MEYRIER, A., D. VALEYRE, R. BOUILLON, F. PAILLARD, J. P. BATTESTI & R. GEORGES. 1985. Resorptive versus absorptive hypercalciuria in sarcoidosis: Correlations with 25-hydroxy vitamin D_3 and 1,25-dihydroxyvitamin D_3 and parameters of disease activity. Q. J. Med. N. Ser. **54:** 269-281.
34. TANAKA, Y. & H. F. DELUCA. 1971. Bone-mineral mobilization activity of 1,25-dihydroxycholecalciferol, a metabolite of vitamin D. Arch. Biochem. Biophys. **146:** 574-578.
35. TANAKA, Y., H. FRANK & H. F. DELUCA. 1972. Role of 1,25-dihydroxycholecalciferol in calcification of bone and maintenance of serum calcium concentration in the rat. J. Nutr. **102:** 1569-1578.
36. RAISZ, L. G., C. L. TRUMMEL, H. F. HOLICK & H. F. DELUCA. 1972. 1,25-Dihydroxycholecalciferol: A potent stimulator of bone resorption in tissue culture. Science **175:** 768-769.
37. WONG, G. L., R. A. LUBEN & D. V. COHN. 1977. 1,25-Dihydroxycholecalciferol and parathormone: Effects on isolated osteoclast-like and osteoblast-like cells. Science **197:** 663-665.
38. MAIERHOFER, W. V., R. W. GRAY, H. S. CHEUNG & J. LEMANN, JR. 1983. Bone resorption stimulated by elevated serum 1,25-$(OH)_2$-vitamin D concentrations in healthy men. Kidney Int. **24:** 555-560.
39. BOUVIER, M., P. QUENEAU & J. BRUN. 1972. Les formes ostéoarticulaires de la sarcoidose. Praxis **61:** 631-646.
40. SHARMA, O. P. 1975. The musculo-skeletal system in sarcoidosis. *In* Sarcoidosis: A Clinical Approach. O. P. Sharma, Ed.: 103-112. Charles C. Thomas. Springfield, IL.
41. NEVILLE, E., L. S. CARSTAIRS & D. G. JAMES. 1976. Bone sarcoidosis. Ann. N.Y. Acad. Sci. **278:** 475-487.
42. HOLICK, M. F. & M. A. HOFFMAN. 1982. A 63-year-old woman with hypercalcemia and facial weakness. N. Engl. J. Med. **307:** 1257-1265.
43. FALLON, M. D., H. M. PERRY III & S. L. TEITELBAUM. 1981. Skeletal sarcoidosis with osteopenia. Metab. Bone Dis. **3:** 171-175.
44. MUNDY, G. R., L. G. RAISZ, R. A. COOPER, G. P. SCHECHTER & S. E. SALMON. 1974. Evidence for the secretion of an osteoclast stimulating factor in myeloma. N. Engl. J. Med. **291:** 1041-1046.

45. Raisz, L. G. 1981. What marrow does to bone. N. Engl. J. Med. **304:** 1485-1486.
46. Mundy, G. R., M. E. Rick, R. Turcotte & M. A. Kowalski. 1978. Pathogenesis of hypercalcemia in lymphosarcoma cell leukemia: Role of an osteoclast activating factor-like substance and a mechanism of action of glucocorticoid therapy. Am. J. Med. **65:** 600-606.
47. Horton, J. E., J. J. Oppenheim, S. E. Mergenhagen & L. G. Raisz. 1974. Macrophage-lymphocyte synergy in the production of osteoclast activating factor. J. Immunol. **113:** 1278-1287.
48. Keogh, B. A., G. W. Hunninghake, B. R. Line & R. G. Crystal. 1983. The alveolitis of pulmonary sarcoidosis. Am. Rev. Respir. Dis. **128:** 256-265.
49. Sandron, D., D. Lecossier, A. Grodet, C. Barbe, G. Basset & J. P. Battesti. 1983. Seric angiotensin-converting enzyme (SACE) and the diffusion of the sarcoid granuloma: Evolutive and therapeutic interest. *In* Sarcoidosis and Other Granulomatous Disorders. J. Chrétien, J. Marsac & J. C. Saltiel, Eds.: 345-348. Pergamon Press. Paris.

Production of 1,25-Dihydroxyvitamin D_3 by Pulmonary Alveolar Macrophages from Patients with Sarcoidosis

JOHN S. ADAMS, MERCEDES A. GACAD, FREDERICK R. SINGER, AND OM P. SHARMA

Bone and Connective Tissue Research Laboratory
Orthopedic Hospital
University of Southern California School of Medicine
Los Angeles, California 90007

INTRODUCTION

In 1954 Henneman *et al.*[1] were the first to suggest that the hypercalcemic/hypercalciuric disturbance in sarcoidosis was related to the endogenous overproduction of vitamin D. Their postulate was supported by data on calcium balance that showed intestinal calcium hyperabsorption,[1,2] and by historical evidence that showed exacerbation of hypercalcemia or hypercalciuria during summer months, when skin is exposed to more ultraviolet light,[3] in patients with sarcoidosis. The observation that patients with sarcoidosis were susceptible to the development of hypercalcemia during treatment with vitamin D,[4] however, prompted Anderson *et al.*[2] and other investigators[5–7] to propose that sensitivity to vitamin D in sarcoidosis was abnormal. The notion that the calcium metabolic disturbance in sarcoidosis resulted from increased end-organ sensitivity to vitamin D persisted until it was recognized that serum levels of 1,25-dihydroxyvitamin D (1,25-$(OH)_2$-D), the active form of the sterol hormone, were elevated in some sarcoidosis patients with hypercalciuria and/or hypercalcemia.[8,9] More recently, an elevated serum concentration of 1,25-$(OH)_2$-D, a metabolite synthesized solely in the kidney in normal, nonpregnant human subjects,[10] was reported in a hypercalcemic, anephric male patient with sarcoidosis.[11] These data support the original postulate of Henneman *et al.* that the hypercalcemia of sarcoidosis is indeed a form of vitamin D intoxication and further suggest that the source of hormone exists at an extrarenal site. The experiments described in the present report point to the pulmonary alveolar macrophage (PAM) in patients with sarcoidosis as the synthetic source of an active vitamin D sterol in this disease and characterize the metabolite as 1,25-$(OH)_2$-D_3.

METABOLISM OF 25-OH-D_3 BY PAM's FROM PATIENTS WITH SARCOIDOSIS

The macrophage is the ubiquitous cellular constituent of the noncaseating granulomas of sarcoidosis. We employed monolayer cultures of PAM's derived from patients with sarcoidosis as a model to study the metabolism of 25-OH-D_3, the naturally occurring precursor of 1,25-$(OH)_2$-D_3, *in vivo.* Primary monolayer cultures of PAM's were established, by standard techniques,[12] from the bronchoalveolar lavage fluid of patients with biopsy-proven sarcoidosis and roentgenographic evidence of diffuse infiltrative pulmonary disease with or without hilar lymphadenopathy (stages II and III, respectively) as well as of patients with roentgenographic evidence of only hilar lymph node involvement (stage I). Lavage specimens were also obtained from individuals with nonsarcoidosis-mediated, diffuse infiltrative pulmonary disease to serve as control cultures. After 7 to 12 days in primary culture, homogeneous macrophage monolayers (confirmed by histochemical staining for nonspecific esterase activity[13]) were subjected to incubation with 5 nM [26,27-*methyl*-^{3}H]25-OH-D_3 as previously described.[14] At the conclusion of a 3-hr incubation period the medium was aspirated,

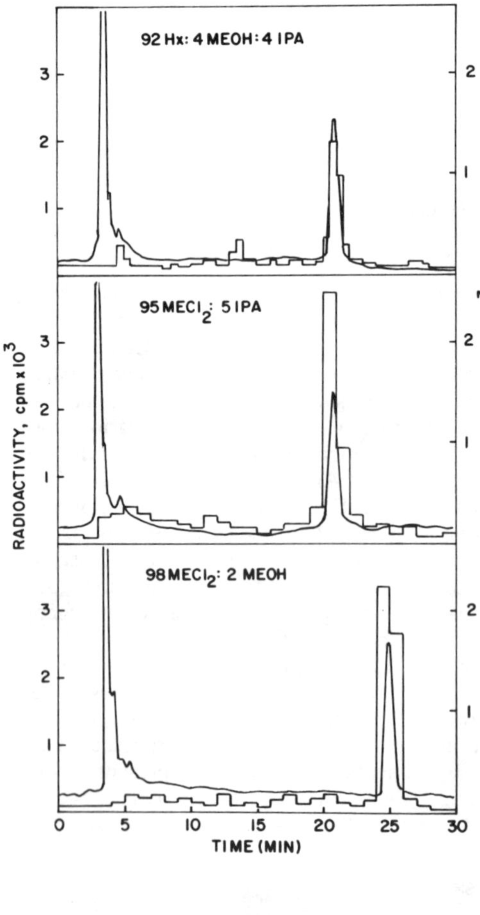

FIGURE 1. PAM's from a patient with sarcoidosis, high-intensity alveolitis, and hypercalcemia were incubated with [^{3}H]25-OH-D, the lipid was extracted, and the extract was purified by Sep-Pak chromatography. (See text for more details.) A portion of the sample was co-chromatographed by normal-phase HPLC with authentic 1,25-$(OH)_2$-D_3 (smooth line) in three different mobile phases. (See reference 14, from which the figure is reproduced, for more details.)

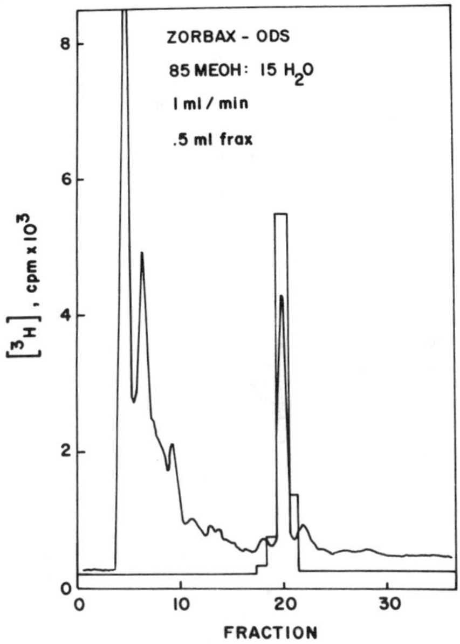

FIGURE 2. Reverse-phase HPLC of the 1,25-$(OH)_2$-D_3-co-chromatographing fractions from normal-phase HPLC shown in FIGURE 1.

and the cell monolayer was harvested by gentle scraping. The lipid was extracted from the cells and medium in methanol-methylene chloride, and the resultant extracts were chromatographed on silica Sep-Pak cartridges.[15] The Sep-Pak fraction containing metabolites more polar than [^{3}H]25-OH-D_3 was then chromatographed by both normal and reverse-phase high performance liquid chromatography (HPLC). The chromatograms of material extracted from cells derived from a sarcoidosis patient with high intensity alveolitis, hypercalcemia, and a high circulating 1,25-$(OH)_2$-D concentration are shown in FIGURES 1 & 2. On normal-phase HPLC there was a homogeneous peak of radiolabeled metabolite that co-chromatographed with authentic 1,25-$(OH)_2$-D_3 in three different mobile phases. Co-chromatography of the PAM metabolite and 1,25-$(OH)_2$-D_3 in a mobile phase containing methylene chloride is of particular interest because this solvent system successfully separates 1,25-$(OH)_2$-D_3 from a [^{3}H]1,25-$(OH)_2$-D_3-like metabolite of [^{3}H]25-OH-D_3 produced by cultured rodent peritoneal macrophages.[16] Therefore, the metabolite produced by rodent macrophages and that of human PAM origin are distinct. Further evidence for the chromatographic identity of the macrophage metabolite as 1,25-$(OH)_2$-D_3 was obtained by reverse-phase HPLC (FIG. 2). No metabolite with the chromatographic mobility of 1,25-$(OH)_2$-D_3 was identified after incubation of nonviable macrophages, cultured intestinal epithelial cells,[17] or culture medium alone with [^{3}H]25-OH-D_3.

In an attempt to functionally characterize the tritiated metabolite, the PAM-derived material was employed as radiolabeled ligand for binding to the specific, high-affinity receptor for 1,25-$(OH)_2$-D_3 (FIG. 3). Displacement of the labeled PAM metabolite and that of commercially available [^{3}H]1,25-$(OH)_2$-D_3 of comparable specific activity by increasing concentrations of radioinert 1,25-$(OH)_2$-D_3 were identical. While these data suggest that the tritiated PAM metabolite is chromatographically and functionally (in terms of receptor binding) identical to [^{3}H]1,25-$(OH)_2$-D_3, they do not provide structural evidence for the identity of the radioinert metabolite.

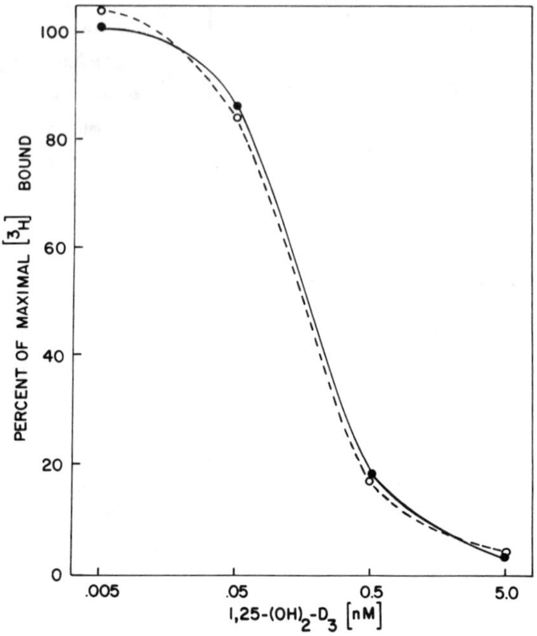

FIGURE 3. Displacement of [^{3}H]1,25-$(OH)_2$-D_3 (●) and the [^{3}H]PAM metabolite (○) from the receptor for 1,25-$(OH)_2$-D_3 by increasing quantities of unlabeled hormone. (See reference 14, from which the figure is reproduced, for more details.)

SYNTHESIS OF THE RADIOINERT PAM METABOLITE

The generation of unlabeled metabolite from 25-OH-D_3 for ligand binding studies and subsequent structural analysis was facilitated by three factors: 1) at least 25% of the metabolite synthesized by PAM monolayers reappears in the incubation medium; 2) the K_m of the *in vitro* conversion reaction is between 50 and 70 nM; and 3) the production of metabolites persists for at least 30 days after establishment of cell monolayers. Thus, it was possible to incubate PAM monolayers derived from two sarcoidosis patients with high-intensity alveolitis and abnormal calcium metabolism with high concentrations of 25-OH-D_3 (200-400 nM) over a sustained incubation period (12 hr) on a repetitive basis and collect the metabolite-containing medium without destroying the synthetic source of the hormone. As shown in FIGURE 4, these experiments led to the production of 0.45 nmoles of the 1,25-$(OH)_2$-D_3-like metabolite, assuming the metabolite possessed the same ultraviolet absorption spectrum as its precursor, 25-OH-D_3. Quantitative serial dilutions of the metabolite were equipotent to authentic 1,25-$(OH)_2$-D_3 in displacing [^{3}H]1,25-$(OH)_2$-D_3 from either the receptor for 1,25-$(OH)_2$-D_3 or from antibody developed against 1,25-$(OH)_2$-D_3. Preliminary data from structural analysis indicate that the PAM metabolite possesses the characteristic ultraviolet spectrum of a carbon 5,7,10 *cis*-triene vitamin D sterol and a mass spectrum indistinguishable from authentic 1,25-$(OH)_2$-D_3. Collectively, these findings suggest that the 25-OH-D_3 metabolite formed *in vitro* by macrophages from patients with sarcoidosis is indeed 1,25-$(OH)_2$-D_3.

CLINICAL CORRELATES WITH THE RATE OF CELLULAR 1,25-$(OH)_2$-D_3 SYNTHESIS

FIGURE 5 depicts the rate of $[^3H]$1,25-$(OH)_2$-D_3 production from $[^3H]$25-OH-D_3 in cell cultures derived from the alveolar lavage of patients with pulmonary sarcoidosis or other infiltrative pulmonary diseases. In the control group, which included three patients with idiopathic pulmonary fibrosis, two patients each with scleroderma and bronchogenic carcinoma, one of whom was hypercalcemic, and one patient with berylliosis, no metabolite with the chromatographic mobility of 1,25-$(OH)_2$-D_3 was detected. In cultures derived from seven patients with pulmonary sarcoidosis limited radiographically to the hilar lymph nodes (stage I), production of $[^3H]$1,25-$(OH)_2$-D_3 occurred in PAM monolayers from only two such patients, and the specific activity of the conversion reaction was low (< 0.1 nmoles/(10^6 cells · min)$^{-1}$). By comparison, PAM cultures derived from patients with diffuse infiltrative pulmonary disease of sarcoidosis (stages II or III) exhibited a broad range in $[^3H]$1,25-$(OH)_2$-D_3-converting activity to values as high as 8.6 nmoles/(10^6 cells · min)$^{-1}$. The specific activity of the conversion reaction also appeared to be greatest in cells from patients with a clinical abnormality in calcium metabolism (especially from those patients with an elevated serum concentration of 1,25-$(OH)_2$-D and elevated serum angiotensin-converting enzyme activity).

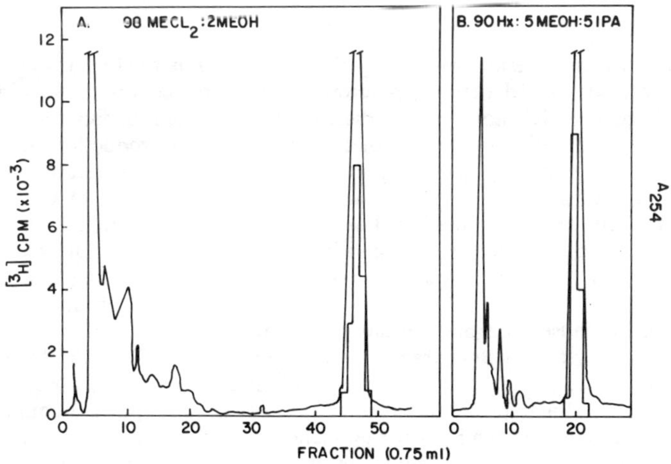

FIGURE 4. The final two sequential purification steps on normal-phase HPLC of the radioinert PAM metabolite of 25-OH-D_3 (smooth line). The macrophage metabolite was co-chromatographed with tracer quantities of authentic, radiolabeled 1,25-$(OH)_2$-D_3.

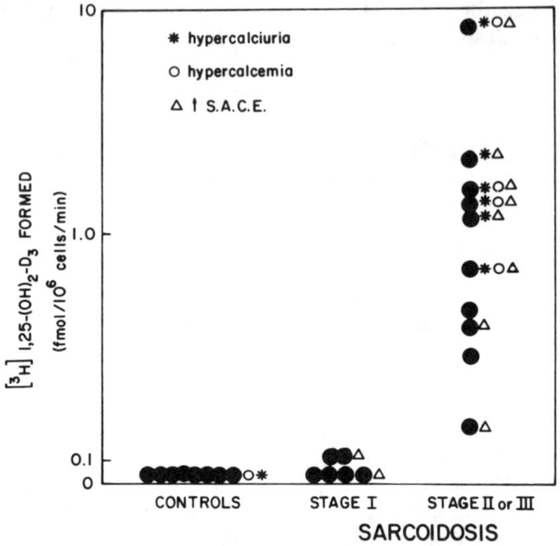

FIGURE 5. Specific activity of the [^{3}H]25-OH-D_3 (5 nM) conversion reaction to [^{3}H]1,25-$(OH)_2$-D_3 in PAM's cultured from patients with nonsarcoidosis-mediated infiltrative pulmonary diseases (controls); patients with pulmonary sarcoidosis confined, according to radiographs, to the hilar lymph nodes (stage I sarcoidosis); and patients with sarcoidosis and infiltrative pulmonary disease evident on radiographs (stage II and stage III sarcoidosis).

CONCLUDING REMARKS

Our experimental results suggest that 1,25-$(OH)_2$-D_3 is the hypercalcemia-causing factor in sarcoidosis and that the macrophage from patients with sarcoidosis is the synthetic source of hormone in the disease. The mechanism and reason for sterol synthesis in sarcoidosis, however, remain unclear. Is the production of 1,25-$(OH)_2$-D_3 purely a pathological process, or, alternatively, is it an exaggerated physiological response on the part of the host to the immunologic challenge of the disease? We tend to favor the latter explanation. For example, it is known that PAM's harvested from patients with sarcoidosis and high-intensity alveolitis spontaneously synthesize interleukin-1 (IL-1),[18] which may be responsible for the spontaneous and prolific production of interleukin-2 (IL-2)[19] in such patients. The overproduction of IL-2, in turn, probably causes the preferential proliferation of thymus-derived (T) helper/effector lymphocytes, which characterize the intraalveolar cellular infiltrate of patients with sarcoidosis and high-intensity alveolitis.[20] If IL-2 production were to proceed unchecked, the cellular proliferative response and its consequences could prove detrimental to the host, particularly if the offending, disease-related stimulus (antigen?) to cellular proliferation is not removed by the host's immune response. Therefore, for the sake of the host, another monokine may be required to "brake" the IL-2-mediated effects and prevent the potential detrimental action of the normal immune response: 1,25-$(OH)_2$-D_3 may be such a monokine.

Evidence supporting a role for 1,25-$(OH)_2$-D_3 in the human immune response includes 1) the presence of receptors for 1,25-$(OH)_2$-D_3 in activated lymphocytes;[21,22] 2) the inhibition of mitogen or specific antigen-induced lymphocyte proliferation and immunoglobulin production by 1,25-$(OH)_2$-D_3;[23] and 3) the reduction in lymphocyte IL-2 production after exposure to 1,25-$(OH)_2$-D_3.[24] Moreover, preliminary results from our laboratory indicate that the specific target for the hormone is the T helper lymphocyte. In sarcoidosis 1,25-$(OH)_2$-D_3 may be called into play as an antagonist to the further proliferation of IL-2-secreting T helper cells. A schema to explain the immunological events in sarcoidosis is shown in FIGURE 6. The "sarcoidosis antigen," whatever it is, interacts with the macrophage and T inducer lymphocytes resulting in activation of the immune cascade. Activation leads to the production of IL-1 and/ or other monokines which induce proliferation and expression of receptors for 1,25-$(OH)_2$-D_3 in T helper cells. The T helper lymphocytes respond by elaboration of lymphokines, including IL-2 and γ-interferon (γ-IFN). IL-2 promotes the proliferation and maturation of bone marrow-derived (B) lymphocytes into immunoglobulin-producing cells. The inability of the host macrophage to metabolize or inactivate the "sarcoidosis antigen" results in perpetuation of the immune cascade and the prolific T helper lymphocyte response seen in the alveolar space of patients with sarcoidosis and extensive infiltrative pulmonary disease.[20] In response to the intensity of the immune stimulus, or possibly under the influence of γ-IFN, the macrophage produces 1,25-$(OH)_2$-D_3. The active vitamin D metabolite binds to its specific intracellular receptor in activated T helper cells and acts to check the overproduction of IL-2, the further proliferation of T effector lymphocytes, and immunoglobulin production by stimulated B cells. The current studies indicate that in sarcoidosis patients with extensive disease and a large "antigen" burden, the local production of 1,25-$(OH)_2$-D_3 is accelerated. This may result in the escape of the sterol into the circulation and induction of hypercalcemia. Experiments are underway to test the validity of this model and to determine whether 1,25-$(OH)_2$-D_3, previously considered to be solely a mediator of mineral ion homeostasis, is an important immunoregulatory hormone.

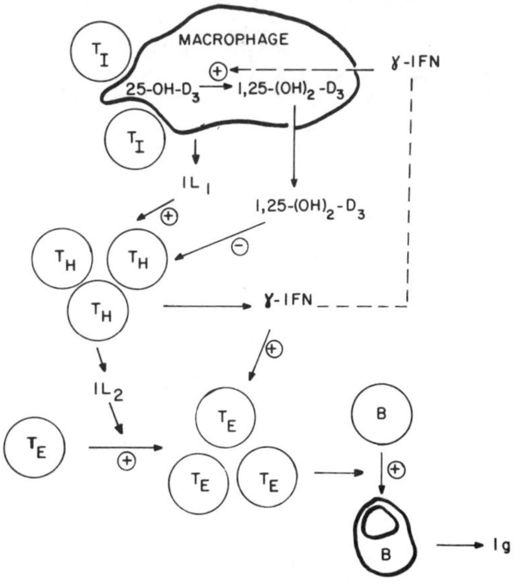

FIGURE 6. Possible role for 1,25-$(OH)_2$-D_3 in the human immune response.

REFERENCES

1. Henneman, P. H., E. F. Dempsey, E. L. Carroll & F. Albright. 1956. J. Clin. Invest. **35:** 1229-1242.
2. Anderson, J., C. Harper, C. F. Dent & G. F. Philpot. 1954. Lancet **ii:** 720-724.
3. Taylor, R. L., H. J. Lynch, Jr. & W. G. Wysor, Jr. 1963. Am. J. Med. **34:** 221-227.
4. Winnacker, J. L., K. L. Becker & S. Katz. 1968. N. Engl. J. Med. **278:** 427-434.
5. Bell, N. H., J. R. Gill, Jr. & F. C. Bartter. 1961. Am. Rev. Respir. Dis. **84:** 27-31.
6. Bell, N. H., J. R. Gill, Jr. & F. C. Bartter. 1964. Am. J. Med. **36:** 500-513.
7. Jackson, W. P. U. & C. Dancaster. 1959. J. Clin. Endocrinol. Metab. **19:** 658-680.
8. Papapoulos, S. E., T. L. Clemens, L. J. Fraher, I. G. Lewin, L. M. Sandler & J. L. O'Riordan. 1979. Lancet **i:** 627-630.
9. Bell, N. H., P. H. Stern, E. Pantzer, T. K. Sinha & H. F. DeLuca. 1979. J. Clin. Invest. **64:** 218-225.
10. DeLuca, H. F. & H. K. Schnoes. 1983. Annu. Rev. Biochem. **52:** 411-439.
11. Barbour, G. L., J. W. Coburn, E. Slatapolsky, A. W. Norman & R. L. Horst. 1981. N. Engl. J. Med. **305:** 440-443.
12. Hunninghake, G. W., J. E. Gadek, S. V. Szapiel, I. J. Strumpf, O. Kawanani, V. J. Ferrans, B. A. Keogh & R. G. Crystal. 1980. Methods Cell Biol. **21A:** 95-112.
13. Koski, I. F., D. G. Poplack & R. M. Blase. 1976. *In In Vitro* Methods in Cell-mediated and Tumor Immunity. B. R. Bloom & J. R. David, Eds.: 369-372. Academic Press. New York, NY.
14. Adams, J. S., O. P. Sharma, M. A. Gacad & F. R. Singer. 1983. J. Clin. Invest. **72:** 1856-1860.
15. Adams, J. S., T. L. Clemens & M. F. Holick. 1981. J. Chromatogr. **226:** 198-201.
16. Gray, T. K., F. W. Maddux, G. E. Lester & M. E. Williams. 1982. Biochem. Biophys. Res. Commun. **109:** 723-729.
17. Quaroni, A. & R. J. May. 1980. Methods Cell Biol. **21B:** 403-427.
18. Hunninghake, G. W. 1984. Am. Rev. Respir. Dis. In press.
19. Pinkston, P., P. B. Bitterman & R. G. Crystal. 1983. N. Engl. J. Med. **308:** 793-800.
20. Crystal, R. G., P. B. Bitterman, S. I. Rennard, A. J. Hance & B. A. Keogh. 1984. N. Engl. J. Med. **310:** 235-244.
21. Bhalla, A. K., E. P. Amento, T. L. Clemens, M. F. Holick & S. M. Krane. 1983. J. Clin. Endocrinol. Metab. **57:** 1308-1310.
22. Provvedini, D. M., C. D. Tsoukas, L. J. Deftos & S. C. Manolagas. 1983. Science (Washington, DC) **221:** 1181-1183.
23. Lemire, J. M., J. S. Adams, R. Sakai & S. C. Jordan. 1984. J. Clin. Invest. **74:** 657-661.
24. Tsoukas, C. D., D. M. Provvedini & S. C. Manolagas. 1984. Science (Washington, DC) **224:** 1438-1440.

Reassessing the Standard Chest Radiograph for Intraparenchymal Activity

CHARLES E. PUTMAN[a]

Department of Radiology
Duke University Medical Center
Durham, North Carolina 27710

BARBARA HOECK

Department of Radiology
National Institutes of Health
Bethesda, Maryland 20205

INTRODUCTION

Despite the recent enthusiasm for better means of determining the extent of the active inflammatory response in the lung parenchyma of sarcoidosis patients, standard chest radiography remains a reliable method of determining staging, and parenchymal activity as well. The chest radiograph is characteristically used to determine the severity and course of sarcoidosis, but most studies imply there are poor correlations between the radiographic opacities and other indicators such as physiological parameters, gallium scans, and computed tomography and bronchoalveolar lavage results.[1-3]

Many authorities concur that the standard radiograph remains the most simple, reproducible, and cost-efficient means of determining the staging of the disease.[4,5] The same authorities would agree that staging has no relationship to activity, even though the ultimate prognosis and course of the disease would have more pragmatic meaning than any determination of activity. Wurm *et al.* reported the best prognosis in patients in stage I, an intermediate prognosis in patients in stage II, and the worst prognosis in patients in stage III.[6] Siltzbach reported the outcomes among 311 patients, noting that 54% of the patients in stage I had disease that became completely resolved, and that only 7% of the patients progressed to stage II. Thirty-one percent of the patients in stage II but only 10% of the patients in stage III returned to normal.[7] A more comprehensive study, which involved 11 university hospitals and 3676 patients, reported resolution of the chest radiograph in 65% of the patients in stage I, 49% of the patients in stage II, and 20% of the patients in stage III.[8] Some would argue that these statistics are meaningless because of poor controls and no criteria for the type,

[a] Address for correspondence: P.O. Box 3808, Department of Radiology, Duke University Medical Center, Durham, North Carolina 27710.

amount, or duration of treatment. We do not promote the naive argument that the standard method of staging sarcoidosis is sufficient to precisely determine activity, but we do believe that standard radiography has become somewhat neglected in favor of other technologies.

In this preliminary communication, we report a new method of determining sarcoidosis activity, as compared to the gallium scan, based solely on the standard chest radiograph. This method is based on the presence or absence of air bronchogram abnormalities, peribronchial cuffing, and subpleural thickening. Adenopathy and linear, reticulonodular, and nodular opacities are not included in our system. In 85 recent studies, which were performed in 51 patients with biopsy-proven sarcoidosis, this staging method agreed with gallium scanning in 68.2% of the patients. This system failed in specific and identifiable subgroups of patients that we will delineate. We will not report the comparative indices with a pulmonary function analysis or bronchoalveolar lavage results. Our database has not been tabulated to conclusively present these results, but it is our belief that this methodology will probably have a better correlation with lavage results and small airway function than would results of gallium scans. Of singular importance is the fact that this method can, with a more than acceptable degree of accuracy, distinguish between "low-intensity" alveolitis and "high-intensity" alveolitis.

MATERIALS AND METHODS

Fifty-one patients that constituted a typical population of sarcoidosis patients in terms of age, sex, race, and symptomatology were evaluated. Out of 29 women and 22 men, 37 patients were black, and 14 patients were white. Ages ranged from 21 to 53 years. Symptoms at initial presentation or during evaluation for exacerbation of pulmonary symptoms covered the spectrum from asymptomatic patients, in whom sarcoidosis was detected by routine radiography, to patients with severe dyspnea on exertion, with fever, with arthralgias, or with a variety of constitutional symptomatologies.

The diagnosis of noncaseating granulomas was established in most patients by transbronchial or open-lung biopsies. The remaining patients had biopsies of several sites including lymph nodes, liver, skin, muscle, or conjunctiva. Patients with concomitant diseases, such as congestive heart failure or acute bacterial pneumonia, were excluded from this study population. This was obviously necessary because the secondary disease process might well have produced air bronchogram abnormalities, peribronchial cuffing, or subpleural thickening. Complicating conditions that would have excluded patients from the study were not found, however.

All patients had multiple bronchoalveolar lavages, gallium-67 scanning, and pulmonary function evaluations, as well as routine chest radiography. Some patients had as many as four separate evaluations during the course of study, resulting in a total of 85 separate determinations. Although a variety of laboratory and clinical parameters could have been determined for most patients, we have only compared our radiographic evaluations to gallium scans.

As mentioned earlier, we believe that lavage and physiologic parameters may be more closely correlated to assessments based on our criteria for reading the standard chest radiograph than to assessments based on gallium scans. It is unfortunate that investigators who are proponents of gallium scanning have such a low regard for the chest radiograph; we therefore feel compelled to address the utility and efficacy of the less expensive chest radiograph. As shown by Johnson *et al.,* gallium scan results are comparable to the results of the other technologies currently being employed.[9]

Each patient had multiple posterior-anterior and lateral chest radiographs taken utilizing a high-kVp (130 to 140) technique. One of the difficulties of previous studies evaluating the chest radiograph is that low-kVp (less than 100) was often utilized. This is particularly true if taken with office equipment of clinicians who often acquire radiographic equipment with poor advice and consultation. We certainly do not believe that our criteria can be applied to suboptimal film technology. Each of the 85 studies were read independently by two chest radiologists without knowledge of any other pertinent data, particularly any derived from gallium scans. A second reading of all cases was performed by one radiologist to determine intraobserver variation (not significant).

Each case was characterized based on the classical staging of adenopathy, linear, reticulonodular, airspace, or fibrotic parenchymal changes. The radiographs were then classified according to Chrétien's staging system: stage 0: a normal chest; stage I: adenopathy; stage IIa: adenopathy with parenchymal opacities; stage IIb: parenchymal opacities only; and stage III: interstitial fibrosis.

All 85 posterior-anterior and lateral high-kVp chest radiographs were then evaluated for the volume of lung exhibiting peribronchial cuffing (beyond third-order bronchi), air bronchogram abnormalities, or subpleural thickening (FIGS. 1-3). Each posterior-anterior radiograph was scored from 0 to 10 with 0 representing a complete absence of the three abnormalities, and 10 representing the presence of these three features throughout the specific lung volume. The lateral view was used as an adjunct to better visualize lung in the most anterior and posterior portions as well as to determine more precisely the accentuation of fissures (subpleural edema).

In order to more easily quantify a primarily subjective analysis of the volume of lung involved in radiographic changes of activity, the lung was visually divided into four quadrants and each quadrant scored independently. The upper lobes and lower lobes were divided by an intercept with the division line between the two upper and lower lobes being at the level of the carina (FIG. 4). Therefore, four separate quadrants were evaluated. A quadrant was scored 0 if no air bronchogram abnormalities, subpleural edema, or peribronchial cuffing was seen in that quadrant. If any or all of these three criteria were met throughout the entire quadrant, a score of 2.5 was given. Scores of 0.5, 1.0, 1.5, or 2.0 were given depending upon the reader's assessment of the volume of the quadrant showing these specific changes. The total score ranging from 0 to 10 was derived from the sum of the four quadrant scores. A total score of 4 or below was classified as representing low-intensity alveolitis; a total score of 4.5 or above, as representing high-intensity alveolitis.

Following an intravenous injection of 5 mCi of gallium-67 citrate, images were obtained with a large-field-of-view scintillation camera. Studies were performed at 24 and/or 48 hr following injection. It should be noted that we have not found any particular difference in the results of our respective studies completed at 24 and 48 hr, despite the theoretical advantage of doing both examinations. A gallium index was determined by comparison of lung to liver activity as described by Johnson *et al.*[9] Out of a maximum of 400, a gallium index of 50 or more was considered indicative of high-intensity alveolitis. Every effort to eliminate as much subjectivity in the evaluation of the gallium scan should be employed. Computer indexing of the gallium scan in our experience is more reliable than the visual index and of course is much more reproducible. Each investigative effort utilizing the gallium scan as the determining factor can alter comparative analysis by having a relatively low or high value for its range of activity. There is often poor quality control relative to the many

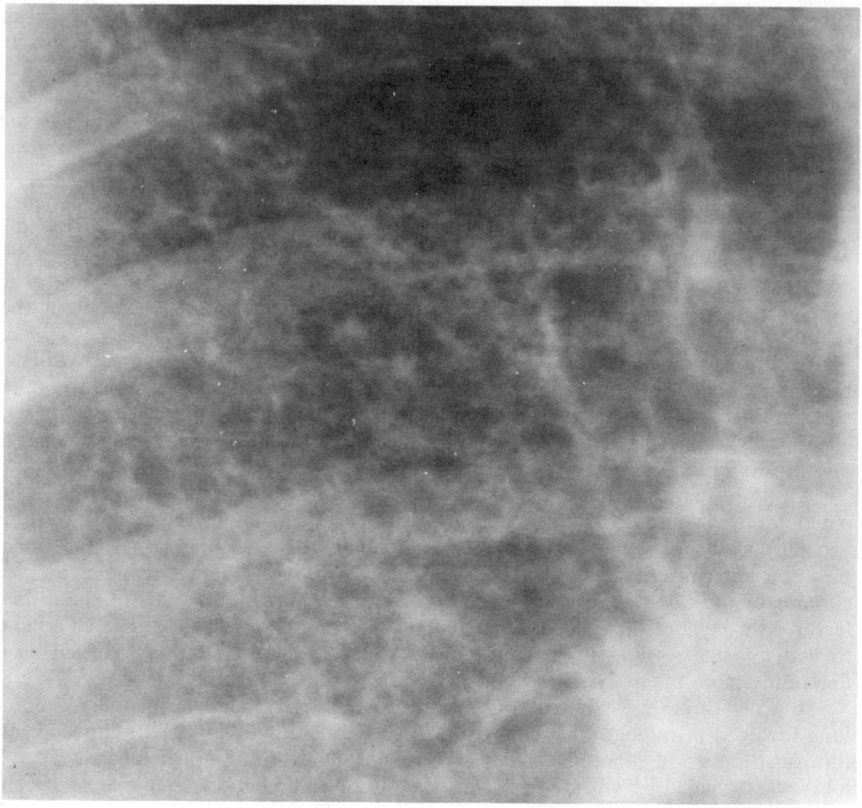

FIGURE 1. Coned posterior-anterior radiograph of the right upper lobe of the lung in a patient with a small high-intensity alveolitis (score: 2.0). Note thickening of minor fissure, moderate peribronchial cuffing, and focal air bronchogram abnormalities.

reported studies utilizing gallium, and, unfortunately, there has been no agreed upon, precise indices for determining activity. At present, each reported study must be evaluated on its own merit rather than applying these results to a different patient population. This is of particular importance in the utilization of gallium in patients with suspected stage III disease. Quantifying the gallium uptake for regional lung analysis is necessary to select focal alveolitis.

RESULTS

The results of the traditional classification and its comparison to the gallium studies can be summarized in the following way: 5% were stage 0 with 3 active gallium scans; 7% were stage I with 1 active gallium scan; 48% were stage IIa with 21 active gallium scans; 34% were stage IIb with 17 active gallium scans; and 6% were stage III with 2 active gallium scans. Distribution of the five classifications as they occurred related to the positive radiographic assessments for high-intensity alveolitis can be classified in the following way: stage 0, 0 of 8; stage I, 1 of 12; stage IIa, 57 of 82; stage IIb, 40 of 58; and stage III, 9 of 10. It is obvious that the majority of the cases (82%) were in stages IIa and IIb; however, these stages showed little correlation between high-intensity alveolitis and low-intensity alveolitis as documented by gallium scan or our standard chest radiographic analyses.

In 68.2% of the cases in our study, the chest radiographic scoring system yielded the same conclusion concerning the activity or inactivity of the alveolitis as did the gallium study. When only positive gallium studies were considered, the percentage of accurate radiographic assessments increased to 83.3%. Of the 54 radiographic interpretations that did not correspond to the gallium results, 40 of these (74%) occurred when the gallium study was negative for activity and the chest radiograph positive.

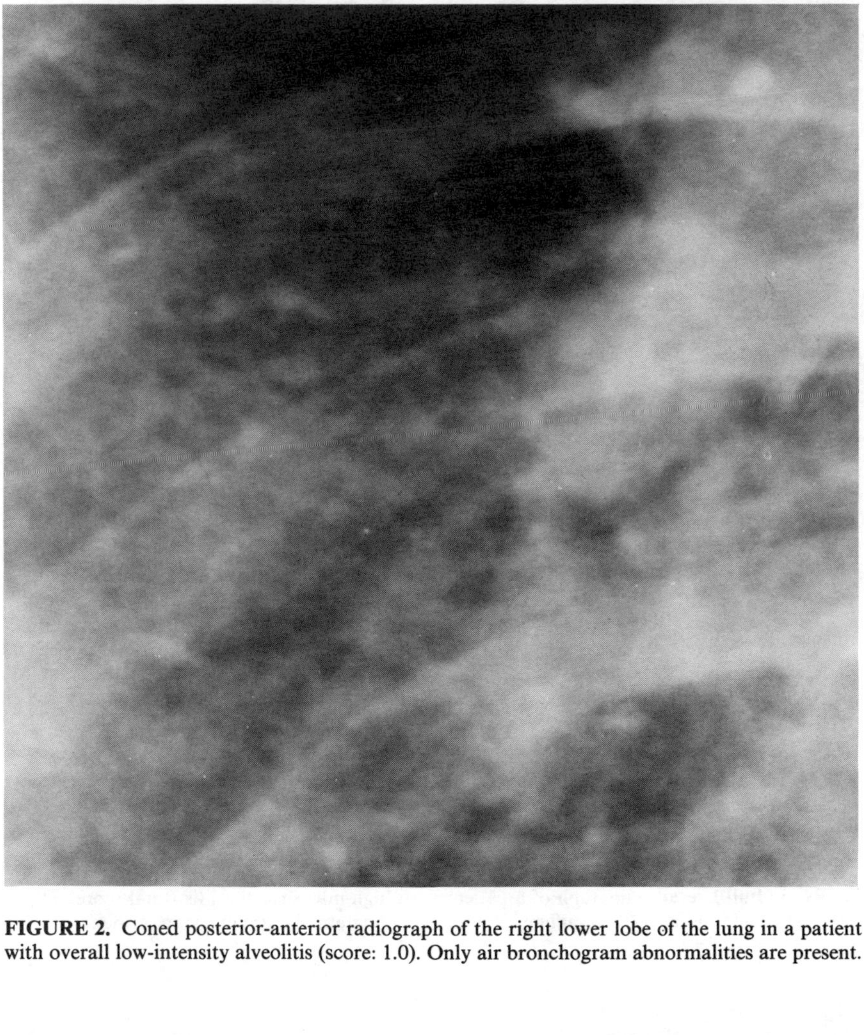

FIGURE 2. Coned posterior-anterior radiograph of the right lower lobe of the lung in a patient with overall low-intensity alveolitis (score: 1.0). Only air bronchogram abnormalities are present.

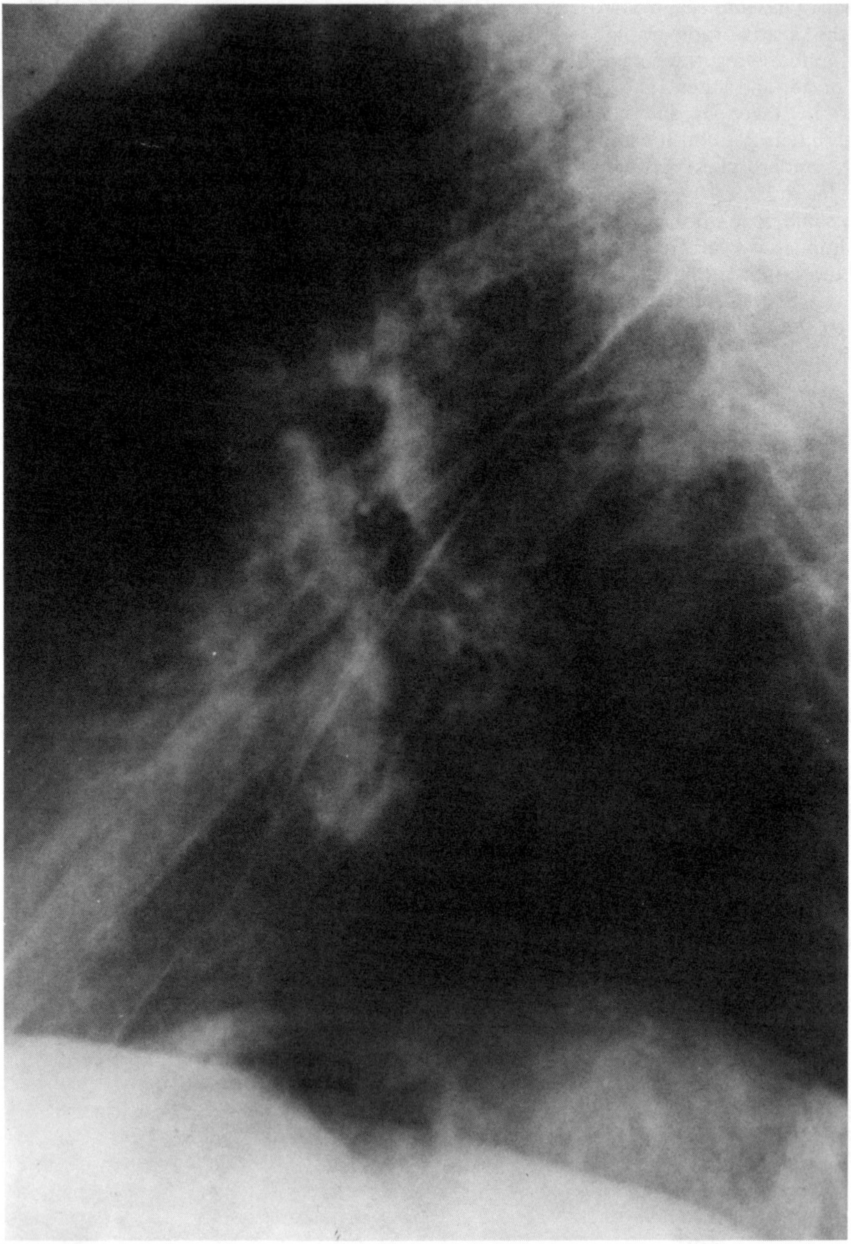

FIGURE 3. Full lateral radiograph of a patient with high-intensity alveolitis (total score: 6.0). Subpleural edema, peribronchial cuffing, and air bronchogram abnormalities are evident.

In our experience, the gallium scan usually lags behind the clearing of the chest radiograph in a variety of situations, including opportunistic infection and chemotherapy directed toward the lung, or in patients with neoplasms such as non-Hodgkin's lymphoma. Therefore, it should not be surprising that differing pathological events responsible for the positive results of the chest radiograph and gallium scan are temporally dependent. Our studies suggest that the chest radiograph might show positivity for high-intensity alveolitis while the gallium indices have returned to normal. Likewise, peribronchial cuffing, subpleural thickening, and air bronchogram abnormalities may be irreversible as they are often seen in patients with stage III disease. Even though physiologic parameters may indicate significant abnormality, the gallium scan and pulmonary lavage results may indicate no evidence of acute activity. In these cases, the chest radiograph indicates a high degree of irreversibility.

Intraobserver variation great enough to change a radiographic interpretation from high-intensity to low-intensity alveolitis, or vice versa, occurred in only 4 of 85 cases. Since the initial readings, we have attempted to minimize the subjectivity of our analysis by dividing each quadrant of the lung into fifths, giving each of these divisions a score of 0.5 if any of our three criteria was met in that section. Again, the total

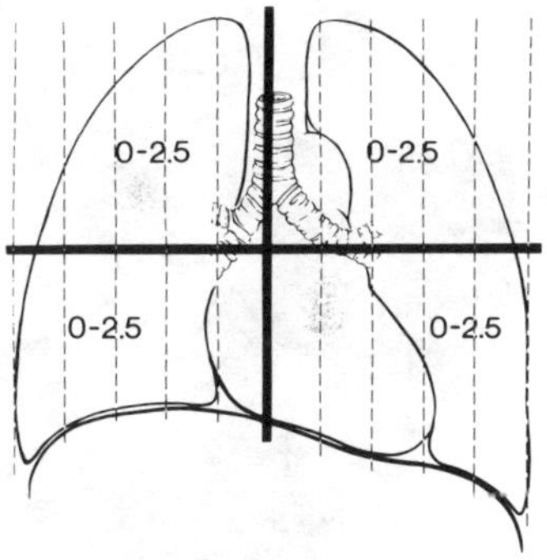

FIGURE 4. Depiction of the quadrant analysis scoring system by area and volume.

possible score for any one quadrant would be 2.5. Utilizing this system in more recent cases, we have not seen any major alteration from our initial statistical analysis. Also, it is interesting to note that if a consensus of opinion of two readers is required to determine activity or inactivity, the accuracy of radiographic scoring rises to 74.5% in comparison to the gallium indices.

DISCUSSION

Over the last several years our group has been employing computed tomography (CT) in studies of a variety of pulmonary diseases.[10–12] Specifically, we have reported the utility of CT for defining both parenchymal disease and adenopathy in patients with sarcoidosis. In addition to quantifying the abnormality, we have determined that essentially all patients with stage 0 disease have detectable mediastinal and parenchymal abnormalities by this sophisticated technology. In other words, our present methods of staging sarcoidosis by standard radiography would be altered considerably by applying CT in all cases. This technique, with its lack of availability and its complexity, is not only impractical but probably cost prohibitive. Data soon to be published from our institution describe the ability of CT to not only quantify but to differentiate between a variety of diffuse interstitial pulmonary diseases. By employing CT in a variety of patients with diffuse parenchymal disease, for example, idiopathic interstitial fibrosis, scleroderma, lymphangitic carcinoma, and sarcoidosis, we hoped to clarify the location and extent of the morphologic abnormality. The CT observations were based upon parenchymal alterations including increased attenuation—nodular, linear, ring-like, and confluent opacities. Decreased attenuation values as well as focal and diffuse bronchovascular distortion were noted. We now have evaluated 60 patients in this fashion and correlated these observations with pathological material. CT ac-

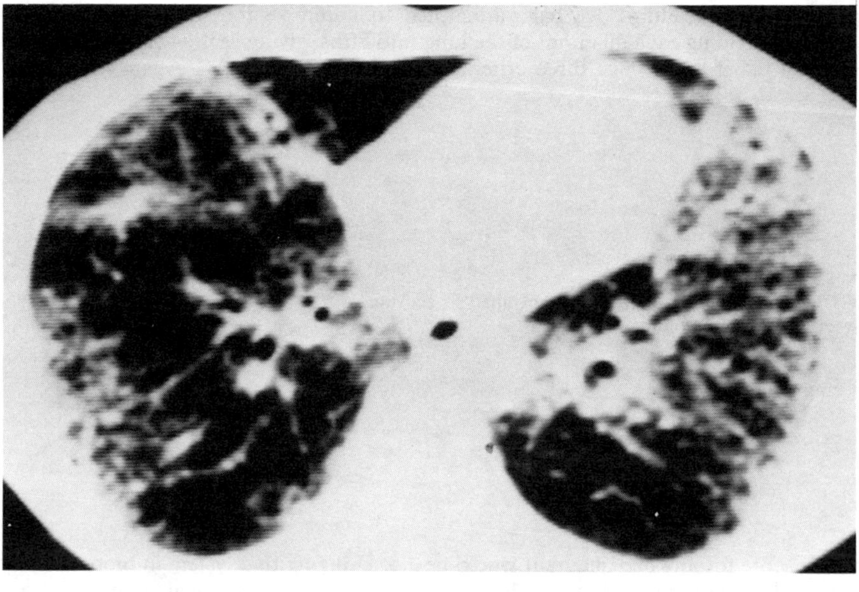

FIGURE 5. CT scan of a patient with stage IIb sarcoidosis. Subpleural opacities, peribronchial cuffing, and air bronchogram abnormalities are obvious. By all criteria, high-intensity alveolitis is evident.

curately reflected the gross pathological process in at least 80% of these diffuse parenchymal entities. Relative to the sarcoidosis cases was the focal and diffuse peribronchial proliferation and the subpleural location of much of the parenchymal abnormality (increased attenuation). This finding is in contrast to that for patients with usual interstitial pneumonitis and fibrosis where bronchi and vessels are distorted with focal decreased attenuation values. Unlike sarcoidosis, there is more subsegmental distribution, but the peribronchial and perivascular connective tissue alteration is less evident. It also was very uncommon to find extensive pleural disease in any of these interstitial diseases except those associated with connective tissue disorders. The so-called pleural thickening identified by standard chest radiography is actually subpleural or parenchymal in location. It is this work that made evident the original premise that standard radiography could be utilized in a much different way to determine the activity of sarcoidosis (FIG. 5).

It is well accepted that the inflammatory reaction and early granuloma formation of sarcoidosis have a predilection for alveolar walls, peribronchial and subpleural spaces, interlobular septae, and perivascular connective tissues. These morphologic changes could be readily identified by CT scans, and would be evident by standard radiography, which would show peribronchial cuffing, air bronchogram abnormalities, and subpleural edema (FIGS. 6 & 7).

Peribronchial cuffing, detected by standard chest radiography as a bronchial wall thickness of greater than 1 mm in bronchi beyond third order, indicates apparent increased thickness of the bronchial wall due to accumulation of interstitial fluid or inflammation.[13] An air bronchogram abnormality is a bronchus outlined as a negative shadow by opaque pulmonary parenchyma.[13] This finding is produced in one of two ways: the air in the alveoli may be replaced by material of water density, or severe interstitial disease in the small airways may encroach on the alveolar air spaces, effectively rendering the alveoli airless. Finally, subpleural edema or thickening is represented by accentuation of the fissures on the plain radiograph.[13] It is caused by disease in the peripheral connective tissue compartment where interstitial transudate secondary to inflammation accumulates under the visceral pleura, creating a band of increased opacity along the fissures. The infiltration of lymphocytes and macrophages into the peripheral interstitium and alveolar walls and the ensuing inflammatory reaction seen with active alveolitis of sarcoidosis can produce all three of these conditions.

Most investigators believe that the intensity of sarcoid alveolitis is the determining factor relative to the functional outcome of the disease. Keogh *et al.* have shown that high-intensity alveolitis over a 6-month period is followed by decreasing pulmonary function that may be irreversible.[1] Obviously, assessment of the activity is necessary for optimal management. If corticosteroids are to have an effect, they should be introduced during the most active phase of the disease. Because the classic radiographic means of staging sarcoidosis are purely based on a descriptive pattern of adenopathy or opacities, these criteria do not obviously determine the presence or absence of alveolitis (FIG. 8). Therefore, several authors have questioned the ability of the standard radiographic staging system to adequately predict the patient's course or to distinguish areas of active inflammation from normal lung or irreversible interstitial fibrosis.[3,14,15] The addition of our methodology, which appears to correlate best with cellular infiltration rather than gross tissue response, could alter the role of standard chest radiography as a prognostic indicator. Acceptance or rejection of our methodology will depend upon other investigator clarification.

The best imaging systems for describing cellular and microscopic pathology could be positron emission tomography and magnetic resonance imaging or spectroscopy. The former, by utilizing cyclotron-generated isotopes and imaging with a machine similar to a CT scanner, can measure intracellular metabolism as well as determine localized regional blood flow. Both functions would not only distinguish the degree of alveolitis, but also enable a direct method of following therapeutic interventions.

Magnetic resonance, by employing techniques to measure hydrogen or protons, may be able to quantify extravascular lung water. Preliminary data from our laboratory give promising results in this regard as well as correlating the water content with focal cellular concentration. Even more exciting is the potential to perform *in vivo* spectoscopy, thereby measuring phosphorus metabolism as well as the other elements of basic energetics. At present, these technologies are limited to a few institutions,

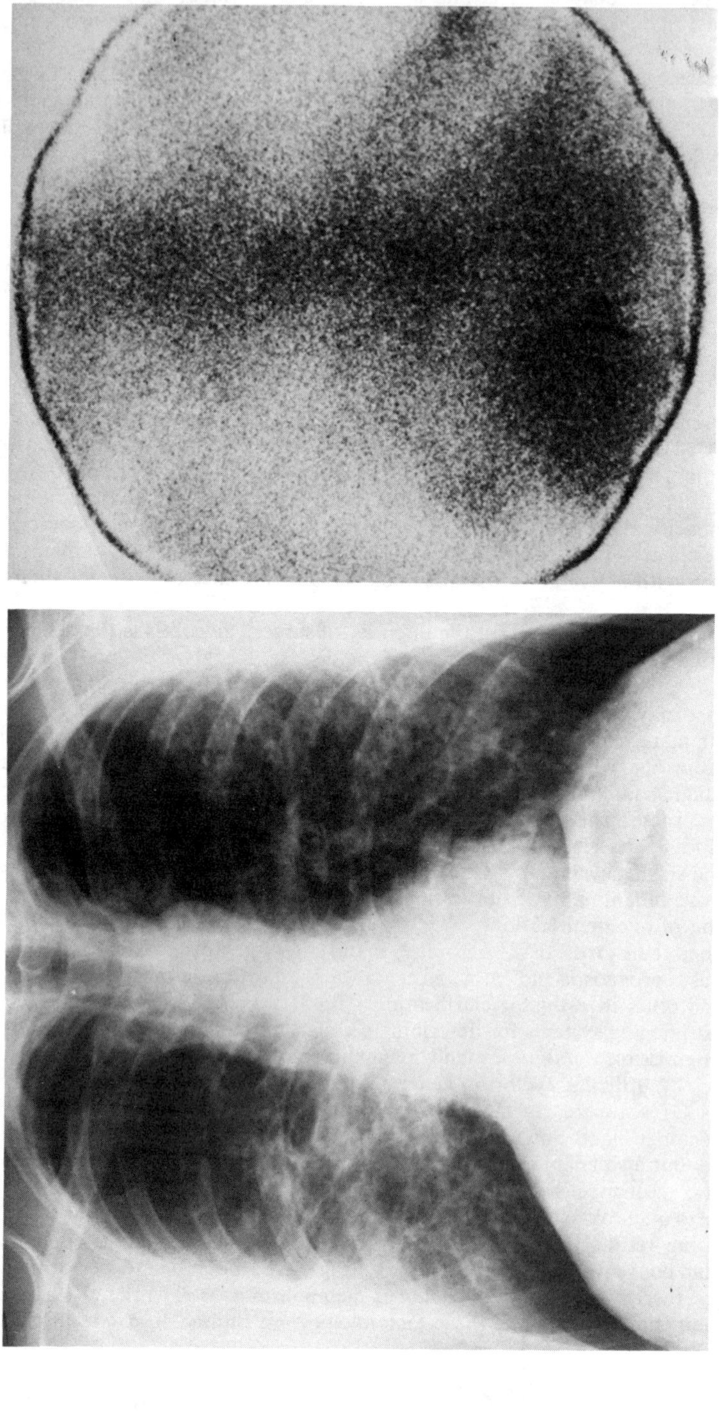

FIGURE 6. A posterior-anterior radiograph of a patient with high-intensity alveolitis (score: 5.0) is shown on the left. A gallium scan, of the same patient, which also detected the alveolitis (gallium index: 80) is shown on the right.

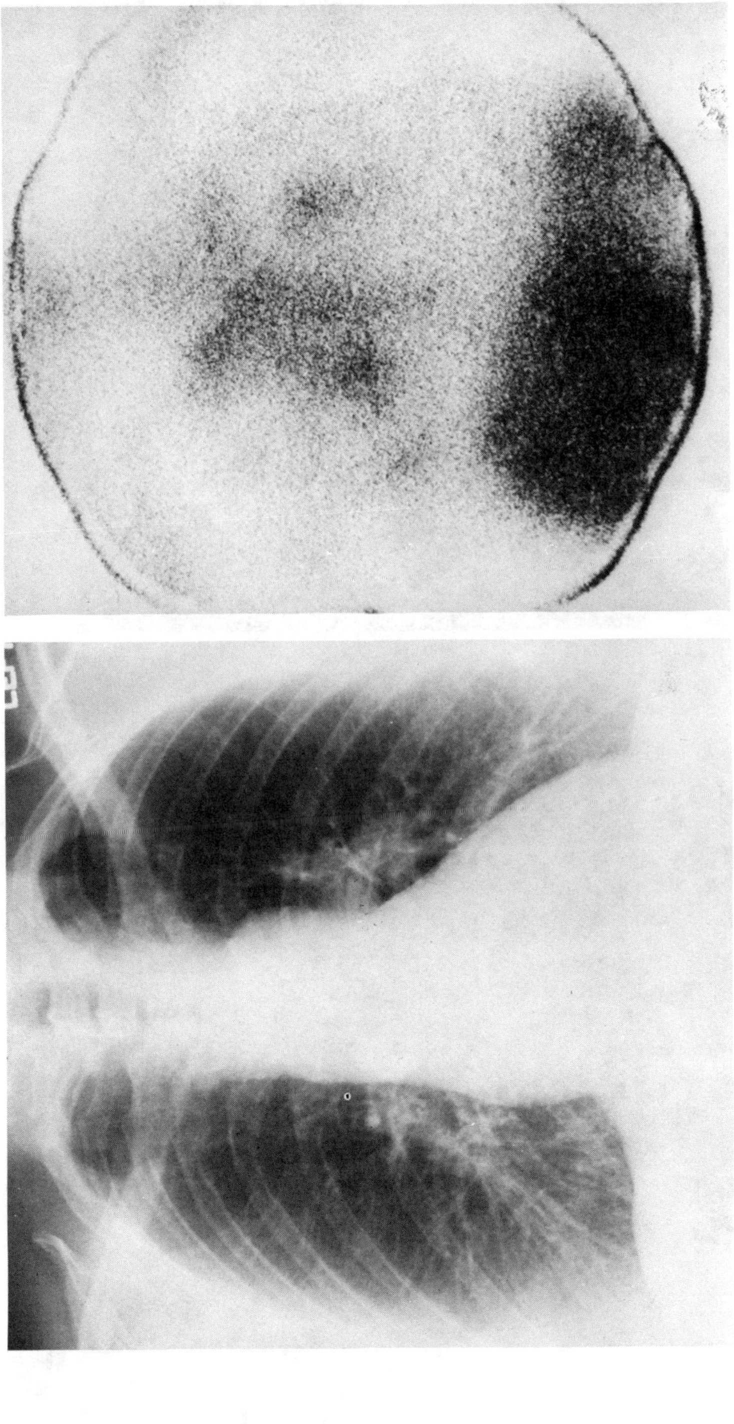

FIGURE 7. A posterior-anterior radiograph of patient with low-intensity alveolitis (score: 2.5) is shown on the left. A gallium scan, of the same patient, which did not detect the alveolitis (gallium index: 35) is shown on the right.

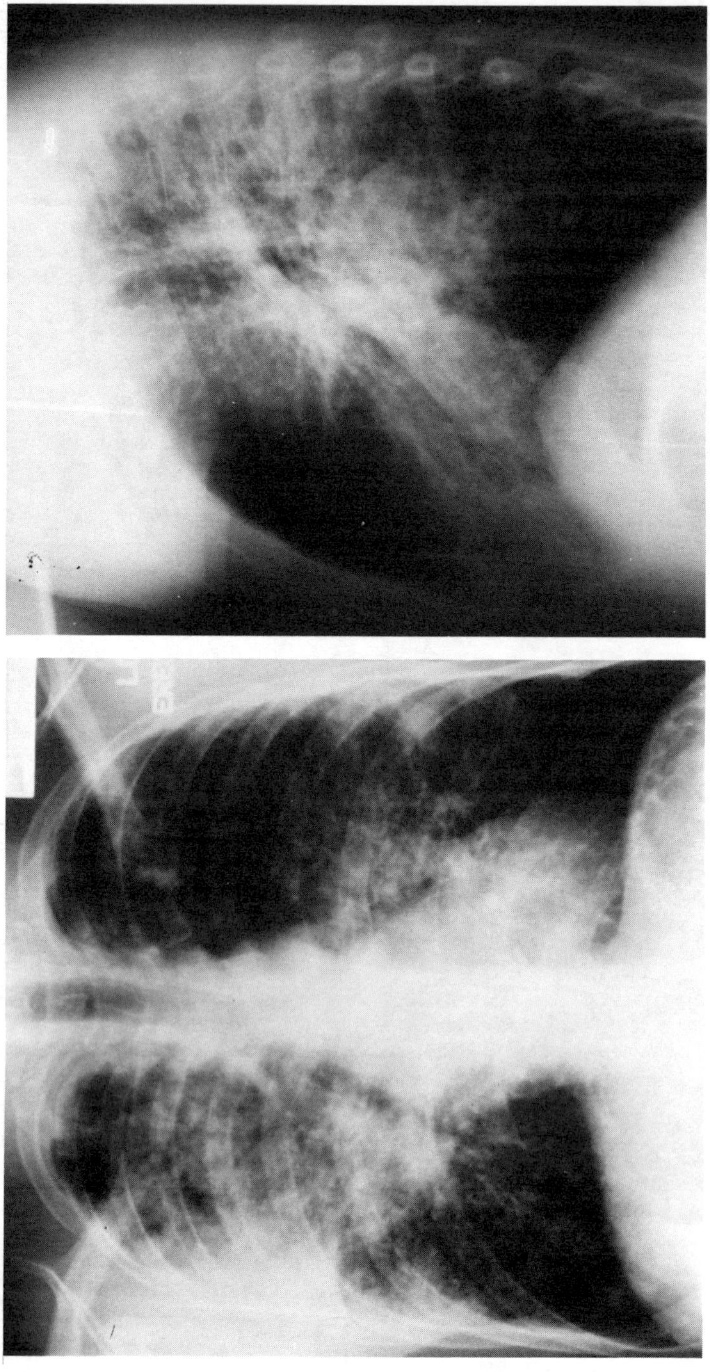

FIGURE 8. A posterior-anterior radiograph of a patient with high-intensity alveolitis (score: 8.0) is shown on the left. A lateral radiograph of the same patient confirming peribronchial cuffing, subpleural edema, and air bronchogram abnormalities is shown on the right.

and the speculation that they can be applied to basic lung pathophysiology is theoretical. Unlike CT scanners of the present generation, both technologies require extensive support personnel as well as cardiac and respiratory gating systems. It is doubtful that either will be more than a basic or clinical research system relative to sarcoidosis. It is very probable, though, that the information gained from this research will indirectly lead to a better interpretation of present studies, including those utilizing standard chest radiography. The role of any of these sophisticated imaging systems will not focus on gross morphology but cellular and subcellular abnormalities.

SUMMARY

The results concerning the activity or inactivity of the alveolitis determined with our proposed scoring system were comparable to those determined with gallium scanning in 68.2% of the patients with biopsy-proven sarcoidosis in our study. Certainly, further evaluation of a larger series of patients over a longer period of time will be required to more adequately evaluate this classification method. We also believe this methodology is reproducible and can be utilized by experienced interpreters of chest radiographs.

If we closely reevaluate the 32% of the cases in which the radiographic results disagreed with the gallium assessment of activity, two points worthy of mention become evident. In one group the gallium indices were borderline for activity whereas in the other group the radiographic criteria were most likely indicative of irreversible parenchymal changes. When the radiographs for the latter group were revaluated for signs of fibrosis such as volume loss, cystic changes, and alteration in vascular patterns, it was possible to delineate a significant false-positive group of patients. We will be reporting the long-term results of our observations over the next several years as well as adding more groups of patients to our initial study analysis. At that time, correlation with all other measurable parameters in determining high-intensity alveolitis versus low-intensity alveolitis will be compared to these new chest radiographic profiles.

REFERENCES

1. KEOGH, B. A., G. W. HUNNINGHAKE, B. R. LINE & R. G. CRYSTAL. 1983. The alveolitis of pulmonary sarcoidosis: Evaluation of natural history and alveolitis-dependent change in lung function. Am. Rev. Respir. Dis. **123:** 256-265.
2. CRYSTAL, R. G., W. C. ROBERTS, G. W. HUNNINGHAKE, J. E. GADEK, J. D. FULMER & B. R. LINE. 1981. Pulmonary sarcoidosis: A disease characterized and perpetuated by activated T-lymphocytes. Ann. Intern. Med. **94:** 73-94.
3. ABE, S., M. MUNAKATA & M. NISHIMURA. 1984. Gallium-67 scintigraphy, bronchoalveolar lavage, and pathologic changes in patients with pulmonary sarcoidosis. Chest **85:** 650-655.
4. DEREMEE, R. A. 1983. The roentgenographic staging of sarcoidosis: Historic and contemporary perspectives. Chest **83:** 128-133.
5. CHRÉTIEN, J., G. STANISLAS-LEGUERN, J. C. SALTIEL, G. HUCHON & J. MARSAC. 1979. Course and treatment of sarcoidosis in 350 patients. *In* Japan Medical Research Foundation. University of Tokyo Press. Tokyo.
6. WURM, K., H. REINDELL & L. HEILMEYER. 1958. Der Lungenboeck in Rontgen bild Stuttgart. Goerg Thieme. Verlag. Stuttgart.

7. SILTZBACH, L. E. 1967. Sarcoidosis: Clinical features and management. Med. Clin. North Am. **51:** 483-502.
8. JAMES, D. G., E. NEVILLE, L. E. SILTZBACH, J. TURIAF, J. P. BATTESTI, O. P. SHARMA, Y. HOSODA, R. MIKAMI, M. ODAKA, T. G. VILLAR, B. DJURIČ, A. C. DOUGLAS, W. MIDDLETON, A. KARLISH, A. BLASI, D. OLIVIERI & P. PRESS. 1976. A worldwide review of sarcoidosis. Ann. N.Y. Acad. Sci. **278:** 321-334.
9. JOHNSON, D. G., S. M. JOHNSON, C. C. HARRIS, C. A. PIANTADOSI, R. A. BLINDER & R. E. COLEMAN. 1984. Gallium-67 uptake in the lung in sarcoidosis. Radiology **150:** 551-555.
10. HEDLUND, L. W., P. VOCK & E. EFFMANN. 1983. Computed tomography of the lung: Densitometric studies. *In* Radiologic Clinics of North America: Cardiopulmonary Imaging. C. E. Putman, Ed. Vol. **21**(4): 775-788. W.B. Saunders. Philadelphia, PA.
11. HEDLUND, L. & C. E. PUTMAN. 1981. Analysis of lung density by computed tomography. *In* Pulmonary Diagnosis, Imaging, and Other Techniques. C. E. Putman, Ed.: 107-123. Appleton-Century-Crofts. New York, NY.
12. PUTMAN, C. E., S. ROTHMAN, M. LITTNER, W. ALLEN, N. SCHACHTER, T. MCLOUD, M. BEIN & B. GEE. 1977. Computerized tomography in pulmonary sarcoidosis. Comput. Tomogr. **1:** 197-209.
13. HEITZMAN, E. R. 1984. The Lung: Radiologic-Pathologic Correlations. 2nd edit. C. V. Mosby. St. Louis, MO.
14. BAUGHMAN, R. P., M. FERNANDEZ, C. H. BOSKEN, J. MANTIL & P. HURTUBISE. 1984. Comparison of gallium-67 scanning, bronchoalveolar lavage, and serum angiotension-converting enzyme levels in pulmonary sarcoidosis: Predicting response to therapy. Am. Rev. Respir. Dis. **129:** 676-681.
15. DEREMEE, R. A. 1984. Letter to the editor. Am. Rev. Respir. Dis. **129:** 343-344.

Factors Affecting Outcome of Sarcoidosis

Influence of Race, Extrathoracic Involvement, and Initial Radiologic Lung Lesions[a]

HAROLD L. ISRAEL,[b] PAUL KARLIN, AND HYMAN MENDUKE

Department of Medicine
Jefferson Medical College
Thomas Jefferson University
Philadelphia, Pennsylvania 19107

OSWALD G. DeLISSER

Data Information Systems Center
University City Sciences Center
Philadelphia, Pennsylvania 19104

The chest roentgenogram has long been used to estimate the severity of sarcoidosis and to follow its course. Some investigators[1] have found it to be superior to gallium scans, bronchoalveolar lavage, and serum angiotensin-converting enzyme levels for this purpose. McLoud *et al.*[2] have described a modification of the International Labor Office/University of Cincinnati (ILO/UC) classification devised for pneumoconiosis and have shown that 64 patients, most of whom were white, displayed, for a mean of 3.4 years in a follow-up study, a correlation between total profusion and physiological changes over time.

In this paper we report observations on 99 black and 53 white patients whose conditions were followed for a mean of 9.3 years after the detection of pulmonary infiltrates. It was considered that after such prolonged observation, recovery could be accurately identified by clinical and radiological criteria to assess the predictive value of the character, extent, and severity of the initial roentgenographic opacities.

[a]This study was aided by a grant from the Chairman's Fund, Department of Medicine, Jefferson Medical College, Thomas Jefferson University, Philadelphia, Pennsylvania 19107.

[b]Address for correspondence: 804 Jefferson Medical College, Philadelphia, Pennsylvania 19107.

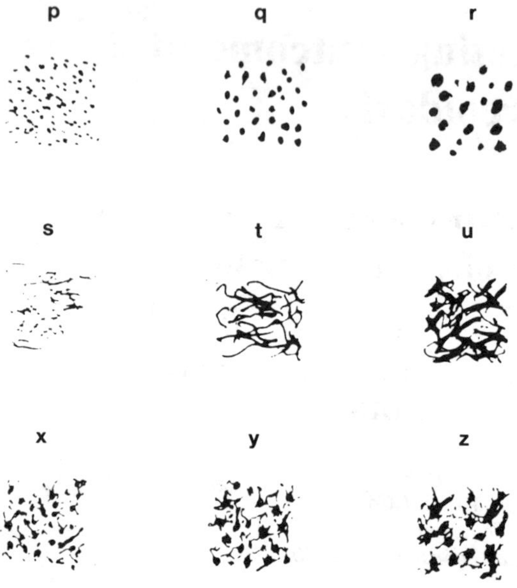

FIGURE 1. Modified ILO/UC classification applies to pulmonary sarcoidosis. Categories x, y, and z describe the reticulonodular opacities commonly seen in sarcoidosis. See the text for more details. Adapted, with permission, from reference 2.

METHODS AND CLINICAL MATERIAL

Patients seen in clinics or in private practice were unselected but for two requirements: patients had to have roentgenographically evident lesions, and had to have had their conditions followed for at least 3 years after the detection of infiltrates. Sarcoidosis patients with type 0 (normal chest roentgenograms) or type 1 (hilar/mediastinal adenopathy alone) disease were not included unless pulmonary opacities developed. In such cases, observations were dated from the time of onset of type 2 (adenopathy plus infiltrates) or type 3 (infiltrates without discernible adenopathy) disease.

As shown in FIGURE 1, pulmonary opacities were classified as being small and round (pqr), small and irregular (stu), or reticulonodular (xyz). The first letter of each classification refers to lesions with diameters up to 1.5 mm; the second, to lesions with diameters exceeding 1.5 mm and up to 3 mm; and the third, to lesions with diameters exceeding 3 mm and up to 10 mm. The term "ground glass" refers to airspace or alveolar patterns.

The severity of the radiographic abnormality was graded separately for the upper, middle, and lower zones of each lung as 0 (normal), 1 (slight), 2 (moderate), and 3 (advanced). The total of these scores represented the overall profusion, which could range from 1 to 18. The extent of the pulmonary densities was indicated by tabulating the number of the six zones involved, thus indicating the number of initial infiltrates confined to a single zone, to a single lung, or to the upper or lower thirds of the lungs. Patients were classified as having achieved radiologic recovery if the end roentgenogram appeared normal, with complete resolution of infiltrates and adenopathy.

Patients classified as having achieved clinical recovery had normal chest roentgenograms except for scars, did not require corticosteroids, and were able to perform normal work or domestic duties. The remaining patients included those still receiving corticosteroids, or who were disabled or dead. Patients with radiologic recovery were not necessarily clinically well, some requiring corticosteroids for extrathoracic disease. Some patients classified as recovered had considerable impairment of pulmonary function, but in each instance, function on the last examination was better than on earlier tests. Note was made of prior or concurrent erythema nodosum and of persistent cutaneous, ocular, hepatic, neural, myocardial, and bone sarcoidosis.

Descriptive data are tabulated separately for white and for black patients in TABLE 1. There was no significant difference in age or in duration of follow-up. The marked female predominance in black patients was similar to that observed in other studies.[3–5] Erythema nodosum occurred in three patients: one young woman with erythema nodosum had massive hilar adenopathy and faint pulmonary nodulation, and two patients had erythema nodosum with type 1 disease 1 and 3 years, respectively, before the development of pulmonary infiltrates.

Corticosteroid therapy was given less often to white (67.9%) than to black (87.9%) patients and was continued as long as palliation of symptoms was demonstrated. Failure of corticosteroids or intolerance of this medication led to use of chlorambucil in 3 white and in 12 black patients. At the end of the observation period, 15.1% of white and 21.3% of black patients were still under treatment.

TABLE 1. Clinical Data on 152 Patients with Roentgenographic Evidence of Pulmonary Sarcoidosis

	Number of Patients Exhibiting the Feature		
Clinical Feature	White ($N = 53$)	Black ($N = 99$)	Significance of Difference
Sex			
Male	26	28	$p < .01$
Female	27	77	
Age (years)			
< 30	32	54	
30-40	17	37	NS
> 40	4	8	
Prednisone therapy			
Present	36	87	$p < .01$
Absent	17	12	
Extrathoracic disease			
Present	12	38	NS
Absent	41	61	
Treatment			
Completed	28	61	NS
Not completed	8	21	

NOTE: The conditions of white and of black patients were followed for means of 9.0 and 9.4 years, respectively. This did not represent a significant difference.

STATISTICAL METHODS

Associations between the variables were examined in contingency tables and the degree of statistical significance indicated by appropriate χ^2 tests. In order to determine which subset of variables could provide good predictors of clinical recovery, a series of stepwise logistic regressions[6,7] was done using the dichotomy—recovered, not recovered—as the dependent variable. A variable was considered as having improved the prediction if the statistical significance, or p, of the test criterion was not greater than .05.

INITIAL PULMONARY RADIOGRAPHIC CHANGES

The initial abnormal roentgenographic changes in black and in white patients are indicated in TABLE 2. No significant ethnic difference was observed in frequency of associated hilar/mediastinal adenopathy, in the extent or location of lesions, the character (pqr, stu, xyz) or size (psx, qty, ruz) of the lesions, or frequency of ground-glass patterns. The severity of disease as indicated by the profusion of densities in the initial abnormal roentgenogram was greater in white patients, but the difference was not significant.

OUTCOME OF DISEASE

Five black patients died of respiratory failure due to sarcoidosis, complicated by pulmonary embolism in one case, and following lobectomy for aspergilloma in another. Clinical recovery was achieved in 71.4% and radiologic recovery in 48% of the patients (TABLE 3). The clinical and radiological outcomes were unrelated to age, sex, and initial roentgenographic appearances, with the sole exception that radiologic recovery was more frequent in the small number of patients with alveolar patterns. Stepwise logistic regression analysis[6,7] demonstrated race and the presence of extrathoracic disease to be the only factors affecting the probability of clinical recovery, which is estimated to be .894 in white patients with disease limited to the chest, .697 in white patients with extrathoracic disease, and .760 in black patients without and .464 in black patients with extrathoracic sarcoidosis (TABLE 4).

Late recurrence of pulmonary sarcoidosis was observed in three women who had had type 1 sarcoidosis years earlier and recovered with normal examinations and roentgenograms 9, 11, and 20 years before type 3 infiltrates appeared.

DISCUSSION

Application of a modified ILO/UC pneumoconiosis classification of pulmonary opacities of sarcoidosis had no value in predicting the ultimate outcome of the disease.

Use of this classification proved most illuminating, however, with respect to the different characteristics and course this disease takes in black and in white patients. It is not surprising that race and extrathoracic disease were important influences affecting the ultimate recovery from sarcoidosis; what is remarkable is the demonstration that the character, extent, and profusion of the initial roentgenographic opacities were identical in black and in white patients and that the severity of the initial roentgenographic changes was unrelated to the probability of clinical recovery.

The present study demonstrates a better prognosis for pulmonary sarcoidosis than other American reports[3] of prolonged observation, probably because of our policy of urging continued surveillance of recovered patients so that our experience is not limited

TABLE 2. Effect of Race on Initial Pulmonary Changes in Sarcoidosis

Clinical Feature	Number of Patients Exhibiting the Feature: White (N = 53)	Black (N = 99)
Hilar/mediastinal adenopathy		
Present	41	69
Absent	12	30
Lung involvement		
One segment	2	4
Unilateral	5	7
Upper third only	2	8
Lower third only	3	3
Lesion character		
pqr	1	5
stu	2	9
xyz	50	85
Lesion size		
psx	24	53
qty	17	34
ruz	12	12
Ground-glass pattern		
Present	5	8
Absent	45	91

NOTE: White patients and black patients had mean profusion scores of 6.8 and 5.8, respectively. No significant differences between white and black patients were found using χ^2 tests.

to patients requiring protracted treatment. It should be emphasized that all studies, American and European, concur that the prognosis is far better in patients with hilar and mediastinal adenopathy alone than in those presenting with radiologic evidence of pulmonary involvement with (type 2) or without (type 3) visible nodal enlargement.

Hillerdal *et al.*[8] followed the progress of patients in Uppsala, Sweden and found radiologic recovery at the end of 5 years in 82.4% of 308 patients with type 1 disease and in 57% of 216 patients with type 2/3 disease. In England, Neville *et al.*[9] observed clinical recovery within 2 years in 73% and radiologic recovery in 59% of type 1 cases, whereas the recovery rates were 34% and 38%, respectively, in patients with type 2 and in patients with type 3 disease. The corresponding rates for radiological recovery at the end of 2 years in a Philadelphia study were 34% for type 1 cases, and 10% for patients presenting with pulmonary infiltrates.[10]

The favorable long-term outcome observed in the present study is therefore more remarkable, since our observations were confined to patients with type 2/3 chest roentgenograms. Ultimate recovery from sarcoidosis in the United States must be considerably higher than the 84.9% we observed in white patients, or the 64.7% we observed in black patients, since approximately half the patients in American studies have onset with type 1 roentgenograms.[4,5,11,12] The frequency of recovery may be surprising to physicians treating patients seriously ill with respiratory or extrapulmonary sarcoidosis who are likely to be impressed with the chronicity and high

TABLE 3. Factors Influencing Clinical and Radiological Recovery in Sarcoidosis

Clinical Feature	Total Number (N = 152)	Patients Exhibiting the Feature: Clinically Recovered Patients: Number (N = 109)	Clinically Recovered Patients: Significance of Difference	Radiologically Recovered Patients: Number (N = 73)	Radiologically Recovered Patients: Significance of Difference
Race					
White	53	45 (84.9)	$p < .025$	31 (58.5)	NS
Black	99	64 (64.7)		42 (42.4)	
Sex					
Male	48	35 (72.9)	NS	21 (43.8)	NS
Female	104	74 (71.2)		52 (50.0)	
Age (years)					
< 30	86	66 (76.7)		44 (51.2)	
30-40	54	35 (64.8)	NS	23 (42.6)	NS
> 40	12	8 (66.7)		6 (50.0)	
Extrathoracic disease					
Present	50	26 (52.0)	$p < .001$	17 (34.0)	$p < .025$
Absent	102	83 (81.4)		56 (54.9)	
Hilar/mediastinal adenopathy					
Present	110	80 (72.7)	NS	56 (50.9)	NS
Absent	42	29 (69.9)		42 (40.5)	
Lung Involvement					
Three regions or less	48	36 (75.0)	NS	19 (39.6)	NS
Four regions or more	104	73 (70.2)		54 (51.9)	
Lesion character					
pqr	135	98 (72.6)		65 (48.2)	
stu	6	3 (50.0)	NS	5 (83.3)	NS
xyz	11	8 (72.7)		3 (27.3)	
Lesion size					
psx	77	56 (72.7)		34 (44.2)	
qty	51	35 (68.6)	NS	24 (47.1)	NS
ruz	24	18 (61.5)		15 (62.5)	
Ground-glass pattern					
Present	13	8 (61.5)	NS	10 (76.9)	$p < .05$
Absent	139	101 (72.7)		63 (45.3)	

NOTE: Percentages are shown in parentheses.

TABLE 4. Estimated Probability of Clinical Recovery according to Race and Extrathoracic Disease

	Probability
White	
No extrathoracic disease	.894
Extrathoracic disease	.697
Black	
No extrathoracic disease	.760
Extrathoracic disease	.464

frequency of relapse of this disease. Nevertheless, we believe our observations reliably reflect the ultimate outcome of the disease. Although a majority (81%) of our patients received prednisone, often for prolonged periods, the usual dosage was low (< 20 mg daily), and the percentage treated was smaller than that of the patients of Johns *et al.* (96%).[3]

The lack of a relationship between the outcome and the initial severity of the roentgenographic changes in the lung is surprising. It is well known that histologic findings, chest roentgenographic changes, bronchoalveolar lavage, and gallium uptake are poorly correlated. There has been general acceptance of the concept that, with occasional exceptions, the chest roentgenograms is a reliable tool for assessing the course of sarcoidosis. Our application of the modified ILO/UC classification indicates that in the long run neither the roentgenographic character of the opacities, their extent, nor their profusion are predictors of the outcome; that is, patients found with extensive pulmonary infiltrates are as likely to recover as those with small focal infiltrates. Only race and the presence of persistent extrathoracic disease affected the outcome: the probability of clinical recovery is estimated to vary from .894 in white patients with no extrathoracic lesions to .464 in black patients with extrathoracic involvement.

An unexpected finding was that the striking difference in outcome of sarcoidosis in black and in white patients is unrelated to the severity of the initial roentgenographic lesions. Few comparisons of the roentgenographic changes in white and in black patients have been reported.[4,10,12] Kirks *et al.*[12] studied 56 white and 94 black patients; found no difference in occurrence of type 1, 2, and 3 disease; and noted the frequency of reticulonodular, fibrotic, acinar, and nodular opacities to be similar in the two races. Review of 258 white and 351 black patients examined in Ohio, South Carolina, and Pennsylvania, however, demonstrated a greater frequency of type 1 and a lower frequency of type 2 onsets in white patients.[4]

Use of the ILO/UC classification for the two races has not previously been reported. McLoud *et al.*[2] studied 211 patients, 64.3% of whom were white, and classified 33% as having pqr (nodular) densities, 19% as having stu (linear) densities, and 35% as having xyz (reticulonodular) densities. Carrington *et al.*[13] applied this classification to the roentgenograms of 43 patients with sarcoidosis (race unspecified) and classified 16% as pqr, 21% as stu, and 53% as xyz. Our classification of xyz opacities in 89% of patients is supported by Kirks *et al.*,[12] who described 82% of the infiltrates in their series has having a reticulonodular configuration, and our identification of an alveolar pattern in 8% is similar to the 4% noted by Battesti *et al.*[14] in their 746 cases.

Analysis of the initial parenchymal changes yielded information of clinical interest. Although the typical distribution of sarcoidosis is bilateral and central, sparing lung apices and bases,[11] atypical presentations were frequent in our patients, 18.4% of whom had infiltrates that were confined to one lung or to lung apices or bases. In six patients the initial discernible lesion was confined to a single third of one lung.

As McLoud *et al.*[2] emphasized, pulmonary function tests are more sensitive than the chest roentgenograms in measuring residual impairment. The degree of permanent impairment may be significant even in patients whose chest roentgenogram has regained a normal appearance. It should also be emphasized that serious extrathoracic disease, whether ocular, myocardial, cutaneous, neural, or hepatic, may be disabling and even fatal in patients whose chest roentgenograms returned to normal.

No long-term studies of large numbers of patients have assessed the frequency of late relapse in patients seemingly recovered from sarcoidosis. We have encountered in the present study three instances of pulmonary infiltrates appearing in patients who had had type 1 sarcoidosis 9, 12, and 20 years earlier with apparent recovery. A new illness appearing in patients recovered from sarcoidosis may represent a relapse but is often of other etiology.

It has long been recognized that the most reliable indicator of rapid recovery from sarcoidosis is onset with erythema nodosum (Löfgren's syndrome). Neville *et al.*[9] observed remission within 2 years in 84% of patients who had erythema nodosum. Since erythema nodosum is usually associated with type 1 disease, this predictor of a favorable outcome was of little use in the patients we observed; erythema nodosum occurred in only one of our patients at the time pulmonary sarcoidosis was found, and two additiional patients had histories of erythema nodosum 1 to 2 years earlier when hilar adenopathy alone had been present. All three patients recovered, but the infrequency of erythema nodosum in American sarcoidosis patients limits its value as a guide to outcome.

If the initial roentgenographic changes have no predictive value regarding the later course of the disease, there is little evidence that other parameters are more reliable. An important recent demonstration has been that 13 of 14 patients whose onset was with erythema nodosum had marked lymphocytosis evident upon bronchoalveolar lavage.[15] The observation of intense initial alveolitis in patients assured of rapid recovery by reason of erythema nodosum indicates that the intensity of initial pulmonary inflammation is not a reliable guide to the outcome of sarcoidosis. We have observed 31 patients for a mean of 6.1 years after gallium scans: clinical recovery was unrelated to pulmonary uptake.[16] There is as yet inadequate evidence for basing therapeutic decisions on initial roentgenographic changes, bronchoalveolar lavage findings, or gallium uptake in the lungs.

The mechanisms which make sarcoidosis a transient illness in most patients and a chronic disabling or fatal one in others are unknown; the evidence that the eventual course depends on the intensity of the early pulmonary reaction is as yet unsubstantial. The study of the genesis and protective action of erythema nodosum in sarcoidosis, the mechanisms of the extrathoracic spread of the disease, and racial differences in the immunologic and histologic alterations in the pulmonary parenchyma is essential if the diverse manifestations of this disease are to be understood. The intensive investigation which pulmonary sarcoidosis has received in recent years should be balanced by greater attention to its systemic aspects which together with race significantly affect the outcome of sarcoidosis.

SUMMARY

Chest roentgenograms of 152 patients with type 2/3 disease observed 3 or more years were reviewed using modified ILO/UC nomenclature. After a mean length of observation of 9.3 years, clinical recovery was observed in 71.7% and radiologic recovery in 48.0% of the patients. Age; duration of observation; mediastinal adenopathy; and character (xyz, pgr, stu), size, extent, and profusion of pulmonary densities were similar in the 53 white and 99 black patients, who differed significantly only in sex distribution. White patients achieved clinical recovery (84.9%) more often than black patients (64.7%) (p=.05). Factors influencing clinical recovery were analyzed by means of stepwise logistic linear regression. The initial roentgenographic features were unrelated to outcome; only race and extrathoracic disease proved to have significant predictive value. The probability of clinical recovery is estimated to be .894 in white patients with disease limited to the chest, .697 in white pateints with extrathoracic disease, and .760 in black patients without and .454 in black patients with extrathoracic sarcoidosis. Recovery appears to be related not to the severity of the initial pulmonary reaction but to racially associated factors that influence extrathoracic dissemination as well as lung damage.

REFERENCES

1. McAllister, W. A. C., P. Haslam, A. Davidson, A. Britten, J. Payne & M. Turner-Warwick. 1983. A longitudinal study of a ^{67}Ga scan, alveolar lavage, and SACE in the assessment of pulmonary sarcoidosis during therapy. Am. Rev. Respir. Dis. **127**(4, 2): 63.
2. McLoud, T. C., G. R. Epler, E. A. Gaensler, G. W. Burke & C. B. Carrington. 1982. A radiographic classification for sarcoidosis: Physiologic correlation. Invest. Radiol. **17:** 129-138.
3. Johns, C. J., J. B. Zachary, M. I. MacGregor, J. L. Curtis, P. P. Scott & P. B. Terry. 1982. The longitudinal study of chronic sarcoidosis. Trans. Am. Clin. Climatatol. Assoc. **94:** 173-181.
4. Israel, H. L. & Y. Kataria. Clinical aspects of sarcoidosis. *In* Sarcoidosis. J. Lieberman, Ed. Grune and Stratton. New York, NY. In press.
5. Ellis, K. & G. Renthal. 1962. Pulmonary sarcoidosis: Roentgenographic observations on course of disease. Radiology **88:** 1070-1083.
6. BMDP Statistical Software. 1981. University of California Press. Los Angeles, CA.
7. SAS Users Guide: Statistics. 1982. SAS Institute. Cary, NC.
8. Hillerdal, G., E. Nou, K. Osterman & B. Schmekel. 1984. Sarcoidosis: Epidemiology and prognosis. Am. Rev. Respir. Dis. **130**.
9. Neville, E., A. N. Walker & D. G. James. 1983. Prognostic factors predicting the outcome of sarcoidosis: An analysis of 818 patients. J. Med. **52:** 525-533.
10. Israel, H. L. & D. J. Washburne. 1980. Characteristics of sarcoidosis in black and in white patients: Analysis of 162 recent cases. *In* Eighth International Conference on Sarcoidosis and Other Ganulomatous Diseases. W. Jones Williams & B. H. Davies, Eds.: 497-507. Alpha Omega. Cardiff.
11. Freundlich, I. M., H. I. Libshitz, L. M. Glassman & H. L. Israel. 1970. Sarcoidosis: Typical and atypical thoracic manifestations and complications. Clin. Radiol. **21:** 376-383.
12. Kirks, D. R., V. D. McCormick & R. H. Greenspon. 1973. Pulmonary Sarcoidosis: Roentgenologic analysis of 150 patients. Am. J. Roentgenol. **117:** 777-786.
13. Carrington, C. B., E. A. Gaensler, J. P. Mikus, A. W. Schachter, G. W. Burke & A. M. Goff. 1976. Structure and function in sarcoidosis. Ann. NY. Acad. Sci. **278:** 265-283.
14. Battesti, J. P., G. Saumon, D. Valeyre, J. Amouróux, B. Pechnick, D. Sandron & R. Georges. 1982. Pulmonary sarcoidosis with an alveolar radiographic pattern. Thorax **37:** 448-452.

15. VALLEYRE, D., G. SAUMON, R. GEORGES, J. L. KEMENY, D. BLADIER, J. AMOURÓUX, J. PRÉ & J. P. BATTESTI. 1984. The relationship between disease duration and noninvasive pulmonary explorations in sarcoidosis with erythema nodosum. Am. Rev. Respir. Dis. **129:** 938-942.
16. ISRAEL, H. L., G. F. GUSHUE & C. H. PARK. 1986. Assessment of gallium-67 scanning in pulmonary and extrapulmonary sarcoidosis. Ann. NY. Acad. Sci. This volume.

Ocular Sarcoidosis

A Case-Control Study among Black Patients

JOHN C. MERRITT,[a,b] DAVID J. BALLARD,[c]
HARVEY CHECKOWAY,[b] PATRICIA MOWER,[b]
AND ROGER GRIMSON[d]

[b] *The University of North Carolina School of Medicine*
Chapel Hill, North Carolina 27514

[c] *Mayo Foundation*
Rochester, Minnesota 55904

[d] *State University of New York*
Stony Brook, New York 11794

INTRODUCTION

Sarcoidosis is a granulomatous disease of unknown etiology that potentially can involve several organs, especially the eye. Epidemiologic surveys have revealed that American blacks, particularly those residing in the Southeastern United States, have among the highest reported incidence and prevalence rates in the world.[1-3] Additionally, ocular involvement has been noted to be about five times more common among black than white sarcoidosis patients.[3] We report, herein, the results of a case-control study of ocular sarcoidosis conducted among blacks in Eastern North Carolina. The hypotheses examined were that exposures to pine tree products and specific occupational exposures, which are common in North Carolina, were related to risk for ocular sarcoidosis.

METHODS

Cases

Forty-four cases of ocular sarcoidosis among blacks were seen at the Glaucoma/Uveitis Clinic of the North Carolina Memorial Hospital during 1980-1981. There

[a] Address for correspondence and reprint requests: Department of Ophthalmology, 617 Burnett/Womack Building 229H, the University of North Carolina School of Medicine, Chapel Hill, North Carolina 27514.

were 29 female and 15 male cases, aged 10 to 57 years. Cases were defined as patients whose clinical presentations (corneal endothelial precipitates, iris nodules, and/or retinal perivasculitis) were observed in the presence of biopsy-positive evidence of noncaseating granulomas consistent with sarcoidosis. All subjects exhibited epithelioid granulomas consistent with sarcoidosis from excised tissues, usually the 1) conjunctiva, 2) lungs, 3) skin, 4) buccal mucosa, and 5) nasal mucosa. Patients with other conditions known to cause granulomatous disease (such as tuberculosis) and other diseases capable of inducing endogenous uveitis in children[4] were screened, and these patients were excluded after their histories, laboratory studies, and physical examinations were evaluated.

Differential diagnoses were used to determine whether the presence of granulomas in a patient could be due to a disease other than sarcoidosis. Common granulomatous diseases other than sarcoidosis that are found in Eastern North Carolina include 1) tuberculosis; 2) leprosy; 3) histoplasmosis, toxoplasmosis, and mycobacteriosis; 4) foreign-body reactions 5) juvenile rheumatoid arthritis syndromes; and 6) Vogt-Koyanagi disease. Patients with such diseases were excluded from this study.

Controls

A control group subject to the same disease exclusion criteria was drawn from a list of black patients attending out-patient clinics at the North Carolina Memorial Hospital during 1980-1981. Initial attempts to match three controls to one case were hampered by matching problems encountered in young male controls at the North Carolina Memorial Hospital. A convenient sample of controls consisted of 110 females and 28 males.

The sex and age distributions of the cases and controls are shown in TABLE 1. Both male and female cases were older than their respective controls, but the differences were not significant.

Ascertainment of Exposure

A questionnaire was administered by a trained interviewer to cases and controls to elicit information on their past histories of inhaling smoke from burning pine, chewing pine products (bark, gum sap, and resin), and employment in the wood and lumber, textile, and tobacco industries. The interviewer was unaware of the study hypotheses; however, she knew the cases from the controls.

Data Analysis

Subjects were considered to have been exposed to a study factor if they gave an affirmative answer to the relevant question. The small sample size precluded a detailed, dose-effect analysis; consequently, exposures were treated as being either present or absent. Relative risks associated with the exposure factors were approximated by the

TABLE 1. Age and Sex Distributions of Cases and Controls

	Females		Males	
Age Group (years)	Number of Cases	Number of Controls	Number of Cases	Number of Controls
10-19	0 (0)	9 (8.2)	5 (33.3)	8 (28.6)
20-29	11 (37.9)	50 (45.5)	5 (33.3)	14 (50.0)
30-39	12 (41.3)	33 (30.0)	3 (20.0)	3 (10.7)
40-49	2 (7.0)	3 (2.7)	2 (13.3)	3 (10.7)
>50	4 (13.8)	15 (13.6)	0 (0)	0 (0)
	29 (100)	110 (100)	15 (100)	28 (100)

NOTE: Percentages are indicated in parentheses, and the totals for each column are shown in the bottom line of the table. The mean ages corresponding to each total, left to right, are 34.5, 31.0, 26.1, and 25.1 years.

odds ratio,[5] with allowance made for age differences between the cases and controls by means of an age-stratified analysis.[6] Two age strata, >35 and <35 years, were defined in the analysis. The statistical significance of the odds ratio was evaluated from inspection of the 95% summary confidence limits which were based on inverse variance estimates derived from the Taylor series.[7] Separate analyses were performed for females and males. Only summary odds ratios, by gender, are shown because the data in the age-gender-specific tables were too sparse to yield reliable relative risk estimates.[8]

RESULTS

The results for the five exposure variables among female cases and controls are given in TABLE 2. The odds ratios were above the expected value of 1.0 for the burning of pine (OR=1.8) and tobacco industry employment (OR=2.0). Neither result was

TABLE 2. Risk Factors for Females with Ocular Sarcoidosis

Factor	Number of Cases Exposed	Number of Controls Exposed	Odds Ratio	Significance[a]	Confidence Interval (95%)
Exposure to burning pine	21	65	1.8	.10	0.7, 4.5
The chewing of pine products[b]	6	29	0.7	.53	0.3, 2.0
Lumber industry employment	4	20	0.7	.58	0.2, 2.3
Textile industry employment	9	28	1.3	.54	0.5, 3.2
Tobacco industry employment	7	15	2.0	.17	0.7, 5.5

[a]Entries in this column represent p values from two-sided tests.
[b]Includes pine bark, gum, and resin.

statistically significant at the conventional 5% probability level as both associated confidence intervals included 1.0.

Among males, the chewing of pine products (OR=3.0) and employment in the lumber (OR=3.6) and textile (OR=9.8) industries were related to an increased risk of contracting ocular sarcoidosis (TABLE 3). None of these findings, however, was statistically significant. Unlike the situation for females where the risk associated with tobacco industry employment was elevated, occupational exposures in this industry were apparently unrelated to ocular sarcoidosis risks among males.

DISCUSSION

A case-control study was used instead of a cohort approach because case-control studies are more practical for investigations of rare diseases. There are, however, numerous potential biases inherent in case-control studies that can result in distorted findings.[9] The most serious of these in the present study is the possibility of biased selection of study subjects. It is possible that the case group may not be representative of all ocular sarcoidosis patients among blacks because of idiosyncratic referral patterns to medical care facilities within North Carolina. Selection bias could have occurred among the controls for a similar reason; however, the exposure of interest probably did not influence the probability of presentation at our hospital clinic.

TABLE 3. Risks Factors for Males with Ocular Sarcoidosis

Factor	Number of Cases Exposed	Number of Controls Exposed	Odds Ratio	Significance[a]	Confidence Interval (95%)
Exposure to burning pine	11	19	1.3	.71	0.3, 5.2
The chewing of pine products[b]	4	3	3.0	.18	0.6, 15.9
Lumber industry employment	10	10	3.6	.06	0.9, 13.5
Textile industry employment	4	1	9.8	.06	0.9, 98.0
Tobacco industry employment	3	8	0.6	.54	0.1, 2.8

[a]Entries in this column represent p values from two-sided tests.
[b]Includes pine bark, gum, and resin.

Errors in the assignment of subjects to exposed and nonexposed categories may have distorted the results, but the "blinding" of the data collectors minimized the possibility for differential misclassification. As a result, if misclassification of exposure had distorted the findings, the bias would have been in a conservative direction; that is, the estimates of relative risk would have been reduced.[10] Bias resulting from differential recall of exposure among cases and controls is another potential source of errors; however, this bias is greatest when instances of the exposure of interest that may be recalled are few and when controls have been drawn from the community.[9]

Inadequate control of confounding variables (factors associated with the exposure and the disease) is another possible source of biases. The confounding variables of gender and age were controlled by means of stratification analysis. Other potential confounding variables which could not be evaluated and controlled because of small numbers are urban or rural residential factors.[3]

Despite these limitations, several of the findings warrant note. Specifically, positive elevations of ocular sarcoidosis risks were detected for exposures to burning pine among females and males. Occupational exposure in the textile, wood, and lumber industries demonstrated positive association for males whereas tobacco industry employment was related to risk among females. The reason for the discrepancy in risk associated with tobacco industry employment for men and women is unknown.

Previous work has revealed no consistent patterns of association between occupation and sarcoidosis.[11] In contrast, the relationship between pine-product exposures and sarcoidosis has engendered considerable controversy. In 1956, Cummings *et al.*[12] postulated that there may be a causal pathway between hypersensitivity induced by pine pollen and sarcoidosis. This hypothesis derived from Cummings' observation that the geographic distribution (birthplace) of 1194 hospitalized sarcoidosis patients was closely correlated with the distribution of pine forests in the United States. Subsequent research yielded conflicting results. Studies conducted in Louisiana[13] and Florida[14] have provided supportive evidence, but investigations carried out in Denmark,[15] Scotland,[16] Switzerland,[17] Japan,[18] and Uruguay[19] did not demonstrate similar correlations.

The results of the present study suggest there may be associations of pine product and occupational exposures with ocular sarcoidosis. A unifying hypothesis that may explain these results for the exposures considered is that the pathogenesis of sarcoidosis is a granulomatous response to incomplete phagocytic digestion of nonbiodegradable foreign bodies (such as pine pollen) and associated macrophage destruction. Definitive confirmation or refutation of these observations and related pathogenetic hypotheses awaits evidence from future investigations involving larger surrounding populations within Eastern North Carolina.

SUMMARY

A case-control study was conducted to investigate possible environmental risk factors for ocular sarcoidosis. The factors studied were exposures to pine products and occupational histories of employment in the tobacco, lumber, and textile industries. The exposure histories of 29 female and 15 male cases, patients with newly diagnosed ocular sarcoidosis that were attending the Glaucoma/Uveitis Clinic of the North Carolina Memorial Hospital, were compared to those of 110 female and 28 male controls selected from out-patient clinics. Elevated risks for sarcoidosis were detected among those females that were exposed to burning pine or were employed in the tobacco industry. For males, positive associations were observed for chewing pine products and for employment in the lumber and textile industries. These preliminary data are consistent with incomplete phagocytic clearance of nonbiodegradable foreign bodies present within our environment that may become antigenic to the immunologically susceptible host. Confirmation or refutation of these hypotheses awaits additional clinical and epidemiological research within the sarcoidosis belt.

REFERENCES

1. GENTRY, J. T., H. M. NITOWSKY & M. MICHAEL. 1955. Studies on the epidemiology of sarcoidosis in the United States: The relationship to soil areas and to urban-rural residence. J. Clin. Invest. **34:** 1839-1856.
2. GUNDELFINGER, B. & S. BRITTEN. 1961. Sarcoidosis in the United States Navy. Am. Rev. Respir. Dis. **84:** 109-115.
3. SARTWELL, P. & L. EDWARDS. 1974. Epidemiology of sarcoidosis in the United States Navy. Am. J. Epidemiol. **99:** 250-257.
4. MERRITT, J. C. 1979. Endogenous uveitis in children. J. Natl. Med. Assoc. **71:** 645-647.
5. MIETTINEN, O. 1976. Estimability and estimation in case-referent studies. Am. J. Epidemiol. **103:** 226-235.
6. MANTEL, N. & W. HAENSZEL. 1959. Statistical aspects of the analysis of data from retrospective studies of disease. J. Natl. Cancer Inst. **22:** 719-748.
7. KLEINBAUM, D. G., L. L. KUPPER & H. MORGENSTERN. 1982. Epidemiologic Research: Principles and Quantitative Methods. Lifetime Learning Publications. Belmont, CA.
8. MANTEL, N. & J. FLEISS. 1980. Minimum expected cell size requirements for the Mantel-Haenszel one-degree-of-freedom chi-square test and a related rigid procedure. Am. J. Epidemiol. **112:** 129-134.
9. SACKETT, D. L. 1979. Bias in analytic research. J. Chronic Dis. **32:** 51-63.
10. COPELAND, K. T., H. CHECKOWAY, A. J. MCMICHAEL & R. H. HOLBROOK. 1977. Bias due to misclassification in the estimation of relative risk. Am. J. Epidemiol. **105:** 488-495.
11. KELLER, A. 1971. Hospital, age, race, occupational, geographical, clinical and survivorship characteristics in the epidemiology of sarcoidosis. Am. J. Epidemiol. **94:** 222-230.
12. CUMMINGS, M. M., E. DUNNER, R. H. SCHMIDT & J. B. BARNWELL. 1956. Concepts of epidemiology of sarcoidosis. Postgrad. Med. J. **19:** 437-446.
13. TERRIS, M., M. M. ZISKIND & C. MCGULL. 1963. Incidence of diagnosed sarcoidosis in Louisiana. Am. Rev. Respir. Dis. **87:** 509-517.
14. MCCUISTON, C., M. MICHAEL & P. C. HUDGINS. 1961. Geographic epidemiology of sarcoidosis in Florida. Am. Rev. Respir. Dis. **84:** 124-129.
15. HOROWITZ, O. 1961. Geographic epidemiology of sarcoidosis in Denmark: 1954-1957. Am. Rev. Respir. Dis. **84:** 135-142.
16. DOUGLAS, A. 1961. Sarcoidosis in Scotland. Am. Rev. Respir. Dis. **84:** 143-147.
17. UEHLINGER, E. 1961. Epidemiology of sarcoidosis in Switzerland. Am. Rev. Respir. Dis. **84:** 153-154.
18. NOBECKI, K. 1961. Epidemiology of sarcoidosis in Japan. Am. Rev. Respir. Dis. **84:** 148-152.
19. PURRIEL, P. & E. NAVARRETTE. 1961. Epidemiology of sarcoidosis in Uruguay and other countries of Latin America. Am. Rev. Respir. Dis. **84:** 155-161.

Reduced Prevalence of Smokers in Sarcoidosis

Results of a Case-Control Study

R. A. HARF,[a,b] C. ETHEVENAUX,[b] J. GLEIZE,[c]
M. PERRIN-FAYOLLE,[b] J. C. GUERIN,[d]
AND C. OLLAGNIER[e]

[b] *Hôpital Sainte-Eugenie*
69230 Saint-Genis-Laval, France

[c] *Check-up Clinics*
69004 Lyons, France

[d] *Hôpital Croix-Rousse*
69004 Lyons, France

[e] *Hôpital Jules Courmont*
69310 Pierre-Benite, France

The definition of sarcoidosis specifies that it is a disease of unknown etiology,[1] and a considerable search has been undertaken to identify the responsible agent(s). The results of this search have, until recently, been disappointing.

Surprisingly, for a disease that in most cases involves the respiratory tract, little attention has been given to the possible role of tobacco smoking. In a recent exhaustive review of the epidemiology of sarcoidosis, Bresnitz and Strom stated that ". . . the results of various studies suggest that, if anything, smoking may have a protective effect for the pathogenesis of sarcoidosis."[2]

In an earlier study we found a smaller percentage of smokers in a cohort of sarcoidosis patients than in the general population.[3] In order to confirm these data, we reinvestigated this point using matched controls.

MATERIALS AND METHODS

All cases of histologically confirmed sarcoidosis recorded between 1 January 1980 and 1 April 1982 in three adult chest clinics located in the township of Lyons, France were reviewed. Recorded data included sex; date and place of birth; profession; date

[a] Address for correspondence and reprint requests: Service de Pneumologie, Hôpital Sainte-Eugenie, 69230 Saint-Genis-Laval, France.

of onset of the disease or symptoms; and, of course, smoking habits (duration and intensity). Each case that smoked at least one cigarette/day and who had not given up smoking for more than 1 year before onset of the disease was considered a smoker. Each case that had never smoked or had given up smoking for more than 1 year before onset of the disease was considered a nonsmoker. The control group comprised healthy volunteers. These controls visited three check-up clinics, which were all located in the same area as the three adult chest clinics, during the same period of time the cases were studied. In France, anyone from 18 to 60 years of age who belongs to the national public health insurance system, which includes about 95% of the population, has the right to visit one of these clinics every 5 years. The check-up includes, besides clinical and paraclinical examinations (such as those involving chest radiography and electrocardiography), a detailed interview that includes questions on smoking habits.

Every case was matched with four controls; that is, a given case and the corresponding controls were all of the same sex, had the same year of birth, and had the same place of birth. Three categories for place of birth were considered: the Rhone Department (the administrative area in which Lyons is located), places in France outside the Rhone Department, and foreign countries.

Statistical analyses were done using the Mantel-Haenszel procedure and the standard chi-square tests.[4]

RESULTS

From 113 eligible sarcoidosis patients, 12 had to be withdrawn: 7 because of insufficient or contradictory data about their smoking habits, 5 because they were too young or too old to be matched.

FIGURE 1 shows age and sex distributions of patients which are very similar to those described in the literature: the sex ratio is about 1, and the highest peak for age is that corresponding to ages between 30 and 35 years.

A comparison of the values for the percentage of smokers between the two groups (TABLE 1) shows a highly significant negative association between sarcoidosis and smoking (odds ratio: 3.8; 95% confidence interval: 2.4, 6.5). This difference is present for both sexes, and the rate for smokers is higher in controls for groups of all ages (FIG. 2). Analysis of professional status did not reveal any differences between the two groups.

DISCUSSION

D. G. James has described sarcoidosis as an iceberg in which the diagnosed cases would represent the emerged part.[5] Although it may not be possible to assume that our cohort is representative of the disease, it must be noticed that our sample has the same clinical features as those described in the literature for patients with sarcoidosis.[6] About 20% of the patients were recruited (from dermatology, rheumatology, or internal medicine departments) because they had extrapulmonary symptoms, and were included in the present series because pulmonary investigation and advice had been required.

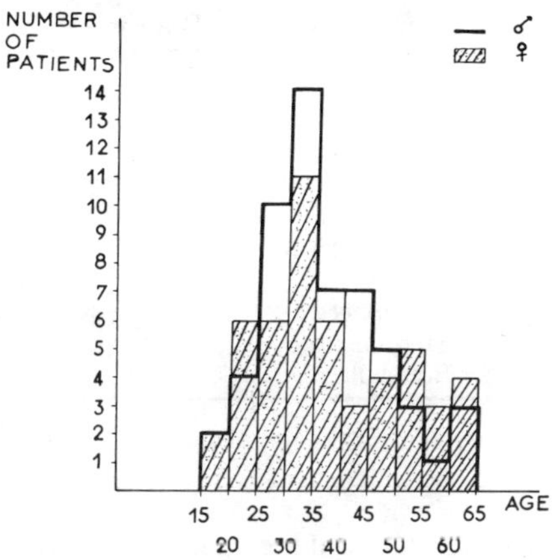

FIGURE 1. Age and sex distributions of patients with sarcoidosis.

Patients were matched with healthy subjects for two reasons: First, because smoking is positively related to numerous pulmonary and extrapulmonary diseases, a difference observed in the smoking percentages of the two groups could be due to an increased proportion of smokers in a hospital control group. Second, in the absence of any known etiological factor, a cohort of patients with sarcoidosis may be considered as a random sample from the general population. Several comparative studies, conducted by the check-up clinics themselves, have shown that volunteer cohorts do not differ from their original group in many respects, and especially not for their smoking habits. Smoking as a major risk factor does not seem to attract or to prevent people from visiting such centers.

It is surprising to find how little attention has been given to smoking in sarcoidosis: Epidemiologic studies have rarely taken this factor into account. A study by Terris and Chaves did, however, and noted that 47% of a group of patients with sarcoidosis and 42% of the corresponding healthy, matched controls had never smoked.[7] Comstock *et al.* found results similar to ours.[8] On the other hand, Warren found the percentage of smokers among patients with sarcoidosis to be identical to that in the general population.[9]

Curiously, authors dealing with pulmonary function in the disease usually do not report smoking data. Recent literature on bronchoalveolar lavage data in sarcoidosis takes this factor into account more frequently. In TABLE 2 we report data that has been taken from studies of larger groups of patients. Although the times and locations

TABLE 1. Smoking Habits of Sarcoidosis Patients and Controls

	Percentage of Smokers			
	Sarcoidosis Patients	Controls	Odds Ratio[a]	Significance
Men	34.0 (18/53)	75.0 (159/212)	5.8	$p<.001$
Women	14.6 (7/48)	34.4 (66/192)	3.1	$p<.01$
Men and women	24.8 (25/101)	55.7 (225/404)	3.8	$p<.001$

[a] Relative risk of being diagnosed for sarcoidosis for a nonsmoker compared to that for a smoker.

TABLE 2. Summary of the Data in the Literature on Smoking and Sarcoidosis

Author	Year	Percentage of Smokers among Sarcoidosis Patients
Young *et al.*	1973	45 (18/40)
Renzi and Dutton	1974	36 (16/44)
Warren	1977	41 (31/75)[a]
Arnoux *et al.*	1980	23 (24/106)
Sandron *et al.*	1983	21 (61/293)
Brambilla *et al.*	1983	13 (8/60)

[a] Fifty percent (22/44) of the men and 29% (9/31) of the women were smokers.

of these studies differ greatly, the proportions of smokers that were observed are comparable to ours.

Recently, major life-threatening risk factors have been reported to be negatively associated with different diseases. Concerning smoking, this situation has been observed in four circumstances: 1) By comparison of cases with matched neighbors, Baumann *et al.*[15] confirmed previous data on reduced mortality rates due to Parkinson's disease in smokers.[15] 2) Warren found a lower reduced incidence of farmer's lung disease among smoking than among nonsmoking farmers.[9] Indirect support of these findings was given by Gruchow *et al.*, who have reported a reduced prevalence of specific precipitating antibodies among smokers in a farming population.[16] 3) More recently, tobacco smoking was recognized as a positive risk factor in ulcerative colitis.[17] Some clinical observations suggest a direct influence of nicotine on the disease. 4) A negative association is also found between tobacco smoking and endometrial cancer. Smoking women have a reduced relative risk for cancer incidence but an increased risk for cancer death.[18] The protective effect is probably due to an earlier menopause induced by smoking.

Although these data are insignificant in terms of public health, they may yet help us understand the mechanisms leading to these diseases.

Regarding sarcoidosis, several hypotheses can be suggested. The first is the possibility that the initial pulmonary symptoms would lead the patient to give up smoking. This possibility was accounted for in the design of the study. Patients who had given

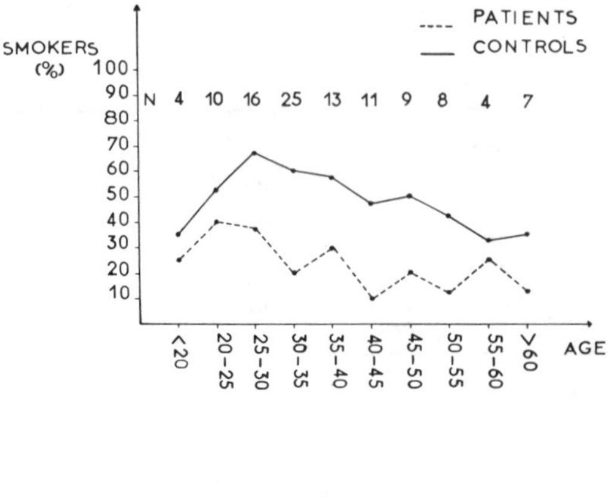

FIGURE 2. Comparison of smoking habits between sarcoidosis patients and healthy controls.

up smoking at least 1 year before onset of the first symptom of the disease were considered nonsmokers.

It can also be postulated that the link between disease and abstinence from smoking is related to a third factor. There is still no evidence, however, for an etiological factor that could be simultaneously related to the onset of sarcoidosis and abstinence from smoking, or that nonsmoking habits make people more prone to encounter (one of) the real causative factor(s) of the disease.

On the other hand, there is growing evidence that tobacco smoke interferes directly with the mechanisms which promote or maintain the disease. In recent years, numerous biological studies, especially those dealing with bronchoalveolar lavage data, have shown that tobacco smoke and sarcoidosis are responsible for opposite disturbances of the immune system within the lungs. Whereas disease is characterized by an activation of macrophages and lymphocytes, tobacco smoke provokes an influx of macrophages with a reduced phagocytic potential associated with an increased number of T suppressor cells. In a recent study we showed that levels of proteins in fluid recovered by bronchoalveolar lavage were increased for smokers that were healthy controls, but were decreased for smokers that had sarcoidosis.[19] We have summarized the available data in TABLE 3.

TABLE 3. The Effect of Sarcoidosis and the Effect of Smoking on the Immune Response

	Sarcoidosis		Smoking	
	Effect	Reference Number	Effect	Reference Number
Lung data				
Lymphocyte:macrophage ratio	↑	20	↓	21
Phagocytic activity of macrophages	↑	22	↓	21
Migration activity of macrophages	↓	23	↑	24
Sensitivity of effector cells to lymphokines	↑	25	↓	21
Number of T helper cells	↑	20		
Number of T suppressor cells			↑	21
Blood data				
Immunoglobulin level	↑	1	↓	26
Number of T cells	↓	20	↑	28

If our results receive further confirmation, tobacco could become the first etiological factor—and, of course, the first negative etiological factor—described for sarcoidosis. In such a case the following possibilities would have to be considered: 1) The lung could be the usual starting point of the disease, and tobacco smoke could interfere with the macrophage-lymphocyte activation process which ends in granuloma formation. The reduced incidence of the disease in smokers could be due either to a true preventive effect or to a reduction in the duration of as well as in the maintenance of abnormalities at an undetectable level. 2) Our results could have a therapeutic implication in the testing of some pharmacological substances present in tobacco smoke (some preliminary results seem to implicate nicotine in the control of ulcerative colitis) or of topical immunosuppressive drugs such as inhaled steroids and other substances capable, like tobacco smoke, of locally and transiently depressing the immune response.

REFERENCES

1. MITCHELL, D. N. & J. G. SCADDING. 1974. Sarcoidosis. Am. Rev. Respir. Dis. **110:** 774-802.
2. BRESNITZ, E. A. & B. L. STROM. 1983. Epidemiology of sarcoidosis. Epidemiol. Rev. **5:** 124-156.
3. HARF, R. & M. PERRIN-FAYOLLE. 1980. Sarcoidosis and smoking. *In* Third European Conference on Sarcoidosis and Other Granulomatous Disorders. Sremska Kamenica. Novi Sad.
4. MANTEL, N. & HAENSZEL. 1959. Statistical aspects of the analysis of data from retrospective studies of disease. J. Natl. Cancer Inst. **22:** 719-748.
5. JAMES, D. G. 1980. Sarcoidosis in perspective. *In* Eighth International Conference on Sarcoidosis and Other Granulomatous Diseases. W. Jones Williams & B. H. Davies, Eds.: xxvii-xxxii. Alpha Omega. Cardiff.
6. JAMES, D. G., E. NEVILLE, L. E. SILZBACH, J. TURIAF, J. P. BATTESTI, O. P. SHARMA, Y. HOSODA, R. MIKAMI, M. ODAKA, T. G. VILLAR, B. DJURIČ, A. C. DOUGLAS, W. MIDDLETON, A. KARLISH, A. BLASI, D. OLIVIER & P. PRESS. 1976. A worldwide review of sarcoidosis. Ann. N.Y. Acad. Sci. **278:** 321-334.
7. TERRIS, M. & A. D. CHAVES. 1966. An epidemiologic study of sarcoidosis. Am. Rev. Respir. Dis. **94:** 50-55.
8. COMSTOCK, G. W., H. KELTZ & D. J. SENCER. 1961. Clay eating and sarcoidosis. Am. Rev. Respir. Dis. **80:** 130-134.
9. WARREN, C. P. W. 1977. Extrinsic allergic alveolitis: A disease commoner in nonsmokers. Thorax **32:** 567-569.
10. YOUNG, R. C., JR., V. E. HEADINGS, S. BOSE, K. A. HERDEN, E. D. CROKETT, JR. & R. L. HACKNEY, JR. 1973. Alpha-antitrypsin levels in sarcoidosis: Relationship to disease activity. Chest **64:** 39-45.
11. RENZI, G. & R. E. DUTTON. 1974. Pulmonary function in diffuse sarcoidosis. Respiration **31:** 124-136.
12. ARNOUX, A., C. MORCAMP, A. B. TONNEL, C. AERTS, J. MARSAC, G. HUCHON, J. C. SALTIEL, J. P. MARTIN, C. VOISIN & J. CHRÉTIEN. 1980. Bronchopulmonary cellular and protein studies in sarcoidosis and hypersensitivity pneumonitis. *In* Eighth International Conference on Sarcoidosis and Other Granulomatous Diseases. W. Jones Williams & B. H. Davies, Eds.: 409-416. Alpha Omega. Cardiff.
13. SANDRON, D., D. LECOSSIER, A. GRODET, C. BARBE, G. BASSET & J. P. BATTESTI. 1983. Serum angiotensin-converting enzyme and the diffusion of the sarcoid granuloma: Evolutive and therapeutic interest. *In* Sarcoidosis and Other Granulomatous Disorders. J. Chrétien, J. Marsac & J. C. Saltiel, Eds.: 345-348. Pergamon Press. Paris.
14. BRAMBILLA, C., L. CHAVEZ, E. BRAMBILLA, F. MOREL, P. GROSLAMBERT, D. MAISONNEUVE, A. VINCENT, A. DAMAK, A. RIGAUD & B. PARAMELLE. 1983. Prognostic value of bronchoalveolar lavage and angiotensin-converting enzyme in sarcoidosis. *In* Sarcoidosis and Other Granulomatous Disorders. J. Chrétien, J. Marsac & J. C. Saltiel, Eds.: 419-423. Pergamon Press. Paris.
15. BAUMANN, R. J., H. D. JAMESON, H. E. MCKEAN, D. G. HAACK & L. M. WEISBERG. 1980. Cigarette smoking and Parkinson's disease: A comparison of cases with matched neighbors. Neurology **30:** 839-843.
16. GRUCHOW, H. W., R. G. HOFFMAN, J. J. MARX, JR., D. A. EMANUEL & A. A. RIMM. 1981. Precipitating antibodies to farmer's lung antigens in a Wisconsin farming population. Am. Rev. Respir. Dis. **124:** 411-415.
17. JICK, H. & E. M. WALKER. 1983. Cigarette smoking and ulcerative colitis. N. Engl. J. Med. **308:** 261-263.
18. BARON, J. A. 1984. Smoking and estrogen-related disease. Am. J. Epidemiol. **119:** 9-22.
19. HARF, R., N. BIOT, A. KHOURY & M. PERRIN-FAYOLLE. Consequences of cigarette smoking on bronchoalveolar lavage data from sarcoidosis patients and healthy controls. First International Conference on Bronchoalveolar Lavage. May 1984. Columbia, MD.
20. HUNNINGHAKE, G. W., J. D. FULMER, R. C. YOUNG, JR., J. E. GADEK & R. G. CRYSTAL.

1979. Localization of the immune response in sarcoidosis. Am. Rev. Respir. Dis. **120:** 49-57.

21. GREEN, G. M., G. J. JAKAB, R. B. LOW & G. S. DAVIS. 1977. Defense mechanisms of the respiratory membrane. Am. Rev. Respir. Dis. **115:** 479-514.
22. GODARD, P., J. CHAINTREUIL, M. DAMON, E. MONNIN, J. TAIB, O. FLANDRE, C. DE PAULET & F. B. MICHEL. 1983. Prostaglandin metabolism in alveolar macrophages in sarcoidosis. *In* Sarcoidosis and Other Granulomatous Disorders. J. Chrétien, J. Marsac & J. C. Saltiel, Eds.: 71-75. Pergamon Press. Paris.
23. LEMARIE, E., M. LAVANDIER, M. F. LEGRAND, P. ANTHONIOZ, M. RENOUX & G. RENOUX. 1983. Alveolar macrophage migration in pulmonary sarcoidosis. *In* Sarcoidosis and Other Granulomatous Disorders. J. Chrétien, J. Marsac & J. C. Saltiel, Eds.: 598-599. Pergamon Press. Paris.
24. WARR, G. A. & R. R. MARTIN. 1974. Chemotactic responsiveness of human alveolar macrophages: Effect of cigarette smoking. Infect. Immun. **9:** 769-778.
25. CRYSTAL, R. G., G. W. HUNNINGHAKE, J. E. GADEK, B. A. KEOGH, S. RENNARD & P. B. BITTERMAN. 1983. The pathogenesis of sarcoidosis. *In* Sarcoidosis and Other Granulomatous Diseases. J. Chrétien, J. Marsac & J. C. Saltiel, Eds.: 13-35. Pergamon Press. Paris.
26. ANDERSEN, P., O. F. PEDERSEN, B. BACH & G. J. BONDES. 1982. Serum antibodies and immuglobulins in smokers and nonsomkers. Clin. Exp. Immunol. **47:** 467-473.
27. DANIELE, R. P., J. H. DAUBER & M. D. ROSSMAN. 1979. Lymphocyte population in the bronchoalveolar air spaces: Bronchoalveolar lavage in man. INSERM **84:** 193-210.
28. GINNS, L. C., P. D. GOLDENHEIM, L. G. MILLER, R. C. BURTON, L. GILLICK, R. B. COLVIN, G. GOLDSTEIN, P. C. KUNG, C. HURWITZ & H. KAZEMI. 1982. T lymphocyte subsets in smoking and lung cancer. Am. Rev. Respir. Dis. **126:** 265-269.

Possible Risk Factors for Sarcoidosis

A Case-Control Study[a]

EDDY A. BRESNITZ,[b,c] PAUL D. STOLLEY,[d]
HAROLD L. ISRAEL,[e] AND KEITH SOPER[d]

[c] *Department of Community and Preventive Medicine*
Medical College of Pennsylvania
Philadelphia, Pennsylvania 19129

[d] *Clinical Epidemiology Unit*
Section of General Medicine
University of Pennsylvania
Philadelphia, Pennsylvania 19104

[e] *Department of Medicine*
Jefferson Medical College
Thomas Jefferson University
Philadelphia, Pennsylvania 19107

INTRODUCTION

Descriptions of sarcoidosis first appeared in the medical literature approximately 100 years ago.[1] During the last 30 years, there have been many epidemiological studies of sarcoidosis that have demonstrated relatively few risk factors for this disease. Accepted facts include a higher incidence of sarcoidosis in the young adult, black population in the United States;[2,3] a clustering of disease in families; and an increased incidence in females. The etiology of the disease, however, remains unknown.[4]

Several groups of investigators have used the case-control method to either generate hypotheses or to test a specific hypothesis of an association between sarcoidosis and a suspected risk factor. In 1961, Comstock *et al.*[5] reported the results of a case-control study that was done to investigate potential etiologic factors for sarcoidosis. Although the study produced no definitive leads, the authors concluded that the case-control research design was a valid method to generate hypotheses concerning the etiology of sarcoidosis.

Interestingly, Comstock *et al.*,[5] in the study cited above, observed that patients with sarcoidosis smoked less than matched controls. The observation persisted when

[a] This work was supported in part by funds from the Andrew W. Mellon Foundation.

[b] Address for correspondence and reprint requests: Department of Community and Preventive Medicine, Medical College of Pennsylvania, 3300 Henry Avenue, Philadelphia, Pennsylvania 19129.

the analysis was adjusted for rural residence. The authors noted this inverse association, however, only among the white subjects in the study. In addition, patients with sarcoidosis may have underreported their smoking habits if they had given up smoking because of respiratory symptoms resulting from undiagnosed sarcoidosis. Thus, the apparent protective effect of smoking may have been due to misclassification bias on exposure. This finding was not investigated further by these researchers.

Recently, two groups of investigators in France[6,7] reported that patients with sarcoidosis were less likely to have been smokers than controls. The magnitude of this apparent protective effect is small but does have some biological plausibility. It is known that there is a decreased proliferative response of lung thymus-derived (T) lymphocytes of cigarette smokers on exposure to various mitogens compared to that of lung T lymphocytes of control subjects.[8] Cigarette smoke also recruits macrophages to the lungs[9] and thus reduces the proportion of lymphocytes in lung secretions. It is possible that this reduction in the activity and number of lymphocytes prevents sufficient interaction with an etiologic, exogenous agent for the development of sarcoidosis.

A similar negative association between smoking and the development of hypersensitivity pneumonitis has been observed recently in farmers. In 1981, Gruchow *et al.*[10] reported that patients with farmer's lung disease smoked less than control patients. In the same descriptive study, these investigators also noted the prevalence of antibodies to *Micropolyspora faeni* among smokers was higher than among nonsmokers (that is, patients who had never smoked) and former smokers. The higher prevalence of these antibodies among smokers could not be attributed to any particular characteristics of farming, such as the size of the dairy herd or the length of time spent farming. The authors postulated a possible protective effect of cigarrette smoking against the development of farmer's lung disease. This potential protective effect among farmers for the development of hypersensitivity pneumonitis, a granulomatous disease with histopathologic and immunopathologic changes similar to sarcoidosis, remains unexplained.

In this paper, we report the results of a multi-institutional case-control study to investigate the hypothesis that a history of smoking decreases the risk of sarcoidosis. In addition, we examined the relationship between other potential risk factors and the development of sarcoidosis.

METHODS

Selection of Cases

The study was based in four hospitals in the center-city area of Philadelphia: the Hospital of the University of Pennsylvania, the Veterans Administration Hospital of Philadelphia, the Presbyterian Hospital, and the Thomas Jefferson University Hospital. Potential subjects between the ages of 18 and 70 were recruited from both in-patient and out-patient services between 1 June 1982 and 31 December 1982. Only newly incident cases, first diagnosed after January 1981, were included in the study. A patient was identified as a case when there was either histological proof of sarcoidosis or a history of bilateral lymphadenopathy without evidence of another granulomatous disease. Cases were identified through daily review of both in-patient hospitalization log books and out-patient appointment schedules. Permission to contact the patient was obtained initially from the resident or attending physician of record. All patients who were identified as cases agreed to participate in the study by informed consent.

Selection of Controls

All control patients were selected from the in-patient and out-patient areas of the Hospital of the University of Pennsylvania (HUP). Potential in-patient controls were identified from the same daily admission sheets from which the cases were identified. Potential out-patient controls were selected from the same out-patient medical service appointment schedule lists. Cases were frequency matched to controls with respect to age (within 5 years), sex, and race. All out-patient controls gave informed consent. Subjects were identified at random from the prepared lists of potential controls. The frequency distribution of the primary diagnosis among the participating controls was similar to that of the potential controls. Information on the patients who refused to participate was not recorded. Most subjects who refused to participate, however, did so because of lack of time.

Potential study subjects, both cases and controls, who had either a history of previous chronic pulmonary disease or another granulomatous disorder listed on the face sheet of the chart were excluded as controls. A small number of interviewed patients, however, subsequently were found to have had a past history of a chronic respiratory disorder such as asthma. These patients were included in the study. A total of 51 cases and 107 controls were eventually recruited into the study.

Data Collection and Analysis

The main source of information was the personal interview. Trained interviewers used pretested, standardized forms. The interview was designed to collect data concerning demographic information, the general health of the subject, a detailed occupational and environmental history, a detailed past medical history with particular emphasis on respiratory disease and smoking information, and other miscellaneous questions. Material from questionnaires developed by the American Thoracic Society—Division of Lung Disease,[11] the Connecticut Tumor Registry,[12] and the American Health Foundation was adapted for use in this study.

Many of the questions on previous health and exposures were phrased to assess what the patient's status was 3 or more years before the diagnosis of his/her illness. This was done to minimize the potential for unmasking bias, a type of selection bias. Unmasking bias has been related to the suspicion of disease that arises when an "innocent exposure . . . causes a sign or symptom which precipitates a search for the disease."[13] For example, as the symptoms of chronic bronchitis may mimic those of sarcoidosis, one would expect that patients with latent sarcoidosis are more likely to be detected if they have a history of bronchitis. This may result in a systematic error; that is, one may detect a more frequent history of bronchitis among sarcoidosis patients than among controls.

Hospital medical records were reviewed in all cases to corroborate the diagnosis of sarcoidosis. To assess the reliability of responses, a random sample of 8% of the study group was called on the telephone within 6 months of the initial interview. Each patient was asked several questions selected from the initial interview. A kappa statistic was calculated to measure the reproducibility of the response to a specific question.[14]

We estimated the relative risk (odds ratio) of sarcoidosis for several different risk factors. Point estimates were derived for both crude and stratified data by the Mantel-Haenszel method.[15] Ninety-five percent confidence intervals were determined using the method based on Miettinen's test.[16] Analyses were performed with the calculator programs developed by Rothman and Boice.[17] We performed a logistic regression analysis to assess the role of several variables as risk factors for the development of sarcoidosis. The LOGIST procedure in the statistical analysis system (SAS) was used to perform the logistic regression analysis.[18]

RESULTS

Forty-nine of the 51 cases had biopsy proof of sarcoidosis. The remaining two cases were diagnosed on the basis of typical radiographic changes. The distribution

TABLE 1. Percent Distribution of Controls by Primary Diagnosis[a]

	Percent Distribution	
Primary Diagnosis[b]	Controls ($N = 104$)	Population ($N = 310$)
Hypertension	37.5	33.9
Gastrointestinal disease	16.4	5.8
Endocrine disease[c]	15.4	25.8
Cardiovascular disease	6.7	6.8
Musculoskeletal system disease	3.9	11.6
Collagen-vascular disease	4.8	3.2
Other[d]	15.3	12.3
Total[e]	100	99.4

[a] Excludes all patients with a respiratory disease as the primary diagnosis.

[b] From the patient chart.

[c] Includes diabetes.

[d] Includes renal disease, ovarian cyst, neurologic disease, gynecologic disease, and hematologic disease.

[e] $p > .05$

of primary diseases of the controls included in the study was similar to the distribution of clinic patients identified as potential controls (TABLE 1). Although the study group had more patients with gastrointestinal disease and the clinic population had more patients with endocrine disease as a primary diagnosis, neither difference was statistically significant ($p > .05$).

TABLE 2 shows the percent distribution of cases and controls by demographic factors. The two groups were similar in their distributions of age, sex, and race, as would be expected by frequency matching. Although they had the same distribution in years of education, the control group had a higher proportion of individuals with low family incomes than did the case group ($\chi^2 = 5.29$; $p < .05$).

TABLE 2. Percent Distribution of Cases and Controls by Sex, Race, Age, Income, and Education[a]

Characteristic	Percent Distribution: Cases ($N = 51$)	Controls ($N = 107$)
Race, Sex		
White		
Male	17.6	14.0
Female	9.8	11.2
Black		
Male	19.6	18.7
Female	52.9	56.1
Age (years)		
20-24	5.9	8.4
25-29	27.4	28.0
30-34	29.4	26.2
35-39	15.7	20.6
≥ 40	21.6	16.8
Income[b]		
< 13,000	27.1	42.0
13,000-19,999	14.6	19.0
20,000-24,999	8.3	11.0
25,000-34,999	22.9	9.0
≥ 35,000	27.1	19.0
Education (years)		
≤ 11	22.9	17.5
12	25.0	24.8
13-16	39.6	42.7
> 16	12.5	15.5

[a] $p > .05$.
[b] $\chi^2 = 5.29$; df = 1. $p < .05$.

TABLE 3. Kappa Statistic for Test of Reliability for Selected Questions[a]

	Kappa Statistic	SEM
Occupation at the time of illness	0.89	0.16
Allergies	0.85	0.26
Smoking status		
Smokers and former smokers	1.00	0.26
Smokers	1.00	0.33
Age when started smoking	0.40	0.19
Cigarette consumption		
Number smoked/day	1.00	0.24
Amount of smoke inhaled	0.43	0.22

[a] A random sample of 8% of the study group was given a second interview.

TABLE 4. Crude, Unadjusted Odds Ratio for Sarcoidosis for Different Factors

Potential Factor	Percentage of Cases (N = 51)	Percentage of Controls (N = 107)	Odds Ratio	Confidence Interval (95%)
Cigarettes[a]	54.9	62.6	0.7	0.4, 1.3
Alcohol	81.4	82.7	1.0	0.7, 1.2
Unprescribed drugs	11.8	17.9	0.9	0.6, 1.2
Pets	68.6	84.1	0.9	0.6, 1.0
Allergies	33.3	33.6	0.9	0.6, 1.1
Hairsprays	58.8	51.4	0.9	0.7, 1.1

[a] Both smokers and former smokers were taken into account.

TABLE 3 shows kappa statistics, for selected questions, as tests of reliability. In general, there was good to excellent agreement between the information obtained in the initial interview and that obtained in the subsequent interview for the selected questions.

The percent distribution for different potenial risk factors in the study groups is shown in TABLE 4. None of the differences were statistically significant. In addition, occupational exposures, home-heating fuel, cooking fuel, state of birth, and rural residence were not associated with an increased risk for the development of sarcoidosis (data not shown).

The crude, unadjusted odds ratio for sarcoidosis was 0.7, with a 95% confidence interval of 0.4 to 1.3, when smokers and former smokers were compared to nonsmokers. The odds ratios for sarcoidosis were 0.7 for smokers versus nonsmokers and 0.9 for former smokers versus nonsmokers (TABLE 5) when the study subjects were grouped according to current smoking status. When subjects were grouped according to the average number of cigarettes smoked each day, there was a trend for an increasingly protective effect of smoking with increasing cigarette consumption (TABLE 6). As indicated by the 95% confidence intervals that included the null value of 1, none of the odds ratios were statistically significant. A logistic regression analysis was done to assess the contribution of smoking to the development of sarcoidosis. When family income, race, and age were included in the model, the smoking history did not add any information.

The risk for developing sarcoidosis was elevated in those who had one or more chest illnesses 3 or more years before the diagnosis of their disease (TABLE 7). The

TABLE 5. Distribution of Cases and Controls according to Smoking Status at the Time of Diagnosis and Estimates of the Odds Ratio

Smoking Status	Number of Cases[a]	Number of Controls[a]	Odds Ratio	Confidence Interval (95%)[b]
Nonsmoker	22 (44)	41 (39)	1.0	
Former smoker	14 (28)	28 (20)	0.9	0.7, 1.1
≤ 3 years	7	7	1.9	0.6, 6.0
> 3 years	7	21	0.6	0.2, 1.7
Smoker	14 (28)	36 (41)	0.7	0.3, 1.6

[a] Percentages are shown in parentheses.
[b] The nonsmokers constituted the reference group.

TABLE 6. Distribution of Cases and Controls according to Smoking History and Estimates of the Odds Ratio

Smoking History (cigarettes smoked/day)	Number of Cases[a]	Number of Controls[a]	Odds Ratio	Confidence Interval (95%)[b]
0	22 (44)	41 (39)	1.0	
1-15	21 (42)	42 (40)	0.9	0.5, 1.7
16-34	6 (12)	16 (15)	0.7	0.3, 1.7
≥ 35	1 (2)	6 (6)	0.3	0.1, 1.8
Total	50 (100)	105 (100)	0.7	0.4, 1.3

[a] Percentages are shown in parentheses.
[b] Nonsmokers constituted the reference group.

illness was characterized as being associated with the production of phlegm and as being severe enough to prevent them from working and to keep them indoors at home or in bed. These illnesses were distinct from episodes of pneumonia and attacks of asthma. There is a potential diagnostic bias, however, in that control patients were more likely to have been under medical care, and to have a diagnosis of bronchitis confirmed by a physician. Thus it is possible that the chest illnesses that the patients with sarcoidosis reported were actually episodes of undiagnosed bronchitis. When a history of bronchitis and a history of previous chest illnesses were combined into a new variable representing acute respiratory illnesses, the odds ratio for sarcoidosis dropped from 4.6 to 1.7, with a 95% confidence interval of 0.8 to 3.8 ($p > .05$). When patients who had a history of either asthma or chronic bronchitis were excluded from the analysis, the odds ratio for sarcoidosis among those with a history of acute respiratory disease (chest illnesses and/or bronchitis) dropped to 1.4 with a 95% confidence interval of 0.6 to 3.4 ($p > .05$).

TABLE 7. Distribution of Cases and Controls according to Previous Respiratory Illnesses

Previous Respiratory Illness[a]	Percentage of Cases ($N = 51$)	Percentage of Controls ($N = 107$)
Bronchitis (ever)	17.7	15.9
Allergies	33.3	33.6
Chest illness	28.0	6.5[b]
Phlegm		
Chronic	8.0	5.8
Daily	12.0	6.7
A.M.	10.0	15.2
Other	8.6	9.6
Hay fever	23.5	23.8
Asthma (ever)	10.0	6.5
Chronic bronchitis	2.0	2.8
Pneumonia (ever)	27.5	11.2

[a] Had to have been present 3 or more years before the diagnosis of the major illness.
[b] $\chi = 3.22$; df = 1. $p < .001$.

DISCUSSION

An inverse association between exposure to cigarette smoke and the development of sarcoidosis has been noted previously in two separate case-control studies.[5,19] This association, however, was limited to specific subgroups of study subjects in both reports. Also, neither the dose-response relationship nor the specific temporal relationship between exposure and the development of sarcoidosis were analyzed. The authors of the above studies discounted their findings on the basis of some of these considerations.

Our study showed a crude, unadjusted odds ratio of 0.7 for sarcoidosis when smokers and former smokers were compared to nonsmokers. This was not statistically significant as shown by the 95% confidence intervals that included the null value of 1. Although our study showed a negative trend with increasing cigarette consumption, this association was confounded by socioeconomic status; that is, patients with sarcoidosis were from a higher socioeconomic group than the control group in this study and would be less likely to have ever smoked. Also, the relative risk of sarcoidosis was close to 1 (the null hypothesis) for both former smokers and smokers compared to nonsmokers when the study groups were stratified according to smoking status at the time of diagnosis.

Recall bias is a potential problem in any case-control study where data is obtained from personal interviews. The reliability as well as the validity of the information is always in question. In this study, the reliability of some of the information was assessed and demonstrated by readministering the questions used in the study. The kappa statistic, which accounts for chance agreement, showed good to excellent agreement of response, especially for questions on current smoking status. We were not able to confirm the information on smoking status (for example, by questioning family members) and therefore could not establish the validity of the study subjects' current smoking status.

Although the sample sizes of the case and control groups were small, the study had an 80% chance of detecting an odds ratio of 0.44, using a two-sided test at the .05 level. (The magnitude of a relative risk of 0.44 is analogous to a positive association of 2.3.) Thus it is unlikely that a clinically significant association was missed because of insufficient study power.

Several hypotheses have been proposed to explain the preponderance of sarcoidosis in the young, black adult population of the United States.[5] These include exposure to pine pollen or clay;[4,20] rural residence;[21,22] infection with unusual microbiologic organisms;[23–25] genetic predisposition;[26–28] and occupational exposures.[22,29,30]

Our study did not show a statistically significant positive association between sarcoidosis and any of the following potential risk factors: a history of allergies; the ingestion of illicit drugs; exposure to pets; the use of hairspray; rural birthplace or residence; and exposure to specific chemicals in the workplace. It should be noted that the power of this study to detect an elevated, statistically significant exposure in patients with sarcoidosis was quite small for some of these variables. For example, the large number of potential workplace exposures resulted in small numbers of subjects within any particular exposure stratum. Also, only the longest job held and the most recent job held for at least 6 months were analyzed. Nevertheless, if there was a real, undetected association between sarcoidosis and a particular occupational exposure, the relative risk for sarcoidosis in those exposed would be quite small.

The lack of an association between the state of birth or rural residence and sarcoidosis is interesting in that some previous studies have reported a positive relationship between the development of sarcoidosis and residence in the Southeastern United States.[21,31,32] In our study only 14% of the cases and 7% of the controls were born in the Southeastern United States ($p = .23$). Clearly this study did not support the hypothesis that those born in the Southeastern United States are at higher risk for the development of sarcoidosis.

The only risk factor in this study that was associated with sarcoidosis was a history of previous chest illnesses that was distinct from a history of bronchitis. This was an unexpected finding and may be due to information bias. The data in this study was historical information obtained through a questionnaire. Patients were asked about their medical history 3 or more years before the diagnosis of their major illness. This was done to avoid including information about symptoms that may have actually reflected an early stage of disease. It is unlikely that chronic symptoms, such as cough or phlegm, would represent latent sarcoidosis that remained undiagnosed for 3 years. Also, the magnitude of the overall relative risk for a previous history of chest illnesses, after adjustment for several confounding variables, ranged from 5.3 to 8.8 (data not shown). When one considers that the control group consisted of individuals with other chronic diseases, it is noteworthy that this risk is so high. We would expect a control group composed of individuals with chronic disease to have had a high prevalence of respiratory illnesses. This, however, was not the case.

It is also unlikely that the association of past chest illnesses and sarcoidosis was confounded by age, sex, race, cigarette smoking, or family income. When this association was adjusted for these variables using the Mantel-Haenszel method, the overall relative risk remained markedly and significantly elevated.

It is possible that these chest illnesses were really episodes of acute bronchitis. In a previous case-control study of United States veterans, Keller found that cases were more likely than controls to have preexisting bronchitis.[31] He did not, however, adjust his analysis for potential confounding variables such as smoking and family income. In addition, the temporal relationship between the history of bronchitis and the development of sarcoidosis was not stated.

One possible explanation for the association of previous chest illnesses and sarcoidosis is that patients with sarcoidosis underreported episodes of diagnosed bronchitis. This is possible in that they may be less likely to see a physician before their disease is diagnosed than patients who are seeing a physician regularly in a general medical clinic. Thus a patient from the control group would have a chest illness diagnosed as bronchitis whereas a patient with a subsequent diagnosis of sarcoidosis would not. When cases were compared to controls for a history of bronchitis and/or previous chest illnesses, the odds ratio for sarcoidosis approached the null value of 1 and was not statistically significant. Thus it is difficult to interpret the nature of the association between sarcoidosis and a history of previous chest illnesses.

In conclusion, smoking does not appear to have a protective effect for the development of sarcoidosis in American patients. An unexpected association of sarcoidosis and a history of previous chest illnesses was observed, but this association may be the result of a diagnostic bias. Further studies of sarcoidosis should focus on this association in more detail.

REFERENCES

1. Buckley, M. P. 1970. Historical aspects of sarcoidosis. Ir. J. Med. Sci. **3**(1): 29-35.
2. Mitchell, D. N. & J. G. Scadding. 1974. Sarcoidosis. Am. Rev. Respir. Dis. **110:** 774-802.
3. James, D. G., E. Neville, L. E. Siltzbach, J. Turiaf, J. P. Battesti, O. P. Sharma, Y. Hosoda, R. Mikami, M. Odaka, T. G. Villar, B. Djurič, A. C. Douglas,

W. Middleton, A. Karlish, A. Blasi, D. Olivieri & P. Press. 1976. A worldwide review of sarcoidosis. Ann. N.Y. Acad. Sci. **278:** 321-324.

4. Bresnitz, E. A. & B. L. Strom. 1983. Epidemiology of sarcoidosis. Epidemiol. Rev. **5:** 124-156.
5. Comstock, G. W., H. Keltz & D. J. Sencer. 1961. Clay eating and sarcoidosis: A controlled study in the state of Georgia. Am. Rev. Respir. Dis. **84**(Suppl.): 130-134.
6. Harf, R., C. Ethevenaux, J. Gleize, M. Perrin-Fayolle, J. C. Guerin & J. C. Ollagnier. 1986. Reduced prevalence of smokers in sarcoidosis: Results of a case-control study. Ann. N.Y. Acad. Sci. This volume.
7. Hance, A. J., F. Basset, G. Saumon, C. Danel, D. Valeyre, J.-P. Battesti, J. Chrétien & R. Georges. 1986. Smoking and interstitial lung disease: The effect of cigarette smoking on the incidence of pulmonary histiocytosis X and sarcoidosis. Ann. N.Y. Acad. Sci. This volume.
8. Daniele, R. P., J. H. Dauber, M. D. Altose, D. T. Rowlands, Jr. & D. J. Gorenberg. 1977. Lymphocyte studies in asymptomatic cigarette smokers. Am. Rev. Respir. Dis. **116:** 997-1005.
9. Dauber, J. H., M. D. Rossman & R. P. Daniele. 1979. Bronchoalveolar cell populations in acute sarcoidosis: Observations in smoking and nonsmoking patients. J. Lab. Clin. Med. **94:** 862-871.
10. Gruchow, H. W., R. G. Hoffman, J. J. Marx, Jr., D. A. Emanuel & A. A. Rimm. 1981. Precipitating antibodies to farmer's lung antigens in a Wisconsin farming population. Am. Rev. Respir. Dis. **124:** 411-415.
11. Ferris, B. G. Epidemiology standardization project. 1978. Am. Rev. Respir. Dis. **118**(2): 10-35.
12. McCrea Curnen, M. G., E. R. Schoenfeld & L. E. Forehand. 1982. Patient Environmental History Questionnaire.
13. Sackett, D. L. 1979. Bias in analytic research. *In* The Case-Control Study: Consensus and Controversy. M. A. Ibraham, Ed. J. Chronic Dis. **32:** 51-63.
14. Fleiss, J. L. 1981. Statistical Methods for Rates and Proportions. 2nd edit. Wiley. New York, NY.
15. Mantel, N. & W. Haenszel. 1959. Statistical aspects of the analysis of data from retrospective studies of disease. J. Natl. Cancer Inst. **22**(4): 719-748.
16. Miettinen, O. S. 1976. Estimability and estimation in case-referent studies. Am. J. Epidemiol. **103:** 226-235.
17. Rothman, K. J. & J. D. Boice, Jr. 1979. Epidemiologic analysis with a programmable calculator. U.S. Department of Health, Education, and Welfare Publication Number 79-1649. U.S. Government Printing Office. Washington, DC.
18. SAS User's Guide. 1982. SAS Institute. Cary, NC.
19. Terris, M. & A. D. Chaves. 1966. An epidemiologic study of sarcoidosis. Am. Rev. Respir. Dis. **94:** 50-55.
20. Horwitz, O. 1961. Geographic epidemiology of sarcoidosis in Denmark. Am. Rev. Respir. Dis. **84**(Suppl.): 130-134.
21. Gentry, J. T., H. M. Nitowsky & M. Michael. 1955. Studies on the epidemiology of sarcoidosis in the United States: The relationship to soil areas and to urban-rural residence. J. Clin. Invest. **34:** 1839-1856.
22. Buck, A. A. & P. E. Sartwell. 1961. Epidemiologic investigations of sarcoidosis. II. Skin sensitivity and environmental factors. Am. J. Hyg. **74:** 152-173.
23. Mankiewicz, E. & M. Van Walbeck. 1962. Mycobacteriophages: Their role in tuberculosis and sarcoidosis. Arch. Environ. Health **5:** 122-128.
24. Mitchell, D. N. & R. J. W. Rees. 1976. The nature and physical characteristics of a transmissible agent from human sarcoid tissue. Ann. N.Y. Acad. Sci. **278:** 233-248.
25. Byrne, E. B., A. S. Evans, D. E. Fouts & H. L. Israel. 1973. A seroepidemilogical study of Epstein-Barr virus and other viral antigens in sarcoidosis. Am. J. Epidemiol. **97:** 355-363.
26. Hedfors, E. & E. Möller. 1973. HL-A antigens in sarcoidosis. Tissue Antigens **3:** 95-98.
27. Al-Arif, L., R. A. Goldstein, L. F. Affronti, B. W. Janicki & J. W. Foellmer. 1980. HLA antigens and sarcoidosis in a North American black population. *In* Eighth

International Conference on Sarcoidosis and Other Granulomatous Diseases. W. Jones Williams & B. H. Davies, Eds.: 206-212. Alpha Omega. Cardiff.
28. NEWILL, C. A., C. J. JOHNS, B. H. COHEN, E. L. DIAMOND & W. B. BIAS. 1983. Sarcoidosis, HLA and immunoglobulin markers in Baltimore blacks. *In* Sarcoidosis and Other Granulomatous Disorders. J. Chrétien, J. Marsac & J. C. Saltiel, Eds.: 253-256. Pergamon Press. Paris.
29. DUNNER, E. & J. H. WILLIAMS, JR. 1961. Epidemiology of sarcoidosis in the United States. Am. Rev. Respir. Dis. **84**(Suppl.): 163-167.
30. KELLER, A. Z. 1971. Hospital, age, racial, occupational, geographical, clinical and survivorship characteristics in the epidemiology of sarcoidosis. Am. J. Epidemiol. **94:** 222-230.
31. KELLER, A. Z. 1973. Anatomic sites, age attributes, and rates of sarcoidosis in U.S. veterans. Am. Rev. Respir. Dis. **107:** 615-620.
32. SARTWELL, P. E. & L. B. EDWARDS. 1984. Epidemiology of sarcoidosis in the U.S. Navy. Am. J. Epidemiol. **99:** 250-257.

Smoking and Interstitial Lung Disease

The Effect of Cigarette Smoking on the Incidence of Pulmonary Histiocytosis X and Sarcoidosis

ALLAN J. HANCE,[a] FRANÇOISE BASSET,[a]
GEORGES SAUMON,[a] CLAIRE DANEL,[b]
DOMINIQUE VALEYRE,[c] JEAN-PAUL BATTESTI,[c]
JACQUES CHRÉTIEN,[b] AND ROBERT GEORGES[a]

[a]*Institut National de la Santé et de la Recherche Médicale Unité 82*
Faculté Xavier Bichat
Paris, France

[b]*Clinique de Pneumophtisiologie*
Hôpital Laennec
Paris, France

[c]*Departement de Pneumologie*
Hôpital Avicenne
Bobigny, France

INTRODUCTION

Although smoking is commonly recognized as a major risk factor in the development of obstructive lung disease,[1] the impact of smoking on the pathogenesis of restrictive lung diseases has received less attention.[2-4] Currently available information, however, suggests that cigarette smoking may influence the development of interstitial lung diseases in two ways. First, interstitial lung diseases are thought to result from the development of an abnormal inflammatory response in the lower respiratory tract.[4] Since cigarette smoking may also produce profound changes in the numbers, types, and activities of immune and inflammatory cells in the lower respiratory tract,[4-23] this preexisting cigarette-induced "alveolitis" could alter the appearance of abnormal immune reactions responsible for initiating interstitial diseases. Second, the lung parenchyma is the site in which the alveolitis of interstitial lung diseases develops. Cigarette smoking also results in a variety of changes to the structure of the lung parenchyma,[1,24] and these cigarette-induced modifications of the lung parenchyma may also influence the frequency and type of abnormal immune responses which can develop in the lower respiratory tract.

Such changes in the immune and inflammatory cells and/or lung parenchyma induced by cigarette smoking could either promote or impede the development of interstitial lung disease. In this context, the incidence of cigarette smoking may be strikingly different in different forms of interstitial lung disease.[2-4] In a recent study, we found that the percentage of patients with histiocytosis X who were smokers was considerably higher than the percentage of patients with sarcoidosis who were smokers.[25] The purpose of this communication is to further explore the relationship between cigarette smoking and these two forms of interstitial lung disease. First, we have compared the levels of tobacco consumption in patients with histiocytosis X and sarcoidosis with that of persons of a similar age in the general population. Second, we have examined the effect of cigarette smoking on the numbers and types of cells recovered by bronchoalveolar lavage from patients with these two interstitial lung diseases. The results indicate that smoking has a significant impact on the pathogenesis of both diseases. Smoking appears to be an important risk factor for the development of histiocytosis X, which may result from cigarette-induced changes in the structure of the lung parenchyma. In contrast, cigarette smokers appear to have a lower incidence of sarcoidosis, which may result from cigarette-induced changes in the balance of immune and inflammatory cells present in the lower respiratory tract.

MATERIALS AND METHODS

Patients with Histiocytosis X

The patients with histiocytosis X were selected from among all patients diagnosed as having histiocytosis X at Avicenne, Bichat, Laennec, Percy, and Salpetrière hospitals between 1976 and 1984. Among this group of patients, 76 individuals were identified who met the following criteria: 1) Clinical findings consistent with pulmonary histiocytosis X. 2) Typical pathological findings on open lung biopsy (62 cases) or the presence of $\geq 2\%$ Langerhans' cells among cells recovered by bronchoalveolar lavage, as determined by indirect immunofluorescence microscopy using monoclonal antibody OKT6 (Ortho Diagnostics, Raritan, NJ) and confirmed by immunoelectron microscopy (14 cases).[26] 3) The availability of detailed information concerning past and present smoking habits.

Patients with Sarcoidosis

The medical records of all patients diagnosed at Hôpital Avicenne between 1976 and 1984 as having sarcoidosis with evidence of pulmonary involvement were reviewed. Among this group of patients, 130 patients were identified who met the following criteria: 1) Clinical findings consistent with pulmonary sarcoidosis. 2) A biopsy of bronchus, of lung parenchymal tissue, or of the site of a Kveim-Siltzbach skin test demonstrating noncaseating granulomas. 3) No evidence of mycobacterial, fungal, or parasitic infections. 4) No history of exposure to agents known to cause granulomatous lung disease. 5) The availability of detailed information concerning past and present smoking habits.

Control Populations

Data concerning tobacco consumption by persons in the general population in France was obtained from a survey conducted between 30 April 1983 and 5 May 1983 by la Société B.V.A. and sponsored by le Comité Français d'Education pour la Santé.[27] The persons interviewed in this survey were representative of the population of France in terms of age, sex, and socioeconomic status. For comparisons made in the present study, only responses by persons between 25 and 49 years of age were considered.

Bronchoalveolar lavage was performed on 13 normal volunteers (8 nonsmokers and 5 smokers). None of these controls had clinical evidence of present or prior pulmonary abnormalities.

Evaluation of Cells Recovered by Bronchoalveolar Lavage

Bronchoscopy and bronchoalveolar lavage were performed as previously described.[15,25,26] In brief, one subsegment, usually the lateral subsegment of the right middle lobe, was lavaged sequentially with five 50-ml aliquots of sterile isotonic saline solution. The fluid was recovered by gentle aspiration, and the volume of fluid recovered was measured. The total number of cells recovered/ml lavage fluid was determined by counting the cells present in a resuspended aliquot of the original lavage fluid.[28] Cytocentrifuge preparations were performed using uncentrifuged lavage fluid and stained with Wright-Giemsa stain; a differential cell count was made by examining at least 500 cells. The total number of each cell type recovered/ml lavage fluid was determined by the following formula: the number of each cell type/ml lavage fluid = (the total cells/ml) $\times$ (the percentage of cell type)/100.

Bronchoalveolar lavage data was available for 123/130 patients with sarcoidosis and for 57/76 patients with histiocytosis X. For the present study, patients who had received corticosteroids within the 6 months before lavage (sarcoidosis, $N=12$) or patients who had previously smoked, but who had discontinued smoking prior to undergoing lavage (sarcoidosis, $N=3$; histiocytosis X, $N=4$), were excluded from the analyses.

Statistical Methods

Comparisons of the prevalence of smoking among patients with histiocytosis X and patients with sarcoidosis and persons in the general population were made using the chi-square distribution.[29] Comparisons of the level of tobacco consumption by patients and the control population were made by placing the populations in ordered categories: 1) nonsmokers, 2) 1-20 cigarettes/day, and 3) > 20 cigarettes/day. Numerical values were then assigned to the groups (1, 2, and 3, respectively), and comparisons between the two populations were made using the two-tailed t test.[29,30] Comparisons of the numbers of cells recovered by lavage were made using Student's t test.

RESULTS

Tobacco Consumption by Patients with Histiocytosis X

The percentage of patients with histiocytosis X who were smokers was higher than the percentage of controls who were smokers ($p<.001$) (TABLE 1). The percentages of men and women with histiocytosis X who were smokers were similar (NS), but this was not the case with the controls ($p<.001$).

Not only were patients with histiocytosis X more likely to smoke, but patients with histiocytosis X who smoked tended to be heavy smokers (TABLE 2). When

TABLE 1. Smokers among Patients with Histiocytosis X and Controls

	Age (years)	Percentage of Smokers		
		Men	Women	All Patients
Patients with histocytosis X	31 ± 11	91	90	91
Controls	25-49	57	35	46

smokers in the control population and the smokers among the patients with histiocytosis X were divided into three groups on the basis of the number of cigarettes smoked/day (1-10, 11-20, and > 20 cigarettes/day) and the numbers of individuals in each group were compared, it became apparent that smokers with histiocytosis X were much more likely to be heavy smokers than persons of the same age in the normal population ($p<.05$). Similarly, the level of tobacco consumption by female smokers with histiocytosis X was significantly higher than that of the female smokers of a similar age in the general population ($p<.05$). Interestingly, the level of tobacco consumption by male smokers with histiocytosis X was similar to that of female smokers with histiocytosis X, but neither group consumed more cigarettes than the male smokers in the general population ($p>.2$ for all comparisons). These findings suggest that smoking is a very strong risk factor for the development of histiocytosis X.

Tobacco Consumption by Patients with Sarcoidosis

In contrast to patients with histiocytosis X, patients with sarcoidosis smoked less than persons of a similar age in the general population ($p<.05$) (TABLE 3). The percentages of men and women with sarcoidosis who were smokers were less than

TABLE 2. Cigarette Consumption by Patients with Sarcoidosis and by Patients with Histiocytosis X

	Age (years)	*N*	Cigarette Consumption (cigarettes/day)			
			0	1-10	11-20	>20
Sarcoidosis						
Men		71	38	9	12	12
Women		59	52	5	1	1
All Patients	33 ± 10	130	90	14	13	13
Histiocytosis X						
Men		56	5	11	26	14
Women		20	2	4	9	5
All Patients	31 ± 11	76	7	15	35	19

those observed in the respective control groups, although the differences between the men with sarcoidosis and the men of a similar age in the general population were not significant at the .05 level. The difference in the percentages of men and women with sarcoidosis who were smokers was significant ($p<.001$); this was also the case with the controls ($p<.05$). Although patients with sarcoidosis were less likely to be smokers than persons in the general population, the level of tobacco consumption by the smokers among the patients with sarcoidosis and smokers in the control population was similar ($p>0.1$ for the following comparisons: patients with sarcoidosis with the control population, males with sarcoidosis with male controls, and females with sarcoidosis with female controls).

The Effect of Cigarette Smoking on the Alveolitis of Pulmonary Histiocytosis X

In order to determine the effect of cigarette smoking on the number of cells of each immune/inflammatory cell type recovered by lavage from patients with histiocytosis X, the patients were divided into three groups on the basis of smoking habits: 1) nonsmokers, 2) moderate smokers (1-20 cigarettes/day), and 3) heavy smokers (>20 cigarettes/day). The average number of cells of each cell type recovered/ml lavage fluid was then determined for each group (TABLE 4). Although bronchoalveolar lavage data is frequently presented in terms of the percentage of each cell type recovered, this form of presentation was avoided because increases in one cell population (that is, a dramatic increase in the number of macrophages) could have reduced the percentage of the other cell populations present, even though the number of these

TABLE 3. Smokers among Patients with Sarcoidosis and Controls

	Age (years)	Percentage of Smokers		
		Men	Women	All Patients
Patients with sarcoidosis	33±10	46	12	31
Controls	25-49	57	35	46

TABLE 4. The Effect of Smoking on the Alveolitis of Pulmonary Histiocytosis X

	Cigarette Consumption (cigarettes/day)		
	0	1-20	>20
Controls			
Number of patients	8	5	—
Number of cells[a]			
Macrophages	176 ± 76	310 ± 93[b]	—
Lymphocytes	17 ± 9	16 ± 6	—
Neutrophils	3 ± 3	8 ± 2[b]	—
Eosinophils	1 ± 1	1 ± 1	—
Patients with histiocytosis X			
Number of patients	6	29	14
Number of cells[a]			
Mononuclear phagocytes	255 ± 155	417 ± 211[b]	820 ± 301[b,c]
Lymphocytes	25 ± 25	46 ± 48	20 ± 16
Neutrophils	16 ± 17[b]	35 ± 3[b]	18 ± 18[b]
Eosinophils	18 ± 23[b]	35 ± 42[b]	23 ± 22[b]

[a] Results are expressed as cells $\times$ 10^{-3}/ml lavage fluid.
[b] $p < .05$ compared to nonsmoking controls.
[c] $p < .05$ compared to nonsmoking patients with histiocytosis X.

other cell types/ml lavage fluid might not have changed or might have actually increased.[16,31]

Alveolar Macrophages

Nonsmoking patients with histiocytosis X did not have an increased number of alveolar macrophages/ml lavage fluid compared to the number recovered from normal individuals ($p > .2$) (TABLE 4). The number of alveolar macrophages/ml lavage fluid, however, was significantly increased in patients with histiocytosis X who smoked. The magnitude of this increase observed in the patients who smoked was dependent upon the number of cigarettes smoked/day ($p < .05$ in comparisons of patients with histiocytosis X who smoked 1-20 cigarettes/day and those who smoked > 20 cigarettes/day), and appeared to be similar to the increase in the number of alveolar macrophages/ml lavage fluid observed in smokers without interstitial lung disease ($p > .2$ in comparisons of patients with histiocytosis X and controls who smoked 1-20 cigarettes/day).

Lymphocytes

The number of lymphocytes recovered/ml lavage fluid from patients with histiocytosis X varied considerably. Although the number of lymphocytes recovered from some patients was clearly elevated (> 40 × 10³ lymphocytes/ml; $N=12$), when histiocytosis X patients were considered as a group, the number of lymphocytes/ml was not significantly different from that of the normals. Furthermore, no significant differences were observed when the number of lymphocytes/ml lavage fluid recovered from the nonsmokers, light smokers, and heavy smokers were compared.

Neutrophils and Eosinophils

Both the number of neutrophils/ml lavage fluid and the number of eosinophils/ml lavage fluid were considerably increased in nonsmoking patients with histiocytosis X. When the numbers of these cells recovered by lavage from smoking and nonsmoking patients were compared, however, no significant differences were found.

Langerhans' Cells

In some cases, the number of mononuclear phagocytes expressing the T6 surface antigen was quantitated. In each case, these $T6^+$ cells were confirmed to be Langerhans' cells (LC's) by electron microscopy. As expected, the number of LC's/ml lavage fluid was increased in patients with histiocytosis X. The number of LC's/ml recovered from patients with histiocytosis X, however, did not follow any obvious trend as a function of cigarette smoking. In any case, the number of patients studied was too small to allow any firm conclusions to be drawn: number of LC's/ml for nonsmokers ($N=1$): 11×10^3; for light smokers ($N=16$): $35 \pm 43 \times 10^3$; and, for heavy smokers ($N=10$): $28 \pm 15 \times 10^3$.

The Effect of Smoking on the Alveolitis of Pulmonary Sarcoidosis

In order to determine the effect of cigarette smoking on the alveolitis of pulmonary sarcoidosis, the number of cells of each inflammatory cell type recovered/ml of lavage fluid was compared in nonsmokers, light smokers, and heavy smokers (TABLE 5).

TABLE 5. The Effect of Smoking on the Alveolitis of Pulmonary Sarcoidosis

	Cigarette Consumption (cigarettes/day)		
	0	1-20	>20
Patients with sarcoidosis			
Number of patients	77	23	8
Number of cells[a]			
Macrophages	119 ± 134	151 ± 115	285 ± 271[b,c]
Lymphocytes	72 ± 61[b]	69 ± 50[b]	63 ± 41[b]
Neutrophils	3 ± 4	3 ± 3	12 ± 20[b,c]

[a] Results are expressed as cells × 10^{-3}/ml lavage fluid.
[b] $p<.05$ compared to nonsmoking controls.
[c] $p<.05$ compared to nonsmoking patients with sarcoidosis.

Alveolar Macrophages

In this series, the nonsmoking patients with sarcoidosis did not have an increased number of alveolar macrophages/ml lavage fluid compared to the number recovered from controls (TABLE 5). Furthermore, the number of alveolar macrophages/ml recovered by lavage from patients with sarcoidosis who were light smokers was not significantly greater than the number of alveolar macrophages recovered from controls who were nonsmokers, and was considerably less than the number of alveolar macrophages recovered from otherwise healthy smokers ($p < .05$ in comparisons of patients with sarcoidosis and controls who smoked 1-20 cigarettes/day). In the few patients with sarcoidosis who were heavy smokers, the number of alveolar macrophages recovered by lavage was greater than that recovered from nonsmoking patients with sarcoidosis and nonsmoking controls. Strikingly, however, even among patients with sarcoidosis who were heavy smokers, the average number of alveolar macrophages recovered by lavage was not increased above that observed in the otherwise healthy moderate smokers.

Lymphocytes

The number of lymphocytes recovered by lavage from nonsmoking patients with sarcoidosis was more than four times greater than that recovered from nonsmoking controls. The number of lymphocytes recovered from moderate or heavy smokers with sarcoidosis, however, was not significantly different compared to the number of lymphocytes recovered from the nonsmoking patients with sarcoidosis (TABLE 5).

Neutrophils and Eosinophils

The number of neutrophils recovered by lavage from nonsmoking patients with sarcoidosis and the number recovered from controls were similar. Although cigarette smoking was associated with an increase in the number of neutrophils recovered by lavage from controls, the number of neutrophils recovered by lavage from smoking patients with sarcoidosis was significantly increased only in the group of heavy smokers (TABLE 5). Most patients with sarcoidosis had very few eosinophils among cells recovered by lavage, and the numbers of eosinophils/ml lavage fluid were not significantly different in the nonsmokers, light smokers, or heavy smokers (data not shown).

DISCUSSION

Cigarette smoking produces profound changes in the structure of the lung parenchyma and in the population of immune and inflammatory cells present in the lower respiratory tract.[1,4–24] The findings in this study suggest that these cigarette-induced abnormalities may profoundly effect the likelihood of the subsequent appearance of two different interstitial lung diseases. Smoking is a strong risk factor for the development of pulmonary histiocytosis X, but appears to reduce the incidence of sarcoidosis. In an effort to understand how cigarette smoking influences the incidence of these two disorders, we compared the numbers and types of inflammatory cells recovered by bronchoalveolar lavage from smokers and nonsmokers with histiocytosis X and sarcoidosis. In patients with histiocytosis X, cigarette smoking resulted in an increase in the number of alveolar macrophages recovered by lavage which was similar in magnitude to that seen in normal smokers. In contrast, the number of macrophages recovered from patients with sarcoidosis who smoked was considerably less than that observed in normal smokers. This difference in the intensity of the cigarette-induced macrophage alveolitis in these two groups of patients may be of importance in explaining the opposite effect of cigarette smoking on the incidence of the two diseases.

Smoking and Histiocytosis X

In our series, the incidence of cigarette smoking is significantly higher among patients with pulmonary histiocytosis X than that observed among persons in the general population, a finding consistent with previous studies.[32–34] Furthermore, since more men than women smoke, this may explain, at least in part, the predominance of males in this series. Interestingly, the levels of cigarette consumption by male and female patients with histiocytosis X were similar, and these levels of consumption were significantly higher than that observed among women in the general population but not significantly higher than that among men in the general population of a similar age. This finding suggests that a certain level of tobacco consumption is necessary to maximize this risk factor. The level of smoking observed among men in the general population, however, is apparently sufficient to maximize the added risk of developing pulmonary histiocytosis X which smoking produces.

The alveolitis of histiocytosis X in nonsmokers was characterized by significantly increased numbers of LC's, neutrophils, eosinophils, and, in some cases, lymphocytes. Interestingly, the number of alveolar macrophages was not significantly increased in nonsmoking patients. In smoking patients with histiocytosis X, there was a significant increase only in the number of alveolar macrophages, an increase that was directly related to the level of tobacco consumption. The magnitude of this increase in the number of alveolar macrophages, however, was similar to that of otherwise healthy smokers. Since an increased number of alveolar macrophages is not an essential feature of the alveolitis of histiocytosis X (for example, the number of alveolar macrophages was normal in most nonsmoking patients), the increase in the number of alveolar macrophages seen in smoking patients is probably not of primary pathogenetic significance in histiocytosis X. Inflammatory changes resulting from this cigarette-induced alveolitis, however, may play a role in the increased incidence of this disorder seen in smokers.

It is possible that histiocytosis X may result from an allergic reaction to a component of cigarette smoke,[4] but several facts argue against this explanation. First, it does not easily explain the simultaneous appearance of lesions in other tissues which occurs in an important percentage of cases. Second, it does not explain why a certain level of cigarette consumption is necessary to maximize the risk of developing histiocytosis X, since allergic reactions are usually not dose related. Third, it does not explain the presence of LC's within the lung. Fourth, it does not explain why nonsmokers may also develop pulmonary histiocytosis X.

A more attractive hypothesis to explain the increased risk of histiocytosis X in heavy smokers takes into consideration the fact that inflammatory changes associated with cigarette smoking may produce squamous metaplasia of the pulmonary epithelium, as well as the fact that LC's are known to be attracted to normal or abnormal squamous epithelium, including areas of squamous metaplasia in the lung.[24,35] According to this hypothesis, two stimuli are required to produce pulmonary histiocytosis X. One stimulus is required to produce squamous metaplasia or other changes in the pulmonary epithelium that secondarily attract LC's to the lung. This stimulus could be provided either by cigarette smoking, a common cause, or by a variety of other insults, such as radiation therapy[36] or occupational exposure.[34] A second stimulus is required to abnormally activate the LC's.[36] In heavy smokers, or individuals who have developed squamous metaplasia (and, therefore, LC infiltration) for other reasons, this would result in the appearance of lesions within the lung, as well as at other sites where LC's are activated.

Smoking and Sarcoidosis

Our findings also suggest that the percentage of patients with sarcoidosis who smoke is significantly less than that observed in the general population. This finding supports the conclusion of Harf and Perrin-Fayolle[3] that cigarette smoking reduces the likelihood of subsequently developing sarcoidosis. This "protection," however, is not complete, and some patients with sarcoidosis were smokers. In this study, the level of daily cigarette consumption by smokers with sarcoidosis was not significantly different from the control population. The number of smoking patients with sarcoidosis, however, was relatively small, and both the light and heavy smokers among the patients with sarcoidosis had smoked fewer total cigarettes than the corresponding smokers with histiocytosis X. Thus, further studies, involving a larger number of patients, are required to determine whether daily cigarette consumption, total cigarette consumption, or other factors modulate the degree to which smoking prevents the appearance of sarcoidosis.

The most striking feature of the results of bronchoalveolar lavage in patients with sarcoidosis who smoked was the relatively small number of alveolar macrophages recovered. The number of alveolar macrophages recovered from patients with sarcoidosis who were moderate smokers was not increased compared to nonsmoking controls or nonsmoking patients with sarcoidosis. The number of macrophages recovered from patients with sarcoidosis who were heavy smokers was increased compared to nonsmoking patients with sarcoidosis. The increase in the number of alveolar macrophages observed in these heavy smokers with sarcoidosis was far less than the increase in the number of macrophages observed in the histiocytosis X patients who were heavy smokers. Our findings are in agreement with those of Dauber *et al.*,[16] who previously noted that the number of macrophages recovered from smoking patients with sarcoidosis is significantly less than that recovered from smoking controls, although other series have not demonstrated such differences.[20,37]

It is possible that the reduced incidence of sarcoidosis observed in smokers is a direct consequence of the macrophage alveolitis induced by cigarette smoking. This theory would explain why only nonsmokers and smokers with sarcoidosis who have developed little or no macrophage alveolitis in response to smoking are more likely to develop sarcoidosis. Additional indirect evidence supports this hypothesis. Sarcoidosis is thought to represent a disorder of unrestrained T lymphocyte proliferation,[4,38,39] a process which may be both stimulated and suppressed by alveolar macrophages.[40]

Smoking, however, has been shown to impair the ability of alveolar macrophages to interact with T lymphocytes[37,41] and to reduce HLA-DR expression by alveolar macrophages.[42] As a consequence of these and perhaps other factors, alveolar macrophages from smokers may have a reduced capacity to stimulate proliferation of autologous T lymphocytes compared to that of normal alveolar macrophages.[43] Furthermore, the increased alveolar macrophage/T lymphocyte ratio present in the lung of most otherwise healthy smokers,[3-23] as well as increased release of a variety of soluble products by these activated alveolar macrophages,[15,18] may increase the ability of alveolar macrophages from smokers to suppress T lymphocyte proliferation.[40,44-47] This shift in the functional capacity of these cells toward suppression may provide partial protection against the development of sarcoidosis. Not all studies, however, have demonstrated that alveolar macrophages from smokers are impaired in their ability to induce T lymphocyte proliferation.[12,48] Therefore, it is possible that other effects of cigarette smoking, such as cigarette-induced changes in the lymphocyte population,[12] play a role in the reduced incidence of sarcoidosis in smokers.

Regardless of the mechanisms involved, these studies demonstrate that cigarette smoking may influence the incidence of histiocytosis X and sarcoidosis. Better understanding of the mechanisms by which cigarette smoking affects the incidence of these disorders may provide insights into the pathogenesis and treatment of these and other interstitial lung diseases.

SUMMARY

Cigarette smoking produces marked alterations in the lung parenchyma and in the population of immune and inflammatory cells present in the lower respiratory tract. These cigarette-induced changes appear to influence the incidence of two different interstitial lung diseases, histiocytosis X and sarcoidosis. Smoking is a strong risk factor for the development of pulmonary histiocytosis X, since the incidence of smoking is very high among patients with histiocytosis X: 90% of the patients with histiocytosis X were smokers; 46% of the controls were smokers ($p < .001$). In contrast, smoking appears to reduce the incidence of sarcoidosis: 31% of the patients with sarcoidosis were smokers ($p < .05$ compared to controls). In an effort to understand how cigarette smoking influences the incidence of these two disorders, we compared the numbers and types of immune and inflammatory cells recovered by bronchoalveolar lavage from nonsmoking and smoking controls and patients with histiocytosis X and sarcoidosis. Although nonsmoking patients with histiocytosis X did not have a significant increase in the number of alveolar macrophages recovered by lavage ($p > .2$ compared to normals), smoking patients had an increase in the number of alveolar macrophages similar to that observed in the control population. In contrast, the number of macrophages recovered from patients with sarcoidosis who smoked was considerably less than that observed in normal smokers ($p < .05$ comparing patients with sarcoidosis and controls who smoked 1-20 cigarettes/day). This difference in the intensity of the cigarette-induced macrophage alveolitis observed in the two patient groups may be important in explaining the opposite effects of cigarette smoking on the incidence of histiocytosis X and sarcoidosis.

ACKNOWLEDGMENTS

The authors thank Drs. Sors, Kermarec, Gallouedec, Marsac, Patte, and Brocard for providing some of the clinical data used in these studies; Mrs. Grandsaigne, Jarland, Mazin, and Wyllie for their skillful technical assistance; and Mrs. Miklovic for her editorial assistance.

REFERENCES

1. United States Department of Health, Education, and Welfare. 1972. The health consequences of smoking: A report of the surgeon general. Publication number: 72-7516. U.S. Government Printing Office. Washington, DC.
2. WARREN, C. P. W. 1977. Extrinsic allergic alveolitis: A disease commoner in nonsmokers. Thorax **32:** 567-569.
3. HARF, R. & M. PERRIN-FAYOLLE. 1982. Sarcoidose et tabac. *In* Proceedings of the Third European Conference on Sarcoidosis and Other Granulomatous Disorders. B. Durič, Ed.: 167-174. Sremska Kamenica. Novi Sad.
4. CRYSTAL, R. G., P. B. BITTERMAN, S. I. RENNARD, A. J. HANCE & B. A. KEOGH. 1984. Interstitial lung diseases of unknown cause: Disorders characterized by chronic inflammation of the lower respiratory tract. N. Engl. J. Med. **310:** 154-166, 235-244.
5. HARRIS, J. O., E. W. SWENSON & J. E. JOHNSON III. 1970. Human alveolar macrophages: Comparison of phagocytic ability, glucose utilization, and ultrastructure in smokers and nonsmokers. J. Clin. Invest. **49:** 2086-2096.
6. PRATT, S. A., M. H. SMITH, A. J. LADMAN & T. N. FINLEY. 1971. The ultrastructure of alveolar macrophages from human cigarette smokers and nonsmokers. Lab. Invest. **24:** 331-338.
7. REYNOLDS, H. Y. & H. H. NEWBALL. 1974. Analysis of proteins and respiratory cells obtained from human lungs by bronchial lavage. J. Lab. Clin. Med. **84:** 559-573.
8. HARRIS, J. O., G. N. OLSEN, J. R. CASTLE & A. S. MALONEY. 1975. Comparison of proteolytic enzyme activity in pulmonary alveolar macrophages and blood leukocytes in smokers and nonsmokers. Am. Rev. Respir. Dis. **111:** 579-587.
9. WARR, G. A., R. R. MARTIN, C. L. HOLLEMAN & B. S. CRISWELL. 1976. Classification of bronchial lymphocytes from nonsmokers. Am. Rev. Respir. Dis. **113:** 96-100.
10. REYNOLDS, H. Y., J. D. FULMER, J. A. KAZMIEROWSKI, W. C. ROBERTS, M. M. FRANK & R. G. CRYSTAL. 1977. Analysis of cellular and protein content of bronchoalveolar lavage fluid from patients with idiopathic pulmonary fibrosis and chronic hypersensitivity pneumonitis. J. Clin. Invest. **59:** 165-175.
11. WARR, G. A., R. R. MARTIN, P. M. SHARP & R. ROSSEN. 1977. Normal human bronchial immunoglobulins and proteins: Effects of cigarette smoking. Am. Rev. Respir. Dis. **116:** 25-30.
12. DANIELE, R. P., J. H. DAUBER, M. D. ALTOSE, D. T. ROWLANDS, JR. & D. J. GORENBERG. 1977. Lymphocyte studies in asymptomatic smokers. Am. Rev. Respir. Dis. **116:** 997-1005.
13. LOW, R. B., G. S. DAVIS & M. S. GIANCOLA. 1978. Biochemical analyses of bronchoalveolar lavage fluids of healthy human volunteer smokers and nonsmokers. Am. Rev. Respir. Dis. **118:** 863-875.
14. WEINBERGER, S. E., J. A. KELMAN, N. A. ELSON, R. C. YOUNG, JR., H. Y. REYNOLDS, J. D. FULMER & R. G. CRYSTAL. 1978. Bronchoalveolar lavage in interstitial lung disease. Ann. Intern. Med. **89:** 459-466.
15. HUNNINGHAKE, G. W., J. E. GADEK, O. KAWANAMI, V. J. FERRANS & R. G. CRYSTAL. 1979. Inflammatory and immune processes in the human lung in health and disease: Evaluation by bronchoalveolar lavage. Am. J. Pathol. **97:** 149-206.

16. DAUBER, J. H., M. D. ROSSMAN & R. P. DANIELE. 1979. Bronchoalveolar cell populations in acute sarcoidosis: Observations in smoking and nonsmoking patients. J. Lab. Clin. Med. **94:** 862-871.
17. HASLAM, P. L., C. W. G. TURTON, A. LUKOSZEK, A. J. SALSBURY, A. DEWAR, J. V. COLLINS & M. TURNER-WARWICK. 1980. Bronchoalveolar lavage fluid cell counts in cryptogenic fibrosing alveolitis and their relation to therapy. Thorax **35:** 328-339.
18. REYNOLDS, H. Y. & W. W. MERRILL. 1981. Airway changes in young smokers that may antedate chronic obstructive lung disease. Med. Clin. North Am. **65:** 667-689.
19. HOIDAL, J. R., R. B. FOX, P. A. LE MARBE, R. PERRI & J. E. REPINE. 1981. Altered oxidative metabolic responses *in vitro* of alveolar macrophages from asymptomatic cigarette smokers. Am. Rev. Respir. Dis. **123:** 85-89.
20. ARNOUX, A., J. MARSAC, G. STANISLAS-LEGUERN, G. HUCHON & J. CHRÉTIEN. 1982. Bronchoalveolar lavage in sarcoidosis: Correlation between alveolar lymphocytosis and clinical data. Pathol. Res. Pract. **175:** 62-79.
21. MARTIN, W. J., II, D. E. WILLIAMS, D. E. DINES & D. R. SANDERSON. 1983. Interstitial lung disease: Assessment by bronchoalveolar lavage. Mayo Clin. Proc. **58:** 751-757.
22. KEOGH, B. A., G. W. HUNNINGHAKE, B. R. LINE & R. G. CRYSTAL. 1983. The alveolitis of pulmonary sarcoidosis: Evaluation of natural history and alveolitis-dependent changes in lung function. Am. Rev. Respir. Dis. **128:** 256-265.
23. HUNNINGHAKE, G. W. & R. G. CRYSTAL. 1983. Cigarette smoking and lung destruction. Am. Rev. Respir. Dis. **128:** 833-838.
24. HEARD, B. E. 1969. Pathology of Chronic Bronchitis and Emphysema. Churchill. London.
25. SOLER, P., F. BASSET, F. MAZIN, M. GRANDSAIGNE & J. BRETON-GORIUS. 1982. Peroxidatic activities of human alveolar macrophages in some pulmonary granulomatous disorders. J. Reticuloendothel. Soc. **31:** 511-521.
26. CHOLLET, S., P. SOLER, P. DOURNOVO, M. S. RICHARD, V. J. FERRANS & F. BASSET. 1984. Diagnosis of pulmonary histiocytosis X by immunodetection of Langerhans cells in bronchoalveolar lavage fluid. Am. J. Pathol. **115:** 225-232.
27. Comité Français d'Education pour la Santé. 1983. Les français et le tabac. Tabac et Santé **52:** 10-13.
28. SALTINI, C., A. J. HANCE, V. J. FERRANS, F. BASSET, P. B. BITTERMAN & R. G. CRYSTAL. 1984. Accurate quantitation of cells recovered by bronchoalveolar lavage. Am. Rev. Respir. Dis. **130:** 650-658.
29. SNEDECOR, G. W. & W. G. COCHRAN. 1967. Statistical Methods. Iowa University Press. Ames, IA.
30. MOSES, L. E., J. D. EMERSON & H. HOSSEINI. 1984. Analyzing data from ordered categories. N. Engl. J. Med. **311:** 442-448.
31. KEOGH, B. A. & R. G. CRYSTAL. 1982. Alveolitis: The key to the interstitial lung disorders. Thorax **37:** 1-10.
32. BASSET, F., B. CORRIN, H. SPENCER, J. LACRONIQUE, C. ROTH, P. SOLER, J.-P. BATTESTI, R. GEORGES & J. CHRÉTIEN. 1978. Pulmonary histiocytosis X. Am. Rev. Respir. Dis. **118:** 811-820.
33. KING, T. E., JR., M. I. SCHWARZ, R. E. DREISIN, D. S. PRATT & A. N. THEOFILOPOULOUS. 1979. Circulating immune complexes in pulmonary eosinophilic granuloma. Ann. Intern. Med. **91:** 397-399.
34. FRIEDMAN, P. J., A. A. LIEBOW & J. SOKOLOFF. 1981. Eosinophilic granuloma of the lung: Clinical aspects of primary pulmonary histiocytosis in the adult. Medicine **60:** 385-396.
35. BASSET, F., P. SOLER & A. J. HANCE. The Langerhans' cell in human pathology. Ann. N.Y. Acad. Sci. This volume.
36. SAJJAD, S. M. & M. A. LUNA. 1982. Primary pulmonary histiocytosis X in two patients with Hodgkin's disease. Thorax **37:** 110-113.
37. YEAGER, H., JR., M. C. WILLIAMS, J. F. BECKMAN, T. C. BAYLY, B. L. BEAMAN & R. J. HAWLEY. 1977. Sarcoidosis: Analysis of cells obtained by lavage. Am. Rev. Respir. Dis. **116:** 951-954.
38. PINKSTON, P., P. B. BITTERMAN & R. G. CRYSTAL. 1983. Spontaneous release of interleukin-2 by lung T lymphocytes in active pulmonary sarcoidosis. N. Engl. J. Med. **308:** 793-800.

39. DANIELE, R. P., J. H. DAUBER & M. D. ROSSMAN. 1980. Immunologic abnormalities in sarcoidosis. Ann. Intern. Med. **92:** 406-416.
40. KALTREIDER, H. B. 1982. Alveolar macrophages: Enhancers or suppressors of pulmonary immune reactivity? Chest **82:** 261-262.
41. LUSSIER, L. M., D. K. F. CHANDLER, A. SYBERT & H. Y. YEAGER, JR. 1978. Human alveolar macrophages: Antigen-independent binding of lymphocytes. J. Appl. Physiol. **45:** 933-938.
42. LAWRENCE, E. C., T. B. FOX, B. T. HALL & R. R. MARTIN. 1983. Deleterious effects of cigarette smoking on expression of Ia antigens by human pulmonary alveolar macrophages. Clin. Res. **31:** 418A.
43. LAUGHTER, A. H., R. R. MARTIN & J. J. TWOMEY. 1977. Lymphoproliferative responses to antigens mediated by human pulmonary alveolar macrophages. J. Lab. Clin. Med. **89:** 1326-1332.
44. METZGER, Z., J. T. HOFFELD & J. J. OPPENHEIM. 1980. Macrophage-mediated suppression. I. Evidence for participation of both hydrogen peroxide and prostaglandins in suppression of murine lymphocyte proliferation. J. Immunol. **124:** 983-988.
45. MCCOMBS, C. C., J. P. MICHALSKI, B. T. WESTERFIELD & R. W. LIGHT. 1982. Human alveolar macrophages suppress the proliferative response of peripheral blood lymphocytes. Chest **82:** 266-271.
46. MAYERNIK, D. G., A. UL-HAG & J. J. RINEHART. 1983. Differentiation-associated alteration in human monocyte-macrophage accessory cell function. J. Immunol. **130:** 2156-2160.
47. TOEWS, G. B., W. C. VIAL, M. M. DUNN, P. GUZZETTA, G. NUNEZ, P. STASTNY & M. F. LIPSCOMB. 1984. The accessory cell function of human alveolar macrophages in specific T cell proliferation. J. Immunol. **132:** 181-186.
48. DE SHAZO, R. D., D. E. BANKS, J. E. DIEM, J. A. NORDBERG, Y. BASER, D. BEVIER & J. E. SALVAGGIO. 1983. Bronchoalveolar lavage cell-lymphocyte interactions in normal nonsmokers and smokers. Am. Rev. Respir. Dis. **127:** 545-548.

Cigarette Smoking and Bronchoalveolar T Cell Populations in Sarcoidosis[a]

E. CLINTON LAWRENCE, TERESA B. FOX,
ROBERT B. TEAGUE, KIM BLOOM,
AND R. KEITH WILSON

Rockwell-Keough Pulmonary Immunology Laboratory
General Clinical Research Center
Methodist Hospital
and
Department of Medicine
Baylor College of Medicine
Houston, Texas 77030

INTRODUCTION

Pulmonary physicians must often deal with patients, including patients with sarcoidosis, who smoke cigarettes. Since changes in local pulmonary immune function have been associated with both sarcoidosis[1–4] and cigarette smoking,[5–10] it is important to distinguish which of these immunological changes in the lungs are due to the disease, which are due to cigarette smoking, and which, perhaps, are due to both.

Abnormally large numbers of helper thymus-derived (T) lymphocytes are found in fluids recovered by bronchoalveolar lavage (BAL) from patients with sarcoidosis.[11] By contrast, normal numbers of lymphocytes are found in BAL fluids from normal cigarette smokers,[6] and lower than normal percentages of the cells in these fluids are lymphocytes.[5,6,10] The effects of smoking on T lymphocyte subpopulations in normal cigarette smokers and on those in patients with sarcoidosis, however, have not been thoroughly characterized.

The purposes of this study, therefore, were 1) to determine the effects of smoking on T lymphocyte subpopulations in BAL fluids from healthy normal volunteers ("normals") and on those in BAL fluids from patients with sarcoidosis ("sarcoids"), and 2) to determine whether comparisons of the T lymphocyte subpopulations of normals and those of sarcoids revealed any effects of cigarette smoking.

[a] This work was supported in part by Grant 1215B from the Council for Tobacco Research, Grant HL-29542 from the National Institutes of Health, and Grant RR-0030 from the General Clinical Research Center.

METHODS

Shown in TABLE 1 are the characteristics of the four populations studied. Eight normals and four sarcoids were nonsmokers, and six normals and six sarcoids were cigarette smokers. The ages were fairly comparable, but the sex and race characteristics of the groups were somewhat divergent. These divergencies probably reflect the small sample size of each respective group. All sarcoids had radiographic stage 2 or stage 3 disease. All had active disease: all had abnormal gallium-67 lung scans or increased angiotensin-converting enzyme levels or both.[12–15] All were untreated at the time of study.

Bronchoscopy and BAL were performed as previously described.[16,17] Briefly, the lingula and/or the right middle lobe were each lavaged with four 30-ml aliquots of normal saline solution: a total of 120 ml was instilled into each respective lobe. Cell recovery prior to washing was determined with a hemacytometer. Cell differentials were determined from Wright-Giemsa and/or esterase stains of cytocentrifuge preparations. Data were expressed as the percentage and total number of recovered cells as well as the number of cells per ml of recovered BAL fluid.[18] Bronchoalveolar lymphocytes were isolated from macrophages by passage over Sephadex G-10 columns.[19] The percent cell recovery from the G-10 column varied greatly between different individuals and groups of subjects (TABLE 2). Recovered bronchoalveolar lymphocytes were incubated with one of the OK series of monoclonal antibodies: OKT3 was used to determine the total number of T cells; OKT4, the number of putative helper T cells; OKT8, the number of putative suppressor/cytotoxic T cells.[20] Bronchoalveolar lymphocytes were incubated with an fluorescein isothiocyanate (FITC)-conjugated goat antimouse IgG, and then the percentage of lymphocytes expressing each marker was determined using a cytofluorograf.

TABLE 1. Characteristics of Study Populations

	Normals		Sarcoids	
	Nonsmokers	Smokers	Nonsmokers	Smokers
Total number	8	6	4	6
Age (years)				
Mean	24.9	30.5	35.5	29.7
Range	21-30	21-49	30-40	23-39
Sex				
Number of males	1	4	4	3
Number of females	7	2	0	3
Race				
Number of blacks	0	1	1	5
Number of whites	8	5	3	1

RESULTS

Shown in FIGURE 1 are the effects of cigarette smoking on bronchoalveolar helper (T4) lymphocytes from both normals and sarcoids. Interestingly, no differences in the

TABLE 2. Percentages of Bronchoalveolar Lymphocytes Recovered from Sephadex G-10 Columns

	Number	Percentage of Lymphocytes Recovered[a] Mean	Range
Normals			
Nonsmokers	5	68	20-100
Smokers	5	81	47-100
Sarcoids			
Nonsmokers	4	48	17-100
Smokers	6	57	5-95

[a] Percentage of lymphocytes recovered = (number of lymphocytes recovered from the column/number of lymphocytes placed over the column) × 100.

expression of T4 were seen between bronchoalveolar lymphocytes from nonsmoking or cigarette smoking sarcoids. By contrast, however, the expression of T4 was reduced in smoking normals to a mean value of 24%, as opposed to 48% for nonsmoking normals (p=.01).

Shown in FIGURE 2 are the effects of cigarette smoking on bronchoalveolar suppressor (T8) lymphocytes in both normals and sarcoids. There were no appreciable differences due to cigarette smoking in either group.

Shown in FIGURE 3 are the effects of cigarette smoking on the bronchoalveolar helper/suppressor (T4/T8) ratio for both normals and sarcoids. Since there were no differences attributed to cigarette smoking in the expression of either T4 or T8 in sarcoids, the T4/T8 ratio was likewise unaffected by cigarette smoking. In the normals, however, the T4/T8 ratio was reduced from 1.7 ± 0.3 in nonsmokers to 0.9 ± 0.2 in cigarette smokers (p = .05) due to the previously shown reduction in T4 expression (FIG. 1). Thus, cigarette smoking had adverse effects on helper T cells, as measured by expression of T4, in normals but had no appreciable deleterious effects in sarcoids.

We next compared normals with sarcoids: both were grouped according to smoking status. FIGURE 4 compares bronchoalveolar helper (T4) lymphocytes in normals to

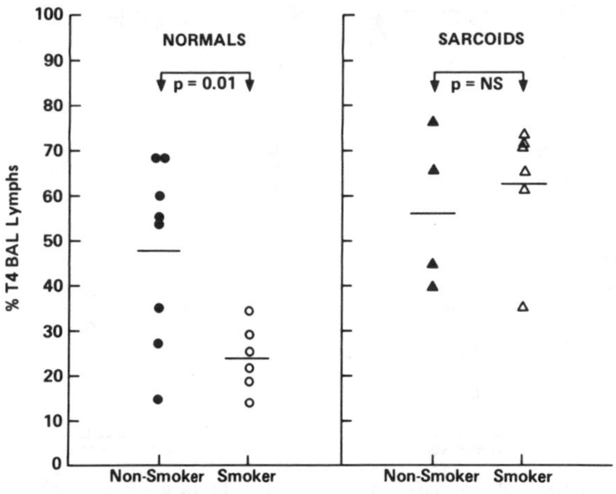

FIGURE 1. Effects of cigarette smoking on T4 lymphocytes in normals and sarcoids.

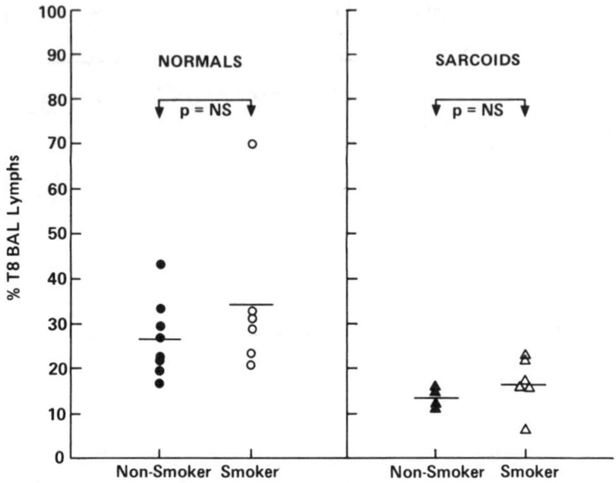

FIGURE 2. Effects of cigarette smoking on T8 lymphocytes in normals and sarcoids.

those in sarcoids. In contrast to previous studies,[11] we found no significant differences in the expression of T4 between normals and sarcoids who were nonsmokers. There was, however, greater expression of T4 by bronchoalveolar lymphocytes from smoking sarcoids than by those from smoking normals: the respective values were 62.6 ± 5.8% and 23.8 ± 3.0% ($p < .001$). As shown earlier, however, this difference was due more to a reduction in T4 expression by bronchoalveolar lymphocytes from smoking normals than to an increase in the number of bronchoalveolar T4 lymphocytes in smoking sarcoids (FIG. 1).

Shown in FIGURE 5 is a comparison of bronchoalveolar T8 lymphocytes in normals to those in sarcoids. There was a reduction in T8 expression by T cells in sarcoidosis in both nonsmokers (26.5 ± 3.1% versus 13.1 ± 1.0%) ($p = .002$) and cigarette smokers (34.2 ± 7.4% versus 16.3 ± 2.4%) ($p = .06$). The latter results, however, were not quite statistically significant.

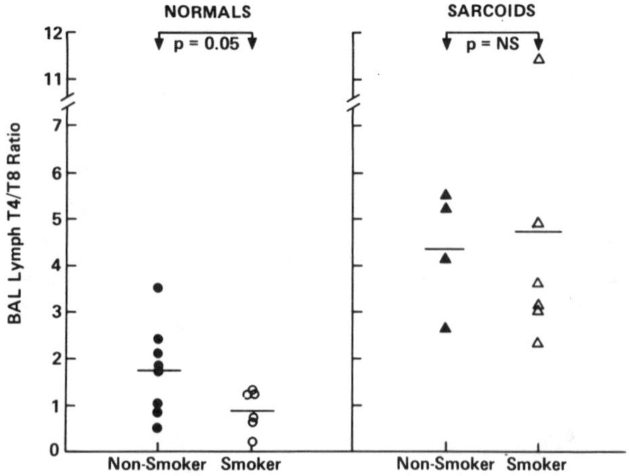

FIGURE 3. Effects of cigarette smoking on T4/T8 ratios in normals and sarcoids.

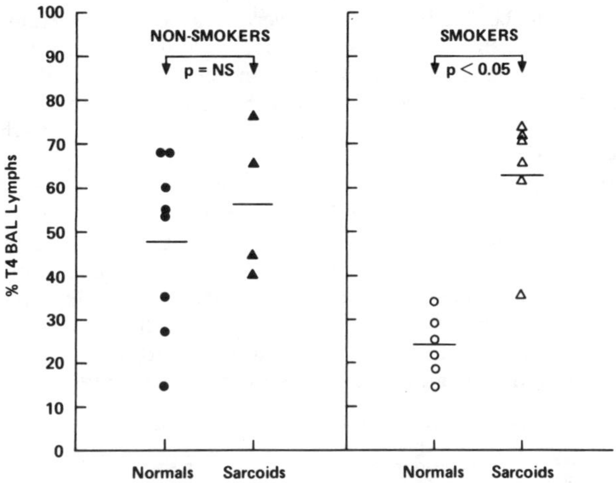

FIGURE 4. Comparison of T4 lymphocytes in normals and sarcoids of similar smoking status.

When all the foregoing observations are collated into a comparison of the helper/suppressor (or T4/T8) ratios in normals and sarcoids, one finds an increase in the ratio in sarcoidosis in both nonsmokers and cigarette smokers compared to normals (FIG. 6). Thus, the T4/T8 ratio was 1.70 ± 0.34 in nonsmoking normals and 4.4 ± 0.7 in nonsmoking sarcoids ($p = .01$). In smoking normals the T4/T8 ratio was 0.9 ± 0.2; in smoking sarcoids, 4.7 ± 1.4 ($p = .02$).

DISCUSSION

Previous studies in sarcoidosis have described increased numbers of bronchoalveolar lymphocytes.[18,21–23] The majority of these cells are T cells,[18,21,22] and these T

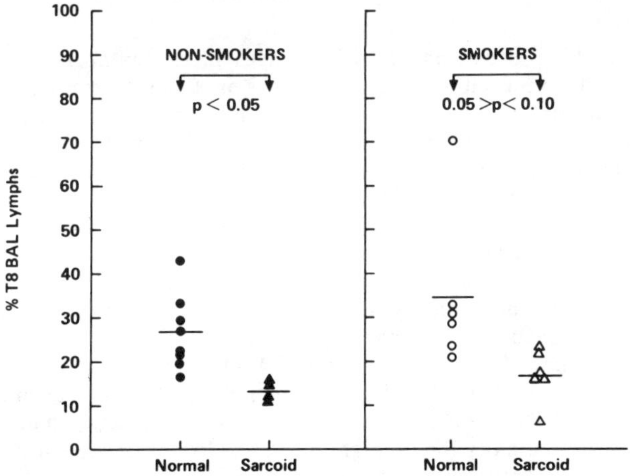

FIGURE 5. Comparison of T8 lymphocytes in normals and sarcoids of similar smoking status.

cells are considered to be "activated" for several reasons.[18,19,24,25] Hunninghake and Crystal have shown that BAL fluid from sarcoids with "high-intensity alveoitis" has an increased T4/T8 ratio due to an increase in the proportion of T4 cells and a decrease in the proportion of T8 cells.[11] Similar findings have been reported by Ceuppens *et al.*[26] Patients in these studies were not subclassified according to their cigarette-smoking status, however, and were compared only to nonsmoking control subjects.

The present study confirmed the previous observations that the T4/T8 ratio is increased in sarcoidosis.[11,26] The mechanisms for this altered ratio, however, differed for nonsmoking and smoking sarcoids. In nonsmoking sarcoids a decreased number of T8 cells accounted for the increase in the ratio whereas in smoking sarcoids a decreased number of T4 cells and an increased number of T8 cells accounted for the decrease in the ratio. Increases in the number of T4 cells in sarcoidosis were not observed in our studies, in contrast to the findings of Hunninghake and Crystal.[11] Whether these are methodological differences or differences due to different patient populations is unclear.

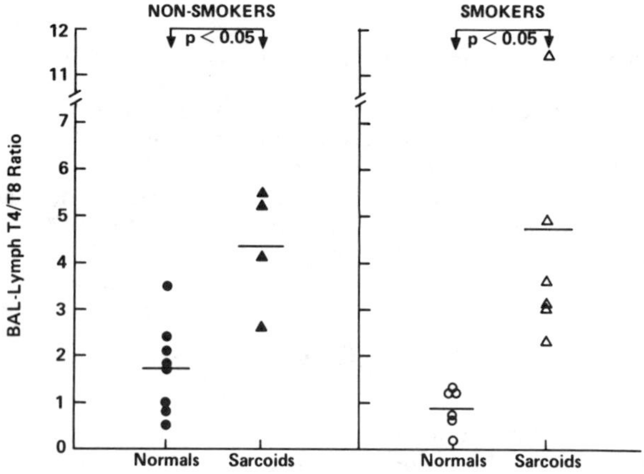

FIGURE 6. Comparison of T4/T8 ratios in normals and sarcoids of similar smoking status.

Cigarette smoking is associated with changes in the numbers of cells and the relative sizes of different subpopulations of cells in fluids recovered by BAL from normals.[5–10] Pulmonary alveolar macrophages are present in abnormally high numbers and constitute an abnormally large portion of the total number of cells in BAL fluid recovered from smoking normals.[5,6] Lymphocytes from smoking normals, on the other hand, are present in numbers no different from those of nonsmoking normals,[6] but constitute an abnormally low portion of the total number of cells.[5,6,10] T lymphocytes may be present in abnormally large number,[6] but do not constitute an abnormally large portion of the total number of cells. The cell-mediated immune response of the T cells of smokers, as measured by *in vitro* responses to the mitogens phytohemagglutinin and concanavalin A, is impaired.[10]

In the present study, decreased numbers of T4 cells were found in smoking normals. Costabel and co-workers have described similar findings for T4 cells and have found increased numbers of T8 cells in smoking normals.[27] This imbalance in local pulmonary helper/suppressor regulatory forces might be implicated in the propensity to infections and malignancy in cigarette smokers.

The present study has investigated the effects of cigarette smoking on T cell populations in both normals and sarcoids. Cigarette smoking profoundly alters these populations, but affects normals and sarcoids differently. We conclude that if helper/suppressor T cell ratios in sarcoidosis are to be properly interpreted, the smoking habits of patients must be taken into account.

ACKNOWLEDGMENTS

The technical assistance of Mrs. Karen Brousseau and Mrs. Diana Flitcraft and the expert typing skills of Mrs. Janice Hodges are greatly appreciated.

REFERENCES

1. Crystal, R. G., J. E. Gadek, J. D. Fulmer, V. J. Ferrans, B. R. Line & G. W. Hunninghake. 1984. Interstitial lung disease: Current concepts of pathogenesis, staging and therapy. Am. J. Med. **70:** 542-568.
2. Crystal, R. G., P. B. Bitterman, S. I. Rennard, A. J. Hance & B. A. Keogh. 1984. Interstitial lung diseases of unknown cause: Disorders characterized by chronic inflammation of the lower respiratory tract. N. Engl. J. Med. **310:** 154-166, 235-244.
3. Daniele, R. P., J. H. Dauber & M. D. Rossman. 1980. Immunologic abnormalities in sarcoidosis. Ann. Intern. Med. **92:** 406-416.
4. Hunninghake, G. W., K. C. Garrett, H. B. Richerson, J. C. Fantone, P. A. Ward, S. I. Rennard, P. B. Bitterman & R. G. Crystal. 1984. Pathogenesis of the granulomatous lung diseases. Am. Rev. Respir. Dis. **130:** 476-496.
5. Reynolds, H. Y. & H. H. Newball. 1974. Analysis of proteins and respiratory cells obtained from human lungs by bronchial lavage. J. Lab. Clin. Med. **84:** 559-573.
6. Warr, G. A., R. R. Martin, C. L. Holleman & B. S. Criswell. 1976. Classification of bronchial lymphocytes from nonsmokers and smokers. Am. Rev. Respir. Dis. **113:** 96-100.
7. Martin, R. R. 1973. Altered morphology and increased acid hydrolase content of pulmonary macrophages from cigarette smokers. Am. Rev. Respir. Dis. **107:** 596-601.
8. Warr, G. A. & R. R. Martin. 1973. *In vitro* migration of human alveolar macrophages: Effects of cigarette smoking. Infect. Immun. **8:** 222-227.
9. Laughter, A. H., R. R. Martin & J. J. Twomey. 1977. Lymphoproliferative responses to antigen mediated by human pulmonary alveolar macrophages. J. Lab. Clin. Med. **89:** 1326-1332..
10. Daniele, R. P., J. H. Dauber, M. D. Altose, D. T. Rowlands, Jr. & D. J. Gorenberg. 1977. Lymphocyte studies in asymptomatic cigarette smokers: Comparison between lung and peripheral blood. Am. Rev. Respir. Dis. **116:** 997-1005.
11. Hunninghake, G. W. & R. G. Crystal. 1981. Pulmonary sarcoidosis: A disorder mediated by excess helper T-lymphocyte activity at sites of disease activity. N. Engl. J. Med. **305:** 429-434.
12. Line, B. R., G. W. Hunninghake, B. A. Keogh, A. E. Jones, G. S. Johnson & R. G. Crystal. 1981. Gallium-67 scanning to stage the alveolitis of sarcoidosis: Correlation with clinical studies, pulmonary function studies, and bronchoalveolar lavage. Am. Rev. Respir. Dis. **123:** 440-446.
13. Lieberman, J. 1975. Elevation of serum angiotensin-converting enzyme (ACE) level in sarcoidosis. Am. J. Med. **59:** 365-372.
14. Keogh, B. A., G. W. Hunninghake, B. R. Line & R. G. Crystal. 1983. The alveolitis of pulmonary sarcoidosis: Evaluation of natural history and alveolitis-dependent changes in lung function. Am. Rev. Respir. Dis. **128:** 256-265.

15. LAWRENCE, E. C., R. B. TEAGUE, M. S. GOTTLIEB, S. G. JHINGRAN & J. LIEBERMAN. 1983. Serial changes in markers of disease activity with corticosteroid treatment in sarcoidosis. Am. J. Med. **74:** 747-756.
16. LAWRENCE, E. C., R. R. MARTIN, R. M. BLASE, R. B. TEAGUE, R. J. AWE, R. K. WILSON, W. J. DEATON, K. BLOOM, S. D. GREENBERG & P. M. STEVENS. 1980. Increased bronchoalveolar IgG-secreting cells in interstitial lung diseases. N. Engl. J. Med. **302:** 1186-1188.
17. LAWRENCE, E. C., R. M. BLASE, R. R. MARTIN & P. M. STEVENS. 1978. Immunoglobulin secreting cells in normal bronchial lavage fluids. J. Clin. Invest. **62:** 832-835.
18. DAUBER, J. H., M. S. ROSSMAN & R. P. DANIELE. 1979. Bronchoalveolar cell populations in acute sarcoidosis: Observations in smoking and nonsmoking patients. J. Lab. Clin. Med. **94:** 862-871.
19. LY, I. & R. I. MISHELL. 1974. Separation of mouse spleen cells by passage through columns of Sephadex G-10. J. Immunol. Methods **5:** 239-247.
20. REINHERZ, E. L. & S. F. SCHLOSSMAN. 1980. Regulation of the immune response-inducer and -suppressor T-lymphocyte subsets in human beings. N. Engl. J. Med. **303:** 370-373.
21. HUNNINGHAKE, G. W., J. D. FULMER, R. C. YOUNG, J. E. GADEK & R. G. CRYSTAL. 1979. Localization of the immune response in sarcoidosis. Am. Rev. Respir. Dis. **120:** 49-57.
22. WEINBERGER, S. E., J. A. KELMAN, N. A. ELSON, R. C. YOUNG, JR., H. Y. REYNOLDS, J. D. FULMER & R. G. CRYSTAL. 1978. Bronchoalveolar lavage in interstitial lung disease. Ann. Intern. Med. **89:** 459-466.
23. ROTH, C., G. J. HUCHON, A. ARNOUX, G. STANISLAS-LEGUERN, J. H. MARSAC & J. CHRÉTIEN. 1978. Bronchoalveolar cells in advanced pulmonary sarcoidosis. Am. Rev. Respir. Dis. **124:** 9-12.
24. PINKSTON, P., P. B. BITTERMAN & R. G. CRYSTAL. 1983. Spontaneous release of interleukin-2 by lung T lymphocytes in active pulmonary sarcoidosis. N. Engl. J. Med. **308:** 793-800.
25. HUNNINGHAKE, G. W., G. N. BEDELL, D. C. ZAVALA, M. MONICK & M. BRADY. 1983. Role of interleukin-2 release by lung T-cells in active pulmonary sarcoidosis. Am. Rev. Respir. Dis. **128:** 634-638.
26. CEUPPENS, J. L., L. M. LACQUET, G. MARIEN, M. DEMEDTS, A. VAN DEN EECKHOUT & E. STEVENS. 1983. Alveolar T-cell subsets in pulmonary sarcoidosis: Correlation with disease activity and effect of steroid treatment. Am. Rev. Respir. Dis. **129:** 563-568.
27. COSTABEL, U., C. REUTER, K. J. BROSS, K. H. RUHLE & H. MATTHYS. 1984. Alterations in immunoregulatory T cells in smoking are more pronounced in bronchoalveolar lavage fluid than in blood. Am. Rev. Respir. Dis. **129:** A17.

Pulmonary Function Tests, Serum Angiotensin-converting Enzyme Levels, and Clinical Findings as Prognostic Indicators in Sarcoidosis[a]

RICHARD FINKEL, ALVIN S. TEIRSTEIN,[b]
REBECCA LEVINE, LEE K. BROWN,
AND ALBERT MILLER

Department of Medicine
Mount Sinai Medical Center
New York, New York 10029

INTRODUCTION

The majority of patients who present with radiographic stage 1 sarcoidosis experience a favorable prognosis, without treatment. Approximately 80% of the chest radiographs of these patients will stabilize or completely clear. Of the remaining 20%, progression to a worse radiographic stage with concomitant impairment of pulmonary function and, in a small number, death due to pulmonary insufficiency, will occur. A reliable prognostic indicator early in the course of the disease which might separate those who deteriorate from those who clear spontaneously would be of great value in monitoring and treatment planning. Such a marker might identify the small cohort of patients who would reap the greatest benefit from aggressive steroid treatment.

To date, many different parameters have been suggested as indicators of eventual outcome in patients with early sarcoidosis. These include pulmonary function tests (PFT's), serum angiotensin-converting enzyme (SACE) levels, bronchoalveolar lavage (BAL) constituents, gallium-67 scans, race, symptoms, and physical findings (particularly evidence of extrathoracic sarcoidosis).

Previous studies from our laboratories have demonstrated a correlation between radiographic staging of sarcoidosis and the pattern of physiologic abnormalities.[1,2] In general, pulmonary function deteriorates from radiographic stage 1 to radiographic stage 3 disease, although pulmonary function abnormalities are not uncommon even in radiographic stage 1 sarcoidosis. It has been proposed that pulmonary dysfunction in this "early" stage may herald a poorer outcome.

SACE levels have been noted to parallel disease "activity" and have been proposed as a guide to therapy. Similarly, an elevated percentage of lymphocytes in the BAL

[a]This work was supported by the Catherine and Henry Gaisman Foundation and the Pulmonary Academic Award HL00985-05.

[b]Address for correspondence: Department of Medicine, Mount Sinai Medical Center, One Gustav L. Levy Place, Annenberg 24-30, New York, New York 10029.

fluid and gallium-67 citrate uptake in the lung parenchyma have been utilized as prognostic indicators. Also, it has been proposed that race may influence prognosis, with blacks exhibiting a more chronic and debilitating course than whites. Finally, the presence of symptoms or sarcoidal involvement of three or more organ systems has been said to be a marker of poor prognosis.

To assess the value of data, easily obtained at the first patient visit, as indicators of prognosis, this study compared the variables of age, sex, race, PFT's, SACE level, clinical symptoms, and presence of extrathoracic sarcoidosis in two groups. Group A consisted of 46 patients with radiographic stage 1 sarcoidosis whose chest radiographs cleared or remained unchanged; group B consisted of 22 patients who progressed from stage 1 to stages 2 or 3. BAL constitutents and gallium-67 scanning were not included in this study.

METHODS

A retrospective study was undertaken of 68 patients with Kveim test- and/or biopsy-proven sarcoidosis attending the out-patient departments of the Mount Sinai Medical Center who initially presented with radiographic stage 1 disease. Radiographic staging was made according to the classic patterns: stage 1, bilateral hilar (and often paratracheal) lymph node enlargement with clear lung fields; stage 2, bilateral hilar adenopathy with lung mottling; stage 3, pulmonary mottling without evidence of hilar adenopathy. A normal chest radiograph was designated as stage 0. All patients had history and physical examinations, PFT's, and chest roentgenographs performed at the time of their first examination. Twenty-two patients had SACE level determinations. Serial examinations and studies were performed for a period of at least 2 years.

Forced vital capacity (FVC); forced expiratory volume in 1 second (FEV_1); forced expiratory flow, 25-75% ($FEF_{25\text{-}75\%}$); and maximum voluntary ventilation (MVV) were obtained by using a Fleisch pneumotachygraph and were plotted against time to obtain a spirographic tracing. Single-breath carbon monoxide diffusion capacity (D_LCO_{SB}) was obtained by a modification of the Ogilvie method.[3] SACE levels were determined in 22 patients by the method of Lieberman.[4] SACE levels above 35 units were considered abnormal.

For pulmonary function, abnormal tests results were defined statistically at the lower 95% confidence limit using the predicted values of Morris as modified by Miller *et al.*[5] for FVC, FEV_1, and $FEF_{25\text{-}75\%}$, and the value of Miller *et al.* for D_LCO_{SB}.[6] For MVV, abnormalities were defined as less than 80% of the predicted values of Baldwin *et al.*[7]

The clinical symptoms, cough, dyspnea (two flights, five blocks), wheezing, and chest pain, were recorded both by the examining physician and by the pulmonary laboratory technician at the time of presentation in 60 of the 68 patients.

STATISTICAL METHODS

Two-sided *t* tests for age and continuous values of the pulmonary function variables (FVC, FEV_1, $FEF_{25\text{-}75\%}$, MVV, FEV_1/FVC, and D_LCO_{SB}) and SACE were done to evaluate the differences between the two groups. A significance level of .01 was used to adjust for multiple testing. The values of the pulmonary function tests were classified as normal or abnormal based on the above criteria for a post-hoc analysis of their individual relationships to stage 2 progression using the chi-square and Fisher's exact tests when appropriate.[8] The same tests were applied to determine the association between ethnic group, sex, the presence of specific symptoms and extrathoracic sarcoidosis, and group membership. The relationship between the presence of any symptom and extrathoracic sarcoidosis and the group was similarly tested. Chi-square tests to find possible trends were done to determine the presence of a gradient in these relationships.[9]

RESULTS

Forty-six of the 68 patients with radiographic stage 1 sarcoidosis at presentation exhibited clearing or stable radiographs throughout the study (group A). The remaining

TABLE 1. Comparison of Sarcoidosis Patients in Groups A and B at Initial Presentation

	Group A[b]			Group B[c]			
Variable[a]	N	Mean	SD	N	Mean	SD	Significance[d]
Age (years)	45	37.0	9.8	22	37.5	9.1	.850
FVC	45	91.7	15.7	21	87.4	14.9	.302
FEV_1	44	92.2	16.6	20	86.6	16.3	.219
$FEF_{25-75\%}$	36	82.2	27.9	16	74.5	27.2	.358
MVV	42	106.6	27.7	16	97.5	24.5	.254
D_LCO	31	82.4	19.8	15	75.6	17.9	.266
FEV_1/FVC	45	80.1	6.5	20	78.4	7.7	.358
SACE (U/ml)	13	37.1	14.8	9	29.6	13.8	.122

[a] The pulmonary function values are expressed as percentages of those that would have been predicted.
[b] Patients who remained in stage 1 or whose radiographs cleared.
[c] Patients who progressed to stage 2 or stage 3.
[d] The p value associated with Student's t test.

22 patients progressed to stage 2 or stage 3 (group B). The two groups showed no significant differences in age, sex, ethnic group, the presence or number of sites of extrathoracic sarcoidosis, SACE level, FVC, FEV_1, $FEF_{25-75\%}$, MVV, or D_LCO_{SB}. Although PFT's and SACE levels tended to be higher in group A, the differences were not significant (TABLES 1-5).

Since many individual variations in PFT's occurred, an analysis of the number of patients with PFT abnormalities in groups A and B was undertaken. This study also failed to reveal a statistical difference in pulmonary function between the two groups.

There was a significant association between the presence of any symptom at presentation and the progression from radiographic stage 1 to radiographic stage 2: 23 out of 39 patients (59%) in group A and 19 out of 21 patients (90%) in group B exhibited symptoms (TABLE 6). The probability of progressing to stage 2 increased significantly with the number of symptoms at presentation (TABLE 7). The presence

TABLE 2. Comparison of Sarcoidosis Patients in Groups A and B by Ethnic Group[a]

	Number of Patients[b]		
	Group A	Group B	Total
White	11 (24.4)	5 (22.7)	16
Black	23 (51.1)	12 (54.6)	35
Hispanic	8 (17.7)	5 (22.7)	13

[a] $\chi_2^2 = 1.65$; $p = 9.21$.
[b] Percentages are shown in parentheses.

TABLE 3. Comparison of Sarcoidosis Patients in Groups A and B by Sex[a]

	Number of Patients[b]		
	Group A	Group B	Total
Male	9 (20.5)	4 (18.2)	13
Female	35 (79.5)	18 (81.8)	53

[a] Fisher's exact test $p = .5523$.
[b] Percentages are shown in parentheses.

TABLE 4. Comparison of Extrathoracic Sarcoidosis in Patients in Groups A and B[a]

	Extrathoracic Sarcoidosis		
	Absent	Present	Total
Number of patients[b]			
Group A	15 (41)	22 (59)	37
Group B	8 (36)	14 (64)	22

[a] $\chi_2^2 = .102$; $p = .750$.
[b] Percentages are shown in parentheses.

TABLE 5. Comparison of the Number of Extrathoracic Sites of Sarcoidosis in Groups A and B[a]

	Number of Extrathoracic Sites				
	None	One	Two	Three or More	Total
Number of Patients					
Group A	15	9	7	6	37
Group B	8	5	8	1	22

[a] χ_1^2 for the trend $= .004$; $p = .9516$.

TABLE 6. Comparison of Sarcoidosis Patients in Groups A and B by Symptoms[a]

	Symptoms		
	Absent	Present	Total
Number of patients[b]			
Group A	16 (41)	23 (59)	39
Group B	2 (10)	19 (90)	21

[a] χ_1^2 $p = .0069$.
[b] Percentages are shown in parentheses.

of cough was the most important single symptom for distinguishing group A from group B (TABLE 8).

DISCUSSION

At the Fifth International Congress on Sarcoidosis, in Prague, we noted that the usual outcome of sarcoidosis was favorable.[10] Sixty-four percent of our first 311 patients improved and 20% remained unchanged; however, 16% worsened and 50% of these died. Many investigators have searched diligently for a marker or markers which would identify those patients at risk for an unfavorable course at the time of their initial presentation. The simple study presented here suggests that demographic data, the presence of extrathoracic disease on physical examination, SACE levels, and initial pulmonary function values offer no clue as to which patient with sarcoidosis presenting with radiographic stage 1 disease will follow a salutory course and which will grow worse.

Israel and Washburne noted more symptoms, impaired vital capacity, a greater prevalence of extrathoracic disease, and a lesser frequency of complete clearing of disease in blacks when compared with whites in Philadelphia.[11] A similar prevalence of extrathoracic sarcoidosis in blacks was noted in New York, but the ultimate outcome in blacks and whites was the same in that study.[12] In the study presented here, there was no greater frequency of progression from stage 1 to stage 2 radiographs among blacks when compared with whites.

The importance of extrathoracic sarcoidosis is still unclear. The concept that single or multiple extrathoracic organ involvement is indicative of a poorer prognosis was

TABLE 7. Comparison of the Number of Symptoms in Groups A and B[a]

	Number of Symptoms				
	None	One	Two	Three	Total
Number of patients					
Group A	16	8	9	6	39
Group B	2	6	6	7	21

[a] χ_1^2 for the trend $= 5.712$; $p = .0168$.

not confirmed by this investigation. Since worsening of disease was defined as radiographic progression, and since progression of sarcoidosis can occur at extrathoracic sites without concomitant worsening of the chest radiograph, it is possible that some patients with advancing sarcoidosis were undetected in this study.

Elevated SACE levels have been heralded as an indicator of "active" sarcoidosis. Numerous studies have emphasized the value of SACE levels as a guide to adrenocorticosteroid therapy in sarcoidosis.[13-16] Since, in those studies, patients with elevated SACE levels have been shown to be susceptible to progression of disease, it is understandable that some physicians interpret an elevated SACE level as an indication for adrenocorticosteroid therapy. However, many patients with "active" sarcoidosis have normal SACE levels. Recognizing this, DeRemee and Rohrbach have proposed that even in patients with normal SACE, levels will become lower in patients undergoing adrenocorticosteroid therapy, and that SACE levels remain a good guide to the efficacy of treatment.[17] Other studies have shown a poor correlation of SACE levels and other indicators of sarcoidosis activity, particularly BAL constituents[18,19] and gallium-67 scans.[20,21] The investigation presented here reveals no correlation between initial SACE levels and radiographic progression of sarcoidosis.

Our finding of an insignificant trend toward worsening pulmonary function in patients who later progressed from stage 1 to stage 2 radiographs follows the general rule that pulmonary dysfunction parallels radiographic progression. There was no significant difference, however, in the initial FVC, FEV_1, FEV_1/FVC, $FEF_{25-75\%}$, D_LCO_{SB}, and MVV values between groups A and B.

TABLE 8. Comparison of the Presence of Cough in Groups A and B[a]

	Cough		
	Absent	Present	Total
Number of Patients			
Group A	29 (74)	10 (26)	39
Group B	7 (33)	14 (67)	21

[a] χ_1^2 p = .0024; p = .0019.

Only the presence of symptoms at initial presentation appeared to be a harbinger of poor prognosis. Fifty-nine percent of the 39 patients whose radiographs did not worsen had the symptoms cough, dyspnea, wheezing, and/or chest pain whereas 19 of the 21 patients whose radiographs progressed had one or more of these complaints (p=.0098). Specifically, the symptom cough was most closely linked to a poorer prognosis (p=.019). In addition, in a test for a trend, an increasing number of symptoms at presentation indicated a poorer prognosis (p=.017). There was a large overlap, however, of individuals with symptoms in both groups obscuring the specificity and sensitivity of symptoms alone as a marker of poor prognosis. Obviously, the prognosis for an individual patient with sarcoidosis cannot be predicted on the basis of symptoms alone.

REFERENCES

1. MILLER, A., M. CHUANG, A. S. TEIRSTEIN & L. E. SILTZBACH. 1976. Pulmonary function in stage I and II pulmonary sarcoidosis. Ann. N.Y. Acad. Sci. **278:** 292-300.

2. MILLER, A., K. EINSTEIN, J. THORNTON, A. S. TEIRSTEIN & L. E. SILTZBACH. 1980. Physiologic classification and staging of intrathoracic sarcoidosis. *In* Eighth International Conference on Sarcoidosis and Other Granulomatous Diseases. W. Jones Williams & B. H. Davies, Eds.: 331-336. Alpha Omega. Cardiff.
3. OGILVIE, C. M., R. E. FORSTER, W. S. BLAKEMORE & J. W. MORTON. 1957. A standardized breath-holding technique for the clinical measurement of the diffusing capacity of the lung for carbon monoxide. J. Clin. Invest. **36:** 1-17.
4. LIEBERMAN, J. 1975. Elevation of serum angiotensin-converting enzyme (ACE) level in sarcoidosis. Am. J. Med. **59:** 365-372.
5. MILLER, A., J. C. THORNTON, H. SMITH, JR. & J. F. MORRIS. 1980. Spirometric "abnormality" in a normal male reference population: Further analysis of the 1971 Oregon survey. Am. J. Ind. Med. **1:** 55-68.
6. MILLER, A., J. C. THORNTON, R. WARSHAW, H. ANDERSON, A. S. TEIRSTEIN & I. J. SELIKOFF. 1983. Single-breath diffusing capacity in a representative sample of the population of Michigan, a large industrial state. Am. Rev. Respir. Dis. **127:** 270-277.
7. BALDWIN, E. DEF., A. COURNAND & D. W. RICHARDS, JR. 1948. Pulmonary insufficiency. I. Physiologic classification, clinical methods of analysis, standard values in normal subjects. Medicine **27:** 243-278.
8. FLEISS, J. L. 1981. Statistical Methods for Rates and Proportions. 2nd edit.: 24-26. Wiley. New York, NY.
9. FLEISS, J. L. 1981. Statistical Methods for Rates and Proportions. 2nd edit.: 143-146. Wiley. New York, NY.
10. TEIRSTEIN, A. S., L. E. SILTZBACH, H. W. BERGER & D. BARTHOLD. 1971. Causes of death in sarcoidosis: The prognostic significance of the presenting chest radiograph. *In* Fifth International Conference on Sarcoidosis. L. Levinsky & F. Macholda, Eds.: 541-545. Universita Karlova Praha. Prague.
11. ISRAEL, H. L. & J. D. WASHBURNE. 1980. Characteristics of sarcoidosis in black and in white patients: Analysis of 162 recent cases. *In* Eighth International Conference on Sarcoidosis and Other Granulomatous Diseases. W. Jones Williams & B. H. Davies, Eds.: 497-507. Alpha Omega. Cardiff.
12. TEIRSTEIN, A. S., L. E. SILTZBACH & H. BERGER. 1976. Patterns of sarcoidosis in three population groups in New York City. Ann. N.Y. Acad. Sci. **278:** 371-376.
13. LIEBERMAN, J., L. A. SCHLEISSNER, A. NOSAL, A. SASTRE & F. S. MISHKIN. 1983. Clinical correlations of serum angiotensin-converting enzyme (ACE) in sarcoidosis: A longitudinal study of serum ACE, gallium scans, chest roentgenograms, and pulmonary function. Chest **84:** 522-528.
14. FANBURG, B. L., M. D. SCHOENBERGER, B. BACHUS & G. L. SNIDER. 1976. Elevated serum angiotensin I-converting enzyme in sarcoidosis. Am. Rev. Respir. Dis. **114:** 525-528.
15. GRÖNHAGEN-RISKA, C., O. SELROOS & M. NIEMSTRO. 1980. Serum levels as monitors of disease activity in corticosteroid-treated sarcoidosis. Eur. J. Respir. Dis. **61:** 113-122.
16. ROULSTON, J. E., G. I. O'MALLEY & J. G. DOUGLAS. 1984. Effects of prednisolone on angiotensin-converting enzyme activity. Thorax **39:** 356-360.
17. DEREMEE, R. A. & M. S. ROHRBACH. 1984. Normal serum angiotensin-converting enzyme activity in patients with newly diagnosed sarcoidosis. Chest **85:** 45-48.
18. CRYSTAL, R. G. 1981. Pulmonary sarcoidosis: A disease characterized and perpetuated by activated lung T-lymphocytes. Ann. Intern. Med. **94:** 73-94.
19. ROSSI, G. A., O. SACCO, E. COSULICH, G. DAMINAI, G. CORTE, A. BARGELLESI & C. RAVAZZONI. 1984. Pulmonary sarcoidosis: Excess of helper T lymphocytes and T cell subset imbalance at sites of disease activity. Thorax **39:** 143-149.
20. LINE, B. R., G. W. HUNNINGHAKE, B. A. KEOGH, A. E. JONES, G. S. JOHNSTON & R. G. CRYSTAL. 1981. Gallium-67 scanning to stage the alveolitis of sarcoidosis: Correlation with clinical studies, pulmonary function studies, and bronchoalveolar lavage. Am. Rev. Respir. Dis. **123:** 440-446.
21. SCHOENBERGER, C. I., B. R. LINE, B. A. KEOGH, G. W. HUNNINGHAKE & R. G. CRYSTAL. 1982. Lung inflammation in sarcoidosis: Comparison of serum angiotensin-converting enzyme levels with bronchoalveolar lavage and gallium-67 scanning assessment of the T lymphocyte alveolitis. Thorax **37:** 19-25.

Elevated Serum Immunoglobulin G Levels and Bronchoalveolar Lymphocytosis as Predictors of Clinical Course in Pulmonary Sarcoidosis[a]

D. Y. BELL,[b,c] S. M. JOHNSON,[d] AND C. A. PIANTADOSI[d]

[c]*Department of Pediatrics*
and
[d]*Department of Medicine*
Duke University Medical Center
Durham, North Carolina 27710

INTRODUCTION

Sarcoidosis is a granulomatous disease which in approximately 90% of cases affects the lung.[1,2] Its cause is undetermined, and its course in individual patients varies widely. Resolution of the disease may be spontaneous, or in association with corticosteroid therapy. In a small number of affected patients, the disease will produce progressive, irreversible deterioration in pulmonary function resulting in permanent impairment or death.[3] In managing patients with sarcoidosis, it would be useful to identify those patients likely to require corticosteroid therapy before permanent loss of pulmonary function and to know when a successful response has occurred. In the past, physicians have made such clinical evaluations based upon a history of symptoms, chest radiographic findings, and the results of pulmonary function tests. More recently, it has been suggested that certain measurements in blood and in fluids obtained by bronchoalveolar lavage (BAL) may provide a more sensitive index of disease activity in a given patient.[4-12] Because the irreversible loss in lung function due to progressive fibrosis is preceded and caused by a period of alveolitis,[13] or active disease, parameters which indicate the presence and intensity of that alveolitis in the lung could provide such a sensitive index. For example, both serum immunoglobulin (Ig)[6-12,14] and an-

[a]This study was supported in part by Grant 5 P50 HL 14212 from the National Heart, Lung, and Blood Institute and by Grant RR-30 from the Division of Research Resources, General Clinical Research Centers Program, of the National Institutes of Health. Data were managed and analyzed using the CLINFO Data Analysis System.

[b]Address for correspondence and reprint requests: Box 3841, Duke University Medical Center, Durham, North Carolina 27710.

giotensin-converting enzyme (ACE)[5,10,12,15,16] levels are increased in many patients with sarcoidosis, and decreases in serum gamma globulin or ACE levels have been shown to correlate with improved pulmonary function in patients.[5,8,9,11,12] This suggests that initial higher values for these measurements in a patient's serum might predict the need for steroid therapy and a positive treatment response. Others have suggested that an increased percentage of lymphocytes[10,17,18] or of a certain lymphocyte subset[4,16,19,20] in a differential count of cells obtained by BAL identified patients likely to deteriorate if untreated. The ability to identify such patients in a population could enable the physician to use corticosteroid therapy more selectively, and to evaluate its effectiveness with greater sensitivity.

METHODS

We report the results of a study to determine the accuracy of two measurements in predicting the clinical course of sarcoidosis: 1) the serum IgG concentration and 2) the lymphocyte percentage (%LYM), that is, the percentage of cells obtained by BAL that were lymphocytes, as determined from a differential cell count. Thirty-three patients underwent initial and serial evaluations (average number of evaluations/patient, 3; average interval between evaluations, 7.2 months). Twenty-seven patients were black, 18 were female. Twenty-six patients were nonsmokers; the remaining seven patients had a mean smoking history of 10.3 pack-years. One patient was already receiving corticosteroid therapy when the study began. Initial and subsequent evaluations included physical examination, pulmonary function testing, and BAL.

Lavage was performed by the instillation of five aliquots of 20 ml of normal saline solution through a fiberoptic bronchoscope wedged in a subsegment of either the right middle lobe (52 cases), right lower lobe (1 case), or lingula (5 cases). Recovery was by gentle suction, and averaged 52 ml. Lavage cell differential counts were obtained from cytocentrifuge preparations after Wilson's staining. Serum was prepared from a blood sample obtained at the time of lavage.

The serum concentration of IgG was measured by radial immunodiffusion in agarose gel,[21] and was expressed as a percentage of total serum protein as determined by a Lowry assay.[22]

In order to test the ability of either serum IgG or %LYM in BAL fluid to predict course, we applied the following criteria to each. Serum IgG was defined as normal ($<20\%$ of total protein) based upon a mean normal value of $14.2 \pm 3.1\%$ established in our laboratory.[23] The %LYM in BAL fluid was considered indicative of low- ($\leq 28\%$) or high- ($>28\%$) intensity alveolitis based upon the findings of others.[17,18]

Pulmonary function was assessed by standard spirometry, helium lung volume, and single-breath carbon monoxide diffusion (DL_{CO}) determinations. Using standard physiologic criteria, 8 patients had normal pulmonary functions, 16 had mild to moderate restrictive impairment, and 9 had severe restrictive impairment. Eleven of 33 had a forced expiratory volume in 1 sec (FEV_1)/forced vital capacity (FVC) ratio indicative of obstruction (<0.72). Changes in DL_{CO}, which was measured as a percentage of the value that would have been predicted, were used to describe course across an interval between evaluations. Positive or negative changes of $>10\%$ were used to define improvement or deterioration, respectively. Patients whose DL_{CO} did not change by $>10\%$ from one evaluation to the next were considered stable.

The decision to treat patients with corticosteroids over an interval between evaluations was made by an attending physician blinded to the results of serum or BAL fluid analyses. No attempt was made to control corticosteroid administration, and both alternate and daily prednisone regimens were used. Of the 55 intervals studied, 15 were completely without corticosteroid treatment while during 40 intervals patients received steroid therapy.

RESULTS AND DISCUSSION

When intervals without corticosteroid therapy were evaluated based upon the change in DL_{CO}, it was found that there were six intervals of improved diffusing capacity, five intervals of stable diffusing capacity, and four intervals of worsened diffusing capacity (TABLE 1). In all stable cases, initial DL_{CO} findings were normal

TABLE 1. Changes in DL_{CO} in Patients during Intervals with and without Corticosteroid Therapy

		Serum IgG Level[b]		%LYM[b]	
Interval Type	DL_{CO}[a]	Normal[c]	High	Low[c]	High
No treatment	Increased	4 (1)[d]	1	2	3 (1)
	Stable	4	1	2	3
	Decreased	3	1	4	0
Treatment	Increased	11 (4)	3 (1)	5 (1)	9 (4)
	Stable	3 (4)	4 (4)	2 (3)	5 (5)
	Decreased	0 (3)	0 (3)	0 (3)	0 (3)

[a] DL_{CO} was considered to have increased or decreased if the experimental values for it, expressed as percentages of the predicted value, rose or fell 10% or more over an interval, respectively.

[b] Values indicate the number of patients that were untreated in the prior interval; values in parentheses, the number of patients that were treated in the prior interval.

[c] Serum IgG values $\leq 20\%$ of the total amount of protein were normal; values $> 20\%$ were high.

[d] The %LYM in BAL was defined as high if $> 28\%$ of all BAL cells were lymphocytes; values $\leq 28\%$ were defined as low.

(mean: 93.2%, range: 87-110%). If changes in DL_{CO} had been predicted based upon the initial serum IgG concentration, 9 of 11 improved or stable intervals (82%) and 1 of 4 periods of decrease (25%) would have been correctly identified. Two patients with high serum IgG concentration did not deteriorate over the interval. One maintained a moderate increase in IgG (24%) and remained stable at good pulmonary function whereas the second improved. In the latter case, serum IgG fell across the interval (28.1 to 21.9%) but did not enter the normal range. Of three patients with normal serum IgG who decreased their DL_{CO} over the interval, two would not have been classified as having deteriorated if other physiologic criteria, changes in FVC or total lung capacity (TLC), had been included in the evaluation. In these two cases, it is unlikely that placement in the group of deteriorated patients is a correct description of course. In all other cases, classification of course did not change when changes in FVC and TLC were considered in addition to those in DL_{CO}. Given 13 intervals of improvement or stability at normal pulmonary function, 11 were correctly predicted (sensitivity: 85%) while 1 of 2 intervals of deterioration was identified (specificity: 50%), for a predictive accuracy for 12 of 15 intervals of 80%.

When the ability of %LYM in BAL fluids was similarly evaluated, it was found that normal initial counts occurred in 4 of 11 cases (36%) where improvement or stability in DL_{CO} was seen. Initial high %LYM's were seen in seven patients who did not deteriorate over the interval between evaluations. Of these seven intervals, three reflected falling counts, three had stable high counts, and in one patient the %LYM increased. In the four cases where counts decreased, none fell to 28% or below. In the four intervals where a marked decline in DL_{CO} occurred, all patients had a normal %LYM at the start of the interval. In two cases, %LYM increased by the end of the interval, and one of the increases moved the count into the high range. In the two cases where the %LYM remained normal, the FVC and TLC findings did not confirm deterioration, as discussed above in consideration of serum IgG. Therefore, in 6 of 13 intervals where patients improved or maintained normal pulmonary function, the %LYM in BAL fluids correctly predicted course (sensitivity: 46%); in two cases of unequivocal deterioration, the %LYM's were normal (specificity: 0%). The %LYM in BAL thus correctly predicted course over 15 untreated intervals in 6 cases, for an accuracy of 40%.

Across treatment intervals ($N=40$), a change in DL_{CO} indicating improved or stable pulmonary function occurred in 34, or 85%. This is similar to the 87% found across intervals with no treatment. For 25 intervals when patients had initial normal serum IgG values, 3 intervals showed deterioration, and across these the serum IgG increased markedly in two cases. Failure to predict deterioration in these three of six intervals of decreased DL_{CO} is similar to the 50% specificity seen for untreated intervals. Twelve intervals began with high serum IgG values but did not result in deterioration. In eight cases, IgG fell markedly (2 cases) or returned to normal (6 cases) across the treatment interval while four IgG concentrations remained high and stable or increased. In two of these four cases, the patients, although they had stable DL_{CO}, were stable with impaired diffusing capacity; that is, they maintained DL_{CO}'s of 59% and 56% of the predicted values, respectively. Of 20 intervals of stable DL_{CO} in the study, only these 2 were rated stable and poor, and indicate a failure of corticosteroid therapy to effect improvement rather than a successful steroid response. In one of the four cases, the patient's disease flared in the subsequent interval in spite of renewed steroid therapy, and IgG remained high. For the one remaining patient with an interval where IgG increased, a subsequent evaluation has not been done.

In the group of 40 treatment intervals, 14 had initial %LYM $\leq$28%. Eleven of these intervals resulted in improved or stable, good pulmonary function. Three of six patients who deteriorated had counts of >28%, for a specificity of 50% (versus 0% in the untreated group). Twenty-six intervals were preceded by %LYM which was $\leq$28%, but in only three cases did the course evaluation indicate deterioration. In the other 23 cases, %LYM fell (13 cases) or returned to $\leq$28% (2 cases) across the treatment interval, while in 8 cases they remained stable high or rose. Of these eight cases, three improved in the next interval, although the %LYM did not decrease, one deteriorated with persistent high %LYM, one remained stable at poor pulmonary function, and three patients have not had a subsequent evaluation.

The persistence of high %LYM in patients who remained stable at good pulmonary function or improved pulmonary function has been noted by others.[1,4] In our study, the average %LYM high value which fell changed 1.5% each month. The 33 intervals which began with high %LYM had a mean initial value of 45.3%. To decrease from that initial level at that rate of change until %LYM $\leq$ 28% would require at least 11.5 months, or 1.5 times the mean interval between evaluations. Slow resolution of the pulmonary lymphocytosis in patients with otherwise good clinical course would produce many false positives if %LYM was used to predict deterioration over untreated intervals.

Because of the accuracy (80%) of serum IgG measurements in predicting change in these patients' intervals, it is likely that there is a much better tracking of IgG levels and alveolitis than is seen with BAL lymphocytes. The model drawn in FIGURE 1 summarizes these findings.

CONCLUSIONS

1. Patients with a normal serum IgG level are unlikely to deteriorate if untreated; however, patients with a normal serum IgG level may improve their DL_{CO} if placed on corticosteroid therapy. This is true whether their initial DL_{CO} indicated poor or good pulmonary function.

2. Patients with a high serum IgG level are at risk to deteriorate over the next interval.

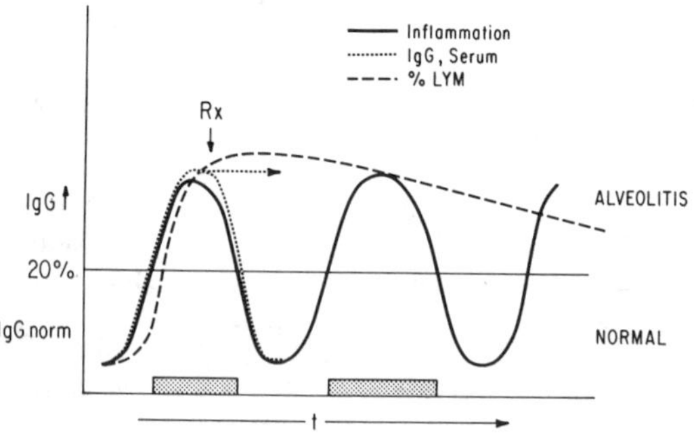

FIGURE 1. A proposed model for the tracking of alveolitis, the serum IgG level, and the %LYM in BAL fluids. The shaded areas under the peaks indicate periods of active disease. As alveolitis increases to a level indicative of active disease, the serum IgG level increases to above normal. The %LYM in BAL fluid increases as well. When disease resolution occurs, the serum IgG level falls to normal; the %LYM in BAL fluid, however, remains markedly abnormal, falling gradually but no longer in phase with either the alveolitis or serum IgG level measurement.

3. Patients with a high serum IgG level who do not deteriorate, whether treated or untreated, tend to have decreases in their serum IgG level over the interval.

4. Patients with a %LYM in their BAL fluid $\leq 28\%$ are at slight risk to deteriorate over the next interval, and may improve their DL_{CO} if treated with corticosteroids.

5. Patients with a higher %LYM in their BAL fluid (>28%) may deteriorate, may remain stable at good or poor pulmonary function, or may improve. Most patients with a high %LYM remain stable at good pulmonary function or improve their pulmonary function whether treated or untreated.

6. Patients with a high %LYM who do not deteriorate tend to decrease their %LYM over the next interval; however, many patients (12/30) maintain or increase their high counts.

REFERENCES

1. MITCHELL, D. N. & J. G. SCADDING. 1974. State of the art: Sarcoidosis. Am. Rev. Respir. Dis. **110:** 774-802.
2. MAYOCK, R. L., P. BERTRAND, C. E. MORRISON & J. H. SCOTT. 1963. Manifestations of sarcoidosis: Analysis of 145 patients with review of nine series selected from the literature. Am. J. Med. **35:** 67-89.

3. ISRAEL, H. L. Prognosis of sarcoidosis. 1970. Ann. Intern. Med. **73:** 1038-1039.
4. CUEPPENS, J. L., L. M. LACQUET, G. MARIËN, M. DEMEDTS, A. VAN DEN EECKHOUT & E. STEVENS. 1983. Alveolar T-cell subsets in pulmonary sarcoidosis. Am. Rev. Respir. Dis. **129:** 563-568.
5. LIEBERMAN, J., A. NOSAL, L. A. SCHLEISSNER & A. SASTRE-FOKEN. 1979. Serum angiotensin-converting enzyme for diagnosis and therapeutic evaluation of sarcoidosis. Am. Rev. Respir. Dis. **120:** 329-335.
6. BELL, D. Y., A. SPOCK, C. A. PIANTADOSI & S. M. JOHNSON. 1983. Serum IgG and ceruloplasmin concentrations as indicators of high intensity alveolitis in the lung in sarcoidosis. Am. Rev. Respir. Dis. **127:** 89.
7. SAINT-REMY, J. M. R., D. N. MITCHELL & P. J. COLE. 1983. Variation in immunoglobulin levels and circulating immune complexes in sarcoidosis. Am. Rev. Respir. Dis. **127:** 23-27.
8. MITCHELL, D. N., J. R. MIKHAIL, M. TURNER-WARWICK & I. SUTHERLAND. 1977. Immunoglobulin levels in patients with sarcoidosis. Z. Erkr. Atmungsorgane **149:** 247-252.
9. CELIKOGLU, S., L. O. VIEIRA & L. E. SILTZBACH. 1971. Serum immunoglobulin levels in sarcoidosis. *In* Fifth International Conference on Sarcoidosis. L. Levinský & F. Macholda, Eds.: 168-170. Universita Karlova. Prague.
10. VALEYRE, D., G. SAUMON, R. GEORGES, J. L. KEMENY, D. BLADIER, J. AMOUROUX, J. PRÉ & J. P. BATTESTI. 1984. The relationship between disease duration and noninvasive pulmonary explorations in sarcoidosis with erythema nodosum. Am. Rev. Respir. Dis. **129:** 938-943.
11. LECLERC, P., D. DUCHASSAING, M. CAMBIELAU, F. CAPRON, B. LEBEAU, M. LECLERC & J. ROCHEMAURE. 1984. Cytology and protein study of broncho-alveolar fluid in predicting sarcoidosis activity. Am. Rev. Respir. Dis. **127:** 63.
12. LAWRENCE, E. C., R. B. TEAGUE, M. S. GOTTLEIB & S. G. JHINGRAN. 1983. Serial changes in markers of disease activity with corticosteroid treatment in sarcoidosis. Am. J. Med. **74:** 747-756.
13. ROSEN, Y., T. J. ATHANASSIADES, S. MOON & H. A. LYONS. 1978. Nongranulomatous interstitial pneumonitis in sarcoidosis: Relationship to the development of epithelioid granulomas. Chest **74:** 122-125.
14. BUCKLEY, C. E., H. NAGAYA & H. O. SIEKER. 1966. Altered immunologic activity in sarcoidosis. Ann. Intern. Med. **64:** 508-520.
15. RADERMECKER, M., M. GUSTIN & P. SAINT-REMY. 1984. Lack of correlation between serum angiotensin-converting enzyme activity and bronchoalveolar lymphocytosis in lung sarcoidosis. Eur. J. Respir. Dis. **65:** 189-195.
16. COSTABEL, U., K. J. BROSS & H. MATTHYS. 1984. Pulmonary sarcoidosis: Assessment of disease activity by lung lymphocyte subpopulations. Klin. Wochenschr. **61:** 349-356.
17. HUNNINGHAKE, G. W., O. KAWANAMI, V. J. FERRANS, R. C. YOUNG, JR., W. C. ROBERTS & R. G. CRYSTAL. 1981. Characterization of the inflammatory and immune effector cells in the lung parenchyma of patients with interstitial lung disease. Am. Rev. Respir. Dis. **123:** 407-412.
18. KEOGH, B. A., G. W. HUNNINGHAKE, B. R. LINE & R. G. CRYSTAL. 1983. The alveolitis of pulmonary sarcoidosis: Evaluation of natural history and alveolitis-dependent changes in lung function. Am. Rev. Respir. Dis. **128:** 256-265.
19. BAUGHMAN, R. P., M. FERNANDEZ, C. H. BOSKEN, J. MANTIL & P. HURTUBISE. 1984. Comparison of gallium-67 scanning, bronchoalveolar lavage, and serum angiotensin-converting enzyme levels in pulmonary sarcoidosis. Am. Rev. Respir. Dis. **129:** 676-681.
20. HUNNINGHAKE, G. W. & R. G. CRYSTAL. 1981. Pulmonary sarcoidosis: A disorder mediated by excess helper T-lymphocyte activity at sites of disease activity. N. Engl. J. Med. **305:** 429-434.
21. MANCINI, G., A. O. CARBONARA & J. F. HEREMANS. 1965. Immunochemical quantitation of antigens by single radial immunodiffusion. Immunochemistry **2:** 235-254.
22. LOWRY, O. H., N. J. ROSEBROUGH, A. L. FARR & R. J. RANDALL. 1951. Protein measurement with the Folin phenol reagent. J. Biol. Chem. **193:** 265-275.
23. BELL, D. Y., J. A. HASEMAN, A. SPOCK, G. MCLENNAN & G. E. R. HOOK. 1981. Plasma proteins of the bronchoalveolar surface of the lungs of smokers and nonsmokers. Am. Rev. Respir. Dis. **124:** 72-79.

Bronchoalveolar Lavage Cell Analysis in Sarcoidosis

A Comparison of Lymphocyte Counts and Clinical Course

S. BUCHALTER, W. APP, L. JACKSON,
D. CHANDLER, R. JACKSON, AND J. FULMER

Department of Medicine
Pulmonary Division
University of Alabama at Birmingham
and
Veterans Administration Medical Center
Birmingham, Alabama 35294

INTRODUCTION

Pulmonary sarcoidosis is a disease of unknown etiology characterized by a mononuclear cell alveolitis and noncaseating granulomata with varying degrees of interstitial fibrosis.[1,2] While granulomata are the histologic hallmark of this disease, current thoughts are that the alveolitis, characterized by activated thymus-derived (T) lymphocytes and alveolar macrophages, precedes and directs the formation of granulomata and fibrosis.[3–5] While most patients with sarcoidosis improve spontaneously with no residual disease, some may develop significant respiratory impairment, and a small number die with ventilatory insufficiency.[6–8] The administration of corticosteroids remains the treatment of choice for patients with sarcoidosis, but variability in the clinical course of this disease makes rational decisions regarding the use of corticosteroids difficult. In this context, a number of indirect measures of disease activity, including clinical, radiographic, and pulmonary physiologic parameters, have been used to judge disease activity and predict natural history, and to thus assess the need for therapy.[2,9] Unfortunately, while general guidelines are established, these measurements are often unreliable in predicting the course of individual patients.

Recently, bronchoalveolar lavage has been suggested as an effective means of assessing disease activity.[10] Since an expanded population of activated lymphocytes appears to be an integral part of the alveolitis of pulmonary sarcoidosis, determination of the proportion of lymphocytes found in bronchoalveolar lavage fluid may be useful in assessing the natural history of this disease and for predicting the need for therapy. The present study was undertaken to address these possibilities. We compared the initial percentage of lymphocytes recovered by bronchoalveolar lavage with the overall change in pulmonary physiology in a group of untreated and treated patients with active pulmonary sarcoidosis. Our findings suggest that the initial proportion of lymphocytes recovered with bronchoalveolar lavage predicts neither evolution of disease nor response to treatment.

METHODS

Study Population

The study population consisted of 29 patients examined by members of the Pulmonary Division at the University of Alabama at Birmingham. All research protocols were approved by the Institutional Review Board, and informed consent was obtained for all procedures. Each patient was required to have clinical and radiographic data consistent with pulmonary sarcoidosis, and a lung biopsy showing noncaseating granulomata without evidence of infection by special stains and culture.[1] All patients were judged to be clinically active based on symptoms.

Bronchoalveolar Lavage

Bronchoalveolar lavage was performed using a fiberoptic bronchoscope with the tip wedged in the lingula or the right middle lobe. Premedication consisted of 0.8 mg of atropine and 50-75 mg of meperidine. A total of 100 ml of saline solution in five 20-ml aliquots was used. Lavage fluid was immediately transported to our laboratories and processed as previously described.[11] Lavage cell differential counts were made by counting 500 cells on a Wright-Giemsa-stained cytocentrifuge preparation.

Study Design

All subjects who met the criteria for inclusion in this study were evaluated at the time of entry with complete pulmonary function studies and with bronchoalveolar lavage. Each subject then had serial measurements of at least three pulmonary function parameters [vital capacity (VC), total lung capacity (TLC), and diffusing capacity for carbon monoxide (DL_{CO})] at intervals of 3-6 months. The DL_{CO} was corrected for alveolar volume and hemoglobin.[11]

All patients were examined by their private physicians within the Pulmonary Division and managed in accord with general principles of patient care. Fourteen of 29 patients were treated symptomatically without corticosteroids. Fifteen of 29 patients had severe impairment because of systemic symptoms or were judged to have clinically worsened so that corticosteroid therapy was indicated. Prednisone ($1\ mg \cdot kg^{-1} \cdot day^{-1}$) for 6 weeks, followed by a gradual taper to 15-20 mg daily for 3-6 months, was routinely used.

TABLE 1. Study Population and Clinical Data

Groups	Average Age (years)	N	Sex (F/M)	Race (B/W)	Lung Function[a] VC (l)	TLC (l)	DL_{CO} ($ml \cdot min^{-1} \cdot mm\ Hg^{-1}$)	Lymphocyte Percentage[a]
No treatment	32.9	14	10/4	11/3	3.1 ± 0.3	4.5 ± 0.3	17.4 ± 1.4	24.0 ± 3.3
Treatment	35.6	15	10/5	14/1	2.9 ± 0.2	4.2 ± 0.3	16.0 ± 1.2	32.0 ± 4.2

NOTE: F: female; M: male; B: black; W: white.
[a] Each value is a mean ± SEM.

Data Analysis

Physiologic data was used to assess the natural history and response to corticosteroid treatment. Two methods were used to assess physiologic changes for each patient: 1) estimation of the rate of change in each functional parameter using the slope of a simple linear regression by the least-squares technique, and 2) calculation of the absolute change in each functional parameter using the following formula: absolute change = (absolute value of the parameter at the end of the study) − (absolute value of the parameter at time of entry).

To determine if lavage lymphocyte counts were of value in patients with active sarcoidosis, Spearman rank correlations were made between the initial percentage of lavage lymphocytes and both the rate of change in physiologic parameters and the absolute change in physiologic parameters. A p value of $<.05$ was considered significant.

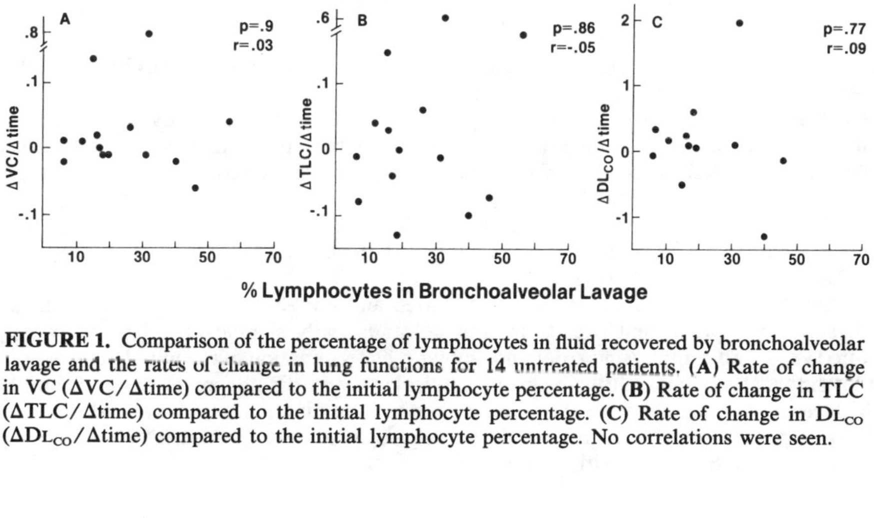

FIGURE 1. Comparison of the percentage of lymphocytes in fluid recovered by bronchoalveolar lavage and the rates of change in lung functions for 14 untreated patients. **(A)** Rate of change in VC (ΔVC/Δtime) compared to the initial lymphocyte percentage. **(B)** Rate of change in TLC (ΔTLC/Δtime) compared to the initial lymphocyte percentage. **(C)** Rate of change in DL_{CO} (ΔDL_{CO}/Δtime) compared to the initial lymphocyte percentage. No correlations were seen.

RESULTS

At the beginning of the study, 29 patients with biopsy-proved sarcoidosis were evaluated with baseline pulmonary function tests and bronchoalveolar lavage cell analysis. The length of time the patients were studied, expressed as a mean ± SEM, was 23.45 ± 4.52 months (range: 2-60 months). Fourteen patients received no treatment whereas 15 patients were treated with prednisone. The two groups could not be distinguished based on age, sex, race, baseline function, or lavage lymphocyte counts ($p>.2$ all comparisons) (TABLE 1).

The 14 untreated patients were studied over an average of 15.57 ± 4.46 months with serial measurements of lung function. When these values were compared with the initial percentage of lavage lymphocytes, no significant correlations were found in the rates of change in VC ($r=.03$; $p=.9$), TLC ($r=-.05$; $p=.86$), or DL_{CO} ($r=.09$; $p=.77$) (FIG. 1). Likewise, the initial percentage of lavage lymphocytes did not cor-

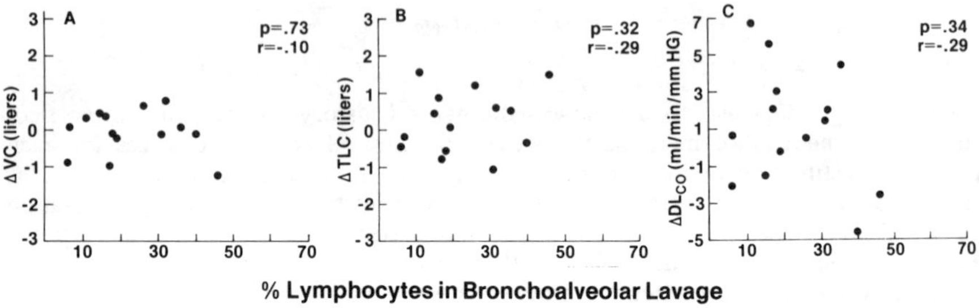

FIGURE 2. Comparison of the percentage of lymphocytes in fluid recovered by bronchoalveolar lavage and absolute changes in lung functions for 14 untreated patients. **(A)** Absolute change in VC (ΔVC) in liters compared to the initial lymphocyte percentage. **(B)** Absolute change in TLC (ΔTLC) in liters compared to the initial lymphocyte percentage. **(C)** Absolute change in DL_{CO} (ΔDL_{CO}) in $ml \cdot min^{-1} \cdot mm\ Hg^{-1}$ compared to the initial lymphocyte percentage. No correlations were seen.

relate with absolute changes over time for VC ($r=-.10$; $p=.73$), TLC ($r=-.29$; $p=.32$), or DL_{CO} ($r=-.29$; $p=.34$) (FIG. 2).

Fifteen patients were treated with prednisone and were studied over an average of 30.8 ± 7.33 months. Among these individuals, there were no significant correlations between the initial proportion of lavage lymphocytes and subsequent rates of change in VC ($r=-.38$; $p=.16$), TLC ($r=-.04$; $p=.98$), or DL_{CO} ($r=-.33$; $p=.23$) (FIG. 3). Additionally, lavage lymphocyte counts did not predict which patients in this group would show improvement in VC ($r=-.16$; $p=.57$), TLC ($r=-.04$; $p=-.90$), or DL_{CO} ($r=-.32$; $p=.27$) (FIG. 4).

On the average, patients in both the treated and untreated groups tended to have physiologic improvement over time, and no statistically significant differences were noted ($p>.2$ all comparisons) (data not shown). Determination of the initial percentage of lymphocytes obtained utilizing bronchoalveolar lavage did not correlate significantly with rates of change or with absolute changes in lung function over time, and did not help to predict which patients would subsequently show improvement in these parameters after treatment with prednisone.

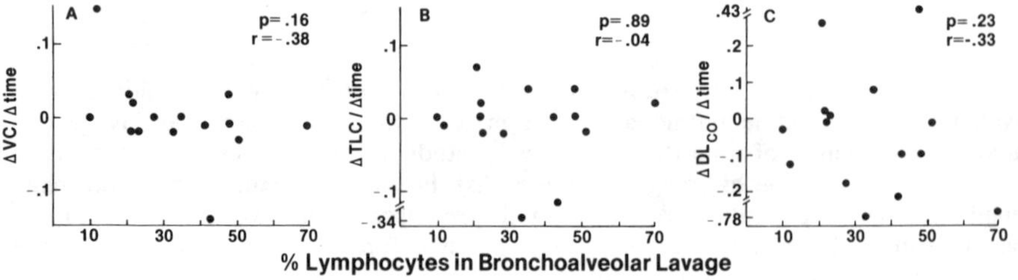

FIGURE 3. Comparison of the percentage of lymphocytes in fluid recovered by bronchoalveolar lavage and the rates of change in lung functions for 15 treated patients. **(A)** Rate of change in VC (ΔVC/Δtime) compared to the initial lymphocyte percentage. **(B)** Rate of change in TLC (ΔTLC/Δtime) compared to the initial lymphocyte percentage. **(C)** Rate of change in DL_{CO} (ΔDL_{CO}/Δtime) compared to the initial lymphocyte percentage. No correlations were seen.

DISCUSSION

The current study was undertaken to determine if initial bronchoalveolar lavage lymphocyte counts are useful in patients with sarcoidosis in predicting the natural history and response of this disease to therapy. A group of 29 patients with active pulmonary sarcoidosis underwent bronchoalveolar lavage and were then studied with pulmonary function testing for up to 5 years. Fourteen of the patients were untreated and 15 were treated with corticosteroids. No correlation was found between the initial lavage lymphocyte counts and either the clinical course or the response to therapy.

Pulmonary sarcoidosis has a variable clinical course, and although most patients develop no or minimal residual disease, a small percentage ultimately die from ventilatory insufficiency. While corticosteroids remain the mainstay of therapy for this disease, their value is unproven. If, however, one could predict which patients would worsen functionally, then a more rational approach to therapy could be established.

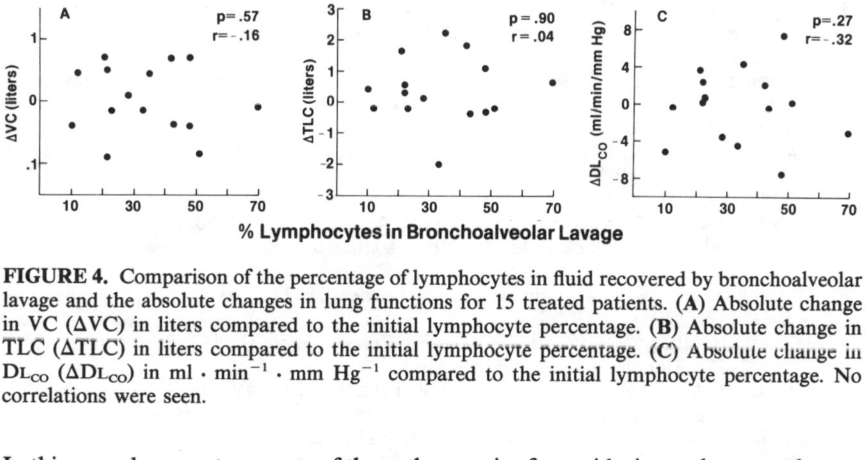

FIGURE 4. Comparison of the percentage of lymphocytes in fluid recovered by bronchoalveolar lavage and the absolute changes in lung functions for 15 treated patients. **(A)** Absolute change in VC (ΔVC) in liters compared to the initial lymphocyte percentage. **(B)** Absolute change in TLC (ΔTLC) in liters compared to the initial lymphocyte percentage. **(C)** Absolute change in DL_{CO} (ΔDL_{CO}) in ml · min^{-1} · mm Hg^{-1} compared to the initial lymphocyte percentage. No correlations were seen.

In this regard, current concepts of the pathogenesis of sarcoidosis are that granulomata are preceded and caused by a mononuclear cell alveolitis. Unchecked, the alveolitis and granulomata lead to fibrosis and end-stage lung disease in some patients. Current data indicate that the alveolitis of sarcoidosis consists mainly of activated T lymphocytes and macrophages.[2,3,10] Since one component of the alveolitis is the T lymphocyte, and the majority of lavage lymphocytes are T cells, it would then be reasonable to hypothesize that the initial lymphocyte counts could predict which patients would show worsening lung function, and which patients would respond to treatment.

In the current study we found no correlation between initial lavage lymphocyte counts and functional outcome or response to treatment. These results confirm and extend the previous observation that lavage lymphocyte counts are of no value in the management of sarcoidosis.[12] In the context of newer concepts concerning the pathogenesis of sarcoidosis, particularly with regard to lymphocyte subtypes and alveolar macrophage synergism, these findings are not unexpected.[2,3,10] Recent data suggests that assessments of both the T lymphocyte and the alveolar macrophage components of the alveolitis are necessary to accurately predict short-term functional changes.[10] Further, current studies also suggest that delineation of more specific lavage lymphocyte subpopulations, such as $OKT4^+$ cells or OKT4/OKT8 ratios, may be better predictors of natural history and response to treatment than are T lymphocytes alone.[12]

In summary, lavage lymphocyte counts from patients with pulmonary sarcoidosis predicted neither the natural history nor the response to therapy over an average of 2 years. These data complement the recent findings of Baughman *et al.*[12] and supports the need for further prospective, longitudinal studies. Bronchoalveolar lavage remains an extremely valuable research tool, but its clinical utility in patients with sarcoidosis has yet to be determined.

REFERENCES

1. MITCHELL, D. N., J. G. SCADDING, R. E. HEART & K. F. W. HINSON. 1977. Sarcoidosis: Histopathological definition and clinical diagnosis. J. Clin. Pathol. **30:** 395-408.
2. CRYSTAL, R. G., J. E. GADEK, V. J. FERRANS, J. D. FULMER, B. R. LINE & HUNNINGHAKE. 1981. Interstitial lung disease: Current concepts of pathogenesis, staging, and therapy. Am. J. Med. **70:** 542-568.
3. CRYSTAL, R. G., W. C. ROBERTS, G. W. HUNNINGHAKE, J. E. GADEK, J. D. FULMER & B. R. LINE. 1981. Pulmonary sarcoidosis: A disease characterized and perpetuated by activated lung T-lymphocytes. Ann. Intern. Med. **94:** 73-94.
4. ROSEN, Y., T. J. ATHANASSIADES, S. MOON & H. A. LYONS. 1978. Nongranulomatous interstitial pneumonitis in sarcoidosis: Relationship to the development of epithelioid granulomas. Chest **74:** 122-125.
5. CARRINGTON, C. B., E. A. GAENSLER, J. P. MIKUS, A. W. SCHACHTER, G. W. BURKE & A. M. GOFF. 1976. Structure and function in sarcoidosis. Ann. N.Y. Acad. Sci. **278:** 265-282.
6. ISRAEL, H. L. 1979. Prognosis of sarcoidosis. Ann. Intern. Med. **73:** 2038-2039.
7. LONGSCOPE, W. T. & D. G. FREIMAN. 1952. A study of sarcoidosis. Medicine (Baltimore) **31:** 1-132.
8. BACHARACH, T. 1961. Sarcoidosis: A clinical review of 111 cases. Am. Rev. Respir. Dis. **84:** 6-12.
9. ISRAEL, H. 1979. Sarcoidosis. *In* Current Pulmonology. D. H. Simmons, Ed. Vol. **1:** 152-182. Houghton Mifflin. Boston, MA.
10. KEOGH, B. A., G. W. HUNNINGHAKE, B. R. LINE & R. G. CRYSTAL. 1983. The alveolitis of pulmonary sarcoidosis: Evaluation of natural history and alveolitis-dependent changes in lung function. Am. Rev. Respir. Dis. **128:** 256-265.
11. WEINBERGER, S. E., J. A. KELMAN, N. A. ELSON, R. C. YOUNG, H. Y. REYNOLDS & R. G. CRYSTAL. 1978. Bronchoalveolar lavage in interstitial lung disease. Ann. Intern. Med. **89:** 459-466.
12. BAUGHMAN, R. D., M. FERNANDEZ, C. H. BOSKEN, J. MANTIL & P. HURTUBISE. 1984. Comparison of gallium-67 scanning, bronchoalveolar lavage, and serum angiotensin-converting enzyme levels in pulmonary sarcoidosis. Am. Rev. Respir. Dis. **129:** 676-681.

Panel Discussion

Bronchoalveolar Lavage: Research or Clinical Tool?[a]

DR. GORDON L. SNIDER (*Boston University School of Medicine, Boston, Massachusetts*): It is clear that in the decade since it was first applied to evaluating diffuse, interstitial lung disease, bronchoalveolar lavage (BAL) has given us important insights into the descriptive biology of sarcoidosis and the other interstitial lung diseases. It has opened up an area that must make investigators of other organs envious. Direct examination of cells and soluble substances from BAL fluid is a much clearer reflection of the inflammatory process in the lungs than can be gained by study of the blood.

As investigators, we realize that our understanding of the pathogenesis of sarcoidosis and the other interstitial lung diseases is preliminary. Nevertheless, we are all subjected to great pressure to turn each new advance in understanding to some practical effect in patient care. The pressure to move as quickly as possible from research to the clinical arena comes from within us as we deal with our sick patients. It also comes from our colleagues, and from the people who grant funds to us. In point of fact, 10 years is not a very long time in the history of a disease, and I believe that we must be cautious in making the jump from the research laboratory to the bedside and the clinic. The high-technology techniques represented by BAL are expensive. Although carrying only minimal risk, they are invasive. They should only be used to evaluate and follow our patients if we are sure that they will influence our decisions in such a way as to favorably affect the outcome of the patients' disease. It is our hope that this panel can serve a useful purpose for clinicians and investigators by clearly enunciating both the areas of agreement and disagreement on BAL in sarcoidosis.

If a technique such as BAL is to be transferred from the research laboratory to the clinic, it is important to know whether the technique has been sufficiently standardized so that many physicians and their laboratories doing the procedure occasionally can get results comparable to those collected in a research laboratory. Can data be interpreted using standards that other laboratories have developed, or must each group develop its own standards? Dr. Jack Fulmer will address these questions.

DR. JACK FULMER (*University of Alabama School of Medicine, Birmingham, Alabama*): In my opinion, BAL is a powerful research tool, but the clinical value of BAL in most diseases remains to be established. Not only are clinical data on the utility of BAL incomplete, but lack of standardization constitutes a major problem. I shall discuss three aspects of this problem.

The first is the question of the anatomical site for lavage. Current data indicate that variations in the lavage site in normals appears to have little influence on differential counts of cells. There is no information on the effects of variations in anatomical site of lavage on the soluble components of the fluid. Current data indicate that in disease states, the site chosen for lavage may have profound influence on both cellular

[a] Correspondence should be addressed to Dr. Gordon L. Snider, who was chairman of the panel, as follows: Pulmonary Section, Veterans Administration Medical Center, 150 South Huntington Avenue, Boston, Massachusetts 02130.

recovery and the differential cell count. Whether one should use a chest roentgenogram or gallium scintiscanning to identify the site of localized disease and lavage is not clear. What is needed is a systematic examination of the effect of lavage site on BAL findings in disease. Several institutions are now engaged in such studies.

The next area I wish to discuss is the volume of lavage fluid. It is clear that the first aliquots instilled mainly sample airway components and subsequent aliquots mainly sample alveoli. Because of this, some investigators actually discard the first aliquot. However, the investigative group at the University of Vermont has shown that the kinetics of cellular recovery in normal volunteers are complex and do not follow simple patterns. The effects of disease are likely even more complex, and are unknown. In studies from the Yale group the kinetics of the soluble components appear to be dilutional in volunteers, but the effects of disease are quite unclear. The effects of dwell time are unknown.

I wish finally to consider the processing and analysis of BAL fluid. It has been indicated that a 2- or 3-hr delay does not affect cellular viability. It is less clear what the effects of delay are on cell differential counts and on soluble components. The cytocentrifuge has been most widely used to prepare microscopic preparations for differential cell count. However, recent data using the millipore filter method suggest that the cytocentrifuge method underestimates the percentage of lymphocytes. If the

TABLE 1. The Clinical Value of BAL

1. BAL results "suggest" diagnosis in interstitial lung disease, in the presence of either abnormal or normal radiographs.
2. In assessing disease activity, BAL is of limited utility, unless further evaluations are performed. Longitudinal studies could prove useful, and BAL fluid could be examined for histamine, complement components, and proteases.
3. BAL may help assess the response to drug therapy. Trials are well underway.
4. BAL may help define inflammatory pathways. Such knowledge could lead to the development of new drugs, which are badly needed.

cytocentrifuge is used, speed of rotation and centrifugation time need to be controlled. The problem of variations due to smoking is also real and troublesome.

It is clear, that until we have better standardization of methods, each laboratory needs to validate its own techniques. All of us need to make a systematic examination of the technical factors that we use, and we should keep them standard until new data from our own or other sources indicate the need for change.

SNIDER: Professor Margaret Turner-Warwick will speak to us on the usefulness of BAL in making the diagnosis of diffuse interstitial lung disease. I have asked her to broaden the topic and to talk about disorders other than sarcoidosis and to summarize her earlier presentation on the value of BAL in predicting the course of sarcoidosis.

DR. MARGARET TURNER-WARWICK (*Brompton Hospital, London, England*): I summarize the points I want to make here in TABLE 1. There is controversy regarding the value of BAL in diagnosis, in assessing activity of disease, and in assessing patients' drug responsiveness. Obviously, everyone agrees that BAL has been most exciting and extremely valuable in research.

Contrary to the views of many, I believe as a practicing physician that the diagnostic value of BAL is very considerable as classified under two headings. One is that BAL certainly does identify certain pathognomonic appearances that can lead to a confident diagnosis and save further investigation. Examples include hemosiderosis, alveolar proteinosis, and certain inorganic-dust diseases. The infections represent a big area where BAL is helpful, particularly with difficult infections such as some chronic infections and with immunosuppressed individuals including the acquired immune deficiency syndrome patient. I do not think there is much difference of opinion in this important area.

Secondly, I think that BAL can be useful for the clinician as a diagnostic screening test. It is probable that only about 10% of the medical laboratory investigations we do are pathognomonic. Nevertheless, we do not discard radiographs, blood tests, or pulmonary function tests because they are not pathognomonic. We use them in the clinical context. We should not expect too much of BAL diagnostically but should evaluate how it may sometimes influence our clinical decisions. An example might be a patient with an atypical chest radiograph showing diffuse lung disease. If the BAL shows a high percentage of lymphocytes, it will obviously direct our thoughts to a relatively short list of differential diagnoses characterized by lavage lymphocytosis. The list would be quite different if the lavage fluid came back showing many neutrophils. In summary, I think the cell counts can be valuable as a screening test, although of course I fully recognize that they are not pathognomonic.

BAL may also be useful in occupational lung disease where simple microscopy and more complicated tests such as X-ray emission spectroscopy may identify various types of particles. There are also some rather special appearances like giant cells seen in hard-metal disease. Studies of BAL fluid may also be useful in that difficult group of patients that have breathlessness with normal lung functions and chest radiographs. It is disconcerting to do a lung biopsy that is subsequently reported as normal lung. Inflammatory cells of any type reported in a lavage strongly suggest that the lungs are really abnormal and justifies further invasive procedures.

We have had a long discussion on the assessment of "activity" of disease and I do not intend to go over that again. The value of following drug therapy in sarcoidosis with BAL has been well covered over the last two days and the general feeling, it seems to me, is that lung lavages are not very useful for that purpose.

The unanswered question I would like to leave with you is, what is the relationship of the alveolitis to the fibrosis in sarcoidosis? I find it very mysterious. The left plate of FIGURE 1 is the chest radiograph of a patient, seen by Professor Scadding in 1963, who had extensive abnormal shadows, but was surprisingly asymptomatic and therefore did not receive treatment. Four years later he reappeared because he was extremely short of breath. His lung function had fallen considerably. His chest radiograph (FIG. 1, right plate) looks much blacker, representing considerable distortion and destruction of his lung. How has this change taken place, and in particular, why is the distribution of abnormal shadows different in the earlier (nonfibrotic) and later (fibrotic) radiographs?

Perhaps, if we studied the relationship between the development of fibrosis and the preceding alveolitis and granuloma (FIG. 1, right plate), we might get better markers for the development of fibrosis and destruction, which is after all the clinically important question. To encourage us that these are worthwhile considerations, I pose the following questions: Why is the distribution of fibrosis so different from the preceding granuloma? What are the linear shadows? Why does the radiographic pattern differ from other widespread, fibrosing interstitial diseases? Is the confluence of granulomata important in the development of the upper lung field fibrosis, and how much does airway involvement contribute? These are questions that might well be worthwhile for consideration at the next international sarcoidosis conference.

SNIDER: Dr. Turner-Warwick has said that she thinks that BAL has an established position in clinical medicine in the investigation of patients who we think clinically might have infections. I would like to ask the other two panelists to indicate how

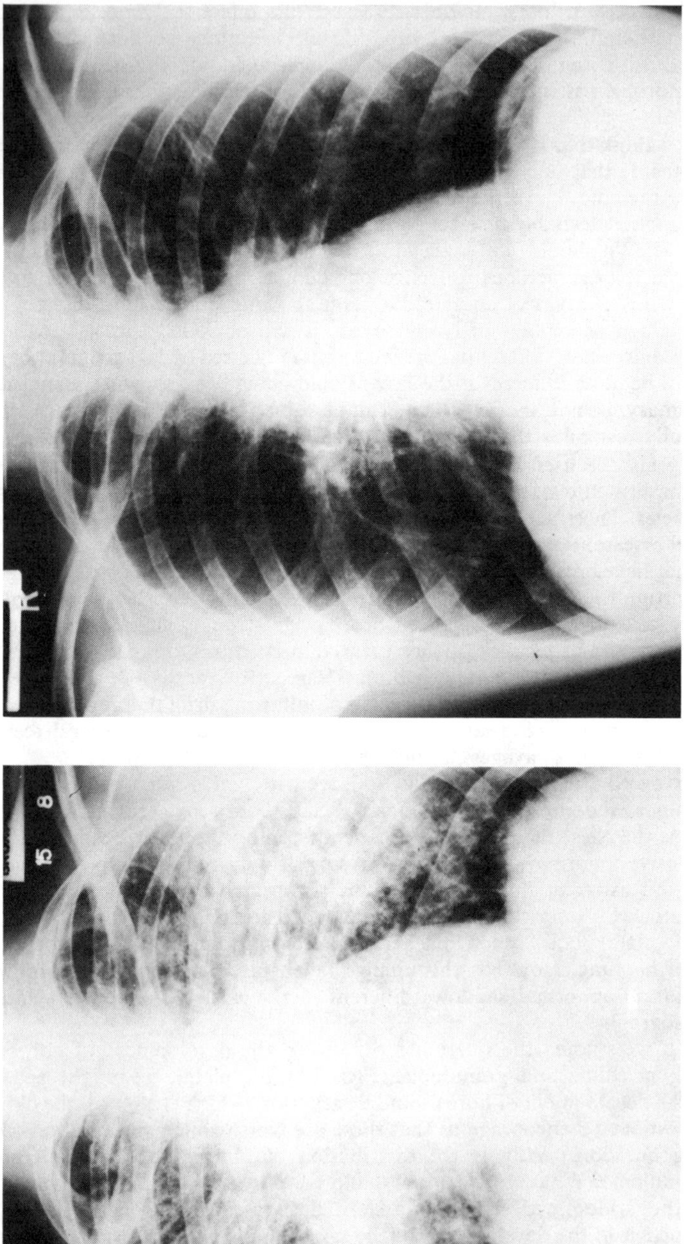

FIGURE 1. Left plate: An asymptomatic patient with extensive lung shadowing in 1963. Right plate: The same patient, who was readmitted because of considerable breathlessness, with extensive scarring in 1967.

they feel about the use of BAL for investigating the immunocompromised host, whether the immunocompromised state be iatrogenic or due to the acquired immunodeficiency syndrome.

FULMER: I agree with Dr. Turner-Warwick. I think that lavage is extremely valuable in the diagnosis of infectious disorders, but it has more value if the laboratory can promptly analyze the specimen, using appropriate techniques. If prompt evaluation cannot be made, I do not think that lavage ought to delay open lung biopsy in someone who is critically ill. I think the same is true of lavage in general. I find that lymphocytosis in a patient with atypical sarcoidosis comforts me. On the other hand, in this time of great efforts to control hospital costs, I am often reluctant to delay biopsy while waiting for lavage data.

DR. CLAUDE PIANTADOSI (*Duke University, Durham, North Carolina*): I agree with what Drs. Turner-Warwick and Fulmer say about infection. Following a general philosophy of moving from less invasive to more invasive diagnostic tests, lavage is certainly something that you ought to do when you are considering infection. The procedure is safe, and if you obtain a diagnosis (pneumocystis is one that we commonly encounter at Duke), then I think you have a positive result that is sufficient in most clinical circumstances. If you do not obtain the diagnosis of a specific infection, and your index of suspicion is still clinically high, you should move on to the more invasive procedures.

SNIDER: Let me ask all three panelists what stains should be done on the BAL specimens in investigating a patient suspected of having an infection?

TURNER-WARWICK: We do cultures as well as special stains. Our practice, when we suspect infection, is to use silver stains and stains for bacteria and fungi as well as Giemsa stains. Electron microscopy results come back very quickly in our hospital.

FULMER: We use the same special stains noted by Professor Turner-Warwick and get them back quite rapidly after lavage. In terms of utility of lavage in diagnosing patients with inorganic-dust disease, I just do not know how many ferruginous bodies are normal. We wash them out of normal patients all the time. The finding is useful in someone that has a chest radiograph or history consistent with asbestosis, but I am not sure what to make of the data in the absence of such findings.

PIANTADOSI. I agree with Dr. Fulmer that demonstration of ferruginous bodies is sometimes helpful in revealing the need for a more careful history.

SNIDER: Am I correct that neither at Birmingham nor at Duke are you using electron microscopy in a routine way?

FULMER AND PIANTADOSI: That is correct.

SNIDER: I would like to put one other question to the panelists before going on. We have heard that BAL often provides supportive or suggestive evidence of a particular clinical diagnosis. What is the relative place of measurement of proteins in the supernatants as opposed to microscopic examination of the cell pellet? The cost of a total and differential cell count is obviously much less than complete BAL evaluation without electron microscopy. Such an analysis might include protein concentrations in the lavage fluid and cell surface markers on lymphocytes in cases where there are enough lymphocytes to do the determination, and might cost as much as 600 to 800 dollars.

TURNER-WARWICK: We are not using the supernatants in any diagnostic way.

PIANTADOSI: We are in the same situation. We do make a large number of research measurements on soluble components of the lavage and of the serum because we are interested in trying to find something useful for monitoring the progress of the disease. However, these data are not available for clinical decision making.

FULMER: I think anything aside from special stains for infectious disorders and perhaps cell counts and differentials constitutes research.

SNIDER: I would now like Dr. Claude Piantadosi to talk to us about the place of BAL in monitoring the progress of corticosteroid therapy and sarcoidosis.

PIANTADOSI: Dr. Turner-Warwick discussed the place of BAL in monitoring sarcoidosis activity yesterday, but I want to address the topic from a slightly different point of view. Because of the time constraints, I am going to make three assumptions: first, that there is a therapeutic role for corticosteroids in the management of sarcoidosis; second, that there is a clinical problem in determining when to begin the steroids and how to taper them; and third, that we can adequately control the variables in performing BAL. I am going to confine my comments to the BAL lymphocyte fraction, the only parameter for which I think there are sufficient data available.

The Duke approach has been a simple one. It is based on the premise that any new index of activity should enhance the accuracy of the existing clinical evaluation. In our institution, disease activity assessment is based on signs and symptoms, pulmonary function data, chest radiographs, and arterial blood gas determinations. We do not routinely use serum angiotensin-converting enzyme levels or serum immunoglobulin G concentrations. Each patient also undergoes BAL and gallium-67 lung scan, but the clinician is not allowed to see these data before he makes the corticosteroid treatment decision. We have standard criteria for treating these patients, and our regimen is very similar to the one that Dr. Turner-Warwick described yesterday.

The first thing I wish to examine is the relation between the clinical decision to give corticosteroids and the BAL lymphocyte fraction in 62 untreated nonsmokers with sarcoidosis grouped according to physiologic function. Category A patients have normal function; category B patients have mild impairment; and category C patients have definite physiological impairment (defined as a total lung capacity and/or a carbon monoxide diffusing capacity of less than 65% of the respective predicted values). I have also identified patients with airflow obstruction. These patients are defined as having values for forced expiratory volume in 1 sec equal to or less than 72% of the predicted value.

We gave corticosteroids to all in category C, the patients with definite lung function impairment. These patients had a wide range of lymphocyte counts, from 12 to 77% of total cell number. Patients in the other categories received steroids about 45% of the time. Once again there was no relation between the treatment decision and the lymphocyte differential count in the BAL fluid. A similar result was obtained in 16 smokers with sarcoidosis.

I would now like to look at the relation between the initial lymphocyte differential count and the course of sarcoidosis, using data from a 6-month follow-up period on 55 of our 78 patients. Thirty-one patients were initially begun on corticosteroids, and this analysis is therefore confined to the 24 patients not initially receiving steroids.

I have classified these 24 patients into those requiring initiation of corticosteroids on clinical grounds during the period of observation and those not requiring initiation of steroid therapy. I shall use 28% as the dividing point for low- versus high-intensity alveolitis as suggested by Hunninghake.[1] Thirteen of these patients had initial lymphocyte counts of less than 28%. Eleven of these did not require initiation of corticosteroid therapy, but two did. There were 11 patients with initial lymphocyte counts of greater than 28%, and all of these remained stable or were improved over the 6-month interval without treatment.

I shall make only a few observations in the corticosteroid-treated group of 31 patients. Six of 11 patients with less than 28% lymphocytes improved clinically. These data suggest that low-intensity alveolitis, as determined by lymphocyte count, is not very reliable as an indicator of response to corticosteroid therapy.

I would also like to present several patterns of change associated with corticosteroid therapy from our series of patients who have been evaluated every 6 to 7 months. I have looked at changes in the BAL lymphocyte percentage, gallium-67 scan activity (scored by the computer technique mentioned by Dr. Putman), and interval change in the forced vital capacity for 31 patients. Less than half the patients whose lung function showed improvement while on corticosteroids went from a high-intensity alveolitis to a low-intensity alveolitis in both gallium-67 scans and BAL lymphocyte counts. The majority of our physiologically improved patients decreased their gallium-67 scores with steroid treatment. They followed one of four lymphocyte BAL patterns: initial high lymphocyte levels, decreasing but remaining high; low lymphocyte levels, decreasing; low lymphocyte levels, staying stable; and initial high lymphocyte levels, staying stable. We conclude from this analysis that we cannot use the lymphocyte count to predict physiologic response to corticosteroid therapy.

The final point to be made from our experience is that we have a considerable number of patients, 11 of 78 (14%), who have low-intensity alveolitis by BAL lymphocyte counts but high-intensity alveolitis by gallium-67 scans. The clinicians, who did not know the results of either the gallium-67 scans or the BAL lymphocyte counts, determined that the disease was active in 9 of these 11 patients. I am not touting the gallium-67 scan as more sensitive than the BAL lymphocyte count, I am only noting the problem that we face of discrepant indices of disease activity.

In summary, I want to say that for an individual patient, a low BAL lymphocyte count does not exclude the possibility of deterioration or a response to corticosteroid therapy, and a high lymphocyte count does not necessarily mean deterioration if the patient is untreated.

SNIDER: We have agreed that BAL clearly has a place in the diagnosis of infectious problems and that findings in the cell pellet may be of help in inorganic-dust diseases. BAL cell counts and differential cell counts may provide information that is helpful in a nonpathognomonic way in interstitial lung diseases. Finally, we have agreed that as of the present time, there is no evidence that BAL can be used to monitor the activity of sarcoidosis, to monitor the course of its therapy with corticosteroids, or to predict the outcome of the disease.

REFERENCE

1. HUNNINGHAKE, G. W. & R. G. CRYSTAL. 1981. Pulmonary sarcoidosis: A disorder mediated by excess helper T-lymphocyte activity at sites of disease activity. N. Engl. J. Med. **305:** 429-434.

International Controlled Clinical Trial of Prednisone Therapy in Pulmonary Sarcoidosis

YUTAKA HOSODA AND RIICHIRO MIKAMI[a]

Sarcoidosis Committee of Japan
Tokyo, Japan

INTRODUCTION

Few of the approximately 200 papers that have been published with the words "corticosteroid therapy" in their titles were controlled therapeutic studies. Corticosteroids in these controlled studies were administered to patients with stage 1 or stage 2 sarcoidosis every day or every other day, and doses of the corticosteroids, in either treatment, were tapered over several months. None of the studies in which long-term observations were conducted could demonstrate whether one treatment was better than the other.

At the Ninth International Conference of Sarcoidosis and Other Granulomatous Disorders, which was held at Paris in 1981, Drs. J. Chrétien and D. G. James organized a commission to establish guidelines for therapeutic trials. The commission issued guidelines based on the commonly used regimens, but the members of the commission hoped to eventually improve on the conventional treatment that was recommended. They gathered again, to grope for more effective corticosteroid regimens, at the Johns Hopkins Hospital in June 1982 in cooperation with Dr. C. J. Johns. The members agreed, after lengthy discussions, to conduct a year-long international controlled study in which 50-mg and 5-mg doses of prednisone would be administered to patients and controls, respectively, every other day. The Epidemiology Committee[b] completed the research protocol at the commission's third meeting, at the Johns Hopkins Hospital in October 1982. The commission members met a fourth time, at Sorrento during the Fourth European Symposium of Sarcoidosis, and the Steering Committee,[c] with the kind assistance of Dr. A. Blasi, decided a placebo group should be included as a second control group in the trials whenever possible. A standard system to record chest radiograph changes was suggested by the Radiography Committee[d] after it had

[a]Yutaka Hosoda and Riichiro Mikami are chairmen of the Sarcoidosis Committee of Japan. Correspondence may be addressed to Yutaka Hosoda as follows: JNR Central Health Institute, Yoyogi 2-1, Shibuya-ku, Tokyo 151.

[b]Epidemiology Committee: C. Newill (Baltimore), K. Nobutomo (Tokyo), and N. Saito (Tokyo).

[c]Steering Committee: R. A. DeRemee (Rochester), A. Douglas (Edinburgh), B. Djurič (Novi Sad), H. Eule (Sommerfeld), Y. Hosoda (Tokyo), H. L. Israel (Philadelphia), T. Izumi (Kyoto), C. J. Johns (Baltimore), J. Meier-Sydow (Frankfurt), R. Mikami (Nara), G. Rizzato (Milan), O. B. Selroos (Lund), O. P. Sharma (Los Angeles), A. S. Teirstein (New York), and M. Yamamoto (Nagoya).

[d]Radiography Committee: O. Doi (Tokyo), R. H. Morgan (Baltimore), H. Rieman (Frankfurt), and A. S. Tuengerthal (Frankfurt).

met three times (in Baltimore, June 1982; in Tokyo, May 1983; and in Sorrento, October 1983). The recording system proposed by this committee has been tested by a few groups to check its practicability. Dr. C. J. Johns kindly arranged for this committee to meet during the conference in which this paper was presented.

SUBJECTS AND METHODS

We set forth a hypothesis: Corticosteroid therapy can arrest irreversible lung damage and stabilize the course of the disease one or more years after cessation of therapy, as evidenced by chest radiographic changes, lung function measurements, clinical symptoms, and angiotensin-converting enzyme activity. It is recognized that continued treatment may be required.

A patient may enter the controlled trial 6 months after his first visit to the sarcoidosis clinic if he meets the following criteria: 1) histologically confirmed sarcoidosis; 2) an age between 20 and 50 years; 3) stage 2 or stage 3 sarcoidosis; 4) no significant breathlessness; 5) no extrapulmonary symptoms requiring orally administered corticosteroids; 6) no other complications requiring treatment; 7) no previous oral corticosteroid therapy for sarcoidosis; and 8) no contraindications to corticosteroids such as diabetes mellitus, peptic ulcer, or serious infection.

If the patient does not appear as scheduled, the clinical status cards should be returned to the central coordinator stating the reasons why.

The assessment variables are chest radiography findings, symptoms and signs, lung function tests (forced vital capacity, forced expiratory volume in 1 sec, and single-breath transpulmonary CO diffusion), and serum angiotensin-converting enzyme levels.

Several area coordinators were designated. These coordinators are to be responsible for listing eligible patients for the trial, assigning each patient into one of the three regimen groups, and following each patient's progress by receiving the clinical status cards from the doctor in charge. Blocked randomization and mailing methods are to be applied to this process.

Prednisone is to be administered orally in 50-mg doses to patients in the treatment group (group A) Monday, Wednesday, and Friday mornings, preferably at 8:00 AM, for 12 months; the doses are then to be tapered over the next 4 months. This schedule is also to be used for the first and second control groups (groups B and C, respectively); however, patients in group B are to receive placebos instead of prednisone (or to receive no administrations at all), and patients in group C are to receive 5-mg instead of 50-mg doses of prednisone (group C is necessary to accommodate those patients whose circumstances require the use of drugs). The steering committee recognized that double-blind tests may sometimes be impossible because of domestic laws.

Breathlessness is to assessed using a Medical Research Council questionnaire. A patient may have considerable breathlessness if he answers yes to the following questions: 1) Are you troubled by shortness of breath when walking quickly on level ground or when walking up a slight incline? 2) Do you get short of breath when walking with people your own age on level ground? 3) Do you have to stop for breath when walking at your own pace on level ground?

RESULTS

The central coordinator received 10 registry cards from Dr. G. Rizzato, the area coordinator of Milano; 10 from Dr. B. Djurič, the area coordinator of Novi Sad; and

10 from Drs. R. Mikami and Y. Hiraga, the area coordinators of Japan. The number of cases is expected to increase, and the progress of the conditions of the patients has been traced.

DISCUSSION

The evaluation of the radiographic changes may be very difficult when the shadows include secondary changes. The Radiography Committee established a system for recording radiographic changes based on the International Labor Office classification scheme.

CONCLUSION

An international controlled clinical trial of prednisone therapy in pulmonary sarcoidosis is being conducted. The regimen in this trial might represent the last challenge of prednisone therapy to sarcoidosis. International cooperation is expected for this trial.

The Possible Influence of Corticosteroid Therapy on the Natural Course of Pulmonary Sarcoidosis

Late Results of a Continuing Clinical Study

H. EULE,[a] A. WEINECKE, AND I. ROTH

Hellmuth Ulrici Klinik
Sommerfeld, German Democratic Republic

H. WUTHE

Forschungsinstitut für Lungenkrankheiten und Tuberkulose
Berlin-Buch, German Democratic Republic

Observations of spontaneous resolution on the one side and of relapse after successful treatment of pulmonary sarcoidosis on the other side are well known. Such experiences have motivated us, since 1967, to conduct a continuing clinical study to evaluate the long-term influence of corticosteroid therapy on the natural course of pulmonary sarcoidosis stage 1 (hilar adenopathy only) and especially stage 2 and stage 3 (pulmonary infiltrates with or without hilar lymph node enlargement, respectively). The diagnosis was histopathologically proven in all patients. They were free of sarcoidosis-related symptoms, had no significant functional impairment, and had no evidence of extrapulmonary manifestations.

The patients were admitted at random to two treatment groups, which differ with respect to the duration of therapy (A_1 and A_2, respectively), and to an untreated control group (B). In the treatment groups 40 mg of prednisolone was given daily for 4 weeks followed by weekly dose reductions of 5 mg until the maintenance dosis (10 mg) was reached. The duration of treatment was 12 months for group A_1 and 6 months for group A_2.

Results of the radiological dynamics and the development of some functional parameters have been published before.[1–3]

Although values of CO transfer and breathing mechanics of our patients at the start of the study were not available, we decided to assess such supplementary functional parameters as diffusing capacity (D_LCO_{SB}), membrane diffusing capacity (DM),

[a] Address for correspondence: Hellmuth Ulrici Klinik, Bezirksfachkrankenhaus für Lungenkrankheiten und Tuberkulose der Hauptstadt der DDR Berlin, 1421 Sommerfeld, German Democratic Republic.

TABLE 1. Duration of Observation

Duration (years)[a]	Number of Patients[b] $A_1 + A_2$	B	Total
5-7	41 (37)	15 (24)	56 (33)
8-10	46 (42)	24 (39)	70 (41)
11-14	23 (21)	23 (37)	46 (26)
	110 (100)	62 (100)	172 (100)

[a]The mean duration was 8.9 years.
[b]Percentages are shown in parentheses.

capillary blood volume (V_c), and compliance (C_{stat}) to get more information on late consequences of possible fibrosing processes.

One hundred seventy-two of 209 patients analyzed in our paper presented during the Eighth International Conference on Sarcoidosis and Other Granulomatous Disorders[3] could be reexamined clinically, radiographically, and functionally. The mean duration after the start of the observation was 8.9 years (TABLE 1).

All patients were examined by body plethysmography and assessment of arterial pressure of O_2 (PaO_2). Because of technical reasons and lack of cooperation, the compliance could be assessed only in half of the treated and in two-thirds of the untreated patients; the D_LCO_{SB} could be assessed in approximately 90% of the patients.

The distribution of patients according to stages and groups is shown in TABLE 2. One hundred five of the total 172 patients had stage 2 or stage 3 disease; two-thirds were treated; and one-third was not treated. The sex ratio was 1:1. Half of the patients were younger than 40 years; one-third were between 40 and 50 years; and the rest were older than 50 years.

RESULTS

The patients were in a good physical condition, felt well generally, and were able to work when reexamined. Eighty-three percent of the treated and 77% of the untreated

TABLE 2. Distribution of Patients

	Number of Patients[a] A_1[b]	A_2[c]	$A_1 + A_2$	B	Total
Stage 1	26	15	41 (37)	26 (42)	67
Stage 2/3	30	39	69 (63)	36 (58)	105
	56	54	110 (100)	62 (100)	172

[a]Percentages are shown in parentheses.
[b]Treated for 12 months.
[c]Treated for 6 months.

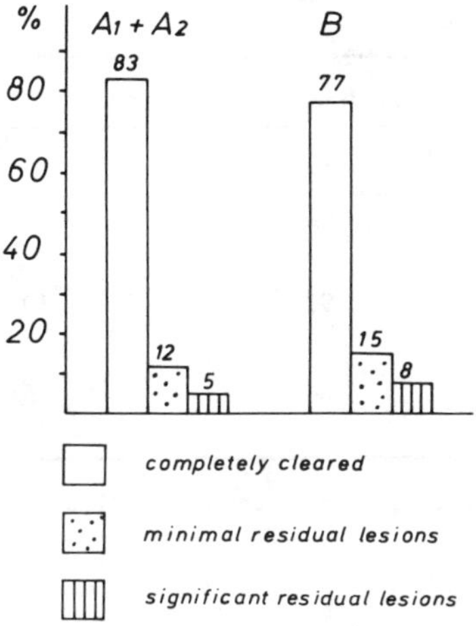

FIGURE 1. Radiographic findings at the end of each observation period. The mean duration of the observation periods was 9 years.

patients showed a complete regression of the radiographic findings, and significant residual lesions were found in 5% and 8%, respectively (FIG. 1). At the time of the last reexamination, a progressive course was observed in 3 of the 110 treated patients (2.7%) but in none of the untreated patients.

During the follow-up period after completing therapy a relapse occurred in 24 of the 110 treated patients (22%). The disease was progressive in 10 of the 62 untreated patients (16%) (TABLE 3). All these patients were immediately and successfully treated by corticosteroids except for two patients of group B (no treatment) who recovered spontaneously.

TABLES 4 & 5 show no differences in the mean percentages of forced ventilatory capacity (FVC) and of forced expiratory volume in 1 sec (FEV_1) related to treatment groups and stages. There were no differences between the groups when assessing PaO_2 at rest, either (TABLE 6).

The results of D_LCO_{SB}, DM, and C_{stat} are demonstrated in TABLES 7, 8 & 9. In 76% of the treated and 86% of the untreated patients with stage 2 or stage 3 sarcoidosis a practically normal value of D_LCO_{SB} was found at reexamination. The difference in stage 1 patients (84% and 65%, respectively) is statistically insignificant.

A reduction of D_LCO_{SB} to less than 70% of predicted was stated no more often in the untreated patients of all stages compared to the treated ones (6% and 11%, respectively). The results are very similar when comparing the percentages of predicted values for DM and for C_{stat} compliance.

TABLE 3. "Relapse" after Completing Therapy or Progressive Course in Untreated Patients

	Percentage of Patients	
	$A_1 + A_2$	B
Stage 1	7	15
Stage 2/3	30	17
All stages	22	16

TABLE 4. FVC Values

	FVC (mean %)[a]		
	A_1	A_2	B
Stage 1			
At start	96	99	100
At end of follow-up	103	97	103
Stage 2/3			
At start	92	99	94
At end of follow-up	93	104	99

[a]FVC values are expressed as percentages of the predicted value. Each entry for FVC above is a mean.

TABLE 5. FEV_1 Values

	FEV_1 (mean %)[a]		
	A_1	A_2	B
Stage 1			
At start	100	102	102
At end of follow-up	98	107	111
Stage 2/3			
At start	96	103	99
At end of follow-up	110	97	102

[a]FEV_1 values are expressed as percentages of the predicted value. Each entry for FEV_1 above is a mean.

TABLE 6. PaO_2 Values

	PaO_2 (torr)[a]		
	A_1	A_2	B
Stage 1			
At start	91 (12.10)	86 (11.44)	85 (11.31)
At end of follow-up	85 (11.31)	86 (11.44)	83 (11.04)
Stage 2			
At start	87 (11.57)	90 (12.00)	88 (11.70)
At end of follow-up	89 (11.84)	89 (11.84)	86 (11.44)

[a]Values in kPa are shown in parentheses.

TABLE 7. $D_L CO_{SB}$ Values at the End of Each Observation Period

	Percentage of Patients			
	Stage 1		Stage 2/3	
$D_L CO_{SB}$ (%)[a]	$A_1 + A_2$ (N = 38)	B (N = 20)	$A_1 + A_2$ (N = 59)	B (N = 28)
≥ 80	84	65	76	86
70-79	11	25	9	10
< 70	5	10	15	4

[a] $D_L CO_{SB}$ values are expressed as a percentage of the predicted value.

TABLE 8. DM Values at the End of Each Observation Period

	Percentage of Patients			
	Stage 1		Stage 2/3	
DM (%)[a]	$A_1 + A_2$ (N = 36)	B (N = 19)	$A_1 + A_2$ (N = 58)	B (N = 29)
≥ 80	81	95	76	79

[a] DM values are expressed as percentages of the predicted value.

TABLE 9. C_{stat} Values at the End of Each Observation Period

	Percentage of Patients			
	Stage 1		Stage 2/3	
C_{stat} (%)[a]	$A_1 + A_2$ (N = 25)	B (N = 15)	$A_1 + A_2$ (N = 37)	B (N = 21)
≥ 80	84	80	68	76
70-79	16	7	24	19
< 70	0	13	8	5

[a] C_{stat} values are expressed as a percentage of the predicted value.

There was no correlation between D_LCO_{SB} and C_{stat} on the one hand and residual radiological alterations on the other hand.

DISCUSSION

Whereas the immediate supressive effect of prednisolone therapy on the granulomatous disorders was clearly demonstrated in our investigations, as has been generally found, the late results after a mean observation of about 9 years have not shown any advantage in favor of the treated patients.

This is true also when supplementary functional parameters considered more suitable for the early detection of fibrosing processes were assessed and the results for treated and untreated patients with stage 1 sarcoidosis, and the results for those with stage 2 and stage 3 sarcoidosis, were compared.

Thus there was no evidence that corticosteroid therapy of the chosen regimen had real influence on the long-term course of sarcoidosis stage 1, 2, or 3.

The different ways to diagnose sarcoidosis disease could be one of the reasons for the disagreement about the needs of and the right time to begin corticosteroid therapy—as discussed recently by DeRemee.[4]

Unlike many other investigators, we detected sarcoidosis in the great majority of our patients in the course of a mass radiographic investigation, or by chance when sarcoidosis was not clinically evident. It is obvious that individuals with radiological findings who did not feel ill came to medical attention and were made patients who otherwise would never have been discovered and who would have recovered spontaneously if they had not attended the mass radiographic investigation. This method of finding cases of other pulmonary diseases was practiced in the German Democratic Republic every year for the whole population aged 16 years or more, but now only for those aged 40 or more.

CONCLUSIONS

As long as reliable markers are not available to identify patients with a high risk of an unfavorable long-term course of the pulmonary sarcoidosis which requires an immediate treatment, we continue to start treatment of functionally unimpaired patients, even those with stage 2 or stage 3 sarcoidosis without extrapulmonary manifestations, only if spontaneous regression does not occur during the 12 months (or 12-18 months) after the initial diagnosis, or if, in this period, the disease shows a progressive course.

REFERENCES

1. Roth, I., I. Ehrke, H. Eule & W. Weinecke. 1975. Erster Bericht über eine kontrollierte klinische Untersuchung zur Prednisolon-Behandlung der thorakalen Sarkoidose. Z. Erkr. Atmungsorgane **142:** 49-58.

2. EULE, H., I. ROTH, I. EHRKE & W. WEINECKE. 1977. Corticosteroid therapy of intrathoracic sarcoidosis stages I and II: Results of a controlled clinical trial. Z. Erkr. Atmungsorgane **149:** 142-147.
3. EULE, H., I. ROTH & W. WEIDE. 1978. Clinical and functional results of a controlled clinical trial of the value of prednisolone therapy in sarcoidosis stages I and II. *In* Eighth International Conference on Sarcoidosis and Other Granulomatous Diseases. W. Jones Williams & B. H. Davies, Eds.: 624-628. Alpha Omega. Cardiff.
4. DEREMEE, R. A. 1977. The present status of treatment of pulmonary sarcoidosis: A house divided. Chest **71:** 388-393.

Longitudinal Study of Chronic Sarcoidosis with Low-Dose Maintenance Corticosteroid Therapy

Outcome and Complications[a]

CAROL J. JOHNS,[b] STEVEN A. SCHONFELD,[b,c] PENELOPE P. SCOTT,[b,c] JIMMY B. ZACHARY,[b] AND M. ISABELLE MACGREGOR[b]

[b]*Department of Medicine*
Johns Hopkins University School of Medicine
and
The Johns Hopkins Hospital
Baltimore, Maryland

[c]*Sinai Hospital*
Baltimore, Maryland

Many studies of sarcoidosis have reviewed the varied manifestations of the disease and some have summarized the occurrence of spontaneous remissions or radiographic clearing with or without treatment.[1–4] Patients with persistent disease over several years are of special concern. The Hopkins group has previously reported a study of changes in pulmonary sarcoidosis during and after long-term corticosteroid treatment.[5,6] Features of chronic sarcoidosis have been noted in other publications.[7–10] Although disease of more than 2 years duration is often described as "chronic" sarcoidosis, the present study selectively directs attention to patients whose clinical evidence of sarcoidosis extends over 5 years or more. A previous report reviewed 101 patients.[11] The present study extends this to include 181 patients. No conclusions can be drawn about the relative frequency of this type of chronic disease as the patients include a highly selected group drawn to the Johns Hopkins Hospital from a wide area. The Sarcoid Clinic and Consultation Service have provided the opportunity to study such patients over a period of many years. Some patients also have been studied at Sinai Hospital of Baltimore and Good Samaritan Hospital.

We have observed that significant numbers of patients do have severe and often progressive disease requiring prolonged treatment. This study addresses the following major questions: What are the patterns of disease in chronic sarcoidosis? Are there differences between white and black patients? Does the major disease feature of the initial presentation predict the nature of further long-term manifestations? What are

[a]This research was supported in part by the Hospital for the Consumptives of Maryland (Eudowood) and by Out-Patient Department Clinical Research Grant 5 MO1 RR 00722 from the United States Public Health Service.

the effects and complications of corticosteroid treatment? How long is treatment required?

RESULTS

The series reported in this paper included 181 patients, 141 (78%) of whom were black and 40 (22%) of whom were white. The series included 125 (69%) women and 56 (31%) men. Sarcoidosis was diagnosed during the third and fourth decade in 75% of the patients (TABLE 1). Eighteen (13%) black patients were diagnosed under the age of 20 with the youngest age 12. This series identified no white patients less than age 20 at the time of diagnosis. Seventy-eight percent of the patients were studied for a minimum of 10 years. The mean period of follow-up was 14 years (TABLE 2).

TABLE 1. Age at Diagnosis

Age (years)	Number of Patients[a]		
	Black	White	Total
<20	18 (13)	0	18 (10)
20-39	105 (74)	32 (80)	137 (75)
40-59	18 (13)	7 (17)	25 (14)
>60	0	1 (3)	1 (<1)
Total	141 (78)	40 (22)	181 (100)

[a]Percentages are shown in parentheses.

TABLE 3 summarizes the manifestations of sarcoidosis in these patients separated according to race. Pulmonary disease was the most frequent and occurred in 88% of the patients. Skin disease was more frequent in the black patients (27%) and tended to be more severe than in white patients (12%) with an overall incidence of 24%. Ocular disease, mucosal and joint disease, and peripheral adenopathy also were more frequent in the black patients. Heart disease and hypercalcemia seemed more frequent in the white patients. Mucosal, parotid, bone, and lacrimal involvement were observed only in the black patients.

Treatment is summarized in TABLE 4. Ninety-four percent of the patients received prednisone (98% of the blacks and 83% of the whites) and 14% (25 blacks) received chloroquine or hydroxychloroquine for severe skin and mucosal involvement. All but two of these patients also received prednisone at some time during their treatment. Eight patients (seven whites and one black) received no specific treatment. One of these patients was felt to have stable, irreversible lung fibrosis. The other seven had mild disease or experienced spontaneous remission and required no treatment. Treatment was usually initiated with prednisone (40 mg daily), the doses of which were

TABLE 2. Years of Follow-up since Diagnosis

Follow-up (years)	Number of Patients[a]		
	Black	White	Total
5-9	31 (22)	10 (25)	41 (22)
10-14	40 (28)	12 (30)	52 (29)
15-19	48 (34)	13 (32)	61 (34)
>20	22 (16)	5 (12)	27 (15)
Total	141 (78)	40 (22)	181 (100)

[a]Percentages are shown in parentheses.

reduced progressively at 2-week intervals to 30, 25, 20, and then to 15 mg daily. Fifty-three percent (91/171) of the treated patients required continued low daily doses of prednisone. This percentage includes five patients who have since died but were receiving prednisone at the time of their deaths.

TABLE 5 shows the duration of prednisone treatment in this series. Only 22% received prednisone for 2 years or less. Sixty-three percent (108/171) required treatment for more than 5 years. The prolonged period of treatment was necessitated by the frequency of relapses which are presented in TABLE 6. Seventy-five percent of patients demonstrated at least one relapse as treatment was withdrawn. These occurred when the dose was below 15 mg and most frequently within 1 to 2 months after cessation of treatment.

TABLE 3. Sarcoidosis Manifestations

	Number of Patients[a]		
	Black (N = 141)	White (N = 40)	Total (N = 181)
Lungs	123 (87)	37 (92)	160 (88)
Skin	38 (27)	5 (12)	43 (24)
Eyes	26 (18)	5 (12)	31 (17)
Mucosa	23 (16)	—	23 (13)
Liver and spleen (hepatosplenomegaly)	15 (11)	1 (2)	16 (9)
Spleen (splenomegaly)	11 (8)	5 (12)	16 (9)
Joints	12 (9)	1 (2)	13 (7)
Peripheral nodes	13 (9)	—	13 (7)
Nervous system	10 (7)	2 (5)	12 (7)
Heart	7 (5)	5 (12)	12 (7)
Hypercalcemia	3 (2)	5 (12)	8 (4)
Parotid glands	6 (4)	—	6 (3)
Erythema nodosum	6 (4)	—	6 (3)
Bone	5 (4)	—	5 (3)
Lacrimal glands	3 (2)	—	3 (2)
Hilar nodes (not pulmonary)	1 (<1)	2 (5)	3 (2)
Muscles	1 (<1)	—	1 (<1)

[a]Percentages are shown in parentheses.

TABLE 4. Treatment

	Number of Patients[a]		
	Treated with Prednisone	Treated with Chloroquine	Never Treated
Black patients (N = 141)			
Continued treatment	74 (52)	7 (5)	
Total treated	138 (98)	25 (18)	1 (<1)
White patients (N = 40)			
Continued treatment	17 (43)	0 (0)	
Total treated	33 (83)	0 (0)	7 (18)
Total (N = 181)			
Continued treatment	91 (50)	7 (4)	
Total treated	171 (94)	25 (14)	8 (4)

[a]Percentages are shown in parentheses.

TABLE 5. Duration of Prednisone Treatment

Duration (years)	Number of Patients[a]
<1	14 (8)
1-2	23 (14)
3-5	26 (15)
6-10	50 (29)
11-15	37 (22)
16-20	14 (8)
>20	7 (4)
Total	171 (100)

[a]Percentages are shown in parentheses.

TABLE 6. Relapses with Prednisone Withdrawal

Number of Relapses	Number of Patients[a]
None	43 (25)
One	41 (24)
Several	87 (51)
Total	171 (100)

[a]Percentages are shown in parentheses.

TABLE 7. Current Prednisone Dose

Dose (mg/day)	Number of Patients[a]
0	74 (45)
≤5	16 (10)
6-10	43 (26)
11-15	24 (14)
16-20	7 (4)
>20	1 (<1)
Total	165 (100)

[a]Percentages are shown in parentheses.

TABLE 7 presents the current prednisone dose in the 165 treated and living patients. Ninety-one percent (83/91) were on daily doses of prednisone of 15 mg or less and 65% (59/91) no more than 10 mg daily. Daily treatment usually has been utilized to facilitate compliance.

Generally, steroid complications were not serious in nature of frequency and are presented in TABLE 8. Sixty-two instances were observed in 53 patients. Weight gain of more than 20 pounds was observed in 41 patients (24%). Diabetes mellitus was observed in 13 patients (8%), several of whom had a strong family history of diabetes. Aseptic necrosis of the hip was encountered in only three patients, and findings of peptic ulcer or mild gastrointestinal bleeding were observed in three patients. Two patients may have developed cataracts related to steroid treatment, but in one it was not clear whether it may have been related to previous uveitis. Psychiatric problems may preclude the use of corticosteroids. One white woman with previous psychotic episodes and recurrent skin lesions and pulmonary infiltrates developed a manic-depressive psychosis requiring withdrawal of corticosteroids. A black woman had schizophrenia which was worsened by prednisone, and she received prednisone only for 10 days.

TABLE 9 presents the initial major disease feature and compares it with the major disease feature at the outcome of disease. The entries in which the column and row headings are identical indicate the number of patients in which there was concordance between the initial major manifestation and subsequent major manifestation. Con-

TABLE 8. Steroid Complications[a]

	Number of Patients[b] ($N = 171$)
Weight gain (>20 lb)	41 (24)
Diabetes mellitus	13 (8)
Aseptic necrosis	3 (2)
Peptic ulcer/gastrointestinal bleeding	3 (2)
Cataract	2 (1)

[a]There were 62 instances in 53 patients.
[b]Percentages are shown in parentheses.

TABLE 9. Initial and Ultimate Major Disease Features

Initial Disease Feature	Ultimate Major Disease Feature[a]					
	Lung	Skin/Mucosa/Joint	Eye	Other	Asymptomatic	Total
Lung	70	2	—	—	49	121 (67)
Skin/mucosa/joint	1	13	—	—	5	19 (10)
Eye	—	1	4	—	5	10 (6)
Other	2	1	1	9	9	22 (12)
Asymptomatic	3	—	1	1	5	9 (5)
Total	76 (42)	17 (9)	6 (3)	10 (6)	73 (40)	181 (100)

[a]Each entry indicates the number of patients with a given initial disease feature and ultimate major disease feature. Percentages are shown in parentheses.

TABLE 10. Pulmonary Function Outcome

FVC[a]	FEV$_1$/FVC[b] ≥ 80	65-79	50-64	< 50	Total Number of Patients[c]
≥ 80	24	29	10	—	63 (35)
65-79	23	28	9	3	63 (35)
50-64	16	15	5	1	37 (20)
< 50	5	5	7	1	18 (10)
Total[b]	68 (38)	77 (42)	31 (17)	5 (3)	181 (100)

[a]Percentage of predicted normal.
[b]Each entry indicates the number of patients with a given percentage of predicted normal FVC and FEV$_1$/FVC.
[c]Percentages are shown in parentheses.

cordance or an asymptomatic outcome was observed in 169 patients (93%). One hundred one patients (56%) showed concordance of the major disease feature initially and at outcome. New "surprise" major manifestations were infrequent. There was an asymptomatic outcome in 73 patients (40%), including 5 who also were asymptomatic initially. Pulmonary manifestations were most frequent and major in 127 patients (70%). The grouping of patients with skin and/or mucosal and/or joint disease identified 23 patients (13%). Eye disease was a major manifestation in 12 patients (7%). The group of "other" patients includes those with significant fever and weight loss, hepatosplenomegaly, and hypercalcemia.

TABLE 10 presents the pulmonary function outcome with the percentages of the predicted forced vital capacity (FVC) along the horizontal and those of the forced expiratory volume in 1 sec (FEV$_1$)/FVC in the vertical columns. TABLES 11 & 12 present the same data by race. The FVC was at least 80% of the predicted normal value in 63 patients (35%), with 38 black patients (27%) and 25 white patients (63%), suggesting that restrictive lung disease is more common in black patients. Forty-eight black patients (34%) but only seven white patients (17%) had a FVC of less than 65%. Interestingly, 13 white patients (33%) showed moderate to severe airway obstruction (FEV$_1$/FVC < 65%) compared to 23 black patients (16%), suggesting a

TABLE 11. Percentage of Predicted Normal FVC Outcome by Race

FVC[a]	Number of Patients[b] Black	White	Total
≥ 80	38 (27)	25 (63)	63 (35)
65-79	55 (39)	8 (20)	63 (35)
50-64	33 (23)	4 (10)	37 (20)
< 50	15 (11)	3 (7)	18 (10)

[a]Percentage of predicted normal.
[b]Percentages are shown in parentheses.

TABLE 12. Percentage of Predicted Normal FEV_1/FVC Outcome by Race

	Number of Patients[b]		
FEV_1/FVC[a]	Black	White	Total
≥80	61 (43)	7 (17)	68 (37)
65-79	57 (40)	20 (50)	77 (43)
50-64	20 (14)	11 (28)	31 (17)
<50	3 (2)	2 (5)	5 (3)

[a]Percentage of predicted normal.
[b]Percentages are shown in parentheses.

tendency to greater airway disease in whites. Fully normal ventilatory function with no restriction or obstruction as measured by figures of at least 80% of the predicted normal value was seen only in 24 patients (13%). Some obstruction with the FEV_1/FVC less than 80% was demonstrated in 113 patients (62%).

TABLE 13 summarizes the symptom outcome of 171 patients treated with prednisone. Forty-seven black patients (34%) and 17 white patients (52%) were asymptomatic. Of the total group, 64 (37%) were asymptomatic. Twenty-eight percent had moderate or severe incapacity. Six patients, four blacks and two whites (4%), died, and five of the six deaths were directly related to sarcoidosis. Four patients (three blacks and one white) died with severe lung disease, including a black male with a massive hemoptysis. One white patient with known recurrent cardiac arrhythmias died suddenly. One black male died with carcinoma of the colon.

Chloroquine or hydroxychloroquine was utilized in 25 black patients because of progressive skin and mucosal changes. This was usually administered in repetitive 6-month courses of chloroquine 250 mg daily after an initial period of 500 mg daily for 14 days. This intermittent therapy was utilized to avoid ocular toxicity. All patients had ophthalmologic consultations before and after receiving chloroquine, and none demonstrated ocular toxicity. Skin and mucosal lesions usually regressed significantly during treatment, but also gradually recurred when chloroquine was withdrawn and improved again when chloroquine was reinstituted. Skin and mucosal changes requiring this treatment were not observed in any of the white patients in this series.

TABLE 13. Outcomes for Patients Treated with Prednisone

	Number of Patients[a]		
Outcome	Black	White	Total
Asymptomatic	47 (34)	17 (52)	64 (37)
Slightly Incapacitated	47 (34)	6 (18)	53 (31)
Moderately Incapacitated	33 (24)	3 (9)	36 (21)
Severely Incapacitated	7 (5)	5 (15)	12 (7)
Dead	4 (3)	2 (6)	6 (4)
Total	138	33	171

[a]Percentages are shown in parentheses.

DISCUSSION

Although spontaneous remissions are frequent in sarcoidosis, chronic persistent disabling disease is also observed. A highly selected group of 181 patients has been reviewed with all of the patients known directly by one of the authors. It had been the original intention to compare equal numbers of white and black patients. Patients fulfilling the 5-year persistent disease criterion for chronic sarcoidosis, however, were black by a 3.5:1 ratio. Therefore, in Baltimore, such chronic sarcoidosis seems more frequent in black patients, but also occurs in white patients. More extensive disease in black patients has been noted in other series.[12] It has been observed that the more extensive and severe the initial disease manifestations, the more likely it is that the disease will persist. An initial presentation of asymptomatic bilateral hilar adenopathy did progress to other disease manifestations in 22 patients (12%) (19 blacks and 3 whites) in this series.

Corticosteroids usually produce prompt clinical improvement with decreased pulmonary infiltrations, improved pulmonary function, and striking remission of symptoms. Therapeutic decisions were based on clinical observations of symptoms, chest roentgenograms, and spirometry. Serial *objective* measurements are essential in assessing the need for continued prednisone treatment. Delayed or interrupted treatment seems to allow progression and/or irreversible disease. Treatment given late in the disease has less benefit, as irreversible fibrosis may have occurred. When significant lung disease is present with no spontaneous remission or with gradual progression within 1 to 2 years, a trial of prednisone treatment should be considered, even though the patient may be relatively asymptomatic. Gradual progression of pulmonary disease with few or no symptoms has been observed more commonly in white patients than in black. Occasionally prednisone is not given when the disease is felt to be old and stable. In some instances, a therapeutic trial to determine reversibility of radiographic and pulmonary function abnormalities is necessary. Objective study of the chest radiographs and spirometry after 2 months of treatment should demonstrate improvement if treatment is to be continued. A previously "normal" vital capacity may have become super-normal, especially in relatively asymptomatic white patients.

Patient compliance is an obvious important factor. This seems to be facilitated with daily treatment rather than alternate-day therapy, according to patient testimony. The advantages and necessity for alternate-day treatment have not been clearly demonstrated when these low doses of prednisone are utilized. Even intelligent, cooperative patients may find it difficult to comply with an alternate-day schedule.

Prolonged periods of treatment are often necessary as relapses are frequent in these patients as treatment is withdrawn. Relapses may occur even after 10-15 years of treated and controlled disease and are usually significantly reversible when treatment is reinstituted. Some deterioration is observed with repeated relapses, especially if prolonged. Repeated pulmonary infections in these abnormal, distorted lungs also predispose them to gradual worsening. Low-dose daily prednisone (5-15 mg) seems to prevent relapses and sustain improvement. Periodic attempts to withdraw treatment are justified. Treatment for 10-20 or more years often is required in these patients, however, and provides beneficial effects and infrequent complications.

Very few patients have later major manifestations of a type different from those at the outset, as 94% show concordance of early and late major manifestations or an asymptomatic outcome. Thus, the pattern of disease in an individual patient is declared early in the course of disease, usually within the first year.

SUMMARY

A series of 181 patients with chronic persistent sarcoidosis for more than 5 years have been reviewed, with a mean follow-up period of 14 years, and 77% followed for more than 10 years. Efforts to identify more white patients meeting the criteria of such persistent disease were unsuccessful. Seventy-eight percent were black, and 69% were women. Pulmonary disease was the major manifestation in 70% and was present in 88%. The early major disease feature predicts the nature of the long-term manifestation in 94%. Ninety-four percent were treated with prednisone, with 63% for more than 5 years. Fifty-three percent required continued treatment, and of those receiving continued treatment, 91% were maintained on doses of no more than 15 mg daily and 65% on no more than 10 mg of prednisone daily. Relapses were frequent as prednisone was withdrawn, occurring at least once in 75% and several times in 51%.

Low-dose prednisone treatment with 5-15 mg daily provides significant benefit. A mean treatment period of 8 years was observed (range: 10 days to 24 years). The benefits of treatment greatly exceed the infrequent complications. In Baltimore, chronic sarcoidosis with persistent disease seems to be more frequently encountered in black patients than in white patients.

ACKNOWLEDGMENTS

The authors wish to express their appreciation to Kelly Manos for her assistance with the patient reviews and to Mardi Frey for her help in preparing the manuscript.

REFERENCES

1. Longcope, W. T. & D. G. Freiman. 1952. A study of sarcoidosis. Medicine **31:** 1-132.
2. Mayock, R. L., P. Bertrand, C. E. Morrison & J. H. Scott. 1963. Manifestations of sarcoidosis: Analysis of 145 patients with a review of nine series selected from the literature. Am. J. Med. **35:** 67-89.
3. Smellie, H. & C. Hoyle. 1960. The natural history of sarcoidosis. Q. J. Med. **29:** 539-559.
4. Wurm, K. & R. Rosner. 1976. Prognosis of chronic sarcoidosis. Ann. N.Y. Acad. Sci. **278:** 732-735.
5. Johns, C. J., J. B. Zachary & W. C. Ball, Jr. 1974. A ten-year study of corticosteroid treatment in pulmonary sarcoidosis. Johns Hopkins Med. J. **134:** 251-270.
6. Johns, C. J., M. I. MacGregor, J. B. Zachary & W. C. Ball, Jr. 1976. Extended experience in the long-term corticosteroid treatment of pulmonary sarcoidosis. Ann. N.Y. Acad. Sci. **278:** 722-731.
7. Johns, C. J., M. I. MacGregor, J. B. Zachary, J. Caplan & J. K. Silverman. 1980. Chronic sarcoidosis: Outcome, unusual features and complications. *In* Eighth International Conference on Sarcoidosis and Other Granulomatous Diseases. W. Jones Williams & B. H. Davies, Eds.: 558-566. Alpha Omega. Cardiff.
8. Kaplan, J. & C. J. Johns. 1979. Mycetomas in pulmonary sarcoidosis: Non-surgical management. Johns Hopkins Med. J. **145:** 157-161.

9. JOHNS, C. J. 1982. Editorial: Management of hemoptysis with pulmonary fungus balls in sarcoidosis. Chest **82:** 400-401.
10. CHRÉTIEN, J., J. MARSAC & J. C. SALTIEL, Eds. 1983. Sarcoidosis and Other Granulomatous Disorders. Pergamon Press. Paris.
11. JOHNS, C. J., J. B. ZACHARY, M. I. MACGREGOR, J. L. CURTIS, P. P. SCOTT & P. B. TERRY. 1982. The longitudinal study of chronic sarcoidosis. Trans. Am. Clin. Climatol. Assoc. **94:** 173-181.
12. SARTWELL, P. E. 1976. Racial differences in sarcoidosis. Ann. N.Y. Acad. Sci. **278:** 368-370.

Use of Budesonide in the Treatment of Pulmonary Sarcoidosis

OLOF B. SELROOS[a]

Department of Pulmonary Medicine
Lund University Hospital
and
Department of Clinical Research
AB Draco
Lund, Sweden

Glucocorticosteroids are the drugs most frequently used for treatment of sarcoidosis in the respiratory tract. The indications for starting therapy have differed from time to time, and have varied between different centers. Today, however, it is generally agreed that patients with enlarged intrathoracic lymph nodes but without radiographic changes of the lung parenchyma (stage 1 disease) should be left untreated. In patients who have parenchymal lesions, with or without enlarged lymph nodes (stage 2 and stage 3 disease, respectively), treatment is indicated if the respiratory symptoms persist, or if the respiratory function is significantly impaired or deteriorates.[1] Generally, an initial observation period without therapy for 6-12 months is recommended.[2] This is done because spontaneous recovery is common, and long-term treatment with steroids may cause side effects.

With the clinical routine described above, however, the therapy may be started too late. Many patients have already developed irreversible lung fibrosis when treatment is instituted after the observation period. Unfortunately, no clinical tests or measurements done at the time of diagnosis can predict the prognosis in the individual patient.[3]

The clinical situation would probably be different if an effective therapy without side effects were available. Such a therapy could be started early—although some patients would be treated unnecessarily. If local inhalation therapy with glucocorticosteroids could be shown to be efficacious this might partly solve the problem.

BUDESONIDE

Budesonide is a nonhalogenated glucocorticosteroid developed for inhalation therapy in patients with bronchial asthma. It has a high local anti-inflammatory potency.[4] Because of its rapid metabolic inactivation in the liver, budesonide has a very favorable ratio of local to systemic glucocorticosteroid effects.[5]

In the treatment of patients with chronic steroid-dependent asthma, budesonide has about the same antiasthmatic efficacy as beclomethasone dipropionate (BDP) per

[a] Address of correspondence: AB Draco, Department of Clinical Research, PB 34, S-221 00 Lund, Sweden.

μg substance. Budesonide is significantly less able, however, to depress the level of plasma cortisol. On all dose levels of BDP, a 70% higher dose of budesonide can be used with the same effect on the pituitary-adrenal axis.[6] All doses of budesonide above the low, standard dose of 400 μg per day, therefore, have obvious advantages. In prednisone-dependent asthmatic patients all the tested doses of budesonide (800, 1600, and 3200 μg per day) have been significantly more efficacious than the 15-, 30-, and 60-mg doses of prednisone, which were given on alternate days,[7] or the 10-, 20-, and 40-mg doses of prednisone given daily.[8]

Budesonide is not metabolized locally in the lungs.[9] *In vitro* studies using an isolated, perfused, and ventilated rat lung model indicate that higher pulmonary tissue concentrations of budesonide can be obtained after intratracheal instillation than after injection of the substance into the circulation.[10] The tissue concentrations have also been high enough to be of therapeutic interest.

It has been found that inhaled budesonide, 1600 μg per day for 8 weeks, significantly reduces the ratio of T helper cells/T suppressor cells in the bronchoalveolar lavage fluid in patients with active sarcoidosis.[11]

The abovementioned properties of budesonide provide the basis for the first open clinical trial with inhaled budesonide in patients with pulmonary sarcoidosis.

PATIENTS AND METHODS

Twenty patients with biopsy-proven sarcoidosis participated in the study. There were 13 female and 7 male patients with a mean age of 47 years (range: 24-68 years). All of them showed pulmonary parenchymal changes (stages 2-3) and an increased serum angiotensin-converting enzyme (ACE) activity. They had been followed for at least 6 months without therapy. Nine of the 20 patients had been treated earlier with oral corticosteroids, but not within the 6 months preceding the study. In all the patients progressive pulmonary disease was noted, and there was an obvious clinical indication for starting treatment with steroids. No extrapulmonary manifestations of sarcoidosis were present that would have made treatment with corticosteroids necessary.

The patients inhaled budesonide (Pulmicort®) instead of taking oral medication. Budesonide was administered from a metered-dose inhaler that delivered 200 μg per actuation. A 32 × 100-mm tube spacer (Inhalet®) was attached to the actuator, thereby reducing the oropharyngeal deposition of the steroid and increasing the deposition in the airways and alveolar spaces.[12]

The initial dose of budesonide was 800 μg, twice daily, in patients with a body weight above 70 kg, and 600 μg, twice daily, if the body weight was below 70 kg. This dose was maintained for 3-6 months, and thereafter was individually reduced to 800 μg per day and, if possible, to 400 μg per day.

The patients were followed at 3-6-month intervals when chest roentgenograms, pulmonary function tests, routine laboratory tests, and serum ACE level determinations were done.

The serum ACE level determinations were done by the spectrophotometric method. The chest roentgenograms were examined independently without knowledge of the clinical findings and therapy.

RESULTS

Subjective Symptoms

Four patients were symptom-free throughout the study. The remaining 16 complained of dyspnea at rest or during exercise. In all the symptomatic patients, except one, subjective improvement was noted within 3 months from the start of therapy.

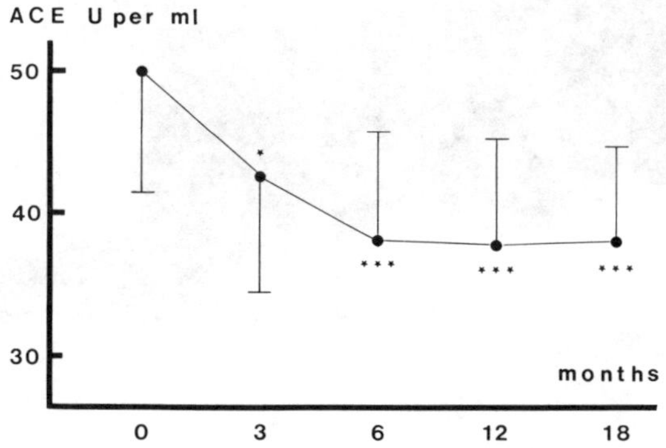

FIGURE 1. Mean values ± SD's of serum ACE levels in 20 sarcoidosis patients treated with inhaled budesonide. The upper limit of the normal range is 40 U/ml. The asterisks indicate statistically significant decreases during treatment: * = $p<.05$; *** = $p<.001$.

Serum ACE

The serum ACE activities are shown in FIGURE 1. According to the inclusion criteria all the patients had an abnormally high ACE activity (above 40 U/ml), the mean value ± SD being 50.0 ± 8.5 U/ml initially. After 3 months a statistically significant ($p<.02$) decrease to 42.8 ± 8.3 U/ml had occurred. At 6, 12, and 18 months the mean values ± SD's were 38.3 ± 7.6, 37.9 ± 7.5, and 38.2 ± 6.6 U/ml, respectively. All these mean values differ significantly ($p<.001$) from the mean value on admission to the study.

Chest Roentgenograms

On the first examination all patients had pulmonary parenchymal changes with or without enlarged hilar lymph nodes (stages 2-3). FIGURE 2 shows the lesions in

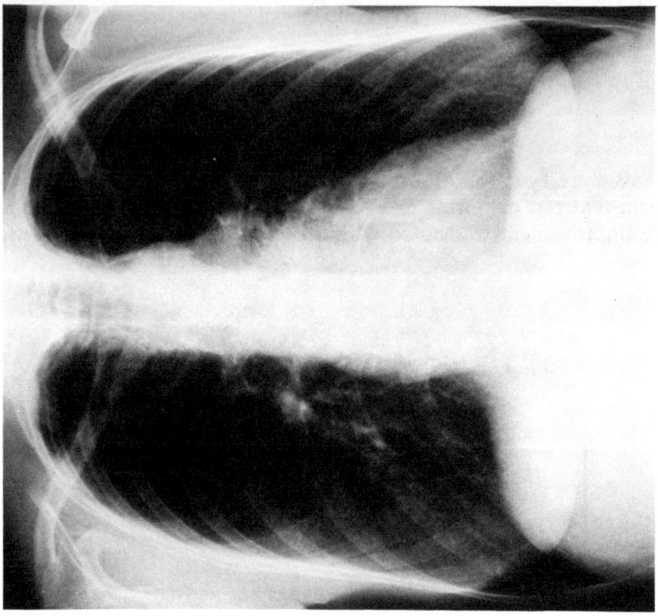

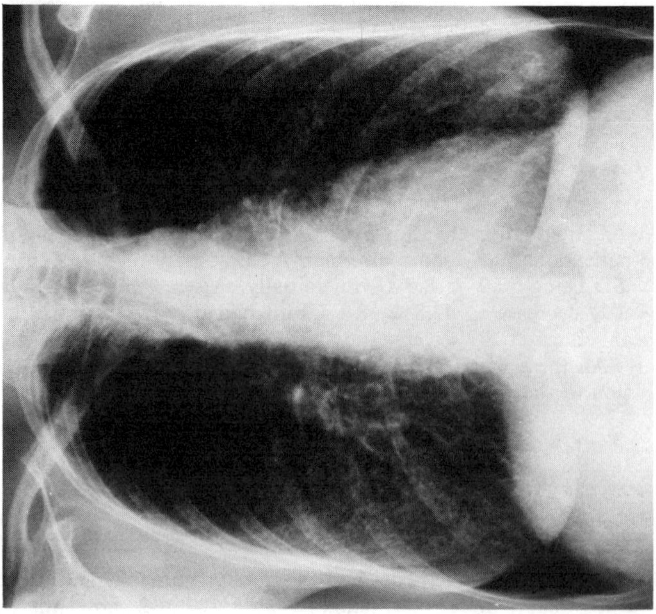

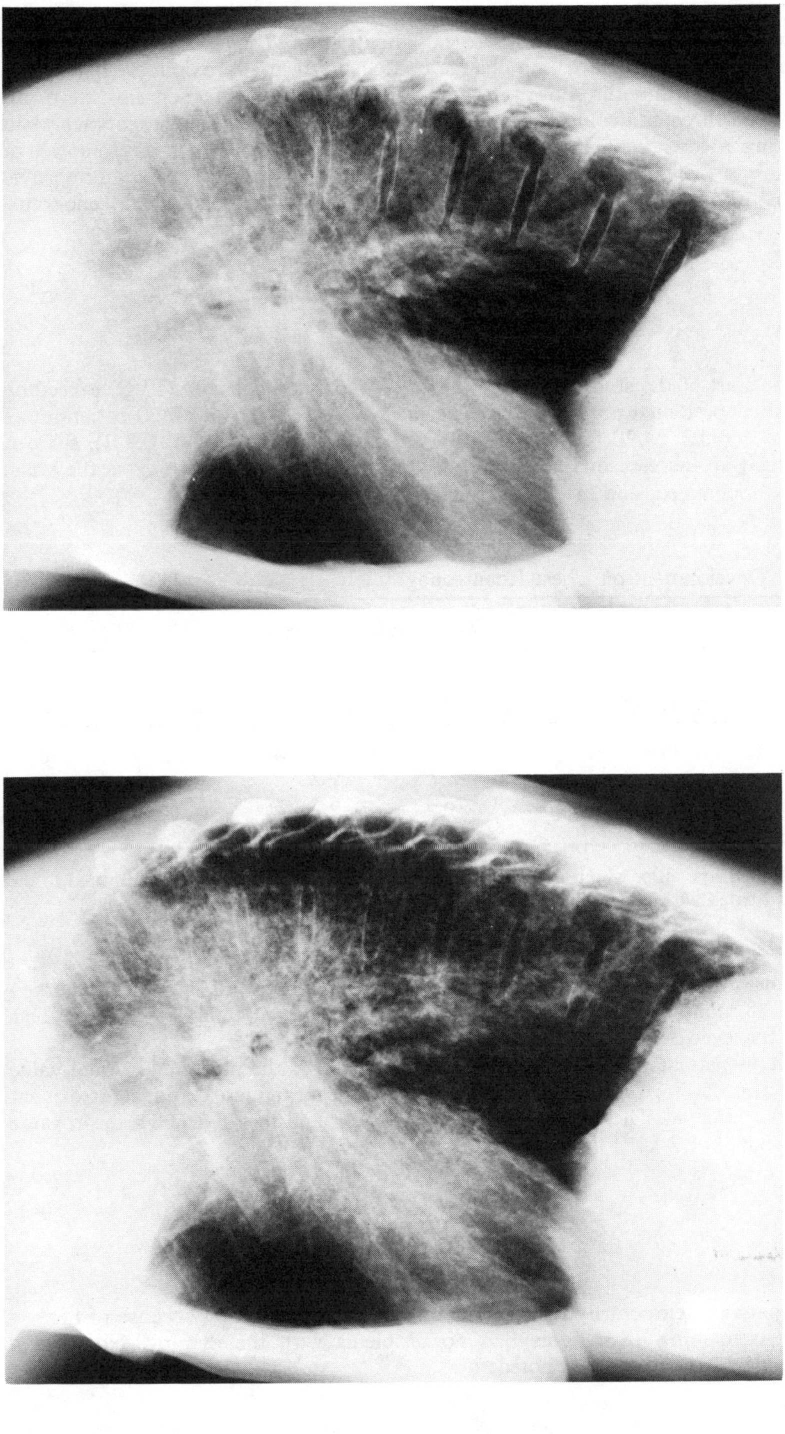

FIGURE 2. Chest roentgenograms of a 40-year-old woman with sarcoidosis. The patient was treated with oral prednisolone for 15 and 46 months after the disease was first active, and after the first relapse, respectively. The roentgenograms on the left were taken during the patient's second relapse; the roentgenograms on the right, after nine months of treatment with budesonide. The improvement is obvious.

one of the patients. The changes in the roentgenographic findings during treatment are shown in TABLE 1. After 3 months, six patients showed some degree of regression of the lesions. After 6 months, no change had occurred in approximately half of the patients. After 12 months, however, only four patients' roentgenograms were unchanged, and three had completely normalized. At 18 months, two patients who had been taking a low, maintenance dose of budesonide, 400 μg per day, showed a progression of their roentgenographic lesions. They subsequently showed an improvement when the dose was increased. Six patients had a normal chest roentgenogram.

Vital Capacity

At the start of the study 12 patients had a forced vital capacity (FVC) exceeding 80% of their predicted normal value. The mean value ± SD for all 20 patients was 3.1 ± 0.9 l (80.2 ± 20.7% of the predicted normal value, 3.9 ± 0.8 l). Sixteen patients had an increase in FVC during budesonide therapy. In two cases the value remained unchanged, and in two other cases it decreased slightly.

TABLE 1. Development on Chest Roentgenograms[a]

Time of Study (months)	Chest Roentgenogram				
	Unchanged	Deteriorated	Slightly Improved	Markedly Improved	Normal
3	13	1	4	2	0
6	9	0	9	2	0
12	4	0	6	7	3
18	3	2	4	5	6

[a]Twenty patients, all of whom had either stage 2 or stage 3 sarcoidosis, were admitted to the study and treated with inhaled budesonide.

The maximum increase, 0.49 ± 0.32 l, was noted after 10 months of therapy (range: 2-18 months), the mean value ± SD after treatment being 3.5 ± 0.9 l. This increase, however, was not statistically significant.

The eight patients with an initial FVC below 80% of the predicted normal value (mean ± SD: 2.5 ± 1.1 l) had approximately the same mean increase during treatment as the other patients. Their mean increase was 0.52 l, and they reached a mean value ± SD of 3.0 ± 1.2 l.

Side Effects

Two patients temporarily interrupted their inhalation therapy because of hoarseness. The remaining 18 patients had no problems with the therapy. No case of oropharyngeal candidiasis was noted.

DISCUSSION

Oral prednisone and prednisolone are the most widely used glucocorticosteroids for the treatment of sarcoidosis. Methylprednisolone has been routinely used in some centers.[13] Recently, it has been shown that methylprednisolone penetrates the lung acini in a greater concentration for a given blood level than does prednisone.[14] In the treatment of patients with steroid-responsive idiopathic lung fibrosis, methylprednisolone has also been more efficacious than prednisone.[15] Therefore, there seems to be a difference in the effects produced by these two corticosteroids in the treatment of respiratory diseases.

Inhalation therapy with corticosteroids has been used almost solely in the treatment of airway diseases. BDP has been given to patients with bronchial sarcoidosis with or without stenosis, but no controlled clinical studies have been carried out. The experience with inhalation steroids in the treatment of pulmonary parenchymal sarcoidosis is scanty, and the results are poor.

The inhalation of budesonide reveals unique properties compared to other steroid inhalation preparations, which have been available for some time. It is not locally metabolized in the lungs, and, after inhalation, it also gives sufficiently high tissue concentrations for the necessary steroid receptor binding. Because of its rapid inactivation in the liver after systemic absorption, systemic bioavailability is low, and high doses can be used with a definitely lower risk of systemic side effects than when oral doses of steroids are given. It is also interesting that inhaled budesonide can cause the same change as oral prednisone in the ratio of T helper cells/T suppressor cells in the bronchoalveolar lavage fluid. This change seems to be more important with regard to therapeutic efficacy than a change in the absolute lymphocyte counts.[16]

The present series of patients had progressive parenchymal lung lesions that had been followed without therapy for at least 6 months. They also had an increased serum ACE activity, and in all cases therapy with corticosteroids was initiated on clinical grounds. It seems likely that without active therapy the lesions would have become worse in most of the patients. With budesonide an improvement was noted. ACE activity was normalized in all patients. The chest roentgenogram remained unchanged in only four patients, and in two of these patients the deterioration was probably due to too low a dose of budesonide. The respiratory function, measured as the FVC, also improved in most of the patients. The study was open and uncontrolled, but the positive effects were too clear to be ascribed to a placebo.

The inhalation therapy was well tolerated, and only two patients complained of temporary hoarseness. No pharyngeal candidiasis was noted. The sparsity of local side effects may be due to the use of the tube spacer. In this study possible systemic side effects were not specifically looked for. Clinical studies in patients with asthma and in healthy subjects have shown that the highest dose of budesonide used in this study, 1600 μg per day, corresponds to 5 mg of oral prednisolone, with respect to its ability to depress the level of plasma cortisol. Treatment with budesonide is therefore much safer than the standard treatment with oral steroids.

The regression of the radiographic lesions, however, seemed to be somewhat slower in this study than that usually seen when treatment with oral steroids is given. This may be because the initial dose of budesonide, 1200-1600 μg per day, was low compared to the usual initial dose of prednisolone, for example. It seems possible that patients with respiratory symptoms and untreated sarcoidosis should initially be treated with a combination of oral methylprednisolone and budesonide. The oral treatment could be administered for 6-12 weeks using an initial dose of only 16-20 mg per day. Such a regimen, however, should be studied in controlled clinical trials.

Inhalation therapy with budesonide can, of course, be efficacious only in the treatment of pulmonary sarcoidosis. Extrapulmonary lesions must be treated with systemically administered drugs. In many cases, however, the pulmonary manifestations represent the only indication to start therapy, and, in such cases, inhaled budesonide seems promising as an additional, and safer, alternative to the usual therapeutic arsenal.

Future clinical studies will determine the place of inhaled budesonide in the treatment of pulmonary sarcoidosis and other inflammatory parenchymal diseases. It will also be interesting—and, indeed, necessary—to find out whether the overall prognosis of sarcoidosis can be influenced by starting treatment with inhaled steroids early, without an initial observation period. The safety of budesonide permits such a clinical approach.

SUMMARY

Twenty patients with active sarcoidosis (increased serum ACE activity) and progressive pulmonary disease (stages 2-3) were treated with inhaled budesonide instead of with oral glucocorticosteroids in an open clinical study. Results after an 18-month treatment are reported.

A general improvement in chest roentgenograms and FVC was noted. Serum ACE activity was normalized.

The results indicate that pulmonary manifestations of sarcoidosis can be treated with the inhaled steroid, budesonide. In this way the risk of systemic side effects is considerably reduced. The final place of inhaled budesonide in the treatment of sarcoidosis must be determined via placebo-controlled and comparative, double-blinded clinical studies in larger series of patients.

REFERENCES

1. DeRemee, R. A. & A. R. Zinsmeister. 1981. State of the art: The treatment of pulmonary sarcoidosis. *In* Sarcoidosis and Other Granulomatous Disorders. J. Chrétien, J. Marsac & J. C. Saltiel, Eds.: 457-464. Pergamon Press. Paris.
2. Turiaf, J., C. J. Johns, A. S. Teirstein, S. Tsuji & K. Wurm. 1976. The problem of the treatment of sarcoidosis: Report of the subcommittee on therapy. Ann. N.Y. Acad. Sci. **278:** 743-750.
3. Selroos, O. 1984. Value of biochemical markers in serum for determination of disease activity in sarcoidosis. Sarcoidosis **1:** 45-49.
4. Brattsand, R., A. Thalén, K. Roempke, L. Källström & E. Gruvstad. 1982. Development of new glucocorticosteroids with a very high ratio between topical and systemic activities. Eur. J. Respir. Dis. **63**(Suppl. 122): 62-73.
5. Andersson, P., S. Edsbäcker, Å. Ryrfeldt & C. von Bahr. 1982. *In vitro* biotransformation of glucocorticoids in liver and skin homogenate fractions from man, rat and hairless mouse. J. Steroid Biochem. **16:** 787-795.
6. Löfdahl, C.-G., T. Mellstrand & N. Svedmyr. 1984. Glucocorticoids and asthma: Studies of resistance and systemic effects of glucocorticoids. Eur. J. Respir. Dis. **65**(Suppl. 136): 69-79.
7. Toogood, J. H., B. Jennings, J. Baskerville, N. M. Lefcoe & S.-Å. Johansson. 1983. Bioequivalent doses of inhaled vs. oral steroids for severe asthma. Chest **84:** 349.

8. TOOGOOD, J. H., B. JENNINGS, J. BASKERVILLE, N. M. LEFCOE & S.-Å. JOHANSSON. 1984. Safe and effective dose limits for budesonide treatment of chronic asthma. Abstract. Canadian Lung Association Annual Scientific Meeting. Edmonton.
9. ANDERSSON, P. & Å. RYRFELDT. 1984. Biotransformation of the topical glucocorticoids budesonide and beclomethasone 17α,21-dipropionate in human liver and lung homogenate. J. Pharm. Pharmacol. **36:** 763-765.
10. RYRFELDT, Å., G. PERSSON, E. NILSSON & O. SELROOS. 1984. Pulmonary disposition of the potent glucocorticoid budesonide evaluated in an isolated, perfused rat lung model. Submitted for publication.
11. SELROOS, O. 1984. Unpublished data.
12. NEWMAN, S. P., F. MORÉN, D. PAVIA, F. LITTLE & S. W. CLARKE. 1981. Deposition of pressurized suspension aerosols inhaled through extension devices. Am. Rev. Respir. Dis. **124:** 317-320.
13. SELROOS, O. & T.-L. SELLERGREN. 1979. Corticosteroid therapy of pulmonary sarcoidosis: A prospective evaluation of alternate day and daily dosage in stage II disease. Scand. J. Respir. Dis. **60:** 215-221.
14. BRAUDE, A. C. & A. S. REBUCK. 1983. Prednisone and methylprednisolone disposition in the lung. Lancet **ii:** 995-997.
15. KEOGH, B. A., J. BERNADO, G. W. HUNNINGHAKE, B. R. LINE, D. L. PRICE & R. G. CRYSTAL. 1983. Effect of intermittent high dose parenteral corticosteroids on the alveolitis of idiopathic pulmonary fibrosis. Am. Rev. Respir. Dis. **127:** 18-22.
16. CEUPPENS, J. L., L. M. LACQUET, G. MARIEN, M. DEMEDTS, A. VAN DEN EECKHOUT & E. STEVENS. 1984. Alveolar T-cell subsets in pulmonary sarcoidosis: Correlation with disease activity and effect of steroid treatment. Am. Rev. Respir. Dis. **129:** 563-568.

Neurosarcoidosis

Presentation and Management

BARNEY J. STERN AND ALLAN KRUMHOLZ

Division of Neurology
Sinai Hospital of Baltimore
and
Department of Neurology
Johns Hopkins University and Hospital
Baltimore, Maryland

CAROL J. JOHNS

Department of Medicine
Johns Hopkins University and Hospital
Baltimore, Maryland

Neurosarcoidosis is a diagnostic consideration in diverse clinical settings. Neurosarcoidosis is often suspected in patients with systemic sarcoidosis who develop neurologic symptoms. Furthermore, sarcoidosis may also be considered in the neurologic evaluation of patients without established systemic sarcoidosis who develop symptoms suggestive of neurosarcoidosis.

Despite the diverse neurologic manifestations of sarcoidosis, a unified concept of neurosarcoidosis can be formulated. Central nervous system (CNS) sarcoidosis may be conceptualized as a disease having a predilection for the meninges.[1] The granulomatous process characteristically infiltrates along the meninges at the base of the brain to involve the cranial nerves. A more extensive spread may disrupt the flow of cerebrospinal fluid (CSF) and cause hydrocephalus. Aseptic meningitis may also reflect extensive meningeal infiltration by granulomas. Lastly, meningeal spread of granulomas along perivascular routes may cause parenchymatous disease such as seizures and mass lesions.

In this study, the neurologic manifestations of sarcoidosis are assessed in a large population. A profile of the neurologic manifestations of sarcoidosis is developed and an approach to the diagnosis and management of patients with suspected neurosarcoidosis proposed. Furthermore, evoked-potential studies and CSF immunologic assays were obtained in some patients with sarcoidosis to investigate the potential value of these newer neurodiagnostic procedures in neurosarcoidosis.

METHODS

Patients with sarcoidosis cared for at the Johns Hopkins Hospital or the Sinai Hospital of Baltimore formed the population base of our investigations. For the first part of our study, the charts of all patients cared for at the Johns Hopkins Hospital Sarcoid Clinic or discharged from the Johns Hopkins Hospital with a diagnosis of sarcoidosis from 1975 to 1980 were identified. Neurologic disease need not have presented during the study period; patients were included in the series if they received care at the Johns Hopkins Hospital during the specified time period.

A patient was considered to have neurosarcoidosis if 1) systemic sarcoidosis was present and the neurologic illness could be reasonably attributed to sarcoidosis while other causes were excluded or 2) other systemic manifestations of sarcoidosis could not be established but pathologic examination at the site of neurologic involvement was consistent with a diagnosis of sarcoidosis and no other cause for the illness could be identified.

Another recent group of patients with sarcoidosis cared for at the Johns Hopkins Hospital or the Sinai Hospital of Baltimore was studied with brainstem auditory and visual evoked potentials. Patients were classified into two groups based on the nature of their clinical involvement with sarcoidosis. The patients were classified as having neurosarcoidosis or systemic manifestations of sarcoidosis without clinical evidence of neurosarcoidosis. Local ocular disease or involvement of the second and/or eighth cranial nerves, the specific cranial nerves tested by evoked-potential studies, was also noted.

Brainstem auditory evoked potentials (BAEP's) and visual evoked potentials (VEP's) were obtained using standard procedures.[2-4] The auditory stimulus was a 65-dB sensation level (SL) click presented at a rate of 10 Hz, and the visual stimulus was a checkerboard pattern with each square subtending an angle of 55 minutes of arc. Limits of normality were defined as three standard deviations above mean values for normal controls in our laboratory.[2,4]

Three patients had an assay of mononuclear cell subpopulations in blood and CSF. All patients had neurosarcoidosis and other systemic manifestations of sarcoidosis. Dr. Diane E. Griffin of the Johns Hopkins Medical Institutions performed the mononuclear cell subpopulation assays. Peripheral blood mononuclear cells were isolated from heparinized venous blood by density-gradient centrifugation. CSF was placed directly into a cytocentrifuge chamber, and the cells were precipitated. Cells were sedimented and fixed in periodate-lysine-paraformaldehyde-glutaraldehyde according to the method of Gendelman *et al.*[5] Immunoperoxidase staining was slightly modified from the avidin-biotin complex method.[6] Slides were incubated with the following primary antibodies to identify the mononuclear cell subpopulations: T11 (total T cells), T8 (cytotoxic/suppressor T cells), T4 (helper/inducer T cells), B1 (B cells), and M1 (monocytes/macrophages).

RESULTS

Six hundred forty-nine patients seen at the Johns Hopkins Hospital had sarcoidosis, and 33 of these patients (5.1%) were judged to have neurosarcoidosis. In this group of 33 patients with neurologic disease, the average age of onset of sarcoidosis was 30.3 years; 64% of the 33 patients were female, and 85% were black. These demographics are similar to the general population of patients with sarcoidosis.

TABLE 1. Neurosarcoidosis: Frequencies of Clinical Manifestations

Clinical Manifestation	Number of Patients Affected ($N = 33$)
Cranial neuropathy	24 (73)
Aseptic meningitis	6 (18)
Hydrocephalus	3 (9)
CNS parenchymatous disease	
Mass or focal lesion	
Hypothalamus	5 (15)
Other intracranial	0
Intraspinal	2 (6)
Encephalopathy/vasculopathy	0
Seizures	0
Myopathy	4 (12)
Peripheral neuropathy	2 (6)

NOTE: Percentages are shown in parentheses.

The presenting manifestation of sarcoidosis was neurologic in 16 of the 33 patients with neurosarcoidosis. An additional eight patients developed neurologic complications within 2 years of developing sarcoidosis. Therefore, three-fourths of the patients who developed neurosarcoidosis did so within the first 2 years of their illness.

More than one manifestation of neurosarcoidosis was present in 30% of the patients (TABLE 1). Cranial neuropathy was the most common problem with involvement in 24 of 33 patients (73%) (TABLE 2). Two-thirds of these patients had multiple cranial nerve lesions. Facial weakness was the only neurologic abnormality in 6 of the 16 patients with a peripheral seventh-nerve palsy.

Other manifestations of neurosarcoidosis included six patients with aseptic meningitis, three with hydrocephalus, four with myopathy, and two with peripheral neuropathy. Five patients had hypothalamic dysfunction, and two patients had intraspinal lesions. No patient had seizures.

The diagnostic evaluation of the 33 patients revealed an abnormality on the initial chest radiograph in 82% and a positive Kveim test in 73% of the 15 patients tested. A biopsy was abnormal and consistent with sarcoidosis in 24 of 28 patients. Other systemic manifestations of sarcoidosis were found in 97% of the patients, typically at intrathoracic (88% of patients) and ocular (55% of patients) sites.

Over one-half of the 30 patients studied had at least one abnormal CSF evaluation. Computed tomography (CT) scans were obtained in 13 patients and were abnormal in 5. CT scan abnormalities included hydrocephalus in three patients, calcification in the right temporal lobe in one patient, and incidentally discovered enhancing nodules in two patients. The electroencephalogram (EEG) was abnormal in 4 of 10 patients tested and revealed generalized or focal slowing. No patient had epileptiform discharges.

The clinical course could be adequately assessed in 25 patients. There were 33 episodes of neurologic dysfunction in these patients, and the clinical outcome was judged to be good in 82% of the cases. Only one patient died of neurologic disease; this patient had progressive hydrocephalus and multiple nodules apparent on CT scan. He was noncompliant in following his prescribed steroid therapy. Steroids were administered to 21 of 25 patients with a documented clinical course. The outcome of the patients treated with steroids was similar to that of the overall group, but only a small number of patients failed to receive steroids, a fact that makes comparison to the treated group difficult.

VEP and BAEP results are summarized in TABLE 3. There were no detectable abnormalities in the nine patients without CNS disease. Among the eight patients with neurosarcoidosis, a single patient with no clinical evidence of ocular or optic nerve disease had an abnormal VEP. Two patients with visual symptoms due to optic nerve disease had abnormal VEP's. The initially abnormal VEP's in these symptomatic patients normalized following steroid therapy.

Mononuclear cell subpopulations were examined in three patients with CNS sarcoidosis (TABLE 4). One patient (number 3) demonstrated an abnormally increased helper/suppressor ratio of 6.8.

DISCUSSION

Analysis of our patients allows some guidelines to be formulated to aid the physician in the evaluation of patients with suspected neurosarcoidosis. In many patients the clinical presentation of sarcoidosis is so classical that there is little doubt as to the correct diagnosis. Other patients, however, present in an atypical manner and create considerable difficulty in establishing a diagnosis. This latter situation is frequently

TABLE 2. Neurosarcoidosis: Cranial Neuropathies

Cranial Nerve	Manifestation	Patients Affected ($N = 24$)
1	Anosmia	
	Unilateral	1
	Bilateral	2
2	Diminished visual acuity	
	Papilledema	2
	Optic neuritis	1
	Indeterminate	1
3	Ophthalmoplegia	1
	Ptosis	1
4	Ophthalmoplegia	1
5	Sensorimotor neuropathy	1
	Hypoesthesia	1
	Neuralgia	1
6	Ophthalmoplegia	3
7	Peripheral palsy	
	Unilateral	11
	Bilateral[a]	5
8	Unilateral dysfunction	1
	Bilateral dysfunction[a]	6
9,10	Bilateral dysfunction	1
11	—	—
12	Unilateral Palsy	1

[a]Three patients had bilateral seventh and eighth nerve dysfunction.

TABLE 3. Sarcoidosis: Evoked Potentials

	Number of Patients	
	Patients without Neurosarcoidosis ($N = 9$)	Patients with Neurosarcoidosis ($N = 8$)
VEP		
Normal	9[a]	5
Abnormal	—	3[b]
BAEP		
Normal	9	6
Abnormal	—	—

[a]Two patients had ocular disease.
[b]Two patients had optic nerve disease.

encountered in neurologic practice. The common presentations of neurosarcoidosis are well known and, with some minor differences, reaffirmed in the present series.[7,8] The absence of patients with epilepsy in our series is of interest and may reflect the low incidence of CNS parenchymatous disease and the overall low morbidity and mortality of our patients.

Neurologic dysfunction was the initial presentation of sarcoidosis in one-half of our patients with neurosarcoidosis. In general, neurologic disease seems to develop early in the course of sarcoidosis. Other systemic disease is usually documented in patients presenting with neurosarcoidosis and is most common at intrathoracic and ocular sites. Because of the high likelihood of documenting systemic disease, an ophthalmologic examination[9] and chest radiograph should be routine in the evaluation of patients with suspected neurosarcoidosis. Our current recommendation for obtaining histologic confirmation of sarcoidosis is to biopsy a palpably enlarged lymph node or an obvious cutaneous or mucosal lesion. A transbronchial biopsy is often helpful, and other procedures such as biopsy of minor salivary glands or conjunctiva are potential diagnostic aids. A Kveim test or liver biopsy may provide useful information.

In general, the neurodiagnostic evaluation should be appropriate to the clinical problem, and, therefore, few specific recommendations can be made. Given the protean nature of sarcoidosis, however, a thorough evaluation of patients with suspected neurosarcoidosis should be undertaken to delineate the full extent of the disease and guide therapy.

A CSF examination should be performed whenever possible in patients with suspected CNS sarcoidosis.[10] In one of three patients with neurosarcoidosis we have shown that the CSF helper/suppressor ratio is abnormal. Although the CSF cellular composition might be expected to reflect disease activity at the site of symptomatic neurologic involvement, this has recently been questioned.[6] The limitations of obtaining biopsy material from the CNS, however, makes the study of CSF worthwhile. Further analysis of CSF mononuclear cell subpopulations will be of interest. In theory an elevated helper/suppressor ratio may identify patients with particularly intense CNS inflammation.[11–13]

A CT scan is particularly helpful in the evaluation of neurosarcoidosis because it may reveal the potentially life-threatening complications of neurosarcoidosis, progressive hydrocephalus and mass lesions. Asymptomatic mass lesions may be more common than previously appreciated and would be demonstrated by CT scan.[14]

A preliminary analysis of our VEP and BAEP results demonstrates abnormalities of the VEP in patients with sarcoidosis of the optic nerves and resolution of these abnormalities following steroid therapy. A single patient with neurosarcoidosis without clinical evidence of ocular or optic nerve disease also had an abnormal VEP. Although our data suggest that evoked potentials may be useful in patients with symptomatic neurosarcoidosis, it does not demonstrate the utility of BAEP or VEP studies in the detection of subclinical neurologic disease in patients without neurosarcoidosis. More patients will need to be examined before a definitive statement is made, but our results differ from others[15] who have found a high incidence of abnormal VEP studies even in patients with no overt neurologic disease.

Given the rarity of neurosarcoidosis, it will be difficult to conduct a controlled treatment trial, and, therefore, large clinical series can help delineate guidelines for therapy. Based on current evidence, we would advocate treating patients with neurologic manifestations of sarcoidosis with steroids and gradually decreasing the dose as the clinical course is monitored. An initial dose of prednisone 40 mg daily is usually sufficient to control the inflammatory reaction, although higher doses are occasionally required for severely ill or deteriorating patients.

In particular, steroid therapy has been found to be beneficial for CNS parenchymatous disease, especially mass lesions.[16,17] We have had personal experience outside this study with five patients with CNS sarcoid mass lesions.[17] In four of these patients

TABLE 4. CNS Sarcoidosis: Mononuclear Cell Subpopulations

Patient Number	Systemic Disease	CNS Disease	Peripheral Mononuclear Cells	CSF Studies[a]	CSF Mononuclear Cells
1	Intrathoracic Ocular Skin Nasal	CN 7	T11 = 68% T4 = 53% T8 = 24% T4/T8 = 2.2	TP = 40 mg/dl glu = 48 mg/dl WBC – 34, 97% mononuclear IgG index = 0.39 OCB (−)	T11 = 63% T4 = 51% T8 = 25% T4/T8 = 2.8
2[b]	Intrathoracic Lymph node	CN 2,8	T11 = 59% T4 = 42% T8 = 17% T4/T8 = 2.5	TP = 83 mg/dl glu = 50 mg/dl WBC = 2, 100% mononuclear IgG index = 0.58 OCB (−)	T11 = 49% T4 = 35% T8 = 13% T4/T8 = 2.7
3	Intrathoracic Ocular Skin Lymph node	CN 5,7,8	T11 = 61% T4 = 46% T8 = 23% T4/T8 = 2.0	TP = 60 mg/dl glu = 58 mg/dl WBC = 10, 96% mononuclear IgG index = 0.64 OCB (−)	T11 = 83% T4 = 75% T8 = 11% T4/T8 = 6.8

NOTE: CN: cranial nerve; TP: total protein; glu: glucose; WBC: white blood cells; and OCB: oligoclonal bands.

[a]The IgG index was normal in all patients.

[b]The patient was treated with 10 mg of prednisone each day.

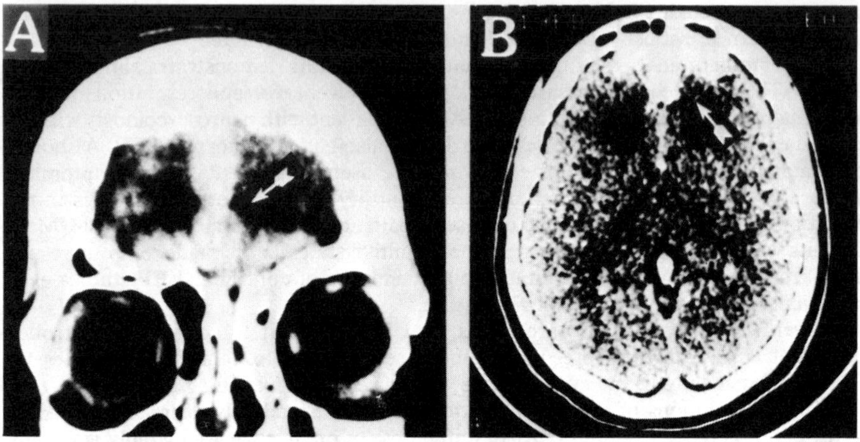

FIGURE 1. A 39-year-old black female developed headaches, anosmia, and progressive bilateral visual loss. A chest radiograph revealed bilateral hilar adenopathy; a nasal mucosal biopsy revealed noncaseating granulomas; and a Kveim test was consistent with sarcoidosis. An enhanced CT scan with coronal (**A**) and axial (**B**) reconstruction revealed a dense plaque-like lesion above the planum sphenodale and in the interhemispheric fissure.

the mass lesions were symptomatic while in one patient the CNS mass was an incidental finding on CT scan. In all of our patients, clinical symptoms and/or CT scan findings demonstrated improvement with steroid therapy (FIGS. 1 & 2). Based on our experience, we recommend that if a patient with systemic sarcoidosis develops a mass lesion consistent with a CNS sarcoid mass lesion, and if there is no evidence of

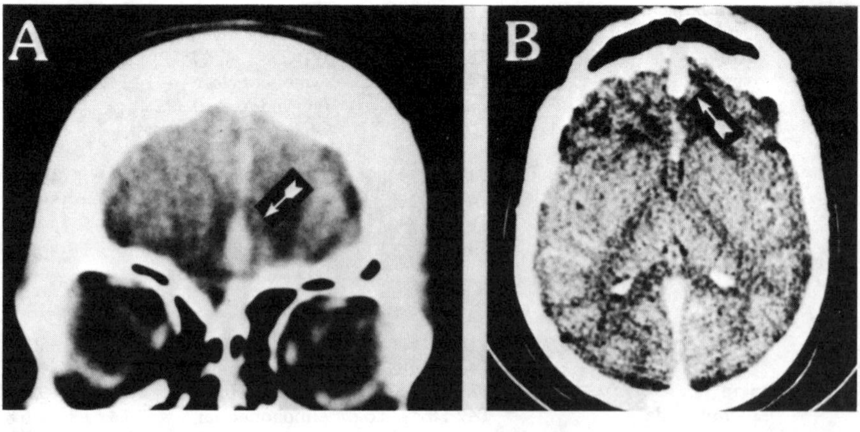

FIGURE 2. The patient depicted in FIGURE 1 was treated with steroids and improved within days. (**A**) A coronal enhanced CT scan after 5 months of prednisone therapy (average daily dose = 30 mg) documents marked improvement in the size of the sarcoid mass lesion. The patient was asymptomatic except for anosmia. (**B**) An axial enhanced CT scan 26 months after presentation documents continued improvement with only a small interhemispheric mass. Continuous steroid therapy (average daily prednisone dose = 15 mg) has been required to keep the patient asymptomatic except for anosmia.

infection, steroid therapy should be initiated. If there is no clinical or CT scan improvement, however, surgery should then be considered. Furthermore, if a patient without known sarcoidosis is found to have noncaseating granulomas on biopsy of a CNS mass, surgical resection should be deferred and a course of steroids begun. The subsequent clinical course would dictate the need for further surgery.

In summary, a thorough investigation of the patient with suspected neurosarcoidosis is indicated to delineate the extent of disease. CSF immunologic assays and evoked-potential studies merit further investigation in patients with neurosarcoidosis. Steroid therapy is indicated to try to impede the development of irreversible fibrosis that may be associated with the inflammatory process. The prognosis, in general, is quite good for most patients with neurosarcoidosis.

ACKNOWLEDGMENTS

Dr. Diane E. Griffin kindly performed the mononuclear cell subpopulation assays. Robert Luke provided research assistance. Carolyn J. Bitzel prepared the manuscript.

REFERENCES

1. WAXMAN, J. S. & J. H. SHER. 1979. The spectrum of central nervous system sarcoidosis: A clinical and pathologic study. Mt. Sinai J. Med. **46:** 309-317.
2. KRUMHOLZ, A., H. S. SINGER, E. NIEDERMEYER, R. BURNITE & K. HARRIS. 1983. Electrophysiological studies in Tourette's syndrome. Ann. Neurol. **14:** 638-641.
3. CHIAPPA, K. H. 1983. Evoked potentials in clinical medicine. Raven Press. New York, NY.
4. STERN, B. J., A. KRUMHOLZ, H. D. WEISS, P. GOLDSTEIN & K. C. HARRIS. 1982. Evaluation of brainstem stroke using brainstem auditory evoked responses. Stroke **13:** 705-711.
5. GENDELMAN, H. E., T. R. MOENCH, D. NARAYAN & D. E. GRIFFIN. 1983. Selection of a fixative for identifying T cell subsets, B cells and macrophages in paraffin embedded mouse spleen. J. Immunol. Methods **65:** 137-145.
6. MOENCH, T. R. & D. E. GRIFFIN. 1984. Immunocytochemical identification and quantitation of the mononuclear cells in the cerebrospinal fluid, meninges, and brain during acute viral meningoencephalitis. J. Exp. Med. **159:** 77-88.
7. WIEDERHOLT, W. C. & R. G. SIEKERT. 1965. Neurological manifestations of sarcoidosis. Neurology **15:** 1147-1154.
8. DELANEY, P. 1977. Neurologic manifestations in sarcoidosis: Review of the literature, with a report of 23 cases. Ann. Intern. Med. **87:** 336-345.
9. CAPLAN, L., J. CORBETT, J. GOODWIN, C. THOMAS, D. SHENKER & N. SCHATZ. 1983. Neuro-ophthalmologic signs in the angiitic form of neurosarcoidosis. Neurology (Cleveland) **33:** 1130-1135.
10. GAINES, J. D., P. B. ECKMAN & J. S. REMINGTON. 1970. Low CSF glucose level in sarcoidosis involving the central nervous system. Arch. Intern. Med. **125:** 333-336.
11. HUNNINGHAKE, G. W. & R. G. CRYSTAL. 1981. Pulmonary sarcoidosis: A disorder mediated by excess helper T-lymphocyte activity at sites of disease activity. N. Engl. J. Med. **305:** 429-434.
12. GROMAN, G. S., R. J. CASTELE, M. D. ALTOSE, J. SCILLIAN, M. E. KLEINHENZ & R. EHLERS. 1984. Lymphocyte subpopulations in sarcoid pleural effusion. Ann. Intern. Med. **100:** 75-76.

13. SEMENZATO, G., A. PEZZUTTO, G. PIZZOLO, M. CHILOSI, E. OSSI, M. R. ANGI & A. CIPRIANI. 1984. Immunohistological study in sarcoidosis: Evaluation at different sites of disease activity. Clin. Immunol. Immunopathol. **30:** 29-40.
14. BROOKS, B. S., T. E. GAMMAL, G. D. HUNGERFORD, J. ACKER, R. P. TREVOR & W. RUSSELL. 1982. Radiologic evaluation of neurosarcoidosis: Role of computed tomography. Am. J. Neuroradiol. **3:** 513-521.
15. STRELETZ, L. J., R. A. CHAMBERS, S. H. BAE & H. L. ISRAEL. 1981. Visual evoked potentials in sarcoidosis. Neurology **31:** 1545-1549.
16. POWERS, W. J. & E. M. MILLER. 1981. Sarcoidosis mimicking glioma: Case report and review of intracranial sarcoid mass lesions. Neurology **31:** 907-910.
17. RECHTHAND, E., B. J. STERN & A. KRUMHOLZ. 1983. Beneficial effects of steroid therapy for intracranial sarcoid mass lesions. Neurology **33**(Suppl. 2): 152.

Fluorescent Bronchial Angiography in Sarcoidosis

YOHMEI HIRAGA, KOHKI KIKUCHI, AND ASAKO YAMAMOTO

Japanese National Railways Sapporo Hospital
Sapporo, Japan

INTRODUCTION

Microangiopathy in sarcoidosis has been found by Kobayashi[1,2] to affect retinal blood vessels; more recently, it has been found by Mikami *et al.*[3] to affect muscle and the kidney, as well as heart muscle and the lung. Further investigations on the bronchial submucosa disclosed that the network of the blood vessels is recognized in this disease[4] but not usually in other diseases. If such a network is formed by the same mechanism that forms the network in the retina,[5] fluorescent bronchial angiography (FBA) would reveal leakage of fluorescent dye from the blood vessels and also the retention of the dye in the walls of the blood vessels. The present study investigates a series of moving fluorescent patterns of blood vessels in the bronchial submucosa, in timely connection with the intravenous injection of fluorescein to patients with sarcoidosis.

SUBJECTS AND METHODS

The study included 18 cases of sarcoidosis that were diagnosed histologically and were accompanied by a high titer of serum angiotensin-converting enzyme (ACE) and lysozyme. All the cases presented with networks in the blood vessels of the submucosa of the bilateral bronchi, and the extent of these networks varied from case to case. Ten cases were male, and eight were female. One case was in his teens, nine were in their 20's, four were in their 30's, and two each were in their 40's and 50's. The duration between the diagnosis and the present examinations was less than 6 months in 14 cases and from 1 to 3 years in 4 cases. The involvements were as follows: bilateral hilar adenopathy (BHL) with no other lesions (two cases); BHL and eye lesions (six cases); BHL and pulmonary lesions (two cases); BHL and pulmonary and eye lesions (three cases); BHL and eye and skin lesions (one case); BHL, eye lesions, and arthralgia (one case); pulmonary lesions only (one case); and pulmonary and eye

[a] Address for correspondence: Japanese National Railways Sapporo Hospital, N3 E1, Chuo-ku, Sapporo, Japan.

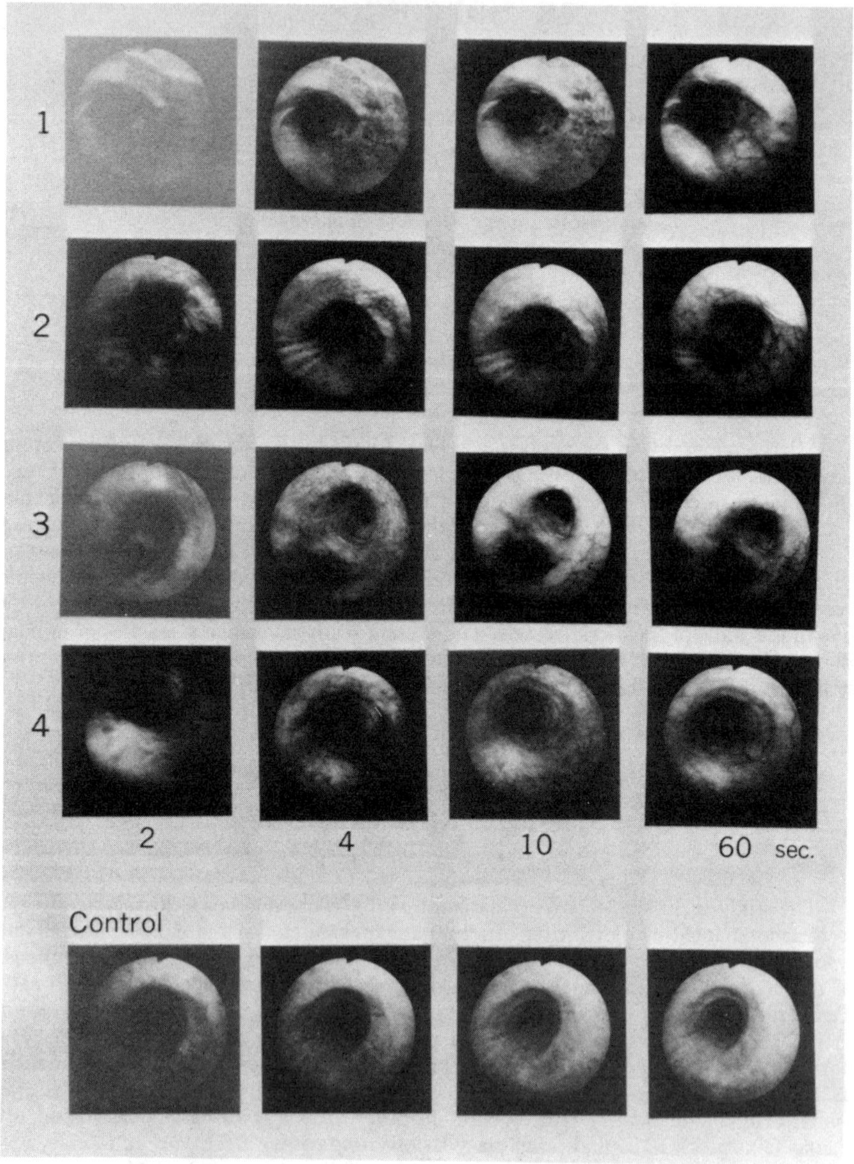

FIGURE 1. Fluorescence of blood vessels and its leakage to the periphery 2, 4, 10, and 60 seconds after the intravenous injection of fluorescein.

lesions (two cases). The tuberculin reaction was negative in 13 cases, equivocal in 3 cases, and positive in 2 cases. The FBA procedure was as follows: a fiberoptic bronchoscope was fixed to the left bronchial trunk; 5 ml of 10% (w/v) diagnostic fluorescein was injected for 3 seconds into the cubital vein;[6] and pictures were taken after the injection for 20 consecutive minutes, according to the Shimizu-Oho[7] method. The filters employed were the Kodak Wratter 12, as a barrier filter (placed at the camera side), and the Kodak Wratter 47, as an exciter filter (placed at the light-source side). At the same time, that is, during or immediately after this procedure, the fundus photographs were taken. Other examinations were gallium-67 citrate scintigraphy and computed tomography (CT) scans of the chest to confirm the grade of peribronchial thickening.

TABLE 1. The Relationship of Vascular Changes to FBA Changes

Vascular Network Formation	Grade of Leakage in FBA			
	+++	++	+	Total
+++	9	2	0	11
++	0	4	0	4
+	0	0	3	3
Total	9	6	3	18

RESULTS

FBA

Two seconds after the injection, the fluorescent dye was detected in some blood vessels, as was its leakage to the periphery. After 10 seconds, the fluorescence became marked on the background, and the network stood out in sharp relief. Large numbers of nodule-like fluorescein accumulations were seen. The fluorescence on the background lasted for more than 20 minutes in most cases. The surface of the bronchial mucosa came to be edematous with increased secretions in about 20 minutes. The above-mentioned findings were more or less commonly visible in all cases (FIG. 1).

Network Formation and FBA

Network formation, as evident by bronchoscopic vascular changes, was marked in 11 cases. Fluorescence was marked in nine and moderate in two of these cases. Network formation was moderate in four and slight in three cases. The degree of leakage in each of these cases corresponded to the degree of network formation (TABLE 1).

TABLE 2. The Relationship of Gallium-67 Accumulation in the Pulmonary Hilar Region to FBA Changes

Gallium Accumulation	Grade of Leakage in FBA			
	+++	++	+	Total
+++	6	3	1	10
++	3	1	1	5
+	0	2	1	3
Total	9	6	3	18

Gallium-67 Accumulation in the Pulmonary Hilar Nodes and FBA

Strong uptake (uptake equivalent to liver uptake) in the pulmonary hilar nodes was found in 10 cases; moderate uptake (uptake weaker than liver uptake) was found in 5 cases; weak uptake (uptake significantly denser than background uptake) was found in 3 cases (TABLE 2).

Peripheral Bronchial Thickening and FBA

Marked bronchial thickening, as evident by CT, was found in four cases. Three of these cases had marked leakage, one had moderate leakage, and one had slight leakage detected by FBA. Slight bronchial thickening was found in four cases; of these four, two had moderate and two had slight leakage (TABLE 3).

Perivasculitis in the Eye Fundus and FBA

Marked retinal perivasculitis was found in 10 cases. Six of these cases had marked leakage, three had moderate leakage, and one had slight leakage detected by FBA. Slight retinal perivasculitis was found in two cases; of these two, one had marked and one had slight leakage. No retinal perivasculitis was found in six cases; of these six, two had marked, three had moderate, and one had slight leakage (TABLE 4).

TABLE 3. The Relationship of Peribronchial Thickening to FBA Changes

Peribronchial Thickening	Grade of Leakage in FBA			
	+++	++	+	Total
+	2	1	1	4
±	2	2	0	4
−	5	4	2	11
Total	9	7	3	19

TABLE 4. The Relationship of Perivasculitis of the Fundus to FBA Changes

	Grade of Leakage in FBA			
Vasculitis	+++	++	+	Total
+	6	3	1	10
±	1	0	1	2
−	2	3	1	6
Total	9	6	3	18

Fluorescent Angiographic Changes of the Fundus and FBA

Fluorescent leakage in the fundus was found in 11 cases. Seven of these cases had marked leakage, three had moderate leakage, and one had slight leakage detected by FBA. No fundus leakage was found in seven cases; of these seven, two had marked, three had moderate, and two had slight bronchial leakage detected by FBA (TABLE 5).

Other Diseases and FBA

Of three cases of diabetes mellitus, one had a slight degree of bronchial fluorescent leakage, and two had no findings. Three healthy controls also showed no findings. A slight degree of leakage was found in a case of juvenile idiopathic bronchial bleeding.

Adverse Side Effects

Of 25 cases examined so far, 7 had adverse side effects. One case had dyspnea, three had abdominal pain, and three had nausea. None of them showed serious side effects.

TABLE 5. The Relationship of Fluorescent Angiographic Changes of the Fundus to FBA Changes

Grade of Fluorescent Angiopathy of the Fundus	Grade of Leakage in FBA			
	+++	++	+	Total
+	7	3	1	11
−	2	3	2	7
Total	9	6	3	18

DISCUSSION

It appears Yamada *et al.*[7] have performed the only other FBA study. They observed intratubular cancer lesions indicated by hyperfluorescence, and concluded that the contour of protuberant cancer lesions was more clearly recognized with this technique than with other conventional techniques. It was difficult for them, however, to distinguish clearly each change through the three phases—arterial, capillary, and venous. They observed blood vessels in a negative fluorescent state, and they gained useful information while the tissue was fluorescently dyed. On the other hand, we used an injection technique and observed blood vessels as fluorescein-positive images, images in which peripheral leakage was evident. We also found that network changes were rare in diabetes mellitus. It was not possible to distinguish plainly each change through the three phases with our technique, either. The network of small blood vessels stood up in a sharp relief against the background, which was also fluorescently dyed. These two findings, leakage and retention, are considered to be characteristic of sarcoidosis. In our study, fluorescent bronchial changes were more frequently and easily seen than changes in perivasculitis were seen with retinography and retinal fluorescent angiography. Such a relationship may lead to a hypothesis that bronchial changes precede retinal changes.

CONCLUSION

Intravenously administered dye and FBA in sarcoidosis revealed fluorescence in some of the blood vessels, leakage from peripheral blood vessels, and large fluorescent foci (nodules). The fluorescent network of blood vessels stood in sharp relief against the background. The retention of fluorescein was observed in the relevant area for a relatively long time. These findings were hardly ever seen in healthy controls or in patients with diabetes mellitus. The FBA changes were well related to the network formation of blood vessels in bronchoscopy and also to the gallium-67 uptake in the pulmonary hilar region, but were not well related to the retinal vascular changes and chest CT changes. These FBA findings suggest a relationship to the development of the disease; that is, they suggest the precedence of bronchial microangiopathic changes over retinal changes.

As for the fundus and the choroidal capillaries, basic morphological problems have been solved, and confirmation has been obtained for how fluorescein infiltrates tissue and through which areas fluorescein passes. On the other hand, many problems have remained unsolved in the bronchial artery and vein systems. Further investigations should be made on the morphology of the bronchial arteries and veins, as well as on the infiltration capacity of fluorescein in the areas through which fluorescein passes.

REFERENCES

1. KOBAYASHI, F. 1971. Supplementary findings on fundus involvement in ocular sarcoidosis. Acta Soc. Ophthalmol. Jpn. **75:** 513-518.

2. KOBAYASHI, F. 1976. On microangiopathy of sarcoid retinopathy. Acta Soc. Ophthalmol. Jpn. **80:** 694-701.
3. MIKAMI, R., Y. SHIMADA & H. YOTSUMOTO. 1977. Microangiopathy in sarcoidosis from the study of muscle biopsy: Vascular lesions of collagen diseases and related conditions. Japanese Medical Research Foundation.
4. KOBAYASHI, T., Y. HIRAGA, M. OGIWARA, M. WASHIZAKI, H. OKANO, Y. RYUJIN, T. KOSUDA, I. MOCHIZUKI, K. OZAWA & R. MIKAMI. 1983. Vascular changes in bronchoscopy in patients with sarcoidosis. Sarcoidosis and Other Granulomatous Diseases. J. Chrétien, J. Marsac & J. C. Saltiel, Eds.: 652-654. Pergamon Press. Paris.
5. SUDO, M. & Y. SATO. 1968. Fluorescein fundus photography of sarcoidosis. Jpn. J. Clin. Ophthalmol. **22:** 167-170.
6. SCHATZ, E., T. BURTON, L. A. YANNUZZI & M. F. RABB. 1978. Interpretation of Fundus Fluorescein Angiography. C. V. Mosby. Saint Louis, MO.
7. YAMADA, R., K. OHO, R. AMEMIYA, T. OHTANI, N. TAKIZAWA, H. TAKAKURA, I. OGAWA & Y. HAYATA. 1982. Comparison of bronchoscopic findings with histological ones. Jpn. J. Chest Dis. **41:** 12-16.

Thermolysin-like Serum Metalloendopeptidase

A New Marker for Active Sarcoidosis That Complements Serum Angiotensin-converting Enzyme[a]

JUNE ALMENOFF,[b] MARY LOU SKOVRON,[c] AND ALVIN S. TEIRSTEIN[b,d]

[b]Department of Medicine
and
[c]Department of Community Medicine
Mount Sinai Medical Center
New York, New York 10029

INTRODUCTION

Assessment of disease activity in sarcoidosis is a persistent challenge faced by clinicians treating this disease. It is not uncommon for patients to be relatively asymptomatic while granulomatous proliferation is causing organ dysfunction. On the other hand, it is difficult to assess worsening symptoms in patients with existing pulmonary disease. These exacerbations may be the result of fresh granulomatous activity that could be suppressed with steroid treatment or may be due to irreversible fibrosis.

Several methods are currently in use for assessment of disease activity in sarcoidosis, each of which may reflect a different aspect of the disease process. Immunocytochemistry of bronchoalveolar lavage fluid has facilitated characterization of the alveolitis of sarcoidosis, and its clinical usefulness is currently being elucidated.[1–3] Gallium-67 scanning is a commonly used method for assessing sarcoid activity. The avidity of granulomas for gallium-67 citrate provides a sensitive method with which to quantitate and localize disease activity. The gallium-67 scan, however, is a relatively nonspecific test.[4,5] In addition, the expense of this test and the exposure of patients to radiation are undesirable features.

A widely used tool for detecting active sarcoidosis is the determination of the serum angiotensin-converting enzyme (SACE) level. This method has the advantage

[a]This work was performed with the support of the Catherine and Henry Gaisman Foundation.

[d]Address for correspondence: Department of Medicine, Annenberg 24-30, Mount Sinai School of Medicine, One Gustav L. Levy Place, New York, New York 10029.

of being noninvasive and inexpensive. Although it has been reported to have specificity as high as 80-90%, it has only moderate sensitivity, in the range of 50-60%.[6-8]

We have recently identified a thermolysin-like neutral metalloendopeptidase (EC 3.4.24.11) in human serum and have shown that its concentration is significantly elevated in sarcoidosis patients as compared with healthy controls.[9] The function of this enzyme is unknown at present. Like the angiotensin-converting enzyme, it is a membrane-bound metallopeptidase that is abundant in lung. The two enzymes, however, are biochemically distinct. In this report, we present a comparison of SACE and thermolysin-like metalloendopeptidase (TME) as markers of clinical activity in sarcoidosis.

METHODS AND MATERIALS

Glutaryl-Ala-Ala-Phe-2-naphthylamide was synthesized as described by Orlowski and Wilk.[10] Aminopeptidase M was obtained from Boehringer-Mannheim Biochemicals (Indianapolis, IN) and further purified on phenylsepharose (Pharmacia Laboratories, Piscataway, NJ) as previously described.[11] Most commercial preparations of aminopeptidase M contain contaminating enzymes that interfere with the assay and must therefore be purified by this method.

Sera were obtained by venopuncture and stored at −20° C. SACE activity was determined by the method of Lieberman[12] in which an SACE level above 35 units was considered elevated.[13] TME activity was determined as described by Almenoff *et al.*[9] in a coupled enzyme assay using glutaryl-Ala-Ala-Phe-2-naphthylamide as the substrate in the presence of excess aminopeptidase M.

$$\text{Glutaryl-Ala-Ala-Phe-2-naphthylamide} \xrightarrow{\text{TME}} \text{glutaryl-Ala-Ala-Phe-2-naphthylamide}$$

$$\text{Phe-2-naphthylamide} \xrightarrow{\text{aminopeptidase M}} \text{Phe} + \text{2-naphthylamine}$$

The 2-naphthylamine formed in the latter reaction is quantitated by diazotization. One unit (U) of TME activity is defined as the amount of enzyme catalyzing the formation of 1 nmole of product $\cdot$ min^{-1} $\cdot$ ml of serum^{-1} under the conditions previously described.[9] The upper limit of normal serum TME was set at 8 U. This value was selected by creating a receiver-operator-characteristic plot to optimize sensitivity and specificity and corresponds to approximately the 95th percentile for healthy controls.[14]

Statistical analyses were performed using CLINFO.[15] Enzyme distributions of the various groups were compared by nonparametric analysis. The level of significance for all statistical tests was .05.

The patients studied were 122 consecutive sarcoidosis patients seen at the Mount Sinai Medical Center on whom complete clinical evaluations and chest roentgenograms were obtained. The diagnosis of sarcoidosis was confirmed with either a positive Kveim test or organ biopsy. Patients with medical illnesses in addition to sarcoidosis were excluded from the study. Clinical assessment by the examining physician was made without knowledge of the patient's TME or SACE activities.

The criteria for active disease listed below are based on the work of Rohatgi and Ryan,[6] and are derived from data easily obtained at clinic visits.

1. Worsening chest radiographs from previous visit.

TABLE 1. Descriptive Statistics of SACE and TME Activities in Sarcoidosis Patients

	Enzyme Activity (U)	
	TME (N = 122)	SACE (N = 122)
Mean	8.24	31.80
Median	4.71	28.50
SD	11.57	14.50
Maximum	74.4	86.2
Minimum	0.4	9.0

2. Extrathoracic manifestations including constitutional symptoms; lymphadenopathy; neurologic, skin, eye, lacrimal, or parotid gland involvement; splenomegaly; and joint or bone involvement.

3. Worsening pulmonary function from previous visit and a 10% or greater decrease in forced vital capacity or diffusing capacity.

4. Onset of breathlessness in a previously healthy, asymptomatic individual.

5. Exacerbation of symptoms upon withdrawal of corticosteroids and improvement upon restarting medication.

Patients whose records revealed one or more of these criteria were classified as "active"; all other patients were considered to have "inactive" disease.

RESULTS

The patients studied included 49 males and 73 females. They ranged in age from 21 to 68 years with a mean age of 40 years. Twenty-four patients were receiving corticosteroid treatment.

The descriptive statistics of TME and SACE activities in this series of patients are given in TABLE 1. The mean and median TME activities were 8.24 U and 4.71 U, respectively, with a minimum of 0.4 U and a maximum of 74.4 U. The mean and median SACE activities were 31.77 U and 28.5 U, respectively, with a minimum of

TABLE 2. Comparison of TME and SACE Activities in Active and Inactive Sarcoidosis

		Enzyme Activity (U)			
		TME		SACE	
Sarcoidosis	Number of Patients	Mean	Median	Mean	Median
Active	67	10.96	5.98	36.7	32.0
Inactive	53	4.69	2.80	25.4	25.0

NOTE: The mean values for both SACE and TME were significantly different ($p < .001$ in the Wilcoxon rank-sum test) for active versus inactive disease.

TABLE 3. Validity of TME Activity as a Marker of Active Disease

	Number of Cases of Sarcoidosis		
TME Activity	Active	Inactive	Total
Elevated	30	9	39
Normal	39	44	83
Total	69	53	122

NOTE: Sensitivity: 43%; specificity: 83%; positive predictive value: 77%.

9.0 U and a maximum of 86.20 U. Both distributions were skewed toward higher values.

Patients were classified as active or inactive as described in the previous section. A comparison of TME and SACE values in these two groups of patients is shown in TABLE 2. The mean TME value for the patients with active disease was 10.96 U (median: 5.98 U) as compared with a mean of 4.69 U (median: 2.80 U) for the inactive group ($p < .001$). These results are consistent with our previous observation on a smaller series of patients.[9] SACE levels in the active patients were significantly higher than those in patients with inactive disease ($p < .001$). These data are consistent with most reports in the literature.[4–8,12,13]

TABLE 3 illustrates the sensitivity and specificity of TME for detection of disease activity. On the basis of the criteria for activity described above, TME has a sensitivity of 43%, a specificity of 83%, and a positive predictive value of 77%. Similar data on SACE are given in TABLE 4. In this series of patients, SACE was found to have a sensitivity of 45%, a specificity of 87%, and a positive predictive value of 82%.

The striking similarity in the sensitivities and specificities of SACE and TME raises the question of whether these enzymes identify similar or different groups of active patients. There was no significant correlation ($r = .15$; $p = .98$) between SACE and TME; this suggests that the enzymes identify different groups of patients.

The validity of TME and SACE used in combination was tested next, as shown in TABLE 5. The combined sensitivity of the enzymes was 68%; the combined specificity, 75%; and the positive predictive value, 78%. Thus, concurrent use of SACE and TME increased the detection of active disease by 50% as compared with either enzyme individually. This was accompanied by a 12% decrease in specificity compared

TABLE 4. Validity of SACE Activity as a Marker of Active Disease

	Number of Cases of Sarcoidosis		
SACE Activity	Active	Inactive	Total
Elevated	31	7	38
Normal	38	46	84
Total	69	53	122

NOTE: Sensitivity: 45%; specificity: 87%; positive predictive value: 82%.

with use of SACE alone, and an 8% decrease in specificity compared with use of TME alone.

DISCUSSION

The present study reveals that serum TME is as sensitive and specific a marker for active sarcoidosis as is SACE. The data indicate that the two enzymes complement each other as markers of active disease. Combined use of the enzymes enhances their respective sensitivities by 50% with minimal compromise in specificity. Thus, TME may ultimately serve as a useful adjunct to SACE in the routine evaluation of sarcoidosis.

TABLE 5. Validity of SACE and TME Activities Used in Combination for Detection of Active Disease

	Number of Cases of Sarcoidosis		
Activity	Active	Inactive	Total
Either SACE or TME elevated	47	13	60
Both SACE and TME normal	22	40	62
Total	69	53	122

NOTE: Sensitivity: 68%; specificity: 75%; positive predictive value: 78%.

Many problems in our understanding of disease activity stem from our inability to precisely define this concept. There are disparities throughout the literature on the validity of SACE and gallium-67 scanning for detection of activity. These disparities result, at least in part, from varying definitions of disease activity. The criteria for activity used here are derived from data that are readily obtainable in an office or clinic visit. More sophisticated data obtained from gallium-67 scans and immunocytochemical analysis of bronchoalveolar lavage fluid provide additional information about the disease process.

In conclusion, TME is a new noninvasive and inexpensive laboratory test that may be useful in the evaluation of sarcoidosis. It has similar sensitivity and specificity to SACE, but it appears to reflect a different aspect of disease activity. Prospective studies on the prognostic significance of TME may provide further insight into its clinical usefulness.

ACKNOWLEDGMENTS

We wish to acknowledge Dr. Marian Orlowski, for his guidance on the biochemical aspects of this work, and Dr. Robert Schneider, who performed the SACE determinations. June Almenoff is a trainee on Medical Scientist Training Grant GM-07280 from the National Institutes of Health. This work was submitted as partial fulfillment of the clerkship requirement in community medicine while June Almenoff was a third-year student at the Mount Sinai School of Medicine.

REFERENCES

1. CRYSTAL, R. G., P. B. BITTERMAN, S. I. RENNARD, A. J. HANCE & B. A. KEOGH. 1984. Interstitial lung disease of unknown cause. Part One. N. Engl. J. Med. **310:** 154-166.
2. CRYSTAL, R. G., P. B. BITTERMAN, S. I. RENNARD, A. J. HANCE & B. A. KEOGH. 1984. Interstitial lung disease of unknown cause. Part Two. N. Engl. J. Med. **310:** 235-244.
3. KEOGH, B. A., G. W. HUNNINGHAKE, B. R. LINE & R. G. CRYSTAL. 1983. The alveolitis of pulmonary sarcoidosis: Evolution of natural history and alveolitis-dependent changes in lung function. Am. Rev. Respir. Dis. **128:** 256-165.
4. KOHN, H., H. KLECH, A. MOSTBECK & F. KUMMER. 1982. ^{67}Ga scanning for assessment of disease activity and therapy decisions in pulmonary sarcoidosis in comparison to chest radiography, serum ACE, and blood lymphocytes. Eur. J. Nuc. Med. **7:** 413-416.
5. KLECH, H., H. KOHN, F. KUMMER & A. MOSTBECK. 1982. Assessment of activity in sarcoidosis: Sensitivity and specificity of ^{67}Ga scintigraphy, serum ACE levels, chest roentgenography, and blood lymphocyte subpopulations. Chest **82:** 732-738.
6. ROHATGI, P. K. & J. W. RYAN. 1980. Simple radioassay for measuring serum angiotensin-converting enzyme in sarcoidosis. Chest **78:** 69-76.
7. ROHRBACH, M. S. & R. A. DEREMEE. 1979. Serum angiotensin-converting enzyme activity in sarcoidosis as measured by a simple radiochemical assay. Am. Rev. Respir. Dis. **119:** 761-767.
8. STUDDY, P. R. & D. G. JAMES. 1981. The specificity and sensitivity of serum angiotensin-converting enzyme in sarcoidosis and other diseases: Experience in twelve centers in six different countries. *In* Sarcoidosis and Other Granulomatous Disorders. J. Chrétien, J. Marsac & J. S. Salteil, Eds.: 332-344. Pergamon Press. Paris.
9. ALMENOFF, J., A. S. TEIRSTEIN, J. C. THORNTON & M. ORLOWSKI. 1984. Identification of a thermolysin-like neutral metalloendopeptidase in serum: Activity in normal subjects and in patients with sarcoidosis. J. Lab. Clin. Med. **103:** 420-431.
10. ORLOWSKI, M. & S. WILK. 1981. Purification and specificity of a membrane-bound metalloendopeptidase from bovine pituitaries. Biochemistry **20:** 4942-4950.
11. ALMENOFF, J. & M. ORLOWSKI. 1983. Membrane-bound kidney neutral metalloendopeptidase: Interaction with synthetic substrates, natural peptides, and inhibitors. Biochemistry **22:** 590-599.
12. LIEBERMAN, J. 1975. Elevation of serum angiotensin-converting enzyme (serum ACE) level in sarcoidosis. Am. J. Med. **59:** 365-372.
13. LAWRENCE, E. C., R. B. TEAGUE, M. C. GOTTLEIB, S. G. JHINGRAN & J. LIEBERMAN. 1983. Serial changes in markers of disease activity with corticosteroid treatment in sarcoidosis. Am. J. Med. **74:** 747-756.
14. GRINIER, P. F., R. J. MAYEWSLI, A. I. MUSHLIN & P. GREENLAND. 1981. Principles of test selection and use. Ann. Intern. Med. **94**(2): 559-570.
15. CLINFO. Clinical Data Management System. 1984. Bolt, Beranek & Newman. Cambridge, MA.

The Kveim Test after Siltzbach[a]

ALVIN S. TEIRSTEIN[b]

Department of Medicine
Mount Sinai Medical Center
New York, New York 10029

In 1985, some of us celebrated the golden anniversary of Williams and Nickerson's description of the appearance of a papule after an intradermal injection of a suspension of sarcoidal tissue in 48 patients with sarcoidosis.[1] In 1941, Nickerson[2] and Kveim[3] independently confirmed the reaction which was then accorded an eponym, the Nickerson-Kveim test. After recording remarkable specificity and sensitivity in large-scale studies of 200[4] and 750[5] patients with sarcoidosis, Siltzbach became the most articulate and ardent supporter of this unique biologic reaction. Numerous reports followed, including a multinational cooperative study of more than 2394 subjects sponsored by the International Committee on Sarcoidosis,[6] which have buttressed confidence in the reliability of the Kveim test in the diagnosis of sarcoidosis. At the Eighth International Congress on Sarcoidosis and Other Granulomatous Diseases, 106 respondents cited the Kveim test as the favored initial diagnostic procedure to be performed in patients with the common stage 1 radiographic presentation.[7] Even when the initial radiograph revealed parenchymal disease, these workers reported that the Kveim test was almost as popular as forceps lung biopsy by fiberoptic bronchoscopy as the first diagnostic study.

Despite these favorable reports of the superb diagnostic accuracy of the Kveim test, Siltzbach was required to devote many months studying, lecturing, and writing in an effort to refute numerous reports of contrary results by the reputable investigators Israel, Daniel and Schneider, Karlish, Bringle, Mitchell, Hirsch, and Chrétien. With the extraordinary assistance of Izumi in Japan and James in England, refute them he did. In almost every instance Siltzbach demonstrated that Kveim suspensions which were not carefully validated and monitored according to the criteria set forth at the Second International Congress on Sarcoidosis[8] were producing an unacceptably high percentage of false-positive results in nonsarcoid patients. To the contrary, in Siltzbach's laboratory, where he maintained strict surveillance and diligently adhered to rules of validation, Kveim suspensions were produced which consistently yielded more than 80% positive reactions in patients with sarcoidosis and less than 0.5% false-positive tests.

It has been suggested that Siltzbach was unique. Perhaps he possessed a particularly potent source of Kveim suspension or was graced with uncanny skill in producing good Kveim material. Siltzbach died on 22 April 1980. At the time of his death, we at the Mount Sinai Medical Center, New York, the home of Siltzbach's laboratory, found ourselves in a similar position to all other centers involved in the study, diagnosis,

[a] This work was supported by the Catherine and Henry Gaisman Foundation.

[b] Address for correspondence: Department of Medicine, Mount Sinai Medical Center, Annenberg 24-30, One Gustave L. Levy Place, New York, New York 10029.

and care of patients with sarcoidosis throughout the world, with regard to the availability of good Kveim material. Could we manufacture Kveim suspensions which would reproduce the specificity and sensitivity of Siltzbach's material? Fortunately, he left us a legacy of 18 frozen sarcoidal spleens and a sarcoidosis out-patient service which served approximately 30 patients a week, including almost 150 new patients each year. This report consists of our experience with new Kveim suspensions produced at the Mount Sinai Medical Center since Siltzbach's death.

The Kveim suspensions tested were produced from seven separate sarcoidal spleens, one inherited from Siltzbach and six acquired at intervals during the past four years. Kveim test suspensions were made according to the published method of Chase and Siltzbach.[8] Injections of 0.15 ml of the test suspension were injected intradermally in tandem with a previously validated suspension according to the published method of Siltzbach.[9] Only after experience with at least 30 patients revealed acceptable results was the test material considered validated. Biopsies were performed 4 weeks after implantation if a nodule appeared at the site of injection. Tissue specimens were fixed in formalin, stained with hematoxylin and eosin, and were read by an experienced pathologist and the author without knowledge of the clinical status of the patients, with the exception that all subjects were suspected of having sarcoidosis.

TABLE 1. Results of the Kveim Test in 747 Patients Suspected of Having Sarcoidosis

	Number of Patients	Kveim Test Positive	Kveim Test Negative
Sarcoid	583	458 (78.6)	125 (21.4)
Nonsarcoid	164	1 (0.07)	164 (99+)

NOTE: Percentages are shown in parentheses.

RESULTS

The results are shown in TABLE 1. From April 1980 to June 1984, 753 patients referred to the Mount Sinai Medical Center with a possible diagnosis of sarcoidosis were tested. Six patients refused biopsy of the Kveim injection sites or were lost during the follow-up period. Of the remaining 747, 164 proved to have diseases other than sarcoidosis during idiopathic pulmonary fibrosis, lymphoma, lung cancer, tuberculosis, rheumatoid arthritis, idiopathic uveitis, cardiomyopathy, various neuromuscular disorders, and hypersensitivity pneumonitis. Five hundred eighty-three patients were accepted as manifesting unequivocal evidence of sarcoidosis on the basis of a typical radiographic and clinical presentation coupled with a positive Kveim test and/or organ biopsy revealing noncaseating epithelioid granulomas. Four hundred fifty-eight of these patients with sarcoidosis had a positive Kveim test (78.6%) and 125 had a negative test (21.4%). One patient with bilateral hilar and right paratracheal lymph node enlargement died of metastatic adenocystic carcinoma within one year of the positive Kveim reaction. No postmortem examination was performed. This patient is considered to have had the only false-positive test among the 164 (0.07%) patients without sarcoidosis who were tested (TABLE 1). In 118 of the 583 patients with sarcoidosis and a positive Kveim test, biopsy of lymph nodes, lung, lacrimal glands, or skin also yielded tissue compatible with sarcoidosis.

Our experience with 78.6% positive Kveim tests in 583 patients with sarcoidosis reveals a rate of positivity almost identical to that reported by Siltzbach. Of the 125 patients with sarcoidosis and a negative Kveim test, 92 had sarcoidosis for more than 2 years. This reaffirms previous studies that described a decreased rate of positivity after the first 2 years of clinical disease. Thirty-three patients had negative Kveim tests, despite apparent recent onset of disease. All but 1 of the 36 patients with erythema nodosum, a fulminant clinical indicator of acute sarcoidosis, had a positive test.

There is good Kveim material and bad Kveim material. In our strict adherence to the guidelines published in the proceedings of previous meetings of the International Congress on Sarcoidosis and consistently reiterated by Siltzbach, we found it necessary to discard batches of Kveim material produced from two of our newly acquired spleens and two lots made from a spleen which previously, and subsequently, was the source of good Kveim material. The bad Kveim material was discarded because of low sensitivity in three instances and the evocation of bizarre, histologically confusing tissue reactions in one.

Siltzbach was not unique in his ability to produce reliable Kveim suspensions. He was a unique, meticulous investigator, scholar, and teacher. The manufacture, validation, and clinical application of the Kveim test in sarcoidosis according to the methods promoted by Siltzbach are reaffirmed by this study of 747 tests performed at the Mount Sinai Medical Center since his death. We applaud those who now refer to this remarkably sensitive and specific biologic test as the Kveim-Siltzbach test.

REFERENCES

1. WILLIAMS, R. H. & D. A. NICKERSON. 1935. Skin reactions in sarcoid. Proc. Soc. Exp. Biol. Med. **33:** 403-405.
2. NICKERSON, D. A. 1941. Sarcoid. Arch. Dermatol. Syphilol. **43:** 172-173.
3. KVEIM, A. 1941. En ny og spesifik Kulan-reackjon ved Boeck's sarcoid. Nord. Med. **9:** 169.
4. SILTZBACH, L. E. & J. C. EHRLICH. 1954. The Nickerson-Kveim reaction in sarcoidosis. Am. J. Med. **16:** 790-803.
5. SILTZBACH, L. E. 1961. The Kveim test in sarcoidosis: A study of 750 patients. J. Am. Med. Assoc. **178:** 476-482.
6. SILTZBACH, L. E. 1967. The international Kveim test study, 1960-1966. *In* Proceedings of the Fourth International Conference on Sarcoidosis. T. Turiaf & J. Chabot, Eds.: 201-213. Masson & Cie. Paris.
7. TEIRSTEIN, A. S., L. E. SILTZBACH & D. DORPH. 1980. Report of international questionnaire regarding diagnostic procedures in sarcoidosis: The subject of fiberoptic bronchoscopy. *In* Eighth International Conference on Sarcoidosis and Other Granulomatous Diseases. W. Jones Williams and B. H. Davies, Eds.: 233-237. Alpha Omega. Cardiff.
8. CHASE, M. W. 1961. The preparation and standardization of Kveim testing antigen. Am. Rev. Respir. Dis. **84**(Part 2): 86-88.
9. SILTZBACH, L. E. 1974. The Kveim test is a reliable means of diagnosing sarcoidosis. *In* Controversy in Internal Medicine. F. J. Ingelfinger, Ed. Vol. **2:** 349-358. W. B. Saunders. Philadelphia, PA.

Index of Contributors

(Italicized page numbers refer to comments in the Panel Discussion)